KU-533-237

DISEASES OF THE LIVER
AND BILIARY SYSTEM

DISEASES OF THE LIVER AND BILIARY SYSTEM

Sheila Sherlock

DBE MD (Edin.), Hon. DSc (Edin., New York, Yale),
Hon. MD (Leuven, Lisbon, Oslo), Hon. LLD (Aberd.),
FRCP, FRCPE, FRACP, Hon. FRCCP,
Hon. FRCPI, Hon. FACP

Professor of Medicine,
Royal Free Hospital School of Medicine,
University of London

EIGHTH EDITION

BLACKWELL SCIENTIFIC PUBLICATIONS

OXFORD LONDON EDINBURGH

BOSTON MELBOURNE

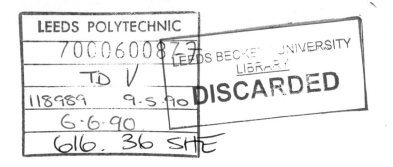

LEEDS POLYTECHNIC

700060008 7 3

TD V

118989   9·5·90

6·6·90

616. 36 SHE

LEEDS BECKET UNIVERSITY
LIBRARY
DISCARDED

© 1963, 1968, 1975, 1981, 1985, 1989
Blackwell Scientific Publications
Editorial offices:
Osney Mead, Oxford OX2 0EL
   (*Orders*: Tel. 0865 240201)
8 John Street, London WC1N 2ES
23 Ainslie Place, Edinburgh EH3 6AJ
3 Cambridge Center, Suite 208
   Cambridge, Massachusetts 02142, USA
107 Barry Street, Carlton, Victoria 3053, Australia

All rights reserved. No part of this publication may be
reproduced, stored in a retrieval system, or transmitted, in
any form or by any means, electronic, mechanical,
photocopying, recording or otherwise without the prior
permission of the copyright owner

First published 1955
Reprinted 1956
Second edition 1958
Reprinted 1959, 1961
Third edition 1963
Reprinted 1965, 1966
Fourth edition 1968
Reprinted 1969, 1971
Fifth edition 1975
Sixth edition 1981
Reprinted 1982, 1983
Seventh edition 1985
Reprinted 1986, 1987
Eighth edition 1989

German third edition 1965
Greek fourth edition 1972
Japanese fourth edition 1973
   fifth edition 1980
Spanish first edition 1956
   third edition 1966
   fifth edition 1976
Portuguese fourth edition 1970
   fifth edition 1978
   seventh edition 1988
Turkish fifth edition 1981

Set by Setrite Typesetters, Hong Kong;
printed and bound in Great Britain
by Wm. Clowes Ltd,
Beccles and London

DISTRIBUTORS

USA
   Year Book Medical Publishers
   200 North LaSalle Street
   Chicago, Illinois 60601
   (*Orders*: Tel. 312 726-9733)

Canada
   The C.V. Mosby Company
   5240 Finch Avenue East
   Scarborough, Ontario
   (*Orders*: Tel. 416 298-1588)

Australia
   Blackwell Scientific Publications
   (Australia) Pty Ltd
   107 Barry Street
   Carlton, Victoria 3053
   (*Orders*: Tel. (03) 347-0300)

British Library
Cataloguing in Publication Data

Sherlock, Sheila, *1918–*
   Diseases of the liver and biliary system.—8th ed.
   1. Man. Biliary tract. Diseases
   I. Title
   616.3'6

   ISBN 0-632-02443-7

Contents

CONTENTS

CONTENTS

CONTENTS

x

Preface to the Eighth Edition

Basic research, particularly biochemical, immunological and virological, is having an accelerated impact on clinical hepatology. The radiologist and endoscopist have lightened the darkness which used to face us in the biliary tract, and they have added fresh dimensions to our investigation and treatment. This has stimulated production of this eighth edition, so that the reader is aware of these new developments.

This edition casts aside what has become obsolete. The book has been completely revised and rewritten. The presentation has been modernized for easy reading; approximately 200 new figures and tables, many in colour, have been introduced, and there are over 1000 new references.

There have been major advances in our understanding of all members of the family of hepatitis viruses and we have a significant breakthrough in the biology and diagnosis of the non-A, non-B group. With some degree of vision, we can foresee the eradication of the major forms of hepatitis as a world problem.

Liver transplantation is becoming as commonplace as its renal counterpart. In 1988, in the United States alone, 2000 liver transplants were performed — six every day. All aspects, including selection of patients, results and complications and their management, are described.

Hepatology, like all aspects of medicine, is to be enjoyed — at the bedside, in the laboratory, in hospital staff meetings, in recording the progress of our patients, and in choosing and evaluating their treatment. This textbook is devised with the hope that it will enhance this enjoyment by simplifying difficult hypotheses, keeping them up to date and illustrating them with fresh tables and figures.

Our daughters, and now a son-in-law, Michael Davis, have all helped in various ways to provide that camaraderie so that hepatology may flourish worldwide.

I owe a great debt to my colleagues, especially to Professor P. J. Scheuer, whose textbook *Liver Biopsy Interprétation* is now in its third edition, and who has generously supplied figures and given much advice. Dr Robert Dick, from his wealth of experience, has kept me up to date on radiological diagnosis and therapy, and he has supplied many of the figures. Professor Howard Thomas has guided me on the molecular biology of the hepatitis viruses. I would also like to express my indebtedness to Dr Andrew Burroughs, Dr James Dooley, Professor Kenneth Hobbs, Dr Aidan McCormack, Professor Neil McIntyre and Dr Roger Williams.

Miss Aileen Duggan has made light of the secretarial burden. Miss Anne Fletcher and her staff at the Royal Free Hospital Library have been meticulous with the bibliography. Miss Janice Cox has contributed her unique brand of artistry.

I am particularly grateful for the editorial assistance of Mrs Elizabeth Healing, of Blackwell Scientific Publications; she has been indefatigable with both manuscript and proofs.

My husband, Dr D. Geraint James, has given his continued and unswerving support in the production of this edition and, indeed, all the others.

SHEILA SHERLOCK
London
February 1989

Preface to the First Edition

My aim in writing this book has been to present a comprehensive and up-to-date account of diseases of the liver and biliary system, which I hope will be of value to physicians, surgeons and pathologists and also a reference book for the clinical student. The modern literature has been reviewed with special reference to articles of general interest. Many older more specialized classical contributions have therefore inevitably been excluded.

Disorders of the liver and biliary system may be classified under the traditional concept of individual diseases. Alternatively, as I have endeavoured in this book, they may be described by the functional and morphological changes which they produce. In the clinical management of a patient with liver disease, it is important to assess the degree of disturbance of four functional and morphological components of the liver—hepatic cells, vascular system (portal vein, hepatic artery and hepatic veins), bile ducts and reticulo-endothelial system. The typical reaction pattern is thus sought and recognized before attempting to diagnose the causative insult. Clinical and laboratory methods of assessing each of these components are therefore considered early in the book. Descriptions of individual diseases follow as illustrative examples. It will be seen that the features of hepato-cellular failure and portal hypertension are described in general terms as a foundation for subsequent discussion of virus hepatitis, nutrition liver disease and the cirrhoses. Similarly blood diseases and infections of the liver are included with the reticulo-endothelial system, and disorders of the biliary tract follow descriptions of acute and chronic bile duct obstruction.

I would like to acknowledge my indebtedness to my teachers, the late Professor J. Henry Dible, the late Professor Sir James Learmonth and Professor Sir John McMichael, who stimulated my interest in hepatic disease, and to my colleagues at the Postgraduate Medical School and elsewhere who have generously invited me to see patients under their care. I am grateful to Dr A. G. Bearn for criticizing part of the typescript and to Dr A. Paton for his criticisms and careful proof reading. Miss D. F. Atkins gave much assistance with proof reading and with the bibliography. Mr Per Saugman and Mrs J. M. Green of Blackwell Scientific Publications have co-operated enthusiastically in the production of this book.

The photomicrographs were taken by Mr E. V. Willmott, FRPS, and Mr C. A. P. Graham from sections prepared by Mr J. G. Griffin and the histology staff of the Postgraduate Medical School. Clinical photographs are the work of Mr C. R. Brecknell and his assistants. The black and white drawings were made by Mrs H. M. G. Wilson and Mr D. Simmonds. I am indebted to them all for their patience and skill.

The text includes part of unpublished material included in a thesis submitted in 1944 to the University of Edinburgh for the degree of M. D., and part of an essay awarded the Buckston—Browne prize of the Harveian Society of London in 1953. Colleagues have allowed me to include published work of which they are jointly responsible. Dr Patricia P. Franklyn and Dr R. E. Steiner have kindly loaned me radiographs. Many authors have given me permission to reproduce illustrations and detailed acknowledgments are given in the text. I wish also to thank the editors of the following journals for permission to include illustrations: *American Journal of Medicine, Archives of Pathology, British Heart Journal, Circulation, Clinical Science, Edinburgh Medical Journal, Journal of Clinical Investigation,*

Journal of Laboratory and Clinical Investigation, Journal of Pathology and Bacteriology, Lancet, Postgraduate Medical Journal, Proceedings of the Staff Meetings of the Mayo Clinic, Quarterly Journal of Medicine, Thorax and also the following publishers: Butterworth's Medical Publications, J. & A. Churchill Ltd, The Josiah Macy Junior Foundation and G. D. Searle & Co.

Finally I must thank my husband, Dr D. Geraint James, who, at considerable personal inconvenience, encouraged me to undertake the writing of this book and also criticized and rewrote most of it. He will not allow me to dedicate it to him.

1 · Anatomy and Function

The liver, the largest organ in the body, weighs 1200–1500 g and comprises one-fiftieth of the total adult body weight. It is relatively larger in infancy, comprising one-eighteenth of the birth weight. This is mainly due to a large left lobe.

Sheltered by the ribs in the right upper quadrant, it is shaped like a pyramid whose apex reaches the xiphisternum (figs 1.1, 1.2, 1.3). The upper border lies approximately at the level of the nipples. There are two anatomical lobes, the right being about six times the size of the left. Lesser segments of the right lobe are the *quadrate lobe*, on its inferior surface, and the *caudate lobe* on the posterior surface. The right and left lobes are separated anteriorly by a fold of peritoneum called the falciform ligament, inferiorly by the fissure for the ligamentum teres, and posteriorly by the fissure for the ligamentum venosum.

The liver has a double blood supply. The *portal vein* brings venous blood from the intestines and spleen and the *hepatic artery*, coming from the coeliac axis, supplies the liver with arterial blood. These vessels enter the liver through a fissure, the *porta hepatis*, which lies

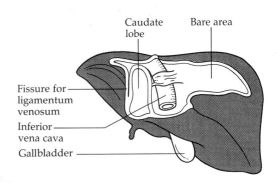

Fig. 1.2. Posterior view of the liver.

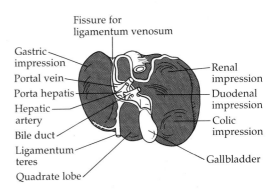

Fig. 1.3. Inferior view of the liver.

far back on the inferior surface of the right lobe. Inside the porta, the portal vein and hepatic artery divide into branches to the right and left lobes, and the right and left hepatic bile ducts join to form the common hepatic duct. The *hepatic nerve plexus* contains fibres from both sympathetic ganglia T7 to T10 which synapse in the coeliac plexus, the right and left vagi and the right phrenic nerve. It accompanies the hepatic artery and bile ducts into their finest ramifications, even to the portal tracts and hepatic parenchyma.

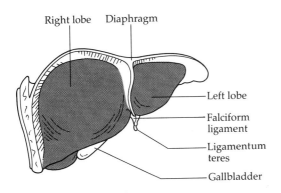

1 **Fig. 1.1.** Anterior view of the liver.

The *ligamentum venosum*, a slender remnant of the ductus venosus of the fetus, arises from the left branch of the portal vein and fuses with the inferior vena cava at the entrance of the left hepatic vein. The *ligamentum teres*, a remnant of the umbilical vein of the fetus, runs in the free edge of the falciform ligament from the umbilicus to the inferior border of the liver and joins the left branch of the portal vein. Small veins accompanying it connect the portal vein with veins around the umbilicus. These become prominent when the portal venous system is obstructed inside the liver.

The venous drainage from the liver is into the *right* and *left hepatic veins* which emerge from the back of the liver and at once enter the inferior vena cava very near its point of entry in the right auricle.

Lymphatic vessels terminate in small groups of glands around the porta hepatis. Efferent vessels drain into glands around the coeliac axis. Some superficial hepatic lymphatics pass through the diaphragm in the falciform ligament and finally reach the mediastinal glands.

Another group accompanies the inferior vena cava into the thorax and ends in a few small glands around the intrathoracic portion of the inferior vena cava.

The *inferior vena cava* makes a deep groove to the right of the caudate lobe about 2 cm from the mid-line.

The *gallbladder* lies in a fossa extending from the inferior border of the liver to the right end of the porta hepatis.

The liver is completely covered with peritoneum except in three places. It comes into direct contact with the diaphragm through the bare area which lies to the right of the fossa for the inferior vena cava. The other areas without peritoneal covering are the fossae for the inferior vena cava and gallbladder.

The liver is kept in position by peritoneal ligaments and by the intra-abdominal pressure transmitted by the tone of the muscles of the abdominal wall.

Segmental and functional divisions (figs 1.4, 1.5)

Segmental anatomy has been defined by injecting vinyl into vessels and bile ducts and preparing casts and also *in vivo* by imaging techniques (CT, magnetic resonance and ultrasound) [16]. The segmental anatomy of the liver is particularly important in planning hepatic resections.

One lobar fissure is in line with the fissure of the inferior vena cava above and the fossa of the gallbladder below. This fissure takes an oblique course from left to right to the porta hepatis and divides the liver into two anatomical left and right lobes (figs 1.2, 1.3). The left segmental fissure divides the two left lobes into medial and lateral segments. The right segmental fissure divides the right lobe into an anterior and a posterior segment.

Three hepatic planes are defined by the hepatic veins.
Plane A indicates the boundary between the right posterior and right anterior segment.
Plane B indicates the boundary between the right anterior and left medial segment.

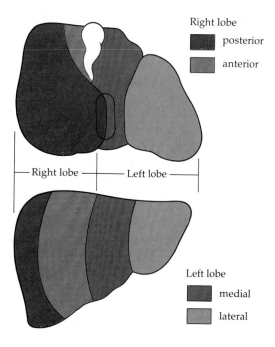

Right lobe
posterior
anterior

Right lobe — Left lobe

Left lobe
medial
lateral

Fig. 1.4. The segments of the human liver (Healey 1970).

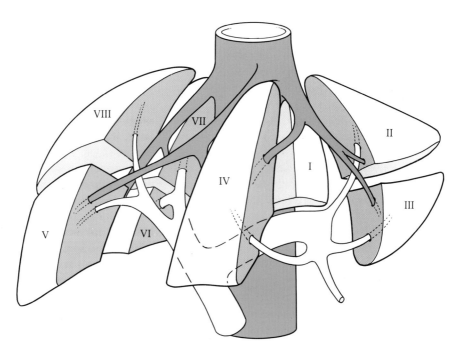

Fig. 1.5. Schematic representation of the functional anatomy of the liver. Three main hepatic veins divide the liver into four sectors, each of them receiving a portal pedicle; hepatic veins and portal veins are intertwined as the fingers of two hands (Bismuth, 1982).

Plane C indicates the boundary between the left medial and left lateral segment.

Each segment has its own major blood supply. There is no anastomosis between macroscopic branches but communications exist at a sinusoidal level. The functional division into right and left lobes with respect to biliary drainage and vascular supply differs from the anatomically accepted right and left lobes. The line of functional division lies to the right of the attachment of the falciform ligament and follows an irregular line from the inferior vena cava obliquely across the upper surface of the liver to the tip of the gallbladder. The functional right and left lobes are supplied by the right and left hepatic ducts and portal venous branches and drained by corresponding hepatic veins.

Anatomy of the biliary tract (fig. 1.6)

3 The *right and left hepatic ducts* emerge from the right and left lobes of the liver and unite in the porta hepatis to form the *common hepatic duct*. This is soon joined by the *cystic duct* from the gallbladder to form the common bile duct.

The *common bile duct* runs between the layers of the lesser omentum, lying anterior to the portal vein and to the right of the hepatic artery. Passing behind the first part of the duodenum in a groove on the back of the head of the pancreas, it enters the second part of the duodenum. The duct runs obliquely through the postero-medial duodenal wall about its middle, usually joining the main pancreatic duct to form the *ampulla of Vater* (1720). The ampulla makes the mucous membrane bulge inwards to form an eminence, the *duodenal papilla*. In about 30% of subjects the bile and pancreatic ducts open separately into the duodenum. The common bile duct, measured at operation, is about 0.5–1.5 cm in diameter.

The duodenal portion of the common bile duct is surrounded by a thickening of both longitudinal and circular muscle fibres derived

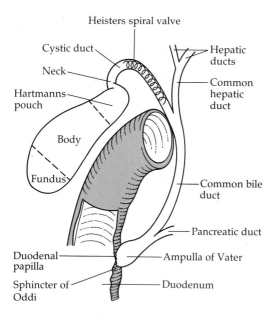

Heisters spiral valve

Cystic duct

Neck

Hartmanns pouch

Body

Fundus

Hepatic ducts

Common hepatic duct

Common bile duct

Pancreatic duct

Duodenal papilla

Ampulla of Vater

Sphincter of Oddi

Duodenum

Fig. 1.6. Gallbladder and biliary tract.

from the intestine. This is called the *sphincter of Oddi* (1887).

The *gallbladder* is a pear-shaped bag 9 cm long with a capacity of about 50 ml. Any decrease in concentrating power is accompanied by a lowering of the powers of expansion. The fundus is the broad end and is directed forward: this is the part palpated when the abdomen is examined. The body extends into a narrow neck which continues into the cystic duct. The *valves of Heister* are spiral folds of mucous membrane in the wall of the cystic duct and neck of the gallbladder. *Hartmann's pouch* is a sacculation at the neck of the gallbladder; this is a common site for a gallstone to lodge.

The wall consists of a musculo-elastic network without definite layers, the muscle being particularly well developed in the neck and fundus. The mucous membrane is in delicate closely woven folds; instead of glands there are deep indentations of mucosa, the *crypts of Luschka*, which penetrate into the muscular layer. There is no submucosa or muscularis mucosae.

The *Rokitansky—Aschoff sinuses* are branching evaginations from the lumen into the mucosa and muscularis of the gallbladder. They play an important part in acute cholecystitis and gangrene of the gallbladder wall.

The gallbladder receives blood from the *cystic artery*. This branch of the hepatic artery is large, tortuous and variable in its anatomical relationships. The bile ducts also have a variable arterial supply [17]. Smaller blood vessels enter from the liver through the gallbladder fossa. The venous drainage is into the *cystic vein* and thence into the portal venous system.

There are many *lymphatic vessels* in the submucous and subperitoneal layers. These drain through the cystic gland at the neck of the gallbladder to glands along the common bile duct, where they anastomose with lymphatics from the head of the pancreas.

Nerve supply. The gallbladder and bile ducts are liberally supplied with nerves, from both the parasympathetic and the sympathetic system.

Development of the liver and bile ducts

The liver begins as a hollow endodermal bud from the foregut (duodenum). The bud separates into two parts. The hepatic section forms the hepatic duct and its branches and the main mass of liver cells. It is met by ingrowing capillary plexuses from the vitelline veins which will form the sinusoids. The biliary part forms the gallbladder and extrahepatic bile ducts.

Anatomical abnormalities of the liver

These are being increasingly diagnosed with more widespread use of CT and ultrasound scanning.

Accessory lobes. The liver of the pig, dog and camel is divided into distinct and separate lobes by strands of connective tissue. Occasionally the human liver may show this reversion and up to sixteen lobes have been reported. This abnormality is rare and without clinical significance. The lobes are small and usually on the

4

under surface of the liver so that they are not detected but noted incidentally at scanning, operation or necropsy. Rarely they are intra-thoracic. An accessory lobe may have its own mesentery containing hepatic artery, portal vein, bile duct and hepatic vein [21]. This may twist and demand surgical intervention.

Riedel's lobe [23] is fairly common and is a downward tongue-like projection of the right lobe of the liver. It is a simple anatomical variation; it is not a true accessory lobe. The condition is more frequent in women. It is detected as a mobile tumour on the right side of the abdomen which descends with the dia-phragm and on respiration. It may come down as low as the right iliac region. It is easily mistaken for other tumours in this area, es-pecially a visceroptotic right kidney. It does not cause symptoms and treatment is not required. Scanning may be used to identify Riedel's lobe and other anatomical abnormalities.

Cough furrows on the liver are parallel grooves on the convexity of the right lobe. They are one to six in number and run antero-posteriorly, being deeper posteriorly. They are said to be associated with a chronic cough.

Corset liver [19]. This is a fibrotic furrow or pedicle on the anterior surface of both lobes of the liver just below the costal margin. Mechanism is unknown, but it affects elderly women who have worn corsets for many years. It presents as an abdominal mass in front of and below the liver and is isodense with the liver. It may be confused with a hepatic tumour.

Atrophy of the left lobe [1, 6]. Severe atrophy confined to the functional left lobe of the liver is not uncommon at post mortem. The lobe is decreased in size, with wrinkling and thick-ening of the capsule, fibrosis and prominent biliary and vascular markings. Histologically, the portal areas seem crowded together.

The usual cause is interference with the left branch of the portal vein. At the time of birth the left lobe loses its blood and oxygen supply when the ductus venosus is obliterated; de-generative changes follow. This atrophy may persist into adult life. Later, compression of the left hepatic duct or the left branch of the portal

vein or the left branch of the hepatic artery, for instance by malignant disease, can result in atrophy of the left lobe.

Agenesis of the right lobe [22]. This rare lesion may be an incidental finding associated, prob-ably coincidentally, with biliary tract disease and also with other congenital abnormalities. It can cause presinusoidal portal hypertension. The other liver segments undergo compensa-tory hypertrophy. It must be distinguished from lobar atrophy due to cirrhosis or hilar cholangiocarcinoma.

Anatomical abnormalities of gallbladder and biliary tract (see Chapter 30).

Surface marking (figs 1.7, 1.8)

Liver. The upper border of the right lobe is on a level with the 5th rib at a point 2 cm medial to the right mid-clavicular line (1 cm below the right nipple). The upper border of the left lobe corresponds to the upper border of the 6th rib at a point in the left mid-clavicular line (2 cm below the left nipple). Here only the diaphragm separates the liver from the apex of the heart.

The lower border passes obliquely upwards from the 9th right to the 8th left costal cartilage.

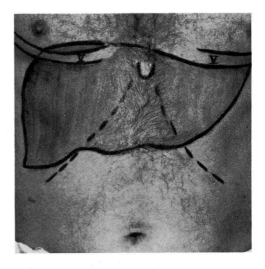

Fig. 1.7. Surface marking of the liver. The 5th ribs are outlined.

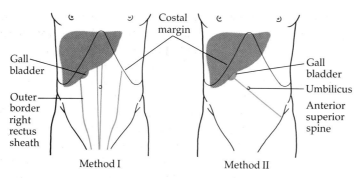

Fig. 1.8. Surface markings of the gallbladder. Method I: the gallbladder is found where the outer border of the right rectus abdominis muscle intersects the 9th costal cartilage. Method II: a line drawn from the left anterior iliac spine through the umbilicus intersects the costal margin at the site of the gallbladder.

In the right nipple line it lies between a point just under to 2 cm below the costal margin. It crosses the mid-line about mid-way between the base of the xiphoid and the umbilicus and the left lobe extends only 5 cm to the left of the sternum.

Gallbladder. The fundus lies at the outer border of the right rectus abdominis muscle at its junction with the right costal margin (9th costal cartilage) (fig. 1.8). In an obese subject it may be difficult to identify the outer border of the rectus sheath and the gallbladder may then be located by the Grey−Turner method. A line is drawn from the left anterior superior iliac spine through the umbilicus; its intersection with the right costal margin indicates the position of the gallbladder.

Methods of examination

Liver. The lower edge should be determined by palpation just lateral to the right rectus muscle. This avoids mistaking the upper intersection of the rectus sheath for the liver edge.

The liver edge moves 1−3 cm downwards with deep inspiration. It is usually palpable in normal subjects inspiring deeply. The edge may be tender, regular or irregular, firm or soft, thickened or sharp. The lower edge may be displaced downwards by a low diaphragm, for instance in emphysema. Movements may be particularly great in athletes or singers. Some patients with practice become very efficient at 'pushing down' the liver. The normal spleen can become palpable in a similar fashion. Common causes of a liver palpable below the um-

bilicus are malignant deposits, polycystic or Hodgkin's disease, amyloidosis, congestive cardiac failure, and gross fatty change. Rapid change in liver size may occur when congestive cardiac failure is corrected, cholestatic jaundice relieved, severe diabetes controlled, or when fat is dispersed. The surface can be palpated in the epigastrium and any irregularity or tenderness noted. An enlarged caudate lobe, as in the Budd−Chiari syndrome or with some cases of cirrhosis, may be palpated as an epigastric mass.

Pulsation of the liver, usually associated with tricuspid valvular incompetence, is felt by manual palpation with one hand over the right lower ribs posteriorly and the other anteriorly on the abdominal wall.

The upper edge is determined by fairly heavy percussion passing downwards from the nipple-line. The lower edge is recognized by very light percussion passing upwards from the umbilicus towards the costal margin. Percussion is a valuable method of determining liver size and is the only clinical method of determining a small liver.

The anterior liver span is obtained by measuring the vertical distance between uppermost and lowermost points of hepatic dullness by percussion in the right mid-clavicular line. This is usually 12−15 cm. Direct percussion is as accurate as ultrasound in estimating liver span [27].

Friction may be palpable and audible, usually due to recent biopsy, tumour or peri-hepatitis [8]. The venous hum of portal hypertension is audible between the umbilicus and the xiphisternum. An arterial murmur over the liver may indicate a primary liver cancer or acute alcoholic hepatitis.

The gallbladder is palpable only when it is distended. It is felt as a pear-shaped cystic mass usually about 7 cm long. In a thin person, the swelling can sometimes be seen through the anterior abdominal wall. It moves downwards on inspiration and is mobile laterally but not downwards. The swelling is dull to percussion and directly impinges on the parietal peritoneum, so that the colon is rarely in front of it. Gallbladder dullness is continuous with that of the liver.

Abdominal tenderness should be noted. Inflammation of the gallbladder causes a positive *Murphy's sign*. This is the inability to take a deep breath when the examining fingers are hooked up below the liver edge. The inflamed gallbladder is then driven against the fingers and the pain causes the patient to catch his breath.

The enlarged gallbladder must be distinguished from a *visceroptotic right kidney*. This, however, is more mobile, can be displaced towards the pelvis and has the resonant colon anteriorly. A *regenerative* or *malignant nodule* feels much firmer.

Imaging. A plain film of the abdomen, including the diaphragms, may be used to assess liver size and in particular to decide whether a palpable liver is due to actual enlargement or to downward displacement. On moderate inspiration the normal level of the diaphragm, on the right side, is opposite the 11th rib posteriorly and the 6th rib anteriorly.

Ultrasound, CT or magnetic resonance can also be used to study liver size, shape and consistence.

Hepatic morphology

Kiernan (1833) introduced the concept of hepatic lobules as the basic architecture. He described circumscribed pyramidal lobules consisting of a central tributary of the hepatic vein and at the periphery a portal tract containing bile duct, portal vein radicle and hepatic artery branch. Columns of liver cells and blood-containing sinusoids extended between these two systems.

Stereoscopic reconstructions and scanning electron microscopy have shown the human liver as columns of liver cells radiating from a central vein, and interlaced in orderly fashion by sinusoids (fig. 1.9).

The liver tissue is pervaded by two systems of tunnels, the portal tracts and the hepatic central canals which dovetail in such a way that they never touch each other; the terminal tunnels of the two systems are separated by about 0.5 mm (fig. 1.10). As far as possible the two systems of tunnels run in planes perpendicular to each other (fig. 1.11). The sinusoids are irregularly disposed, normally in a direction perpendicular to the lines connecting the central veins. The terminal branches of the portal vein discharge their blood into the sinusoids and the direction of flow is determined by the higher pressure in the portal vein than in the central vein.

The *central hepatic canals* contain radicles of the hepatic vein and their adventitia. They are surrounded by a limiting plate of liver cells.

The *portal triads* (syn. portal tracts, Glisson's capsule) contain the portal vein radicle, the hepatic arteriole and bile duct with a few round cells and a little connective tissue (fig. 1.12). They are surrounded by a limiting plate of liver cells.

The liver has to be divided *functionally*. Traditionally the unit is based on a central hepatic vein and its surrounding liver cells. However, Rappaport [23] envisages a series of functional acini, each centred on the portal triad with its terminal branch of portal vein, hepatic artery and bile duct (zone 1) (figs 1.13, 1.14). These interdigitate, mainly perpendicularly, with terminal hepatic veins of adjacent acini. The circulatory peripheries of acini (adjacent to terminal hepatic veins) (zone 3) suffer most from injury whether viral, toxic or anoxic. Bridging necrosis is located in this area. The regions closer to the axis formed by afferent vessels and bile ducts survive longer and may later form the core from which regeneration

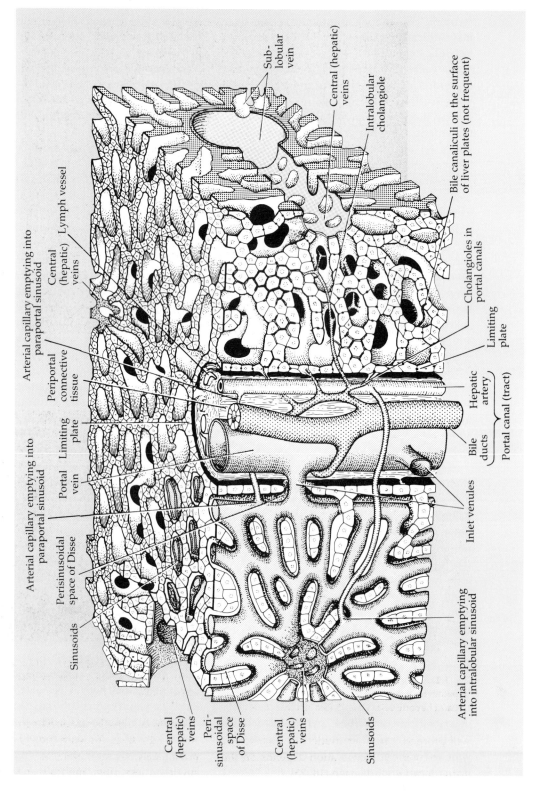

Sub-lobular vein

Central (hepatic) veins

Intralobular cholangiole

Bile canaliculi on the surface of liver plates (not frequent)

Cholangioles in portal canals

Limiting plate

Hepatic artery

Bile ducts

Portal canal (tract)

Inlet venules

Arterial capillary emptying into intralobular sinusoid

Sinusoids

Central (hepatic) veins

Peri-sinusoidal space of Disse

Central (hepatic) veins

Sinusoids

Perisinusoidal space of Disse

Portal vein

Limiting plate

Periportal connective tissue

Central (hepatic) veins

Lymph vessel

Arterial capillary emptying into paraportal sinusoid

Limiting plate

Arterial capillary emptying into paraportal sinusoid

Fig. 1.9. The structure of the normal human liver.

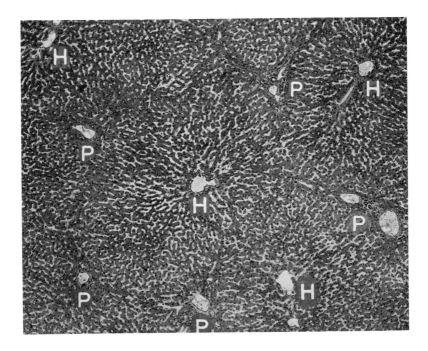

Fig. 1.10. Normal hepatic histology. H = terminal hepatic vein; P = portal tract. (Stained H & E, ×60.)

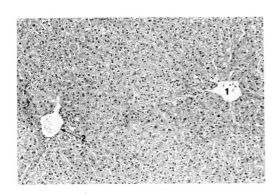

Fig. 1.11. Normal liver shows columns of hepatocytes extending between portal zone (tract) to left and hepatic vein to right. (Stained H & E, ×40.)

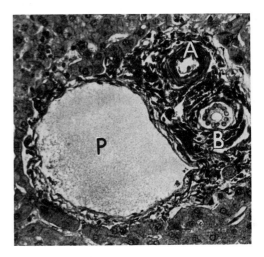

Fig. 1.12. Normal portal tract. B = bile duct; P = portal vein; A = hepatic artery. (Stained elastic tissue, ×220.)

will proceed. The contribution of each acinar zone to liver cell regeneration depends on the acinar location of damage [18, 23].

The liver cells (*hepatocytes*) comprise about 60% of the liver. They are polygonal and approximately 30 µm in diameter. The nucleus is single or, less often, multiple and divides by

9

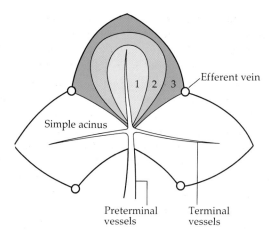

Fig. 1.13. The complex acinus according to Rappaport. Zone 1 is adjacent to the entry (portal venous) system. Zone 3 is adjacent to the exit (hepatic venous) system.

mitosis. The lifespan of liver cells is about 150 days in experimental animals. The hepatocyte has three surfaces: one facing the sinusoid and space of Dissë, the second facing the canaliculus and the third facing neighbouring hepatocytes. There is no basement membrane.

The walls of the sinusoids consist of endothelial and phagocytic cells of the reticuloendothelial system. The flat cell components are known as *Kupffer cells.*

There are approximately 202×10^3 cells in each milligramme of normal human liver, of which 171×10^3 are parenchymatous and 31×10^3 littoral (sinusoidal including Kupffer cells) [9].

The *space of Dissë* is a tissue space between hepatocytes and sinusoidal lining cells. The

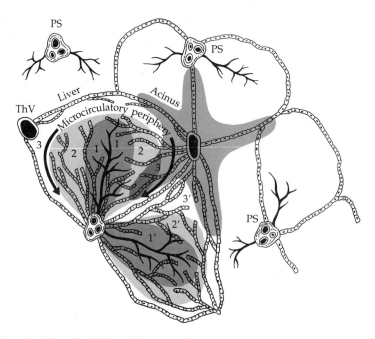

Fig. 1.14. Blood supply of the simple liver acinus, zonal arrangements of cells and the microcirculatory periphery. The acinus occupies adjacent sectors of neighbouring hexagonal fields. Zones 1, 2 and 3 respectively represent areas supplied with blood of first, second and third quality with regard to oxygen and nutrient contents. These zones centre about the terminal afferent vascular branches, bile ductules, lymph vessels and nerves (PS) and extend into the triangular portal field from which these branches crop out. Zone 3 is the microcirculatory periphery of the acinus since its cells are as remote from their own afferent vessels as from those of adjacent acini. The *perivenular* area is formed by the most peripheral portions of zone 3 of several adjacent acini. In injury progressing along this zone, the damaged area assumes the shape of a seastar (heavy, cross-hatching around a ThV in the centre). 1, 2, 3 = microcirculatory zones; 1′, 2′, 3′ = zones of neighbouring acinus; ---- afferent vessels of acini outlining the hexagons (Rappaport 1976).

hepatic lymphatics are found in the peri-portal connective tissue and are lined throughout by endothelium. Tissue fluid seeps through the endothelium into the lymph vessels.

The branch of the *hepatic arteriole* forms a plexus around the bile ducts and supplies the structures in the portal tracts. It empties into the sinusoidal network at different levels. There are no direct hepatic arteriolar–portal venous anastomoses.

The excretory system of the liver begins with the *bile canaliculi* (figs 7.6, 13.3). These have no walls but are simply grooves on the contact surfaces of liver cells. Their surfaces are covered by microvilli. The plasma membrane is reinforced by microfilaments forming a supportive cytoskeleton (fig. 13.1). The canalicular surface is sealed from the rest of the intercellular surface by junctional complexes including tight junctions, gap junctions and desmosomes. The intralobular canalicular network drains into thin-walled terminal bile ducts or ductules (cholangioles, canals of Hering) lined with cuboidal epithelium. These terminate in larger (interlobular) bile ducts in the portal canals. They are classified into small (less than 100 μm in diameter) medium (±100 μm), and large (more than 100 μm).

Electron microscopy and hepato-cellular function (figs 1.15, 1.16)

The liver cell margin is straight except for a few anchoring pegs (desmosomes). From it equally sized and spaced microvilli project into the lumen of the bile canaliculi. Along the sinusoidal border, irregularly sized and spaced microvilli project into the perisinusoidal tissue space. The microvillous structure indicates active secretion or absorption, mainly of fluid.

The *nucleus* contains deoxyribonucleo-protein. Human liver after puberty also contains tetraploid nuclei and, at about age 20, in addition, octoploid nuclei are found. Increased polyploidy has been regarded as precancerous. In the chromatin network one or more nucleoli are embedded. The nucleus has a double con-tour with pores allowing interchange with the surrounding hyaloplasm.

The *mitochondria* also have a double membrane, the inner being invaginated to form grooves or cristae. An enormous number of energy-providing processes take place within them, particularly those involving oxidative phosphorylation. They contain many enzymes, particularly those of the citric acid cycle and those involved in β-oxidation of fatty acids. They can transform energy so released into ADP. Haem synthesis occurs here.

The *rough endoplasmic reticulum* (RER) is seen as lamellar profiles lined by ribosomes. These are responsible for basophilia under light microscopy. They synthesize specific proteins, particularly albumin, those used in blood coagulation and enzymes. They may adopt a helix arrangement, as polysomes, for coordination of this function. Glucose-6-phosphatase is synthesized. Triglycerides are synthesized from free fatty acids and complexed with protein to be secreted by exocytosis as lipoprotein. The RER may participate in glycogenesis.

The *smooth endoplasmic reticulum* (SER) forms tubules and vesicles. It contains the microsomes. It is the site of bilirubin conjugation and the detoxification of many drugs and other foreign compounds. Steroids are synthesized. These include cholesterol and the primary bile acids which are conjugated with the amino acids glycine and taurine. The SER is increased by enzyme inducers such as phenobarbital.

Peroxisomes are distributed near the SER and glycogen granules. Their function is unknown.

The *lysosomes* are peri-canalicular dense bodies adjacent to the bile canaliculi. They contain many hydrolytic enzymes which, if released, could destroy the cell. They are probably intracellular scavengers which destroy organelles with shortened lifespans. They are the site of deposition of ferritin, lipofuscin, bile pigment and copper. Pinocytic vacuoles may be observed in them. Some peri-canalicular dense bodies are termed *microbodies*.

The *Golgi apparatus* consists of a system of particles and vesicles again lying near the cana-liculus. It may be regarded as a 'packaging' site

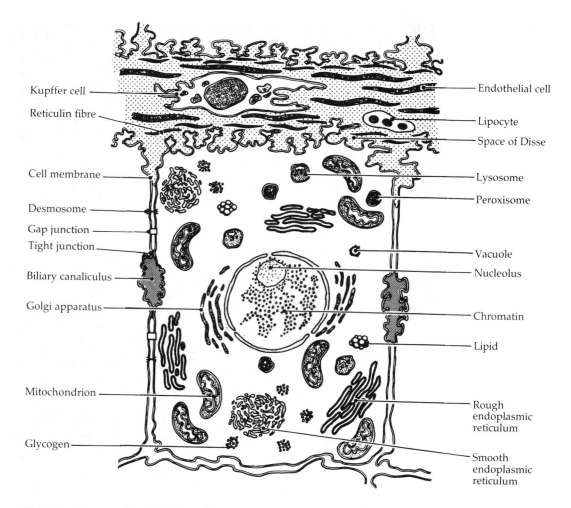

Kupffer cell
Reticulin fibre
Cell membrane
Desmosome
Gap junction
Tight junction
Biliary canaliculus
Golgi apparatus
Mitochondrion
Glycogen

Endothelial cell
Lipocyte
Space of Disse
Lysosome
Peroxisome
Vacuole
Nucleolus
Chromatin
Lipid
Rough endoplasmic reticulum
Smooth endoplasmic reticulum

Fig. 1.15. The organelles of the liver cell.

for excretion into the bile. This entire group of lysosomes, microbodies and Golgi apparatus is a means of sequestering any material which was ingested and has to be excreted, secreted or stored for metabolic processes in the hyaloplasm. The Golgi apparatus, lysosomes and canaliculi are concerned in cholestasis (Chapter 13).

The intervening *hyaloplasm* contains granules of glycogen, lipid and fine fibrils.

Microtubules and microfilaments (fig. 13.1) provide a supporting cytoskeleton. They are contractile, the microtubule containing tubulin and the microfilament F actin. They control subcellular motility, vesicle movements and cell shape. Canalicular motility and bile flow may depend on microfilament function [20].

Sinusoidal cells

The sinusoidal cells (endothelial cells, Kupffer cells, fat storing cells and pit cells) form a functional and histological unit together with the sinusoidal aspect of the hepatocyte [29] (figs 1.14, 1.16). The Kupffer cells and endothelial cells are littoral cells in contact with the lumen of the sinusoids. The fat storing cells (Ito cells) lie in the space of Dissë between the hepatocytes and the endothelial cells. *Dissë space* contains tissue fluid which flows outwards into

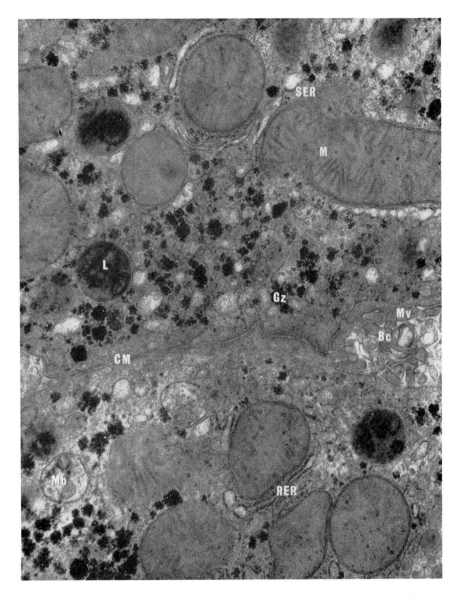

Fig. 1.16. Electron microscopic appearances of a normal human liver cell: the zone around the bile canaliculus. ×102 000. M = mitochondria; L = lysosome; Mb = microbody; Bc = bile canaliculus; CM = cell membrane; Mv = microvillus; Gz = Golgi zone; SER = smooth endoplasmic reticulum; RER = rough endoplasmic reticulum (Krustev 1967).

lymphatics in the portal zones. When sinusoidal pressure rises, lymph production in Dissë space increases and this plays a part in ascites formation where there is hepatic outflow (zone 3) obstruction.

Kupffer cells. These are highly mobile macrophages attached to the endothelium. They are peroxidase staining and have a nuclear envelope. They phagocytose large particles and contain vacuoles and lysosomes. They

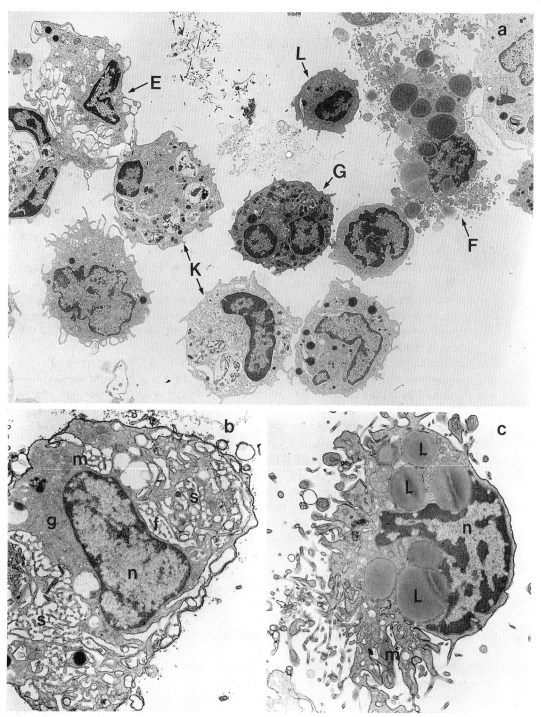

Fig. 1.17. Transmission electron micrographs of freshly isolated human sinusoidal liver cells. (a) Overview of a sinusoidal liver cell fraction showing the different cell types: K = Kupffer cell; E = endothelial cell; F = fat-storing cell; L = lymphocyte; G = granulocyte. (×3600). (b,c) Higher magnification of (b) an endothelial cell with sieve plates (×6800) and (c) a fat-storing cell (×8800) displaying the most prominent cellular characteristics. S = sieve plates; F = fenestrations; N = nucleus, L = lipid droplets; G = Golgi complex; M = mitochondria. (Brouwer *et al.* 1988).

are derived from blood monocytes and have only limited capabilities of division. They phagocytose by endocytosis (pinocytosis or phagocytosis) which may be absorptive (receptor-mediated) or fluid phase (non-receptor-mediated). Kupffer cells endocytose old cells, foreign particles, tumour cells, bacteria, yeasts, viruses and parasites. They attach denatured proteins and fibrin in disseminated intravascular coagulation.

The Kupffer cell has specific membrane receptors, including ligands for the Fc portion of immunoglobulin and C3b component of complement, which are important for antigen presentation.

With generalized infections or trauma, Kupffer cells become activated. They specifically endocytose endotoxin and in response, secrete a series of factors such as tumour necrosing factor (TNF), interleukins, collagenase and lysosomal hydrolases. These increase discomfort and sickness. The toxicity of endotoxin is caused by the secretory products of Kupffer cells as endotoxin itself is not toxic.

The Kupffer cell secrete arachidonic acid metabolites including prostaglandins [5].

The Kupffer cell has specific membrane receptors for insulin, glucagon and lipoproteins. The carbohydrate receptor, which recognizes N-acetyl glucosamine, mannose and galactose may mediate the pinocytic uptake of certain glycoproteins, particularly lysosomal hydrolases. It also mediates the uptake of IgM-containing immune complexes.

Kupffer cells have erythroblastoid function in fetal liver.

Opsonins, plasma fibronectin and immunoglobulins promote recognition and speed of endocytosis by Kupffer cells.

Endothelial cells. These sessile cells form a continuous wall to the lumen of the sinusoid. Fenestrae (0.1 μm in diameter) (sieve plates) determine the exchange of fluids and size of particulate matter to and from the space of Dissë and the hepatocyte [29]. Endothelial cells have lobular gradients. Scanning electron microscopy has shown, particularly in zone 3 in alcoholic patients, a striking reduction in the number of fenestrae with formation of a basal lamina [15]. Endothelial cells also have Fc receptors and may participate with K cells in binding IgG opsonized material in sinusoidal blood (25). They play a role in defence of the liver against viral infection.

Fat storing (Ito) cells. These stellate sessile cells lie within the space of Dissë. They may contain fat. When empty, ultrastructurally they resemble fibroblasts. They store excess vitamin A and other retinoids [14], also other fat soluble vitamins. In the presence of hepatocyte damage, Ito cells migrate to zone 3 where they change into myofibroblasts which secrete collagen types I, III, IV and laminin. They may regulate sinusoidal blood flow and hence contribute to portal hypertension [2]. Collagenization of the space of Dissë results in decreased access of protein-bound substrates to the hepatocyte [28].

Pit cells. These are highly mobile, natural killer lymphocytes attached to the endothelium. They show characteristic granules and rod cored vesicles. Pit cells show spontaneous cytotoxicity against tumour and virus infected hepatocytes.

Altered hepatic microcirculation and disease [28]

In liver disease, particularly in the alcoholic, the liver microcirculation may be altered by collagenization of the space of Dissë, formation of a basal lamina beneath the endothelium and modification of the endothelial fenestrations [15]. All these processes are maximal in zone 3. They contribute to deprivation of nutriments intended for the hepatocyte and to the development of portal hypertension.

Functional heterogeneity

The relative functions of cells in the circulating periphery of acini (zone 3) adjacent to terminal hepatic veins are different from those in the circulatory area adjacent to terminal hepatic arteries and portal veins (zone 1) (figs 1.14, 1.15) (table 1.1) [1.0].

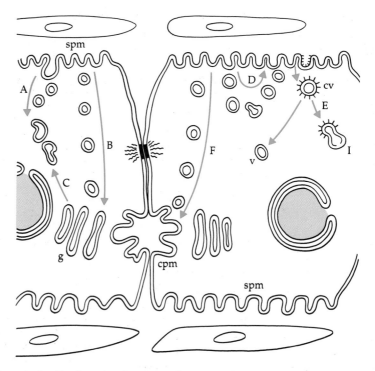

Fig. 1.18. Traffic routes leading from the plasma membrane into the hepatocyte interior. A = Receptor-mediated uptake direct route from the sinusoidal plasma membrane (spm) region to the lysosomes (l). B = Receptor-mediated uptake route from the sinusoidal plasma membrane region to the Golgi apparatus region (G). C = Route from Golgi apparatus region to lysosomes. D = Receptor-mediated uptake route involving recycling from and to the blood–sinusoidal plasma membrane region. E = Receptor-mediated internalization route involving coated pit formation at the blood–sinusoidal plasma membrane region followed by internalization of a coated vesicle (cv) which may interact with lysosomes or migrate further having lost its coat (v). F = Receptor-mediated internalization route involving transfer of ligands contained within vesicles from blood–sinusoidal to the bile canalicular plasma membrane regions (cpm) for release into bile. Transit times vary from about 2 to 60 min. (Evans 1981).

Table 1.1. Metabolism related to the zonal location of the hepatocyte whether zone 3 (central, acinar inlet) or zone 1 ('peri-portal' acinar outlet) (Gumucio & Miller 1981)

	Zone 1	Zone 3
Carbohydrates	Gluconeogenesis	Glycolysis
Proteins	Albumin ⎫ synthesis Fibrinogen ⎭	Albumin ⎫ synthesis Fibrinogen ⎭
Cytochrome P-450	+	++
after phenobarbital	+	++++++++
Glutathione	++	−
Oxygen supply	+++	+
Bile formation		
Bile salt-dependent	++	−
Non-bile salt-dependent	−	++
Sinusoids	Small	Straight
	Highly anastomotic	Radial

Krebs cycle enzymes (urea synthesis and glutaminase) are found in highest concentration in zone 1 whereas glutamine synthetase is peri-venous [12].

Oxygen supply is an obvious difference, cells in zone 3 receive their oxygen supply last and are particularly prone to anoxic liver injury.

The drug-metabolizing P-450 enzymes are present in greater amounts in zone 3. This is particularly so after enzyme induction, for instance with phenobarbital. Hepatocytes in zone 3 receive a higher concentration of any toxic product of drug metabolism. They also have a reduced glutathione concentration. This makes them particularly susceptible to hepatic drug reactions.

Hepatocytes in zone 1 receive blood with a high bile salt concentration and therefore are particularly important in bile salt-dependent bile formation. Hepatocytes in zone 3 are important in non-bile salt-dependent bile formation. There are also zonal differences in the hepatic transport rate of substances from sinusoids to canaliculus [26].

Plasma membrane and membrane traffic

Plasma membrane consists of a receptor-rich and metabolically dynamic blood-sinusoidal domain which is separated from the bile canalicular domain by a lateral domain which participates in cell—cell interactions [7].

The sinusoidal plasma membrane domain has a large number of specific binding sites for hormones and metabolites. Most molecules enter the hepatocyte through receptor-mediated binding and subsequent uptake of the membrane ligand. Passive transfer into the hepatocyte is much less important. The paracellular shunt pathway into bile is confined mainly to small ions and water. Traffic routes from the plasma membrane vary (fig. 1.18). Sequestration inside lysosomes leads to discharge of products into blood. There may be a direct route from the sinusoidal membrane to the biliary pole and hence discharge into bile. Transport of ligands across the hepatocyte may be vesicular.

References

1 Benz EJ, Baggenstoss AH, Wollaeger EE. Atrophy of the left lobe of the liver. *Arch. Path.* 1952; **53**: 315.

2 Bhathal PS, Grossman HJ. Reduction of the increased portal vascular resistance of the isolated perfused cirrhotic rat liver by vasodilators. *J. Hepatol.* 1985; **1**: 325.

3 Bismuth H. Surgical anatomy and anatomical surgery of the liver. *World J. Surg.* 1982; **6**: 3.

4 Bismuth H, Houssin D, Ornowski J *et al.* Liver resections in cirrhotic patients: a Western experience. *World J. Surg.* 1986; **10**: 311.

5 Brouwer A, Barelds RJ, de Leeuw AM *et al.* Isolation and culture of Kupffer cells from human liver. *J. Hepatol.* 1988; **6**: 36.

6 Emery JL. Degenerative changes in the left lobe of the liver in the newborn. *Arch. Dis. child.* 1952; **27**: 558.

7 Evans WH. Membrane traffic at the hepatocyte's sinusoidal and canalicular surface domains. *Hepatology* 1981; **1**: 452.

8 Fred HL, Brown GR. The hepatic friction rub. *N. Engl. J. Med.* 1962; **266**: 554.

9 Gates GA, Henley KS, Pollard HM *et al.* The cell population of human liver. *J. Lab. clin. Med.* 1961; **57**: 182.

10 Gumucio JJ, Miller DL. Functional implications of liver cell heterogeneity. *Gastroenterology* 1981; **80**: 393.

11 Gumucio JJ, May M, Dvokak C *et al.* The isolation of functionally heterogeneous hepatocytes of the proximal and distal half of the liver acinus in the rat. *Hepatology* 1986; **6**: 932.

12 Haussinger D, Sies H, Gerok W. Functional hepatocyte heterogeneity in ammonia metabolism. The intracellular glutamine cycle. *J. Hepatol.* 1984; **1**: 3.

13 Healey JE Jr. Vascular anatomy of the liver. *Ann. NY Acad. Sci.* 1970; **170**: 8.

14 Hendriks HFJ, Brouwer A, Knook DL. The role of hepatic fat-storing (stellate) cells in retinoid metabolism. *Hepatology* 1987; **7**: 1368.

15 Horn T, Christoffersen P, Henriksen JH. Alcoholic liver injury: defenestration in non-cirrhotic livers. A scanning microscopic study. *Hepatology* 1987; **7**: 77.

16 Mukai JK, Stack CM, Turner DA *et al.* Imaging of surgically relevant hepatic vascular and segmental anatomy; Part 1: Normal anatomy. *Am. J. Roent.* 1987; **149**: 287.

17 Northover JMA, Terblanche J. A new look at the arterial supply of the bile duct in man and its surgical implications. *Br. J. Surg.* 1979; **66**: 379.

18 Nostrant TT, Miller DL, Appelman HD *et al.* Acinar distribution of liver cell regeneration after

selective zonal injury in the rat. *Gastroenterology* 1978; **75**: 181.

19 Philips DM, La Brecque DR, Shirazi SS. Corset liver. *J. clin. Gastroenterology* 1985; **7**: 361.

20 Phillips MJ, Oshio C, Miyairi M *et al.* What is actin doing in the liver cell? *Hepatology* 1983; **3**: 433.

21 Pujari BD, Deodhare SG. Symptomatic accessory lobe of liver with a review of the literature. *Postgrad. med. J.* 1976; **52**: 234.

22 Radin DR, Colletti PM, Ralls PW *et al.* Agenesis of the right lobe of the liver. *Radiology* 1987; **164**: 639.

23 Rappaport AM. The microcirculatory acinar concept of normal and pathological hepatic structure. *Beitr. Path.* 1976; **157**: 215.

24 Reitemeier RJ, Butt HR, Baggenstoss AH. Riedel's lobe of the liver. *Gastroenterology* 1958; **34**: 1090.

25 Shaw RG, Johnson AR, Schulz WW *et al.* Sinusoidal endothelial cells from normal guinea pig liver: isolation, culture and characterization. *Hepatology* 1984; **4**: 591.

26 Sherman IA, Fisher MM. Hepatic transport of fluorescent molecules: *in vivo* studies using intravital TV microscopy. *Hepatology* 1986; **6**: 444.

27 Skrainka B, Stahlhut J, Fullbeck CL *et al.* Measuring liver span. Bedside examination versus ultrasound and scintiscan. *J. clin. Gastroenterol.* 1986; **8**: 267.

28 Villeneuve J-P, Huet P-M. Microcirculatory abnormalities in liver diseases. *Hepatology* 1987; **7**: 186.

29 Wissë E, De Zanger RB, Charels K *et al.* The liver sieve: considerations concerning the structure and function of endothelial fenestrae, the sinusoidal wall and the space of Dissë. *Hepatology* 1985; **5**: 683.

2 · Assessment of Liver Function

Selection of biochemical tests

Tests are needed for accurate diagnosis, to estimate the severity, to assess prognosis and to evaluate therapy (table 2.1). There is no 'magic' test and a large number of methods are unnecessary. The more investigations are multiplied, the greater chance there is of a biochemical deficiency being demonstrated. This type of 'shotgun' investigation adds to the confusion. A few simple tests of established value should be used.

If an abnormality is found it may need to be confirmed by a repeat estimation to show that it is real and not a laboratory error.

Tests most useful in the *diagnosis of jaundice* (Chapter 12) are the serum alkaline phosphatase level, and serum transaminase values. An iso-

lated rise in serum unconjugated bilirubin suggests Gilbert's syndrome or haemolysis.

Assessment of the *severity of liver cell damage* is done by serial serum total bilirubin, albumin, transaminase and prothrombin after vitamin K estimations.

The diagnosis of *minimal hepato-cellular damage*, due to well-compensated cirrhosis or alcoholic liver damage, may be attempted by noting minimally elevated serum bilirubin and serum transaminase values. Similar changes will be seen in conditions such as fever or circulatory failure. Serum γ-glutamyl transpeptidase (γ-GT) may be useful for diagnosing minimal alcoholic liver damage.

Hepatic infiltrations such as primary or secondary cancer, amyloid disease or the reticu-

Table 2.1. Essential serum methods in hepato-biliary disease

Test	Normal range	SI units	Value
Bilirubin			
Total	0.3−1.0 mg/dl	5−17 mmol	Diagnosis jaundice. Assess severity
Conjugated	<0.3 mg/dl	<5 mmol	Gilbert's disease, haemolysis
Alkaline phosphatase		35−130	Diagnosis jaundice, hepatic infiltrations
Aspartate transaminase (AST SGOT)		5−40	Early diagnosis of hepato-cellular disease, follow progress
Alanine transaminase (ALT SGPT)		5−35	ALT relatively lower than AST in alcoholism
γ-glutamyl transpeptidase		10−48	Diagnosis alcohol abuse, marker biliary cholestasis
Albumin	3.5−5.0 g/dl	35−50 g	Assess severity
γ-globulin	0.5−1.5 g/dl	5−15 g	Diagnosis chronic hepatitis and cirrhosis—follow course
Prothrombin time (PTT) (after vitamin K)	12−16 sec		Assess severity

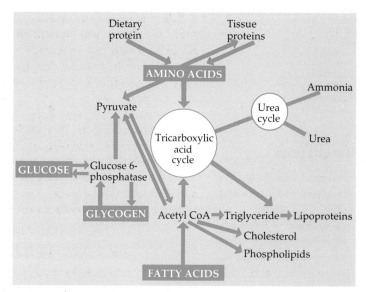

Fig. 2.1. The important metabolic pathways of protein, carbohydrate and fat in the liver.

loses are suggested by an elevated serum alkaline phosphatase value without jaundice.

Fibrosis may be estimated by the serum procollagen type III peptide (Chapter 19).

Conventional tests are being gradually reduced by more specific methods such as viral hepatitis markers and immunological tests such as the mitochondrial antibody for primary biliary cirrhosis and by more accurate anatomical localization by ultrasonography and CT scanning.

Quantitative assessment of hepatic function

Chronic liver diseases pass through a long period of minimum non-specific symptoms ('compensated') until the final stage of ascites, jaundice, encephalopathy and pre-coma ('decompensated'). Serial estimates of quantitative liver function in the early stages would be helpful both in monitoring treatment and in prognosis but are of no value in diagnosis. Such tests, however, suffer from the drawback of their complexity.

In the rat model of biliary cirrhosis, serial breath tests allow prediction of the time of death from cirrhosis [5]. Such tests may be useful in the evaluation of patients for hepatic transplantation.

GALACTOSE ELIMINATION CAPACITY

Galactose is pharmacologically safe and can be injected intravenously in a dose sufficient to saturate the enzyme system responsible for its elimination [2]. The rate limiting step is the initial phosphorylation by galactokinase. Account must be taken of the substantial fraction of the dose eliminated extra-hepatically (fig. 2.2). This test seems to reflect hepatocellular function fairly accurately but requires multiple determinations over a two hour period.

BREATH TESTS

Aminopyrine is metabolized (*N*-demethylated) by the cytochrome p-450 (microsomal) system to carbon dioxide. It has many of the characteristics of an ideal breath test substance for the measurement of hepatic function [1, 4, 8]. The aminopyrine is labelled with ^{14}C and given by mouth. Samples of $^{14}CO_2$ are collected from the breath for intervals over two hours. The expired $^{14}CO_2$ correlates with the rate of disappearance of radioactivity from the plasma. The test reflects the residual functional microsomal mass and viable hepatic tissue. Results in cirrhotic rats suggest that reduced *N*-demethylation is due to loss of liver cell volume. The function

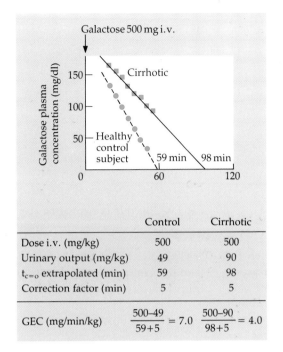

Galactose 500 mg i.v.

	Control	Cirrhotic
Dose i.v. (mg/kg)	500	500
Urinary output (mg/kg)	49	90
$t_{c=0}$ extrapolated (min)	59	98
Correction factor (min)	5	5
GEC (mg/min/kg)	$\dfrac{500-49}{59+5} = 7.0$	$\dfrac{500-90}{98+5} = 4.0$

Fig. 2.2. The method for the calculation of the galactose elimination capacity (GEC) consists of the intravenous administration of a dose of 0.5 g/kg of galactose, followed by an extrapolation of the zero order elimination to obtain the time theoretically needed for the complete elimination of the injected galactose. For the calculation of the GEC, the administered dose (in the numerator) is corrected for the amount of galactose lost in urine, and the extrapolated time (in the denominator) is augmented by a term (5 minutes) correcting for unequal distribution of galactose within the organism. It should be noted, that extra-hepatic tissues eliminate galactose at a rate of approximately 2.5 mg/min/kg. This value may therefore be regarded as zero liver function. The average value in normal volunteers (7.5 mg/min/kg) may be assumed to correspond to a 'functioning liver cell mass' of 100%, with a lower limit of reference range of 70%. According to this interpretation, the examples illustrate a normal control subject and a cirrhotic patient with an estimated functioning liver cell mass of 90% and 30% respectively (Bircher 1983).

per hepatocyte remains constant [9]. It is of value in prognosis and to assess therapy rather than for screening or diagnosis. It may be useful to assess the effect of drugs on the hepatic microsomal enzyme function.

^{14}C-caffeine and phenacetin [3] have been used as breath test substances. The ^{14}C-galactose breath test measures cytosolic function. All breath tests are complex and costly. They are unlikely to achieve general popularity.

Salivary caffeine clearance. Caffeine is metabolized almost exclusively in the hepatic microsomal enzyme system. Plasma clearance is a reliable indicator of severity of liver disease but is complicated to perform. A test calculating caffeine clearance from salivary levels, obtained overnight after oral caffeine, may be a useful quantitative test of hepatic function [7].

EXCRETORY CAPACITY (: BROMSULPHALEIN)

The old intravenous bromsulphalein disappearance technique allowed an estimate of the storage capacity of the hepatocyte (S) and its excretory function (Tm). It was abandoned because of its complexity, its cost and the untoward reactions to BSP [6].

References

1 Baker AL, Kotake AN, Schoeller DA. Clinical utility of breath tests for the assessment of hepatic function. *Semin. Liv. Dis.* 1983; **3**: 318.
2 Bircher J. Quantitative assessment of deranged hepatic function: a missed opportunity? *Semin. Liv. Dis.* 1983; **3**: 275.
3 Breen KJ, Bury RW, Calder IV *et al.* A [^{14}C]phencetin breath test to measure hepatic function in man. *Hepatology* 1984; **4**: 47.
4 Galizzi J, Long RG, Billing BH *et al.* Assessment of the (^{14}C)aminopyrine breath test in liver disease. *Gut* 1978; **19**: 40.
5 Gross JB Jr, Reichen J, Zeltner TB *et al.* The evolution of changes in quantitative liver function tests in a rat model of biliary cirrhosis: correlation with morphometric measurement of hepatocyte mass. *Hepatology* 1987; **7**: 457.
6 Hacki W, Bircher J, Presig R. A new look at the plasma disappearance of sulfobromophthalein (BSP): correlation with the BSP transport maximum and the hepatic plasma flow in man. *J. Lab. clin. Med.* 1976; **88**: 1019.
7 Jost G, Wahll Ander A, von Mandach U, Preisig R. Overnight salivary caffeine clearance: a liver function test suitable for routine use. *Hepatology* 1987; **7**: 338.

8 Monroe PS, Baker AL, Schneider JF *et al.* The aminopyrine breath test and serum bile acids reflect histologic severity in chronic hepatitis. *Hepatology* 1982; **2**: 317.

9 Reichen J, Arts B, Schafroth U *et al.* Aminopyrine N-demethylation by rats with liver cirrhosis. Evidence for the intact cell hypothesis. A morphometric-functional study. *Gastroenterology* 1987; **93**: 719.

Bile pigments

BILIRUBIN

Bilirubin metabolism is described in detail in Chapter 12 (fig. 2.3.).

Serum bilirubin estimations are based on the van den Bergh diazo reaction. A direct reaction at 10 minutes gives an estimate of the conjugated bilirubin present. The total bilirubin is determined in the presence of an accelerator such as caffeine-benzoate or methanol. An approximate value for the unconjugated (indirect) bilirubin is obtained by subtracting the value for conjugated from that for the total bilirubin.

These diazo reactions are subject to error and diagnosis should not be based solely upon them [4]. Other more accurate methods for estimation such as thin layer chromotography, high performance gas liquid chromotography and alkaline methanolysis are available but are too elaborate to be clinically useful [2].

Inspection of *faeces* is an important investigation in jaundice. Clay-coloured stools indicate biliary obstruction or, rarely, very severe bilirubin glucuronyl-transferase deficiency.

Bilirubin cannot be detected in the *urine* of normal subjects or patients with unconjugated hyperbilirubinaemia. In cholestatic patients a small fraction of the conjugated bilirubin in plasma is dialysable and filtered by the glomerulus, some is re-absorbed by the tubules, the remainder gives the dark colour to the urine.

'Dipsticks' are commercially available, easy to use and give satisfactory results for the detection of conjugated *bilirubin* in urine.

Uses. In acute virus hepatitis bilirubin appears in the urine before urobilinogen or before

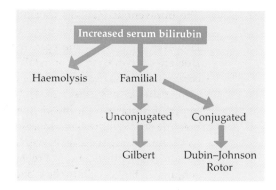

Fig. 2.3. Algorithm for managing a patient with an isolated increase in serum total bilirubin.

jaundice. In an undiagnosed febrile illness, bilirubinuria favours the diagnosis of hepatitis.

UROBILIN(OGEN)

An increase of urobilinogen in the urine is found when hepato-cellular function is inadequate to re-excrete all bilirubin absorbed from the intestines. It is therefore a sensitive index of *hepato-cellular dysfunction*, often when other tests are normal. It is a good indication of alcoholic liver damage, well-compensated cirrhosis or malignant disease of the liver. It is also raised in pyrexia, circulatory failure and haemolytic disease.

In *virus hepatitis* the early appearance of urobilinogen in the urine represents liver cell dysfunction. At the height of the jaundice urobilinogen disappears from the urine. Convalescence is heralded by its reappearance, and complete recovery by its final disappearance.

In *cholestatic jaundice* urobilinogen disappears from the urine; prolonged absence strongly suggests complete biliary obstruction due to malignant disease. Partial obstruction due to gallstones or biliary stricture is usually associated with intermittent urobilinogenuria.

Bromsulphalein

The dye bromsulphalein (BSP) is rapidly removed by the liver and excreted in the bile.

The intravenous test was used to assess liver dysfunction in the absence of jaundice. However, in view of the cost, the occasional side-effects (which may be fatal), and the inconvenience it is rarely performed nowadays.

In patients suspected of Dubin—Johnson hyperbilirubinaemia a blood sample is taken not only at 45 minutes after injection but also at two hours. A higher level at two hours than at 45 minutes is diagnostic and reflects release of conjugated BSP back into the bloodstream after a normal initial uptake [3].

Indocyanine green

This dye is removed from the circulation by the liver. It is not conjugated and there is no extra-hepatic removal or entero-hepatic circulation. It is safer, more expensive and more specific than BSP. It is used for liver blood flow studies [1].

References

1 Caesar J, Shaldon S, Chiandussi L *et al*. The use of indocyanine green in the measurement of hepatic blood flow and as a test of hepatic function. *Clin. Sci.* 1961; **21**: 43.

2 Fevery J, Blanckaert N. What can we learn from analysis of the serum bilirubin? *J. Hepatol.* 1986; **2**: 113.

3 Mandema E, DeFraiture WH, Nieweg HO *et al*. Familial chronic idiopathic jaundice (Dubin—Sprinz disease) with a note on bromsulphalein metabolism in this disease. *Am. J. Med.* 1960; **28**: 42.

4 Rosenthal P. The laboratory method as a variable in the diagnosis of hyperbilirubinemia. *Am. J. Dis. Child.* 1987; **141**: 1066.

Lipid and lipoprotein metabolism [1, 2]

Several types of lipid are carried in plasma in relatively large amounts—cholesterol and cholesterol esters, phospholipids and triglycerides.

Cholesterol is found in cell membranes and is a precursor of bile acids and steroid hormones. It is synthesized in the liver, small intestine and in other tissues. Synthesis takes place mainly from acetate in the microsomal fraction and in cytosol (fig. 2.4). Hepatic synthesis is inhibited by cholesterol feeding and by fasting, and is increased by a biliary fistula or bile duct ligation and also by an intestinal lymph fistula. The rate-limiting step is the conversion of HMG-CoA to mevalonate by the enzyme HMG CoA reductase. The mechanism controlling this process is uncertain. Cholesterol in membranes and in bile is present almost exclusively as free cholesterol. In plasma and in certain tissues such as the liver, adrenal and skin, cholesterol esters (cholesterol esterified with long-chain fatty acids) are also found. Cholesterol esters are more non-polar than free cholesterol and therefore even less soluble in water. Esterification is carried out in plasma by the enzyme lecithin cholesterol acyl transferase (LCAT) which is synthesized in the liver.

Phospholipids are a heterogeneous group of compounds. They contain one or more phosphoric acid groups and another polar group. This may be a heterogeneous base such as choline or ethanolamine. In addition there are one or more long-chain fatty acid residues. The phospholipids are much more complex in terms of chemical reactivity than cholesterol and

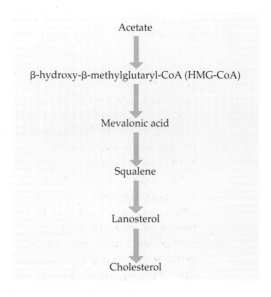

Fig. 2.4. Cholesterol biosynthesis.

cholesterol esters. They are important constituents of cell membranes and take part in a large number of chemical reactions. The most abundant phospholipid in plasma and most cellular membranes is phosphatidyl choline or lecithin.

Triglycerides are simpler compounds than the phospholipids. They have a backbone of glycerol, the hydroxy groups of which have been esterified with fatty acids. Naturally occurring triglycerides contain a variety of fatty acids; they act as a store of energy and also a method of transport of energy from the gut and liver to peripheral tissues.

Lipoproteins [1]. Cholesterol, phospholipids and triglycerides are insoluble in water and would not exist in plasma in free solution. Three major groups of lipoproteins are involved in lipid transport. One migrates in an electrical field with α_1-globulins (HDL) and another with β-globulins (LDL). A third fraction, very low density lipoprotein (VLDL), is also recognized. It is rich in triglyceride and is synthesized by the liver. The fourth type of lipoprotein is the chylomicron which is a large triglyceride-rich particle originating from the gut and appearing in plasma after the ingestion of a fatty meal. The chemical and physical differences between the various lipoproteins are due partly to their differing lipid composition and partly to variations in their protein content. LDL and VLDL remnants are removed by the liver. The fate of HDL is unknown.

A number of different protein sub-units are present in plasma lipoproteins; in their delipidated form they are called apoproteins. Apoprotein APO-A1 activates plasma LCAT; apoprotein APO-C11 activates lipoprotein lipase.

Changes in liver disease (fig. 2.5)

The increase in total serum cholesterol level in cholestasis is not due simply to the retention of cholesterol normally excreted in the bile. The mechanism is uncertain but it might be related to regurgitation into plasma of biliary phos-

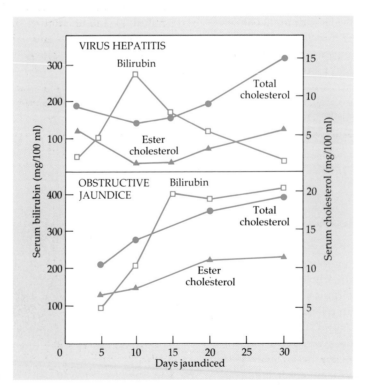

Fig. 2.5. Serum ester and total cholesterol levels in virus hepatitis and cholestasis.

pholipid [2]. Whereas slight increases to 1.5–2 times normal are sometimes seen in acute cholestasis, very high values are found in chronic conditions, especially post-operative stricture and primary biliary cirrhosis. Values of over five times the upper limit of normal are associated with skin xanthomas. Malnutrition lowers the serum cholesterol so that values may be normal in carcinomatous biliary obstruction. Increased values are seen during recovery from virus hepatitis, in fatty liver and in some patients with gallstones.

In cirrhosis total serum cholesterol values are usually normal. Low results indicate malnutrition or decompensation.

In hepato-cellular disease and in obstructive jaundice the plasma triglycerides tend to be increased, the excess being found in the low density lipoprotein (LDL) fraction. In both conditions the percentage of cholesterol esters is decreased due to LCAT deficiency related to impaired formation and, in obstructive jaundice, due to a marked increase in free cholesterol. Lipoprotein electrophoresis shows absence
of pre-β and a wide, deeply staining β band.

In *cholestasis* an abnormal lipoprotein, lipoprotein X, very rich in free cholesterol and lecithin, is found which appears on electron microscopy as bilamellar discs (Chapter 13).

LCAT deficiency is a marked feature, perhaps due to decreased synthesis. This would result in a rise in free cholesterol with a reduction in the esters.

The haematological changes of cholestasis can be related to abnormalities in cholesterol and lipoprotein.

Failure of hepatic apoprotein synthesis leads to difficulty in export of triglyceride from the liver as VLDL and hence to fatty liver in such conditions as hepato-cellular failure and tetracycline toxicity.

Serum cholesterol esters, lipoproteins, LCAT and lipoprotein X are not estimated routinely.

References

1 Cooper AD. Role of the liver in the degradation of lipoproteins. *Gastroenterology* 1985; **88**: 192.
2 McIntyre N. Plasma lipids and lipoproteins in liver disease. *Gut* 1978; **19**: 526.

Bile acids

Bile acids are synthesized only in the liver, 250–500 mg being produced and lost in the faeces daily (Chapter 29). The primary bile acids, cholic acid and chenodeoxycholic acid, are formed from cholesterol (fig. 2.6). Synthesis is controlled by the amount of bile acid returning to the liver in the entero-hepatic circulation. On contact with colonic bacteria the primary bile acids undergo 7α-dehydroxylation with the production of the secondary bile acids, deoxycholic and a very little lithocholic acid. Tertiary bile acids, largely ursodeoxycholic acid, are formed in the liver by epimerization of secondary bile acids. In human bile the

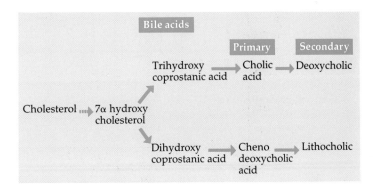

Fig. 2.6. Production of primary and secondary bile acids.

amount of the trihydroxy acid (cholic acid) roughly equals the sum of the two dihydroxy acids (chenodeoxycholic and deoxycholic).

The bile acids are conjugated in the liver with the amino acids glycine or taurine. This prevents absorption in the biliary tree and small intestine but permits conservation by absorption in the terminal ileum. Sulphation and glucuronidation (as a detoxifying mechanism) may be increased with cirrhosis or cholestasis when these conjugates are found in excess in the urine and also in bile [9]. Bacteria can hydrolyse bile salts to bile acid and glycine or taurine.

Bile salts are excreted into the biliary canaliculus against an enormous concentration gradient between liver and bile. This depends on a carrier-mediated, active transport system. Local areas of high fluidity exist in the bile canalicular membrane and bile acids may intercalate there and form vesicles which are shed into the bile canalicular lumen. The bile salts enter into micellar and vesicular associ-

ation with cholesterol and phospholipids (fig. 2.7). In the upper small intestine the bile salt micelles are too large and too polar to be absorbed. They are intimately concerned with the digestion and absorption of lipids. When the terminal ileum and proximal colon are reached absorption takes place by a transport process found only in the ileum. Non-ionic passive diffusion occurs throughout the whole intestine and is most efficient for unconjugated, dihydroxy glycine conjugates.

The absorbed bile salts enter the portal venous system and reach the liver where they are taken up with great avidity by the hepatocytes using a sodium-dependent bile acid co-transport system. Synthesis is under negative feed-back control. Little is known of how the bile acids traverse the liver cell from sinusoid to bile canaliculus but cytosolic bile-acid proteins have been identified in rat liver and may play a part [10]. The bile acids are reconjugated and re-excreted into the bile by a carrier-mediated but not sodium dependent mech-

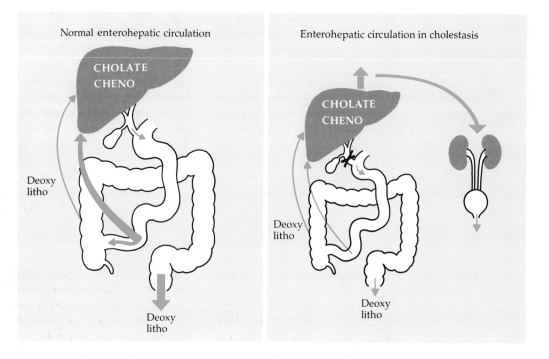

Normal enterohepatic circulation

CHOLATE
CHENO

Deoxy
litho

Deoxy
litho

Enterohepatic circulation in cholestasis

CHOLATE
CHENO

Deoxy
litho

Deoxy
litho

26 **Fig. 2.7.** The entero-hepatic circulation of bile acids in normal subjects and in cholestasis.

anism. Lithocholic acid is not re-excreted. This entero-hepatic circulation of bile salts takes place 2 to 15 times daily (fig. 2.7). Because absorption efficiency varies among the individual bile acids they have different synthesis and fractional turnover rates.

In cholestasis bile acids are excreted in the urine by active transport and passive diffusion. They tend to be sulphated and these conjugates are actively secreted by the renal tubule [11].

Changes in disease

Bile salts increase the biliary excretion of water, lecithin, cholesterol and conjugated bilirubin (fig. 13.7).

Altered biliary excretion with defective biliary micelle formation is important in the pathogenesis of gallstones (Chapter 31). It also leads to the steatorrhoea of cholestasis [2].

They form a micellar solution with cholesterol and monoglyceride or fatty acid, so allowing cholesterol to be absorbed.

Bile salts help to emulsify dietary fat and probably also play a part in the mucosal phase of absorption. Diminished secretion leads to steatorrhoea (fig. 2.8). They assist pancreatic lipolysis. They release gastrointestinal hormones.

Disordered intra-hepatic metabolism of bile salts may be important in the pathogenesis of cholestasis (Chapter 13). They may have a role in the causation of the pruritus of cholestasis, although this has never been confirmed.

They may be responsible for target cells in the peripheral blood of jaundiced patients (Chapter 12) and for the secretion of conjugated bilirubin in urine.

When deconjugated or dehydroxylated by intestinal bacteria, bile acids are ineffective in absorption. This may partly explain the malabsorption complicating diseases with stasis and bacterial overgrowth in the small intestine.

Removal of the terminal ileum interrupts the entero-hepatic circulation and allows large amounts of primary bile acids to reach the colon and to be dehydroxylated by bacteria, thus reducing the body's bile salt pool. The

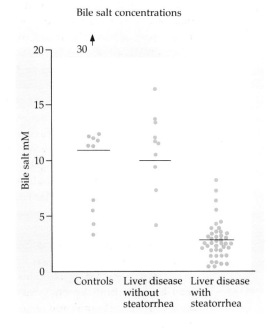

Fig. 2.8. Patients with chronic, non-alcoholic liver disease and steatorrhoea show a reduced bile salt concentration in their aspirated intestinal contents compared with control subjects and patients with chronic liver disease without steatorrhoea (Badley *et al.* 1970).

altered bile salts in the colon excite a profound electrolyte and water loss with diarrhoea.

Lithocholic acid is mostly excreted in the faeces and only slightly absorbed. It is cirrhogenic to experimental animals and can be used to produce experimental gallstones. Taurolithocholic acid can also cause intra-hepatic cholestasis perhaps by interfering with the bile-salt independent fraction of bile flow.

Serum bile acids

Gas−liquid chromatography allows individual bile acids to be distinguished, but the method is time consuming and the equipment expensive.

Enzymatic assays are based on the use of bacterial 3-hydroxysteroid dehydrogenase. The use of a bioluminescence assay, capable of detecting bile salts in the picomole range, has brought the sensitivity of this enzymatic technique up to that of radio-immunoassay [8]. The method is simple and inexpensive if the equipment is available. Radio-immunoassay techniques can also measure individual bile acids. Commercial kits are available.

The concentration of total serum bile acids indicates the fraction re-absorbed from the intestine, but which has escaped extraction on its first passage through the liver. The value reflects the instantaneous balance between intestinal absorption and hepatic uptake. Intestinal load is more important than hepatic extraction in regulating peripheral serum bile acid levels.

Raised levels of serum bile acids are specific for hepato-biliary disease [3]. Sensitivity of serum bile acid estimations is less than originally thought for detecting hepato-cellular damage in viral hepatitis or chronic liver disease. It is, however, better than the serum albumin or the prothrombin time because the value depends not only on hepatic injury, but also on excretory function and portal systemic shunting [6]. It may be useful in determining prognosis. Normal serum bile acids are found in Gilbert's syndrome [12].

The addition to the fasting serum bile acid value of a two-hour post-prandial level adds little in sensitivity [5].

Estimations of individual bile acids are not diagnostic. In cholestasis the ratio of serum trihydroxy to dihydroxy acid increases [7]. Patients with hepato-cellular failure usually have a low ratio, the main bile acid being chenodeoxycholic acid. This is due to a reduction in the activity of the 12 α-hydroxylase enzyme in the hepatocyte.

Amino acid conjugation is preserved even with severe hepato-cellular damage [1].

Serum conjugated cholic acid, measured by radio-immunoassay, may be the best screening method for liver disease [4].

In cholestasis bile acids are excreted in the *urine* by active transport and passive diffusion. The pattern is similar to that in the serum, but sulphate esters account for a larger proportion of the total bile acids [11].

References

1 Arisaka M, Arisaka O, Nittono H *et al.* Conjugating ability of bile acids in hepatic failure. *Acta Paediatr. Scand.* 1986; **75**: 875.
2 Badley BWD, Murphy GM, Bouchier IAD *et al.* Diminished micellar phase lipid in patients with chronic nonalcoholic liver disease and steatorrhea. *Gastroenterology* 1970; **58**: 781.
3 Ferraris R, Colombatti G, Florentini MT *et al.* Diagnostic value of serum bile acids and routine liver function tests in hepatobiliary diseases: sensitivity, specificity, and predictive value. *Dig. Dis. Sci.* 1983; **28**: 129.
4 Ferraris R, Florentini T, Galatola G *et al.* Diagnostic value of serum immunoreactive conjugated cholic or chenodeoxycholic acids in detecting hepatobiliary diseases. Comparison with levels of 3 alpha-hydroxy bile acids determined enzymatically and with routine liver tests. *Dig. Dis. Sci.* 1987; **32**: 817.
5 Greenfield SM, Soloway RD, Carithers RL Jr. *et al.* Evaluation of postprandial serum bile acid response as a test of hepatic function. *Dig. Dis. Sci.* 1986; **31**: 785.
6 Hofmann AF. The aminopyrine demethylation breath test and the serum bile acid level: nominated but not yet elected to join the common liver tests. *Hepatology* 1982; **2**: 512.
7 Osborn EC, Wootton IDP, da Silva LC *et al.* Serum bile-acid levels in liver disease. *Lancet* 1959; **ii**: 1049.
8 Roda A, Kricka LH, DeLuca M *et al.* Bioluminescence measurement of primary bile acids using immobilized 7 alpha-hydroxysteroid dehydrogenase: application to serum bile acids. *J. Lipid Res.* 1982; **23**: 1354.
9 Stiehl A, Raedsch R, Rudolph G, Gundert-Remy U *et al.* Biliary and urinary excretion of sulfated, glucuronidated and tetrahydroxylated bile acids in cirrhotic patients. *Hepatology* 1985; **5**: 492.
10 Stolz A, Sugiyama Y, Kuhlenkamp J *et al.* Cytosolic bile acid binding protein in rat liver: radioimmuno assay, molecular forms, developmental characteristics and organ distribution. *Hepatology* 1986; **6**: 433.
11 Summerfield JA, Cullen J, Barnes S *et al.* Evidence for renal control of urinary excretion of bile acids and bile acid sulphates in the cholestatic syndrome. *Clin. Sci. mol. Med.* 1977; **52**: 51.
12 Vierling JM, Berk PD, Hofmann AF *et al.* Normal fasting-state levels of serum cholyl-conjugated bile acids in Gilbert's syndrome: an aid to diagnosis. *Hepatology* 1982; **2**: 340.

Amino acid metabolism

Amino acids derived from the diet and from tissue breakdown reach the liver for metabolism. Some are transaminated or deaminated to keto-acids which are then metabolized by many pathways including the tricarboxylic acid cycle (Krebs–citric acid cycle). Others are metabolized to ammonia and urea (Krebs–Henseleit urea cycle). The maximal rate of urea synthesis in chronic liver disease is markedly reduced [7]. However, experimentally, at least 85% of liver must be removed before this mechanism fails significantly and before blood and urinary amino acid levels increase. A low blood urea concentration is a rare accompaniment of fulminant liver failure. A rise in blood ammonia level also represents a failure of the Krebs–Henseleit cycle and this increase has been related to hepatic encephalopathy.

CLINICAL SIGNIFICANCE

A generalized or selective amino aciduria is a feature of hepato-cellular disease. In patients with severe liver disease the usual picture is an increase in the plasma concentration of the aromatic amino acids, tyrosine, phenylalanine and methionine and a reduction in the branched-chain amino acids valine, leucine and isoleucine (fig. 2.9) [4]. The changes are explained by impaired hepatic function, portal–systemic shunting of blood and hyperinsulinaemia and hyperglucagonaemia. Patients with minimal liver disease also show changes, particularly a reduction in plasma proline, perhaps reflecting increased collagen production. There is no difference in the ratio between branched-chain and aromatic amino acids whether or not the patients show hepatic encephalopathy.

In fulminant hepatitis there is marked generalized aminoaciduria involving particularly cystine and tyrosine and this carries a bad prognosis.

Plasma proteins

The plasma proteins produced by the hepatocyte are synthesized on polyribosomes bound to the rough endoplasmic reticulum, from which they are discharged into the plasma [9]. Falls in concentration usually reflect decreased hepatic synthesis although changes in plasma volume and losses, for instance into gut or urine, may contribute.

The hepatocyte makes albumin, fibrinogen, α_1-antitrypsin, haptoglobin, caeruloplasmin, transferrin and prothrombin (table 2.2). Some liver-produced proteins are acute phase reactors and rise in response to tissue injury such as inflammation (table 2.2). These include fibrinogen, haptoglobin, α_1-antitrypsin, C_3 component of complement and caeruloplasmin. An acute phase response may contribute to well maintained or increased serum concentrations of these proteins, even with hepato-cellular disease.

The *immunoglobulins* IgG, IgM and IgA are synthesized by the B cells of the lymphoid system.

Some 10 g *albumin* is synthesized by the normal liver daily, whereas those with cirrhosis can only synthesize about 4 g. In liver disease,

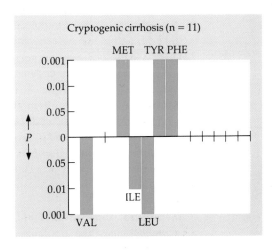

Fig. 2.9. The plasma amino acid pattern in cryptogenic cirrhosis (mean of 11 patients). The aromatic amino acids are increased while the branched chain ones are decreased. Blocks represent increases or decreases in amino acid values. MET = methionine, TYR = tyrosine, PHE = phenyl alanine, VAL = valine, ILE = isoleucine, LEU = leucine (Morgan *et al.* 1980).

Table 2.2. Serum (plasma) proteins synthesized by the liver

	Normal concentration	
	Traditional	SI units
Albumin	4–5 g/100 ml	40–50 g/l
α₁-antitrypsin*	200–400 mg/100 ml	2–4 g/l
α-fetoprotein	less than 30 mg/ml	
α₂-macroglobulin	220–380 mg/100 ml	2.2–3.8 g/l
Caeruloplasmin*	27–39 mg/100 ml	0.3–0.4 g/l
Complement components (C3, C6 & C1)		
Fibrinogen*	200–600 mg/100 ml	2–6 g/l
Haemopexin	80–100 mg/100 ml	0.8–1.0 g/l
Prothrombin (Factor II)†		
Transferrin		2–3 g/l

* Acute phase proteins.

† Vitamin K dependent; also factors VII and X.

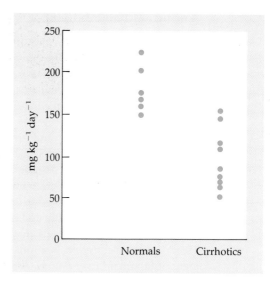

Fig. 2.10. The absolute synthesis of serum albumin (^{14}C carbonate method) in cirrhosis is reduced (Tavill *et al.* 1971).

the fall in serum albumin concentration is slow, for the half-life of albumin is about 22 days. Thus a patient with fulminant liver failure may die with a virtually normal serum albumin value. A patient with decompensated cirrhosis would be expected to have a low level (figs 2.10, 2.11).

α₁-antitrypsin deficiency is genetically determined.

Haptoglobin is a glycoprotein composed of two types of polypeptide chains, alpha and beta, which are covalently associated by disulphide bonds. Haptoglobin is largely synthesized by the hepatocyte. Hereditary deficiencies are frequent in American blacks. Low values are found in severe chronic hepatocellular disease and in haemolytic crises.

Caeruloplasmin is the major copper-containing protein in plasma and is responsible for the oxidase activity. A low concentration is found in 95% of those who are homozygous and about 10% of those heterozygous for Wilson's disease [8]. Caeruloplasmin increases to normal if a patient with Wilson's disease has a hepatic transplant. One must estimate caeruloplasmin in all patients with chronic active hepatitis so

that Wilson's disease, with its mandatory penicillamine therapy, may be diagnosed. However, low values are also found in very severe decompensated cirrhosis which is not due to Wilson's disease. High values are found in pregnancy, following oestrogen therapy and with large bile duct obstruction.

Transferrin is the iron transport protein. The plasma transferrin is more than 90% saturated with iron in patients with untreated idiopathic haemochromatosis. Reduced values may be found with cirrhosis.

The C_3 *component of complement* tends to be reduced in cirrhosis, normal in chronic active hepatitis and increased in compensated primary biliary cirrhosis. Low values in fulminant hepatic failure reflect reduced hepatic synthesis and increased consumption due to activation of the complement system [5]. Transient reductions are found in the early 'immune complex' stage of acute hepatitis B.

Alpha-fetoprotein is a normal component of plasma protein in human fetuses older than six weeks, and reaches maximum concentration at between 12 and 16 weeks of fetal life. A few

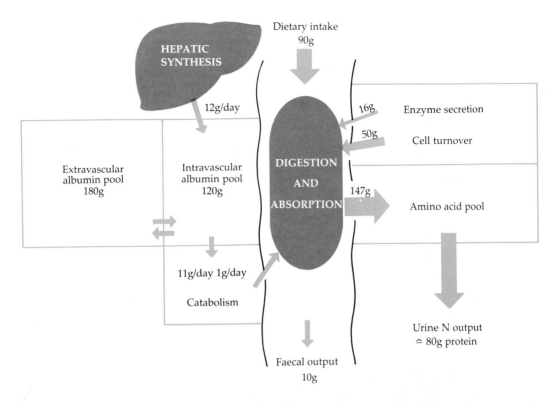

Fig. 2.11. The turnover of plasma albumin in a 70 kg adult seen in the context of the daily protein economy of the gastro-intestinal tract and overall nitrogen balance. The total exchangeable albumin pool of about 300 g is distributed between the intravascular and extravascular compartments in a ratio of approximately 2:3. In this simplified schema the balance sheet is expressed in terms of g of protein ($=6.25 \times$ g of N). Losses do not include relatively minor routes, e.g. 2 g per day from the skin (Tavill 1972).

weeks after birth it disappears from the circulation but reappears in the blood of patients with primary liver cancer and can be shown in the tumour by indirect immunofluorescence. Raised values are also found with embryonic tumours of ovary and testis and in embryonic hepatoblastoma. It may also be present with carcinomas of the gastrointestinal tract with hepatic secondaries. Raised values are also found in hepatitis B surface-antigen-negative, chronic, active hepatitis and during acute viral hepatitis where they may indicate hepato-cellular regeneration. However, very high values are virtually confined to primary liver cancer. In a hepatitis B positive patient, rising values are of particular significance as an indicator of the development of hepato-cellular carcinoma (see Chapter 28).

Electrophoretic pattern of the serum proteins

Electrophoresis is used to determine the proportions of the various serum proteins [11].

In cirrhosis, albumin is reduced and in acute hepatitis these changes are much less conspicuous. Plasma prealbumin may be a very sensitive index of hepatic functional capacity [6].

The α_1-globulins contain glycoproteins and hormone-binding globulins. They tend to be low in hepato-cellular disease, falling in parallel with the serum albumin. An increase accompanies acute febrile illnesses and malignant disease. Ninety per cent of α_1-globulin consists of α_1-antitrypsin and an absent α_1-globulin may indicate α_1-antitrypsin deficiency.

The α_2- and β-globulins include lipoproteins. In cholestasis the increase in α_2- and β-globulin components correlates with the height of serum lipids. This pattern may be useful in distinguishing biliary from non-biliary cirrhosis. High lipoprotein components strongly support a biliary aetiology.

The γ-globulins rise in hepatic cirrhosis due to increased production. The increased numbers of plasma cells in marrow, and even in the liver itself, may be the source. The γ-globulin peak in hepato-cellular disease shows a wide base (*polyclonal gammopathy*). *Monoclonal gammopathy* is rare and may be age rather than chronic liver disease-related. The dip between β- and γ-globulins tends to be bridged.

Immunoglobulins. IgG is markedly increased in chronic active hepatitis and cryptogenic cirrhosis. There is a slow and sustained increase in viral hepatitis and it is also increased in cirrhosis of the alcoholic [1].

IgM is markedly increased in primary biliary cirrhosis and to a lesser extent in viral hepatitis and cirrhosis, whether chronic active or cryptogenic.

IgA is markedly increased in cirrhosis of the alcoholic but also in primary biliary and cryptogenic cirrhosis.

The increase in serum secretory IgA, the predominant immunoglobulin in bile, may be related to communication of the bile canaliculus with the space of Dissë and/or through the bile duct into the portal blood vessels [2].

In chronic active hepatitis and cryptogenic cirrhosis the pattern is surprisingly similar, with increases in IgG, IgM and to a lesser extent IgA [1].

About 10% of patients with chronic cholestasis due to large bile duct obstruction show increases in all three main immunoglobulins.

Patterns are not diagnostic of any one disease but only give suggestive evidence.

References

1 Feizi T. Serum imunoglobulins in liver disease. *Gut* 1968; **9**: 193.
2 Fukuda Y, Nagura H, Asai J *et al.* Possible mechanisms of elevation of serum secretory immunoglobulin A in liver disease. *Am. J. Gastroenterol.* 1986; **81**: 315.
3 Lee FI. Immunoglobulins in viral hepatitis and active alcoholic liver-disease. *Lancet* 1965; **ii**: 1043.
4 Morgan MY, Marshall AW, Milsom JP *et al.* Plasma amino-acid patterns in liver disease. *Gut* 1982; **23**: 362.
5 Potter BJ, Trueman AM, Jones EA. Serum complement in chronic liver disease. *Gut* 1973; **14**: 451.
6 Rondana M, Milani L, Merkel C *et al.* Value of prealbumin plasma levels as a liver test. *Digestion* 1987; **37**: 72.
7 Rudman D, Difulco TJ, Galambos JT *et al.* Maximal rates of excretion and synthesis of urea in normal and cirrhotic subjects. *J. clin. Invest.* 1973; **52**: 2241.
8 Scheinberg IH, Sternieb I. *Wilson's disease.* W.B. Saunders, Philadelphia, 1983.
9 Tavill AS. The synthesis and degradation of liver-produced proteins. *Gut* 1972; **13**: 225.
10 Tavill AS, Craigie A, Rosenoer VM. The measurement of the synthetic rate of albumin in man. *Clin. Sci.* 1968; **34**: 1.
11 Wolf PL. Interpretation of electrophoretic patterns of serum proteins. *Clin. Lab. Med.* 1986; **6**: 441.

Serum enzyme tests

These tests will usually diagnose the type of liver injury, whether hepato-cellular or cholestatic, but cannot be expected to differentiate one form of hepatitis from another or to determine whether cholestasis is intra- or extra-hepatic. Only a few tests are necessary and the combination of a serum aspartate transaminase (AST formerly SGOT) and alkaline phosphatase (with occasionally serum alanine transaminase, ALT formerly SGPT) is adequate.

Alkaline phosphatase

The level rises in cholestasis and to a lesser extent when liver cells are damaged (fig. 2.12) [4]. The mechanisms of the increase are complex [5]. Hepatic synthesis of the alkaline phosphatase by the hepatocyte is increased and this depends on intact protein and RNA synthesis. Secretion into the bile may rise through leakage from canaliculus into the sinusoid because of leaky tight junctions. Increased secretion of phosphatase into sinusoids from the hepatocyte plasma membranes may contribute.

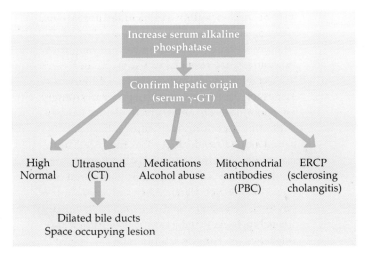

Fig. 2.12. Algorithm for managing a patient with an isolated increase in serum alkaline phosphatase or serum gamma glutamyl transpeptidase (γ-GT).

Serum hepatic alkaline phosphatase may be distinguished from bony phosphatase by fractionation into iso-enzymes, but this is not routinely carried out.

Raised levels are sometimes observed with primary or secondary tumours, even without jaundice or involvement of bone. Increased values without a rise in serum bilirubin are also found with other space-occupying lesions, such as amyloid, abscess, leukaemia or granulomas. Non-specific mild elevations are seen in a variety of conditions including Hodgkin's disease and heart failure. The cause is presumably focal, intra-hepatic, bile duct obstruction caused by these lesions.

Gamma glutamyl transpeptidase (γ-GT) [7]

Serum values are increased in cholestasis and hepato-cellular disease. Levels parallel serum alkaline phosphatase in cholestasis and may be used to confirm that a raised serum phosphatase is of hepato-biliary origin. Levels are increased with hepatic metastases, not consistently but more so than for alkaline phosphatase.

Serum levels are raised in patients with alcohol abuse even without liver disease. Increases may be due to microsomal enzyme induction by alcohol.

Unfortunately many factors influence the level so that increases are non-disease-specific. Disorders include hepato-biliary disease, alcoholism, concomitant drug administration for instance with barbiturates or phenytoin [6]. Screening with serum γ-GT may have led to more alcohol abusers being identified although in a third of these abusers the serum γ-GT does not rise. The finding of increased levels, however, often leads to over-investigation of an elevated level in an innocent person who has never taken alcohol or a social drinker who has never abused alcohol.

Amino transferases

Glutamic oxalo-acetic transaminase (GOT, aspartate transaminase) is a mitochondrial enzyme present in large quantities in heart, liver, skeletal muscle and kidney and the serum level increases whenever these tissues are acutely destroyed, presumably due to release from damaged cells.

Glutamic pyruvic transaminase (GPT, alanine transaminase) is a cytosolic enzyme also present in liver. Although the absolute amount is less than SGOT, a greater proportion is present in liver compared with heart and skeletal muscles. A serum increase is therefore more specific for liver damage than SGOT.

Transaminase determinations are useful in the early diagnosis of virus hepatitis. Measurements must be made early, for normal values may be reached within a week of the onset. The patient may develop fatal acute hepatic necrosis in spite of falling transaminase values. Serial estimations are essential.

Very high levels may be seen in the early stages of acute cholestasis particularly choledocholithiasis [2], and with circulatory failure.

Routine screening may show unexpectedly raised amino transferase levels (fig. 2.13). These are often due to obesity, diabetes mellitus, alcohol abuse, an hepatic drug reaction or circulatory failure. Rarer causes include α_1-antitrypsin deficiency and haemochromatosis. Liver biopsy is usually necessary to make the diagnosis [3]. However, this should be delayed if the patient is asymptomatic and the increase in transaminase is modest. The value should be monitored.

Results vary in cirrhosis, and are particularly high in chronic active hepatitis. Very high levels are unusual in alcoholic liver disease. A high ratio of SGOT or SGPT (greater than two) may be useful in diagnosing alcoholic hepatitis and cirrhosis [1]. This is due not only to hepatocyte damage but to pyridoxal 5-phosphate (vitamin B6) deficiency.

Other serum enzymes

None of these have gained acceptance for routine use.

Lactic dehydrogenase (LDH) is a relatively insensitive index of hepato-cellular injury, but marked increases are found in patients with neoplasms, especially with hepatic involvement.

Cholinesterase is a non-specific esterase synthesized by the liver. Decreases in hepato-cellular disease, especially cirrhosis, reflect diminished synthesis and also poor nutrition. In malnutrition, the serum level parallels that in the liver. Decreases may be useful in detecting hepatotoxicity due to chemicals.

References

1 Cohen JA, Kaplan MM. The SGOT:SGPT ratio—an indicator of alcoholic liver disease. *Dig. Dis. Sci.* 1979; **24**: 835.
2 Fortson WC, Tedesco FJ, Starnes EC *et al.* Marked elevation of serum transaminase activity associated with extrahepatic biliary tract disease. *J. clin. Gastroenterol.* 1985; **7**: 502.
3 Hultcrantz R, Glaumann H, Lindberg G *et al.* Liver investigation in 149 asymptomatic patients with moderately elevated activities of serum aminotransferases. *Scand. J. Gastroenterol.* 1986; **21**: 109.
4 Kaplan MM. Alkaline phosphatase. *Gastroenterology* 1972; **62**: 452.
5 Kaplan MM. Serum alkaline phosphatase—another piece is added to the puzzle. *Hepatology* 1986; **6**: 526.
6 Penn R, Worthington DJ. Is serum gamma glutamyltransferase a misleading test? *Br. med. J.* 1983; **286**: 531.
7 Rosalki SB. Gamma-glutamyl transpeptidase. *Adv. clin. Chem.* 1975; **17**: 53.

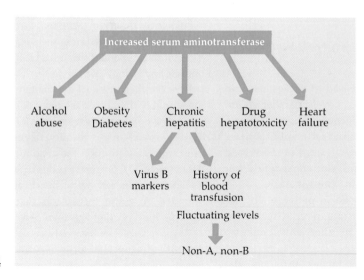

Fig. 2.13. Algorithm for managing a patient with an isolated increase in serum aminotransferase. PBC: primary biliary cirrhosis. ERCP: endoscopic cholangio-pancreatography.

Carbohydrate metabolism

The liver occupies a key position in carbohydrate metabolism (fig. 2.2) [1, 2].

In fulminant acute hepatic necrosis the blood glucose level may be low. This is rare in chronic liver disease. The oral and intravenous glucose tolerance tests may, however, show impairment and there is relative insulin resistance (Chapter 22).

Galactose tolerance is also impaired in hepatocellular disease and oral and intravenous tests have been devised. Results are independent of insulin secretion. Galactose removal by the liver has been used to measure hepatic blood flow.

References

1 Samols E, Holdsworth D. Disturbances in carbohydrate metabolism: liver disease. In *Carbohydrate metabolism*, vol. 2, p. 289, eds F. Dickens, P.J. Randle, & W.J. Whelan. Academic Press, New York, 1968.
2 Sherlock S. Carbohydrate changes in liver disease. *Am. J. clin. Nutr.* 1970; **23**: 462.

Effects of ageing on the liver [2, 3]

The liver weight decreases with ageing. Liver blood flow is reduced and there is compensatory hypertrophy of hepatocytes [4]. Routine biochemical tests are similar to those of the general population.

First-pass metabolism of drugs is reduced and drugs handled in this way have a greater effect. There is a reduction in metabolism of drugs handled by oxidation but not by acetylation. More fatal reactions to halothane and drugs such as benoxyprofen are found in the elderly. The elderly are also liable to have adverse reactions related to the multiplicity of drugs they are taking.

Cholesterol saturation of bile increases with age due to enhanced hepatic secretion of cholesterol and decreased bile acid synthesis [1]. This may explain age as a risk factor for cholesterol gallstones.

References

1 Einarsson K, Nilsell K, Leijd B *et al.* Influence of age on secretion of cholesterol and synthesis of bile acids by the liver. *N. Engl. J. Med.* 1985; **313**: 277.
2 Mooney H, Roberts R, Cooksley WGE *et al.* Alterations in the liver with ageing. *Clin. Gastroenterol.* 1985; **14**: 757.
3 Popper H. Aging and the liver. In *Progress in Liver Diseases VIII* p.659, eds. Popper H, Schaffner F. Grune and Stratton, Orlando 1986.
4 Rawlins MD, James OFW, Williams FM *et al.* Age and the metabolism of drugs. *Q. J. Med.* 1987; **64**: 545.

3 · Needle Biopsy of the Liver

A needle biopsy of the liver was said to have been first performed by Paul Ehrlich in 1883 (table 3.1) [9] in a study of the glycogen content of the diabetic liver, and later in 1895 by Lucatello [19] in Italy, for the diagnosis of tropical liver abscess. The first published series was by Schüpfer (1907) [34] in France, where the technique was used for the diagnosis of cirrhosis and hepatic tumours. The method, however, never achieved early popularity until the 1930s when it was used for general purposes by Huard and co-workers [11] in France, and by Baron [3] in the United States. The last World War saw a rapid increase in the use of liver biopsy, largely to investigate the many cases of non-fatal viral hepatitis which were affecting the armed forces of both sides [14, 38].

Now, in the course of his training, almost every junior doctor will have learnt to perform needle liver biopsy, under supervision. The indications and techniques have changed, the complications are better recognized and the risks have decreased. Interpretation of the biopsy is an important part of a histopathologist's training.

Selection and preparation of the patient

The patient is usually admitted to hospital [39]. The one-stage prothrombin time should not be more than three seconds prolonged over control values after 10 mg vitamin K intramuscularly. The platelet count should exceed 80 000.

In thrombocytopenic patients the risk of haemorrhage depends on the function of the platelets rather than their numbers. A patient with 'hypersplenism' and a platelet count of less than 60 000 is much less likely to bleed than one with leukaemia who has a similar platelet count. This distinction particularly arises in

Table 3.1. History of liver biopsies [40]

Author	Date	Country	Purpose
Erhlich	1883	Germany	Glycogen
Lucatello	1895	Italy	Tropical
Schüpfer	1907	France	Cirrhosis
Huard et al.	1935	France	General
Baron	1939	USA	General
Iversen & Roholm	1939	Denmark	Hepatitis
Axenfeld & Brass	1942	Germany	Hepatitis
Dible et al.	1943	UK	Hepatitis

patients with haematological problems or after organ transplants where the effects on the liver of cytotoxic therapy, viruses and other infective agents and of the graft-versus-host reaction have to be resolved. In such patients, if the platelet count can be raised to greater than 60 000 by platelet infusion, biopsy seems to be safe [37]. Care should also be taken in recently imbibing alcoholic patients who may have reduced platelet counts and platelet dysfunction, especially if acetyl salicylic acid has been consumed. In such patients the platelet count may be 100 000 and the prothrombin time only three seconds prolonged over control values, yet the bleeding time may be 25 minutes.

The patient's blood group should be known and facilities for blood transfusion must always be available.

Biopsy should not be done with tense ascites as a specimen will not be obtained.

Clinically significant haemorrhage complicated 12.5% of 155 liver biopsies in haemophiliacs [1]. Liver biopsy should not be performed in haemophilia A unless there are very definite indications when the factor VIII level should be raised, and maintained, to about

50% for at least 48 hours. This requires 12 hourly infusions for about four doses.

Anatomical abnormalities are common and liver size varies. A small liver may not be penetrated by the needle and distortion may result in puncture of the gallbladder or large blood vessels in the hilum. If possible, before the biopsy, ultrasound or CT scanning should be done and attention paid to liver size, the site of the gallbladder and any anatomical abnormality [7].

Liver biopsy is safe in patients with extra-hepatic bile duct obstruction even if deeply jaundiced [23]. Nowadays, however, the diagnosis is reached more exactly and safely by imaging or by endoscopic or percutaneous cholangiography. Hydatid disease is an absolute contraindication. Suspected amyloid disease is not a contraindication.

In the last 14 years, some 8000 needle biopsies of the liver have been performed at the Royal Free Hospital with only two deaths, one in a haemophiliac and one in a patient with acute virus hepatitis [40]. Some 40 patients had an intraperitoneal haemorrhage requiring transfusion. Patients presented mainly hepatological problems. If more haematological patients had been included a higher complication rate might have been expected. Nonetheless, liver biopsy must only be performed where the patient can be expected to benefit from the information and where it cannot be obtained by less invasive means. Haemorrhage usually develops when least expected and when, at the time of biopsy, the risk seemed small. It might be related to factors other than peripheral clotting, for instance the concentration of clotting factors in hepatic parenchyma and to failure of mechanical compression of the needle tract by elastic tissue [8]. The occasional laceration of a major intra-hepatic vessel cannot be avoided. Known vascular lesions such as haemangioma should not be biopsied.

Out-patients selected must not be jaundiced or show any sign of liver failure such as ascites or encephalopathy. Out-patient biopsy should be avoided in known cirrhotic patients or in those with tumours [26]. Out-patient biopsy is indicated for various reasons, usually the patient's preference and reduction of cost. The patient is admitted to a supervised day ward at 9.00 a.m. The biopsy is never done later than 11.00 a.m. During the first hour post-biopsy, the pulse and blood pressure are taken every 15 minutes and then every 30 minutes for the next two hours. The patient remains recumbent until 4.00 p.m., is seen at 4.30 p.m. by the physician and allowed to go home at 5.00 p.m., accompanied and being driven. The patient stays in his home, a hotel or with friends, not more than 30 minutes away from the hospital by car. The patient should not be alone and must have a telephone available. The usual indication is the diagnosis and management of chronic hepatitis, cirrhosis or in alcoholic liver disease.

Techniques

The Menghini needle obtains a specimen by aspiration (fig. 3.1) [21]. The sheathed 'Trucut' is a modification of the old Vim—Silverman needle. It is of particular value in cirrhotic patients. Fragmentation of the biopsy is greater with the Menghini technique but the procedure is quicker, easier and the costs of the needle less. Complications are less than with the Trucut procedure [26].

Menghini 'one second' needle biopsy (figs 3.1, 3.2). The 1.4 mm diameter needle is used routinely. A short needle is available for paediatric use. The tip of the needle is oblique and slightly convex towards the outside. This results in an excellent cut of the biopsy specimen without any need to rotate the needle. The needle is also fitted within its shaft with a blunt nail, 3 cm long and 0.2 mm diameter smaller than the internal diameter of the cannula. The diameter of the flattened head of the nail is larger than that of the cannula and also than that of the internal diameter of the insertion of the aspirating syringe, thus preventing the nail from falling into the cannula and also from being aspirated into the syringe. This internal block prevents the biopsy from being fragmented or distorted by violent aspiration into the syringe.

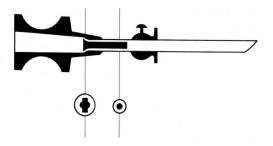

Fig. 3.1. Longitudinal section of the Menghini liver biopsy needle. Note the nail in the shaft of the needle (Menghini 1958).

Three ml of sterile solution are drawn into the syringe which is inserted through the anaesthetized track down to but not through the intercostal space. Two ml of solution are injected to clear the needle of any skin fragments. Aspiration is now commenced and maintained. This is the slow part of the procedure. With the patient holding his breath in expiration, the needle is rapidly introduced perpendicular to the skin into the liver substance and extracted. This is the quick part of the procedure. The tip of the needle is now

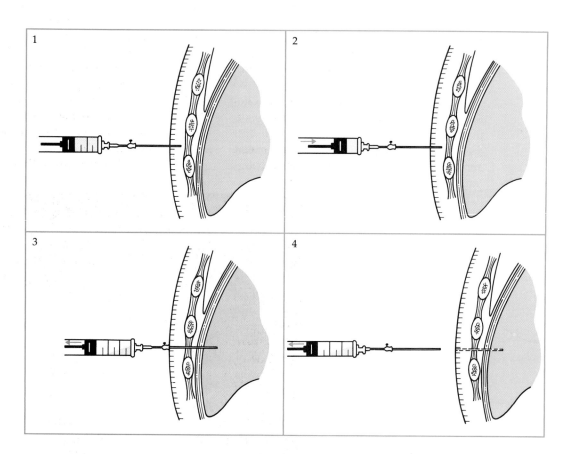

Fig. 3.2. Stages of needle biopsy of the liver using the Menghini technique (Menghini 1958).
1 The biopsy needle with attached syringe is pushed into the subcutaneous tissue.
2 1 ml of saline is injected to expel any tissue fragments from the needle.
3 While aspiration is maintained and the patient holds his breath in expiration, the needle is quickly inserted through the intercostal space and into the liver.
4 Aspiration being maintained, the needle is quickly withdrawn.

placed under saline in a flat-bottomed glass receptacle. It may be necessary gently to inject a little of the remaining saline from the syringe to free the biopsy.

Sedation is not routinely given before biopsy as it may interfere with the patient's co-operation. However, diazepam, 10 mg i.m. is given routinely after the procedure.

The intercostal technique is the most frequent method (fig. 3.2) [40].

It rarely fails, provided care is taken to assess liver size carefully by light percussion. A preliminary ultrasound or CT scan is useful. A small fibrotic liver is a contraindication to the procedure. After adequate local anaesthesia, the needle is inserted in the 8th or 9th intercostal space in the mid-axillary line at the end of expiration with the patient breathing quietly. The direction is slightly posterior and cranial which helps to avoid the gallbladder. If an epigastric mass is present or imaging indicates left lobe disease, an anterior approach is made.

Transvenous (transjugular) liver biopsy. This is done by inserting the special Trucut needle through a catheter placed in the hepatic vein via the jugular vein. The needle is then introduced into the liver tissue by transfixing the hepatic venous wall (fig. 3.3). The technique has the advantage that it can be used in those with abnormal clotting [17]. It is also valuable for patients who are uncooperative or who have very small livers. Another advantage is that wedged and free hepatic venous pressure may be measured at the same time. The procedure may be attempted after percutaneous biopsy has failed (table 3.2). In a French series [17], hepatic tissue was obtained in 1000 out of 1033 attempts and permitted histological diagnosis in 64% of patients with cirrhosis or liver fibrosis, and in 99% of those with non-fibrotic liver lesions. Complications were few, but one patient died from intra-peritoneal bleeding due to a perforation of the liver capsule. The disadvantage is its greater complexity compared with the percutaneous approach. Use of a modified Trucut needle may result in less technical difficulty and larger, less fragmented biopsies. Although usually successful, the liver fragments are sometimes very small.

Directed (guided) liver biopsy with or without

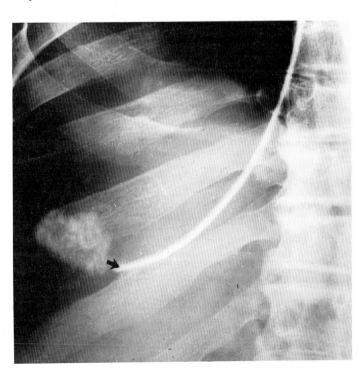

Fig. 3.3. Transvenous liver biopsy. The catheter is in the hepatic vein and contrast has been injected to show the wedged position. The Trucut needle is taking the liver biopsy (arrow).

Table 3.2. Indications for transvenous (transjugular) liver biopsy

Coagulation defects
Measurement wedged hepatic venous pressure
Failed percutaneous biopsy
Small liver
Uncooperative patient

inspection of the liver surface gives a higher percentage of positives than the blind percutaneous technique. This is at the expense of greater cost and complexity. The overall accuracy of diagnosis for chronic liver disease using the 'blind' technique is approximately 81%, but this can be raised to 95% if a directed form of liver biopsy is used [25].

The biopsy TM gun uses a modified 18- or 14-gauge Trucut needle and is operated with one hand. It is fired by a fast and powerful spring mechanism. It allows precise positioning of the needle and is less painful than the manual procedure [10]. It is particularly useful for focal lesions such as tumours, or abscesses [43].

Fine-needle guided biopsy using a 22 swg (0.7 mm) needle adds to the safety. It may provide adequate material for histology and is particularly useful for the diagnosis of tumours [18, 10].

Imaging adds to diagnostic accuracy. A lesion is recognized under imaging and, assuming coagulation and other conditions are satisfactory, a Trucut biopsy needle is advanced into it. On only one of 34 occasions has a focal lesion not been successfully biopsied and the failure was in a patient with an hepatic arterial aneurysm. The method of imaging includes ultrasound [30, 35], computerized tomography [12], and hepatic angiography (fig. 3.4). In those with poor coagulation, a gelfoam plug may be injected through the outer cannula of the Trucut needle after the inner cutting needle, with its contained specimen, has been removed [29]. This is effective in preventing major bleeding after image-guided biopsies.

After-care. The pulse rate is charted hourly for the first 24 hours. Routine visits should be paid four and eight hours after biopsy. A very careful watch must be kept on the patient. Rest in bed is essential for 24 hours.

During the puncture the patient may complain of a drawing feeling across the epigastrium. Afterwards, some patients have a slight ache in the right side for about 24 hours and some complain of pain referred from the diaphragm to the right shoulder.

Difficulties

Failures arise in patients with cirrhosis, especially with ascites, for the tough liver is difficult to pierce and a few liver cells may be extracted, leaving the fibrous framework be-

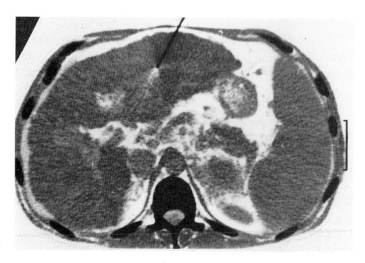

Fig. 3.4. CT of male, age 45, with hepatitis B positive cirrhosis. An irregular liver outline and splenomegaly are clearly seen. Directed biopsy of suspected neoplasm of the left lobe of liver diagnosed hepatocellular carcinoma.

hind. Another source of difficulty may be pulmonary emphysema; the liver is then pushed downwards by the low diaphragm so that the trocar passes above it.

Failure is often due to the needle not being sharp enough to penetrate the capsule. Disposable needles are an advantage for they are sharp.

The percentage of successes increases with diameter of the needle used but so does the complication rate and one must be weighed against the other. The 1-mm Menghini needle, for instance, which is extremely safe, often fails to procure adequate hepatic tissue for diagnosis. The Trucut needle causes more haemorrhages.

Liver biopsy in paediatrics

The Menghini technique may be employed. In infants a local anaesthetic, with 15–60 mg pentobarbital 30 minutes before the biopsy, is adequate. The child is restrained by adhesive strapping across the upper thighs and chest and the subcostal approach used. If the liver is small then the intercostal route is employed, the assistant compressing the chest at the end of expiration to arrest respiration.

In older children general anaesthesia is generally preferred, depending on the co-operation of the child. If splenic venography is necessary, the two procedures can be performed under the same anaesthetic.

Risks and complications

The mortality from various large combined series is about 0.01% (table 3.3). Deaths from haemorrhage are usually in those with a hopeless prognosis. Mortalities are least if the Menghini method is used.

Pleurisy and perihepatitis. A friction rub caused by fibrinous perihepatitis or pleurisy may be heard on the next day. It is of little consequence and pain subsides with analgesics. Chest X-ray may show a small pneumothorax.

Haemorrhage. Bleeding from the puncture wound usually consists of a thin trickle lasting 10–60 seconds and the total blood loss is only

Table 3.3. Fatalities from needle liver biopsy

Source	Date	Reference	Biopsies	Mortality%
USA	1953	(1, 2)	20 016	0.17
Europe combined	1964	(3)	23 382	0.01
Germany	1967	(4)	80 000	0.015
Italy	1986	(5)	68 276	0.009

1 Zamcheck. *N. Eng. J. Med.* 1953; **249**: 1020.
2 Zamcheck. *N. Eng. J. Med.* 1953; **249**: 1062.
3 Thaler. *Wein. Klin. Wchschr.* 1964; **29**: 533.
4 Lindner. *Dtsch. Med. Wschr.* 1967; **92**: 1751.
5 Piccinino. *J. Hepatol.* 1986; **2**: 165.

5–10 ml. Serious haemorrhage is usually intraperitoneal but may be intrathoracic from an intercostal artery. The bleeding results from perforation of distended portal or hepatic veins or aberrant arteries. In some cases a tear of the liver follows deep breathing during the intercostal procedure.

Perforation of the capsule with intraperitoneal haemorrhage may follow transvenous biopsy [5].

Spontaneous recovery may ensue, otherwise angiography followed by transcatheter embolization is usually successful (figs 3.5, 3.6).

Severe haemothorax usually responds to blood transfusion and chest aspiration.

Haemorrhage is rare in the non-jaundiced.

Intra-hepatic haematomas. Ultrasound shows intra-hepatic haematomas in 23% of patients the day after liver biopsy; they are usually asymptomatic [22]. They can cause fever, rises in serum transaminases, a fall in haematocrit and, if large, right upper quadrant tenderness and an enlarging liver. They are usually detected by scanning. They may be seen in the arterial phase of a dynamic CT scan as triangular hyperdense segments. Sometimes a distal portal vein branch may be noted during the arterial phase. Occasionally haematomas are followed by delayed haemorrhage [28].

Haemobilia follows rupture of an intra-hepatic haematoma into a bile duct (fig. 3.7). It is marked by biliary colic with enlargement and

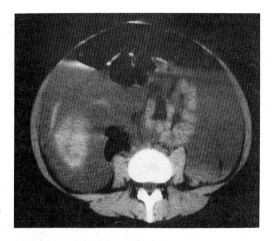

Fig. 3.5. CT scan taken four hours post-biopsy in a patient with hepatic metastases and jaundice shows haemorrhage around and into the liver (arrow).

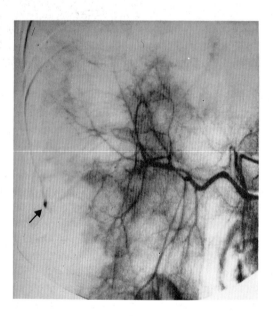

Fig. 3.6. Same patient. Hepatic arteriography (DSA technique) shows blood beside the liver (arrow). The bleeding point was later successfully embolized via the hepatic artery.

tenderness of the liver and sometimes the gall-bladder [24]. The diagnosis is confirmed by ultrasound or ERCP. It may be treated by hepatic arterial embolization however spontaneous recovery is usual.

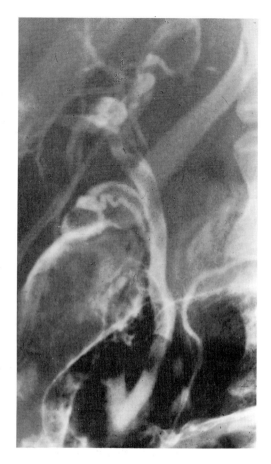

Fig. 3.7. Haemobilia following needle liver biopsy. ERCP shows linear filling defects in the common bile duct.

An arteriovenous fistula, shown by hepatic arteriography, follows 5.4% of liver biopsies (figs 3.8, 3.9) [24]. It may close spontaneously, otherwise it can be treated by direct hepatic arterial catheterization and embolization of the feeding artery.

Biliary peritonitis. This is the second commonest complication after haemorrhage. It was seen 49 times in 123 000 biopsies with 12 deaths [44]. The bile usually comes from the gall-bladder, which may be in an unusual position, or from dilated bile ducts. Surgical management is usually necessary although conservative measures with intravenous fluids, anti-

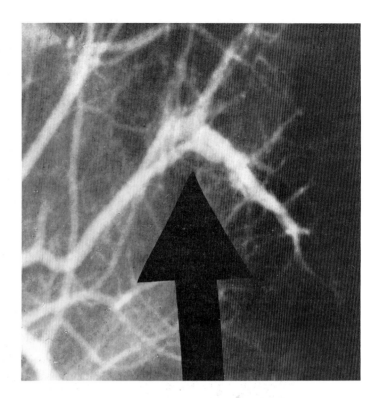

Fig. 3.8. Hepatic arteriography taken post-liver biopsy shows an anteriovenous fistula (arrow).

biotics and intensive care monitoring may be successful [31].

Puncture of other organs such as the kidney or colon is rarely clinically significant.

Infection. Transient bacteriaemia is relatively common, particularly in patients with cholangitis. Septicaemia is rarer; blood cultures are usually positive for *E. coli* [42].

Sampling variability

It is surprising that such a small biopsy should so often be representative of changes in the whole liver. Cholestasis, steatosis, virus hepatitis and the reticuloses are fortunately diffuse. This is also true of most cirrhoses, although in macronodular cirrhosis it is possible to aspirate a large nodule and find normal architecture. There is sampling variability in the diagnosis of cirrhosis in the presence of acute hepatitis or chronic active hepatitis. The focal granulomatous diseases such as sarcoidosis, tumours, deposits and abscesses may be missed, this is infrequent if serial sections are cut.

Misdiagnosis is often due to smallness of sample, especially failure to obtain portal zones, to the focal nature of the disease process and particularly to the inexperience of the interpreter.

The diagnostic yield may be improved if three consecutive samples are obtained by re-directing the biopsy needle through a single entry site [20].

Fibrous tissue is increased under the capsule in operative biopsies and this may give a false impression of the liver as a whole.

Operative biopsies may also show artefactual changes such as patchy loss of glycogen, haemorrhages, polymorph infiltration and even focal necrosis. These are presumably related to the effects of trauma and circulatory changes and hypoxia accompanying surgery.

Naked eye appearances

A satisfactory biopsy is 1–4 cm long and weighs 10–50 mg.

The cirrhotic liver tends to crumble into fragments of irregular contour. The fatty liver has a

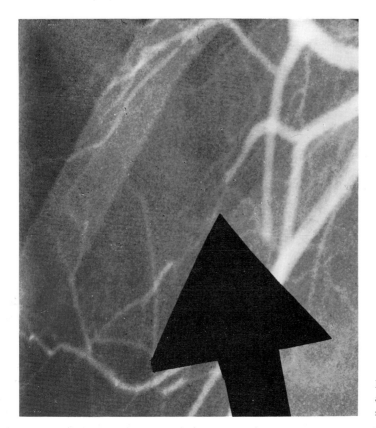

Fig. 3.9. Same patient. The arteriovenous fistula has been successfully embolised (arrow).

pale greasy look and floats in the formol—saline fixative. The liver containing malignant deposits is dull white in colour. The liver from a patient with Dubin—Johnson hyperbilirubinaemia is diffusely chocolate-coloured (fig. 13.10).

In cholestatic jaundice, the greenish central areas contrast with the less green periphery. The vascular centres of lobules in hepatic congestion may be obvious.

Preparation of the specimen

The biopsy is usually fixed in 10% formol—saline. The time taken for such a small piece is less than for a larger specimen. Routine stains include haematoxylin and eosin and a good stain for connective tissue. All specimens are stained for iron by the diastase PAS method. Orcein staining is also useful [33]. This shows hepatitis B surface antigen in the hepatocyte as a uniform, finely granular, brown material. It also stains copper-associated protein in lysosomes as black-brown granules, usually in the periportal area (zone 1). This is a useful indicator of cholestasis and is also sometimes found in Wilson's disease [15].

Specimens for electron microscopy are fixed within seconds in glutaraldehyde and preserved at 4°C until processed. Electron microscopy is particularly valuable for diagnosis of tumours of uncertain origin and storage disorders, including Wilson's disease, Niemann—Pick disease and the Dubin—Johnson syndrome. Micro-enzyme analysis includes the measurement of glucuronyl transferase activity in patients with suspected Gilbert's disease.

Serial sections are important for the diagnosis of lesions such as granulomas which may be scattered through the liver.

Cytological preparations are made by smearing the aspirated tissue core on a slide. These are useful in the diagnosis of cancer.

Interpretation

This depends on skill and experience. The specimen should preferably be at least 2 cm in length with four portal zones if a reliable opinion is to be given. Much smaller specimens may of course sometimes be diagnostic, for instance in hepatocellular carcinoma. Sampling variability is particularly frequent in chronic hepatitis and cirrhosis. The chances of diagnosing hepatic granulomas increases in proportion to the number of sections cut.

Normal histological appearances

The portal zones bear a regular relation to the central areas. This may be difficult to establish in small biopsies especially if no portal zones have been obtained, but this orientation is an essential first step. Each portal zone consists of one or two bile ductules, a branch of the hepatic artery and of the portal vein, a few mononuclears and an occasional fibroblast. The liver cell plates are one cell thick and contain abundant glycogen. Mitoses are not seen in the liver cells which are usually mononucleate and of regular size. The sinusoids are lined by Kupffer cells and can be seen converging upon the central vein.

Isolated sinusoidal dilatation prompts a search for a tumour or a disease associated with granulomas [6].

Table 3.4. Indications for needle liver biopsy

Acute and chronic jaundice
Acute hepatitis and its sequelae
Cirrhosis and portal hypertension
Drug-related liver disease
Liver disease in the alcoholic
Unexplained hepatomegaly or abnormalities of liver function
Storage diseases
Infective and other systemic diseases
Screening of relatives of patients with familial diseases
Space-occupying lesions

Indications (table 3.4) [40]

Between 1960 and 1983, the number of needle liver biopsies performed in the Royal Free Hospital, together with the number referred to the Department of Histopathology for a consultant opinion increased steadily (fig. 3.10). The peak was in 1979, and the last six years has seen a small reduction. This can be attributed to the increasing diagnostic use of percutaneous and endoscopic cholangiography and of imaging procedures. The fall has been most marked in patients with biliary obstruction where imaging procedures are particularly valuable (fig. 3.11).

Despite the advent of specific diagnostic tests for hepatitis A and B, the number of biopsies performed for acute viral hepatitis has been

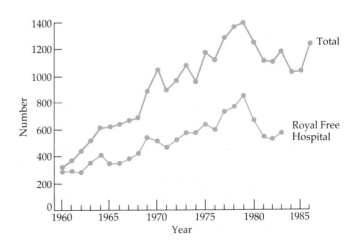

Fig. 3.10. Liver biopsies reviewed by the Histopathology Department at the Royal Free Hospital, 1960–1985. The lower line shows biopsies actually performed in the hospital.

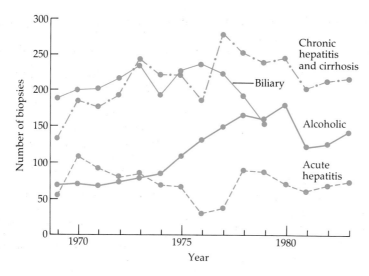

Fig. 3.11. The major indications for liver biopsies performed at the Royal Free Hospital 1969–83 (Sherlock *et al.* 1984).

maintained. This may be due to the inclusion in the group of drug-related hepatitis and of complicated instances of cholestatic viral liver disease. There is no indication nowadays for liver biopsy in most patients with acute hepatitis of type A or type B. Appearances of non-A, non-B hepatitis are suggestive but not specific.

The increase in alcoholism is reflected by the increased number of needle biopsies performed not only to diagnose alcoholic liver disease and for prognosis, but as a deterrent to further consumption.

Chronic hepatitis with or without cirrhosis remains the most important indication. It is in this group that there is most confusion [4]. The distinction between primary biliary cirrhosis and chronic hepatitis leads to errors, particularly as a chronic hepatitis-like picture can be a feature of some stages of primary biliary cirrhosis [13].

Drug-related acute liver disease can be difficult to identify and the history is essential. Sometimes the distinction from acute viral hepatitis is impossible.

Connective tissue stains are important for establishing a diagnosis of cirrhosis [32].

In chronic hepatitis particularly, serial liver biopsy appearances are often the basis of patient management.

Infections. These include tuberculosis, bru-

cellosis, syphilis, histoplasmosis, coccidioidomycosis, pyogenic infection, leptospirosis icterohaemorrhagica and amoebiasis. When indicated, the appropriate stains for the causative organism should be applied and a portion of the biopsy cultured.

Storage diseases. These include amyloidosis and glycogen disease (Chapter 23).

Assessment of therapy, for instance, antivirals corticosteroids, venesection in haemochromatosis.

Other indications include obscure hepatomegaly or splenomegaly, abnormal biochemical tests of liver function of uncertain cause and in the elucidation of chronic sequelae of viral hepatitis.

Space-occupying lesions are diagnosed by direct biopsy under imaging.

Needle liver biopsy in clinical research

Histochemical techniques have been widely applied. Bile canaliculi may be shown by staining for adenosine triphosphatase (ATPase), and staining for glucose-6-phosphatase may be used. Conjugated and unconjugated bilirubin my be shown by a modified diazo technique [27]. Electron microscopy may be combined with histochemistry. ATPase is localized to the microvilli of the canaliculi and 5-nucleotidase to the microvilli of the sinusoidal border. Acid phosphatase is found in Kupffer cells, degenerating foci and regenerating nodules; alkaline phosphatase defines cholangioles.

Hepatic lymphoid malignancies may be characterized by monoclonal antibodies on snap-frozen hepatic tissue [41].

The distribution of hepatitis viral and Delta antigens may be shown by appropriate staining and immunofluorescent methods [4].

Quantitative analysis of liver biopsy specimens is plagued by sampling difficulties and by failure to find a suitable standard of reference. In the liver with normal structure, results are reasonably reliable. For instance, the glycogen content of the diabetic liver has been shown to be normal. The lipid composition can be estimated [16]. Difficulties arise particularly in biopsies from cirrhotic livers where the proportion of fibrous tissue is uncertain. DNA, which is confined to the nucleus, is probably the best reference base although this may be valueless where the proportion of cells of different types is variable. Alternatively the substance being investigated may be referred to dry weight or to total nitrogen content of the biopsy.

Many quantitative studies of hepatic enzymes have been made. The enzymes of mitochondrial, lysosomal, membrane-bound and cytoplasmic fractions of the biopsy can be estimated [36].

References

1 Aledort LM, Levine PH, Hilgartner M *et al.* A study of liver biopsies and liver disease among hemophiliacs. *Blood* 1985; **66**: 367.

2 Axenfeld H, Brass K. Klinische und bioptische Untersuchungen über den sogenannten Icterus catarrhalis. *Frankfurt. Z. Pathol.* 1942; **57**: 147.

3 Baron E. Aspiration for removal of biopsy material from the liver. *Arch. intern. Med.* 1939; **63**: 276.

4 Blum HE, Haase AT, Vyas GN. Molecular pathogenesis of hepatitis B virus infection: simultaneous detection of viral DNA and antigens in paraffin-embedded liver sections. *Lancet* 1984; **ii**: 771.

5 Braillon A, Revert R, Remond A *et al.* Transcatheter embolization of liver capsule perforation

during transvenous liver biopsy. *Gastrointest. Radiol.* 1986; **11**: 277.

6 Bruguera M, Aranguibel F, Ros E *et al.* Incidence and clinical significance of sinusoidal dilatation in liver biopsies. *Gastroenterology* 1978; **75**: 474.

7 Dixon AK, Nunez DK, Bradley JR *et al.* Failure of percutaneous liver biopsy: anatomical variation. *Lancet* 1987; **2**: 437.

8 Ewe K. Bleeding after liver biopsy does not correlate with indices of peripheral coagulation. *Dig. Dis. Sci.* 1981; **26**: 388.

9 Frerichs FT von. *Über den Diabetes.* Hirschwald, Berlin, 1884.

10 Hall-Craggs MA, Lees WR. Fine needle biopsy: cytology, histology or both? *Gut* 1987; **28**: 233.

11 Huard P, May JM, Joyeux B. La ponction biopsie du foie et son utilté dans le diagnostique des affections hépatiques. *Ann. Anat. Path. Anat. norm. Méd-chir* 1935; **12**: 1118.

12 Husband JE, Golding SJ. The role of computed tomography-guided needle biopsy in an oncology service. *Clin. Radiol.* 1983; **34**: 255.

13 International Group. Histopathology of the intrahepatic biliary tree. *Liver* 1983; **3**: 161.

14 Iversen P, Roholm K. On aspiration biopsy of the liver, with remarks on its diagnostic significance. *Acta. med. Scand.* 1939; **102**: 1.

15 Jain S, Scheuer PJ, Archer B *et al.* Histological demonstration of copper-associated protein in chronic liver diseases. *J. clin. Pathol.* 1978; **31**: 784.

16 Judmaier G, Kathrein H. Ultraschallunterstützte perkutane Leber-'blind'-Punktion. *Ultraschall. Med.* 1983; **4**: 81.

17 Kaye R, Koop CE, Wagner BM *et al.* Needle biopsy of the liver. An aid in the differential diagnosis of prolonged jaundice in infancy. *Am. J. Dis. Child.* 1959; **98**: 699.

18 Laurell S, Lundquist A. Lipid composition of human liver biopsy specimens. *Acta med. Scand.* 1971; **189**: 65.

19 Lebrec D, Goldfarb G, Degott C *et al.* Transvenous liver biopsy—an experience based on 1000 hepatic tissue samplings with this procedure. *Gastroenterology* 1982; **83**: 338.

20 Maharaj B, Maharaj RJ, Leary WP *et al.* Sampling variability and its influence on the diagnostic yield of percutaneous needle biopsy of the liver. *Lancet* 1986; **i**: 523.

21 Menghini G. One-second needle biopsy of the liver. *Gastroenterology* 1958; **35**: 190.

22 Minuk GY, Sutherland LR, Wiseman DA *et al.* Prospective study of the incidence of ultrasound-detected intrahepatic and subcapsular hematomas in patients randomized to 6 or 24 hours of bed rest after percutaneous liver biopsy. *Gastroenterology* 1987; **92**: 290.

23 Morris JS, Gallo GA, Scheuer PJ *et al.* Percutaneous

liver biopsy in patients with large bile duct obstruction. *Gastroenterology* 1975; **68**: 750.

24 Okuda K, Musha H, Nakajima Y *et al.* Frequency of intrahepatic arteriovenous fistula as a sequela to percutaneous needle puncture of the liver. *Gastroenterology* 1978; **74**: 1204.

25 Pagliaro L, Rinaldi F, Craxi A *et al.* Percutaneous blind biopsy versus laparoscopy with guided biopsy in diagnosis of cirrhosis: a prospective, randomised trial. *Dig. Dis. Sci.* 1983; **28**: 39.

26 Piccinino F, Sagnelli E, Pasquale G *et al.* Complications following percutaneous liver biopsy. A multicentre retrospective study on 68 276 biopsies. *J. Hepatol.* 1986; **2**: 165.

27 Raia S. Histochemical separation of conjugated and unconjugated bilirubin and its assessment by thin layer chromatography. *J. Histochem. Cytochem.* 1970; **18**: 153.

28 Reichert CM, Weisenthal LM, Klein HG. Delayed hemorrhage after percutaneous liver biopsy. *J. clin. Gastroenterol.* 1983; **5**: 263.

29 Riley SA, Ellis WR, Irving HC *et al.* Percutaneous liver biopsy with plugging of needle track: a safe method for use in patients with impaired coagulation. *Lancet* 1984; **ii**: 436.

30 Rosenblatt R, Kutcher R, Moussouris HF *et al.* Sonographically guided fine-needle aspiration of liver lesions. *J. Am. med. Assoc.* 1982; **248**: 1639.

31 Ruben RA, Chopra S. Bile peritonitis after liver biopsy: nonsurgical management of a patient with an acute abdomen: a case report with review of the literature. *Am. J. Gastroenterol.* 1987; **82**: 265.

32 Scheuer PJ. Progress report: liver biopsy in the diagnosis of cirrhosis. *Gut* 1970; **11**: 275.

33 Scheuer PJ. *Liver Biopsy Interpretation*, 4th edn. Baillière-Tindall, London, 1988.

34 Schüpfer F. De la possibilité de faire 'intra vitam' un diagnostic histo-pathologique précis des maladies du foie et de la rate. *Sem. Méd.* 1907; **27**: 229.

35 Schwerk WB, Schmitz-Moormann P. Ultrasonically guided fine-needle biopsies in neoplastic liver disease: Cytohistologic diagnoses and echo pattern of lesions. *Cancer* 1981; **48**: 1469.

36 Seymour CA, Peters TJ. Enzyme activities in human liver biopsies: assay methods and activities of some lysosomal and membrane-bound enzymes in control tissue and serum. *Clin. Sci. mol. Med.* 1977; **52**: 229.

37 Sharma P, McDonald GB, Banaji M. The risk of bleeding after percutaneous liver biopsy: relation to platelet count. *J. clin. Gastroenterol.* 1982; **4**: 451.

38 Sherlock S. Aspiration liver biopsy, technique and diagnostic application. *Lancet* 1945; **ii**: 397.

39 Sherlock S. Needle biopsy of the liver: a review. *J. clin. Pathol.* 1962; **15**: 291.

40 Sherlock S, Dick R, van Leeuwen DJ. Liver biopsy today. The Royal Free Hospital experience. *J. Hepatol.* 1984; **1**: 75.

41 Verdi CJ, Grogan TM, Protell R *et al.* Liver biopsy immunotyping to characterize lymphoid malignancies. *Hepatology* 1986; **6**: 6.

42 Vicente VFM, Ranz FMF, del Arbol LR *et al.* Septicaemia as a complication of liver biopsy. *Am. J. Gastroenterol.* 1981; **76**: 145.

43 Whitmire LF, Galambos JT, Phillips VM *et al.* Imaging guided percutaneous hepatic biopsy: diagnostic accuracy and safety. *J. clin. Gastroenterol.* 1985; **7**: 511.

44 Yoshida J, Donahue P, Nyhus LM. Hemobilia: review of recent experience with a worldwide problem. *Am. J. Gastroenterol.* 1987; **82**: 448.

4 · The Haematology of Liver Disease

Hepato-cellular failure, portal hypertension and jaundice may affect the blood picture. Chronic liver disease is usually accompanied by 'hyper-splenism'. Diminished erythrocyte survival is frequent. In addition both parenchymal hepatic disease and cholestatic jaundice may be associated with blood coagulation defects. Dietary deficiencies, alcoholism, bleeding and difficulties in hepatic synthesis of proteins used in blood formation or coagulation add to the complexity of the problem.

Spontaneous bleeding, bruising and purpura together with a history of bleeding after minimal trauma such as venepuncture are more important indications of a bleeding tendency in patients with liver disease than are laboratory tests.

BLOOD VOLUME

Plasma volume is frequently increased in patients with cirrhosis, especially with ascites and also with long-standing obstructive jaundice or with hepatitis. This hypervolaemia may partially, and sometimes totally, account for a low peripheral haemoglobin or erythrocyte level. Total circulating haemoglobin is reduced in only about half the patients.

Erythrocyte changes

The red cells are usually *hypochromic*. This is often due to gastro-intestinal bleeding. In portal hypertension anaemia follows gastro-oesophageal bleeding and is enhanced by thrombocytopenia and disturbed blood coagulation. In cholestasis or cirrhosis of the alcoholic, haemorrhage may be from an ulcer or gastritis. Epistaxis, bruising and bleeding gums add to the anaemia.

The erythrocytes are usually *normocytic*. This is a combination of the microcytosis of chronic blood loss and the macrocytosis inherent in patients with liver disease. *Spherocytes* represent increased splenic sequestration. The ratio of red cell membrane cholesterol to phospholipids (CP ratio) is changed and this results in various morphological abnormalities including thin macrocytes, target cells and spur cells [6].

Thin macrocytes are frequent and associated with a macronormoblastic marrow. These resolve when liver function improves.

Target cells are also thin macrocytes. They are found in both hepato-cellular and cholestatic jaundice. They are flat, macrocytic and have an increased surface area and increased resistance to osmotic lysis. They are particularly prominent in cholestasis where a rise in bile acids may contribute by inhibiting lecithin cholesterol acyl transferase (LCAT) activity [5]. The membrane LCAT activity is decreased.

Spur cells are cells with unusual thorny projections. They are also termed *'burr' cells* or *acanthocytes*. They are associated with far advanced liver disease usually in alcoholics. Severe anaemia and haemolysis is also found [9, 10]. Their appearance is a bad prognostic sign. The membrane CP ratio is markedly increased due to increased membrane cholesterol; total phospholipid remains normal. They have a shortened survival. Their rigid membranes make them particularly susceptible to being filtered in the spleen.

Alcoholics show genuine *thick macrocytes* probably related to the toxic effect of alcohol on the bone marrow. Folic acid and B_{12} deficiency may contribute.

Erythrocytosis may complicate primary liver cancer (Chapter 28).

Bone marrow of chronic hepato-cellular failure is hyperplastic and macronormoblastic. In spite of this, erythrocyte volume is depressed and the marrow therefore does not seem able to compensate completely for the anaemia (*relative marrow failure*).

Folate and B_{12} metabolism

The liver stores folate and converts it to its active storage form, tetrahydrofolate [4]. Folate deficiency may accompany chronic liver disease, usually in the alcoholic. This is largely due to dietary deficiency. Serum folate levels are low. Folate therapy is useful. The liver also stores vitamin B_{12}. Hepatic levels are reduced in liver disease. When hepatocytes become necrotic the vitamin is released into the blood and high serum B_{12} levels are recorded. This is shown in hepatitis, active cirrhosis and with primary liver cancer. Values in cholestatic jaundice are normal.

The blood levels of vitamin B_{12} and folate correlate with the hepatic content. Megaloblastic anaemia is rare with chronic liver disease and vitamin B_{12} therapy is rarely needed.

Erythrocyte survival and haemolytic anaemia

Increased red cell destruction is almost constant in hepato-cellular failure and jaundice of all types [21]. This is reflected in erythrocyte polychromasia and reticulocytosis.

The mechanism is extremely complex. The major factor is hypersplenism with destruction of red blood cells in the spleen. Also spur cells have membrane defects, particularly decreased fluidity, and this with altered architecture exacerbates splenic destruction. In many instances, however, the spleen is not the site of erythrocyte destruction. Splenectomy or corticosteroid therapy have little effect [21].

Haemolysis may be acute in patients with alcoholic hepatitis who also have hypercholesterolaemia (*Zieve's syndrome*) [30].

Very rarely an auto-immune haemolytic anaemia with a positive Coombs' test is seen in chronic active hepatitis and primary biliary cirrhosis.

Aplastic anaemia is a rare complication of acute virus hepatitis, usually type non-A, non-B [28]. It carries a very bad prognosis and has been treated by bone marrow transplantation [27]. It may follow liver transplantation for fulminant non-A, non-B hepatitis.

Hepatitis B virus positive serum inhibits a normal human marrow cell [29].

Changes in the leucocytes and platelets

Leucopenia and thrombocytopenia are commonly found in patients with cirrhosis, usually with a mild anaemia ('*hypersplenism*').

LEUCOCYTES

The leucopenia is of the order of 1500–3000 cells per mm^3, the depression mainly affecting polymorphs. Occasionally it may be more severe.

Leucocytosis accompanies cholangitis, fulminant hepatitis, alcoholic hepatitis, hepatic abscess and malignant disease. Atypical lymphocytes are found in the peripheral blood in virus infections such as infectious mononucleosis and virus hepatitis.

Patients with very high serum globulin values show plasmacytosis of the bone marrow.

PLATELETS

Abnormalities in platelet numbers, structure and function are common in patients with all forms of liver disease.

Reduced numbers, rarely severe, are due to increased splenic sequestration. This is related to a greatly increased splenic platelet pool. Increased destruction of platelets is minimal. Platelet half-life is normal. Platelet volume is low [13]. These changes are also found in other diseases with splenomegaly. Similar haematological changes occur with thrombosis of the portal vein.

Abnormal platelet aggregation, due to disseminated intravascular consumption, may be important in severe liver failure.

Platelet associated antibodies are found particularly in patients with chronic active hepatitis [20].

Qualitatively, the platelets may be inadequate due to reduced availability of arachidonic acid for prostaglandin production [19].

Reduced platelet aggregation follows reduction in the numbers of larger, more haemostatically active platelets [24].

Decreased production of platelets from the bone marrow follows alcohol excess, folic acid deficiency and viral hepatitis.

The thrombocytopenia (usually 60 to 90 000 per mm^3) of chronic liver disease is extremely frequent and is largely due to hypersplenism. It is very rarely of clinical significance. Unless the patient is actually *suffering* from the leucopenia or thrombocytopenia the spleen should *not* be removed; mere demonstration of a low platelet or leucocyte count is not sufficient. The circulating platelets and leucocytes, although in short supply, are, in contrast to those of leukaemia, functioning well. Splenectomy is contra-indicated. The mortality in patients with liver disease is high and the operation is liable to be followed by splenic and portal vein thrombosis which preclude later operations on the portal vein and may make hepatic transplantation more difficult.

The liver and blood coagulation

Disturbed blood coagulation in patients with hepato-biliary disease is particularly complex (table 4.1) [14, 15]. It has now become clear, particularly as a result of isolated hepatocyte and hepatoma cell culture studies, that the liver is the principle site of synthesis of all the coagulation proteins with the exception of the von Willebrand factor and the fibrolytic proteins [7, 15]. The liver also synthesizes protease inhibitors which modulate and coagulation cascade, such as antithrombin 111 (AT111), protein C, and heparin co-factor 11

Table 4.1. Coagulation factors: all those synthesized by the liver may be reduced in acute and chronic hepato-cellular disease especially if severe

Factors	Notes
Fibrinogen	Hepatic synthesis Abnormal polymerization in cirrhosis and hepato-cellular carcinoma
Prothrombin time and VII, IX, X	Hepatic synthesis Vitamin K dependent
V	Hepatic synthesis
VIII & VWF*	Normal in hepato-cellular and cholestatic disease
XI, XII	Hepatic synthesis Reduced severe disease
Antithrombin III	Hepatic synthesis Consumed DIC
Plasminogen	Hepatic synthesis Increased turnover and catabolism
α_2-antiplasmin	Hepatic synthesis

* VWF = Von Willebrand's factor

Table 4.2. Routine before invasive techniques (including surgery)

Measure	Prothrombin time (PT) Partial thromboplastin time (PTT) Platelet count
Routine	Abstain from alcohol for one week Vitamin K$_1$ 10 mg intramuscular Oral folic acid
If necessary	Fresh frozen plasma Platelet infusion

(figs 4.1, 4.2). Homozygous protein C deficiency has been cured by hepatic transplantation [3].

Failure of bile salt secretion into the intestine results in inadequate vitamin K absorption. The liver also clears activated clotting factors from the blood. Disseminated intravascular coagulation can follow acute hepato-cellular necrosis (fig. 4.1). Finally these coagulation

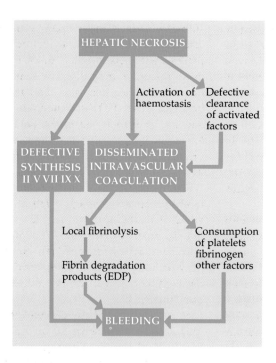

Fig. 4.1. Bleeding in hepato-cellular failure. Hepatic necrosis leads to defective synthesis of clotting factors II, V, VII, IX and X. Disseminated intravascular coagulation can follow activation of haemostasis by cell necrosis and defective clearance of activated factors by the necrotic liver. Platelets, fibrinogen and other factors are consumed and local fibrinolysis leads to fibrin degradation products (FDP). Bleeding is the end result.

difficulties are often combined with thrombocytopenia and an elevated portal venous pressure which predispose to gastrointestinal bleeding.

The liver synthesizes fibrinogen and the vitamin K-dependent factors II, VII, IX and X, also labile factor V, factor VIII, contact factors XI and XII, and fibrin stabilizing factor XIII. The half-life of all these clotting proteins is very short and hence reductions can follow very rapidly on acute hepato-cellular necrosis (fig. 4.1).

The vitamin K-dependent proteins are manufactured in the rough endoplasmic reticulum. They all have a unique amino acid, gamma-carboxyglutamic acid (Gla) on their amino-terminal portion [8, 17]. Vitamin K is necessary for the carboxylation of these blood-clotting proteins, so facilitating the conversion of prothrombin to thrombin. Disorders of this hepatic vitamin K-dependent carboxylation system may be congenital or acquired.

In liver disease, structurally and functionally inadequate clotting factors may be produced. For instance, non-functional, des, gamma-carboxy forms of the vitamin K-dependent coagulation proteins such as abnormal prothrombin, may be formed. Patients with hepato-cellular carcinoma may secrete an abnormal prothrombin (des, gamma-carboxy prothrombin) and this has been used as a serum marker for the disease [17].

In hepato-cellular disease the factors most likely to be affected are VII, followed by II and X. IX is the last to be reduced. Synthesis of factors V and fibrinogen may be decreased but are less easily depressed than the others.

In addition the liver clears active clotting factors from the circulation and this includes thromboplastin. In hepato-cellular disease, failure of this process adds to the bleeding.

Finally the liver cell is concerned with fibrinolysis (fig. 4.2). Plasminogen is probably synthesized by the liver cells and plasmin activator cleared by the liver. Antiplasmin is made by the liver. Primary fibrinolysis may develop in patients with cirrhosis although it is difficult to distinguish from secondary fibrinolysis due to disseminated intravascular coagulation.

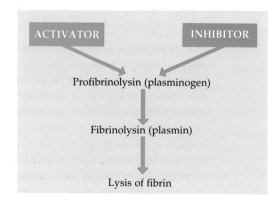

Fig. 4.2. Fibrinolytic enzyme system.

Dysfibrinogenaemia is particularly frequent in cirrhosis, chronic active hepatitis and acute liver failure. It is probably due to hepatic synthesis of an abnormal fibrinogen molecule. It accounts for the prolongation of the thrombin time in many patients with liver disease. It should be suspected if the partial thromboplastin time is increased but fibrinogen is normal and fibrinogen degradation products (FDP) are not increased. Abnormal fibrinogens, resembling those of the fetus, can be found with hepato-cellular carcinoma.

The pathogenesis of *disseminated intravascular coagulation (DIC)* in acute hepatic necrosis is multifactorial and includes the release of tissue thromboplastin from liver cells, reduced clearance of activated coagulation proteins, reduced synthesis of inhibitors (such as ATIII and protein C) and circulating endotoxin [15, 16, 20, 26]. This coagulopathy is marked by depression of plasma fibrinogen, reduced survival of circulating fibrinogen [22], reduced clotting factors and low platelets. Intravascular microthrombi form and circulating FDPs can be shown. Activation of the fibrinolysis system is marked by low plasminogen activator and plasminogen levels. Such changes have been demonstrated in patients with fulminant hepatitis and drug-related acute hepatic necrosis [22]. In most instances the defect is a mild one, platelets are usually above 100 000, FDP only moderately increased and fibrinogen only slightly reduced [12]. Moreover, examination of liver biopsy material shows only slight deposition of fibrin and this is related much more to areas of necrosis than to intravascular deposition. The severity of the bleeding seems unrelated to the degree of coagulopathy.

Ascitic fluid usually contains fibrin monomer, fibrin degradation products and low levels of fibrinogen. This indicates intraperitoneal coagulation. Fibrinolysis, induced by infusion of plasminogen activators, accounts for the coagulopathy [25] which complicates intravenous infusion of ascitic fluid.

TESTS OF COAGULATION

The prothrombin time (PT) before and after 10 mg vitamin K intramuscularly is the most satisfactory test for a coagulation defect in patients with hepato-biliary disease. It is also a most sensitive indication of hepato-cellular necrosis and/or prognosis. The partial thromboplastin time (PTT) is sometimes performed and is slightly more sensitive than the PT. Prolongation indicates not only deficiency of the prothrombin complex but also factors XI and XII.

Estimation of individual clotting factors is rarely necessary although a fall of factor VII, which has the shortest half-life (about six hours), holds a particularly bad prognosis in fulminant hepatic failure [11]. Antithrombin III, plasminogen and α_2-antiplasmin are synthesized by the liver and low values predict a bad outcome [23].

Fibrinolysis and disseminated intravascular coagulation are diagnosed by marked prolongation of the PT, fibrinogen levels below 1.0 g per litre, FDPs greater than 100 g per litre and thrombocytopenia less than 100×10^9 per litre.

Management of coagulation defect

Vitamin K_1 should be given to all patients with a prolonged one-stage prothrombin time. The usual course is 10 mg vitamin K_1 by intramuscular injection for three days. This is effective in about three hours and will correct hypoprothrombinaemia related to bile salt deficiency. Defects predominantly due to hepato-cellular disease will not be restored by the vitamin K_1 treatment. Nevertheless, even in patients with predominantly hepato-cellular jaundice there may be a component of bile salt secretory failure and the prothrombin time often improves by a few seconds. A prolongation of the one-stage prothrombin time of more than three seconds after intramuscular vitamin K_1 contraindicates such procedures as liver biopsy, splenic venography, percutaneous cholangiography or laparotomy. If such procedures are essential, the clotting defect may be corrected by fresh-frozen plasma which corrects the defect for a few hours (table 4.2).

In general, apart from vitamin K_1 therapy, it is not necessary to restore blood coagulation to normal in patients with liver disease unless there is active bleeding. Stored blood transfusion will supply prothrombin, VII, VIII and X. Fresh blood also supplies factor V and platelets. Fresh-frozen plasma is a good source of clotting factors, especially V [18].

Desmopressin (DDAVP), a vasopressin analogue, causes transient shortening of the bleeding time and PTT (but not PT) with increases in factor VIII and von Willebrand factor. Infusions may be helpful for the control of bleeding in patients with chronic liver disease [2].

Disseminated intravascular coagulation is treated by control of trigger factors such as infection, shock and dehydration. Fresh blood is most useful but, if unavailable, fresh-frozen plasma and packed red blood cells may be used. DIC is never severe enough to merit heparin therapy.

Platelet-rich plasma concentrates are used if thrombocytopenia is a problem and may be given to cover a procedure such as liver biopsy in a severely thrombocytopenic patient.

Hepatic transplantation

Pre-operative coagulation defects are due to the diseased liver. This and operative blood loss indicate replacement usually with about 20 units red blood cells and 15 units platelets. Prognosis is related to the amount of blood and blood products required [1]. During surgery, coagulation and fibrolysis are activated. In the anhepatic phase there is reduced clearance of activated proteins and inhibitors. The state of preservation of the donor liver determines postoperative coagulation problems. Revascularization of a compromised liver may lead to extensive defibrination and uncontrolled bleeding.

References

1 Bontempo FA, Lewis JH, Van Thiel DH *et al.* The relation of preoperative coagulation findings to diagnosis, blood usage, and survival in adult liver transplantation. *Transplantation* 1985; **39**: 532.

2 Burroughs AK, Matthews K, Qadiri M *et al.* Desmopressin and bleeding time in patients with cirrhosis. *Br. med. J.* 1985; **291**: 1377.

3 Casella JF, Lewis JH, Bontempo FA *et al.* Successful treatment of homozygous protein C deficiency by hepatic transplantation. *Lancet* 1988; **i**: 435.

4 Chanarin I, Hutchinson M, McLean A *et al.* Hepatic folate in man. *Br. med. J.* 1966; **1**: 396.

5 Cooper RA, Arner EC, Wiley JS *et al.* Modification of red cell membrane structure by cholesterol-rich lipid dispersions: a model for the primary spur cell defect. *J. clin. Invest.* 1975; **55**: 115.

6 Cooper RA, Diloy-Puray M, Lando P *et al.* An analysis of lipoproteins, bile acids, and red cell membranes associated with target cells and spur cells in patients with liver disease. *J. clin. Invest.* 1972; **51**: 3182.

7 Fair DS, Marlar RA. Biosynthesis and secretion of factor VII, protein C, protein S, and the protein C inhibitor from a human hepatoma cell line. *Blood* 1986; **67**: 64.

8 Friedman PA. Vitamin K-dependent proteins. *N. Engl. J. Med.* 1984; **310**: 1458.

9 Gisselbrecht C, Metreau J-M. Dhumeaux D *et al.* L'acanthocytose au cours des cirrhoses. *Gastroenterol. clin. Biol.* 1977; **1**: 621.

10 Grahn EP, Dietz AA, Stefani SS *et al.* Burr cells, hemolytic anemia and cirrhosis. *Am. J. Med.* 1968; **45**: 78.

11 Green G, Poller L, Thomson JM *et al.* Factor VII as a marker of hepatocellular synthetic function in liver disease. *J. clin. Path.* 1976; **29**: 971.

12 Hillenbrand P. Parbhoo SP, Jedrychowski A *et al.* Significance of intravascular coagulation and fibrinolysis in acute hepatic failure. *Gut* 1974; **15**: 83.

13 Jørgensen B, Fischer E, Ingeberg S *et al.* Decreased blood platelet volume and count in patients with liver disease. *Scand. J. Gastroenterol.* 1984; **19**: 492.

14 Kelly DA, Tuddenham EGD. Haemostatic problems in liver disease. *Gut* 1986; **27**: 339.

15 Kelly DA, Summerfield JA. Hemostasis in liver disease. *Semin. Liv. Dis.* 1987; **7**: 182.

16 Knot E, Ten Cate JW, Drujfhout HR *et al.* Antithrombin III metabolism in patients with liver disease. *J. clin. Path.* 1984; **37**: 523.

17 Liebman HA, Furie BC, Furie B. Hepatic vitamin K-dependent carboxylation of blood-clotting proteins. *Hepatology* 1982; **2**: 488.

18 National Institutes of Health Consensus Conference. Fresh-frozen plasma. Indications and risks. *J. Amer. med. Ass.* 1985; **253**: 551.

19 Owen JS, Hutton RA, Day RC *et al.* Platelet lipid composition and platelet aggregation in human liver disease. *J. Lipid Res.* 1981; **22**: 423.

20 Pfueller SL, Firkin BG, Kerlero de Rosbo N *et al.* Association of increased immune complexes,

platelet IgG and serum IgG in chronic active hepatitis. *Clin. exp. Immunol.* 1983; **54**: 655.

21 Pitcher CS, Williams R. Reduced red cell survival in jaundice and its relation to abnormal glutathione metabolism. *Clin. Sci.* 1963; **24**: 239.

22 Rake MO, Flute PT, Pannell G *et al.* Intravascular coagulation in acute hepatic necrosis. *Lancet* 1970; **i**: 533.

23 Rodzynek JJ, Urbain D, Leautaud P *et al.* Antithrombin III, plasminogen and alpha₂ antiplasmin in jaundice: clinical usefulness and prognostic significance. *Gut* 1984; **25**: 1050.

24 Rubin MH, Weston MJ, Langley PG *et al.* Platelet function in chronic liver disease: relationship to disease severity. *Dig. Dis. Sci.* 1979; **24**: 197.

25 Schölmerich J, Zimmerman U, Köttgen E *et al.* Proteases and antiproteases released to the coagulation system in plasma and ascites. Prediction of coagulation disorder in ascites retransfusion. *J. Hepatol.* 1988; **6**: 359.

26 Wion KL, Kelly DA, Summerfield JA *et al.* Distribution of factor VIII mRNA and antigen in human liver and other tissues. *Nature* 1985; **317**: 726.

27 Witherspoon RP, Storb R, Shulman H *et al.* Marrow transplantation in hepatitis-associated aplastic anemia. *Am. J. Hematol.* 1984; **17**: 269.

28 Young N, Mortimer P. Viruses and bone marrow failure. *Blood* 1984; **63**: 729.

29 Zeldis J, Mugishima H, Steinberg H *et al.* In vitro hepatitis B virus infection of human bone marrow cells. *J. clin. Invest.* 1986; **78**: 411.

30 Zieve L. Hemolytic anemia in liver disease. *Medicine (Baltimore)* 1966; **45**: 497.

Haemolytic jaundice

Haemoglobin is released in excessive amounts, increasing from the normal of 6.25 g to as much as 45 g daily. Consequently there is an increase in the serum bilirubin, 85% of which is unconjugated. The rise in conjugated bilirubin is probably due to retention.

Even if bile pigment production reaches its maximum of 1500 mg daily (six times normal) serum, bilirubin rises only to about 2−3 mg/100 ml. This is because of the great capacity of the liver to handle pigment. If patients with haemolytic jaundice show serum bilirubin values greater than 4−5 mg/100 ml there is probably the additional factor of hepato-cellular dysfunction or kidney failure. Anaemia itself will, of course, depress liver function.

Unconjugated bilirubin is not water-soluble and does not pass into the urine. A little bilirubin may be detected in the urine by sensitive tests if the conjugated level in the blood rises to values which are unusually high for haemolysis.

Bile pigment excretion is greatly increased and large quantities of stercobilinogen are found in the stools. Each milligramme of stercobilinogen corresponds to the breakdown of 24 mg haemoglobin. This estimate can only be approximate, for a significant proportion of the faecal haem pigment is derived from sources other than haemoglobin of mature erythrocytes.

PATHOLOGICAL CHANGES

The breakdown of haemoglobin yields iron. *Tissue siderosis* is a feature of most types of haemolytic anaemia.

The *liver* is normal sized and is reddish-brown due to increased amounts of iron. Histology shows iron in Kupffer cells, large macrophages of the portal tracts, and to a lesser extent in hepatic parenchyma (fig. 4.3). In the

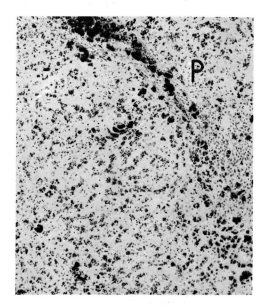

Fig. 4.3. Haemolytic jaundice. The hepatic architecture is normal. Increased amounts of iron are seen in the liver cells. Kupffer cells and especially the large macrophages of the portal tracts (P). (Stained ferro-cyanide, ×90.)

severely anaemic, there is centrizonal sinusoidal distension with fatty change. Focal areas of liver cell necrosis are attributed to vascular obstruction of sinusoids by impacted cells undergoing lysis or to the direct effect of haemolysis on the liver cells. The Kupffer cells are generally swollen and hyperplastic: foci of erythropoiesis are uncommon. The *gallbladder* and *bile passages* contain dark viscid bile. Calcium bilirubinate pigment calculi are found in half to two-thirds of patients. Secondary cholecystitis may be followed by crops of multiple, faceted, mixed gallstones.

The *spleen* is enlarged, fleshy and packed with erythrocytes. The *red bone marrow* is hyperplastic.

CLINICAL FEATURES

The picture varies with the cause, but certain symptoms and signs are common to all forms of haemolysis.

Anaemia depends on the rate of destruction compared with regeneration of red blood cells. It increases rapidly with crises where the patient becomes ill with aching pains in the abdomen and limbs, fever, headache and sometimes even a fall in blood pressure and collapse.

Jaundice is usually mild and lemon yellow. It increases rapidly with haemolytic crises or if there is a coincidental difficulty in biliary excretion such as virus hepatitis or choledocholithiasis or if the kidney fails.

Pigment *gallstones* may be associated with the features of chronic cholecystitis. Stones in the common bile duct may cause obstructive jaundice, and the co-existence of two types of jaundice provides a confusing clinical picture. Gallstones in children always suggest a haemolytic aetiology.

Splenomegaly is present in the chronic forms.

Ulcers or pigmentation from healed ulcers, usually over the internal or external malleoli, occur in some types.

HAEMATOLOGICAL CHANGES

Anaemia is variable and the peripheral blood shows active regeneration. Reticulocytes are increased to 20%. Leucocytes are usually increased.

The sternal marrow is hyperplastic and the proportion of erythroid to leucopoietic cells rises.

The survival of labelled erythrocytes is reduced and increased uptake can be shown in the spleen.

FAECES AND URINE

The faeces are dark and stercobilinogen is increased. Urobilinogen is increased in the urine. Bilirubin is detected in the urine only rarely, when jaundice is deep. When blood destruction is rapid, free haemoglobin may be found in the urine and microscopy reveals pigmented casts.

SERUM BIOCHEMISTRY

Serum unconjugated bilirubin levels are raised but conjugated bilirubin is only slightly increased.

The serum alkaline phosphatase, albumin and globulin concentrations are normal. Serum haptoglobins are diminished. The serum cholesterol level is low.

If haemolysis is particularly acute, methaemalbumin can be detected in the serum. Serum ferritin is increased. Free haemoglobin may be detected.

DIFFERENTIAL DIAGNOSIS

The diagnosis of haemolytic from other forms of jaundice is usually easy. The absence of pain and pruritus and the dark colour of the stools are points of difference from cholestatic jaundice. The absence of other stigmata of hepatocellular disease, the normal serum alkaline phosphatase and protein values distinguish it from virus hepatitis and cirrhosis.

Distinction from the congenital unconjugated hyperbilirubinaemias may be difficult, particularly as many patients with Gilbert's disease show a decreased erythrocyte survival.

The liver in haemolytic anaemias

HEREDITARY SPHEROCYTOSIS

Jaundice is rarely noticed before school age or adolescence. Deep jaundice may, however, develop in the neonatal period and be associated with incipient kernicterus. All grades of severity occur but deep jaundice is rare; the mean serum bilirubin level is 2.0 mg (range 0.6−5.7 mg/100 ml). The spleen is enlarged.

Gallstones are related to age and are rare at less than 10 years old. They are symptomatic in about half the patients. The stones are usually removed at the time of splenectomy.

Hereditary elliptocytosis is usually a harmless trait, the haemolysis being compensated. It may occasionally develop into active decompensated haemolytic anaemia.

VARIOUS ENZYME DEFECTS

Many of the hereditary non-spherocytic anaemias are now known to be due to various defects in the metabolism of the red cells. They include deficiency of pyruvate kinase or triosephosphate isomerase or deficiency in the pentose phosphate pathway such as glucose-6-phosphate dehydrogenase. These conditions may be of particular importance in the aetiology of neonatal jaundice.

Viral hepatitis can precipitate destruction of *glucose-6-phosphate dehydrogenase* deficient cells and so cause acute haemolytic anaemia.

Sickle-cell disease

The abnormal haemoglobin crystallizes in the erythrocytes when the oxygen tension is reduced. There are crises of blood destruction with acute attacks of pain.

Acute liver failure, usually with cholestasis, is rare. Jaundice is very deep with a markedly increased prothrombin time and encephalopathy but with only modestly increased serum transaminases. Liver biopsy shows the changes of sickle-cell disease with marked zone 2 necro-sis and cholestasis. The diagnosis of hepatic crisis from viral hepatitis is difficult. In general, in viral hepatitis pain is less, jaundice deeper and transaminase elevations more prolonged. Liver biopsy and hepatitis viral markers usually help to make the distinction.

Jaundice accompanying sickle-cell disease is always particularly deep, the high serum bilirubin levels being related to the combination of haemolysis and impaired hepato-cellular function. Depth of jaundice *per se* should not be regarded as an indication of severity. Concomitant viral hepatitis or obstructed bile ducts lead to exceptionally high serum bilirubin values. Similarly, very high levels are seen when viral hepatitis complicates *glucose-6-PD deficiency*[2].

Gallstones are found in 50 to 70% of adults with homozygous sickle-cell disease and are symptomatic in two-thirds of adults [1]. About 55% are radio-opaque. The stones are usually in the gallbladder and duct calculi are rare. Gallstones in the gallbladder are shown by ultrasound in about a quarter of homozygous children. Acute cholecystitis and choledocholiasis may simulate hepatic crisis or viral hepatitis. Percutaneous or endoscopic cholangioraphy are helpful investigations in excluding biliary obstruction. Complications after cholecystectomy are common, and this is indicated only if there is great difficulty in making a distinction from abdominal crisis or where symptoms are clearly related to gallbladder disease. Pre-operative exchange transfusion may lessen later complications [1].

Leg ulcers are frequent. The upper jaw is protuberant and hypertrophied. The fingers are clubbed. Bone deformities seen radiologically include rarefaction and narrowing of the cortex of the long bones and a 'hair-on-end' appearance in the skull.

Hepatic histology

Active and healed areas of necrosis may have followed anoxia due to vascular obstruction by impacted sickle cells or by Kupffer cells swollen with phagocytosed erythrocytes following intra-hepatic sickling. The widened sinusoids show a foam-like fibrin reticulum within their lumen. This intra-sinusoidal fibrin may later result in fibre deposition in the space of Dissë and narrowed sinusoids. Bile plugs are prominent. Fatty change is related to anaemia and haemosiderosis to multiple transfusions.

The classical findings are of intra-sinusoidal sickling, Kuppfer cell erythrophagocytosis and ischaemic necrosis. It is difficult to explain the severe liver dysfunction on these histological findings [5]. These changes have been reported largely on autopsy specimens. In biopsies, the histological picture is more likely to be that of a complicating disease such as septicaemia or concurrent viral hepatitis [8].
The hepatic infarcts may become infected with abscess formation or may fill with bile forming a cyst ('biloma') [7]. The excessive bilirubin load induces bilirubin conjugating enzymes.

Electron microscopy

The changes are those of hypoxia. There are sinusoidal aggregates of sickled erythrocytes, fibrin and platelets with increased collagen and occasional basement membranes in the space of Dissë.

Clinical features

Asymptomatic patients commonly have raised serum transaminases and hepatomegaly [9].

In about 10% the crisis selectively affects the liver. It lasts two to three weeks. It is marked by abdominal pain, fever, jaundice, an enlarged tender liver and a rise in serum transaminases. In some patients the crisis is precipitated by salmonella infections or by folic acid deficiency.

THALASSAEMIA

Crises of blood destruction and fever and the reactionary changes in bone are similar to those seen in sickle-cell disease. The liver shows siderosis and sometimes fibrosis. The haemosiderosis may progress to an actual haemochromatosis and indicate treatment by

continuous desferrioxamine therapy (see Chapter 21). The stainable iron in the liver cells may be greater in those who have lost the spleen as a storage organ for iron. Episodes of intra-hepatic cholestasis of uncertain nature can also develop. Gallstones may be a complication.

Treatment

This may include folic acid, blood transfusion, pneumococcal vaccination and occasionally splenectomy. Bone marrow transplantation must be considered.

PAROXYSMAL NOCTURNAL HAEMOGLOBINURIA

This rare disease is due to an unknown defect in the red cells, which are sensitive to lysis when the pH of the blood becomes more acid during sleep.

Acutely the patients show a dusky, reddish jaundice and the liver enlarges. Liver histology shows some centrizonal necrosis and siderosis.

Hepatic vein thrombosis may be a complication.

ACQUIRED HAEMOLYTIC ANAEMIA

The haemolysis is due to extra-corpuscular causes. Spherocytosis is slight and osmotic fragility only mildly impaired.

The patient is moderately jaundiced. The increased pigment is unconjugated, but in severe cases conjugated bilirubin increases and appears in the urine. This may be related to bilirubin overload in the presence of liver damage. Blood transfusion accentuates the jaundice, for transfused cells survive poorly.

The haemolysis may be *idiopathic*. The increased haemolysis is then due to auto-immunization. Coombs' test is positive.

The *acquired* type may complicate other diseases, especially those involving the reticulo-endothelial system. These include Hodgkin's disease, the leukaemias, reticulosarcoma, carcinomatosis and uraemia. The anaemia of hepato-cellular jaundice is also partially hae-molytic. Coombs' test is usually negative.

Auto-immune haemolytic anaemia is a rare complication of chronic active hepatitis and primary biliary cirrhosis.

Wilson's disease may present as a haemolytic crisis.

HAEMOLYTIC DISEASE OF THE NEWBORN (Chapter 24)

INCOMPATIBLE BLOOD TRANSFUSION

Chills, fever and backache are followed by jaun-dice. Urobilinogen is present in the urine. Liver function tests give normal results. In severe cases free haemoglobin is detected in blood and urine. Diagnostic difficulties arise when a patient suffering from a disease that may be complicated by hepato-cellular failure or biliary obstruction becomes jaundiced soon after a blood transfusion.

References

1 Bond LR, Hatty SR, Horn MEC et al. Gallstones in sickle cell disease in the United Kingdom. Br. med. J. 1987; **295:** 234.
2 Chan TK, Todd D. Haemolysis complicating viral hepatitis in patients with glucose-6-phosphate de-hydrogenase deficiency. Br. med. J. 1975; **i:** 131.
3 Croom RD III, McMillan CW, Sheldon GF et al. Hereditary spherocytosis. Recent experience and current concepts of pathophysiology. Ann. Surg. 1986; **203:** 34.
4 Johnson FL, Look AT, Gockerman J et al. Bone-marrow transplantation in a patient with sickle-cell anemia. N. Engl. J. Med. 1984; **311:** 780.
5 Johnson CS, Omata M, Tong MJ et al. Liver involve-ment in sickle cell disease. Medicine 1985; **64:** 349.
6 Maddrey WC, Cukier JO, Maglalang AC et al. Hepatic bilirubin UDP-glucuronyl-transferase in patients with sickle cell anemia. Gastroenterology 1978; **74:** 193.
7 Middleton JP, Wolper JC. Hepatic biloma compli-cating sickle cell disease: a case report and review of the literature. Gastroenterology 1984; **86:** 743.
8 Omata M, Johnson CS, Tong M et al. Pathological spectrum of liver diseases in sickle cell disease. Dig. Dis. Sci. 1986; **31:** 247.
9 Schubert TT. Hepatobiliary system in sickle cell disease. Gastroenterology 1986; **90:** 2013.

The liver and diseases of the reticulo-endothelial system

The reticulo-endothelial system produces re-ticulin fibres and forms an endothelial lining for blood spaces (see Chapter 1). The com-ponents in the liver are the primitive reticulum cells in the portal tracts and sinusoidal walls which differentiate into the following.

Kupffer cells, which line the sinusoidal wall and are phagocytic. They are flat cells with large pale nuclei and abundant cytoplasm, sometimes extending into a star shape. Similar rounded macrophages are found in the portal spaces. Some differentiate into reticulin fibres which extend along the sinusoids and around the liver cords, giving them support. Under the electron microscope they show tube-like pro-cesses and have peroxidase activity.

Free, rounded *stem cells* in the sinusoidal wall and portal tracts. These are potential pre-cursors of the red and white blood series. Under the electron microscope these show pinocytic vesicles.

The *lymphoid tissue* of the liver which is located in the portal tracts.

Lipocytes (Ito cells) which are fat-storing cells in the sinusoids.

The cells are sources of serum immuno-globulins.

The reticulo-endothelial system in the liver is involved in the primary reticuloses, diseases with excessive demand for new blood, reticulo-endothelial storage diseases, fibrosis (where Ito cells are concerned) and chronic hepatitis and infectious diseases which excite a reticulo-endothelial reaction.

Primary reticuloses

The liver is involved to a variable extent. Liver biopsies are helpful for diagnosis. As involve-ment may be focal, serial sections should be cut and guided biopsy gives a higher percentage of positive results. Monoclonal studies on liver biopsies is used to determine the type of reticulosis.

Fulminant liver failure can complicate lymphoreticular malignancy [13], monoblastic hepatic infiltration [31], malignant histocytosis [7] or non-Hodgkin's lymphoma [9]. The extent of liver involvement may be mild compared with the severity of the clinical picture. Küppfer cell failure with endotoxaemia might be causative.

Multiple transfusions are a frequent cause of viral hepatitis, both non-A, non-B, and to a lesser extent B. This is usually mild in the immunocompromised host.

Patients with the myeloproliferative diseases, leukaemia or lymphoma may suffer gastro-intestinal haemorrhage. In some, this is due to peptic ulceration or gastro-intestinal erosions. In others, it is secondary to hepatic, portal or splenic vein thrombosis related to the coagulopathy. Occasionally, the portal hypertension is presinusoidal and seems to be secondary to infiltrative lesions in the portal zones and sinusoids. In others, increased flow due to splenomegaly may be important. If the wedged hepatic venous pressure is increased and the gradient with the intra-splenic pressure is normal, splenectomy may be indicated [28].

In systemic mastocytosis [12] and myeloid-metaplasia [34] new fibre formation in the sinusoids may contribute. Portal and centrizonal fibrosis can be related to cytotoxic therapy.

More aggressive chemotherapy has increased hepatotoxic drug reactions.

Hepatitis B may be reactivated.

Leukaemia

Myelogenous

The enlarged liver is smooth and firm, and the cut section shows small, pale nodules.

Microscopically (figs 4.4, 4.5) both tracts and sinusoids are infiltrated with immature and mature cells of the myeloid series. The immature cells lie outside the sinusoidal wall.

The portal tracts are enlarged, with myelocytes and polymorphs, both neutrophil and eosinophil; round cells are also conspicuous.

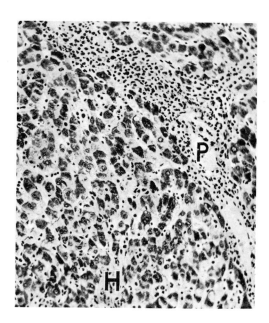

Fig. 4.4. Myelogenous leukaemia. Essential hepatic architecture is normal, but the sinusoids and a portal tract (P) contain increased numbers of cells of the myeloid series. H = hepatic venule. (Stained Best's carmine, ×70.)

The liver cell cords are compressed by the leukaemic deposits.

Lymphocytic

Macroscopically, the liver is moderately enlarged, with pale areas on section.

Microscopically (fig. 4.6) the leukaemic infiltration involves only the portal tracts, the normal sites of lymphoid tissue in the liver. They are enlarged and contain both mature and immature cells of the lymphatic series. The sinusoids are not affected. The liver cells are normal.

Hairy cell leukaemia

The liver is usually involved although specific clinical and biochemical features are rare. Sinusoidal and portal infiltration with mono-

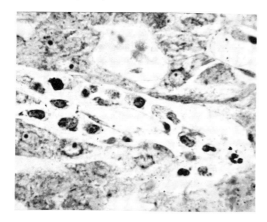

Fig. 4.5. Myelogenous leukaemia. Lining the sinusoid wall, but outside the endothelial lining, can be seen various cells of the myeloid and lymphocytic series. (Stained Leishman, ×350.)

nuclear 'clear' cells is seen with sinusoidal congestion and beading [42]. Angiomatous lesions, usually periportal, consist of blood spaces lined by hairy cells. Methacrylate embedded liver biopsy sections show tartrate-resistant acid phosphatase activity in the hairy cells [42].

BONE MARROW TRANSPLANTATION [30]

Chemotherapy and radiation following bone marrow transplant leads to veno-occlusive disease of the liver in about 20% [30]. Graft-versus-host disease can develop and even proceed to the picture of chronic intra-hepatic biliary obstruction (see Chapter 35) [25].

Opportunist infections are frequent following intensive chemotherapy or marrow transplant (see Chapter 27).

Prolonged chemotherapy with methotrexate and 6-mercapto-purine over many years has been associated with hepato-cellular carcinoma [17].

Lymphoma

Hepatic involvement occurs in about 70% and immediately puts the patient into grade IV [21]. Hepatic involvement may be seen as diffuse infiltrates, as focal tumour-like masses, as portal zone cellularity, as an epithelioid cell reaction or as lymphoid aggregates [12].

In *Hodgkin's disease*, typical tissue is seen spreading out from the portal tracts, with

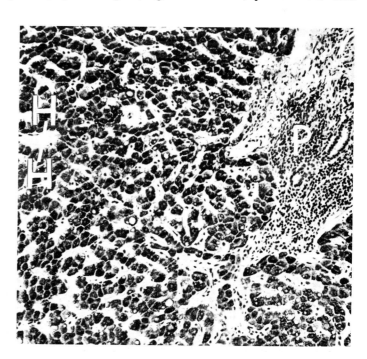

Fig. 4.6. Lymphocytic leukaemia. Essential hepatic architecture is normal, but a portal tract contains many cells of the lymphocyte series. The sinusoids are not affected. (Stained Best's carmine, ×70.)

lymphocytes, large pale epithelioid cells, eosinophils, plasma cells and giant cells of the Dorothy Reed type (fig. 4.7). Later, fibroblasts are found in a supporting connective tissue reticulum. Occasionally, only focal accumulations of Kupffer cells are seen. More usually, the picture is pleomorphic.

In *non-Hodgkin's lymphoma*, the portal zones are usually involved. In small lymphocytic lymphoma, a dense, monotonous proliferation of normal appearing lymphocytes are seen. The more aggressive lymphomas also involve portal zones and form large tumour nodules.

In *histocytic medullary reticulosis*, large numbers of reticulum cells fill the sinusoids and portal tracts. Occasionally, the deposits may be single and large.

Liver granulomas with or without hepatic involvement are found with most lymphomas [2].

Paraproteinaemia and amyloidosis may be complications.

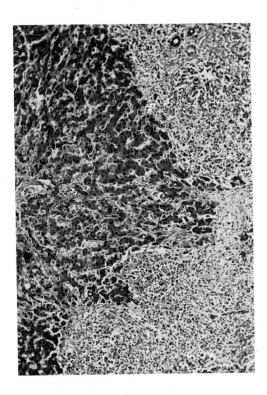

Fig. 4.7. Hodgkin's disease. The portal zones are infiltrated by Hodgkin's tissue. (Stained H & E, ×70.)

DIAGNOSIS OF HEPATIC INVOLVEMENT

Detection of hepatic involvement can be extremely difficult. It is unlikely if hepatomegaly is not found. Fever, jaundice and splenomegaly increase the likelihood. Increases in serum γ-GT and transaminase values are suggestive, although often non-specific [4].

Focal defects may be shown by ultrasound. CT scanning has the additional advantage of showing enlarged abdominal lymph nodes. Magnetic resonance is highly sensitive in detecting hepatic lymphoma by finding high Tl values [33].

Needle liver biopsy rarely reveals Hodgkin's tissue if the CT scan is normal. Laparotomy, peritoneoscopy, or directed ultrasound or CT liver biopsy add to the chances of obtaining Hodgkin's tissue. Needle biopsy does not exclude hepatic involvement if only an epithelioid histiocyte reaction is seen. Sinusoidal dilatation in zone 2 and 3 is found in 50% and may give a clue to the diagnosis [10].

Presentation as jaundice may provide great diagnostic difficulties (table 4.3) Lymphoma should always be considered in patients with jaundice, fever and weight loss.

JAUNDICE IN THE LYMPHOMAS (table 4.3) [8]

Hepatic infiltrates may be massive or present as space-occupying lesions. Large intra-hepatic deposits are the commonest cause of deep jaundice. Histological evidence is essential for diagnosis.

Biliary obstruction is more frequent with non-Hodgkin's lymphoma than with Hodgkin's disease. It is usually due to hilar glands which are less mobile than those along the common bile duct which can be pushed aside. Occasionally the obstructing glands are peri-ampullary. Diagnosis from other causes of extra-hepatic biliary obstruction is difficult and investigations may include percutaneous or endoscopic cholangiography.

Occasionally, a most obscure intra-hepatic, usually cholestatic, jaundice may be seen [27]. It is unrelated to deposits in liver or bile duct

Table 4.3. Jaundice in lymphoma

Related lymphoma	Notes
Hepatic infiltrates Massive Tumour-mass	Scans. Liver biopsy
Biliary obstruction	Usually hilar Investigate percutaneous or endoscopic cholangiography Non-Hodgkin's usually
Intra-hepatic cholestasis	Rare Liver biopsy 'pure' cholestasis Usually Hodgkin's
Haemolysis	Autoimmune haemolytic anaemia Positive Coombs' test

Related therapy	Notes
Chemotherapy	High dose can cause fulminant liver failure (See Chapter 18)
Hepatic irradiation	More than 3000 rads (See Chapter 18)
Post-transfusion (non-A, non-B hepatitis)	(See Chapter 16)
Hepatitis B reactivation	(See Chapter 16)
Opportunist infections	(See Chapter 27)

compression. Hepatic histology shows only canalicular stasis. It is unrelated to therapy. The diagnosis is extremely difficult; it is made by exclusion after fullest possible investigation.

Haemolysis rarely results in deep jaundice. It may be due to Coombs' positive autoimmune haemolytic anaemia. Jaundice is exacerbated by bilirubin overload following blood transfusion.

Chemotherapy may cause jaundice. Almost all the cytotoxic drugs can be incriminated if given in sufficient dose. Common culprits include methotrexate, 6-mercaptopurine, cytosine arabinoside, procarbazine and vincristine. A death has been reported in a patient given ABVD [23]. Hepatic irradiation in a dose usually exceeding 3500 rads may cause jaundice.

Post-transfusion viral hepatitis non-A, non-B, or B, may affect the immunocompromised patient. Opportunist infections are also encountered.

Primary hepatic lymphoma

This rare lymphoma affects only the liver [15]. Histologically it is of large cell type, a non-Hodgkin's lymphoma of B-cell origin. The prognosis is excellent. It has been reported in association with AIDS [11] suggesting an analogy with Burkitt's lymphoma and Epstein–Barr virus. It presents as predominant liver disease with marked hepatomegaly, but without lymphadenopathy [20], or as a large hepatic mass [3].

Treatment of hepatic involvement

More aggressive combination chemotherapy has considerably improved the prognosis of intra-hepatic Hodgkin's deposits causing jaundice. Treatment is the same as for other stage V patients regardless of the jaundice [8]. Similarly, those with 'idiopathic' cholestasis should receive the therapy appropriate for their lymphoma. If MOPP has failed ABVD should be tried. If jaundice is persistent, some palliation may be achieved by moderate local irradiation.

Extra-hepatic biliary obstruction is treated by external radiation and if necessary, the insertion of internal stents by the percutaneous or endoscopic route.

If drug toxicity is the cause, treatment may have to be changed or doses reduced.

Treatment for non-Hodgkin's lymphoma causing jaundice is the same as that for Hodgkin's disease.

Primary hepatic lymphoma is treated by chemotherapy or occasionally by lobectomy [35, 36].

Lymphosarcoma

Nodules of lymphosarcomatous tissue may be found in the liver, especially in the portal tracts. Macroscopically they resemble metastatic carcinoma. The liver may also be involved in giant follicular lymphoma.

Multiple myeloma

The liver may be involved in plasma cell myeloma, the portal tracts and sinusoids being filled with plasma cells. Associated amyloidosis may involve the hepatic arterioles.

Angio-immunoblastic lymphadenopathy

This resembles Hodgkin's disease. The liver shows a pleomorphic portal zone infiltrate (lymphocytes, plasma cells and blast cells) without histiocytes or Dorothy Reed cells [18].

Myeloid metaplasia

The primitive reticulum cells of hepatic sinusoids and portal tracts possess the potential capacity to mature into adult erythrocytes, leucocytes or platelets. If the stimulus to blood regeneration is sufficiently strong, this function can be resumed. This is rare in the adult although myeloid metaplasia in the liver of the anaemic infant is not unusual. In the adult, it occurs with bone marrow replacement or irritation, and especially in association with secondary carcinoma of bone, myelofibrosis, myelosclerosis, multiple myeloma, and the marble bone disease of Albers—Schoenberg. It complicates all conditions associated with a leucoerythroblastic anaemia.

The condition is well exemplified by myelofibrosis and myelosclerosis, where the liver is enlarged, with a smooth firm edge. The spleen is enormous, and its removal results in even greater enlargement of the liver [38].

Microscopic features

The conspicuous abnormality is a great increase in the cellular content, both in the portal tracts and in the distended sinusoids (fig. 4.8). The cells are of all types and varying maturity. Myeloblasts and myelocytes are prominent. There are many reticulum cells and these may

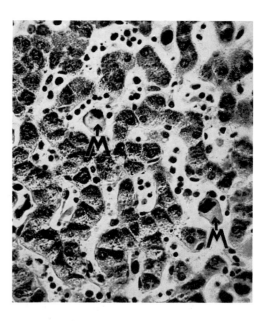

Fig. 4.8. Myeloid metaplasia secondary to bone marrow fibrosis. Giant cells resembling megakaryocytes (M), late erythroblasts, normoblasts and polymorphs are seen in the hepatic sinusoids. (Stained Best's carmine, ×300.)

be converted into giant cells. The haemopoietic tissue may form discrete foci in the sinusoids.

Peri-sinusoidal fibrosis may be a feature with collagen bundles in Dissë's space [34].

Electron microscopy shows haematological cells in the sinusoids with transformation of peri-sinusoidal cells into fibroblasts and myofibroblast-like cells.

Portal hypertension. This may be due to portal vein thrombosis or sinusoidal infiltration with haemopoieitic cells. Dissë space fibrosis contributes [14]. Nodular regenerative hyperplasia may also cause portal hypertension [14].

Systemic mastocytosis

This can present with hepatosplenomegaly [12]. Liver biopsy, stained with haematoxylin and eosin, shows peri-portal, polygonal cells with eosinophil granules. On staining with Giemsa and toluidine blue, the typical metachromatic cytoplasmic granules may be identified.

Lipoid storage diseases

The lipoidoses are disorders in which abnormal amounts of lipids are stored in the cells of the reticulo-endothelial system. They may be classified according to the lipid stored (table 4.4).

PRIMARY AND SECONDARY XANTHOMATOSIS

Cholesterol is stored mainly in the skin, tendon sheaths, bone and blood vessels. The liver is rarely involved but there may be isolated nests of cholesterol-containing foamy histiocytes in the liver. Investigation of the liver is of little diagnostic value.

Diffuse hepatic involvement may be seen in fatal childhood Letterer—Siwe's disease. In Hand—Schuller—Christian disease, multifocal eosinophil granulomas may sometimes be found. These rarely involve the common bile duct causing obstructive jaundice [24].

HISTIOCYTOSIS X

Granulomatous formation with infiltration and proliferation of histiocytes may be associated with marked hepatic sinusoidal dilatation in the absence of obstruction to major hepatic veins [16].

Cholestasis is due to sclerosing cholangitis. The intra-hepatic ducts are markedly distorted with a patent extra-hepatic biliary system [26]. Portal zones are fibrosed but usually without histiocytic infiltration.

CHOLESTERYL ESTER STORAGE DISEASE [5]

This rare, recessive, relatively benign disease is associated with acid cholesteryl ester hydrolase deficiency. It presents with symptomless hepato-splenomegaly. The liver is orange in colour and hepatocytes contain excess cholesteryl ester and neutral fat. A septate fibrosis is also present. The defect is in lysosomal acid lipase.

Gaucher's disease

This rare, familial disease affects mainly Ashkenazi Jews [13]. It is due to a deficiency of lysosomal β-glucocerebrosidase so that the substrate β-glucocerebroside accumulates in the reticulo-endothelial system throughout the body, particularly liver, bone marrow and spleen.

Three types are recognized:

Type 1 has a gene frequency of 1:2500. Sufferers lead a relatively normal life.

Type 2 is marked by hepato-splenomegaly and death in infancy.

Table 4.4. The lipid storage diseases

Disease	Storage material	Liver involvement in lipid storage
I Xanthomatosis	Cholesterol	
Primary essential		
Hyper-cholesterolaemic		Rare
Normo-cholesterolaemic		Rare
(Hand—Schuller—Christian)		
Secondary		
Essential hyperlipaemia		Rare
Diabetes mellitus		Rare
Obstructive jaundice		Rare
II Gaucher's disease	Cerebroside	Constant
III Niemann—Pick disease	Sphingomyelin (phospholipid)	Constant

Type 3 is a predominantly neurological disease of adults.

The various forms represent allelic disorders with different mutations in the structural gene for the glucocerebrosidase locus. This gene has now been cloned [6].

The characteristic Gaucher cell is approximately 70−80 μm in diameter, oval or polygonal in shape and with pale cytoplasm. It contains two or more peripherally placed hyperchromatic nuclei between which fibrils pass parallel to each other (fig. 4.9). It is quite different from the foamy cell of xanthomatosis or Niemann−Pick's disease.

Electron microscopy. The accumulated β-glucocerebroside formed from degraded cell membranes precipitates within the lysosomes and forms long (20−40 nm), rod-like tubules. These are then seen by light microscopy. A somewhat similar cell is seen in chronic myeloid leukaemia and in multiple myeloma due to increased turnover of β-glucocerebroside.

CHRONIC ADULT FORM (TYPE 1)

This is the common type. It is of variable severity and age of onset but usually commences insidiously before the age of 30 years. It is very chronic and may be recognized in quite old people. It is inherited as an autosomal recessive.

The mode of presentation is variable, with unexplained hepato-splenomegaly (especially in children), spontaneous bone fractures, or bone pain with fever. Alternatively there may be a bleeding diathesis, with non-specific anaemia.

The clinical features include pigmentation which may be generalized or a patchy, brownish tan. The lower legs may have a symmetrical pigmentation, leaden grey in colour and containing melanin. The eyes show yellow pingueculae (fig. 4.10).

The spleen is enormous and the liver is moderately enlarged, smooth and firm. Superficial lymph glands are not usually involved.

Portal hypertension may be associated with ascites and bleeding oesophageal varices [1].

Bone X-rays. The long bones, especially the lower ends of the femora, are expanded, so that the waist normally seen above the condyles disappears. The appearance has been likened to that of an Erlenmeyer flask or hock bottle.

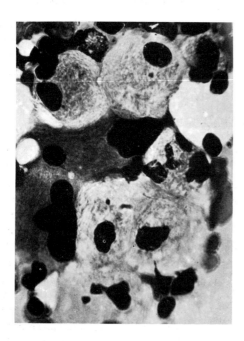

Fig. 4.9. Gaucher's disease. Smears of sternal marrow show large pale Gaucher cells with fibrillary cytoplasm and eccentric hyperchromatic nuclei. (Stained Leishman, ×600.)

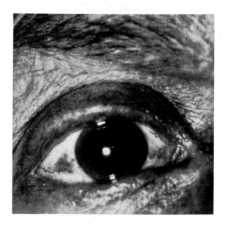

Fig. 4.10. Gaucher's disease. On either side of the pupil are wedge-shaped pingueculae consisting of yellow thickenings, fatty in appearance.

Sternal marrow shows the diagnostic Gaucher cells (fig. 4.9).

Aspiration liver biopsy should be performed if sternal puncture has yielded negative results. The liver is diffusely involved (fig. 4.11).

Peripheral blood changes. With diffuse bone marrow involvement, a leucoerythroblastic picture may be seen. Alternatively leucopenia and thrombocytopenia with prolonged bleeding time may be associated with only a moderate hypochromic microcytic anaemia [37].

Diagnosis may be made by measuring β-glucocerebrosidase in mixed mononuclear cells obtained from venous blood.

Blood biochemical changes. Serum alkaline phosphatase is usually increased, sometimes with a rise in transaminase [22]. Serum cholesterol is normal.

Treatment

There is no specific therapy. Splenectomy is indicated for the very large spleen causing abdominal discomfort, and occasionally for thrombocytopenia or an acquired haemolytic anaemia.

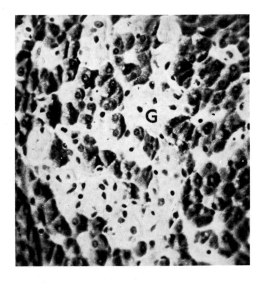

Fig. 4.11. Gaucher's disease. Liver sections show areas between the liver cell cords filled with large pale cells (G) with small dark nuclei. (Stained Best's carmine, ×250.)

Intravenous infusion of normal glucocerebrosidase, sometimes encapsulated in liposomes, leads to biochemical changes but not to clinical improvement.

Bone involvement may be improved by bone marrow transplantation [32] but the risks are difficult to justify in patients with type 1 disease. Somatic gene therapy is being explored.

Acute infantile Gaucher's disease

This acute form of the disease presents within the first six months of life and is usually fatal before two years. The child appears normal at birth. There is cerebral involvement, progressive cachexia and mental deterioration. The liver and spleen are enlarged and superficial lymph glands may also be palpable.

Autopsy shows Gaucher cells throughout the reticulo-endothelial system. They are, however, not found in the brain.

Niemann–Pick disease

This rare, familial disease, inherited as a recessive, mainly affects the Jewish race. The deficiency is in the enzyme sphingo-myelinase in the lysosomes of the reticulo-endothelial system. This results in the lysosomal storage of sphingomyelin. The liver and spleen are predominantly involved.

The characteristic cell is pale, ovoid or round, 20–40 μm in diameter. In the unfixed state it is loaded with granules; when fixed in fat solvents the granules are dissolved, giving a vacuolated and foamy appearance. There are usually only one or two nuclei. Electron microscopy shows lysosomes as laminated myelin-like figures. These contain the abnormal lipid.

Niemann–Pick disease occurs in infants, who die before the age of two years. The condition starts in the first three months, with anorexia, weight loss and retardation of growth. The liver and spleen enlarge, the skin becomes waxy and acquires a yellowish-brown coloration on exposed parts. The superficial lymph glands are enlarged. The patient is blind and deaf. In the terminal stages there is fever.

The fundus oculi may show a cherry-red spot at the macula.

Plain X-ray may show punctuate calcifications scattered throughout the liver and lung [41].

The peripheral blood shows a microcytic anaemia and in the later stages the foamy Niemann−Pick cell may be found.

The disease may present as *neonatal cholestatic jaundice* which remits. Inactive cirrhosis develops slowly. Progressive neurological deterioration appears in late childhood [40].

A further *type B* is associated with neonatal cholestasis which remits but later death occurs from cirrhosis.

Diagnosis is made by marrow puncture, which reveals characteristic Niemann−Pick cells or by finding a low level of sphingomyelinase in leucocytes.

Bone marrow transplant has been done for patients with early severe liver disease. Sphingomyelin disappears slowly from the liver but with a substantial reduction from the spleen and bone marrow [39].

SEA-BLUE HISTIOCYTE SYNDROME

This rare condition is characterized by histiocytes staining a sea-blue colour with Wright or Giemsa stain in bone marrow and in reticuloendothelial cells of the liver. The cells contain deposits of phosphosphingolipid and glucosphingolipid. Clinically the liver and spleen are enlarged. The prognosis is usually good although thrombocytopenia and hepatic cirrhosis have been reported. It probably represents adult Niemann−Pick disease [29] which can involve the liver.

References

1 Aderka D, Garfinkel D, Rothem A *et al.* Fatal bleeding from esophageal varices in a patient with Gaucher's disease. *Am. J. Gastroenterol.* 1982; **77**: 838.

2 Aderka D, Kraus M, Avidor I *et al.* Hodgkin's and non-Hodgkin's lymphomas masquerading as 'idiopathic' liver granulomas. *Am. J. Gastroenterol.* 1984; **79**: 642.

3 Aghai E, Quitt M, Lurie M *et al.* Primary hepatic lymphoma presenting as symptomatic immune thrombocytopenic purpura. *Cancer* 1987; **60**: 2308.

4 Bagleyk CM Jr, Roth JA, Thomas LB *et al.* Liver biopsy in Hodgkin's disease. Clinicopathologic correlations in 127 patients. *Ann. intern. Med.* 1972; **76**: 219.

5 Beaudet AL, Ferry GD, Nichols BL Jr *et al.* Cholesterol storage disease: clinical, biochemical and pathological studies. *J. Paediat.* 1977; **90**: 910.

6 Beaudet AL Gaucher's disease. *New Engl. J. Med.* 1987; **316**: 619.

7 Beaugrand M, Trinchet JC, Callard P *et al.* Malignant histocytosis presenting as a fulminant hepatic disease. *Gastroenterology* 1983; **84**: 447.

8 Birrer MJ, Young RC. Differential diagnosis of jaundice in lymphoma patients. *Sem. Liv. Dis.* 1987; **7**: 269.

9 Braude S, Gimson AES, Portmann B *et al.* Fulminant hepatic failure in non-Hodgkin's lymphoma. *Postgrad. med. J.* 1982; **58**: 301.

10 Bruguera M, Caballero T, Carreras E *et al.* Hepatic sinusoidal dilatation in Hodgkin's disease. *Liver* 1987; **7**: 76.

11 Caccamo D, Pervez NK, Marchevsky A. Primary lymphoma of the liver in the acquired immunodeficiency syndrome. *Arch. Path. Lab. Med.* 1986; **110**: 553.

12 Capron J-P, Lebrec C, Degott C *et al.* Portal hypertension in systemic mastocytosis. *Gastroenterology* 1978; **74**: 595.

13 Colby JV, LaBrecque DR. Lymphoreticular malignancy presenting as fulminant hepatic disease. *Gastroenterology* 1982; **82**: 339.

14 Degott C, Capron J-P, Bettan L *et al.* Myeloid metaplasia, perisinusoidal fibrosis, and nodular regenerative hyperplasia of the liver. *Liver* 1985; **5**: 276.

15 DeMent SH, Mann RB, Staal SP *et al.* Primary lymphomas of the liver. Report of six cases and review of the literature. *Am. J. clin. Path.* 1987; **88**: 255.

16 Fiorillo A, Migliorati R, Vajro P *et al.* Hepatic sinusoidal dilation in the course of histocytosis X. *J. pediatr. Gastroenterol. Nutr.* 1983; **2**: 332.

17 Fried M, Kalra J, Ilardi CF *et al.* Hepatocellular carcinoma in a longterm survivor of acute lymphocytic leukemia. *Cancer* 1987; **60**: 2548.

18 Frizzera G, Moran EM, Rappaport H. Angioimmunoblastic lymphadenopathy: diagnosis and clinical course. *Am. J. Med.* 1975; **59**: 803.

19 Gaucher E. De l'epithélioma primitif de la rate. *Thèse de Paris* 1882.

20 Gaulard P, Zafrani ES, Mavier P *et al.* Peripheral T-cell lymphoma presenting as predominant liver disease: a report of three cases. *Hepatology* 1986; **6**: 864.

21 Jaffe ES. Malignant lymphomas: pathology of hepatic involvement. *Semin. Liv. Dis.* 1987; **7**: 257.

22 James SP, Stromeyer FW, Chang C *et al*. Liver abnormalities in patients with Gaucher's disease. *Gastroenterology* 1981; **80**: 126.

23 Joensuu H, Söderström K-O, Nikkaen V. Fatal necrosis of the liver during ABVD chemotherapy for Hodgkin's disease. *Cancer* 1986; **58**: 1437.

24 Jones MB, Voet R, Pagani J *et al*. Multifocal eosinophilic granuloma involving the common bile duct: histologic and cholangiographic findings. *Gastroenterology* 1981; **80**: 384.

25 Knapp AB, Crawford JM, Rappaport JM *et al*. Cirrhosis as a consequence of graft-versus-host disease. *Gastroenterology* 1987; **92**: 513.

26 Leblanc A, Hadchouel M, Jehan P *et al*. Obstructive jaundice in children with histiocytosis X. *Gastroenterology* 1981; **80**: 134.

27 Lieberman DA. Intrahepatic cholestasis due to Hodgkin's disease. *J. clin. Gastroenterol.* 1986; **8**: 304.

28 Lindor K, Rakela J, Perrault J *et al*. Non-cirrhotic portal hypertension due to lymphoma. Reversal following splenectomy. *Dig. Dis. Sci.* 1987; **32**: 1056.

29 Long RG, Lake BD, Pettit JE *et al*. Adult Niemann–Pick disease: its relationship to the syndrome of the sea-blue histiocyte. *Am. J. Med.* 1977; **62**: 627.

30 McDonald GB, Sharma P, Matthews DE *et al*. Veno-occlusive disease of the liver after bone marrow transplantation: diagnosis, incidence, and predisposing factors. *Hepatology* 1984; **4**: 116.

31 Ondreyco SM, Kjeldsberg CR, Fineman RM, *et al*. Monoblastic transformation in chronic myelogenous leukemia: presentation with massive hepatic involvement. *Cancer* 1981; **48**: 957.

32 Rappaport JM, Ginns El. Bone-marrow transplantation in severe Gaucher's disease. *N. Engl. J. Med.* 1984; **311**: 84.

33 Richards MA, Webb JAW, Reznek RH *et al*. Detection of spread of malignant lymphoma to the liver by low field strength magnetic resonance imaging. *Br. Med. J.* 1986; **293**: 1126.

34 Roux D, Merlio JP, Quinton A *et al*. Agnogenic myeloid metaplasia, portal hypertension and sinusoidal abnormalities. *Gastroenterology* 1987; **92**: 1067.

35 Ryan J, Straus DJ, Lange C *et al*. Primary lymphoma of the liver. *Cancer* 1988; **61**: 370.

36 Ryoo JW, Manaligod JR, Walker MJ. Primary lymphoma of the liver. *J. Clin. Gastroenterol.* 1986; **8**: 308.

37 Sherlock SPV, Learmonth JR. Aneurysm of the splenic artery; with an account of an example complicating Gaucher's disease. *Br. J. Surg.* 1942; **30**: 151.

38 Towell BL, Levine SP. Massive hepatomegaly following splenectomy for myeloid metaplasia. Case report and review of the literature. *Am. J. Med.* 1987; **82**: 371.

39 Vellodi A, Hobbs JR, O'Donnell NM *et al*. Treatment of Niemann–Pick disease type B by allogeneic bone marrow transplantation. *Brit. Med. J.* 1987; **295**: 1375.

40 Wenger DA, Barth G, Githens JH. Nine cases of sphingomyelin lipidosis, a new variant in Spanish-American children. Juvenile variant of Niemann–Pick disease with foamy and sea-blue histiocytes. *Am. J. Dis. Child.* 1977; **131**: 955.

41 Wilson JAP, Raufman J-P. Case report: hepatic failure in adult Niemann–Pick disease. *Am. J. med. Sci.* 1986; **29**: 168.

42 Yam LT, Janckila AJ, Chan CH *et al*. Hepatic involvement in hairy cell leukemia. *Cancer* 1983; **51**: 1497.

5 · Ultrasound (US), Computerized Axial Tomography (CT) and Magnetic Resonance Imaging (MRI)

Radio-isotope scanning

The isotope may be taken up by the reticulo-endothelial system (e.g. ^{99m}technetium) or alternatively by the liver cells and excreted in the bile (e.g. ^{131}I Rose Bengal) [5].

^{99m}Technetium (^{99m}Tc) is a gamma emitter with a short half-life and gives a clear scan. Normal liver shows even activity and the scintiscan gives a good index of liver size and shape unless there are infiltrative lesions invading its borders. Primary or secondary tumours, cysts or abscesses larger than 2 cm appear as space-occupying lesions. Anterior lesions are more easily shown than posterior ones. Extrinsic lesions may be suggested, such as a subphrenic abscess.

Cirrhosis or any generalized hepato-cellular disorder such as viral hepatitis or alcoholic hepatitis is suggested by generalized decrease in uptake, an irregular pattern and uptake of isotope by the spleen and bone marrow (fig. 5.1). Metastases may produce a somewhat similar pattern, but without splenic uptake.

With severe hepato-cellular disease, the blood containing the isotope shunts past the reticulo-endothelial cells. In these circumstances, space-occupying lesions cannot be identified.

Obstruction to the hepatic veins may be shown by preferential uptake by the caudate lobe (fig. 11.10).

^{67}Gallium citrate accumulates in tissues that are actively synthesizing protein. Lesions such as cysts show as cold areas. Hepato-cellular cancer or liver abscess is cold with technetium but takes up gallium. The isotope is expensive, has to be specially obtained and has a relatively short half-life.

Radio-isotopic scanning has been largely

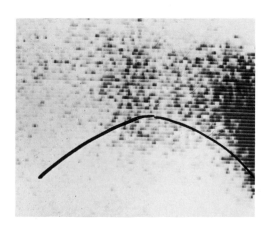

Fig. 5.1. In severe alcoholic hepatitis uptake of ^{99m}technetium by the liver may be negligible. Only splenic uptake is seen.

overtaken by other imaging methods superior for the detection of space-occupying lesions.

Single Photon Emission Computerized Tomography (SPECT)

Following an intravenous bolus of a suitable radio-pharmaceutical agent, serial axial scans allow computerized reconstruction of slices through the liver. By integrating the slices, liver volume and uptake per unit volume may be calculated. Small focal lesions may be detected with slightly more success than with ultrasound or CT. Kupffer cell function may be assessed by using an isotope, such as technetium, which is taken up by reticulo-endothelial cells and liver cell function is measured by using an isotope, such as ^{99}Tc HIDA, which is taken up by hepatocytes. The procedure demands complex apparatus and is not generally available.

Positron-Emission Tomography (PET)

This requires a cyclotron and is based on the principle that a positron emitted from a radio-active substance combines with an electron to form two photons travelling in opposite directions and that these can be localized by confidence detection. Positron-emitting radio elements include ^{15}O, ^{13}N and ^{11}C, and these can be used to study regional blood flow and metabolism. This technique has been largely applied to regional cerebral blood flow and only recently to the liver [15].

Biliary Scanning see Chapter 29

Ultrasound [12] (see also Chapter 29)

B-mode grey scale contact compound scanning is used in most imaging departments. The real-time linear probe technique has the advantage of a relatively inexpensive apparatus, ease in learning and taking only 3–5 minutes to perform. It can be used as an emergency and in routine out-patient clinics by residents who are not specialists in ultrasound. If necessary, the static B mode scan is used for confirmation; this shows lesions of 1 mm in diameter.

Ultrasound enables the consistency of lesions, whether cystic or solid, to be evaluated. However, it does demand experience and it is easy to over-interpret the appearances. Ultrasound scanning may fail with a high diaphragm, low ribs or excessive upper abdominal gas.

A normal ultrasound scan shows the liver to have mixed echogenicity. The portal vein, inferior vena cava and aorta are shown (fig. 5.2). The normal intra-hepatic bile ducts are thin, and run parallel to large portal vein branches. The right and left hepatic ducts are 1–3 mm in diameter and the proximal and distal extra-hepatic ducts range between 2 and 5 mm.

Ultrasonography is a screening investigation in patients with cholestasis and the gallbladder is an ideal organ for sonography.

The portal vein lies at the junction of the superior mesenteric and splenic veins, anterior to the vena cava and slightly to the left of it (fig. 5.2). An obstructed portal vein may be visualized or, alternatively, dilatation may be noted [16]. Ultrasound is a useful first investigation in a patient with bleeding oesophageal varices to determine patency of the portal vein. Patency of a portal–systemic shunt can also be confirmed.

In heart failure, a dilated hepatic vein and inferior vena cava can be observed (fig. 5.3). The hepatic artery is not well seen unless there is aneurysm formation.

Focal lesions are better visualized than diffuse. Under ideal circumstances, lesions down to 1 cm in diameter can be identified [13]. Appearances however are non-specific. Metastases may be well circumscribed, or infiltrative, dense, lucent or bulls-eye-like. The appearances are irrespective of the site of primary or of cell type. Necrotic neoplasms may mimic cysts.

Compared with CT, ultrasound never finishes the race first, and occasionally finishes last [17].

Needle biopsy under sonographic guidance is useful to clarify the nature of a focal lesion.

Ultrasound is a useful screening procedure for hepato-cellular cancer and may be used to follow therapy (fig. 5.4) (Chapter 28). Hepatic cysts or abscesses may be identified and drained under ultrasound guidance (fig. 5.5). Ultrasonography demonstrates ascites (fig. 5.3).

In children, ultrasound has the advantage that ionizing radiation is not given. Focal and diffuse hepato-cellular disease is recognized with only fair activity. Cirrhosis is suggested by dense reflective areas of irregular distribution and increased attenuation, but this is not a reliable method for diagnosing cirrhosis. Fatty change is shown by high levels of echoes with near-normal attenuation.

Echogenic masses may be discovered in an asymptomatic patient during an ultrasound examination. They are usually haemangiomas and these are confirmed by an enhanced (dynamic) CT scan [2, 3].

The use of biliary ultrasound is discussed in Chapter 29.

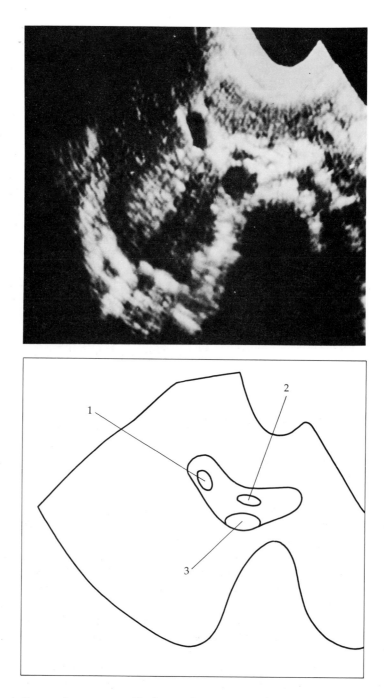

Fig. 5.2. Normal ultrasound appearances. The liver is shown as a large trans-sonic area. The portal vein (1), inferior vena cava (2) and aorta (3) are shown. The normal biliary system is not seen.

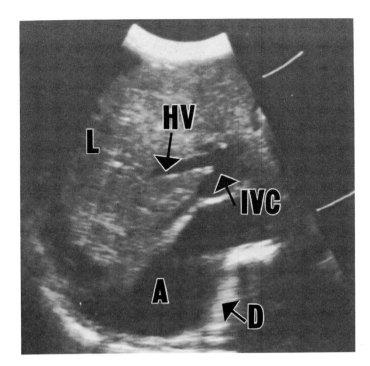

Fig. 5.3. Ultrasonography in congestive cardiac failure shows liver (L) with dilated hepatic vein (HV) and inferior vena cava (IVC). Ascites (A) and the diaphragm (D) are also shown.

Computerized axial tomography (CT scan) [7, 11, 17]

The liver is envisaged as a series of sequential, contiguous, cross-sectional images, each representing a slice of tissue of a specified thickness (fig. 5.6). Typically, 10–12 images are needed to examine the entire liver. A three-dimensional picture of a lesion is built up and can be related to other structures such as dilated ducts, veins in the porta hepatis or lesions in adjacent organs. Fourteen 'cuts' give a surface radiation of 3 rads.

The CT scan demonstrates detailed anatomy across the whole abdomen at the level of the slice (fig. 5.6). The identification of anatomical structures may be facilitated by giving oral contrast material to define the stomach and duodenum, or intravenous contrast enhancement to show blood vessels, kidneys or bile ducts. As with ultrasound, normal-sized bile ducts are not shown. The CT scan has an advantage over ultrasound in the obese and where bowel gas is excessive.

The shape of the liver and any nodules on the surface may be noted. Liver volume can be calculated by obtaining the area of each of ten cross-sectional images. This represents the area of a slice of tissue of a specific thickness. Multiplying the area by the slice thickness gives slice volume, and finally a sum of the values of the slices gives liver volume [8]. Mass is obtained by multiplying liver volume by liver density.

Much that has been described concerning ultrasound applies to CT scanning. In most instances however, apart from non-radio-opaque gallstones, CT scan has the edge (table 5.1). It is safe and the scans are easy to interpret.

CT gives good visualization of adjacent organs particularly kidneys, pancreas, spleen and retroperitoneal lymph nodes (fig. 5.7). Invasion of stomach, anterior abdominal wall and lung bases can be shown. The method is useful in surgical planning and in determining operability; radiotherapy can be planned. CT scanning is, however, more costly than ultrasound. CT scanning is a valuable aid in abdominal

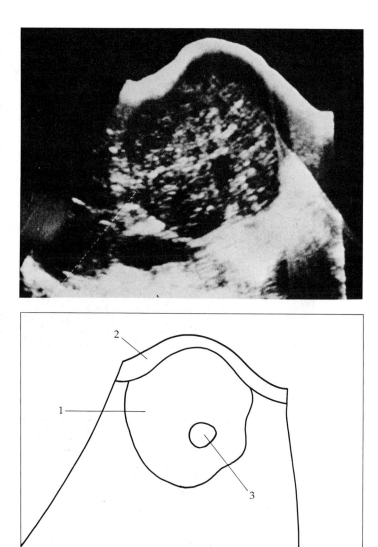

Fig. 5.4. Ultrasonography shows a large, round primary liver cancer (1) pushing out the anterior abdominal wall (2). A central necrotic cavity is seen.

trauma, the size of any laceration may be noted, and the extent of any haemoperitoneum (fig. 5.8) [19].

The use of CT scanning in cholestatic jaundice and in the investigation of the biliary system is discussed in Chapter 29.

CT scanning is the best initial screening procedure for space-occupying lesions. An abscess appears as a well-defined low attenuation mass with concentric walls. Cysts may be ident-

ified (fig. 5.9). Diagnosis is confirmed by aspiration at the time of the scan. Metastases and hepatocellular carcinomas are less dense than normal liver tissue and can usually be identified if 2 cm in diameter or more (fig. 5.10). Again, the lesion can be biopsied under direct CT guidance. The CT scan underestimates the size of a tumour compared with angiography. Enhancement, using intravenous contrast, is of value as normal liver tissue be-

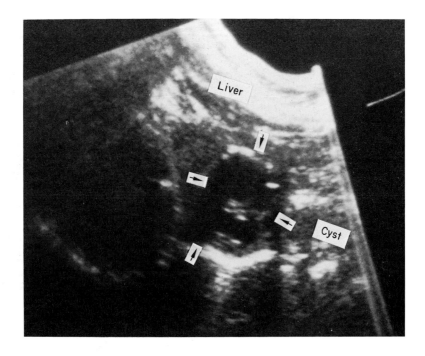

Fig. 5.5. Ultrasound shows multiple cysts in the liver.

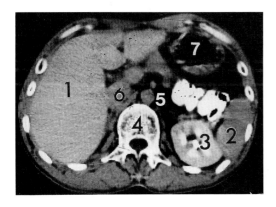

Fig. 5.6. CT scan (enhanced by contrast) showing liver (1), spleen (2), kidney (3), vertebral body (4), aorta (5), pancreas (6) and stomach (7).

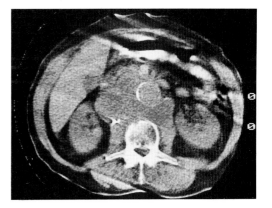

Fig. 5.7. CT scan showing enlarged retro-peritoneal nodes in a patient with Hodgkin's disease.

comes denser than neoplastic. The enhancement pattern is not typical of any particular tumour histology [3]. Infusion of contrast into the hepatic artery during CT scanning adds to the identification of tumour masses.

A haemangioma in the non-enhanced scan shows as a low density mass in the liver. With enhancement the mass fills with contrast from the periphery (fig. 5.11), and with later views it fills in completely becoming isodense with the liver.

Hepatic adenomas and focal nodular hyper-

Table 5.1. Imaging in hepato-biliary disease

	Isotope	Ultrasound	CT scan
Operator skill	Minimal	Great	Moderate
Interpretation	Easy	Complex	Straightforward
Anatomical detail	Fair	Good	Excellent
Localization and disease spread	Poor	Good	Excellent
Dilated bile ducts	No	Excellent	Excellent
Gallstones	Never directly shown	Excellent	Excellent
Acute cholecystitis	Very good*	Good	Fair
Patent biliary−enteric shunts	Very good*	No	Very good
Portal and hepatic veins	No	Good	Good
Patent portal−systemic shunts	No	Fair	Very good
Cysts	Fair	Very good	Excellent
Liver iron and fat	No	Fair	Excellent
Hepato-cellular disease	Good in later disease	Fair	Good
Calcification	No	Good	Excellent
Tumours (>2.5 cm)	Very good	Very good	Very good

* Biliary imaging

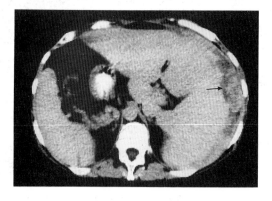

Fig. 5.8. CT scan (enhanced by contrast) in a patient with haemoperitoneum (arrowed) complicating liver biopsy.

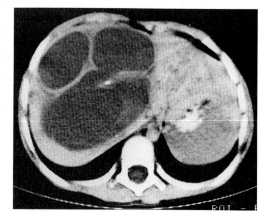

Fig. 5.9. CT scan (enhanced by contrast) showing simple cysts in the liver.

plasia can be missed by both CT and ultrasound because their density is similar to that of normal liver tissue.

CT is useful in diagnosing cirrhosis by showing the size and shape of the liver, any irregularity of the surface especially nodules, the presence of ascites and splenomegaly and of any complicating space-occupying lesion (figs 5.10, 5.12). CT is of particular value in suspected cirrhosis when clotting deficiencies preclude liver biopsy. The portal vein is demonstrated after contrast enhancement as a tubular structure in the hilum of the liver; the splenic vein is visualized at the same time. Portal systemic collaterals around the spleen or perioesophageal region are shown. A single, spontaneous large shunt may also be visualized adding weight to a diagnosis of portal−systemic encephalopathy (fig. 5.13).

In the Budd−Chiari syndrome an enlarged

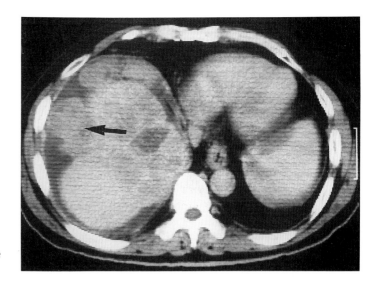

Fig. 5.10. CT scan in primary liver cancer in a cirrhotic liver shows multiple filling defects and rupture of the tumour through the peritoneum (arrow).

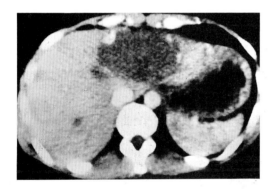

Fig. 5.11. Haemangioma. This is shown anteriorly. After contrast, pools of contrast are noted at its periphery and in delayed films the lesion is filled with contrast.

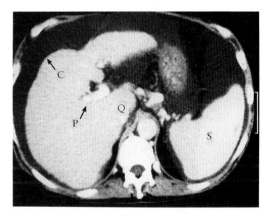

Fig. 5.12. CT enhanced with intravenous contrast in cirrhosis shows irregular surface of a small liver (C), patent portal vein (P), enlarged caudate lobe (Q), ascites (A), and splenomegaly (S).

caudate lobe may be seen with low attenuation frequencies representing regional sinusoidal stasis. There may be patchy enlargement with intravenous contrast. The hepatic vein is not visualized.

CT scanning is particularly valuable in detecting calcium, for instance fine calcification in colonic metastases, calcified glands or pancreatic calcification.

The fatty liver shows a lower radiological density than normal. Mono-energetic CT scan may be used to assess liver fat content in alcoholic subjects. Results agree with chemical and hepatic histological assessment of liver fat. The method may be useful in diagnosing fatty liver when liver biopsy is contraindicated.

Hepatic density, determined by CT, is increased in iron overload (fig. 5.14). The CT scan shows relatively low density branching portal veins highlighted against the higher density liver. Hepatic CT numbers normally vary between 35 and 65. A higher value accompanied by an increased serum ferritin level is diagnostic of increased iron stores. If dual (or tri) energy

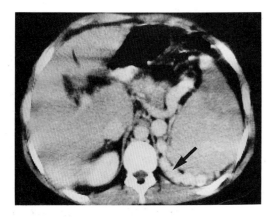

Fig. 5.13. CT enhanced with intravenous contrast in cirrhosis shows large retro-splenic portal-systemic collaterals (arrow).

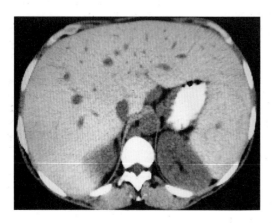

Fig. 5.14. Unenhanced CT scan of secondary haemosiderosis in thalassaemia major. The liver shows increased density greater than that of the kidney. Portal vein radicles are very prominent.

CT is available hepatic iron concentration may be measured. Unfortunately, this technique is not generally available. Liver copper usually has normal liver attenuation values on CT.

Magnetic resonance imaging (MRI) [1, 7, 14]

The technique is non-invasive and harmless. The apparatus is costly and its practical application to hepatology is not established. Physi-

ological motion (respiration especially) is a problem in causing image artefact.

The spin relaxation times (T_1 and T_2) depend on the characteristics of individual tissues. However, the increase tends to be non-specific in many conditions such as acute or chronic hepatitis or steatosis.

Inversion recovery scans (T_1-dependent) show hepatic vein, inferior vena cava, portal vein and bile ducts as dark structures against the much lighter liver parenchyma (fig. 5.15). The spleen appears darker than the liver. Dilated bile ducts are clearly visualized [6].

Steatosis is shown by a rather white liver with a normal parenchymal relaxation time. MRI does not add to the value of a CT scan but may be particularly useful in detecting metastases in a fatty liver.

Short T_1 values are seen in haemochromatosis, Wilson's disease and primary biliary cirrhosis and may be related to deposits of iron or copper. MRI may be useful in the distinction of these from other forms of cirrhosis. MRI may also be useful in portal hypertension in differentiating between hepato-fugal and hepato-pedal flow in the portal vein.

CT is generally believed preferable to MRI for the detection of hepatic metastases [9]. However, with appropriate techniques (PR-TE, T_1-weighted spin echo imaging) imaging time

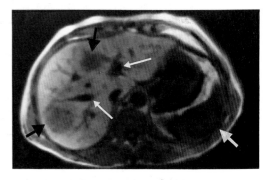

Fig. 5.15. NMR scan (T_1) of the liver in a patient with metastatic deposits. The deposits are well circumscribed and dark grey (black arrows). The bile ducts and portal veins are black (small white arrows). The spleen is also shown (large white arrow) (courtesy R.E. Steiner).

and motion artefacts are reduced and metastases more clearly shown [7].

Small cavernous haemangiomas over 1 cm in diameter are visualized as high intensity areas with spin-relaxation time (T_2) prolonged greater than 80 msec [10]. This contrasts with primary and secondary liver cancers where T_2 rarely exceeds 8 msec.

The application of MRI to hepatic metabolism has so far only been explored in experimental animals [4]. Contrast agents are also being developed . At present, the clinical hepatologist need not feel deprived if he does not have access to abdominal MRI. This view may change in the future with improved techniques.

Conclusions

Choice of a technique for hepato-biliary imaging depends on the availability of the appropriate apparatus, the interpreter and the problem which has to be solved (table 5.1).

In general, radionuclide (isotope) scanning is of particular value in screening for space-occupying lesions and for hepato-cellular disease. Weaknesses are the high false-positive or equivocal rate. Ultrasound is used to confirm and characterize equivocal isotope scan appearances.

CT scanning confirms isotope or ultrasound appearances and shows fatty liver, perihepatic abscess, porta hepatis masses and defines tumour extent. The main disadvantages are the cost and the small ionizing radiation involved. In more affluent centres it has become the primary procedure.

For the diagnosis of jaundice, ultrasound is the preferred screening investigation. If necessary this may be followed by CT scanning to help in the diagnosis of the cause of cholestasis and to show spread of disease.

For the diagnosis of gallstones, ultrasound is the primary method of choice. CT scanning is of little value in gallbladder disease.

HIDA scans provide a non-invasive method of determining bile duct patency in the presence of deep jaundice and for the diagnosis of acute cholecystitis.

References

1 Aisen AM, Martel W, Glazer GM *et al.* Hepatic imaging: positron emission tomography, digital angiography and nuclear magnetic resonance imaging. *Hepatology* 1983; **3**: 1024.

2 Bree RL, Schwab RE, Neiman HL. Solitary echogenic spot in the liver: is it diagnostic of a hemangioma? *Am. J. Roentgenol.* 1983; **140**: 41.

3 Burgener FA, Hamlin DJ. Contrast enhancement of focal hepatic lesions in CT: effect of size and histology. *Am. J. Roentgenol.* 1983; **140**: 297.

4 Cohen SM. Application of nuclear magnetic resonance to the study of liver physiology and disease. *Hepatology* 1983; **3**: 738.

5 Dooley J, Dick R, Viamonte M *et al.* (eds) *Imaging in Hepatobiliary Disease.* Blackwell Scientific Publications, Oxford 1987.

6 Dooms GC, Fisher MR, Higgins CB *et al.* MR imaging of the dilated biliary tract. *Radiology* 1986; **158**: 337.

7 Ferrucci JT. MR imaging of the liver. *Am. J. Roentgenol.* 1986; **147**: 1103.

8 Fritschy P, Robotti G, Schneckloth G *et al.* Measurement of liver volume by ultrasound and computed tomography. *J. clin. Ultrasound* 1983; **11**: 299.

9 Glazer GM, Aisen AM, Francis IR *et al.* Evaluation of focal hepatic masses: a comparative study of MRI and CT. *Gastrointestinal Radiol.* 1986; **11**: 263.

10 Itai Y, Ohtomo K, Furui S *et al.* Non-invasive diagnosis of small cavernous hemangioma of the liver. Advantage of MRI. *Am. J. Roentgenol.* 1985; **145**: 1195.

11 Moon KL, Federle MP. Computed tomography in hepatic trauma. *Am. J. Roentgenol.* 1983; **141**: 309.

12 Okuda K. Advances in hepatobiliary ultrasonography. *Hepatology* 1981; **1**: 662.

13 Shinagawa T, Ohto M, Kimura K *et al.* Diagnosis and clinical features of small hepatocellular carcinoma with emphasis on the utility of real-time ultrasonography: a study in 51 patients. *Gastroenterology* 1984; **86**: 495.

14 Steiner RE. State of the art: magnetic resonance imaging in liver disease. In *Imaging in Hepatobiliary Disease*, p.71, eds J.S. Dooley, R. Dick, M. Viamonte *et al.* Blackwell Scientific Publications, Oxford 1987.

15 Van Heertum RL, Brunetti JC, Yudd AP. Abdominal SPECT imaging. *Sem. nucl. Med.* 1987; **17**: 230.

16 Webb LJ, Berger LA, Sherlock S. Grey-scale ultrasonography of portal vein. *Lancet* 1977; **ii**: 675.

17 Zeman RK, Lee C, Stahl RS *et al.* Ultrasonography and hepatobiliary scintigraphy in the assessment of biliary-enteric anastomoses. *Radiology* 1982; **145**: 109.

6 · Hepato-cellular Failure

Hepato-cellular failure can complicate almost all forms of liver disease. It may follow virus hepatitis, or the cirrhoses, fatty liver of pregnancy, hepatitis due to drugs, overdose with drugs such as acetaminophen (paracetamol), ligation of the hepatic artery near the liver, or occlusion of the hepatic veins. The syndrome does not complicate portal venous occlusion alone. Circulatory failure, with hypotension, may precipitate liver failure, especially in the cirrhotic.

It may be terminal in chronic cholestasis, such as primary biliary cirrhosis or surgical cholestatic jaundice associated with malignant replacement of liver tissue or acute cholangitis. It should be diagnosed cautiously in a patient suffering from acute biliary obstruction, and certainly not until other possible complications have been excluded.

It might be questioned whether so many different conditions should be included under one heading. Although the clinical features may differ, the overall picture and treatment are similar, irrespective of the aetiology. Acute hepato-cellular failure (fulminant hepatic necrosis) poses special problems and will be considered in Chapter 8.

There is no constant hepatic pathology and in particular necrosis is not always seen. The syndrome is therefore a functional rather than an anatomical one. It comprises some or all of the following features.

General failure of health.
Jaundice.
Circulatory changes and cyanosis.
Fever.
Neurological changes (hepatic encephalopathy) (Chapters 7, 8).
Ascites (Chapter 9).
Changes in nitrogen metabolism.

Skin and endocrine changes.
Disordered blood coagulation (Chapter 4).

General failure of health

The most conspicuous feature is weakness and easy fatiguability. Loss of flesh can be related to difficulty in synthesizing tissue proteins. Anorexia and poor dietary habits add to the malnutrition.

Jaundice

Jaundice is largely due to failure of the liver cells to metabolize bilirubin, so it is some guide to the severity of liver cell failure.

In acute failure, due to such causes as virus hepatitis, jaundice parallels the extent of liver cell damage. This is not so evident in cirrhosis, where jaundice may be absent or mild. This is due to the balance achieved between hepatic necrosis and regeneration. When present it represents active hepato-cellular disease and indicates a bad prognosis. Diminished erythrocyte survival adds a haemolytic component to the jaundice.

Circulatory and pulmonary changes

HYPERKINETIC CIRCULATION

This is associated with all forms of hepato-cellular failure. It is shown by flushed extremities, bounding pulses and capillary pulsations. Peripheral blood flow is increased and this is due mainly to increased skin blood flow [19]. Splenic flow is increased [7]. Renal blood flow, and particularly renal cortical perfusion, is reduced [13]. Cardiac output is raised [14, 22] and this is evidenced by tachycardia,

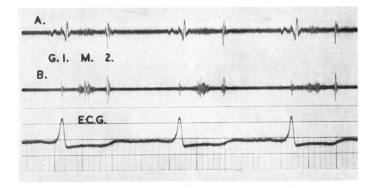

Fig. 6.1. Cirrhosis. Phonocardiogram at apex (A) and base (B) show ejection-type systolic murmur (M) and an auricular sound (presystolic gallop) (G) (Murray *et al.* 1958).

an active precordial impulse and frequently an ejection systolic murmur (figs 6.1, 6.2). These circulatory changes only rarely result in heart failure.

The blood pressure is low and, in the terminal days, further reduces kidney function. At this stage the impaired liver blood flow contributes to hepatic failure and the fall in cerebral blood flow adds to the mental changes [8]. Such hypotension is ominous and attempts at elevation by raising circulatory volume by blood transfusion or by such drugs as dopamine are of only temporary benefit (fig. 9.12) [7]

Liver cell failure is the major factor in causation. Although more common in patients with an extensive portal–collateral circulation, this is of secondary importance, for the cardiac output is raised in fulminant virus hepatitis without major collaterals and is normal in patients with extra-hepatic portal venous obstruction and a large collateral circulation [22].

Vasomotor tone is decreased as shown by reduced vasoconstriction in response to mental exercise, the Valsalva manoeuvre and tilting from horizontal to vertical (fig. 6.3) [18, 19]. The circulation resembles that found in systemic arteriovenous fistulae. It seems possible that large numbers of normally present, but functionally inactive, arteriovenous anastomoses have opened under the influence of a vasodilator substance. The diseased liver might produce such a vasodilator or fail to metabolize one formed elsewhere.

Ferritin is a candidate. Plasma vasoactive

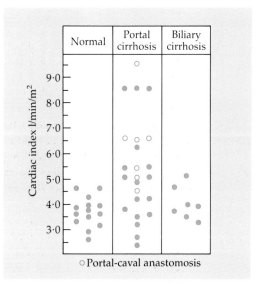

Fig. 6.2. The cardiac output is raised in many patients with hepatic cirrhosis but within normal limits in biliary cirrhosis. Mean normal cardiac index is 3.68 ± 0.60 l/min.$^{-1}$/m^{-2}. Mean in hepatic cirrhosis is 5.36 ± 1.98 l/min.$^{-1}$/m^{-2} (Murray *et al.* 1958).

intestinal peptide is increased but its role in the circulatory changes is uncertain [9].

The sympathetic nervous system is overactive in cirrhosis [1, 10]. This may be a response to blood volume expansion with consequent baroreceptor mediated modulation of sympathoadrenergic activity. This is particularly so with ascites (see chapter 9) but also before ascites develops [1]. These patients show loss of the circadian rhythm of urinary

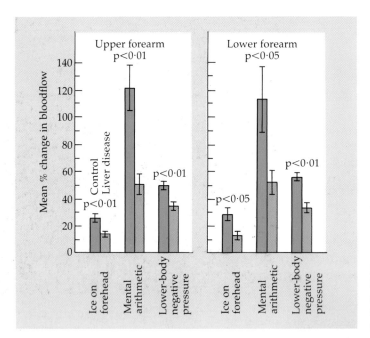

Fig. 6.3. Change in the forearm blood flow in response to autonomic stimuli in control subjects and patients with liver disease (Lunzer *et al.* 1975).

noradrenaline and of arterial blood pressure [1].

The portal circulation is also hyperdynamic with increased portal blood flow (see chapter 10). Again the nature of the portal vasodilator remains unknown.

LUNG CHANGES (HEPATO-PULMONARY SYNDROME)

About a third of patients with decompensated cirrhosis have reduced arterial oxygen saturation and are sometimes cyanosed [24]. This is probably due to intrapulmonary shunting through microscopic arteriovenous fistulae. Injection studies of the pulmonary artery in cirrhotic patients have shown a marked arterial dilatation in fine peripheral branches of the pulmonary artery both within the respiratory parts of the lung and on the pleura where spider naevi are sometimes seen (fig. 6.4) [2]. Rarely, actual pulmonary arterio-venous shunts have been demonstrated by pulmonary angiography including angioscintography (fig. 6.5) [32]. Cardiac catherization studies in one cyanosed patient with cirrhosis showed a right-to-left shunt with an arterial oxygen saturation

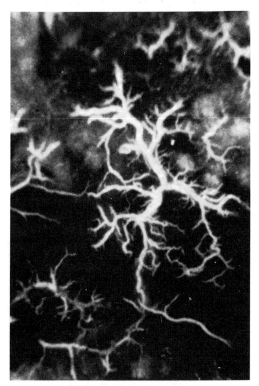

Fig. 6.4. Cirrhosis. Macroscopic appearances of the pleura showing dilated pleural vessels resembling a spider naevus (Berthelot *et al.* 1966).

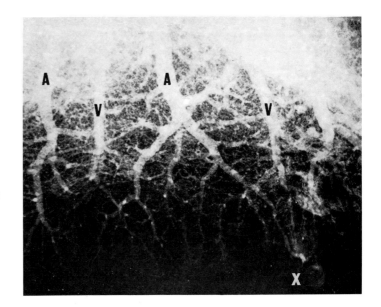

Fig. 6.5. Arteriogram from a patient with cirrhosis showing a slice of the basal region of the left lung. Arteries (A) and veins (V) alternate: X is the site of the arteriovenous shunting, into which a large arterial branch can be directly traced. The injection medium was barium suspension (Berthelot *et al.* 1966).

of 91% falling to 68% on exercise [12]. In another, the right-to-left shunt was estimated at 42% of the cardiac output [11]. Such shunts may be confirmed by infusions of micropaque gelatin into the pulmonary vascular tree at autopsy [4]. The picture at angiography is of a spongy appearance of the basal pulmonary vessels corresponding to the infiltrates seen on chest X-rays in patients with chronic liver disease [26].

Reduction of diffusing capacity is present without a restrictive ventilatory defect (31). This is likely to be due to dilatation of small pulmonary blood vessels, a complication both of advanced cirrhosis and fulminant hepatic failure [2, 29, 34]. A reduction in transfer factor is a consistent finding, perhaps related to thickening of the walls of the small veins and capillaries by a layer of collagen [29].

Lung perfusion studies by scanning or radionuclide methods show dilated pulmonary capillaries and/or arteriovenous communications [35].

The pulmonary vasodilatation is associated with a low pulmonary vascular resistance which fails to respond to hypoxia [5]. This also leads to failure of the lung to match perfusion with ventilation [6, 25]. Even in those who retain hypoxic pulmonary vasoconstriction, the pulmonary artery pressure is low in the face of hypoxia and a raised carbon dioxide.

Porto—pulmonary anastomoses have been demonstrated but are unlikely to contribute to arterial oxygen desaturation as the portal vein has a high oxygen content [27]. Moreover, the flow from them is probably small.

Finally, pulmonary function in cirrhotics may be reduced by a high diaphragm (secondary to hepatomegaly or massive ascites) a pleural effusion or the chronic lung disease of the heavy smoking alcoholic.

Finger clubbing is a frequent but not constant association of the cyanosis and increased cardiac index [30].

The most profound cyanosis and clubbing are associated with chronic active hepatitis and long-standing cirrhosis. Improvement in liver function is associated both with lessening of the cyanosis and the nodularity seen on the chest radiograph [30].

The pulmonary changes of hepato-cellular failure may be summed up as pulmonary vasodilatation with pulmonary arterio-venous shunting combined with ventilation—perfusion inequality (fig. 6.6, table 6.1) [15, 36]. The mechanisms remain uncertain. A pulmonary

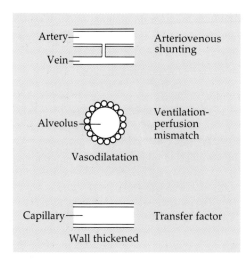

Fig. 6.6. Pulmonary changes in liver failure.

Table 6.1. Pulmonary changes complicating chronic hepato-cellular disease

Hypoxia
Intrapulmonary shunting
Ventilation—perfusion mismatch
Reduced transfer factor
Pleural effusion
Raised diaphragms
Basal atelectasis
Primary pulmonary hypertension
Porto—pulmonary shunting
Chest X-ray mottling

vasodilator is probably responsible but whether this is related to failure of production by the diseased liver or failure of metabolism is unknown. False sympathetic neurotransmitters, coming from the gut and bypassing the diseased liver, have been incriminated. However, although there is substantial sympathetic innervation in the pulmonary vasculature, endogenous noradrenaline has little effect on resting pulmonary vascular tone. Circulating false neurotransmitters would thus be unlikely to lower pulmonary artery pressures or to interfere with hypoxic pulmonary vasoconstriction [23]. Endotoxin inhibits pulmonary hypoxic vasoconstriction in the experimental animal [21].

84   The endogenous prostaglandins contribute

to the increased cardiac output and general diminished vascular resistence observed in cirrhosis [3]. There have been few studies of levels of possible vasodilator substances in cirrhotic patients with pulmonary changes. However, in two patients with cirrhosis and hypoxia due to pulmonary arterio-venous shunting, hormone levels (sex hormones, serotonin, prostaglandins and intestinal) were normal and treatment with oestrogens, CPD choline and indomethacin was ineffective [3].

PULMONARY HYPERTENSION

Primary pulmonary hypertension is a rare complication of cirrhosis [17]. It has been associated with severe hepato-cellular disease with or without a portal—systemic shunt. It can accompany extra-hepatic portal hypertension with portal—systemic shunting [4]. Histometric study of the muscular pulmonary arteries shows dilatation and thickening of the wall and, rarely, thrombi [20]. Plexogenic pulmonary arteriopathy, involving arteries 10 to 200 μm in diameter, and once thought to be diagnostic of pulmonary hypertension, has been found at autopsy in patients with cirrhosis [20].

Chest X-rays from patients with clinical pulmonary hypertension show dilatated pulmonary arteries [17]. The pulmonary hypertension may be part of the high cardiac output and general hyperdynamic circulatory state of cirrhosis. Diversion of splenic blood into the pulmonary circulation may contribute [17].

Pulmonary hypertension can also follow multiple tumour emboli to the pulmonary microvasculature in patients with hepatocellular carcinoma [34].

HYPOXAEMIA AND LIVER
TRANSPLANTATION

Hypoxaemia is considered a contra-indication to transplantation [16] because of the increased morbidity and mortality of the underlying pulmonary problems. However, after liver transplantation hypoxaemia should improve if it is attributable to ventilation—perfusion mismatch but not if it is due to fixed pulmonary vascular abnormalities [16]. Indeed, after hepatic transplantation, the intrapulmonary shunting and ventilation—perfusion mismatch (hepato—pulmonary syndrome) does reverse.

The mechanism of hypoxia must be carefully assessed in candidates for transplant. Measurement of oxygen saturation by oximetry alone is unsatisfactory because of interference by bilirubin pigments. Full arterial blood gasses are necessary. If a severe hypoxaemia is confirmed, echocardiography, radionucleotide scanning and pulmonary angiography should be done.

References

1 Bernardi M, Trevisani F, De Palma R *et al.* Chronobiological evaluation of sympathoadrenergic function in cirrhosis. Relationship with arterial pressure and heart rate. *Gastroenterology* 1987; **93**: 1178.

2 Berthelot P, Walker JG, Sherlock S *et al.* Arterial changes in the lungs in cirrhosis of the liver—lung spider nevi. *N. Engl. J. Med.* 1966; **274**: 291.

3 Bruix J, Bosch J, Kravetz D *et al.* Effects of prostaglandin inhibition on systemic and hepatic hemodynamics in patients with cirrhosis of the liver. *Gastroenterology* 1985; **88**: 430.

4 Cohen MD, Rubin LJ, Taylor WE *et al.* Primary pulmonary hypertension: an unusual case associated with extrahepatic portal hypertension. *Hepatology* 1983; **3**: 588.

5 Daoud FS, Reeves JT, Schaefer JW. Failure of hypoxic pulmonary vasoconstriction in patients with liver cirrhosis. *J. clin. Invest.* 1972; **51**: 1076.

6 Furukawa T, Hara N, Yasumoto K *et al.* Arterial hypoxemia in patients with hepatic cirrhosis. *Am. J. med. Sci.* 1984; **287**: 10.

7 Gitlin N, Grahame GR, Kreel L *et al.* Splenic blood flow and resistance in patients with cirrhosis before and after portacaval anastomoses. *Gastroenterology* 1970; **59**: 208.

8 Hecker R, Sherlock S. Electrolyte and circulatory changes in terminal liver failure. *Lancet* 1956; **ii**: 1121.

9 Henriksen JH, Staun-Olsen P, Fahrenkrug J *et al.* Vaso active intestinal polypeptide (VIP) in cirrhosis: arteriovenous extraction in different vascular beds. *Scand. J. Gastroenterol.* 1980; **15**: 787.

10 Henriksen JH, Ring-Larsen H, Kanstrup IL *et al.* Splanchnic and renal elimination and release of catecholamines in cirrhosis. Evidence of enhanced sympathetic nervous activity in patients with decompensated cirrhosis. *Gut* 1984; **25**: 1034.

11 Hutchison DCS, Sapru RP, Sumerling MD *et al.* Cirrhosis, cyanosis and polycythaemia: multiple pulmonary arteriovenous anastomoses. *Am. J. Med.* 1968; **45**: 139.

12 Karlish AJ, Marshall R, Reid L *et al.* Cyanosis with hepatic cirrhosis: a case with pulmonary arteriovenous shunting. *Thorax* 1967; **22**: 555.

13 Kew MC, Varma RR, Williams HS *et al.* Renal and intrarenal blood-flow in cirrhosis of the liver. *Lancet* 1971; **ii**: 504.

14 Kowalski HJ, Abelmann WH. The cardiac output at rest in Laennec's cirrhosis. *J. clin. Invest.* 1953; **32**: 1025.

15 Krowka MJ, Cortese DA. Pulmonary aspects of chronic liver disease and liver transplantation. *Mayo Clinic Proc.* 1985; **60**: 407.

16 Krowka MJ, Cortese DA. Severe hypoxemia associated with liver disease: Mayo Clinic experience and the experimental use of almitrine bismesylate. *Mayo Clinic Proc.* 1987; **62**: 164.

17 Lebrec D, Capron J-P, Dhumeaux D *et al.* Pulmonary hypertension complicating portal hypertension. *Am. Rev. respir. Dis.* 1979; **120**: 849.

18 Lunzer MR, Manghani KK, Newman SP *et al.* Impaired cardiovascular responsiveness in liver disease. *Lancet* 1975; **ii**: 382.

19 Lunzer MR, Newman SP, Sherlock S. Skeletal muscle blood flow and neurovascular reactivity in liver disease. *Gut* 1973; **14**: 354.

20 Matsubara O, Nakamura T, Uehara T *et al.* Histometrical investigation of the pulmonary artery in severe hepatic disease. *J. Pathol.* 1984; **143**: 31.

21 McDonnell PJ, Toye PA, Hutchins GM. Primary pulmonary hypertension and cirrhosis: are they related? *Am. Rev. respir. Dis.* 1983; **127**: 437.

22 Murray JF, Dawson AM, Sherlock S. Circulatory changes in chronic liver disease. *Am. J. Med.* 1958; **24**: 358.

23 Naeije R, Melot C, Hallemans R *et al.* Pulmonary hemodynamics in liver cirrhosis. *Semin. resp. Med.* 1985; **7**: 164.

24 Rodman T, Sobel M, Close HP. Arterial oxygen unsaturation and the ventilation perfusion defect of Laennec's cirrhosis. *N. Engl. J. Med.* 1960; **263**: 73.

25 Ruff F, Hughes JMB, Stanley N *et al.* Regional lung function in patients with hepatic cirrhosis. *J. clin. Invest.* 1971; **50**: 2403.

26 Sang Oh K, Bender TM, Bowen A *et al.* Plain radiographic, nuclear medicine and angiographic observations of hepatogenic pulmonary angiodysplasia. *Pediatr. Radiol.* 1983; **13**: 111.

27 Shaldon S, Caesar J, Chiandussi L *et al.* The demonstration of porta-pulmonary anastomoses in portal cirrhosis with the use of radioactive krypton (Kr[85]). *N. Engl. J. Med.* 1961; **265**: 410.

28 Sherlock S. The liver—lung interface. *Semin. Resp. Med.* 1988; **9**: 247.

29 Stanley NN, Williams AJ, Dewar CA *et al.* Hypoxia and hydrothoraces in a case of liver cirrhosis: correlation of physiological, radiographic, scintigraphic and pathological findings. *Thorax* 1977; **32:** 457.

30 Stanley NN, Woodgate DJ. The circulation, the lung, and finger clubbing in hepatic cirrhosis. *Br. Heart J.* 1971; **33:** 469.

31 Stanley NN, Woodgate DJ. Mottled chest radiograph and gas transfer defect in chronic liver disease. *Thorax* 1972; **27:** 315.

32 Vergnon JM, de Bonadona JF, Riffat J *et al.* Techniques d'exploration des shunts artério-veineux pulmonaires au cours des cirrhoses hépatiques. *Rev. Mal. Resp.* 1986; **3:** 145.

33 Willett IR, Sutherland RC, O'Rourke MF *et al.* Pulmonary hypertension complicating hepatocellular carcinoma. *Gastroenterology* 1984; **87:** 1180.

34 Williams A, Trewby P, Williams R *et al.* Structural alterations to the pulmonary circulation in fulminant hepatic failure. *Thorax* 1979; **34:** 447.

35 Wolfe JD, Tashkin DP, Holly FE *et al.* Hypoxemia of cirrhosis: detection of abnormal small pulmonary vascular channels by a quantitative radionuclide method. *Am. J. Med.* 1977; **63:** 746.

36 Yao EH, Kong BC, Hsue GL *et al.* Pulmonary function changes in cirrhosis of the liver. *Am. J. Gastroenterol.* 1987; **82:** 352.

Fever and septicaemia

About a third of patients with active, advanced cirrhosis show a continuous low-grade fever which rarely exceeds 38°C. The pyrexia is unaffected by antibiotics or by altering the protein content of the diet. It seems to be attributable to the liver disease alone. It is frequent in alcoholics.

Intercurrent infections, often with coliform organisms, are common. The human liver is bacteriologically sterile and the portal venous blood only rarely contains organisms. Such organisms could, however, reach the general circulation either by passing through a faulty hepatic filter or through portal—systemic collaterals [1]. Patients with cirrhosis have been shown to develop Gram-negative bacteraemia in this way. Positive blood cultures were found in 6.4% of cirrhotic patients (both biliary and non-biliary) [3]. The mortality of those with hepato-cellular disease was 59% and the organisms were frequently Gram-positive, especially pneumococci. This compared with 29%

of those with predominantly biliary disease in which infection was often with Gram-negative organisms.

Septicaemia is frequent in terminal hepato-cellular failure. Clinical features may be atypical with inconspicuous fever, no rigors and only slight leucocytosis. Spontaneous bacterial peritonitis may be a complication (Chapter 9) and also pneumococcal endocarditis and meningitis. These patients have often been receiving previous corticosteroid or neomycin therapy.

Bacterial infections are frequently found in patients with hepato-cellular failure [8]. Multiple factors contribute to this 'spontaneous' bacteraemia. Organisms which cause serious infections must first be coated (opsonized) with complement and/or IgG before they can be engulfed and killed by phagocytic cells. Complement deficiency in liver disease predisposes to bacterial infection [2]. Neutrophil phagocytosis and intracellular killing of organisms is defective in alcoholic cirrhosis and hepatitis [5]. Reticulo-endothelial function is defective with impaired ability to clear the blood of particles [6]. This is particularly true of advanced cirrhosis. Cirrhotic rats inoculated with pneumococci have more frequent bacteraemia, more prolonged antigenaemia and greater mortality than normal rats [4]. These factors contribute to febrile, blood culture-positive episodes and are particularly important in causing spontaneous bacterial peritonitis in patients with ascites where recurrence is very common (69%) and frequently fatal (31%) (see Chapter 9) [7]. In patients with cirrhosis, prophylactic antibiotics must be given during invasive practical procedures. Parenteral broad-spectrum antibiotics should be commenced when infection is suspected.

References

1 Caroli J, Platteborse R. Septicémie porto-cave. Cirrhosis du foie et septicémie a colibacille. *Sem. Hôp. Paris* 1958; **34:** 472.

2 Fox RA, Dudley FJ, Sherlock S. The serum concentration of the third component of complement β_{1C}/β_{1A} in liver disease. *Gut* 1971; **12:** 574.

3 Jones EA, Crowley N, Sherlock S. Bacteraemia in association with hepato-cellular and hepatobiliary disease. *Postgrad. med. J.* 1967; **43**: suppl. 7–11.

4 Mellencamp MA, Preheim LC. Effect of cirrhosis on bacteriemia and capsular antigenemia during experimental pneumococcal pneumonia. *Proc. 26th Interscience Conference on Antimicrobial Agents and Chemotherapy.* 1986; p. 283 (Abstract).

5 Rajkovic IA, Williams R. Abnormalities of neutrophil phagocytosis, intracellular killing, and metabolic activity in alcoholic cirrhosis and hepatitis. *Hepatology* 1986; **6**: 252.

6 Rimola A, Soto R, Bory F *et al.* Reticuloendothelial system phagocytic activity in cirrhosis and its relation to bacterial infections and prognosis. *Hepatology* 1984; **4**: 53.

7 Tito L, Rimola A, Gines P *et al.* Recurrence of spontaneous bacterial peritonitis in cirrhosis: frequency and predictive factors. *Hepatology* 1988; **8**: 27.

8 Wyke RJ. Problems of bacterial infection in patients with liver disease. *Gut* 1987; **28**: 623.

Fetor hepaticus

This is a sweetish, slightly faecal smell of the breath which has been likened to that of a freshly opened corpse, or mice. It complicates severe hepato-cellular disease and especially with an extensive collateral circulation. It is presumably of intestinal origin, for it becomes less intense after defaecation or when the gut flora is changed by wide-spectrum antibiotics. Methyl mercaptan has been found in the urine of a patient with hepatic coma who exhibited fetor hepaticus [1]. This substance can be exhaled in the breath and might be derived from methionine, the normal demethylating processes being inhibited by liver damage.

In patients with acute liver disease, fetor hepaticus, particularly if so extreme that it pervades the room, is a bad omen and often precedes coma. It is very frequent in patients with an extensive portal collateral circulation, when it is not such a grave sign. Fetor may be a useful diagnostic sign in patients seen for the first time in coma.

Reference

1 Challenger F, Walshe JM. Fœtor hepaticus. *Lancet* 1955; **i**: 1239.

Changes in nitrogen metabolism

Ammonia metabolism (Chapter 9). The failing liver is unable to convert ammonia to urea.

Urea production is impaired, but the reserve powers of synthesis are so great that the blood urea concentration in hepato-cellular failure is usually normal. Low values may be found in fulminant hepatitis. Maximal rate of urea synthesis is a good measure of hepato-cellular function, but is too complicated for routine use [3].

Amino acid metabolism. An almost constant excess is present in the urine [4]. In both acute and chronic liver disease a common pattern of plasma amino acids is found. The aromatic amino acids, tyrosine and phenylalanine, are raised together with methionine. The concentration of the three branched-chain amino acids, valine, isoleucine and leucine, is reduced [2]. This results in a lowering of the ratio of branched-chain to aromatic amino acids and this is irrespective of the presence or absence of hepatic encephalopathy (fig. 2.9) [1].

Serum albumin level falls in proportion to the degree of hepato-cellular failure and its duration. The protein is absorbed and retained, but is not used for serum protein manufacture. The low serum protein values may also reflect an increased plasma volume.

Plasma prothrombin falls with the serum protein levels. The consequent prolonged prothrombin time is not restored to normal by vitamin K therapy. Other proteins concerned in blood clotting may be deficient (fig. 4.0). In terminal liver failure the bleeding diathesis may be so profound that the patient is exsanguinated by such simple procedures as a paracentesis abdominis (see Chapter 4).

References

1 Morgan MY, Milsom JP, Sherlock S. Plasma ratio of valine, leucine and isoleucine to phenylalanine and tyrosine in liver disease, *Gut* 1978; **19**: 1068.

2 Morgan MY, Milsom JP, Sherlock S. Plasma amino acid patterns in liver disease. *Gut* 1982; **23**: 362.

3 Rudman D, Di Fulco TJ, Galambos JT. *et al.* Maximal rates of excretion and synthesis of urea in normal and cirrhotic subjects. *J. clin. Invest.* 1973; **52**: 2241.

4 Walshe JM. Disturbances of amino-acid metabolism following liver injury. *Q.J. Med.* 1953; **22**: 483.

Skin changes

An older Miss Muffett
Decided to rough it
And lived upon whisky and gin.
Red hands and a spider
Developed outside her—
Such are the wages of sin. [5]

Vascular spiders [5, 16, 18]

Synonyms: arterial spider, spider telangiectasis,
spider angioma

Arterial spiders are found in the vascular territory of the superior vena cava and very rarely below a line joining the nipples. Common sites are the necklace area, the face, forearms and dorsum of the hand (fig 6.7). They are rarely found in the mucous membrane of the nose, mouth and pharynx. They fade after death.

An arterial spider is so-called because it consists of a central arteriole, radiating from which are numerous small vessels resembling a spider's legs (fig. 6.8). It ranges in size from a pinhead to 0.5 cm in diameter. When sufficiently large it can be seen or felt to pulsate,

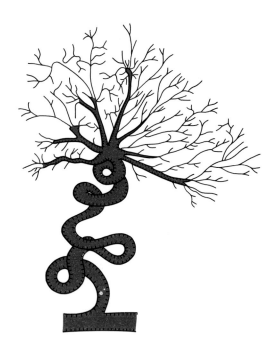

Fig. 6.8. Schematic diagram of an arterial spider (Bean 1953).

and this effect is enhanced by pressing on it with a glass slide. Pressure on the central prominence with a pinhead causes blanching of the whole lesion, as would be expected from an arterial lesion.

Arterial spiders may disappear with im-

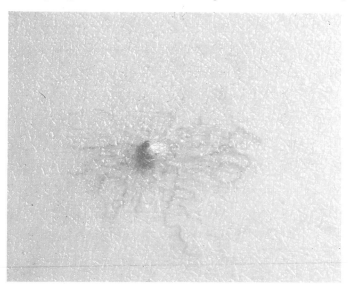

Fig. 6.7. A vascular spider. Note the elevated centre and radiating branches.

proving hepatic function, whereas the appearance of fresh spiders is suggestive of progression of liver damage. The spider may also disappear if the blood pressure falls due to shock or haemorrhage. Spiders can bleed profusely.

In association with vascular spiders, and having a similar distribution, numerous small vessels may be scattered in random fashion through the skin, usually on the upper arms. These resemble the silk threads in United States dollar bills and the condition is called *paper money skin*.

A further association is the appearance of *white spots* on arms and buttocks on cooling the skin [17]. Examination with a lens shows that the centre of each spot represents the beginnings of a spider.

Vascular spiders are most frequently associated with cirrhosis, especially of the alcoholic. They may appear transiently with viral hepatitis. Rarely they are found in normal persons, especially children. During pregnancy, they appear between the second and fifth months, disappearing within two months of delivery. A few spiders should not be sufficient to diagnose liver disease, but many new ones, with increasing size of old ones, arouse suspicion.

DIFFERENTIAL DIAGNOSIS

Hereditary haemorrhagic telangiectasis. The lesions are usually on the upper body. Mucosal ones are common inside the nose, on the tongue, lips, palate, in the pharynx, oesophagus and stomach. The nail beds, palmar surfaces and fingers are frequently involved. Visceral angiography usually shows lesions elsewhere.

The telangiectasis is punctiform, flat or a little elevated, with sharp margins. It is connected with a single vessel, or with several, which makes it resemble the vascular spider. Pulsation is difficult to demonstrate.

The lesion is a thinning of the telangiectatic vessel but the veins show muscular hypertrophy [18].

Telangiectasia may be associated with cir-

rhosis. Calcinosis, Raynaud's phenomenon, sclerodactyly and telangiectasia (*CRST syndrome*) may be found in patients with primary biliary cirrhosis.

Campbell de Morgan's spots are very common, increasing in size and number with age. They are bright red, flat or slightly elevated and occur especially on the front of the chest and the abdomen.

The venous star is found with elevation of venous pressure. It usually overlies the main tributary to a vein of large size. It is 2–3 cm in diameter and is not obliterated by pressure; the blood flow is from the periphery to the central collecting vein (opposite to that of the vascular spider). Venous stars are seen on the dorsum of the foot, legs, back and on the lower border of the ribs.

Palmar erythema (liver palms)

The hands are warm and the palms bright red in colour, especially the hypothenar and thenar eminences and pulps of the fingers (fig. 6.9). Islets of erythema may be found at the bases of the fingers. The soles of the feet may be similarly affected. The mottling blanches on pressure and the colour rapidly returns. When a glass slide is pressed on the palm it flushes synchronously with the pulse rate. The patient may complain of throbbing, tingling palms.

Palmar erythema is not so frequently seen in cirrhosis as are vascular spiders. Although both may be present, they may appear independently, making it difficult to define a common aetiology. Many normal people have *familial palmar flushing*, unassociated with liver disease.

A similar appearance may be seen in prolonged rheumatoid arthritis and in *pregnancy*, with chronic febrile diseases, with chronic leukaemia and with thyrotoxicosis.

Unilateral naevoid telangiectasia

This is a very rare accompaniment of chronic liver disease which is probably related to hereditary telangiectasia [7].

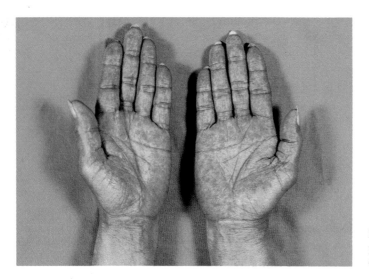

Fig. 6.9. Palmar erythema ('liver palms') in a patient with hepatic cirrhosis.

White nails

White nails, due to opacity of the nail bed, were found in 82 of 100 patients with cirrhosis and occasionally in certain other conditions (fig. 6.10) [16]. A pink zone is seen at the tip of the nail and in a severe example the lunula cannot be distinguished. The lesions are bilateral, thumb and index being especially involved.

Mechanism of the skin changes

The selective distribution of vascular spiders is not understood. Exposure of upper parts of the body to the elements may damage the skin so that it becomes susceptible to the development of spiders when the appropriate internal stimulus exists. Children may develop the lesion on the knees and one nudist with cirrhosis was said to be covered with vascular spiders. The number of arterial spiders does not correlate with the hyperdynamic circulation, although when the cardiac output is very high the spiders pulsate particularly vigorously.

The vascular spiders and palmar erythema have been traditionally attributed to oestrogen excess. They are also seen in pregnancy when circulating oestrogens are increased. Oes-

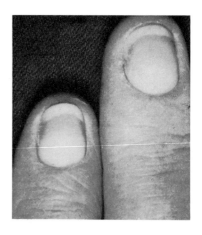

Fig. 6.10. White nails in a patient with hepatic cirrhosis.

trogens have an enlarging, dilating effect on the spiral arterioles of the endometrium, and such a mechanism may explain the closely similar cutaneous spiders [5]. Oestrogens have induced cutaneous spiders in man [5] although this is not usual when such therapy is given for prostatic carcinoma. The liver certainly inactivates oestrogens. However, spider naevi and palmar erythema appear and disappear irrespective of changes in plasma oestradiol.

The aetiology of the other skin lesions remains unknown.

Endocrine changes

Endocrine changes may be found in association with chronic hepato-cellular failure (cirrhosis). They are more common in cirrhosis of the alcoholic and if the patient is in the active, reproductive phase of life. In the male, the changes are towards feminization. In the female the changes are less and are towards masculinization or gonadal atrophy. Very few studies have been made in females.

Hypogonadism

Diminished libido and potency are frequent in men with active cirrhosis and a large number are sterile. The impotence and its severity are greater if the cirrhotic patient is alcoholic [8]. Patients with well-compensated disease may have large families.

The testes are soft and small. Seminal fluid is abnormal in some.

Secondary sexual hair is lost and men shave less often. Prostatic hypertrophy has a lower incidence in men with cirrhosis [6]. Incidence of metaplasia of the prostatic glandular and ductal epithelium is increased.

In the female, gonadal changes are not conspicuous for the patients are usually post-menopausal and any breast or uterine atrophy is of little significance. In younger patients, libido is lowered and the patient is usually infertile; menstruation is erratic, diminished or absent but rarely excessive. The breasts usually atrophy, although an occasional patient develops cystic hyperplasia. The uterus is atrophic.

Feminization

Gynaecomastia, sometimes unilateral, occasionally complicates cirrhosis usually in alcoholics (fig. 6.11), but also in young men with chronic active hepatitis. The breasts may be tender. It is caused by hyperplasia of the glandular elements [6].

Spironolactone therapy is the commonest cause of gynaecomastia in cirrhotic patients. This decreases serum testosterone levels and reduces hepatic androgen receptor activity [10].

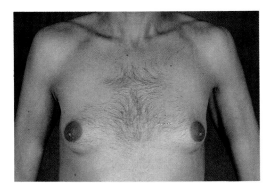

Fig. 6.11. Gynaecomastia in a patient with cirrhosis.

Other signs include female body habitus and a female escutcheon. The changes of feminization are particularly common in alcoholics.

RELATION TO ALCOHOL

It is difficult to disentangle the hypothalamic-pituitary-gonadal dysfunction in patients with chronic liver disease from the aetiology of the liver disease and particularly from the effects of alcohol [11].

Feminization is more frequent with alcoholic cirrhosis than with other types. Acute administration of alcohol to normal men increases the hepatic metabolism of testosterone.

The hepatic uptake of sex steroids depends on liver function. Chronic administration of alcohol raises serum hormone binding globulin (SHBG) so reducing the free fraction of plasma testosterone and the amount presented to the liver [12]. However, low dehydroepiandosterone with raised oestradiol and androstenedione are found in patients with non-alcoholic liver disease [3]. The direct effect of alcohol on the testes may add to the general effects of liver disease. Acutely, alcohol also raises plasma gonadotrophins. Impotence and its severity are greater if the cirrhotic patient is alcoholic [8].

MECHANISM

The three principal unconjugated oestrogens (oestrone, oestradiol and oestriol) are found in the plasma of normal men. They are produced by the testes and adrenals and also from peripheral conversion of major circulating androgens. Oestradiol is the most biologically potent oestrogen. It is bound to SHBG and to albumin. The biologically active unbound form has been reported as marginally raised in patients with cirrhosis [1]. The total is only minimally raised. Levels of oestrone—the precursor of oestradiol but only weakly feminizing—and oestriol, which is also biologically relatively inactive, are increased in cirrhotic patients. The increase in plasma oestrogens is insufficient to account for the degree of feminization. The human liver has both androgen and oestrogen receptors which render it sensitive to androgens and oestrogens [21]. In cirrhosis, the end organ sensitivities to sex hormones may be changed [9]. Hepatic androgen receptors fall and hepatic oestrogen receptor concentrations increase [21, 22]. Alcohol may play a part, for the liver of a male rat with chronic alcohol ingestion shows a decrease in androgen receptor sites [9].

Primary liver cancer occasionally presents with feminization [14]. Serum oestrone levels are high and can return to normal when the tumour is removed. The tumour can be shown to function as trophoblastic tissue.

Hypothalamic—pituitary function

Plasma gonadotrophins are usually normal although a minority of cirrhotic patients have high values. These normal levels in spite of testicular failure suggest either a primary testicular defect or a failure of the pituitary—hypothalamus. Impaired release of luteinizing hormone suggests a possible hypothalamic defect, at least in those with alcoholic liver disease [2].

Basal plasma prolactin levels are generally normal or occasionally raised [19]. It is unlikely that prolactin plays any role in the feminization of liver disease.

Metabolism of hormones [13]

A reduced rate of hormonal metabolism might be related to a decrease in hepatic blood flow, to shunting of blood through or around the liver or to an increase in plasma protein binding globulin (SHBG) which would reduce the free diffusible fraction of circulating hormone [12].

Steroid hormones are made more polar by conjugation in the liver. Derivatives of oestrogens, cortisol and testosterone are conjugated as a glucuronide or sulphate and so excreted in the bile or urine. There seems to be little difficulty in the process even in the presence of hepato-cellular disease. The conjugated hormones excreted in the bile undergo an enterohepatic circulation. In cholestasis the biliary excretion of oestrogens and especially of polar conjugates is greatly reduced. There are changes in the urinary pattern of excretion. Any failure of hormone metabolism results in a rise in blood hormone levels. This alters the normal homeostatic balance between secretion rates of hormones and their utilization. These feedback mechanisms between plasma hormone levels and hormone secretion prevent any but temporary rises in circulating levels. This may explain some of the difficulty in relating plasma hormone levels to clinical features.

Testosterone is converted to a more potent metabolite—dihydrotestosterone. It is degraded in the liver and conjugated for urinary excretion as 17-oxysteroids. Microsomes from cirrhotic animals show an impaired activity of the individual P^{450} concerned with testosterone 17 α-hydroxylation [20].

Oestrogens are metabolized and conjugated for excretion in urine or bile.

Cortisol in degraded primarily in the liver by a ring reduction to tetrahydrocortisone and subsequently conjugated with glucuronic acid (fig. 6.12).

Prednisone is converted to prednisolone.

The liver extracts aldosterone from the blood and converts it to tetrahydroaldosterone [15].

References

1 Baker HWG, Burger HG, De Kretser DM et al. A study of the endocrine manifestations of hepatic cirrhosis. Q. J. Med. 1976; 45: 145.

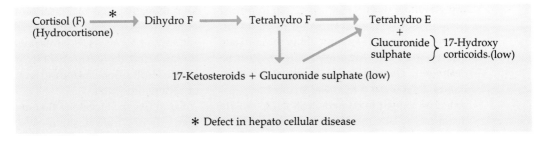

Cortisol (F) $\overset{*}{\longrightarrow}$ Dihydro F $\longrightarrow$ Tetrahydro F $\longrightarrow$ Tetrahydro E
(Hydrocortisone)   +
                                                                         Glucuronide $\Big\}$ 17-Hydroxy
                                                                         sulphate corticoids.(low)

17-Ketosteroids + Glucuronide sulphate (low)

* Defect in hepato cellular disease

Fig. 6.12. The metabolism of cortisol by the liver. In hepato-cellular disease there is difficulty in reducing the 4—3 ketonic group but not in conjugation. Urinary 17-ketosteroids and 17-hydroxycorticoids are therefore reduced.

2 Bannister P, Handley T, Chapman C *et al.* Hypogonadism in chronic liver disease: impaired release of luteinising hormone. *Brit. Med. J.* 1986; **293:** 1191.

3 Bannister P, Oakes J, Sheridan P *et al.* Sex hormones changes in chronic liver disease: a matched study of alcoholic versus non-alcoholic liver disease. *Q. J. Med.* 1987; **63:** 305.

4 Bannister P, Losowsky MS. Sex hormones and chronic liver disease. *J. Hepatol* 1988; **6:** 258.

5 Bean WB. *Vascular Spiders and Related Lesions of the Skin.* Blackwell Scientific Publications, Oxford 1959.

6 Bennett HS, Baggenstoss AH, Butt HR. The testis, breast and prostate of men who die of cirrhosis of the liver. *Am. J. clin. Pathol.* 1950; **20:** 814.

7 Capron J-P, Kantor G, Dupas J-L *et al.* Unilateral nevoid telangiectasia and chronic liver disease. *Am. J. Gasteroenterol.* 1981; **76:** 47.

8 Cornely CM, Schade RR, Van Thiel DH *et al.* Chronic advanced liver disease and impotence: cause and effect? *Hepatology* 1984; **4:** 1227.

9 Eagon PK, Willett JE, Seguiti SM *et al.* Androgen-responsive functions of male rat liver. Effect of chronic alcohol ingestion. *Gastroenterology* 1987; **93:** 1162.

10 Francavilla A, Di Leo A, Eagon PK *et al.* Effect of spironolactone and potassium canrenoate on cytosolic and nuclear androgen and estrogen receptors of rat liver. *Gastroenterology* 1987; **93:** 681.

11 Galvao-Teles A, Monteiro E, Gavaler JS *et al.* Gonadal consequences of alcohol abuse: lessons from the liver. *Hepatology* 1986; **6:** 135.

12 Guechot J, Vaubourdolle M, Ballet F *et al.* Hepatic uptake of sex steroids in men with alcoholic cirrhosis. *Gastroenterology* 1987; **92:** 203.

13 Johnson PJ. Sex hormones and the liver. *Clin. Sci.* 1984; **66:** 369.

14 Kew MC, Kirschner MA, Abrahams GE *et al.* Mechanism of feminization in primary liver cancer. *N. Engl. J. Med.* 1977; **296:** 1084.

15 Lester R, Eagon PK, Van Thiel DH. Feminization of the alcoholic: the estrogen/testosterone ratio (E/T). *Gastroenterology* 1979; **76:** 415.

16 Lloyd CW, Williams RH. Endocrine changes associated with Laennec's cirrhosis of the liver. *Am. J. Med.* 1948; **4:** 315.

17 Martini GA. Über Gefässveränderungen der Haut bei Leberkranken. *Z. klin. Med.* 1955; **150:** 470.

18 Martini GA, Straubesand J. Zur Morphologie der Gefässpinnen. ('vascular spiders') in der Haut Leberkranker. *Virchows Arch.* 1953; **324:** 147.

19 Morgan MY, Jakobovits AW, Gore MBR *et al.* Serum prolactin in liver disease and its relationship to gynaecomastia. *Gut* 1978; **19:** 170.

20 Murray M, Zaluzny L, Farrell GC. Impaired androgen 16 α-hydroxylation in hepatic microsomes from carbon tetrachloride-cirrhotic male rats. *Gastroenterology* 1987; **93:** 141.

21 Porter LE, Elm MS, Van Thiel DH *et al.* Hepatic estrogen receptor in human liver disease. *Gastroenterology* 1987; **92:** 735.

22 Villa E, Baldini G, Di Stabile S *et al.* Human liver estrogen receptors (ER) in health and disease. Evidence for an induction by alcohol abuse. *Hepatology* 1985; **5:** 984.

General treatment

Results are at the same time depressing and encouraging. Once the liver is disorganized, as in cirrhosis, it will never regain normal structure. Much can be achieved by symptomatic measures. The liver cells retain such an enormous regenerative capacity that, even though liver structure may not return to normal, functional compensation may be attained.

Precipitating factors

Any factor depressing hepato-cellular function may throw the patient with a hitherto compensated liver disease into failure. Gastrointestinal haemorrhage or the fall in blood pressure following surgical operation may necessitate blood transfusion. An acute infection must be dealt with along general lines and by antibiotics. If failure has followed an alcoholic episode, the patient is denied alcohol. Electrolyte disturbances, whether diuretic-induced or due to some other factor such as vomiting or diarrhoea must be corrected.

General measures

Bed rest reduces the functional demands on the liver. In the acute case, it is advisable; in the subacute and chronic, bed rest is continued while improvement is maintained. If, after four weeks' bed rest, the condition remains static, the patient should be allowed moderate activity.

Diet. A high protein diet may be of particular value in the alcoholic. In most cirrhotic patients 80–100 g protein and 2500 calories suffice. Fat need not be restricted within the calorie total. Folic acid may be deficient. Meals must be attractively presented—the patient with hepato-cellular failure has a fickle appetite, but if he can be persuaded to eat well clinical improvement will follow.

Diet is more important in the alcoholic who has been depriving himself of food than in the non-alcoholic who has usually been eating well.

Dietary supplements. Methionine, choline and amino acid supplements do not increase the rate of recovery. Very high methionine and cystine levels are found in the plasma in severe hepatitis and cirrhosis. There is no deficiency but rather difficulty in utilization.

Alcohol. Patients with acute hepato-cellular failure should abstain from all alcohol for six months to one year after recovery. If alcoholism can be incriminated the patient should, if possible, become a total and lifelong abstainer. If the chronic liver disease is non-alcoholic, one glass of wine or of beer daily will not be harmful.

Anaemia. The haemoglobin level must be kept above 10 g/100 ml. The anaemia may remit only when liver function improves.

Corticoid hormones. Prednisolone and ACTH do not affect the basic cirrhotic process. They have complications including an increased risk of serious infection.

Sex hormones. Hormone therapy to impotent men suffering from alcoholic cirrhosis may lead to the plasma hormone levels returning to normal but normal sexual potency is not restored. General health and psychosexual problems are more important. Cessation of alcohol and attention to social problems are more important than hormone therapy.

Oral testosterone has no beneficial effect in alcoholic cirrhosis other than to cause a slight decrease in gynaecomastia [1]. Mortality is increased.

Sedatives (Chapter 18). Morphine is very likely to precipitate coma. Paraldehyde may also precipitate coma and should be avoided.

Barbiturates vary in their mode of excretion. The long-acting, short-chain barbiturates such as barbitone or phenobarbitone are excreted largely by the kidney and small doses are reasonably well tolerated by the patient with cirrhosis. The short-acting, long-chain barbiturates such as pentobarbitone and the thiobarbitones such as pentothal are metabolized largely by the liver and should be avoided. If a barbiturate is used, the initial dose must be small.

Chlordiazepoxide (Librium) may lead to over-sedation in patients with liver disease [2]. The disposition of oxazepam is normal and this may be the drug of choice in cirrhosis [3].

References

1 Copenhagen Study Group for Liver Diseases. Testosterone treatment of men with alcoholic cirrhosis: a double blind study. *Hepatology* 1986; **6:** 807.
2 Roberts RK, Wilkinson GR, Branch RA *et al.* Effect of age and parenchymal liver disease on the disposition and elimination of chlordiazepoxide (Librium). *Gastroenterology* 1978; **75:** 479.
3 Shull HJ, Wilkinson GR, Johnson R *et al.* Normal disposition of oxazepam in acute viral hepatitis and cirrhosis. *Ann. intern. Med.* 1976; **84:** 420.

7 · Hepatic Encephalopathy

The relationship of the liver to mental function has been recognized from earliest times. The Babylonians (*circa* 2000 BC) attributed powers of augury and divination to the liver, designating it by the term also used for 'soul' or 'mood'. In the medicine of ancient China (Neiching 1000 BC) the liver was regarded as the storer of blood containing the soul. Hippocrates (460–370 BC) described a patient with hepatitis who 'barked like a dog, could not be held and said things which could not be comprehended'. Frerichs, the father of modern hepatology, described the terminal mental changes in patients with liver disease [21].

'Cases have occurred to me in which individuals who for a long period have suffered from cirrhosis of the liver have suddenly presented a series of morbid symptoms which are foreign to that disease. They have become unconscious, and have been afterwards seized with noisy delirium, from which they passed into deep coma and in this state have died.'

It is now recognized that a neuropsychiatric syndrome of the same basic pattern may complicate liver disease of almost all types. It can culminate in coma and death.

The syndrome of hepatic encephalopathy is difficult to synthesize into an entity. A spectrum of syndromes exists (table 7.1). In acute (fulminant) hepatic failure the syndrome is not simply an encephalopathy but a virtual hepatectomy (Chapter 8); mortality is very high. The encephalopathy of cirrhosis has portal–systemic shunting as a component but hepato-cellular damage is also important; various precipitating factors play a part. Chronic neuropsychiatric states exist, usually in those with chronic portal–systemic shunting, and these may be associated with irreversible brain damage. In these cases the hepato-cellular disease is relatively mild.

Clinical features [1, 16, 57]

The picture is complex and affects all parts of the brain. The disorder is an organic mental reaction associated with a neurological disturbance. Variability is a marked feature, par-

Table 7.1. Factors in hepatic encephalopathy

Type of encephalopathy	% survival	Aetiological factors
Chronic portal–systemic encephalopathy	100	Portal–sytemic shunting Dietary protein intake Intestinal bacteria
Cirrhosis with precipitant	70–80	Diuresis Haemorrhage Paracentesis Diarrhoea and vomiting Surgery Alcoholic excess Sedatives Infections
Acute liver failure	20	Viral hepatitis Alcoholic hepatitis Drug reactions and overdose

ticularly in the more chronic forms. The features depend on the nature and intensity of aetiological and precipitating factors. Children show a particularly acute reaction, often with mania.

Disturbed consciousness with disorder of sleep is usual. Hypersomnia appears early and progresses to inversion of the sleep rhythm. Reduction of spontaneous movement, a fixed stare, apathy and slowness and brevity of response are early signs. Further deterioration results in reaction only to intense or noxious stimuli. Coma at first resembles normal sleep, but progresses to complete unresponsiveness. Deterioration may be arrested at any level. Rapid changes in the level of consciousness are accompanied by delirium.

Personality changes are most conspicuous with chronic liver disease. These include childishness, irritability and loss of concern for family. Even in remission the patient may present similar personality features suggesting frontal lobe involvement. They are usually cooperative, pleasant people with an ease in social relationships and frequently a jocular, euphoric mood.

Intellectual deterioration varies from slight impairment of organic mental function to gross confusion. Focal defects appearing in a setting of clear consciousness relate to disturbances in visual spatial gnosis. These are most easily elicited as constructional apraxia, shown by inability to reproduce simple designs with blocks or matches (fig. 7.1). The *Reitan trail-making test* (fig. 7.2) may be used serially to assess progress [12]. Writing is oblivious of rulings and a daily writing chart is a good check of progress (fig. 7.1). Failure to distinguish objects of similar size, shape, function and position leads to symptoms such as micturating and defaecating in inappropriate places. Insight into such anomalies of behaviour is frequently preserved.

Speech is slow and slurred and the voice is monotonous. In deep stupor, dysphasia becomes marked and is always combined with perseveration.

The most characteristic neurological abnormality is the 'flapping' tremor ('*asterixis*'). This is due to impaired inflow of joint and other afferent information to the brain-stem reticular formation resulting in lapses in posture. It is

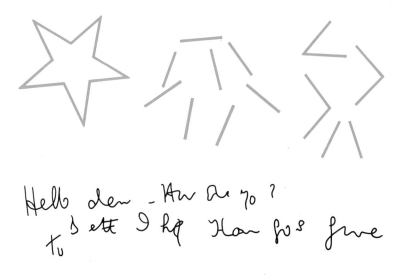

Fig. 7.1. Focal disorders in chronic portal systemic encephalopathy elicited in patients with full consciousness and minimal intellectual defect, in the absence of gross tremor or visual disorder. *Above* Constructional apraxia. *Below* Writing difficulty. 'Hello dear. How are you? Better I hope. That goes for me too.' (Davidson & Summerskill 1956.)

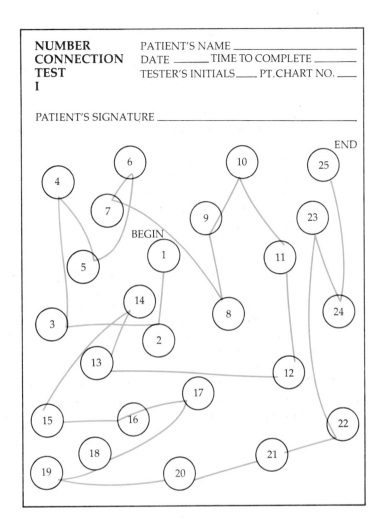

NUMBER CONNECTION TEST I

PATIENT'S NAME _____

DATE _____ TIME TO COMPLETE _____

TESTER'S INITIALS ____ PT.CHART NO. ____

PATIENT'S SIGNATURE _____

Fig. 7.2. The Reitan number connection test.

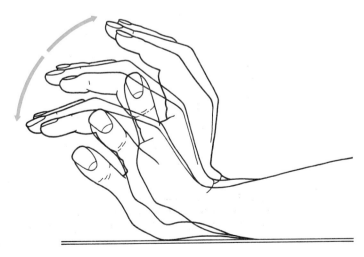

Fig. 7.3. 'Flapping' tremor elicited by attempted dorsiflexion of the wrist with the forearm fixed.

97

demonstrated with the patient's arms outstretched and fingers separated or by hyperextending the wrists with the forearm fixed (fig. 7.3). The rapid flexion–extension movements at the metacarpophalangeal and wrist joints are often accompanied by lateral movements of the digits. Sometimes arms, neck, jaws, protruded tongue, retracted mouth and tightly closed eyelids are involved and the gait is ataxic. Absent at rest, mitigated by intentional movement and maximum on sustained posture, the tremor is usually bilateral, although not bilaterally synchronous, and one side may be affected more than the other. In coma the tremor disappears. It may be appreciated by gentle elevation of a limb or by the patient gripping the physician's hand. A 'flapping' tremor is not specific for hepatic pre-coma. It can also be observed in uraemia, in respiratory failure and in severe heart failure. Deep tendon reflexes are usually exaggerated although patients during coma become flaccid and lose their reflexes. Increased muscle tone is present at some stage and rigidity usually persists through passive flexion and extension. Sus-

tained ankle clonus is often associated with rigidity. The plantar responses are usually flexor becoming extensor in deep stupor or coma. Hyperventilation and hyperpyrexia may be terminal. The diffuse nature of the cerebral disturbance is further shown by excessive appetite, muscle twitchings, grasping and sucking reflexes, and disorders of vision.

The clinical course is very fluctuant, and frequent observation of the patient is necessary. Clinical grading should be used:

Grade 1. Confused. Altered mood or behaviour. Psychometric defects.

Grade 2. Drowsy. Inappropriate behaviour.

Grade 3. Stuporous but speaking and obeying simple commands. Inarticulate speech. Marked confusion.

Grade 4. Coma.

Grade 5. A very severe grade with deep coma and no response to painful stimuli.

Cerebrospinal fluid

This is usually clear and under normal pressure. Patients in hepatic coma may show an in-

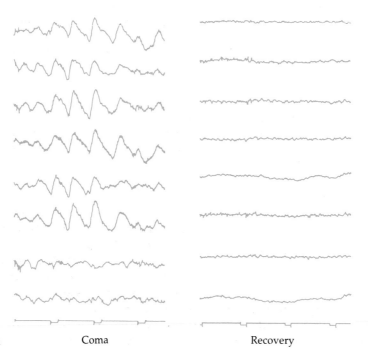

Coma   Recovery

Fig. 7.4. Hepatic cirrhosis with encephalopathy. During coma the EEG tracing shows large bilaterally synchronous slow waves maximal in the frontal and central regions. After recovery (only two days later) a normal alpha rhythm is seen.

creased CSF protein concentration, but the cell count is normal. Glutamic acid and also glutamine may be increased.

Electroencephalogram [45]

There is a slowing of the frequency from the normal alpha range of 8–13 cps right down to the delta range of below 4 cps (fig. 7.4). This is best graded using frequency analysis. Alerting stimuli, such as opening the eyes, fail to reduce the background rhythmic activity. The change commences in the frontal or central region and progresses posteriorly.

This technique is useful for diagnosis and to assess treatment (fig. 8.2). Borderline changes may be clarified by exacerbations produced by high protein feeding.

In very chronic cases with permanent neuronal damage the tracing may be slow or rapid and flat. Such changes may be 'fixed' and unaltered by diet.

EEG changes occur very early even before psychological or biochemical disturbances. They are non-specific, being found also in conditions such as uraemia, CO_2 retention, vitamin B_{12} deficiency or hypoglycaemia. These changes, however, in a conscious patient with liver disease are virtually diagnostic.

Visually evoked potential [72]

This is an expression of postsynaptic cellular potential activity. A flash of light elicits changes in subcortical and cortical neurones through stimulation of visual areas. Latency and wave forms are constant. It is a useful method for differentiating the degree of encephalopathy and more sensitive than the trail test in identifying the neuro-psychological abnormalities that may predict those at risk of developing encephalopathy [16, 72].

Cranial CT scans

These show cerebral atrophy even with apparently well compensated cirrhosis and results are related to the severity of the liver dysfunction. Atrophy is particularly marked in those with chronic persistent encephalopathy and may be potentiated by alcoholism [73]. The CT scan can be quantitated to show cerebral oedema and cortical atrophy even in those with subclinical portal systemic encephalopathy [7].

Neuropathological changes [1, 66]

Grossly, the brain may be normal. About half, usually the younger patients dying with prolonged, deep coma, show cerebral oedema (fig. 8.4); the pathogenesis is unknown. In some, positive pressure ventilation may contribute.

Microscopically, the characteristic changes are increase in number and enlargement of the astrocytes. The commonest is the Alzheimer type 2 change. The Alzheimer type 1 is rarer. The change is diffusely found in the grey matter of cerebrum, cerebellum and in the putamen and globus pallidus. The nerve cells show relatively minor alterations. This combination, and the extent, seem virtually specific for liver disease. The changes bear a rough relationship to the duration and severity of coma and develop within a few days [63].

Early astrocyte changes are probably reversible. In a very long-standing case the structural changes are irreversible and unresponsive to treatment of the liver disease. The cortex is thinned; neurones and fibres are lost. The deep layers of cortex may show laminar necrosis. The cerebellum and basal ganglia are also involved. Demyelination in the pyramidal tracts is associated with spastic paraplegia.

Experimental hepatic coma

The blood–brain barrier shows increased permeability with specific alterations in transport systems [23, 71].

However, in recent studies, using galactosamine-induced hepatic failure in rats, the blood–brain barrier showed no generalized increase in the pre-comatosed animal [32]. There are obvious difficulties in equating animal models with man.

Mechanisms [13, 14, 74]

The essentially reversible nature of the cerebral disturbance, at least in the early stages, and the diffuse involvement suggest that the change is a metabolic one. Research has proceeded to determine firstly the nature of the toxic metabolite(s), secondly the route by which it reaches the brain, and thirdly other possible disturbances of cerebral metabolism which might develop in the presence of a failing liver (table 7.2).

Table 7.2. The cause(s) of chronic hepatic encephalopathy must be

Of colonic origin
Nitrogenous
Produced by intestinal bacteria
Present in the portal blood
Metabolized by the liver
Able to pass the blood−brain (? defective) barrier
Able to disturb cerebral metabolism

PORTAL−SYSTEMIC ENCEPHALOPATHY

Every patient with hepatic pre-coma or coma has a circulatory pathway through which portal blood may enter the systemic veins and reach the brain without being metabolized by the liver [48].

In patients with poor hepato-cellular function, such as acute hepatitis, the shunt is through the liver itself. The damaged cells are unable to metabolize the contents of the portal venous blood completely so that they pass unaltered into the hepatic veins (fig. 7.5).

In patients with more chronic forms of liver disease, such as cirrhosis, the portal blood bypasses the liver through large natural 'collaterals'. The portal−hepatic vein anastomoses, developing around the nodules in a cirrhotic liver, may also act as internal shunts. The picture is a common complication of portacaval anastomosis. The condition is analogous to the neuropsychiatric disturbance devel-

oping in the dog with an Eck fistula if it is fed meat.

Encephalopathy is unusual if liver function is adequate. In hepatic schistosomiasis where the collateral circulation is great and liver function adequate, coma is rare. If shunting is sufficiently great, however, encephalopathy may develop in the absence of obvious liver disease, for instance in extra-hepatic portal hypertension.

Patients going into hepatic coma are suffering from cerebral intoxication by intestinal contents which have not been metabolized by the liver (*portal−systemic encephalopathy*) [57]. The nature of the cerebral intoxicant is nitrogenous. A picture indistinguishable from impending hepatic coma can be induced in some patients with cirrhosis by the oral administration of a high-protein diet, ammonium chloride, urea, or methionine [47, 48, 57].

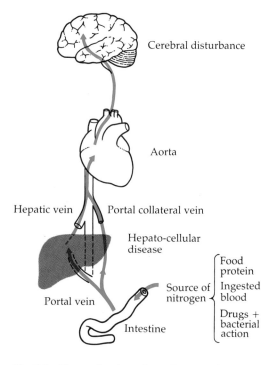

Fig. 7.5. The mechanism of portal−systemic encephalopathy (Sherlock *et al.* 1954).

INTESTINAL BACTERIA

Symptoms can often be relieved by oral antibiotics. The intoxicant therefore seems to be produced by intestinal bacteria. Other measures which diminish the colonic flora, for instance colonic exclusion or purgation, may also be effective. Moreover, urea-splitting bacteria and the small intestinal flora generally are increased in patients with liver disease [36].

AMMONIA TOXICITY

Ammonia has been the most widely investigated toxic substance. The syndrome may be reproduced in some patients by ammonium salts given orally or intravenously and arterial ammonium levels may be high in patients in hepatic coma. Ammonium can be derived from the nitrogenous contents of the intestine by bacterial action. It is present in high concentration in portal blood and is metabolized by the liver to urea [69]. The failing liver cell may also be unable to metabolize ammonium formed by the kidney and, in the terminal stages of hepatic coma, by the peripheral tissues and brain [60]. Gastric urease is another source of ammonia.

Theoretically ammonium intoxication could interfere with cerebral metabolism. This could be by two mechanisms: increased glutamine synthesis and reductive amination of ketoglutarate (fig. 7.5). The increase in glutamine and ketoglutarate in the cerebrospinal fluid in hepatic coma suggests that combination of

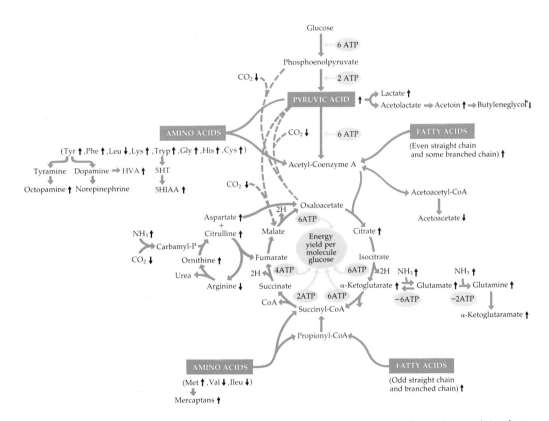

Fig. 7.6. Map of metabolic abnormalities in hepatic coma. Vertical heavy arrows indicate abnormalities that have been observed in blood (Zieve 1974).

ammonium with glutamic acid is increased.

Combination of ammonium with α-ketoglutarate to form glutamic acid removes an important link in the Krebs' citric acid cycle. The brain depends for most of its activity on aerobic glycolysis and this cycle. Experimentally, ammonia can depress cerebral blood flow and glucose metabolism. Ammonia also has a direct effect on the neuronal membrane. Diversion of α-ketoglutarate to glutamate and glutamine would reduce the energy available for oxidative cell metabolism (fig. 7.6). The diminished oxygen consumption of the brain in hepatic coma and the increased blood and cerebrospinal fluid pyruvic acid concentrations [17] would support this hypothesis.

There are, however, points that suggest hepatic coma and ammonium intoxication cannot be equated. The brain in hepatic coma does not always remove ammonium from the blood but may in fact occasionally add to it, the jugular vein concentration exceeding that in an artery.

When ammonium citrate was used to induce a high blood ammonia in patients with liver disease the EEG changed in only one of 19 patients although the arterial and venous ammonia levels were often high [10]. The raised blood ammonium level in hepatic coma may well be more a non-specific indicator of disturbed brain metabolism than the toxic causative factor.

Unfortunately, there is no clear evidence associating the amounts of ammonia in the *brain* and the mental state.

Blood ammonia levels. The estimation must be performed immediately. The upper limit of normal is 0.8−1 µg/ml blood.

Levels usually correlate with severity, but 10% of values are in the normal range regardless of the depth of coma. Estimations in terminal hepatic coma show wide fluctuations. Some patients, particularly after porta-caval anastomosis, may seem normal with raised blood ammonium levels. Levels rise after gastrointestinal bleeding. The level does not relate to prognosis. Blood ammonium values are not necessary for routine use.

CSF glutamine is a sensitive index of hepatic encephalopathy but is not usually necessary.

OTHER NITROGENOUS SUBSTANCES

Pharmacologically active amines can be formed by intestinal bacteria acting on protein and are present in portal blood. They are difficult to estimate in biological fluids.

Methionine precipitates hepatic coma without rises in blood ammonia levels [47]. Tetracycline is preventative. This effect might be related to mercaptans which are derived by bacterial metabolism of methionine and are extremely toxic. They are usually removed by the liver. Raised blood mercaptan levels are found in portal−systemic encephalopathy but not in all patients.

The cerebral disturbance might be related to failure of the liver to add an essential substance, such as cytidine or uridine, to the circulation. However, as judged by brain function in hepatectomized rats perfused with blood from normal donors, this theory is unlikely [52].

AMINO ACID IMBALANCE AND FALSE NEUROTRANSMISSION

Neurotransmitter synthesis is controlled by the brain concentration of the precursor amino acids (fig. 7.6). The aromatic amino acids, tyrosine, phenylalanine and tryptophan, are increased in liver disease, perhaps due to failure of hepatic deamination. The branched-chain amino acids, valine, leucine and isoleucine, are decreased, perhaps due to increased catabolism by skeletal muscle and kidneys secondary to the hyperinsulinism of chronic liver disease (fig. 7.6). The aromatic amino acids could have a profound affect on cerebral metabolism. For instance tryptophan is metabolized to serotonin and phenylalanine and tyrosine are precursors of catecholamines.

A reduced ratio between branched-chain and aromatic amino acids has been related to the development of hepatic encephalopathy [27]. However, in a large group of cirrhotic patients the ratio was reduced both in those with and without encephalopathy (fig. 7.9) [40].

The colon may be a source of false neurotransmitters (fig. 7.7) such as octopamine, formed by bacterial action which might function as week neurotransmitters replacing the true transmitters, noradrenaline and dopamine [20]. Serum and urinary octopamine levels are increased in hepatic encephalopathy [35]. However, intraventricular infusion of enormous quantities of octopamine, with resulting depression of brain dopamine and adrenaline, failed to cause coma in normal rats. Moreover, where brain catecholamines were measured *post mortem* in cirrhotic patients with encephalopathy, no reduction in adrenaline or noradrenaline concentration was found and octopamine levels were decreased compared with cirrhotics who were not encephalopathic at the time of death [15].

The amino acid imbalance, false neurotransmission hypothesis for hepatic encephalopathy remains difficult to establish.

NEUROTRANSMITTER RECEPTOR AND GABA CHANGES

A change in cerebral neuroreceptors has been incriminated in the coma of the rabbit model with galactosamine-induced fulminant hepatic failure [28, 55].

Studies on this model of fulminant hepatitis suggested that gamma-aminobutyric acid (GABA), an inhibitory neurotransmitter present in 30 to 50% of all cerebral synapses, was responsible for the features of hepatic encephalopathy [28]. It is produced by bacterial action in the gut and concentrations are increased in the blood of patients with hepatic encephalopathy. There are difficulties in accepting this hypothesis [58]. The methodology for measuring serum GABA is suspect as other substances, including glutamine, may also be estimated [19]. Furthermore, estimations of GABA have given various results. In one study, mean plasma and CSF fluid GABA levels were not different in patients with or without encephalopathy

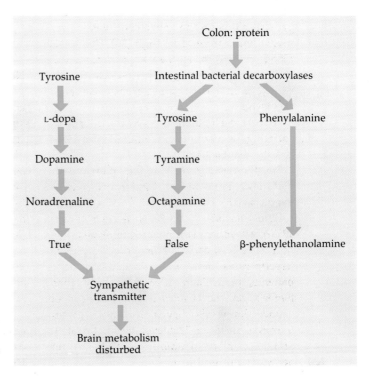

Fig. 7.7. The possible role of false sympathetic neurotransmitters in the disturbed cerebral metabolism in liver disease.

103

and did not change during the course [41]. Using gas liquid chromatography others have confirmed raised GABA levels in the plasma of patients with liver disease and hepatic encephalopathy [30]. GABA may not pass the human blood—brain barrier into the CSF although increased permeability of the blood—brain barrier in experimental hepatic coma has been shown.

An increased number of binding sites for GABA can be shown in the brains of the galactosamine model of fulminant hepatitis although this is not consistent [5]. An increased number of binding sites for benzodiazepines are also found but such an increase is not shown in the thioacetamide model in rats [34]. Autopsy results in man have given conflicting results.

However, positron emission tomography has shown a two to threefold increase in benzodiazepine-receptor density in four individuals who had suffered recent bouts of encephalopathy [54]. Clinically, increased sensitivity to benzodiazepines is well known in cirrhosis and this is now being confirmed and shown to be due not only to impaired drug elimination but also to hypersensitivity of the brain [3]. Gamma GABA and benzodiazepines share the same terminals promoting chloride conductance across the post-synaptic neuromembrane so increasing membrane depolymerization and inhibiting post-synaptic potential. Benzodiazepine antagonists have therefore been suggested for the treatment of hepatic encephalopathy. Indeed in the rabbit model of fulminant

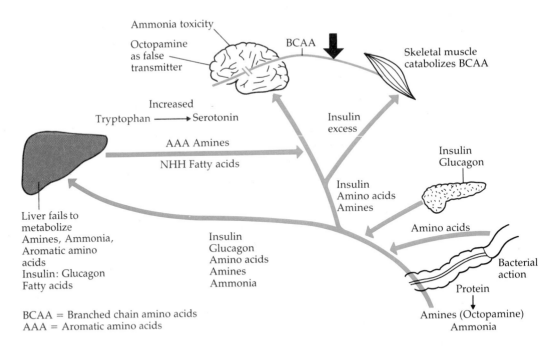

Fig. 7.8. The factors concerned in hepatic encephalopathy. Important concepts illustrated are:
1 Failure of hepatic cellular function.
2 Portal—systemic bypassing.
3 Failure to metabolize insulin and glucagon coming from the pancreas.
4 Increase in false neurochemical transmitters arising from the colon.
5 Amino acid imbalance.
6 Increased change from tryptophan to serotonin in the brain.

hepatic failure, a GABA-benzodiazepine receptor antagonist (flumazenil, R Glow 15—1788) did ameliorate hepatic encephalopathy [6]. Clinical and electrophysiological remission has been reported following flumazenil given to patients with hepatic encephalopathy [4, 24].

As a further twist to the GABA story, benzodiazepine-binding activity has been found in the cerebro-spinal fluid of rabbits and humans with hepatic encephalopathy. This has led to the view that GABA-ergic tone may be increased in hepatic encephalopathy because of the interaction of an *endogenous* benzodiazepine agonist with benzodiazepine receptors [43].

OTHER METABOLIC ABNORMALITIES

These patients are often alkalotic. This may result from toxic stimulation of the respiratory centre by ammonium, from administration of alkalis such as citrate in transfusions or with potassium supplements, or from hypokalaemia.

Hypoxia increases cerebral sensitivity to ammonia. The stimulation of the respiratory centre results in increase in depth and rate of respiration. Hypocapnia follows and this reduces cerebral blood flow. The increase in the blood organic acids (lactate and pyruvate) is correlated with the reduction in CO_2 tension.

Any potent diuretic can precipitate hepatic coma. This may be related to hypokalaemia [40] and to readier penetration of ammonium ion through the blood—brain barrier in the presence of alkalosis. In addition to hypokalaemia, other electrolyte disturbances or a profound diuresis seem to initiate encephalopathy.

CHANGES IN CARBOHYDRATE METABOLISM

The hepatectomized dog dies in hypoglycaemic coma. Hypoglycaemic episodes are rare in chronic liver disease but may complicate fulminant hepatitis (Chapter 8).

Alpha-ketoglutaric and pyruvic acids are transported from the periphery to the metabolic pool in the liver, and blood levels increase as the neurological state deteriorates [17]. These probably reflect severe liver damage. The fall in blood ketones also reflects severity of hepatic dysfunction. There is progressive impairment of intermediate carbohydrate metabolism as the liver fails.

SYNERGISTIC TOXIC SUBSTANCES

Various toxic substances might act together to induce the altered cerebral metabolism. One combination might be ammonia with mercaptans and short- and medium-chain fatty acids which are known to be increased in the blood in hepatic failure [75]. Phenol, another substance that increases in the blood in liver failure, might be another synergistic factor. Such a hypothesis is difficult to prove or dis-

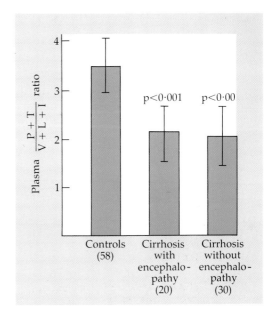

Fig. 7.9. The plasma $\dfrac{V + L + I}{P + T}$ ratio in control subjects and in patients with cirrhosis with and without hepatic encephalopathy. $\bar{\text{I}}$ = mean ratio ± s.d.; p = student's t test. V = valine, L = leucine, I = isoleucine, P = phenylalanine, T = tyrosine (Morgan *et al.* 1978).

prove. In any individual patient the role of one toxin cannot easily be dissected from that of a combination.

Conclusions (fig. 7.10)

The brain of the patient with liver disease seems unduly sensitive to insults that would be without effect in the normal. A small dose of morphine (8 mg) will induce EEG changes in a patient who has experienced pre-coma but not in one who has not [29]. A similar sensitivity is shown to electrolyte imbalance. Indeed, whether cause or effect, cerebral metabolism is undoubtedly abnormal in liver disease. In the chronic case, actual structural changes in the brain can be demonstrated and the EEG is fixed and abnormal and unresponsive to changes in dietary protein or to neomycin.

The role of increased GABA-ergic neurotransmission remains uncertain.

Such factors as infection, hypotension or anoxia act both on liver and brain. Multiple factors may operate; for instance the addition of protein to the diet will increase and the giving of neomycin will decrease the EEG response to morphine in susceptible cirrhotic subjects.

The picture of hepatic pre-coma and coma is non-specific. The organic psychosis, the 'flapping' tremor, the EEG changes and the raised blood ammonium values may be encountered, in whole or in part, in other disturbances such as uraemia, or respiratory failure. There is no sure laboratory method of diagnosis, and recognition depends on clinical acumen with the association of other features of liver disease such as fetor hepaticus, jaundice or ascites. The syndrome is not *only* due to the passage of toxic substances of intestinal origin to the

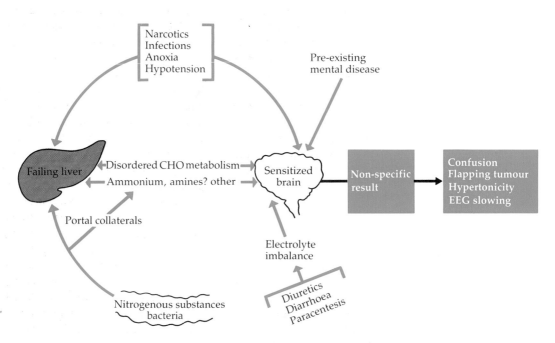

Fig. 7.10. The pathogenesis of a hepatic coma. Many factors affecting hepatic or cerebral function, or both, can lead to the picture of hepatic pre-coma in a patient with liver disease. The brain in such subjects may be particularly sensitive to these factors (Sherlock 1961).

brain. Many other metabolic events occur when the liver fails. The causes of this complex clinical picture are in most part unknown. No one cause has been found. Interactions between various factors are likely. Moreover some events, such as depression of cerebral oxygen and glucose metabolism, may be, in part, effects of the coma rather than primary.

Clinical associations

The syndrome is most frequently associated with *virus hepatitis* (Chapter 16) and *cirrhosis*. Fetor hepaticus is usually present.

Hepatic cirrhosis

PRE-CLINICAL

Clinically inapparent impairment in mental functions, sufficient to cause disruption in the routine of everyday living, is frequent in patients with cirrhosis [62]. The picture is of the type associated with lesions of the fronto-parietal regions of the brain. About three-quarters of patients with cirrhosis and seemingly normal neurological and mental status fail psychometric tests, impairment of performance being more marked than for verbal skills [22].

In Germany only 15% of patients with chronic liver disease and portal hypertension, clinically not encephalopathic, were judged fit to drive a car [56].

ACUTE TYPE

The syndrome may appear spontaneously, without a precipitant, usually in a deeply jaundiced patient with ascites and in the terminal stages. Precipitating factors act by depressing liver cell or cerebral function, increasing nitrogenous material in the intestine, or raising the portal—collateral flow (table 7.3).

The commonest precipitant is a brisk response to a potent *diuretic*. Large *paracenteses*

Table 7.3. Precipitants of acute hepatic encephalopathy in cirrhotic patients

Infection
  Spontaneous bacterial peritonitis
  Urinary
  Chest

Bleeding
  Oesophageal and gastric varices
  Gastro-duodenal erosions
  Mallory—Weiss tear

Electrolyte imbalance
  Diuretics
  Vomiting
  Diarrhoea

Constipation

Large protein meal

Alcohol withdrawal

may also precipitate coma; the mechanism is uncertain. Electrolyte imbalance following removal of large quantities of electrolytes and water, changes in hepatic circulation and hypotension may contribute. Other causes of fluid and electrolyte depletion, such as *diarrhoea* or *vomiting*, may be precipitants.

Gastrointestinal haemorrhage, usually from oesophageal varices, is another common precipitant. Coma is precipitated by the large protein meal (as blood) in addition to the depression in hepato-cellular function due to anaemia and reduction in liver blood flow.

Surgical procedures are tolerated extremely poorly. Hepatic function is depressed by the blood loss, anaesthesia and 'shock'.

Acute alcoholism precipitates coma both by depressing cerebral function and by the associated acute alcoholic hepatitis. *Morphia* [29], *benzodiazepines* and *barbiturates* depress cerebral function and have a prolonged action when hepatic detoxication is delayed.

Infections, especially with bacteraemia and including 'spontaneous' bacterial peritonitis, may be the precipitant.

Coma may occasionally be initiated by a large *protein meal* or severe *constipation*.

CHRONIC TYPE

The portal—systemic collateral circulation is particularly extensive. This may consist simply of the myriad of small anastomotic vessels developing in the cirrhotic patient or, more often, one major collateral channel, such as the spleno-renal, gastro-renal [61], umbilical vein or inferior mesenteric vein, predominates.

Fluctuations are related to dietary protein and diagnosis can be confirmed by noting the effect clinically and on the EEG of a precipitant such as a high-protein diet or by demonstrating improvement by protein withdrawal. Clinical and biochemical evidence of liver disease may be equivocal or absent, and the neuropsychiatric disorder may dominate the picture.

The intermittent neuropsychiatric disturbance may continue for as long as six years [60] and the diagnosis is very liable to fall between various specialist interests. The psychiatrist is interested in the non-specific organic reaction and may not consider underlying liver disease. The neurologist focuses attention on the neurological features, while the hepatologist, recognizing the cirrhosis, fails to elicit the neurological signs or assumes that the patient is just 'odd' or an alcoholic. The patient may be seen for the first time in coma or in remission, adding to the diagnostic difficulty.

The acute psychiatric states often present shortly (two weeks to eight months) after porta-caval anastomosis as a paranoid-schizophrenic picture or as hypomania [51]. 'Classical' portal—systemic encephalopathy, with EEG slowing, is usually present in addition. Formal psychiatric treatment may be required in addition to that of the hepatic encephalopathy.

More persistent neuropsychiatric syndromes are probably related to organic changes in the central nervous system, not only in the brain but also in the spinal cord [66]. Progressive *paraplegia* may commence insidiously in those with a large portal—systemic collateral circulation. The encephalopathy is not severe. The spinal cord shows demyelination. The paraplegia is progressive and the usual treatment for portal—systemic encephalopathy is ineffective.

Chronic cerebellar and *basal ganglia signs* with Parkinsonism, the tremor being unaffected by intention, may develop after some years of chronic hepatic encephalopathy [51, 66]. Permanent cerebral damage is probably present, for treatment has little effect on the tremor. *Focal cerebral symptoms*, epileptic attacks and dementia have also been noted [51].

These persistent neuropsychiatric changes are presumably due to some unknown central nervous system poison which passes through a large portal—systemic shunt in the presence of liver disease.

Differential diagnosis

A *low sodium state* can develop in cirrhotic patients on a restricted sodium diet and having diuretics and abdominal paracenteses. This is shown by apathy, headache, nausea and hypotension. The diagnosis is confirmed by finding low serum sodium levels with a rise in blood urea concentration. The condition may be combined with impending hepatic coma.

Acute alcoholism [16] provides a particularly difficult problem especially as the two syndromes may co-exist (see Chapter 20). Many symptoms attributed to alcoholism may be due to portal—systemic encephalopathy. Delirium tremens is distinguished by the continuous motor and autonomic over-activity, total insomnia, terrifying hallucinations and a finer, more rapid tremor. The patient is flushed, agitated, inattentive and perfunctory in his replies. Tremor, absent at rest, becomes coarse and irregular on activity. Profound anorexia, often with retching and vomiting, is common.

Portal—systemic encephalopathy in an alcoholic has similar features to that in the non-alcoholic except for the frequent absence of rigidity, hyperreflexia and ankle clonus due to concomitant peripheral neuritis. An EEG is helpful, as is the observation of a favourable response to dietary protein withdrawal and neomycin.

Wernicke's encephalopathy is common with profound malnutrition and with alcoholism.

Hepato-lenticular degeneration (Wilson's disease) is found in young people, often with a family history. The symptoms do not fluctuate, the tremor is choreo-athetoid rather than 'flapping', the Kayser—Fleischer corneal ring is seen and disturbances in copper metabolism can usually be demonstrated.

Latent *functional psychoses* such as depression or paranoia are frequently released by impending hepatic coma. The type of reaction is related to the previous personality, and to intensification of personality traits. The psychiatric importance of the syndrome is emphasized by such patients often being admitted to mental hospitals. Conversely a chronic psychiatric state in patients with known liver disease may not be related to the liver dysfunction. In such patients investigations are designed to demonstrate the chronic syndrome and in particular a large collateral circulation by venography or by CT scanning after intravenous contrast enhancement. Clinical and EEG changes induced by high and low protein feeding may also be useful.

Prognosis

Prognosis depends on the extent of liver cell failure. The chronic group with relatively good liver function but with an extensive collateral circulation combined with increased intestinal nitrogen have the best prognosis and the acute hepatitis group the worst. In cirrhosis, the outlook is poor if the patient has ascites, jaundice and a low serum-albumin level—all indicative of liver failure. If treatment is begun early in the precomatose state, the chances of success are increased. The prognosis is better if the precipitant can be treated, for instance infection, diuretic overdose or haemorrhage.

Assessment of therapy is made difficult by fluctuations in the clinical course. The value of any new method can only be assessed after large numbers of patients have been treated by controlled regimes. Results in patients with

chronic encephalopathy (largely related to portal—systemic shunting), with recovery as the rule, must be separated from acute hepatocellular failure in which recovery is rare.

Older patients have the added disadvantage of cerebral vascular disease. Children with portal vein obstruction having a portal—systemic shunt develop no intellectual or psychological side-effects [2].

Treatment of hepatic pre-coma and coma

The factors acting in the particular patient must be defined and treated (table 7.4) [14]. The major ones are toxic nitrogenous substances formed in the intestine by bacterial action on proteins.

Diet

All dietary protein is stopped. At least 1600 calories are supplied daily as glucose drinks or as 20% glucose through a gastric drip. Twenty per cent or 40% dextrose is given via ante-

Table 7.4. Treatment of hepatic pre-coma and coma

Acute
1 Identify precipitating factor
2 Empty bowels of nitrogen-containing materials
   (a) Stop nitrogen-containing drugs
   (b) Phosphate enema
3 Protein-free diet
   Raise dietary protein slowly with recovery
4 Antibiotic
   Neomycin 1 g 4 times a day by mouth for 1 week
5 Maintain calorie, fluid and electrolyte balance
6 Stop diuretics, check serum electrolyte levels

Chronic
1 Avoid nitrogen-containing drugs
2 Protein, largely vegetarian intake, at limit of tolerance (about 50 g daily)
3 Ensure at least two free bowel movements daily
4 Lactulose or lactilol
5 If symptoms worsen adopt a regime for acute coma
6 Consider trial of bromocriptine

cubital or femoral vein into the innominate vein or vena cava.

During recovery, protein is added in 20 g increments on alternate days. The protein is divided between four meals. Any relapse is treated by a return to the former regime. In patients with an acute episode of coma, a normal protein intake is soon achieved. In the chronic group, permanent protein restriction is needed to control mental symptoms [60]: the limits of tolerance are usually 40–60 g per day.

Vegetable protein is tolerated better than animal [41]. It is less ammoniagenic and contains small amounts of methionine and aromatic amino acids. It is also more laxative and increases the intake of dietary fibre with increased incorporation and elimination of nitrogen contained in faecal bacteria [68]. It is difficult to take because of flatulence, diarrhoea and bulk.

An exacerbation of symptoms is treated by rest and abstention from protein.

In the acute cases, a few days' to a few weeks' deprivation of protein does not prove harmful and, even in the chronic group in whom dietary protein has to be restricted for many months, clinical protein malnutrition is rare. Protein restriction is indicated only in patients showing signs of encephalopathy. Others with liver disease may benefit by high protein feeding.

ANTIBIOTICS

Tetracyclines are effective for short periods. Neomycin, given orally, is very effective in decreasing gastrointestinal ammonium formation [18]. Little is absorbed from the gut although blood levels have been detected. Impaired hearing or deafness follow its long-term use. In the acute case 4–6 g are given daily in divided doses. The EEG improves, blood ammonium levels fall and fetor hepaticus goes. Clinical improvement is difficult to correlate with the changes in faecal flora [18].

Metronidazole (0.2 g four times per day) seems to be as effective as neomycin [37]. Because of dose-related central nervous system toxicity, it should not be used long-term.

In acute hepatic coma, neomycin is the antibiotic of choice, although lactulose can also be given. Surprisingly the two drugs seem to act synergistically [67], perhaps because of action on different bacterial populations.

LACTULOSE (fig. 7.11) [8] AND LACTILOL (table 7.5)

The human intestinal mucosa does not produce a lactulose to split this synthetic disaccharide. When given by mouth the *lactulose* reaches the caecum where it is broken down by bacteria to fatty acids. The faecal pH drops. The growth of lactose-fermenting organisms is favoured and organisms such as bacteroides, which are ammonia formers, are suppressed. It may 'detoxify' short-chain fatty acids produced in the presence of blood and proteins. The colonic fermentative bacteria prefer lactulose to blood when both are present [42]. It may be of particular value in hepatic encephalopathy induced by bleeding. The osmotic volume of the colon is increased.

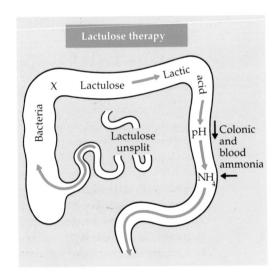

Fig. 7.11. Lactulose reaches the colon unsplit. It is then converted by bacteria to organic acids and an acid stool test results. This may also affect the ionization of ammonia in the colon and reduce its absorption.

The mode of action is uncertain. Faecal acidity would reduce the ionization of ammonia and hence absorption of ammonia (also amines and other toxic nitrogenous compounds); faecal ammonia is not increased. Lactulose more than doubles the colonic output of bacterial mass and 'soluble' nitrogen [68]. This is no longer available for absorption as ammonia and a reduced urea production results [68].

The aim of therapy is to produce acid stools without diarrhoea. The dose is 10–30 ml three times a day and is adjusted to produce two semi-solid stools daily.

Side-effects include flatulence, diarrhoea and intestinal pain. Diarrhoea can be so profound that serum sodium increases to over 145 meq/l, serum potassium falls and alkalosis develops. The blood volume falls so impairing renal function. These side-effects are particularly likely if the daily dose exceeds 100 ml. Some of the side-effects may be related to contamination of lactulose syrup with other sugars, principally galactose and lactulose. Crystalline lactulose may have less toxicity.

Table 7.5. The effects of lactilol compared with lactulose

Colonic effects similar
As effective in encephalopathy
Quicker action
More convenient (powder)
Less sweet
Less diarrhoea and flatulence

Lactilol (β-galactoside sorbitol) is a second generation disaccharide easily produced in chemically pure, crystalline form and can be dispensed as a powder. It is not broken down or absorbed in the small intestine, but is metabolized by colonic bacteria [46]. As a powder, it is more convenient than the liquid lactulose and can easily be used as a sweetening agent. It is more palatable (tasting less sugary). It is given in a dose of approximately 30 g daily. Three controlled trials have been reported comparing lactulose and lactilol. Lactilol seems to be equally as effective as lactulose in chronic [38, 39] and acute [25] portal systemic encephalopathy. Patients respond considerably more quickly to lactilol than lactulose [39], and there is less diarrhoea and flatulence [38, 39].

Purgation. Hepatic encephalopathy follows constipation, and remissions are associated with free bowel action. The value of enemas and purgation with magnesium sulphate in patients with hepatic coma must be emphasized. Lactulose or lactose enemas may be used and are superior to water [65]. All enemas must be neutral or acid to reduce ammonium absorption. Magnesium sulphate enemas can cause dangerous hypermagnesaemia [11]. Phosphate enemas are safe.

OTHER PRECIPITATING FACTORS

Patients in impending coma are extremely sensitive to sedatives and whenever possible these are avoided. If an overdose is suspected, the appropriate antagonist should be given. If the patient is uncontrollable and some sedation is necessary, a small dose of temazepam or oxazepam is given; morphine and paraldehyde are absolutely contraindicated. Diazepoxide or heminevrin is valuable in the alcoholic with impending hepatic coma. Drugs known to induce hepatic coma such as oral amino acids and diuretics are disallowed.

Potassium deficiency can be treated by fruit juices or by effervescent or slow-release potassium chloride. If it is urgent, 0.1% potassium chloride may be incorporated in an infusion.

The possibility of delirium tremens should not tempt the clinician to give alcohol to an alcoholic patient in impending hepatic coma.

LEVODOPA AND BROMOCRIPTINE

If portal–systemic encephalopathy is related to a defect in dopaminergic neurotransmission then replenishment of cerebral dopamines should be beneficial. Dopamine does not pass the blood–brain barrier, but its precursor, levodopa, does and can cause temporary arousal in acute hepatic encephalopathy [33]. However, only a few patients benefit. Nausea and psychiatric disturbances are side-effects.

Bromocriptine is a specific dopamine receptor agonist with a prolonged action. In a dose of up to 15 mg daily it causes clinical, psychometric and electroencephalographic improvement in patients with chronic portal–systemic encephalopathy. Cerebral blood flow, oxygen and glucose consumption increase. Bromocriptine treatment should be considered in the rare patient with chronic portal–systemic encephalopathy and good, stable liver function resistant to dietary protein restriction and lactulose.

BRANCHED-CHAIN AMINO ACIDS

A reduced ratio of branched-chain to aromatic amino acids has been related to the development of hepatic encephalopathy. Infusions of solutions containing a high concentration of branched-chain amino acids have been used to treat the acute and chronic hepatic encephalopathy. Results have been extremely conflicting, perhaps related to differences in the nature of the amino acid solutions, the ways of administration and the patients studied.

Controlled trials of intravenous branched-chain amino acids in acute hepatic encephalopathy have been summarized [53]. In two trials, the patients woke up more quickly. Survival was improved but was not significantly different in the treated group. Trials of oral supplements to prevent recurrent encephalopathic episodes are largely uncontrolled and include cirrhotic patients of different aetiologies but the incidence of hepatic encephalopathy did seem to be reduced. Considering the high cost of intravenous amino acid mixtures, it is difficult to justify their use in acute hepatic encephalopathy where branched-chain amino acid blood levels are high anyway. If used, 53% or 35% branched-chain amino acids are preferable to 100% which increase protein breakdown [70].

SHUNT OCCLUSION

Surgical shunt occlusion can reverse the severe portal–systemic encephalopathy following a porta-caval anastomosis. This may be preceded by an oesophageal transection to avoid the risk of re-bleeding [9]. Alternatively the shunt may be occluded by invasive radiology with the insertion of a balloon [49].

TEMPORARY HEPATIC SUPPORT

Complicated methods of temporary hepatic support are not, in general, applicable to hepatic coma in the cirrhotic. Such a patient is either terminal or can be expected to come out of coma without them. They are discussed under acute hepatic failure (Chapter 9).

HEPATIC HOMOTRANSPLANTATION

This may be the ultimate answer to the problem of chronic hepatic encephalopathy. One such patient with a history of three years showed marked improvement lasting nine months following transplantation [44]. (See also Chapter 8.)

References

1 Adams RD, Foley JM. The neurological disorder associated with liver disease. *Res. Publ. Assn. Res. nerv. ment. Dis.* 1953; **32**: 198.

2 Alagille D, Carlier J-C, Chiva M *et al.* Long-term neuropsychological outcome in children undergoing portal–systemic shunts for portal vein obstruction without liver disease. *J. Pediat. Gastroenterol. Nutr.* 1986; **5**: 861.

3 Batki G, Fisch HU, Karlaganis G *et al.* Mechanism of the excessive sedative response of cirrhotics to benzodiazepines. Model experiments with triazolam. *Hepatology* 1987; **7**: 629.

4 Bansky G, Meier PJ, Riederer E *et al.* Effect of a benzodiazepine antagonist in hepatic encephalopathy in man. *Hepatology* 1987; **7**: 1103.

5 Baraldi M, Zeneroli ML. Experimental hepatic encephalopathy: changes in the binding of gamma-aminobutyric acid. *Science* 1982; **216**: 427.

6 Bassett ML, Mullen KD, Skolnick P *et al.* Amelioration of hepatic encephalopathy by pharmacologic antagonism of the GABA-benzodiazepine receptor complex in a rabbit model of fulminant hepatic failure. *Gastroenterology* 1987; **93**: 1069.

7 Bernthal P, Hays A, Tarter RE *et al.* Cerebral CT scan abnormalities in cholestatic and hepatocellular disease and their relationship to neuropsychologic test performance. *Hepatology* 1987; **7**: 107.

8 Bircher J, Haemmerli UP, Scollo-Lavizzari G *et al.* Treatment of chronic portal−systemic encephalopathy with lactulose. *Am. J. Med.* 1971; **51**: 148.

9 Bismuth H, Houssin D, Grange D. Suppression of the shunt and esophageal transection: a new technique for the treatment of disabling postshunt encephalopathy. *Am. J. Surg.* 1983; **146**: 392.

10 Cohn R, Castell DO. The effect of acute hyperammoniemia on the electroencephalogram. *J. Lab. clin. Med.* 1966; **68**: 195.

11 Collinson PO, Burroughs AK. Severe hypermagnesaemia due to magnesium sulphate enemas in patients with hepatic coma. *Brit. Med. J.* 1986; **293**: 1013.

12 Conn HO. Trailmaking and number-connection tests in the assessment of mental state in portal systemic encephalopathy. *Am. J. dig. Dis.* 1977; **22**: 541.

13 Conn HO, Leevy CM, Vlahcevic ZR *et al.* Comparison of lactulose and neomycin in the treatment of chronic portal−systemic encephalopathy. *Gastroenterology* 1977; **72**: 573.

14 Crossley IR, Wardle EN, Williams R. Biochemical mechanisms of hepatic encephalopathy. *Clin. Sci.* 1983; **64**: 247.

15 Cuilleret G, Pomier-Layrargues G, Pons F *et al.* Changes in brain catecholamine levels in human cirrhotic hepatic encephalopathy. *Gut* 1981; **21**: 565.

16 Davidson EA, Summerskill WHJ. Psychiatric aspects of liver disease. *Postgrad. med. J.* 1956; **32**: 487.

17 Dawson AM, De Groote J, Rosenthal WS *et al.* Blood pyruvic-acid and alpha-keto glutaric-acid levels in liver disease and hepatic coma. *Lancet* 1957; **i**: 392.

18 Dawson AM, McLaren J, Sherlock S. Neomycin in the treatment of hepatic coma. *Lancet* 1957; **ii**: 1263.

19 Ferenci P, Ebner J, Zimmermann C *et al.* Overestimation of serum concentrations of gamma aminobutyric acid in patients with hepatic encephalopathy by the gamma-aminobutyric acid-radioreceptor assay. *Hepatology* 1988; **8**: 69.

20 Fischer JE, Baldessarini RJ. False neurotransmitters and hepatic failure. *Lancet* 1971; **ii**: 75.

21 Frerichs FT. *A Clinical Treatise on Diseases of the Liver*, Vol. I, p. 241 Translated by C Murchison. New Sydenham Society, London, 1960.

22 Gitlin N, Lewis DC, Hinkley L. The diagnosis and prevalence of subclinical hepatic encephalopathy in apparently healthy, ambulant non-shunted patients with cirrhosis. *J. Hepatol.* 1986; **3**: 75.

23 Goldstein GW. The role of brain capillaries in the pathogenesis of hepatic encephalopathy. *Hepatology* 1984; **4**: 565.

24 Grimm G, Ferenci P, Katzenschlager R *et al.* Improvement of hepatic encephalopathy with flumazenil. *Lancet* 1988; **ii**: 1392.

25 Heredia D, Caballeria J, Arroyo V *et al.* Lactilol versus lactulose in the treatment of acute portal systemic encephalopathy. *J. Hepatol.* 1987; **4**: 293.

26 Horst D, Grace ND, Conn HO *et al.* Comparison of dietary protein with an oral-branched chain-enriched amino acid supplement in chronic portal-systemic encephalopathy: a randomized controlled trial. *Hepatology* 1984; **4**: 279.

27 James JH, Ziparo V, Jeppson B *et al.* Hyperammonaemia, plasma amino acid imbalance, and blood−brain amino acid transport: a unified theory of portal-systemic encephalopathy. *Lancet* 1979; **ii**: 772.

28 Jones EA, Schafer DF, Ferenci P *et al.* The neurobiology of hepatic encephalopathy. *Hepatology* 1984; **4**: 1235.

29 Laidlaw J, Read AE, Sherlock S. Morphine tolerance in hepatic cirrhosis. *Gastroenterology* 1961; **40**: 389.

30 Levy LJ, Leek J, Losowsky MS. Evidence for gamma aminobutyric acid as the inhibitor of gamma aminobutyric acid binding in the plasma of humans with liver disease and hepatic encephalopathy. *Clin. Sci.* 1987; **73**: 531.

31 Levy LJ, Bolton RP, Losowsky MS. The use of visual evoked potential (VEP) in delineating a state of subclinical encephalopathy. A comparison with the number connection test (NCT). *J. Hepatol.* 1987; **5**: 211.

32 Lo WD, Ennis SR, Goldstein GW, *et al.* The effects of galactosamine-induced hepatic failure upon blood−brain barrier permeability. *Hepatology* 1987; **7**: 452.

33 Lunzer M, James IM, Weinman J *et al.* Treatment of chronic hepatic encephalopathy with levodopa. *Gut* 1974; **15**: 555.

34 Maddison JE, Dood PR, Johnston GAR *et al.* Brain gamma-aminobutyric acid receptor binding is normal in rats with thioacetamide-induced hepatic encephalopathy despite evaluated plasma gamma-aminobutyric acid-like activity. *Gastroenterology* 1987; **93**: 1062.

35 Manghani KK, Lunzer MR, Billing BH *et al.* Urinary and serum octopamine in patients with portal systemic encephalopathy. *Lancet* 1975; **ii**: 943.

36 Martini GA, Phear EA, Ruebner B *et al.* The bacterial content of the small intestine in normal and cirrhotic subjects: relation to methionine toxicity. *Clin. Sci.* 1957; **16**: 35.

37 Morgan MH, Read AE, Speller DCE. Treatment of hepatic encephalopathy with metronidazole. *Gut* 1982; **23**: 1.

38 Morgan MY, Hawley KM. Lactilol versus lactulose in the treatment of acute hepatic encephalopathy in cirrhotic patients: a double-blind, randomized trial. *Hepatology* 1987; **7**: 1278.

39 Morgan MY, Hawley KE, Stambuk D. Lactilol versus lactulose in the treatment of chronic hepatic encephalopathy. A double-blind, randomized cross-over study. *J. Hepatol.* 1987; **4**: 236.

40 Morgan MY, Milsom JP, Sherlock S. Plasma ratio of valine, leucine and isoleucine to phenylalanine and tyrosine in liver disease. *Gut* 1978; **19**: 1068.

41 Moroni F, Riggio O, Carla V *et al.* Hepatic encephalopathy: lack of changes of gamma aminobutyric acid content on plasma and cerebrospinal fluid. *Hepatology* 1987; **7**: 816.

42 Mortensen PB, Rasmussen HS, Holtug K. Lactulose detoxifies *in vitro* short-chain fatty acid production in colonic contents induced by blood: implications for hepatic coma. *Gastroenterology* 1988; **94**: 750.

43 Mullen KD, Marin JV, Mendelson WB *et al.* Could an endogenous benzodiazepine ligand contribute to hepatic encephalopathy? *Lancet* 1988; **1**: 457.

44 Parkes JD, Murray-Lyon IM, Williams R. Neuropsychiatric and electroencephalographic changes after transplantation of the liver. *Q. J. Med.* 1970; **39**: 515.

45 Parsons-Smith BG, Summerskill WHJ, Dawson AM *et al.* The electroencephalograph in liver disease. *Lancet* 1957; **ii**: 867.

46 Patil DH, Westaby D, Mahida YR *et al.* Comparative modes of action of lactilol and lactulose in the treatment of hepatic encephalopathy. *Gut* 1987; **28**: 255.

47 Phear EA, Ruebner B, Sherlock S *et al.* Methionine toxicity in liver disease and its prevention by chlortetracyline. *Clin. Sci.* 1955; **15**: 93.

48 Phillips GB, Schwartz R, Gabuzda GJ Jr *et al.* The syndrome of impending hepatic coma in patients with cirrhosis of the liver given certain nitrogenous substances. *N. Engl. J. Med.* 1952; **247**: 239.

49 Potts JR III, Henderson JM, Millikan WJ Jr *et al.* Restoration of portal venous perfusion and reversal of encephalopathy by balloon occlusion of portal systemic shunt. *Gastroenterology* 1984; **87**: 208.

50 Read AE, Laidlaw J, Haslam RM *et al.* Neuropsychiatric complications following chlorothiazide therapy in patients with hepatic cirrhosis: possible relation to hypokalaemia. *Clin. Sci.* 1959; **18**: 409.

51 Read AE, Sherlock S, Laidlaw J *et al.* The neuropsychiatric syndromes associated with chronic liver disease and an extensive portal–systemic collateral circulation. *Q. J. Med.* 1967; **36**: 135.

52 Roche-Sicot J, Sicot C, Peignoux M *et al.* Acute hepatic encephalopathy in the rat: the effect of cross-circulation. *Clin. Sci. molec. Med.* 1974; **47**: 609.

53 Rossi-Fanelli F, Cascino A, Cangiano C. Branched-chain amino acids in the management of hepatic encephalopathy. *J. clin. Nutr. Gastroenterol.* 1987; **2**: 44.

54 Samsou Y, Bernuau J, Pappata S *et al.* Cerebral uptake of benzodiazepine measured by positron emission tomography in hepatic encephalopathy (Letter). *N. Engl. J. Med.* 1987; **316**: 414.

55 Schafer DF, Jones EA. Hepatic encephalopathy and the gamma aminobutyric-acid neurotransmitter system. *Lancet* 1982; **i**: 18.

56 Schomerus H, Hamster W, Blunck H *et al.* Latent portal systemic encephalopathy, I. Nature of cerebral functional defects and their effect on fitness to drive. *Dig. Dis. Sci.* 1981; **26**: 622.

57 Sherlock S, Summerskill WHJ, White LP *et al.* Portal–systemic encephalopathy: neurological complications of liver disease. *Lancet* 1954; **ii**: 453.

58 Sherlock S. Chronic portal systemic encephalopathy: update 1987. *Gut* 1987; **28**: 1043.

59 Silk DBA. Branched chain amino acids in liver disease: fact or fantasy? *Gut* 1986; **27**: S1, 103.

60 Summerskill WHJ, Davidson EA, Sherlock S *et al.* The neuropsychiatric syndrome associated with hepatic cirrhosis and an extensive portal collateral circulation. *Q. J. Med.* 1956; **25**: 245.

61 Takashi M, Igarashi M, Hino S *et al.* Portal hemodynamics in chronic portal–systemic encephalopathy. Angiographic study in seven cases. *J. Hepatol.* 1985; **1**: 467.

62 Tarter RE, Hegedus AM, van Thiel DH *et al.* Non-alcoholic cirrhosis associated with neuropsychological dysfunction in the absence of overt evidence of hepatic encephalopathy. *Gastroenterology* 1984; **86**: 1421.

63 Tarter RE, Hays AL, Sandford SS *et al.* Cerebral morphological abnormalities associated with non-alcoholic cirrhosis. *Lancet* 1986; **ii**: 893.

64 Uribe M, Marquez A, Garcia Ramos G *et al.* Treatment of chronic portal–systemic encephalopathy with vegetable and animal protein diets: a controlled crossover study. *Dig. Dis. Sci.* 1982; **27**: 1109.

65 Uribe M, Campoll O, Vargas F *et al.* Acidifying enemas (lactilol and lactulose) versus nonacidifying enemas (tapwater) to treat acute portal–systemic encephalopathy: a double-blind, randomised clinical trial. *Hepatology* 1987; **7**: 639.

66 Victor M, Adams RD, Cole M. The acquired (non-Wilsonian) type of chronic hepatocerebral degeneration. *Medicine (Baltimore)* 1965; **44**: 345.

67 Weber FL, Fresard KM, Lally BR. Effects of lactulose and neomycin on urea metabolism in cirrhotic subjects. *Gastroenterology* 1982; **82**: 213.

68 Weber FL, Banwell JG, Fresard KM, *et al.* Nitrogen in fecal bacterial fiber, and soluble fractions of patients with cirrhosis: effects of lactulose and lactulose plus neomycin. *J. Lab. clin. Med.* 1987; **110:** 259.

69 White LP, Phear EA, Summerskill WHJ *et al.* Ammonium tolerance in liver disease: observations based on catheterization of the hepatic veins. *J. clin. Invest.* 1955; **34:** 158..

70 Wright PD, Holdsworth JD, Dionigi P *et al.* Effect of branched chain amino acid infusions on body protein metabolism in cirrhosis of the liver. *Gut* 1986; **27:** S1, 96.

71 Zaki AEO, Ede RJ, Davis M *et al.* Experimental studies of blood brain barrier permeability in acute hepatic failure. *Hepatology* 1984; **4:** 359.

72 Zeneroli ML, Pinelli G, Gollini G *et al.* Visual evoked potential: a diagnostic tool for the assessment of hepatic encephalopathy. *Gut* 1984; **25:** 291.

73 Zeneroli ML, Cioni G, Vezzelli C *et al.* Prevalence of brain atrophy in liver cirrhosis patients with chronic persistent encephalopathy. Evaluation by computed tomography. *J. Hepatol.* 1987; **4:** 283.

74 Zieve L. The mechanism of hepatic coma. *Hepatology* 1981; **1:** 360.

75 Zieve L, Doizaki WM. Brain and blood methanethiol and ammonia concentrations in experimental hepatic coma and coma due to injections of various combinations of these substances. *Gastroenterology* 1980; **79:** 1070.

8 · Acute (Fulminant) Hepatic Failure

This is defined as a clinical syndrome resulting from massive necrosis of liver cells or sudden and severe impairment of liver function. Preceding liver disease is absent and, in the case of viral hepatitis, the syndrome should have developed within eight weeks of the onset of symptoms.

The problem is not only that of hepatic encephalopathy. Virtual hepatectomy does not lead only to portal−systemic bypassing of nitrogenous products coming from the gastrointestinal tract—although these play a part.

The prognosis is much worse than that of chronic liver failure, but the hepatic lesion is potentially reversible, and survivors usually recover completely. This makes intensive care and temporary hepatic support vitally important.

Causes

The most frequent cause is virus hepatitis A, B and non-A, non-B [19]. The proportion of the different types varies on the location, being about equal in areas such as the United Kingdom [18], compared with a high proportion of hepatitis B in countries such as Greece where the carriage of hepatitis B is higher [38]. In about 50% of hepatitis B positive patients, the fulminant course is precipitated by another factor, usually acute or superinfection with delta virus but sometimes a presumptive non-A, non-B virus infection [44]. In hepatitis B positive patients receiving chemotherapy for a coincidental malignancy the hepatitis B may reactivate and become fulminant.

Other viruses can cause a fatal hepatic necrosis in an immunocompromised individual. These include herpes simplex, [45] cytomegalovirus, adenoviruses [41], Epstein−Barr and varicella.

Hepatotoxic drug reactions comprise the next largest group. The most frequent culprits are anaesthetic agents, non-steroidal anti-inflammatory drugs, anti-depressants and isoniazid given with rifampicyn.

Carbon tetrachloride poisoning usually causes more kidney than hepatic damage. This is true of most industrial poisons although fulminant hepatic failure can follow occupational exposure to the solvent 2-nitropropane [21].

Acetaminophen (paracetamol) self-poisoning has a high mortality from acute hepatic necrosis (Chapter 18).

Acute alcoholic hepatitis can present with a picture of fulminant liver failure particularly in combination with therapeutic quantities of acetaminophen.

Mushroom poisoning is common in France and in areas where unusual fungi are gathered and eaten.

At full-term, pregnant women may develop fulminant hepatic necrosis due to eclampsia or fatty liver (See Chapter 25).

Vascular causes include an episode of low cardiac output in a patient with underlying cardiac disease, acute Budd−Chiari syndrome, and surgical shock with or without Gram negative septicaemia.

Massive infiltration of the liver with blast cells, as with malignant histiocytosis, can lead to fulminant hepatic failure [6, 54].

Acute Wilson's disease must always be excluded in any patient who is less than 35 years old.

Prognosis and causes of death

The survival of a patient with fulminant hepatitis reaching grade 4 or 5 coma is about

14–20% [15]. The variability reflects the number of patients studied: the smaller the series the better the prognosis for good results are likely to be reported. If only grade 1 or 2 coma is reached, 66% survival is expected. Early recognition is important.

Age greater than 30 years and the co-existence of other diseases worsens the prognosis. The outlook is best in children.

If any precipitant can be identified, particularly the administration of sedatives and tranquillizers, the prognosis is better. The patient improves as the sedative is eliminated.

The prognosis depends on the cause of the fulminant hepatic failure. If grade 3 and worse patients are considered, 40% of those with virus A, 15% with virus B, 10% with non-A, non-B, and 5% with drug-related disease will survive. The prognosis is best for the acetaminophen (paracetamol) overdose group.

The prognosis can be related to the time between onset of illness and coma. The outlook is poor if this is less than three weeks. With increasing duration of coma the chances of recovery become less. If recovery follows a course of less than four weeks, clinical normality can ultimately be expected. Prognosis depends on the capacity of the liver to regenerate. Those who survive do not develop cirrhosis [24].

Unfavourable clinical signs include a small liver [26] and ascites. Unfavourable laboratory tests include a prothrombin time exceeding 25 seconds at 48 hours and 39 seconds at 72 hours, a serum bilirubin greater than 22 mg/dl and hypoglycaemia.

Decerebrate rigidity, with loss of the oculo-vestibular reflex, and respiratory failure are particularly ominous features. Such patients if they survive may, rarely, be left with residual brain-stem and cerebral cortical injury [34].

Bleeding precludes liver biopsy. However, if essential, it may be performed by the transjugular route. Histology shows that the extent of hepato-cellular necrosis and of interlobular confluent necrosis are critical in determining outcome [14]. No single histological feature allows certain prediction.

The causes of death are bleeding, respiratory and circulatory failure, cerebral oedema, renal failure, infection, hypoglycaemia and pancreatitis.

Clinical picture

The neuropsychiatric picture is of stimulation of the reticular system of the brain followed by terminal depression of brain-stem function.

One of the earliest signs is change in personality. The patient may show anti-social behaviour or character disturbance. Nightmares, headaches and dizziness are other inaugural, non-specific symptoms. Delirium, mania and fits indicate stimulation of the reticular system. Uncooperative behaviour often continues while consciousness is clouded. The delirium is of the noisy, restless variety and attacks of screaming are spontaneous or induced by light stimuli. Violent behaviour is common. 'Flapping' tremor may be transient and overlooked. Fetor hepaticus is usually present.

In the later stages the picture is that of decerebrate rigidity with spasticity, extension and hyperpronation of the arms, extension of the legs and plantar flexor responses. Fits may occur. The plantar responses remain flexor until very late. Dysconjugate eye movements and skew positions of the eyes may be seen. Pupillary reflexes usually persist until very late. Respiratory and circulatory failure with hypotension, cardiac arrhythmias and respiratory arrest are other indications of depressed brain-stem function.

In the early stages jaundice bears little relation to the neuropsychiatric changes which may even develop before jaundice. Later, jaundice is deep. Liver size is usually small.

Vomiting is common but abdominal pain is rare. Tachycardia, hypertension, hyperventilation and fever are late features. The clinician must be alert to the delay in recognizing liver damage following acetaminophen overdose which may present after a period of two to three days or apparent clinical recovery.

Focal neurological signs, high fever or a slow response to conventional treatment should prompt a search for alternative causes of encephalopathy.

DISTINCTION FROM CHRONIC LIVER DISEASE (table 8.1)

A note should be made of any history of liver disease, duration of symptoms, the presence of a hard liver, marked splenomegaly and vascular spiders on the skin. A problem arises in the alcoholic where recent heavy drinking adds acute hepatitis to underlying chronic liver disease. In these circumstances the liver is large. Potential reversibility of acute alcoholic hepatitis merits more supportive effort in these patients than could be given to the usual end-stage cirrhosis where the liver would not be expected to regenerate.

Table 8.1. Fulminant hepatic failure: distinction between acute and acute-on-chronic types

	Acute	Acute-on-chronic
History	Short	Long
Nutrition	Good	Poor
Liver	±	+Hard
Spleen	±	+
Spiders	0	++

Investigations (table 8.2)

VIROLOGICAL MARKERS

Acute hepatitis A should be diagnosed by a serum IgM anti-A. Serum hepatitis B surface antigen is checked, but the IgM core antibody is necessary for certain diagnosis. HBsAg may have been cleared and HBsAb may not have appeared. Such rapid clearance indicates a favourable prognosis, perhaps because it implies a good immune response to the hepatitis B virus [5]. In those positive for hepatitis B, serum anti-delta should be sought.

Table 8.2. Investigations of acute hepato-cellular failure

Essential
Electro-encephalogram, electrocardiogram, X-ray of chest and abdomen, fluid intake and output

Biochemical
Store 8 ml serum for later use. Blood glucose (urgent), serum bilirubin, aspartate transaminase, albumin, globulin, immunoglobulins
Serum urea, sodium, potassium, bicarbonate, chloride, calcium, phosphate, alkaline phosphatase
Serum amylase

Haematology
Haemoglobin, platelets, WBC, prothrombin, blood group

Microbiology
Hepatitis B antigen and IgM anticore
Hepatitis A (IgM) antibody
Serum anti-delta
Blood culture aerobic and anaerobic. Sputum, urine, stool (culture and microscopy)
Store serum for virological studies

Additional (not always necessary)
Blood alcohol or other drug level
Cerebro-spinal fluid cells, protein and culture
Urine electrolyte concentration
Plasma fibrin split products, euglobulin lysis time
Hepatic scan

BIOCHEMICAL TESTS

Serum bilirubin level is measured as a baseline and to check progress. Of various biochemical variables, a serum bilirubin level exceeding 23 mg is the best predictor of non-survival [12].

Serum aspartate transaminase is measured initially but is of little prognostic value. Levels tend to fall as the patient's condition worsens.

Serum albumin is usually initially normal, but later a low albumin reflects a poor prognosis (fig. 8.1). In the recovery stage infusions of salt-poor albumin may hasten liver regeneration. Serum α-fetoprotein falls, rising with regeneration. The C_3 component of complement falls progressively.

Actin release follows hepatocyte necrosis.

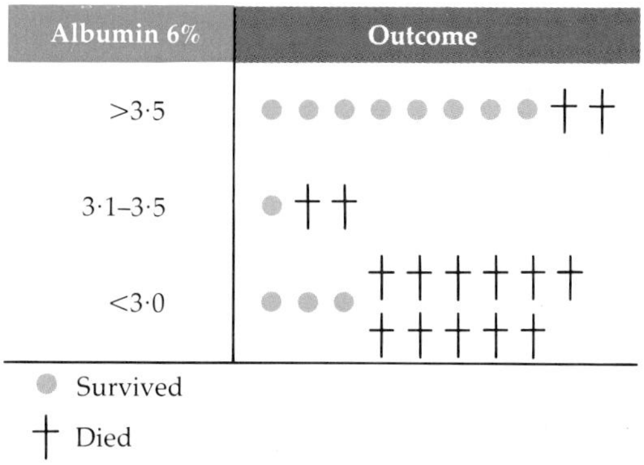

Albumin 6%	Outcome
>3·5	● ● ● ● ● ● ● ● ● ┼ ┼
3·1–3·5	● ┼ ┼
<3·0	● ● ● ┼ ┼ ┼ ┼ ┼ ┼ / ┼ ┼ ┼ ┼ ┼

● Survived

┼ Died

Fig. 8.1. Serum albumin levels related to prognosis in acute hepatic failure. Survivors usually showed more than 3.5 g serum albumin per 100 ml whereas fatalities often showed less than 3 g serum albumin per 100 ml. The patients with the lowest levels tended to have a longer history and to be in coma longer (Hillenbrand *et al.* 1973).

Serum monomeric G-actin, which forms high affinity complexes with group specific component protein is increased [28].

CEREBRO-SPINAL FLUID

Unless the diagnosis is in doubt a lumbar puncture is not necessary. Cerebro-spinal fluid glutamine levels are usually increased.

ELECTRO-ENCEPHALOGRAM (fig. 8.2)

This should be performed as often as possible. It may be used to assess the clinical state and to determine prognosis [25]. Normally the EEG correlates well with the clinical state, although early on it may be more severe than the clinical picture suggests and later may be abnormal for some weeks despite the patient's level of consciousness being normal.

Stage A is normal and the patient is alert. From stages B to D the EEG shows increasing amplitude while frequency decreases. The patient passes from drowsiness to coma. At stage D triphasic waves appear. These carry a poor prognosis. They are never seen in patients under the age of 20 years and are uncommon under 30. In the younger patient stage D abnormality is shown as high voltage, diffuse, slow activity. Beyond this stage recovery is unlikely. The amplitude decreases and the frequency does not change. Finally at stage F there is absence of rhythmic activity.

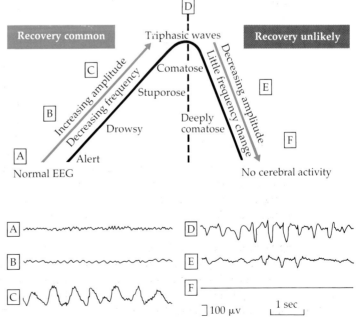

Fig. 8.2. Evolution of the EEG in liver failure. The progression from grade A to D is marked by increasing amplitude, decreasing frequency and increasing drowsiness. At D, triphasic waves appear and the interrupted line indicates the limit beyond which recovery is unlikely. From E to F amplitude decreases with little frequency change and at F there is no cerebral activity (Kennedy *et al.* 1973).

SCANNING

An isotope scan may show virtually no uptake by the liver. A CT scan shows a reduced liver volume. Localized low density areas correspond to necrosis.

Management (table 8.3)

Improvement in survival of patients with fulminant hepatitis in deep coma has come from attention to the details of good supportive care combined with better knowledge of the most important functions lost when the liver cell fails. These patients are rare and should, if at all possible, be treated in a special unit experienced in their management. The recommendations below apply to grade 4 or 5 coma and must be modified for the lower grades. Their early institution may prevent a less serious grade passing to a worse one.

Table 8.3. Management of acute hepato-cellular failure with coma

Problem	Treatment
Portal–systemic encephalopathy	No protein by mouth Neomycin 1 g orally four times a day Phosphate enema, then twice daily bowel washouts using 1% dextrose No sedation
Cerebral oedema	i.v. mannitol (100 g bolus) Continuous haemofiltration
Hypoglycaemia	100 ml 50% glucose if blood glucose falls below 100 mg Up to 3 litres 10% glucose per 24 hours 120–200 mEq KC1 daily (if normal urine output) Check blood glucose hourly
Hypocalcaemia	10 ml 10% calcium gluconate i.v. daily
Renal failure	i.v. salt-poor albumin Dialysis
Respiratory failure	Intubation (*not* tracheostomy) Ventilator Oxygen Maintain normal blood gases
Infection	No inguinal i.v. catheters No routine antibiotics Specific antibiotics only
Bleeding	No arterial puncture Cimetidine or ranitidine i.v. Fresh frozen plasma and platelets

GENERAL

The usual measures for the unconscious patient are adopted. The patient is barrier nursed. Attendants wear gloves, gowns and masks, and should be educated concerning personal hygiene and should have been vaccinated against hepatitis B.

Because of the risk of fluid overload the patient should preferably be nursed in a bed that can be weighed. They should be placed on fluid intake and output balance.

A large-bore catheter is introduced via the right arm into the right atrium. This is used for manometry, blood sampling and feeding. Arterial sampling should not be performed because of the risk of continued bleeding from the puncture site.

A nasogastric tube is passed. Because of the risk of mucosal erosion the stomach should not be actively aspirated but kept empty by gravity drainage.

All comatose patients should have an indwelling urinary catheter.

CLINICAL

The grade of coma (see Chapter 7) must be charted two-hourly.

Temperature, pulse and blood pressure should be recorded at least hourly and preferably continuously. In the later stages hypothermia may be due to brain-stem involvement.

Liver size is determined daily by percussion and the lower margin marked on the abdominal wall (fig. 8.3).

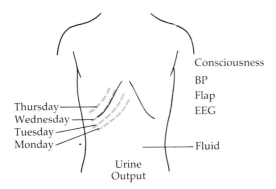

Fig. 8.3. Clinical daily check in patients with fulminant hepatic failure.

HEPATIC ENCEPHALOPATHY AND CEREBRAL OEDEMA

In contrast to the coma of cirrhotic patients, portal−systemic encephalopathy is of minor importance in patients with fulminant hepatitis. Blood ammonium (and presumably amine) levels are increased but do not correlate with the depth of coma or with the prognosis. Such estimates are not necessary for management. The routine treatment for acute portal−systemic encephalopathy is, however, given (table 7.4).

Sedation must be avoided if at all possible. If the patient is uncontrollable by physical means,

a small dose of lorazepam or temazepam may be given. All sedatives, however, are liable to increase the depth of coma.

Cerebral oedema, usually with brain-stem or cerebellar coning, is present at autopsy in about 80% (fig. 8.4). In a rabbit model of fulminant hepatic failure, brain-water increases in the cortical grey matter [46]. Astrocytes swell, but the blood−brain barrier remains impermeable to larger molecules [47]. In patients, the P_a co_2 rises and cerebral blood flow increases. Manometry shows a precipitous rise in intracranial pressure [16]. Death may be related to interruption of the vascular supply to vital brain-stem structures.

Clinically, cerebral oedema is predicted by poorly reacting pupils, paroxysmal hypertension and decerebrate posturing, all indications of brain-stem dysfunction. Monitoring of intra-cranial pressure is no longer performed, but at the earliest sign of brain-stem dysfunction a rapid intravenous infusion of hypertonic mannitol 50 to 100 ml (total 400 ml daily, maximum 200 ml per hour) should be given. If urine flow is not adequate, arteriovenous haemofiltration, preferably continuous, should be given [13].

When neurological features are fixed, CT is useful to diagnose cerebral oedema or intracranial haemorrhage.

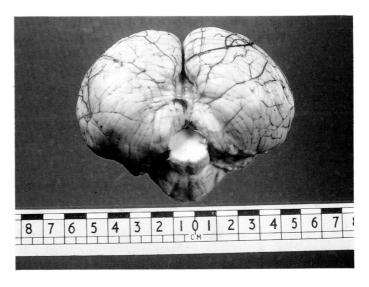

Fig. 8.4. Cerebral oedema in a patient who died in hepatic coma. Note the indented cerebellum.

Approximately 40–45 g protein daily are needed to prevent progressive depletion of body proteins which would lower resistance to infection. Production of neurotoxic amines such as tyramine may be suppressed by glucose feeding.

AMINO ACIDS

Amino aciduria is a feature of massive hepatic necrosis [51] and urinary tyrosine and leucine crystals are classical associations of 'acute yellow atrophy'.

The increase in plasma involves the aromatic amino acids, methionine, tyrosine and phenylalanine with low levels of the branched-chain ones (leucine, isoleucine and valine). The tyrosine increase is due to increased tissue protein breakdown and decreased hepatic oxidation [36].

Infusion of branched-chain amino acids has been recommended but is not of proven value.

HYPOGLYCAEMIA AND LACTIC ACIDOSIS

Frank hypoglycaemia is rare in fulminant hepatitis but can occur, especially in children. It may be persistent and intractable [43]. Plasma insulin levels are high. Hypoglycaemia can cause sudden death in these patients and is one aspect of the condition which can be treated satisfactorily.

If it is necessary to move a patient from one centre to another a 20% glucose infusion should be given during the journey.

On arrival the blood glucose is estimated by a quick procedure such as 'Dextrostix'. One hundred millilitres 50% glucose is given orally or intravenously if the blood glucose level is less than 100 mg/100 ml. Subsequently Dextrostix are used every hour and 50% glucose is again given if the blood glucose level is 90 mg/100 ml or less.

Ten per cent glucose is given continuously, up to 3 litres daily with added potassium chloride. Ascorbic acid 500 mg is given daily in the infusion.

Lactic acidosis develops in about half the patients reaching grade 3 coma. It is related to inadequate tissue perfusion due to arteriovenous shunting. Survival is reduced in patients with hyperlactataemia and metabolic acidosis.

ELECTROLYTES

Serum sodium levels tend to be low, falling markedly in the terminal stages. Persistent hyponatraemia reflects impending cell death. It should not be corrected with hypertonic sodium chloride unless there is clear evidence of a profound loss of sodium from the body.

Serum potassium tends to fall related to urinary losses, poor intake and high glucose feeding. A metabolic alkalosis follows and this potentiates ammonium toxicity. Potassium chloride supplements must be given both orally and intravenously. If urinary output is normal at least 120 mEq daily are needed. Later renal failure leads to hyperkalaemia.

Serum calcium values tend to be low and may reflect pancreatitis and hypoalbuminaemia. Ten millilitres 10% calcium gluconate daily are added to the intravenous infusion and another 10 ml for every unit of citrated blood transfused.

RENAL FAILURE

In the early stages blood urea levels may be reduced due to failure of Krebs' cycle enzymes in the liver. Later azotaemia is progressive. Many factors contribute and include jaundice, infection and haemorrhage—especially gastrointestinal.

Some 55% of patients develop functional renal failure with or without acute tubular necrosis [42]. It is marked by renal vasoconstriction and reduced renal prostaglandin excretion, indicative of an imbalance between vasoactive forces (fig. 8.5) [20]. If hyperkalaemia reaches dangerous levels haemodialysis should be performed.

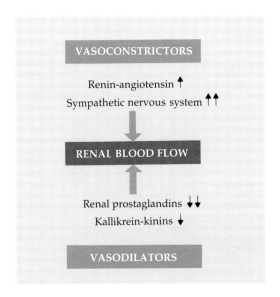

Fig. 8.5. Renal changes in functional renal failure.

Kupffer cell function may be reduced with failure to clear gut-derived endotoxins and these may contribute to the renal failure [11].

RESPIRATORY AND CIRCULATORY FAILURE

Early stimulation of medullary vital centres causes over-breathing, but later, depression of brain-stem function leads to respiratory arrest. Aspiration of gastric contents and haemorrhage into the lungs with infection add to the problems.

The respiratory alkalosis with low P_aCO_2 seems to be in some way beneficial, for coma increases if carbon dioxide is given. Metabolic alkalosis is added due to hypokalaemia, continuous gastric aspiration, and accumulation of basic compounds in the circulation.

Chest X-rays show abnormalities in over a half [48]. These include lobar collapse, patchy consolidation, aspiration bronchopneumonia and in a quarter non-cardiogenic pulmonary oedema.

An airway or endotracheal tube and a mechanical respirator should be employed at the first sign of an impaired 'gag' reflex. Tracheo-

stomy is not advisable. Hypoxaemia may be related to intrapulmonary shunting and to pulmonary oedema [48]. Oxygen by mask should be given routinely to the unconscious patient. Early ventilation should be considered to prevent pulmonary oedema.

Until terminally, the circulation is hyperdynamic and the cardiac output increased, due to a low peripheral resistance and increased arterio-venous shunting. Later, depression of brain-stem function leads to circulatory failure [52]. Bradycardia is ominous, and finally there is cardiac arrest. Arrhythmias and circulatory failure are frequent, especially with acetaminophen overdose.

An electrocardiograph should be taken and cardiac monitoring should be performed if possible.

Volume depletion should be guarded against as it enhances circulatory failure.

BLEEDING (fig. 4.1) (Chapter 4)

Bleeding is a frequent cause of death. It is shown by spontaneous bruising, bleeding from mucous membranes, from the gastrointestinal tract and into the brain. The patient often dies bleeding from everywhere and in spite of all therapeutic efforts. Portal hypertension may contribute [27].

Local trauma is avoided. Arterial punctures are not performed, the stomach is not aspirated, corticosteroids are not given.

Although it will not completely correct the bleeding tendency, vitamin K_1 10 mg is given daily, intravenously.

The prothrombin index is an excellent prognostic guide (figs 8.6, 8.7) [12]. Defects in clotting factors are repaired by fresh frozen plasma, fresh blood and platelets. Intravascular coagulation should be diagnosed only if fibrin split products are found in the blood and there is thrombocytopenia. Acute gastric erosions are frequent and prophylactic intravenous cimetidine or ranitidine should be given in full dosage [31].

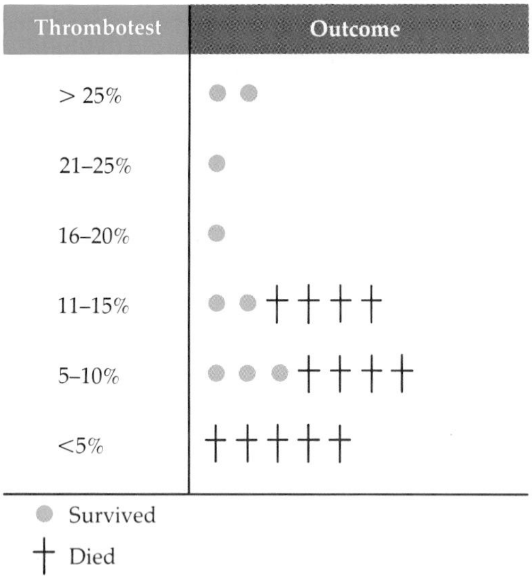

Thrombotest	Outcome
> 25%	● ●
21–25%	●
16–20%	●
11–15%	● ● † † † †
5–10%	● ● ● † † † †
<5%	† † † † †

● Survived
† Died

Fig. 8.6. Thrombotest before intramuscular vitamin K$_1$ related to outcome. Patients with less than 10% thrombotest usually died (Hillenbrand *et al.* 1974).

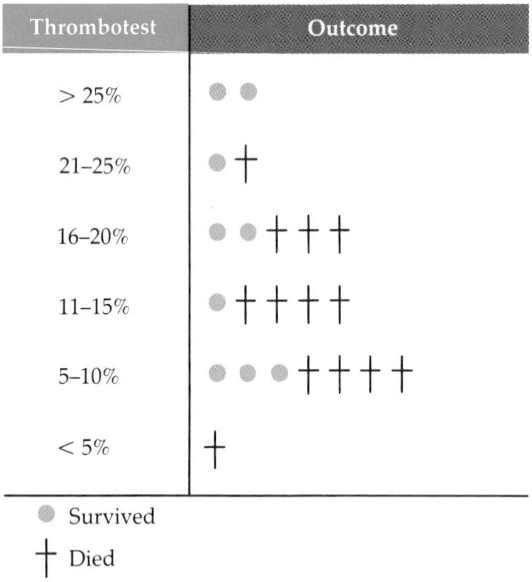

Thrombotest	Outcome
> 25%	● ●
21–25%	● †
16–20%	● ● † † †
11–15%	● † † † †
5–10%	● ● ● † † † †
< 5%	†

● Survived
† Died

Fig. 8.7. Thrombotest after intramuscular vitamin K$_1$ related to outcome. Despite the severe hepato-cellular failure many patients improved their thrombotest after treatment, but prognosis was still very poor in those with less than 20% (Hillenbrand *et al.* 1974).

FIBRONECTIN

This is a glycoprotein, synthesized by the hepatocyte, important as a non-specific opsonin for circulating micro-particles and involved in the formation of the haemostatic plug and in the integrity of the cytoskeleton. Low plasma values are found in fulminant hepatic failure, probably due to failure of hepatic synthesis and to consumption in the phagocytic process [3]. In the rat model of galactosamine-induced liver failure, early administration of fibronectin improved survival rate [33]. This treatment has not yet been applied to man.

INFECTION

Infection is frequent, particularly respiratory, urinary or related to intravenous therapy. Multiple venous catheters should be avoided. It may be Gram-negative or -positive and is an important contributory cause of death. Opportunistic infections such as aspergillosis may be followed by focal neurological defects and pneumonia in those receiving corticosteroids and intravenous antibiotics [50].

Susceptibility to infection may be related in part to deficiency of complement, or serum opsonization and/or chemotaxis [53]. Neutrophil adherence is reduced and contributes to the susceptibility to infection [4].

Potential pathogens were isolated from the inguinal area in 85% of patients with acute hepatic failure and this part should be avoided for intravenous catheterization.

Routine antibiotics should not be given, for these favour skin colonization with potential pathogens. Appropriate antibiotics are given when evidence of infection exists.

Betalactam antibiotics may cause convulsions. Aminoglycosides must be carefully monitored because of renal failure.

A blood culture is performed and repeated particularly while intravenous therapy is being given and the patient is comatose. Septicaemia is often clinically latent. Sputum, urine and stools should also be examined bacteriologically. All catheter tips are cut off and put into culture media.

CORTICOSTEROID THERAPY

Controlled trials have failed to show benefit for large doses of corticosteroids in fulminant hepatic failure; they may even be of negative value [15]. The complications include infections, gastric erosions and pancreatitis.

ACUTE PANCREATITIS [2]

Acute haemorrhagic and necrotic pancreatitis is frequent in patients dying with fulminant massive hepatic failure. It is difficult to recognize in the comatose patient but, rarely, it may be the cause of death. Serum amylase levels are raised in about a third of patients and these should be repeated frequently.

Aetiological factors include 'duodenitis' found with fulminant hepatitis, haemorrhage into and around the pancreas, the causative virus, corticosteroid therapy and shock.

Prevention includes cimetidine, the avoidance of corticosteroid therapy and keeping the stomach empty.

PROSTAGLANDINS

The liver can cyclo-oxygenate arachidonic acid leading to the formation of prostaglandins, thromboxanes and prostacyclin. Experimentally, exogenously administered prostaglandins can protect the liver both *in vitro* and *in vivo* against damage by such agents as carbon tetrachloride, galactosamine, acetaminophen and endotoxin [1]. Preliminary, uncontrolled observations suggest that infusions of 16−16-dimethyl prostaglandin E_2 are useful for fulminant hepatitis in man [30], but the treatment is extremely costly and not generally available.

Artificial hepatic support

There is no controlled evidence that any therapy, other than transplant, now in use for patients with acute hepatic necrosis in coma, is of value in salvaging life [7]. Supportive measures are of value. Many procedures lead to the patient

waking up, but only temporarily. Such measures apply only to patients with potentially reversible acute hepato-cellular failure. They cannot be considered for temporary resuscitation of an otherwise moribund cirrhotic patient, who would succumb within the next few months. Eventually they may have a wider application in preparing for hepatic transplantation.

The aim is to remove toxic metabolites and to keep the patient alive until his own liver can function satisfactorily. Results therefore depend on the capacity of the liver to regenerate. The factors controlling this process remain unknown.

Exchange blood or plasma [29] *transfusion* removes protein-bound, non-dialysable, toxic substances from the blood, or possibly adds essential substances made by the normal liver. Consciousness is often regained, but the overall mortality is unaffected.

Cross-circulation from a donor may not be ethically justifiable [10]. The treatment and benefit are only short-term.

Charcoal haemoperfusion. Blood from patients with fulminant hepatic failure is perfused over charcoal to remove circulating toxins. If perfusion is done early (in grade 2 coma) it seems to reduce cerebral oedema and increase survival [17]. However, at this stage, it is uncertain how many patients will in fact progress to grade 3 and worse. Controlled trials of these methods of artificial support have never been performed.

Rhone−Poulene haemodialysis system has a highly permeable polyacrylonitrile membrane which removes middle-sized substances (up to molecular weight 5000). Significant improvements in consciousness may follow its use, but percentage survival does not improve [37].

TREATMENT OF THE CAUSE

Any potentially hepatotoxic drugs should be stopped. Antidotes to acetaminophen should be given if indicated (see Chapter 18).

Interferon is *not* indicated for fulminant acute hepatitis B or Delta as the virus will have al-

125

ready been eliminated and the progression of hepatocyte necrosis is immunologically mediated.

Hepatic transplantation

Hepatic transplantation should be considered for patients reaching grade 3 and 4 coma due to acute fulminant liver disease. This depends on the local availability of the procedure and on the supply of a suitable donor at short notice. Fulminant hepatic failure is, fortunately, a rare condition and where possible, sufferers should be referred to a specialist liver unit which has access to liver transplantation.

It is difficult to judge the right time for transplant. If too early, transplantation may be unnecessary but the patient will be committed to life-time immunosuppression. If too late, the chances of success are reduced. The shorter the coma, and the less time on a respirator, the better the results [39]. Decerebration is the major obstacle to transplant and the major cause of failure [8].

A suitable candidate should be less than 55 years of age, have reached grade 4 coma, have increasing requirements of intravenous dextrose and fresh frozen plasma and no evidence of cerebral oedema or brain-stem involvement. A plasma factor V level less than 20% of normal together with grade 3 coma, predicts 95% mortality [5]. The patient should not have self-inflicted poisoning.

In one centre, the delay from decision to transplant to the actual operation was an average of 1.9 days [8]. This short time means use of donor livers which are not ideal, for instance, with incompatible blood groups, steatotic or enlarged. This worsens the results. Technically the operation is less difficult than that for chronic liver disease as collateral veins are not present and coagulation defects can be controlled with plasma derivatives and platelets.

Results from five centres show an overall survival of 65% compared with 20% in patients with fulminant hepatic failure who are not transplanted (table 8.4). Results in patients with hepatitis B are particularly satisfactory as the disease does not recur in the transplanted liver. However, several transplanted for putative non-A, non-B hepatitis have suffered acute hepatitis four to six weeks after the transplant but have survived without progressive hepatic disease [32]. Aplastic anaemia has also been a complication. Hepato-toxic drug reactions and acute Wilson's disease are the other major indications.

References

1 Abecassis M, Falk JA, Makowka L *et al.* 16, 16 dimethyl prostaglandin E2 prevents the development of fulminant hepatitis and blocks the induction of monocyte/macrophage procoagulant activity after murine hepatitis virus strain 3 infection. *J. clin. Invest.* 1987; **80:** 881.

2 Achord JL. Acute pancreatitis with infectious

Table 8.4 Hepatic transplantation for fulminant hepatic failure

Ref.	Number	Alive	A	B*	Non-A, non-B	Drug	Other
O'Grady	8	5					
Peleman *et al.*	12[†]	7		1	3	4	4[§]
Vickers *et al.*	16	9		1	11	1	3[¶]
Bismuth *et al.*	23	17	1	8	7	7	
Brems *et al.*	6	4	1	1	2	1	1
Total:	65	42 (65%)					

* Includes Delta virus superinfection.
† Includes subacute liver failure.

§ Acute Wilson's disease.
¶ Acute Budd–Chiari syndrome.

hepatitis. *J. Am. med. Assoc.* 1968; **205**: 129.

3 Almasio PL, Hughes RD, Williams R. Characterisation of the molecular forms of fibronectin in fulminant hepatic failure. *Hepatology* 1986; **6**: 1340.

4 Altin M, Rajkovic IA, Hughes RD *et al.* Neutrophil adherence in chronic liver disease and fulminant hepatic failure. *Gut* 1983; **24**: 746.

5 Bernuau J, Goudeau A, Poynard T *et al.* Multivariate analysis of prognostic factors in fulminant hepatitis B. *Hepatology* 1986; **6**: 648.

6 Beaugrand M, Trinchet JC, Callard P *et al.* Malignant histocytosis presenting as a fulminant hepatic disease. *Gastroenterology* 1983; **84**: 447.

7 Berk PD. Artificial liver: a baby delivered prematurely. *Gastroenterology* 1978; **74**: 789.

8 Bismuth H, Samuel D, Guggenheim J *et al.* Emergency liver transplantation for fulminant hepatitis. *Ann. intern. Med.* 1987; **107**: 337.

9 Brems JJ, Hiatt JR, Ramming KP *et al.* Fulminant hepatic failure: the role of liver transplantation as primary therapy. *Am. J. Surg.* 1987; **154**: 137.

10 Burnell JM, Dawborn JK, Epstein RB *et al.* Acute hepatic coma treated by cross-circulation or exchange transfusion. *N. Engl. J. Med.* 1967; **276**: 935.

11 Canalese J, Gove CD, Gimson AES *et al.* Reticuloendothelial system and hepatocyte function in fulminant hepatic failure. *Gut* 1982; **23**: 265.

12 Christensen E, Bremmelgaard A, Bahnsen M *et al.* Prediction of fatality in fulminant hepatic failure. *Scand. J. Gastroenterol.* 1984; **19**: 90.

13 Davenport A, Will EJ, Losowshy MS *et al.* Continuous arteriovenous haemofiltration in patients with hepatic encephalopathy and renal failure. *Brit. med. J.* 1987; **295**: 1028.

14 Desmet VJ, De Groote J, Van Damme B. Hepatocellular failure: A study of 17 patients with exchange transfusion. *Hum. Pathol.* 1972; **3**: 167.

15 EASL Study Group. Randomised trial of steroid therapy in acute liver failure. *Gut* 1979; **20**: 620.

16 Ede RJ, Gimson AES, Bihari D *et al.* Controlled hyperventilation in the prevention of cerebral oedema in fulminant hepatic failure. *J. Hepatol.* 1986; **2**: 43.

17 Gimson AES, Braude S, Mellon PJ *et al.* Earlier charcoal haemoperfusion in fulminant hepatic failure. *Lancet* 1982; **ii**: 681.

18 Gimson AES, Tedder RS, White YS *et al.* Serological markers in fulminant hepatitis B. *Gut* 1982; **24**: 615.

19 Gimson AES, White YS, Eddleston ALWF *et al.* Clinical and prognostic differences in fulminant hepatitis type A, B, and non-A, Non-B. *Gut* 1983; **24**: 1194.

20 Guarner F, Hughes RD, Gimson AES *et al.* Renal function in fulminant hepatic failure: haemodynamics and renal prostaglandins. *Gut* 1987; **28**: 1643.

21 Harrison R, Letz G, Pasternak G *et al.* Fulminant hepatic failure after occupational exposure to 2-nitropropane. *Ann. intern. Med.* 1987; **107**: 466.

22 Hecker R, Sherlock S. Electrolyte and circulatory changes in terminal liver failure. *Lancet* 1956; **ii**: 1121.

23 Hillenbrand P, Parbhoo SP, Jedrychowski A *et al.* Significance of intravascular coagulation and fibrinolysis in acute hepatic failure. *Gut* 1974; **15**: 83.

24 Karvountzis GG, Redeker AG, Peters RLL. Long term follow-up studies of patients surviving fulminant viral hepatitis. *Gastroenterology* 1974; **67**: 870.

25 Kennedy J, Parbhoo SP, MacGillivray B *et al.* Effect of extracorporeal liver perfusion on the electroencephalogram of patients in coma due to acute liver failure. *Q. J. Med.* 1973; **42**: 549.

26 Komori H, Hirasa M, Takakuwa H *et al.* Concept of the clinical stages of acute hepatic failure. *Am. J. Gastroenterol.* 1986; **81**: 544.

27 Lebrec D, Nouel O, Bernuau J *et al.* Portal hypertension in fulminant viral hepatitis. *Gut* 1980; **21**: 962.

28 Lee WM, Emerson DL, Young WO *et al.* Diminished serum Gc (vitamin D-binding protein) levels and increased Gc: G actin complexes in a hamster model of fulminant hepatic necrosis. *Hepatology* 1987; **7**: 825.

29 Lepore MJ, Martel AJ. Plasmapheresis with plasma exchange in hepatic coma. *Ann. intern. Med.* 1970; **72**: 165.

30 Levy GA. Use of prostaglandin E2 in fulminant liver failure. 1988 in press.

31 Macdougall BRD, Williams R. H2-receptor antagonist in the prevention of acute upper gastrointestinal failure in fulminant hepatic hemorrhage. *Gastroenterology* 1978; **74**: 464.

32 Maddrey WC, Van Thiel DH. Liver transplantation: an overview. *Hepatology* 1988; **8**: 948.

33 Moriyama T, Aoyama H, Ohnishi S *et al.* Protective effects of fibronectin in galactosamine-induced liver failure in rats. *Hepatology* 1986; **6**: 1334.

34 O'Brien CJ, Wise RJS, O'Grady JG *et al.* Neurological sequelae in patients recovered from fulminant hepatic failure. *Gut* 1987; **28**: 93.

35 O'Grady JG, Williams R, Calne RY. Transplantation in fulminant hepatic failure. *Lancet* 1986; **2**: 1227.

36 O'Keefe SJD, Abraham R, El-Zayadi A *et al.* Increased plasma tyrosine concentrations in patients with cirrhosis and fulminant hepatic failure associated with increased tyrosine flux and reduced hepatic oxidation capacity. *Gastroenterology* 1981; **81**: 1017.

37 Opolon P, Denis P, Darnis F. Assistance extracorporelle par hémofiltration continue au cours

des hépatites graves. *Nouv. Presse Med.* 1978; **7:** 2473.

38 Papaevangelou G, Tassopoulos N, Roumeliotou-Karayannis A *et al.* Etiology of fulminant viral hepatitis in Greece. *Hepatology* 1984; **4:** 369.

39 Peleman RR, Gavaler JS, Van Thiel DH *et al.* Orthotopic liver: transplantation for acute and subacute hepatic failure in adults. *Hepatology* 1987; **7:** 484.

40 Posner JB, Plum F. The toxic effects of carbon dioxide and acetazolamide in hepatic encephalopathy. *J. clin. Invest.* 1960; **39:** 1246.

41 Purtilo DT, White R, Filipovich A *et al.* Fulminant liver failure induced by adenovirus after bone marrow transplantation. *N. Engl. J. Med.* 1985; **312:** 1707.

42 Ring-Larsen H, Palazzo U. Renal failure in fulminant hepatic failure and terminal cirrhosis: a comparison between incidence, types and prognosis. *Gut* 1981; **22:** 585.

43 Samson RI, Trey C, Timme AH *et al.* Fulminanting hepatitis with recurrent hypoglycemia and hemorrhage. *Gastroenterology* 1967; **53:** 291.

44 Saracco G, Macagno S, Rosina F *et al.* Serologic markers with fulminant hepatitis in persons positive for hepatitis B surface antigen. A worldwide epidemiologic and clinical survey. *Ann. intern. Med.* 1988; **108:** 380.

45 Taylor RJ, Saul SH, Dowling JN *et al.* Primary disseminated herpes simplex infection with fulminant hepatitis following renal transplantation. *Arch. intern. Med.* 1981; **141:** 1519.

46 Traber PG, Ganger DR, Blei AT. Brain edema in rabbits with galactosamine-induced fulminant hepatitis. Regional differences and effects on intracranial pressure. *Gastroenterology* 1986; **91:** 1347.

47 Traber PG, Dal Canto M, Ganger DR *et al.* Electron microscopic evaluation of brain edema in rabbits with galactosamine-induced fulminant hepatic failure: ultrastructure and integrity of the blood–brain barrier. *Hepatology* 1987; **7:** 1272.

48 Trewby PN, Warren R, Contini S *et al.* Incidence and pathophysiology of pulmonary edema in fulminant hepatic failure. *Gastroenterology* 1978; **74:** 859.

49 Vickers C, Neuberger J, Buckels J *et al.* Transplantation of the liver in adults and children with fulminant hepatic failure. *J. Hepatol.* 1988; **7:** 143.

50 Walsh TJ, Hamilton SR. Disseminated aspergillosis complicating hepatic failure. *Arch. intern. Med.* 1983; **143:** 1189.

51 Walshe JM. Observations on the symptomatology and pathogenesis of hepatic coma. *Q. J. Med.* 1951; **20:** 421.

52 Weston MJ, Talbot IC, Howorth PJN *et al.* Frequency of arrhythmias and other cardiac abnormalities in fulminant hepatic failure. *Br. Heart J.* 1976; **38:** 1179.

53 Wyke RJ, Canalese JC, Gimson AES *et al.* Bacteraemia in patients with fulminant hepatic failure. *Liver* 1982; **2:** 45.

54 Zafrani ES, Leclercq B, Vernant J-P *et al.* Massive blastic infiltration of the liver: a cause of fulminant hepatic failure. *Hepatology* 1983; **3:** 428.

9 · Ascites

MECHANISMS OF ASCITES FORMATION

In 1896 Starling [67] suggested that the inter-change of fluid between the blood and the tissue spaces is controlled by the balance between the capillary blood pressure, forcing fluid into the tissue spaces, and the osmotic pressure of the plasma proteins, retaining fluid in the vascular compartment. There are thus two important factors in the formation of ascites, the plasma colloid osmotic pressure and the portal venous pressure (fig. 9.1). In cirrhosis, albumin synthesis is decreased. In many instances, osmotic pressure provides an accurate discriminant between those with cirrhosis and ascites and those without. Portal venous pressure is not so directly related to ascites. Patients with obstructed portal veins but a normal liver rarely suffer from ascites unless there is a co-incident gastro-intestinal haemorrhage or if for some other reason the plasma protein level falls [71]. The portal hypertension serves to localize the fluid retention in the peritoneal cavity rather than in the peripheral tissues [18].

Once formed, ascitic fluid can exchange with blood through an enormous capillary bed under the visceral peritoneum. This plays a vital, dynamic role, sometimes actively facilitating transfer of fluid into the ascites and sometimes retarding it. Ascites is continuously circulating, about half entering and leaving the peritoneal cavity every hour, there being a rapid transit in both directions. The constituents of the fluid are in dynamic equilibrium with those of the plasma.

In the dog, ascites can be produced by obstruction to hepatic venous outflow by constricting the inferior vena cava above the entry of the hepatic veins [11]. Hepatic lymph production increases and this extravasates into the peritoneal cavity. In cirrhosis, obstruction to hepatic blood flow by regenerating nodules on hepatic veins produces a post-sinusoidal obstruction and increased hepatic lymph production. In severe alcoholic liver disease, there may be actual sclerosis of the central hepatic veins. Some of the hepatic lymph enters the

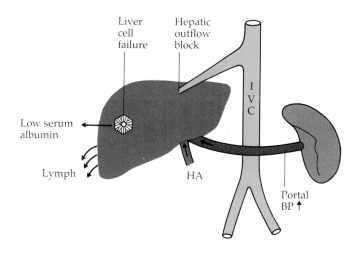

Fig. 9.1. Important factors for ascites production in cirrhosis are liver cell failure leading to a low serum albumin level, portal venous obstruction (pre-sinusoidal, sinusoidal and post-sinusoidal) and hepatic outflow block with over-production of hepatic lymph.

ascitic fluid, particularly when the transport capacity of the hepatic lymph system is exceeded [74]. Subcapsular and hilar lymphatics are increased in patients with ascites [4].

Renal changes

Cirrhotic patients with ascites retain sodium avidly, urinary sodium excretion being less than 5 mEq daily. Serum sodium levels are somewhat reduced. This does not reflect sodium deficiency for, because of the greatly expanded extracellular sodium space, the actual body stores of sodium are increased.

The mechanisms for the renal sodium retention are complex (fig. 9.2) [23].

Underfill theory. Traditionally, the kidney is believed to be responding to a contraction of the effective circulating plasma volume (that part of the total circulating volume that is effective in stimulating volume receptors). High portal venous pressure, the dilatation of the splenic vascular bed, hypoalbuminaemia and peripheral vasodilatation associated with arterio-venous shunting all combine to sequester fluid away from the central arterial tree. The kidney therefore behaves as if it thinks

Decreased cortical perfusion

Na+
Sodium retaining hormone

Reduced free water

Renin → Aldosteronism

Na+
K+

Collecting ducts ADH + H₂O

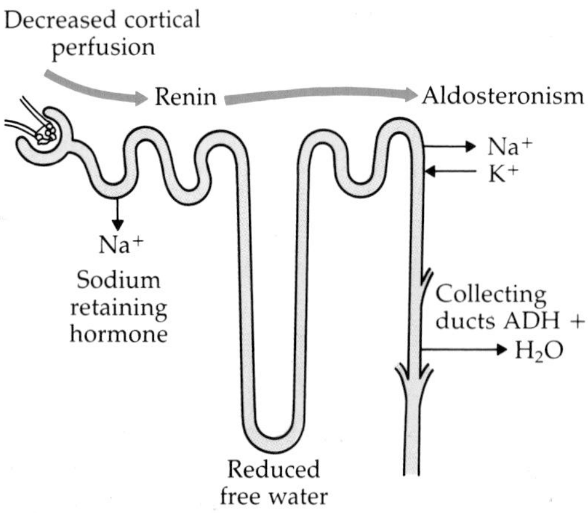

Fig. 9.2. Renal changes in ascites. Decreased renal cortical perfusion leads to renin release with aldosterone excess. Reduced extracellular fluid volume leads to sodium re-absorption. 'Free' water clearance is reduced. ADH plays a minor role.

its owner is underfilled and needs more salt and water [20]. Confirmation of this view has always been difficult as accurate measurements of effective circulating plasma volume in cirrhotic patients is not possible. Indirect confirmation comes from measuring the hormonal correlates of a reduced effective plasma volume. Such a reduction would initiate a baroreceptor reflex and plasma norepinephrine, a marker of peripheral sympathetic activity, would rise. This has been shown in cirrhotic patients who were unable to excrete a water load normally [8]. Plasma vasopressin levels are also increased, presumably related to baroreceptor stimuli related to volume [7]. Increasing the effective plasma volume by body immersion [22] or by peritoneo-venous shunting [56] may induce a diuresis.

Reduction of the effective plasma volume has various consequences (fig. 9.3). The renin–angiotensin II system is stimulated with release of aldosterone.

The sympathetic nervous system is enhanced with increased plasma noradrenaline levels. This may be responsible for renal vasoconstriction and some of the circulatory changes seen in cirrhosis [4, 34].

Non-steroidal anti-inflammatory drugs, such as indomethacin, which inhibit prostaglandin synthesis (cycloxygenase activity) are contra-indicated for they reduce glomerular filtration rate and renal water transport and lead to oliguria [23, 46]. Conversely, infusion of arachidonic acid increases medullary blood flow by enhancing renal prostaglandin production (fig. 9.11).

Bradykinin and other kinins synthesized in the kidney modulate intrarenal blood flow and renal sodium handling. Plasma prekallikrein levels are low in patients with cirrhosis and this may contribute to renal sodium retention [50].

Atrial natriuretic peptides are stored in atrial monocytes. They are released in response to expansion of the extracellular volume and/or a rise in right atrial pressure. Their role in ascites formation in cirrhosis remains unclear. Plasma levels have been reported as highly increased,

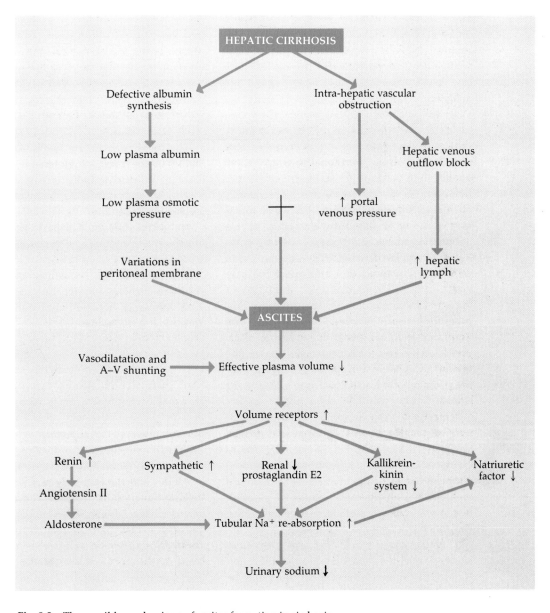

Fig. 9.3. The possible mechanisms of ascites formation in cirrhosis.

moderately raised [25, 29] and normal [73]. Cir-rhotics having head out water immersion, which increases effective plasma volume, show smaller (but insignificant) increases in plasma natriuretic hormone than normal [24]. It is poss-ible that cirrhotic patients fail to elaborate natriuretic hormone when the extracellular fluid volume rises.

Overfill theory. This propounds that inap-propriate renal sodium retention with ex-pansion of the plasma volume is the primary event in ascites formation [42]. As the portal blood pressure is high and the serum colloid osmotic pressure is low, the excess fluid is localized to the peritoneal cavity. This theory seems unlikely as volume expansion seems to

131

improve rather than impair urinary sodium and water clearance in cirrhotic patients with ascites.

However, it is possible that this overfill view is correct in the early stages when general and splanchnic vasodilatation results in increased vascular capacitance, arteriolar, capillary and venous. The mechanism of this circulatory change is uncertain. Secondary compensatory stimulation of the hormonal-pressor system would then attempt to maintain circulatory homeostasis in the presence of a tendency to hypotension [64]. Sodium and water retention would be an appropriate response to this stimulation which could be mediated by intra-hepatic baroreceptors stimulated by the rise in intra-hepatic venous and sinusoidal pressure [72].

Water excretion is defective because proximal tubular re-absorption of sodium is so great that none passes to the distal 'loop' site to allow 'free' water to be generated. It can be treated by giving an osmotic diuretic which flushes sodium distally and so allows free water to be cleared.

Serum potassium is normal or slightly depressed but the body's exchangeable potassium is decreased [16]. This is not only due to excessive loss of the ion from secondary aldosteronism but to failure of the cells to maintain their potassium content (cellular depletion). Reduction in total muscle mass is contributory. Diarrhoea is a factor in alcoholics.

A normal renal circulation and glomerular filtration rate are necessary for sodium excretion. In patients with cirrhosis they may be depressed by intensive diuretic therapy, by complicating renal disease, by increased abdominal pressure of tense ascites on the renal veins, by altered distribution of intrarenal flow [39], or chronic liver failure with hypotension [33].

Summary (figs 9.1, 9.3)

The two most important factors in the development of ascites are failure of the liver to synthesize albumin and hence a lowered plasma osmotic pressure, and portal venous hypertension. More fluid enters the peritoneal cavity than leaves it and ascites develops. This results in depletion of the effective intravascular volume which causes the renal tubules to retain sodium and water. Body fluids are again replete, more ascites is formed, and the whole cycle starts again.

The renal changes are mediated by stimulation of the renin—angiotensin—aldosterone system, an increase in sympathetic function, a rise in prostaglandin E2; the role of natriuretic peptide is uncertain.

An active role of the peritoneal capillary membrane in controlling the passage of fluid is possible.

The increase in intrasinusoidal pressure found in cirrhosis and hepatic venous obstruction stimulates hepatic lymph formation and this adds to the ascites.

Clinical features

ONSET

Ascites may appear suddenly or develop insidiously over the course of months with accompanying flatulent abdominal distension.

Ascites may develop suddenly when hepatocellular function is reduced, for instance by haemorrhage, 'shock', infection or an alcoholic debauch. This might be related to the fall in serum albumin values and/or to intravascular fluid depletion. Occlusion of the portal vein may precipitate ascites in a patient with a low serum albumin level.

The insidious onset proclaims a worse prognosis, possibly because it is not associated with any rectifiable factor. There is gradually increasing abdominal distension and the patient may present with dyspnoea.

EXAMINATION

The patient is sallow and dehydrated. Sweating is diminished. Muscle wasting is profound. The thin limbs with the protuberant belly lead to the description of the patient as a 'spider man'.

The abdomen is distended not only with fluid but also by air in the dilated intestines. The fullness is particularly conspicuous in the flanks. The umbilicus is everted and the distance between the symphysis pubis and umbilicus seems diminished.

The increased intra-abdominal pressure favours the protrusion of hernias in the umbilical, femoral or inguinal regions or through old abdominal incisions. Scrotal oedema is frequent.

Distended abdominal wall veins may represent portal—systemic collateral channels which radiate from the umbilicus and persist after control of the ascites. Inferior vena caval collaterals result from a secondary, functional block of the inferior vena cava due to pressure of the peritoneal fluid. They commonly run from the groin to the costal margin or flanks and disappear when the ascites is controlled and intra-abdominal pressure is reduced. Abdominal striae may develop.

Dullness on percussion in the flanks is the earliest sign and can be detected when about two litres are present. The distribution of the dullness differs from that due to enlargement of the bladder, to an ovarian tumour or a pregnant uterus when the flanks are resonant to percussion. With tense ascites, it is difficult to palpate the abdominal viscera, but with moderate amounts of fluid the liver or spleen may be balloted.

A fluid thrill means much free fluid; it is a very late sign of fluid under tension.

Secondary effects

A *pleural effusion* is found in about 6% of cirrhotics and in 67% of these it is right-sided. It is due to defects in the diaphragm allowing ascites to pass into the pleural cavity (fig. 9.4). This can be shown by introducing ^{131}I albumin or air into the ascites and examining the pleural fluid afterwards. A left-sided pleural effusion may indicate tuberculosis [44].

Right hydrothorax may be seen in the ab-

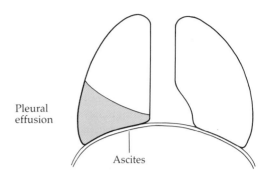

Fig. 9.4. A right-sided pleural effusion may accompany ascites and is related to defects in the diaphragm.

sence of ascites due to the negative intrathoracic pressure during breathing, drawing the peritoneal fluid through the diaphragmatic defects into the pleural cavity [57].

The pleural fluid is in equilibrium with the ascites and control depends on medical control of the ascites. Thoracentesis is followed by rapid filling up of the pleural space by ascitic fluid. Occasionally recurrent pleural effusions demand obliteration of the pleural space.

The lung bases may be dull to percussion due to elevation of the diaphragm.

Oedema usually follows the ascites and is related to hypoproteinaemia. A functional inferior vena caval block due to pressure of the abdominal fluid is an additional factor.

The *cardiac apex beat* is displaced up and out, by the raised diaphragm.

The *neck veins* are distended. This is secondary to the increase in right atrial pressure and intrapleural pressure which follows tense ascites and a raised diaphragm. A persisting increase in jugular venous pressure after ascites is controlled implies a cardiac cause for the fluid retention.

Ascitic fluid

Diagnostic paracentesis (of about 50 ml) is always performed however obvious the cause of the ascites. Complications, including bowel perforation and haemorrhage, can develop, rarely, after paracentesis in patients with cirrhosis [43].

Protein concentration rarely exceeds 1–2 g/100 ml. Higher values suggest infection. Obstruction to the hepatic veins (Budd–Chiari syndrome) is usually, but not always, associated with a very high ascitic fluid protein. Pancreatic ascites is also found with a high ascitic protein value. *Electrolyte concentrations* are those of other extracellular fluids.

Ascitic fluid protein and white cell count, but not polymorph concentration, increase during a diuresis [35].

Fluid appears clear, green, straw-coloured or bile-stained. The volume is variable and up to 70 litres have been recorded. A blood-stained fluid indicates malignant disease or a recent paracentesis or invasive investigation, such as liver biopsy, splenic venography or transhepatic cholangiography.

The *volume* of the ascitic fluid can be approximately estimated by a dilution method, but this is not usually necessary.

The *protein content* and *white cell count* should be measured and a *film* examined for organisms. Aerobic and anaerobic *cultures* should be performed.

The percentage of positive cultures can be markedly increased if ascitic fluid is inoculated directly into blood culture bottles at the bedside [63].

Tuberculous peritonitis should be suspected, particularly in the severely malnourished alcoholic. The patient is usually pyrexial. The cell count in the ascitic fluid is usually mononuclear. The deposit must always be stained for tubercle bacilli and suitable cultures set up.

Cytology of ascitic fluid is of little value. The normal endothelial cells in the peritoneum resemble malignant cells, so leading to an overdiagnosis of cancer.

The *rate of accumulation of fluid* is variable and depends on the dietary intake of sodium and the ability of the kidney to excrete it. Rate of fluid reabsorption is limited to 700–900 ml daily.

The *pressure* exerted by the ascitic fluid rarely exceeds 10 mmHg above the right atrium. At high pressures discomfort makes paracentesis obligatory. Vasovagal fainting may follow too rapid release of ascites.

A *low sodium state* may follow paracentesis, especially if the patient has been on a restricted sodium intake. Approximately 1000 mEq of sodium are lost in every seven litres of ascites. This is rapidly replenished from the blood and the serum sodium level falls. Water may be retained in excess of sodium. The patient collapses with weakness, abdominal distension, cramps, falling blood pressure, a low serum sodium and a raised blood urea level [43]. This syndrome is treated by 200 ml hypertonic (5%) sodium chloride intravenously.

Urine

The urine volume is diminished, deeply pigmented and of high osmolarity.

The daily urinary output of sodium is greatly reduced, usually less than 5 mEq and in a severe case less than 1 mEq.

Radiological features

Plain X-ray of the abdomen shows a diffuse ground-glass appearance. Distended loops of bowel simulate intestinal obstruction. Ultrasound and CT scans show a space around the liver and these can be used to demonstrate quite small amounts of fluid (fig. 9.5) [17].

Differential diagnosis

Malignant ascites. There may be symptoms and localizing signs due to the primary tumour. After paracentesis, the liver may be enlarged and nodular. The peritoneal fluid may be characteristic with a high protein content. A high serum-ascites albumin gradient exceeding 1.1 suggests malignancy. Lactic acid dehydrogenase levels may be high in the fluid. Ascitic cholesterol values exceeding 48 mg/dl suggest malignant ascites (37).

Tuberculous ascites. Abdominal distension is rarely great. After paracentesis lumps of matted omentum can be palpated. The ascitic fluid is

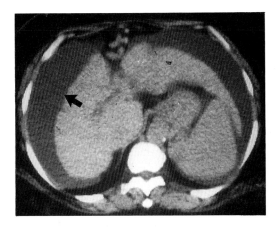

Fig. 9.5. CT scan showing an irregular cirrhotic small liver, splenomegaly and ascites (arrow).

of high protein content, usually with many lymphocytes and sometimes polymorphs. Tubercle bacilli may be cultured.

Constrictive pericarditis. Diagnostic points include the very high jugular venous pressure, the paradoxical pulse, the radiological demonstration of a calcified pericardium and the characteristic electrocardiogram and echocardiograph.

Hepatic venous obstruction (Budd–Chiari syndrome) must be considered, especially if the protein content of the ascitic fluid is high.

Ovarian tumour is suggested by resonance in

the flanks. The maximum bulge is anteroposterior and the maximum girth is below the umbilicus.

Pancreatic ascites. This is rarely gross. It develops as a complication of acute pancreatitis. The amylase content of the ascitic fluid is very high.

Bowel perforation, with infected ascites, is shown by a low glucose and high protein concentration in the fluid [58].

Spontaneous bacterial peritonitis

Infection of the ascitic fluid is very common. This may be spontaneous or follow a previous paracentesis. The spontaneous type develops in about 8% of cirrhotic patients with ascites. It is particularly frequent if the cirrhosis is severely decompensated. In most cases the complication develops *after* the patient is admitted to hospital. These patients are more likely to have gastrointestinal bleeding and renal failure and to require invasive procedures or therapy [15].

The infection is blood-borne, and in 90% monomicrobial (fig. 9.6). Patients with cirrhosis are predisposed to bactiuremia (see page 86). Ascitic fluid favours bacterial growth, opsonic activity is low, and resolution of infection by peritoneal macrophages fails [59]. Deficient

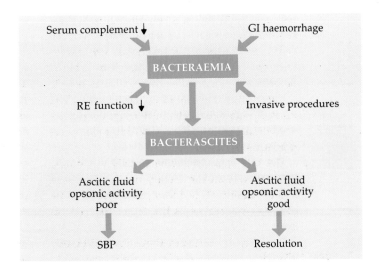

Fig. 9.6. The pathogenesis of spontaneous bacterial peritonitis (SBP) in patients with cirrhosis (Runyon 1987).

ascitic opsonins also lead to defective coating of bacteria which are indigestible by polymorphs. The opsonic activity of the ascitic fluid is proportional to its protein concentration and spontaneous bacterial peritonitis is more likely if ascitic fluid protein is less than 1 gm/dl [60]. It may be increased by diuresis [62].

Infection with more than one organism is likely to be associated with abdominal paracentesis, colonic perforation [58], dilatation [61] or any intra-abdominal source of infection.

Spontaneous bacterial peritonitis is defined as infected ascitic fluid in the absence of a recognizable secondary cause of peritonitis [36]. The ascitic polymorph count exceeds 250 cells per mm^3 and culture is positive. It should be suspected if a patient with known cirrhosis deteriorates, particularly with encephalopathy. It can develop in a fulminant form in a patient who previously had no ascites. Pyrexia, local abdominal pain and tenderness and systemic leucocytosis may be noted. These features, however, may be absent and the diagnosis is made on the index of suspicion with examination of the ascitic fluid. Broad-spectrum antibiotics should be begun (1) in all ascitic cirrhotic patients with a typical clinical picture of spontaneous bacterial peritonitis, (2) in those with greater than 250 polymorphs per mm^3 and the clinical picture compatible with spontaneous bacterial peritonitis, and finally (3) in those with greater than 500 polymorphs per mm^3 even in the absence of symptoms or signs of spontaneous bacterial peritonitis [19].

An easier diagnostic method is said to be finding an ascitic fluid pH of less than 7.3 [32]. The association of a pH less than or equal to 7.34 with a polymorph count greater than 500 per mm^3 is virtually diagnostic of spontaneous bacterial peritonitis [68]. Values less than 7.15 are associated with rapid death [2].

The infecting organisms are usually Gram-negative coliforms or streptococci. Other causes include meningococci [5], *Campylobacter fetus* [69] and organisms of the pasteurella group [30]. Anaerobic bacteria are conspicuous by their absence. Opportunist organisms are identified in the immunosuppressed.

Prognosis. This is grave, and depends on the severity of the underlying liver disease and of the additional acute hepatic deterioration resulting from the infection. This deterioration is shown by marked increases in serum bilirubin and creatinine and by a very high white cell count in the blood [35].

Only 21−38% of patients with spontaneous bacterial peritonitis who leave hospital will survive one year, and half of these will have a recurrence and half again will die of it [36].

Treatment. Monomicrobial infections will respond to cefoxitin, a second generation cephalosporin, for four days. A third generation, cefotaxime covers 98% of the causative flora without nephrotoxicity [24].

Treatment

Indications

The availability of so many potent diuretics and of the patient with obvious ascites who will respond to them may seem a challenge to the physician. Therapy is positive and the results are apparent to one and all. The initial gratitude of the patient and his family may be overwhelming. Nevertheless, although the initial response may be excellent, the ultimate result can be a patient in renal failure or hepatic encephalopathy, 'dry and demented' rather than 'wet and wise'. Indications for therapy must always be clear cut and caution must always be the working rule in deciding therapy.

The mere presence of ascites does not merit active treatment. Indications include:

Uncertain diagnosis. Control of ascites may allow such procedures as better abdominal examination, needle biopsy or venography to be performed.

Gross ascites, causing abdominal pain and/or dyspnoea.

Tense ascites so that an umbilical hernia has ulcerated and is near to rupture. This complication has a very high mortality. The patient may develop shock and pass into renal failure.

Cosmetic reasons are only relative.

Management

Unless the ascites is very slight the patient will have to be admitted to hospital for diagnosis and treatment. The control of ascites in patients with cirrhosis is more difficult than in other forms of fluid retention. Diuretic therapy is liable to be followed by electrolyte disturbances, encephalopathy and renal failure [1].

Restriction of physical activity reduces metabolites which have to be handled by the liver. Portal venous blood flow and renal perfusion increase in recumbency. The patient is weighed daily at the same time. Urine volume and body weight provide a satisfactory guide to progress. Urinary electrolyte determinations are helpful, but not essential. Abdominal girth is unreliable for gaseous distension is common. Serum electrolytes are measured twice weekly while in hospital.

The cirrhotic patient who is accumulating ascites on an unrestricted sodium intake excretes less than 10 mEq (0.2 g) sodium daily in the urine. Extra-renal loss is about 0.5 g. Sodium taken in excess of 0.75 g will result in ascites, every gram retaining 200 ml fluid. If the ascites is to be absorbed the daily intake of sodium must be restricted to less than 22 mEq (0.5 g) daily and even to less than 10 mEq daily. Fluid intake is restricted to one litre daily.

Diet: general remarks

1 Food to be cooked without added salt. No salt on table. Use salt substitute.
2 Use *salt-free* bread, crispbread, crackers or Matzos and *salt-free* butter or margarine—as much as you like.
3 Seasonings such as lemon juice, orange peel, onion, vinegar, garlic, salt-free ketchup and mayonnaise, pepper, mustard, sage, parsley, thyme, marjoram, bay leaves, cloves or low-salt yeast extract, help to make salt-free foods more palatable.
4 Omit anything containing baking powder or baking soda. This includes pastry, biscuits, cake, self-raising flour and ordinary bread.
5 Omit pickles, olives, ham, bacon, corned beef, tongue, oyster, shellfish, canned fish and meat, chutney, salad cream, meat and fish paste, bottled sauces, sausages, kippers and all cheese and ice cream.
6 Omit dry cereals, except shredded wheat, puffed wheat or sugar puffs. **Omit** salted canned foods. Regular canned fruit may be used in place of fresh fruit.
7 Meat or poultry, rabbit, tripe, sweetbreads or fish—4 oz (100 g) daily and one egg. Egg may be used as substitute for 2 oz (50 g) meat.
8 Do not use more than 10 oz (½ pint, ¼ litre) of milk daily. Heavy (double) cream is allowed.
9 Boiled rice (without salt) is permissible.
10 Eat fresh and home cooked fruit and vegetables of all kinds.
11 No candy, pastilles or milk chocolate.

Most protein-containing foods, such as meat, eggs and dairy produce, have a high sodium content and, to maintain a good protein intake, a low-sodium protein supplement should be taken, e.g. Casilan, Edosol or Lanolac. Salt-free bread and butter is used and all cooking is done without added salt. Many low-sodium foods are now available including soups, ketchups and crackers. It is possible to give a diet containing 1500–2000 calories, 70 g protein and only 22 mEq sodium (table 9.1). The patient should be virtually vegetarian.

Failure to adhere to a low-sodium diet is the usual reason for ascites to be termed 'resistant' or 'refractory'. In a severe case, even combinations of the newer diuretics in huge doses will not compensate for a high dietary sodium intake.

The patient may respond rapidly to this regime without the need for diuretics. Such *easy responders* are liable to be those:
● with ascites and oedema presenting for the first time—'virgin' ascites;
● with a 24-hour urine sodium excretion of more than 10 mEq;
● with a normal glomerular filtration rate (creatinine clearance);
● with underlying reversible liver disease such as fatty liver of the alcoholic;
● in whom the ascites has developed acutely in response to a treatable complication such as infection or bleeding;

Table 9.1. Specimen salt-free diet

Calories 2000–2200. Protein 70 g (approx)
Sodium 380–450 mg (18–20 mEq)

Breakfast
Shredded wheat with cream and sugar or stewed
    fruit
2 oz (60 g) salt-free bread or Matzos or salt-free
    Ryvita, unsalted butter, marmalade or jelly or
    honey
1 egg or 2 oz white fish
Tea or coffee with milk from allowance

Lunch
2 oz meat or poultry or 3 oz white fish
Potatoes
Green vegetables or salad
Fresh or stewed fruit

Tea
2 oz salt-free bread or Matzos
Unsalted butter, jam, honey or tomato
Tea or coffee with milk from allowance

Supper
Grapefruit or salt-free soup
Meat, fish or poultry as for lunch
Potatoes
Green vegetables or salad·
Fresh or stewed fruit or jelly made with fruit juice
    and gelatine
Heavy cream
Coffee or tea with milk from allowance

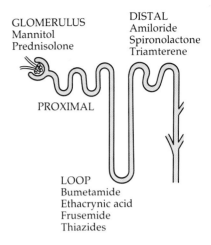

Fig. 9.7. The site of action of diuretics.

Table 9.2. Diuretics for ascites

Urine loss

Loop			
Na++	K++		Frusemide
			Bumetamide
			Muzolimine
Distal			
Na+	K		Spironolactone
			Triamterene
			Amiloride

● with ascites following excessive sodium intake, such as in sodium-containing antacids or purgatives, or spa waters with a high sodium content.

Diuretics

These should be given only if the weight loss is less than 2 lb (1 kg) after four days on the dietetic and fluid restriction regime alone. The dose and frequency of administration must be calculated for each individual patient.

Therapy is aimed at blocking all the renal sodium-conserving mechanisms. Diuretics can be divided into two main groups (fig. 9.7) (table 9.2). The first group comprises the thiazides, frusemide, bumetamide, muzolimine and ethacrynic acid. These are powerful natriuretic agents, but also powerful kaliuretics. Potassium chloride supplements are always necessary when these diuretics are given alone to cirrhotic patients. Loop diuretics increase renal prostaglandin synthesis and cause natriuresis and renal artero-dilatation with increased renal blood flow [52].

The second group comprises spironolactone (an aldosterone antagonist), amiloride and triamterene. These are weakly natriuretic but conserve potassium. When they are combined with a group I diuretic, the potassium chloride supplements are reduced and may even become unnecessary. In general it is advisable to start with one of these diuretics and then add a first group diuretic as required (fig. 9.8) (table 9.3).

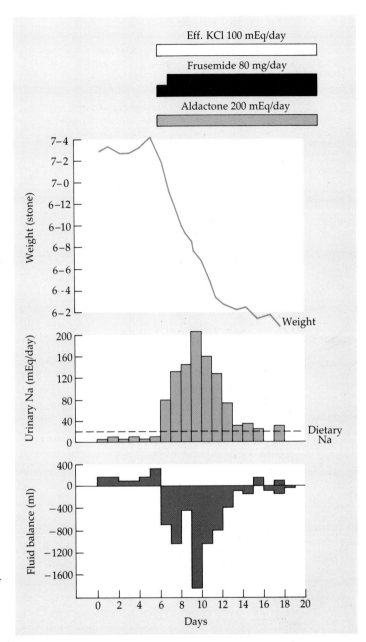

Fig. 9.8. Before treatment this patient with hepatic cirrhosis and ascites excreted less than 10 mEq sodium daily in the urine and was in positive fluid balance. He was treated with frusemide 80 mg and aldactone 200 mg a day with extra potassium chloride 100 mEq a day. A marked natriuresis ensued. Fluid balance became negative and body weight dropped 15 lb (33 kg) in two weeks.

The ease of control and choice of diuretics can be related to the 24-hour urinary sodium content on admission to hospital (table 9.3).

The choice of a diuretic from the first group depends on effectiveness, length of action, incidence of complications and cost. The longer acting diuretics, such as the thiazides and ethacrynic acid, have disadvantages in patients with liver disease because the action may continue when electrolyte disturbances have already developed. The patient may thus continue to lose urinary potassium and become more alkalotic even after stopping the diuretic.

A start is usually made with spironolactone

Table 9.3. Treatment of ascites related to 24-hour urinary sodium excretion

24-hour urinary sodium (mE)	Treatment
< 5	Distal and loop diuretic
5–25	Distal diuretic
> 25	Low sodium diet only

150 mg daily, and this usually induces a diuresis [51]. Long-term spironolactone causes painful gynaecomastia in cirrhotic males and should be replaced by 10–15 mg amiloride daily. Then, if necessary, frusemide or bumetamide are added.

Frusemide may be ineffective in the presence of marked hyperaldosteronism when sodium not reabsorbed in the loop of Henle is taken up by the distal nephron [51].

Satisfactory control is usual and failures are in those with very poor hepato-cellular function who are usually dead within six months of starting therapy (table 9.4). In such refractory patients diuretics have eventually had to be withdrawn because of intractable uraemia, hypotension or encephalopathy.

Complications are avoided by treating the ascites slowly and allowing at least two weeks in hospital. From time to time diuretics need to be stopped for a few days. The rate of ascitic fluid reabsorption is limited to 700–900 ml a day.

If a diuresis of some 3 l is induced, much of the fluid must have come from non-ascitic, extra-cellular fluids including oedema fluid and the intravenous compartment. This is safe as long as oedema persists. Indeed diuresis may be rapid (greater than 2 kg daily) until oedema disappears [53]. If the diuresis continues and exceeds the limits of ascites absorption in the

Table 9.4. Dietetic and diuretic control of ascites

No. patients	Controlled
157	148 (94%]
Failures all dead in 6 months	

absence of oedema, plasma volume will fall. Renal perfusion is reduced and the stage is set for the development of functional renal failure (hepato-renal syndrome).

In a few patients, on discharge from hospital, diuretics are no longer required. In the majority, however, the diuretic and dietetic regime has to be continued according to the individual needs.

COMPLICATIONS (table 9.6)

Encephalopathy

This follows any profound diuresis (table 9.6). It is usually associated with hypokalaemia [55]. There is an overall correlation with any form of electrolyte imbalance in patients with cirrhosis and perhaps most closely with hypochloraemic alkalosis.

Encephalopathy should be recognized early by daily examination for confusion and 'flapping' tremor. The diuretic is then stopped, serum electrolyte levels are checked, dietary protein is withdrawn and a purge given.

Electrolyte disturbances

These are frequent [65]. The development of a profound serum electrolyte abnormality with azotaemia indicates a very poor prognosis. This probably reflects the severity of the underlying liver disease. Large doses of potent diuretics in seriously ill patients with cirrhosis and ascites may induce a diuresis, but the 'hepato-renal syndrome' may be precipitated.

Hypokalaemia reflects not only diuretic effect but also secondary hyperaldosteronism. It is reduced by adding a potassium-sparing diuretic (table 9.4). The serum potassium level is an inaccurate but simple estimate of body potassium, particularly so in liver disease. Levels of less than 3.1 mEq/l indicate severe potassium depletion. Such levels necessitate stopping the diuretic and giving potassium *chloride* supplements.

Hyponatraemia reflects urinary excretion of sodium in excess of water in patients on a

Table 9.5. General management of ascites

1 Bed rest. 22 mEq Na diet. Restrict fluids to 1 litre daily
Check serum (if possible urinary) electrolytes
Weigh daily. Measure urinary volume
Add KC1 100 mEq daily

2 After four days if weight loss less than 1 kg start spironolactone 150 mg or amiloride 10 mg daily
Reduce KC1 to 50 mEq daily

3 After two more days check serum electrolytes
Add frusemide 80 mg or bumetamide 1 mg daily as required

4 After four more days check serum electrolytes. If weight loss less than 2 kg, amiloride 10 mg twice daily or spironolactone 300 mg daily

5 If necessary increase frusemide to 120 mg daily
Stop diuretic drugs if pre-coma ('flap'), hypokalaemia, azotaemia or alkalosis or weight loss more than 0.5 kg daily

6 Consider 5 l paracentesis repeated if necessary (table 9.7)

Table 9.6. Diuretics in cirrhosis—percentage of complications

	No.	Hepatic encephalo-pathy	Serum[†] K	Na	Urea
Chlorothiazide	31	22	55	40	22
+K sparer*	39	28	16	49	31
Frusemide	17	26	64	43	43
+K sparer*	24	4	16	40	40

* Spironolactone or amiloride.
[†] Serum potassium level <3.1 mEq/l, serum sodium level <130 mEq/l, blood urea level >40 mg/dl.

greatly restricted sodium intake. In the particularly ill terminal patient it may also indicate the passage of sodium into the cells. When combined with other electrolyte abnormalities it indicates a particularly bad prognosis and has similar significance to the terminal hyponatraemic state [33]. It is treated by stopping the diuretic and restricting fluid intake to 500 ml or even less per day. Alternatively, mannitol (2 litres 10% intravenously) will act as an osmotic diuretic and increase free water clearance.

The clinician may be tempted to give sodium supplements. In fact body stores of sodium and water are excessive and giving more sodium will only lead to gain in weight and pulmonary oedema. It is therefore contraindicated.

Hypochloraemic alkalosis complicates treatment with potent diuretics such as frusemide and ethacrynic acid given alone. It is due to urinary sodium and chloride loss with normal tubular reabsorption of bicarbonate. Hypokalaemia is not a necessary accompaniment. This complication can be treated only by chloride replacement.

Hyperchloraemic acidosis can complicate spironolactone therapy in alcoholic cirrhosis [27].

Azotaemia in cirrhotic patients reflects altered renal circulation (fig. 9.9) [39]. A brisk diuresis results in contraction of the extracellular fluid volume and accentuates this tendency. The greater the potency of the diuretic, the greater the azotaemia. When azotaemia is part of a profound electrolyte disturbance the prognosis is poor. Many of these patients will progress to the hepato-renal syndrome.

Follow-up advice

On leaving hospital the patient should adhere to the strict low sodium diet as far as possible. He should purchase bathroom scales and weigh himself daily, nude. A daily record should be kept and brought to the physician at each visit.

Diuretics should be continued. The dose depends on the severity of the liver disease. A usual routine is 100–200 mg spironolactone or 10–20 mg amiloride daily with frusemide 40–80 mg every other day. Potassium chloride supplements, about 50 mEq potassium daily, are given. Serum electrolytes, blood urea nitrogen and liver function tests are monitored every four weeks. As liver function improves it may become possible to stop first the frusemide and then the spironolactone or amiloride. Finally the low-sodium diet is relaxed, first to 'no added salt' and then to a normal diet.

Therapeutic abdominal paracentesis

In the 1950s paracentesis was the accepted treatment for tense ascites causing symptoms. In the 1960s it was abandoned because of the fear of complications which included the precipitation of hepatic encephalopathy, acute renal failure, symptomatic hyponatremia and acute renal failure. Moreover, the loss of approximately 50 protein in a 5 litre paracentesis led to the patients becoming severely malnourished. Most of these observations were not adequately controlled and confirmed and renewed interest came with the observation that a 5 litre paracentesis was safe in fluid and salt restricted patients with ascites *and peripheral oedema* [38]. No significant change in serum sodium, urea, haematocrit or blood pressure was noted. After 48 hours serum creatinine rose significantly. There was no change in plasma volume. This work was extended to daily 4–6 litre paracentesis with 40 g salt-poor albumin infused intravenously over the same period [54]. Paracentesis has been compared with spironolactone plus frusemide in a controlled trial [31]. The paracentesis group did not show significant changes in renal or hepatic function, plasma volume or other circulatory changes. The paracentesis group spent a mean of 11.7 days in hospital compared with 31 days for the diuretic group. Probability of requiring re-admission to hospital, survival probability and causes of death did not differ significantly between the paracentesis and diuretic groups.

A single large paracentesis, about 10 l in one hour given with intravenous salt-pure albumin (6 g/l ascites removed), may be equally effective (table 9.7) [70]. The albumin replacement is essential to maintain renal function and restore the decreased plasma volume [66]. It must be emphasized that the patients treated had fairly stable cirrhosis and 15 of 20 had peripheral oedema. This procedure should not be attempted in grade C cirrhotic patients or in

those with serum bilirubin greater than 10 mg/dl, prothrombin time less than 40%, platelets less than 40 000, creatinine greater than 3 and urine sodium less than 10 mEq per 24 hours (table 9.7).

Conclusions

Paracentesis is a safe, cost-effective treatment for cirrhotic ascites. It must not be done in end-stage cirrhotic patients or in those with renal failure. Intravenous salt-poor albumin replaces the protein lost in the ascitic fluid. Haemocell, an inexpensive, synthetic plasma expander may replace the albumin.

Sufficient ascitic fluid is removed to give the patient a flaccid, but not ascites-free abdomen. The paracentesis must be followed by a good salt-free dietary and diuretic regime.

Table 9.7. Therapeutic paracentesis

Selection:	Tense ascites
	Preferably with oedema
	Child's grade B
	Prothrombin > 40%
	Serum bilirubin < 10 mg/dl
	Platelets > 40 000/mm^3
	Serum creatinine < 3 mg/dl
	Urinary sodium > 10 mEq/24 hours
Routine:	In hospital
	Volume removed 5–10 litres
	IV salt-poor albumin 10 g/l removed

Refractory ascites

The majority of patients will respond to the dietary diuretic regime (table 9.5). Failures indicate either failure to comply or such severe liver failure that the patient is terminal. In some patients, however, ascites is gross and diuretics have to be pushed to extreme doses in an attempt to produce a diuresis. In such refractory patients there is particular danger of depletion of the intravascular compartment and the development of the hepato-renal syndrome.

In these resistant cases alternative therapy must be considered. The infusion of salt-poor albumin or ascitic fluid itself expands the plasma volume and may initiate diuresis, albeit temporarily.

Ascites ultrafiltration and re-infusion [49]

The automated ultrafiltration apparatus (Rhodiascit) removes ascitic fluid via a peritoneal dialysis catheter and passes it over an ultrafilter which selects molecules of less than 50 000. The concentrate, which contains 2−4 times as much protein as the ascitic fluid, is returned to the patient intravenously. Up to 13 litres of ascites can be removed in 24 hours. Weight loss is greater than would be accounted for by the volume of fluid ultrafiltered because the urine flow increases during and afterwards. The procedure is costly, but this must be weighed against the price of a longer stay in hospital.

LE VEEN SHUNT

The peritoneal venous shunt system gives continuous treatment over many months [41]. The aim is to produce sustained expansion of the circulating blood volume by continuous passage of ascitic fluid from the peritoneal cavity to the general circulation. The expanded blood volume is confirmed by the fall in plasma levels of renin, angiotensin, noradrenalin and antidiuretic hormone [19]. Renal function and nutrition improved [9, 14].

The peritoneal cavity is drained by a long, perforated, plastic tube that reaches into the pelvis. This connects with a pressure-sensitive valve lying extra-peritoneally and deep through the abdominal muscles. This again connects with a silicone rubber tube which passes subcutaneously from the abdominal wound towards the neck and so into the internal jugular vein. The end of the tube is left in position in the superior vena cava. The operation is performed under antibiotic cover with light general anaesthetic. As the diaphragm descends during inspiration the intra-peritoneal fluid pressure rises whereas that in the intrathoracic superior vena cava falls. This results in a pressure differential of about 5 cm H_2O. Respiration provides the force which opens the valve and propels the fluid into the superior vena cava. The venous tube remains patent only when its interior contains ascitic fluid. The specially designed pressure-sensitive valve totally prevents entry of blood into the venous tubing.

In a few patients the technique undoubtedly controls ascites for long periods. However, there are many complications. The operative mortality is about 13%. Shunt patency may be assessed by injecting isotopic contrast material into the ascitic fluid and following its passage into the neck but only 25−50% remain patent at one year. Disseminated intravascular coagulation always occurs and may be severe and fatal. It may be due to ascitic pro-coagulants and even collagen [3] in the ascitic fluid. Removal of ascites and replacement with saline before introducing the shunt may be a useful preventative measure. Other early complications include ascitic leaks and peritonitis. Bleeding from oesophageal varices and pulmonary oedema may develop. Later about a quarter develop infections of all types including right-sided endocarditis. Shunt dysfunction with occlusion and thrombosis leads to many hospital admissions [21]. The intra-peritoneal tube may produce sufficient peritoneal fibrosis to cause intestinal obstruction. The procedure is of no value in the hepato-renal syndrome [21].

In a multi-centre controlled study, treatment by the Le Veen shunt was not superior to paracentesis with or without diuretics [12]. At one month the Le Veen shunt was more effective treatment, but survival was reduced. At one year reduction of ascites and survival were the same for both groups. The Le Veen shunt is not a panacea for treating ascites [21]. It should only be considered in those with truly refractory ascites who have failed to respond to conventional management. Grade C (advanced) patients are not suitable.

Prognosis

Despite modern dietetic and diuretic measures the prognosis is always grave after ascites develops in a patient with cirrhosis. It is better if the ascites has accumulated rapidly, especially if there is a well defined precipitating factor such as gastrointestinal haemorrhage.

Even with adequate treatment, a patient with cirrhosis developing ascites has only a 40% chance of being alive two years later. Much depends on the major factor in the aetiology of the fluid retention. If liver cell failure, evidenced by jaundice and hepatic encephalopathy, is severe, the prognosis is poor. If the major factor is a particularly high portal pressure, the patient may respond well to treatment. The prognosis is also inversely proportional to the ability to excrete a water load [64].

Ascites cannot be divorced from the underlying liver disease that caused it and, although it may be controlled, the patient is still liable to die from another complication such as haemorrhage, hepatic coma or primary liver cancer. It is questioned whether control of ascites *per se* increases lifespan. It certainly makes the patient more comfortable.

Functional renal failure ('hepato-renal syndrome')

Renal failure in patients with hepato-cellular failure may be due to primary kidney disease or acute tubular necrosis due to haemorrhage or infection. However, in most instances the uraemia and oliguria arise either spontaneously or in response to changes in blood volume or shifts of fluid within body compartments. The histology of the kidney is virtually normal and the failure is a functional one. Such kidneys have even been successfully transplanted when they functioned normally [40]. Conversely, apparently moribund patients with this syndrome have returned to normal kidney function after liver transplantation.

The syndrome is marked by renal failure with normal tubular function in a patient with chronic liver disease (table 9.8). It usually, but

Table 9.8. Diagnosis of hepato-renal syndrome

Chronic liver disease with ascites
Slow onset azotaemia (plasma creatinine > 1.5 mg/dl)
Tubular function good
    Urine to plasma osmolarity ratio > 1.0
    Urine to plasma creatinine ratio > 30
    Urine sodium concentration < 10 mEq/dl
No sustained benefit by expansion of intravascular space

not always, affects patients with alcoholic cirrhosis. The patient is seldom admitted with the hepato-renal syndrome, but it develops probably due to events in hospital acting as precipitants.

The renal failure is often initiated by reduction in the intravascular volume due to over-vigorous diuretic therapy, paracentesis or diarrhoea. It may develop without a precipitant. The classical features of uraemia are usually absent. The syndrome is particularly common in patients with end-stage alcoholic cirrhosis. The prognosis is extremely grave.

In the mildest pre-azotaemic stage, renal dysfunction is shown by failure to excrete a water load, reduction in urinary sodium excretion and hyponatraemia. Hepatic dysfunction is usually severe and ascites is usual.

The more advanced stages are characterized by progressive azotaemia, usually with hepatic failure and ascites difficult to control. The patient complains of anorexia, weakness and fatigue. The blood urea concentration is raised. Hyponatraemia is invariable. Sodium is avidly re-absorbed by the renal tubules and urine osmolarity is increased. Fluid accumulates in spite of a normal urinary volume, dietary sodium restriction and diuretic therapy. In the later stages nausea, vomiting and thirst are added. The patient is drowsy. The picture may be indistinguishable from that of hepatic encephalopathy.

The serum urea and creatinine levels rise progressively. The serum sodium is usually less than 120 mEq/l. Urinalysis is virtually normal. Urinary sodium excretion is very low.

Acute tubular damage may co-exist and urinary $\beta 2$ microglobulin may be a useful diagnostic test [13]. Ascites is refractory. Terminally, coma deepens, blood pressure drops and urine volume falls even more. The terminal stages last from a few days to more than six weeks.

It may be difficult to distinguish hepatic from renal failure although the patients die with biochemical azotaemia rather than the full clinical picture of kidney failure. Death is due to liver failure; survival depends on the reversibility of the *liver* disease.

Iatrogenic renal failure in a cirrhotic patient must be diagnosed from genuine hepato-renal syndrome as the prognosis is different and effective treatment is possible (table 9.9). The causes include diuretic overdose and severe diarrhoea due, for instance, to lactulose [47]. Non-steroidal anti-inflammatory drugs reduce renal prostaglandin production so reducing glomerular filtration rate and free water clearance [28]. Nephrotoxic drug effects, due to such drugs as cyclosporin, the aminoglycosides or dimeclocycline, are diagnosed by measuring urinary β_2 microglobulins [13]. Glomerular mesangial IgA deposits, accompanied by complement deposition, complicate cirrhosis, usually in the alcoholic. They are diagnosed by finding proteinuria with microhaematuria and casts [48].

Table 9.9. Iatrogenic hepato-renal syndrome

Drugs	Treat
Diuretics	Volume expansion
Lactulose	Volume expansion
NSAIF (prostaglandin inhibition)	Stop drug
Aminoglycosides	Diagnose urine β_2-microglobulins
Cyclosporin	Haemodialysis

Mechanisms

Renal failure is related to a reduction of effective renal circulation (see fig. 9.9). Cardiac output is normal or even increased but is distributed to skin, splanchnic area, spleen and brain so that renal plasma flow is reduced. Changes in intrarenal circulation are of great importance. An increased pre-glomerular vascular resistance leads to reduced glomerular filtration rate and plasma renin rises. Blood flow is thus diverted away from the renal cortex (see fig. 9.10) [39]. This change in intrarenal distribution of blood flow can be shown even in well-

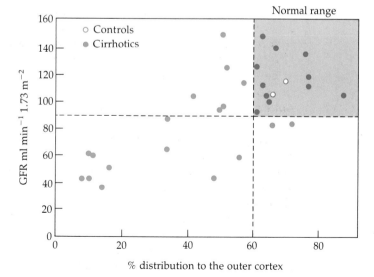

Fig. 9.9. Distribution of renal blood flow measured by injection of ^{133}xenon into the renal artery and external counting. Cirrhotic patients tend to have reduced distribution of renal blood to the outer cortex and this may be present with a normal creatinine clearance (GFR) (Kew *et al.* 1971).

compensated cirrhotic patients. It may explain their susceptibility to develop oliguric renal failure after haemorrhage not sufficiently large to reduce the blood pressure or after minor shifts of fluid within body compartments, such as with abdominal paracentesis or diuretic therapy. Reduced effective plasma volume may be a factor. Volume expansion may increase renal blood flow and institute a diuresis, but the response is not maintained and variceal haemorrhage may be precipitated.

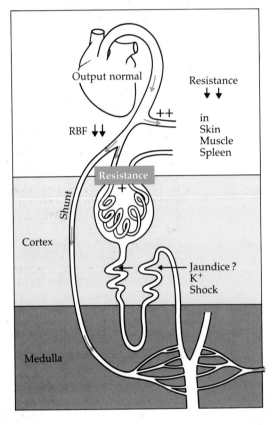

Fig. 9.10. Factors contributing to renal failure in cirrhosis ('hepato-renal syndrome').

The cause of the increased pre-glomerular vascular resistance is unknown. Hepato-renal syndrome can be regarded as an imbalance between systemic vasodilators and renal vaso-constricting mechanisms (fig. 9.11).

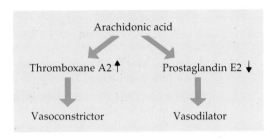

Fig. 9.11. Urinary changes in the hepato-renal syndrome.

Thromboxane A2, a metabolite of arachidonic acid, is a potent vasoconstrictor. Its metabolite thromboxane B2, is markedly increased in the urine of patients with the hepato-renal syndrome. Prostaglandin E2, another metabolite of arachidonic acid, is a vasodilator, and urinary excretion of this is decreased. An imbalance of the renal kallikrein−kinin system may also be involved in the maintenance of renal blood flow in cirrhotic patients with ascites. Impaired renal production of kallikrein and prostaglandins in the setting of activation of the renin−angiotensin and sympathetic nervous systems may lead to functional renal failure [50].

Treatment

The syndrome is prevented by avoiding diuretic overdose, by treating ascites slowly and by early recognition of any complication such as electrolyte imbalance, haemorrhage or infection. The conservative management is that of renal and hepatic failure whatever the cause. Hepatic failure holds the key to the problem and must be treated. Conservative measures include restriction of fluids, sodium, potassium and protein, and withdrawal of potentially nephrotoxic drugs such as the aminoglycosides. Blood cultures should be taken and any septicaemia treated appropriately. Mannitol is useless and may lead to intracellular acidosis. High doses of frusemide are unavailing. Renal dialysis does not improve survival and may precipitate gastrointestinal haemorrhage and shock.

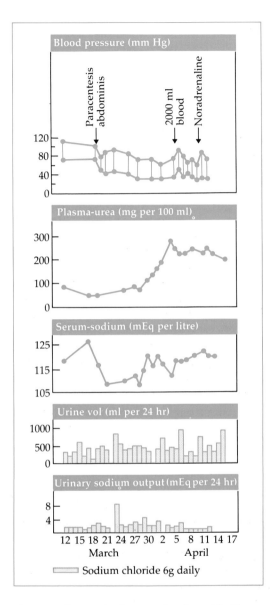

Fig. 9.12. Terminal sub-acute virus hepatitis. Note the low blood pressure which was only temporarily increased by blood transfusion and noradrenaline. Serum sodium values and urinary sodium excretion were profoundly depressed and were uninfluenced by oral sodium chloride. Blood urea rose progressively in the last two weeks (Hecker & Sherlock 1956).

The renal cortical circulatory failure has been related to the action of false neurotransmitter amines of intestinal origin [26]. This has led to the administration of such drugs as L-dopa or metaraminol; they have not been successful.

Terminal hyponatraemia [33] is in part dilutional (over-hydration), in part due to over-administration of diuretics and in part to redistribution of sodium, a raised proportion occurring in the intracellular compartments. It should not be treated with intravenous hypertonic sodium chloride as pulmonary oedema will develop and death will be accelerated (fig. 9.12).

The final combination of azotaemia, hyponatraemia and hypotension is terminal and quite unresponsive to all forms of therapy.

References

1 Arroyo V, Gines P, Rodès J. Treatment of ascites in patients with cirrhosis of the liver. *J. Hepatol.* 1986; **2:** 504.

2 Attali P, Turner K, Pelletier G *et al.* pH of ascitic fluid: diagnostic and prognostic value in cirrhotic and non-cirrhotic patients. *Gastroenterology* 1986; **90:** 1255.

3 Baele G, Rasquin K, Barbier F. Coagulant, fibrinolytic, and aggregating activity in ascitic fluid. *Am. J. Gastroenterol.* 1986; **81:** 440.

4 Baggenstoss AH, Cain JC. The hepatic hilar lymphatics of man. *N. Engl. J. Med.* 1957; **256:** 531.

5 Bar-Meir S, Chojkier M, Groszmann RJ *et al.* Spontaneous meningococcal peritonitis; a report of two cases. *Am. J. dig. Dis.* 1978; **23:** 119.

6 Bernardi M, Trevisani C, Santini C *et al.* Plasma norepinephrine, weak neurotransmitters and renin activity during active tilting in liver cirrhosis; relationship with cardiovascular homeostasis and renal function. *Hepatology 1983;* **3:** 56.

7 Bichet D, Szatalowicz V, Chaimovitz C *et al.* Role of vasopressin in abnormal water excretion in cirrhotic patients. *Ann. intern. Med.* 1982; **96:** 413.

8 Bichet DG, Van Putten VJ, Schrier RW. Potential role of increased sympathetic activity in impaired sodium and water excretion in cirrhosis. *N. Engl. J. Med.* 1982; **307:** 1552.

9 Blendis LM, Harrison JE, Russell DM *et al.* Effects of peritoneovenous shunting on body composition. *Gastroenterology* 1986; **90:** 127.

10 Blendis LM, Sole MJ, Campbell P *et al.* The effect of peritoneovenous shunting on catecholamine metabolism in patients with hepatic ascites. *Hepatology* 1987; **7:** 143.

11 Bolton C. The pathological changes in the liver resulting from passive venous congestion ex-

perimentally produced. *J. Path. Bact.* 1914; **19:** 258.

12 Bories P, Compean DG, Bourel M *et al.* Treatment of cirrhotic refractory ascites. (RA) by LeVeen shunt (a national multicenter controlled study of 57 patients). *J. Hepatol.* 1985 Suppl. 1, S23 (Abstr.)

13 Cabrera J, Arroyo V. Ballesta AM *et al.* Aminoglycoside nephrotoxicity in cirrhosis: value of urinary β_2 microglobulin to discriminate functional renal failure from acute tubular damage. *Gastroenterology* 1982; **82:** 97.

14 Campbell P, Blendis LM. Physiological consequences of peritoneovenous shunting (PVS) in patients with refractory ascites secondary to chronic liver disease: implications for the pathogenesis of ascites. *J. clin. Nutr. Gastroenterol.* 1986; **1:** 159.

15 Carey WD, Boayke A, Leatherman J. Spontaneous bacterial peritonitis: clinical and laboratory features with reference to hospital-acquired cases. *Am. J. gastroenterol.* 1986; **81:** 1156.

16 Casey TH, Summerskill WHJ, Orvis AL. Body and serum potassium in liver disease. I. Relationship to hepatic function and associated factors. *Gastroenterology* 1965; **48:** 198.

17 Cattau EL, Benjamin SB, Knuff TE. The accuracy of the physical examination in the diagnosis of suspected ascites. *J. Am. med. Assoc.* 1982; **247:** 1164.

18 Cherrick GR, Kerr DNS, Read AE *et al.* Colloid osmotic pressure and hydrostatic pressure relationships in the formation of ascites in hepatic cirrhosis. *Clin. Sci.* 1960; **19:** 361.

19 Conn HO. Acidic ascitic fluid: a leap forward (or a step?). *Hepatology* 1982; **2:** 507.

20 Epstein FH. Underfilling versus overflow in hepatic ascites. *N. Engl. J. Med.* 1982; **307:** 1577.

21 Epstein M. Peritoneovenous shunt in the management of ascites and the hepatorenal syndrome. *Gastroenterology* 1982; **82:** 790.

22 Epstein M. Derangements of renal water handling in liver disease. *Gastroenterology* 1985; **89:** 1415.

23 Epstein M. The sodium retention of cirrhosis: a reappraisal. *Hepatology* 1986; **6:** 312.

24 Felisart J, Rimola A, Arroyo V *et al.* Cefotaxime is more effective than ampicillin-tobramycin in cirrhosis with severe infections. *Hepatology* 1985; **5:** 457.

25 Fernandez-Cruz A, Marco J, Cuadrado LM *et al.* Plasma levels of atrial natriuretic peptide in cirhotic patients. *Lancet* 1985; **ii:** 1439.

26 Fischer JE, James JH. Treatment of hepatic coma and hepatorenal syndrome: mechanism of action of L-dopa and Aramine. *Am J. Surg.* 1972; **123:** 222.

27 Gabow PA, Moore S, Schrier RW. Spironolactone-induced hyperchloremic acidosis in cirrhosis. *Ann. intern. Med.* 1979; **90:** 338.

28 Garella S, Matarese RA. Renal effects of prostaglandins and clinical adverse effects of nonsteroidal anti-inflammatory agents. *Medicine (Baltimore)* 1984; **63:** 165.

29 Gerbes AL, Arendt RM, Paumgartner G. Atrial natriuretic factor—possible implication in liver disease. *J. Hepatol.* 1987; **5:** 123.

30 Gerding DN, Khan MY, Ewing JW *et al. Pasturella multocida* peritonitis in hepatic cirrhosis with ascites. *Gastroenterology* 1976; **70:** 413.

31 Gines P, Arroyo V, Quintero E *et al.* Comparison of paracentesis and diuretics in the treatment of cirrhotics with tense ascites. Results of a randomized study. *Gastroenterology* 1987; **93:** 234.

32 Gitlin N, Stauffer JL, Silvestri RC. The pH of ascitic fluid in the diagnosis of spontaneous bacterial peritonitis in alcoholic cirrhosis. *Hepatology* 1982; **2:** 408.

33 Hecker R, Sherlock S. Electrolyte and circulatory changes in terminal liver failure. *Lancet* 1956; **ii:** 1121.

34 Henriksen JH, Ring-Larsen H, Christensen NJ. Sympathetic nervous activity and renal and systematic hemodynamics in cirrhosis. A survey of plasma catecholamine studies. *J. Hepatol.* 1984; **1:** 55.

35 Hoefs JC. Increase in ascites white blood cell and protein concentrations during diuresis in patients with chronic liver disease. *Hepatology* 1981; **1:** 249.

36 Hoefs JC, Canawati HN, Sapico FL *et al.* Spontaneous bacterial peritonitis. *Hepatology* 1982; **2:** 399.

37 Jungst D, Gerbes AL, Martin R *et al.* Value of ascitic lipids in the differentiation between cirrhotic and malignant ascites. *Hepatology* 1986; **6:** 239.

38 Kao HW, Rakov HE, Savage E *et al.* The effect of large volume paracentesis on plasma volume—a cause of hypovolemia? *Hepatology* 1985; **5:** 403.

39 Kew MC, Brunt PW, Varma RR *et al.* Renal and intrarenal blood-flow in cirrhosis of the liver. *Lancet* 1971; **ii:** 504.

40 Koppel MH, Coburn JW, Mims MM *et al.* Transplantation of cadaveric kidneys from patients with hepatorenal syndrome. *N. Engl. J. Med.* 1969; **280:** 1367.

41 LeVeen HH, Wapnick S, Grosberg S *et al.* Further experience with peritoneovenous shunt for ascites. *Ann. Surg.* 1976; **184:** 574.

42 Lieberman FL, Ito S, Reynolds TB. Effective plasma volume in cirrhosis with ascites: evidence that a decreased value does not account for renal sodium retention, a spontaneous reduction in glomerular filtration rate (GFR), and a fall in GFR during drug-induced diuresis. *J. clin. Invest.* 1969; **48:** 975.

43 Mallory A, Schaeffer JW. Complications of diagnostic paracentesis in patients with liver disease. *J. Am. med. Assoc.* 1978; **239**: 628.

44 Martini GA, Raush-Stroomann JG. Das hyponatriämiesyndrom nach kochsalzfreier Kost, erzwungener Diurese und/oder Ascitesponktion bei chronischer Leberinsuffizienz. *Klin. Wschr* 1959; **37**: 835.

45 Mirouze D, Juttner H-U, Reynolds TB. Left pleural effusion in patients with chronic liver disease and ascites: prospective study of 22 cases. *Dig. Dis. Sci.* 1981; **26**: 984.

46 Mirouze D, Zipser RD, Reynolds TB. Effect of inhibitors of prostaglandin synthesis on induced diuresis in cirrhosis. *Hepatology* 1983; **3**: 50.

47 Nelson DC, McGrew WRG Jr, Hoyumpa AM Jr. Hypernatremia and lactulose therapy *J. Am. med. Assoc.* 1983; **249**: 1295.

48 Newell GC. Cirrhotic glomerulonephritis incidence, morphology, clinical features, and pathogenesis. *Am. J. Kidney Dis.* 1987; **9**: 183.

49 Parbhoo SP, Ajdukiewicz A, Sherlock S. Treatment of ascites by continous ultrafiltration and reinfusion of protein concentrate. *Lancet* 1974; **i**: 949.

50 Perez-Ayuso RM, Arroyo V, Camps J *et al.* Renal kallikrein excretion in cirrhotics with ascites: relationship to renal hemodynamics. *Hepatology* 1984; **4**: 247.

51 Perez-Ayuso RM, Arroyo V, Planas R *et al.* Randomized comparative study of efficacy of furosemide versus spironolactone in nonazotemic cirrhosis with ascites. *Gastroenterology* 1983; **84**: 961.

52 Planas R, Arroyo V, Rimola A *et al.* Acetylsalicylic acid suppresses the renal hemodynamic effect and reduces the diuretic action of furosemide in cirrhosis with ascites. *Gastroenterology* 1983; **84**: 247.

53 Pockros PJ, Reynolds TB. Rapid diuresis in patients with ascites from chronic liver disease: the importance of peripheral oedema. *Gastroenterology* 1986; **90**: 1827–1833.

54 Quintero E, Gines P, Arroyo V *et al.* Paracentesis versus diuretics in the treatment of cirrhotics with tense ascites. *Lancet* 1985; **i**: 611.

55 Read AE, Laidlaw J, Haslam RM *et al.* Neuropsychiatric complications following chlorothiazide therapy in patients with hepatic cirrhosis: possible relation to hypokalaemia. *Clin. Sci.* 1959; **18**: 409.

56 Reznick RK, Langer B, Taylor BR *et al.* Hyponatremia and arginine vasopressin secretion in patients with refractory hepatic ascites undergoing peritoneovenous shunting. *Gastroenterology* 1983; **84**: 713.

57 Rubinstein D, McInnes IE, Dudley FJ. Hepatic hydrothorax in the absence of clinical ascites: diagnosis and management. *Gastroenterology* 1985; **88**: 188.

58 Runyon BA, Hoefs JC. Ascitic fluid analysis in the differentiation of spontaneous bacterial peritonitis from gastrointestinal tract perforation into ascitic fluid. *Hepatology* 1984; **4**: 447.

59 Runyon BA, Morrissey RL, Hoefs JC *et al.* Opsonic activity of human ascitic fluid: a potentially important protective mechanism against spontaneous bacterial peritonitis. *Hepatology* 1985; **5**: 634.

60 Runyon BA. Low-protein-concentration ascitic fluid is predisposed to spontaneous bacterial peritonitis. *Gastroenterology* 1986; **91**: 1343.

61 Runyon BA. Fatal bacterial peritonitis secondary to non-obstructive colonic dilatation (Ogilvie's syndrome) in cirrhotic ascites. *J. clin. Gastroenterol.* 1986; **8**: 687.

62 Runyon BA, Van Epps DE. Diuresis of cirrhotic ascites increases its opsonic activity and may help prevent spontaneous bacterial peritonitis. *Hepatology* 1986; **6**: 396.

63 Runyon BA, Umland ET, Merlin T. Inoculation of blood culture bottles with ascitic fluid; improved detection of spontaneous bacterial peritonitis. *Arch. intern. Med.* 1987; **147**: 73.

64 Schrier RW, Caramelo C. Hemodynamics and hormonla alterations in hepatic cirrhosis in *The Kidney in Liver Disease* ed. Epstein M. Williams & Wilkins, New York, 3rd edn. 1988.

65 Sherlock S, Senewiratne B, Scott A *et al.* Complications of diuretic therapy in hepatic cirrhosis. *Lancet* 1966; **i**: 1049.

66 Simon DM, McGain JR, Bonkovsky HL *et al.* Effects of therapeutic paracentesis on systemic and hepatic hemodynamics and on renal and hormonal function. *Hepatology* 1987; **7**: 423.

67 Starling EH. On the absorption of fluids from the connective tissue spaces. *J. Physiol. (Lond.)* 1896; **19**: 312.

68 Strassen WN, McCullough AJ, Bacon BR *et al.* Immediate diagnostic criteria for bacterial infection of ascitic fluid. Evaluation of ascitic fluid polymorphonuclear leukocyte count, pH, and lactate concentration, alone and in combination. *Gastroenterology* 1986; **90**: 1247.

69 Targan SR, Chow AW, Guze LB. Spontaneous peritonitis of cirrhosis due to *Campylobacter fetus*. *Gastroenterology* 1976; **71**: 311.

70 Tito L, Gines P, Panes J *et al.* Total paracentesis plus i.v. albumin infusion in the treatment of cirrhotics with tense ascites. *J. Hepatol.* 1987; **5**, Supl. 1: S67.

71 Webb L, Sherlock S, The aetiology, presentation and natural history of extra-hepatic portal venous obstruction. *Q. J. Med.* 1979; **48**: 627.

72 Unikowsky B, Wexler MJ, Levey M. Dogs with experimental cirrhosis of the liver but without intra-hepatic hypertension do not retain sodium or form ascites. *J. clin. Invest.* 1983; **72**: 1594.

73 Wernze H, Burghardt W. Artial natriuretic peptide, the sympathetic nervous system, and decompensated cirrhosis. *Lancet* 1986; **1**: 331.

74 Zimmon DS, Oratz M, Kessler R *et al*. Albumin to ascites: demonstration of a direct pathway bypassing the systematic circulation. *J. clin. Invest.* 1969; **48**: 2074.

75 Zipser RD, Radvan GH, Kronborg IJ *et al*. Urinary thromboxane B2 and prostaglandin E2 in the hepatorenal syndrome: evidence for increased vasoconstrictor and decreased vasodilator factors. *Gastroenterology* 1983; **84**: 697.

10 · The Portal Venous System and Portal Hypertension

The portal system includes all veins which carry blood from the abdominal part of the alimentary tract, the spleen, pancreas and gallbladder. The portal vein enters the liver at the porta hepatis in two main branches, one to each lobe; it is without valves in its larger channels (fig. 10.1) [47].

The *portal vein* is formed by the union of the superior mesenteric vein and the splenic vein just posterior to the head of the pancreas at about the level of the second lumbar vertebra. It extends slightly to the right of the mid-line for a distance of 5.5–8 cm to the porta hepatis. The portal vein has a segmental intra-hepatic distribution.

The *superior mesenteric vein* is formed by tributaries from the small intestine, colon and

head of the pancreas, and irregularly from the stomach via the right gastro-epiploic vein.

The *splenic veins* (5–15 channels) originate at the splenic hilum and join near the tail of the pancreas with the short gastric vessels to form the main splenic vein. This proceeds in a transverse direction in the body and head of the pancreas, lying below and in front of the artery. It receives numerous tributaries from the head of the pancreas, and the left gastro-epiploic vein enters it near the spleen. The *inferior mesenteric vein* bringing blood from the left part of the colon and rectum usually enters its medial third. Occasionally, however, it enters the junction of superior mesenteric and splenic veins.

Portal blood flow in man is about 1000–1200 ml/min.

Portal oxygen content. The fasting arterio-portal oxygen difference is only 1.9 volumes per cent (range 0.4–3.3 volumes per cent) and the portal vein contributes 40 ml/min or 72% of the total oxygen supply to the liver.

During digestion, the arterio-portal venous oxygen difference increases due to increased intestinal utilization.

Stream-lines in the portal vein. There is no consistent pattern of hepatic distribution of portal inflow. Sometimes splenic blood goes to the left and sometimes to the right lobe. Crossing-over of the bloodstream can occur in the human portal vein. Flow is probably stream-lined rather than turbulent.

Portal pressure is about 7 mmHg in normal man.

Collateral circulation

When the portal circulation is obstructed, whether it be within or outside the liver, a

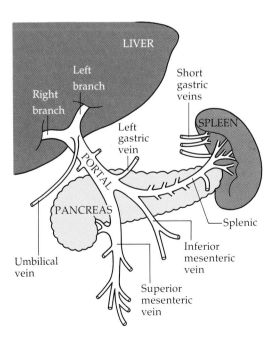

151   **Fig. 10.1.**   The anatomy of the portal venous system.

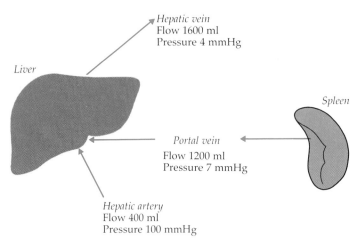

Fig. 10.2. The flow and pressure in the hepatic artery, portal vein and hepatic vein.

remarkable collateral circulation develops to carry portal blood into the systemic veins (figs 10.3, 10.22).

Intra-hepatic obstruction (cirrhosis)

Normally 100% of the portal venous blood flow can be recovered from the hepatic veins whereas in cirrhosis only 13% is obtained [101]. The remainder enters collateral channels which form four main groups.

Group I: Where protective epithelium adjoins absorptive epithelium:

(*a*) At the cardia of the stomach, where the left gastric vein and short gastric veins of the portal system anastomose with the intercostal, diaphragmo-oesophageal and azygos minor veins of the caval system. Deviation of blood into these channels leads to varicosities in the submucous layer of the lower end of the oesophagus and upper part of the stomach.

(*b*) At the anus the superior haemorrhoidal vein of the portal system anastomoses with the middle and inferior haemorrhoidal veins of the caval system. Deviation of blood into these channels may lead to rectal varices.

Group II: In the falciform ligament through the para-umbilical veins, relics of the umbilical circulation of the fetus (fig. 10.4).

Group III: Where the abdominal organs are in contact with retro-peritoneal tissues or adherent to the abdominal wall. These collaterals include veins from the liver to the diaphragm, veins in the lieno-renal ligament and omentum, lumbar veins and veins developing in the scars of previous laparotomies.

Group IV: Portal venous blood is carried to the left renal vein. This may be through blood entering directly from the splenic vein or via diaphragmatic, pancreatic, left adrenal or gastric veins.

Blood from gastro-oesophageal collaterals, retro-peritoneal and venous systems of the abdomen ultimately reaches the superior vena cava via the azygos or hemiazygos systems. A small volume enters the inferior vena cava. Collaterals running to the pulmonary veins have also been described.

Extra-hepatic obstruction

With extra-hepatic portal venous obstruction, additional collaterals form attempting to bypass the block and return blood *towards* the liver. These enter the portal vein in the porta hepatis beyond the block. They include the veins at the hilum, venae comitantes of the portal vein and hepatic arteries, veins in the suspensory ligaments of the liver and diaphragmatic and omental veins. Lumbar collaterals may be very large.

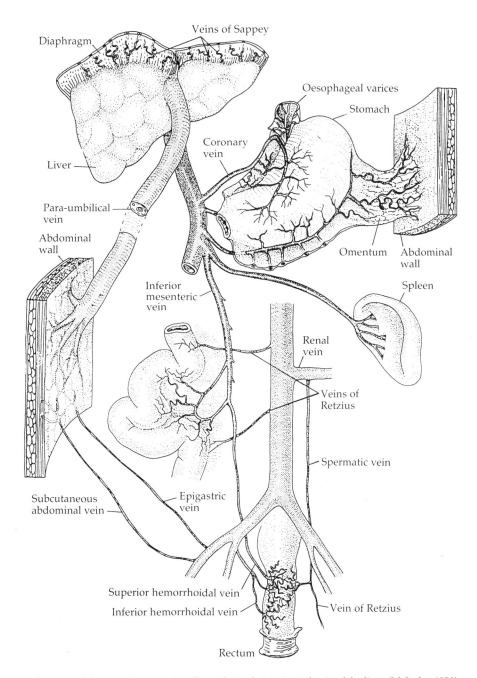

Fig. 10.3. The sites of the portal–systemic collateral circulation in cirrhosis of the liver (McIndoe 1928).

Effects

When the liver is cut off from portal blood by the development of the collateral circulation it **153** depends more and more on blood from the hepatic artery. It shrinks and shows impaired capacity to regenerate. This might be due to lack of hepato-trophic factors, including insulin and glucagon, which are of pancreatic origin.

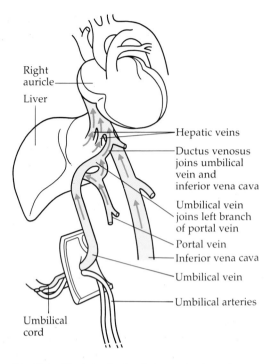

Fig. 10.4. The hepatic circulation at the time of birth.

bodies are inconspicuous. Histologically [102] sinusoids are dilated and lined by thickened epithelium (fig. 10.5). Histiocytes proliferate in the sinusoids with occasional erythrophagocytosis. Peri-arterial haemorrhages may progress to siderotic, fibrotic nodules.

Splenic and portal vessels. The splenic artery and portal vein are enlarged and tortuous and may be aneurysmal. The portal and splenic vein may show endothelial haemorrhages, mural thrombi and intimal plaques and may calcify (fig. 10.13). Such veins are usually unsuitable for portal surgery.

In 50% of cirrhotics small, deeply placed splenic arterial aneurysms are seen [105].

Hepatic changes depend on the cause of the portal hypertension.

The height of the portal venous pressure correlates poorly with the apparent degree of cirrhosis and in particular of fibrosis. There is a much better correlation with the degree of nodularity.

Collaterals usually imply portal hypertension, although occasionally if the collateral circulation is very extensive portal pressure may fall. Conversely, portal hypertension of short duration can exist without a demonstrable collateral circulation.

A large portal—systemic shunt may lead to hepatic encephalopathy, septicaemias due to intestinal organisms, and other circulatory and metabolic effects.

Pathology of portal hypertension

Collateral venous circulation is disappointingly insignificant at autopsy. This is particularly true of oesophageal varices which collapse.

The spleen is enlarged and tough with a thickened capsule. The surface oozes dark blood (*fibro-congestive splenomegaly*). Malpighian

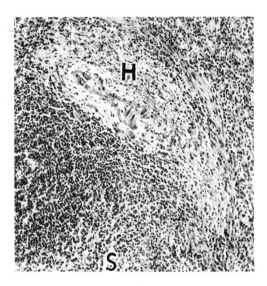

Fig. 10.5. The spleen in portal hypertension. The sinusoids (S) are congested and the sinusoidal wall is thickened. A haemorrhage (H) lies adjacent to an arteriole of a Malpighian corpuscle. (Stained H & E, ×70.)

Varices

Oesophageal

If oesophago-gastric varices did not form and bleed portal hypertension would be of virtually no clinical significance. The major blood supply to oesophageal varices is the left gastric vein. The posterior branch usually drains into the azygos system, whereas the anterior branch communicates with varices just below the oesophageal junction and forms a bundle of thin parallel veins that run in the junction area and continue in large tortuous veins in the lower oesophagus [170]. There seem to be four layers of veins in the oesophagus (fig. 10.6) [82]. *Intra-epithelial veins* may correlate with the red spots seen on endoscopy and which predict variceal rupture [167]. The *superficial venous plexus* drains into larger, *deep intrinsic veins*. *Perforating veins* connect the deeper veins with the fourth layer which is the adventitial plexus. Typical large varices arise from the main trunks of the deep intrinsic veins and these communicate with gastric varices.

The connection between portal and systemic circulation at the gastro-oesophageal junction is extremely complex [184]. Its adaptation to the cephalad and increased flow of portal hypertension is ill-understood. A palisade zone is seen between a gastric zone and the perforating zone (fig. 10.7). In the palisade zone flow is bidirectional and this area acts a water shed between portal and azygos systems. Turbulent flow in perforating veins between the varices and the peri-oesophageal veins at the lower end of the stomach may explain why rupture is frequent in this region [98]. Recurrence of varices after endoscopic sclerotherapy may be related to the communications between various venous channels or perhaps to enlargement of veins in the superficial venous plexus. Failure of sclerotherapy may also be due to failure to thrombose the perforating veins.

Gastric

These are largely supplied by the short gastric veins and drain into the deep intrinsic veins of the oesophagus. They are particularly prominent in patients with extra-hepatic portal obstruction.

In portal hypertension, the gastric vascularity is abnormal showing increased sub-mucosal

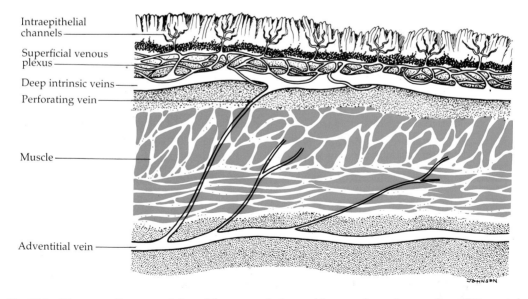

Intraepithelial channels

Superficial venous plexus

Deep intrinsic veins

Perforating vein

Muscle

Adventitial vein

Fig. 10.6. Diagrammatic representation of the venous drainage of the oesophagus in normal man (Kitano *et al.* 1986).

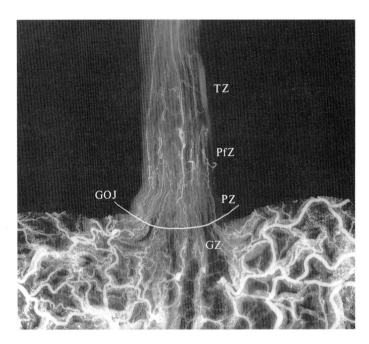

Fig. 10.7. Radiograph of a specimen injected with barium-gelatine, opened along the greater curvature. Four distinct zones of normal venous drainage are identified: gastric zone (GZ), palisade zone (PZ), perforating zone (PfZ), and truncal zone (TZ). A radiopaque wire demarcates the transition between the columnar and stratified squamous epithelium. (GOJ, gastroesophageal junction). (Vianna *et al.* 1987).

arterio-venous communications between the muscularis mucosa and dilated pre-capillaries and veins—a vascular ectasia [138]. This has been termed *congestive gastropathy* [99]. Gastric mucosa may be at particular risk of bleeding and of damage, for instance, by aspirin or non-steroidal anti-inflammatory drugs. Endoscopy shows a beefy red appearance, patechial haemorrhages and a reticular, mosaic pattern of red and yellow mucosa [99, 130]. Bleeding can occur from the gastric red spots [138]. These gastric changes may be increased after successful oesophageal sclerotherapy. They are relieved only by reducing the portal pressure.

Others

If portal hypertension is present, portal systemic collaterals form in relation to bowel—abdominal wall adhesions secondary to previous surgery or pelvic inflammatory disease. Varices also form at muco-cutaneous junctions for instance, at the site of an ileostomy or colostomy.

Duodenal

These may show as filling defects in the bulb and duodenal sweep.

Colonic

These develop secondary to inferior mesenteric—internal iliac venous collaterals [67]. They may present with haemorrhage. They are visualized by colonoscopy. ^{99m}Technetium tagged red blood cell scans are useful for localizing bleeding. Colonic varices may become more frequent after successful oesophageal sclerotherapy.

Rectal

These are collaterals between the superior haemorrhoidal (portal) veins and the middle and inferior haemorrhoidal (systemic) veins. They are visualized with a sigmoidoscope and may bleed. They must be distinguished from simple haemorrhoids which are prolapsed vascular cushions and which do not communicate with the portal system [194].

Common bile duct

These may be life threatening at surgery [41].

Haemodynamics of portal hypertension

This has been considerably clarified by the development of animal models such as the rat with a ligated portal vein or bile duct or carbon tetrachloride-induced cirrhosis [64].

The fundamental haemodynamic abnormality is an increased resistance to portal flow. This may be intra-hepatic as in cirrhosis or due to an obstructed portal vein (fig. 10.3). As the portal venous pressure is lowered by the development of collaterals deviating portal blood into systemic veins the portal hypertension is maintained by increasing the blood flow in the portal system which thus becomes hyperdynamic (figs 10.8, 10.9). This increased flow is achieved by raising cardiac output and by splanchnic vasodilatation. These findings have been confirmed in the rat model and in cirrhotic patients by Doppler ultrasound [148]. The portal vein radicles show hypertrophy of their walls. The increased portal flow probably increases the variceal transmural pressure. The increased flow refers to *total* portal flow (hepatic

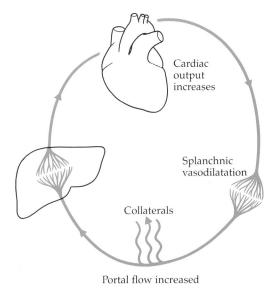

Fig. 10.9. Forward flow theory of portal hypertension.

and collaterals). The actual portal flow reaching the liver is, of course, reduced. Various factors have been suggested as splanchnic vasodilators. They include gut hormones, bile acids, prostaglandins [23] and hepatic anoxia but none is confirmed.

An alternative backward flow view states that, as the portal venous pressure is lowered by the formation of collaterals, hepatic resistance increases to maintain perfusion. The portal venous system thus becomes congested and splenic and systemic circulation hypodynamic. This view does not agree with reports of increased splenic and portal vein flow in patients with cirrhosis.

Clinical features of portal hypertension

HISTORY AND GENERAL EXAMINATION
(table 10.1)

Hepatic cirrhosis is the commonest cause of portal hypertension. Any possible aetiological factor such as alcoholism or past hepatitis

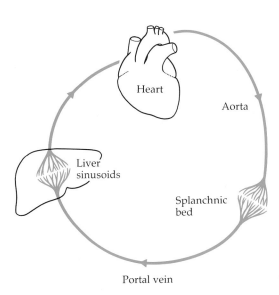

Fig. 10.8. Normal portal circulation.

Table 10.1. Investigation of a patient with suspected portal hypertension

History
Relevant to cirrhosis or chronic hepatitis (Chapter (19)
Gastrointestinal bleedings: number, dates, amounts, symptoms, treatment
Results of previous barium series examinations and endoscopies
P/H: Alcoholism, blood transfusion, hepatitis B, intra-abdominal, neonatal or other sepsis, oral contraceptives, myeloproliferative disorder.

Examination
Signs of hepato-cellular failure
Abdominal wall veins:
   site
   direction of blood flow
Splenomegaly
Liver size and consistency
Ascites
Oedema of legs

Rectal examination

Endoscopy of oesophagus, stomach and duodenum

Additional investigations
Barium series
Aspiration liver biopsy
Hepatic vein catheterization
Selective splanchnic arteriography
Hepatic ultrasound or CT scan

should be considered. Past abdominal inflammation, especially in the neonatal period, is particularly important in the aetiology of extra-hepatic portal block. Clotting diseases and some drugs such as sex hormones conduce to portal and hepatic venous thrombosis.

Haematemesis is the commonest presentation. The number and severity of previous haemorrhages should be noted together with their immediate effects, whether there was associated confusion or coma and whether blood transfusion was required. Melaena, without haematemesis, may result from bleeding varices. The absence of dyspepsia and epigastric tenderness and a previously normal barium meal or endoscopy help to exclude haemorrhage from peptic ulcer.

The stigmata of cirrhosis include jaundice, vascular spiders and palmar erythema. Anaemia and the prodromata of coma should be noted.

ABDOMINAL WALL VEINS

In intra-hepatic portal hypertension, some blood from the left branch of the portal vein may be deviated via para-umbilical veins to the umbilicus, whence it reaches veins of the caval system (fig. 10.10). In extra-hepatic portal obstruction, dilated veins may appear in the left flank.

Distribution and direction. A number of prominent collateral veins radiating from the umbilicus is termed *caput Medusae.* This is rare and usually only one or two veins, frequently epigastric, are seen (figs 10.10, 10.11). The blood flow is away from the umbilicus, whereas in inferior vena caval obstruction the collateral venous channels carry blood upwards to reach the superior vena caval system (fig. 10.10). Tense ascites may lead to functional obstruction of the inferior vena cava and cause difficulty in interpretation.

Abdominal veins can be visualized by *infra-red photography* (fig. 10.12).

Murmurs. A venous hum may be heard, usually in the region of the xiphoid process or umbilicus, occasionally radiating to the praecordium, sternum or over the liver [90]. A thrill, detectable by light pressure, may be felt at the site of the maximum intensity. The sound may be accentuated during systole, in inspiration or in the erect or sitting positions. It is due to blood rushing through a large umbilical or para-umbilical channel in the falciform ligament from the left branch of the portal vein to the superior epigastric, internal mammary or inferior epigastric veins in the abdominal wall. A venous hum may also occasionally be heard over other large collaterals such as the inferior mesenteric vein or after a successful or even unsuccessful porta—caval anastomosis. An arterial systolic murmur usually indicates primary liver cancer or alcoholic hepatitis.

The association of dilated abdominal wall

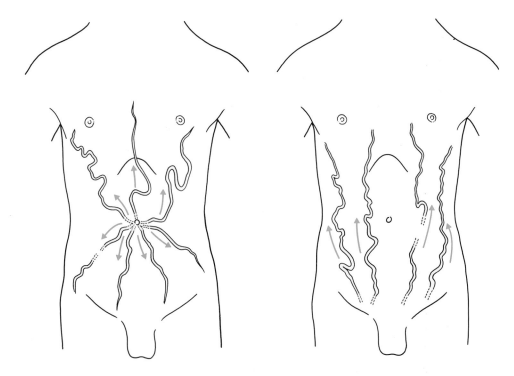

Fig. 10.10. Distribution and direction of blood flow in anterior abdominal wall veins in portal venous obstruction (left) and in inferior vena caval obstruction (right) (Sherlock 1950).

veins and a loud abdominal venous murmur at the umbilicus is termed the *Cruveilhier–Baumgarten* syndrome [9, 39]. This was originally believed to be due to congenital failure of obliteration of the umbilical vein with subsequent hepatic atrophy. In fact, it is usually due to cirrhosis with a congenitally patent umbilical vein.

The para-xiphoid umbilical hum and *caput Medusae* indicate the presence of portal obstruction beyond the origin of the umbilical veins from the left branch of the portal vein. They therefore indicate intra-hepatic portal venous hypertension (cirrhosis).

SPLEEN

The spleen enlarges progressively. The edge is firm. Size bears little relation to the portal pressure. It is larger in young people and in macronodular rather than micronodular cirrhosis.

An enlarged spleen is the single most important diagnostic sign of portal hypertension. If the spleen cannot be felt or is not enlarged on imaging, the diagnosis of portal hypertension is questionable.

The *peripheral blood* shows a pancytopenia associated with an enlarged spleen whatever the cause (*secondary 'hypersplenism'*). This is related more to the reticulo-endothelial hyperplasia than to the portal hypertension and is unaffected by lowering the pressure by porta–caval anastomosis.

LIVER

A small liver may be as significant as a large one, and the size should be evaluated by careful percussion. Liver size correlates poorly with the height of the portal venous pressure, although high pressures are more often found with the small, contracted, fibrotic liver.

Liver consistency, tenderness or nodularity

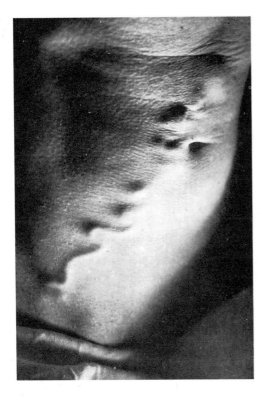

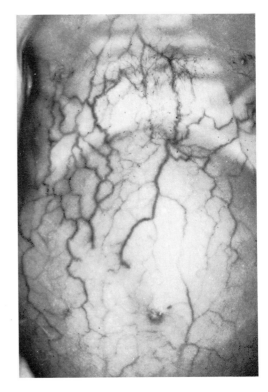

Fig. 10.11. Anterior abdominal wall vein in patient with cirrhosis of the liver (Sherlock & Walshe 1946).

Fig. 10.12. Infra-red photograph of a patient with cirrhosis and ascites. The portal collateral circulation is demonstrated. Note the everted umbilicus.

should be recorded. A soft liver suggests extrahepatic portal venous obstruction. A firm liver supports cirrhosis.

ASCITES

This is rarely due to portal hypertension alone although a particularly high pressure may be a major factor. The portal hypertension raises the capillary filtration pressure, increases the quantity of ascitic fluid and determines its localization to the peritoneal cavity. Ascites in cirrhosis always indicates liver cell failure in addition to portal hypertension.

X-RAY OF THE ABDOMEN
AND CHEST

160   This is useful to delineate liver and spleen

shape and size. Rarely, a calcified portal vein may be shown (fig. 10.13).

Branching, linear, gas-shadows in the portal vein radicles, especially near the periphery of the liver and due to gas-forming organisms, may rarely be seen in adults with intestinal infarction or infants with enterocolitis. Portal gas may be associated with disseminated intravascular coagulation [158].

CT and ultrasound may detect portal gas more often, for instance, in suppurative cholangitis when the prognosis is not so grave [45].

Tomography of the azygos vein may show enlargement (fig. 10.14) the bulk of the collateral flow enters the azygos system.

A widened left paravertebral shadow may be due to lateral displacement of the pleural reflection between aorta and vertebral column by a dilated hemiazygos vein.

(a)

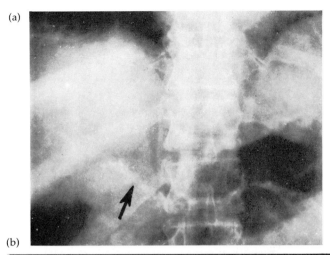

(b)

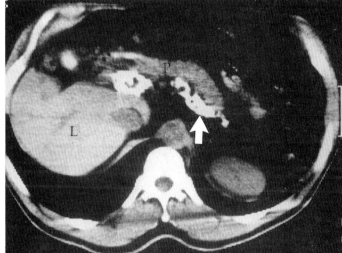

Fig. 10.13. (a) Plain X-ray of the abdomen. Calcification is seen in the line of the splenic and portal vein (arrow). (b) CT shows calcium in the splenic and portal veins (arrow).

Massively dilated para-oesophageal collaterals may be seen on the plain chest radiograph as a retrocardiac posterior mediastinal mass.

BARIUM STUDIES

These have been largely outmoded by upper endoscopy. For the oesophagus, small volumes of barium are required and if negative a further study should be done after paralysis of the oesophagus with intravenous buscopan (hyoscine-*N*-butyl bromide) or, preferably,

intravenous glucagon (fig. 10.15). The stomach and duodenum must also be studied.

Normal oesophageal mucosa shows long, thin, evenly spaced lines. Varices show as filling defects in the regular contour of the oesophagus (fig. 10.15). They are most often seen in the lower third but may spread upwards so that the entire oesophagus is involved. Widening and finally gross dilatation are helpful signs.

Oesophageal varices are nearly always accompanied by gastric varices which pass through the cardia, line the fundus in a worm-like fashion and may be difficult to distinguish

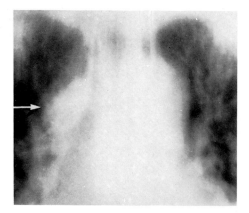

Fig. 10.14. Tomography of the mediastinum of a patient with large portal–systemic collaterals shows enlargement of the azygos vein (marked with arrow).

from mucosal folds. Occasionally gastric varices show as a lobulated mass in the gastric fundus simulating a carcinoma. Portal venography is useful in differentiation.

ENDOSCOPY

This is the best method of visualizing oeso-phageal and gastric varices. The size and distri-bution should be noted. Colour is extremely important [164]. Varices usually appear white and opaque (fig. 10.16). Red colour correlates with blood flow through dilated sub-epithelial and communicating veins [98]. Dilated sub-epithelial veins may appear as raised cherry red spots and red weal markings (fig. 10.17). These lie on top of large sub-epithelial vessels. The haematocystic spot is approximately 4 mm in diameter and represents blood coming from the deeper extrinsic veins of the oesophagus straight out toward the lumen through a com-municating vein into the more superficial sub-mucosal veins. Red colour is usually associated with larger varices. All these colour changes and particularly the red colour sign predict variceal bleeding [117].

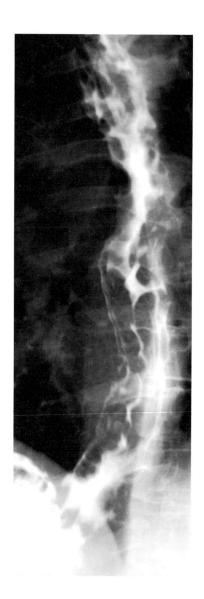

Fig. 10.15. Barium swallow X-ray shows a dilated oesophagus. The margin is irregular. There are multiple filling defects representing oesophageal varices.

Imaging the portal venous system (table 10.2)

Non-invasive

The patency of the portal vein and the nature and extent of any collateral circulation must

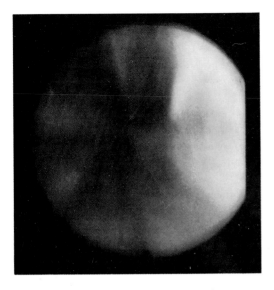

Fig. 10.16. Endoscopy. White opaque varices are seen at the gastro-oesophageal junction.

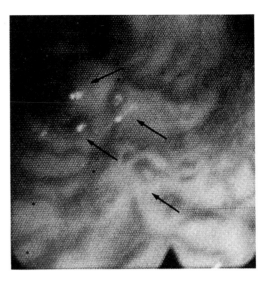

Fig. 10.17. Endoscopic view of cherry-red spots on oesophageal varices (arrows).

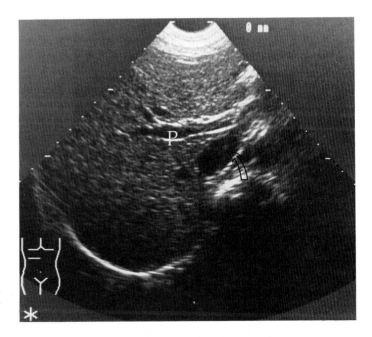

Fig. 10.18. Transverse ultrasound shows patent portal vein (P) arrow indicates inferior vena cava.

be established. Any space-occupying lesion should be identified. The simpliest initial investigation is ultrasound and/or CT. This can be followed by more definitive vascular imaging.

ULTRASOUND

Longitudinal scans at the sub-costal margins and transverse scans at the epigastrium are essential (fig. 10.18). The portal and superior

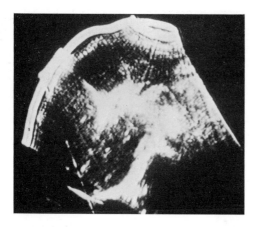

Fig. 10.19. Transverse ultrasound scan through porta hepatis showing a thrombosed portal vein with surrounding scar tissue (Webb *et al.* 1977).

mesenteric veins can always be seen. The normal splenic vein may be more difficult [183].

A large portal vein suggests portal hypertension, but this is not diagnostic. If collaterals are seen, this confirms portal hypertension. Portal vein thrombosis is accurately diagnosed (fig. 10.19) and echogenic areas can sometimes be seen within the lumen [183].

Ultrasound has the advantage over CT in that any number of axes can be used.

CT SCAN

This allows better definition of the portal vein. After enhancement, retroperitoneal, perivisceral and para-oesophageal varices may be visualized (fig. 10.20). Oesophageal varices may be shown as a scalloped contour with intraluminal protrusions enhancing after contrast [7]. The umbilical vein can be seen (fig. 10.21). Gastric varices are shown as rounded or tubular structures indistinguishable from the gastric wall [6].

MAGNETIC RESONANCE

This gives excellent depiction of blood vessels as regions of absent signal. It may be used to study vessels in a similar fashion to digital subtraction angiography. It has been used to show shunt patency [12] and may in future be used to study portal blood flow.

Venography

In a patient with cirrhosis, if the portal vein is

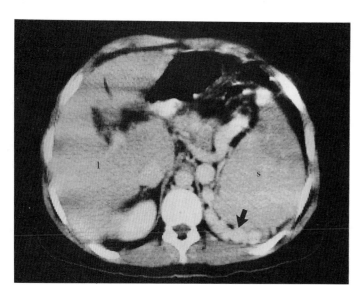

Fig. 10.20. Contrast enhanced CT scan in a patient with cirrhosis and a large retroperitoneal retrosplenic collateral circulation (arrow). s is spleen, l is liver.

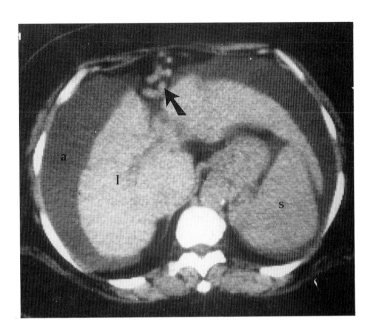

Fig. 10.21. CT scan (after enhancement) of a cirrhotic liver shows patency of the umbilical vein (arrow). l is liver, s is spleen, a is ascites.

patent by scanning, confirmation by venography is not necessary unless portal surgery or hepatic transplantation is being considered. In the case of a probable thrombosed portal vein scanning is not enough and confirmation will have to be sought by venography.

Patency of the portal vein can be established, and this is important particularly in the diagnosis of splenomegaly in childhood and in excluding invasion by a hepato-cellular carcinoma in a patient with cirrhosis.

Anatomy of the portal venous system must be known before such operations as portal systemic shunt or hepatic transplantation. The patency of a surgical shunt may be confirmed.

Flow patterns may be demonstrated in the portal vein. If the liver opacifies prominently, hepatic blood flow is maintained. If flow is predominantly hepato-fugal, flow is probably retrograde.

The demonstration of a large portal collateral circulation is essential for the diagnosis of chronic hepatic encephalopathy (figs 10.20, 10.22). Its absence excludes it.

A filling defect in the portal vein or in the liver due to a space-occupying lesion may be demonstrated.

Venographic appearances

When the portal circulation is normal, the splenic and portal veins are filled but no other vessels are outlined (fig. 10.23). A filling defect may be seen at the junction of splenic and superior mesenteric veins. The size and direction of the splenic and portal veins are very variable. The intra-hepatic branches of the portal vein show a gradual branching and reduction in calibre. Later the liver becomes opaque due to sinusoidal filling. The hepatic veins may rarely be seen in later films.

In cirrhosis, the venogram varies widely. It may be completely normal or may show filling of large numbers of collateral vessels with gross distortion of the intra-hepatic pattern ('tree in winter' appearance) (fig. 10.24).

In extra-hepatic portal or splenic vein obstruction, large numbers of vessels run from the spleen and splenic vein to the diaphragm, thoracic cage and abdominal wall (fig. 10.25). Intra-hepatic branches are not usually seen although, if the portal vein block is localized, para-portal vessels may short-circuit the lesion and produce a delayed but definite filling of the vein beyond.

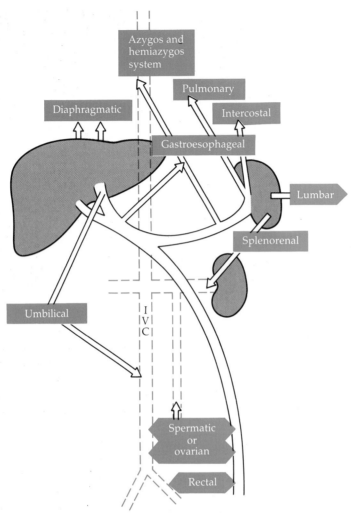

Fig. 10.22. The sites of the collateral circulation in the presence of intra-hepatic portal vein obstruction.

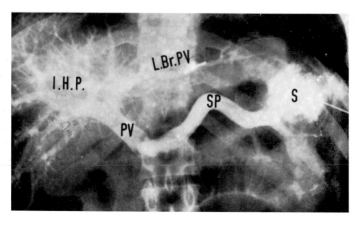

Fig. 10.23. Normal portal venogram obtained by percutaneous splenic puncture. All the dye injected into the spleen passes through the splenic and portal vein into the liver. S = pool of dye in spleen; SP = splenic vein; PV = portal vein; L.Br.PV = left branch of right portal vein; I.H.P. = intra-hepatic pattern.

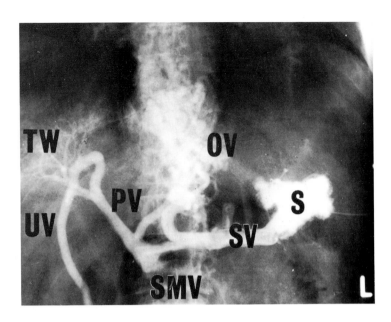

Fig. 10.24. Splenic venogram from a patient with cirrhosis of the liver. The gastro-oesophageal collateral circulation can be seen and the intra-hepatic portal vascular tree is distorted ('tree in winter' appearance). S = splenic pulp; SV = splenic vein; SMV = superior mesenteric vein; PV = portal vein; OV = oesophageal vein; UV = umbilical vein; TW = 'tree in winter' appearance.

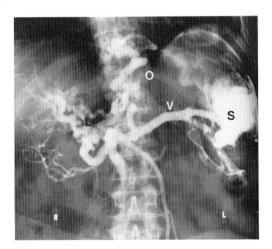

Fig. 10.25. Splenic venogram showing extra-hepatic portal venous obstruction. The portal vein is replaced by numerous small channels. S = spleen; V = splenic vein; L = leash of small collaterals; O = oesophageal collateral circulation.

INDIRECT ANGIOGRAPHY

This technique is safe and is the one most commonly used for portal venography [46]. Safety has increased with the use of smaller (French 5) arterial catheters. Contrast of low osmolarity is painless so that only local anaesthesia is needed. These new contrast materials are less toxic to kidneys and other tissues and hypersensitivity reactions are rare.

The coeliac axis is catheterized via the femoral artery with a preformed opaque catheter and 50–60 ml contrast is injected. The contrast material that flows into the splenic artery returns through the splenic and portal veins and produces a splenic and portal venogram. Similarly, a bolus of contrast introduced into the superior mesenteric artery returns through the superior mesenteric and portal veins which can be seen in radiographs exposed at the appropriate intervals (fig. 10.28).

Visceral angiography has the advantage that the hepatic arterial system can be seen, so allowing space-filling lesions in the liver to be identified. A tumour circulation may diagnose hepato-cellular cancer or another tumour.

The markedly enlarged hepatic artery in a patient with cirrhosis carries a good prognosis compared with those showing a reduction in both hepatic arterial and portal venous flow. Knowledge of splenic and hepatic arterial anatomy is useful if surgery is contemplated. Haemangiomas, other space-occupying lesions and aneurysms may be identified. The portal

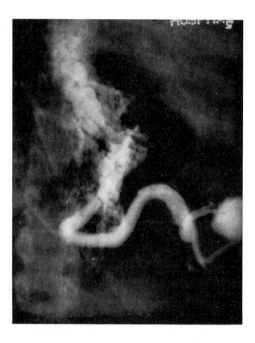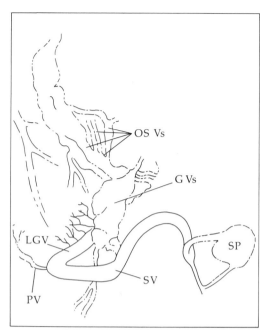

Fig. 10.26. Female patient with portal cirrhosis. Splenic venogram. The bulk of the contrast medium is diverted through the gastric and oesophageal veins and only a trickle enters the portal vein. The portal vein was patent.

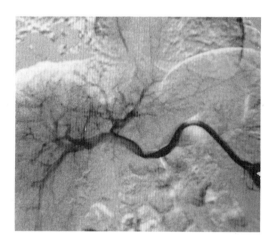

Fig. 10.27. Digital subtraction angiography shows a normal portal venous system.

vascular tree is not so well visualized as in splenic venography.

The portal vein may not opacify if flow in it is hepato-fugal or if there is 'steal' by the spleen or by large collateral channels (fig. 10.26). A superior mesenteric angiogram will confirm that the portal vein is in fact patent.

DIGITAL SUBTRACTION ANGIOGRAPHY

The contrast is given as a central venous injection with immediate subtraction of images [20]. Less material is needed than for the arterial technique and smaller catheters are used. The portal system is very well visualized, free of other confusing images (fig 10.29) [53]. Spatial resolution is poorer than with conventional film-based angiography. The technique is particularly valuable for the parenchymal phase of hepatic angiography and for the diagnosis of vascular lesions such as haemangiomas or arterio-venous malformations [52].

SPLENIC VENOGRAPHY

Contrast material, injected into the pulp of the

R   L

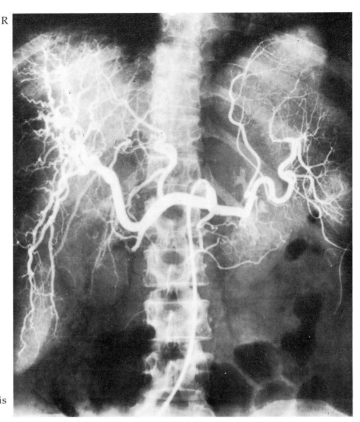

Fig. 10.28. Selective coeliac angiogram shows intra-hepatic arterial pattern. A Riedel's lobe is shown.

spleen, is absorbed into the portal bloodstream with sufficient rapidity to outline the splenic and portal veins [180].

The collateral circulation is particularly well visualized (fig. 10.25) and it is the procedure of choice where extrahepatic portal venous obstruction is suspected.

A fine catheter (0.75 mm outside diameter), fitted with a stilette, is inserted in the mid-axillary line, usually in the 8th or 9th intercostal space with its tip directed at an angle of 45° to the transverse plane. After penetrating 2 cm into the spleen, the stilette is removed.

The intra-splenic pressure is measured and contrast injected. The use of a fine catheter, which can move freely within the spleen, increases the safety of the procedure. After removal of the catheter the exit tract is plugged with pledgets of gel foam [21].

The procedure may be combined with digital subtraction angiography. Prothrombin time should be normal and deep jaundice is a contra-indication, even with a normal prothrombin time. The platelet count should exceed 80 000 per mm^3.

Serious complications are rare provided a careful technique is employed. The most serious is haemorrhage. Bleeding usually ceases and, although blood transfusion may be necessary, splenectomy is indicated rarely. Haemorrhage may be delayed for five days after the puncture. Extra-splenic injection of contrast material causes pain, both local and referred to the left shoulder.

TRANS-HEPATIC PORTOGRAPHY [162]

This technique gives excellent visualization of the portal and splenic veins and the portal–systemic collateral circulation. It is, however,

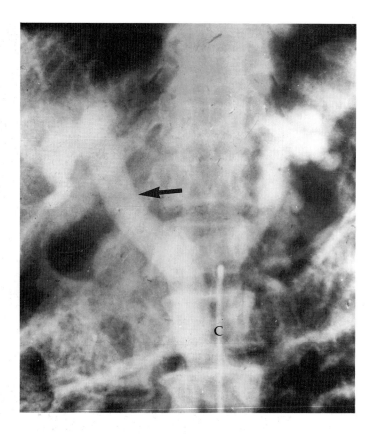

Fig. 10.29. Venous phase of selective coeliac angiogram shows a patent portal (arrow) and splenic veins. C is for catheter in coeliac artery.

technically difficult and carries a greater risk than other procedures. It may precede transhepatic obliteration of varices (fig. 10.30) [174].

Portal venous pressure [61]

WEDGED HEPATIC VENOUS PRESSURE [61]

A balloon catheter is introduced into a hepatic venous radicle via the femoral vein until it can go no further (fig. 10.31). It now prevents blood from flowing through the hepatic vein radical. The pressure measured represents that at the next point of free communication with the hepatic circulation and so measures the sinusoidal venous pressure. The catheter is properly wedged if the pressure tracing shows regular oscillations related to transmission of hepatic arterial pressure and, finally, a small amount of contrast material injected is seen to pass against the predominant flow into the sinusoidal bed. Measurements are then taken with the balloon deflated and reflect the free hepatic venous pressure.

The difference between 'wedged' and 'free' pressure is the portal (sinusoidal) venous pressure. The normal is 5–6 mm Hg and values of about 20 mm Hg are found in patients with cirrhosis. In alcoholic cirrhosis a gradient of 12 mm Hg or greater is a requirement for the development of varices and hence haemorrhage [55].

The wedged hepatic venous pressure does not reflect portal venous pressure in presinusoidal portal hypertension. It may underestimate the true portal venous pressure [181].

The technique is relatively easy, safe, and can be performed in patients with a bleeding

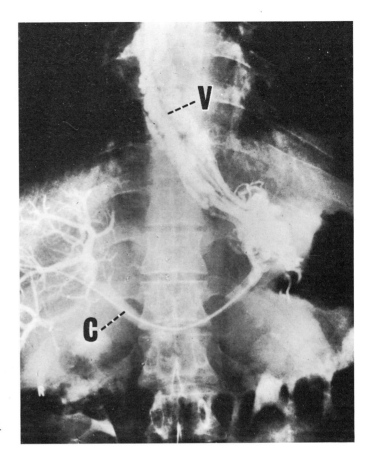

Fig. 10.30. Trans-hepatic portogram shows cannula passed through liver and portal vein into the left gastric vein. Contrast material has been injected and massive oesophageal varices filled. C = cannula, V = varices.

tendency or with ascites. It allows portal pressure to be measured in the splenectomized. Serial estimations are of value in detecting the effect of drugs on the portal system.

TRANS-HEPATIC

This is safe if a 25-gauge needle is used under ultrasound guidance, the needle being replaced by a 5-French catheter which is placed in the main portal vein [140].

INTRASPLENIC PUNCTURE

171 This is the most convenient technique [3].

OPERATIVE

These measurements are unreliable, as they are affected by the anaesthetic, blood loss, position of the patient and duration of the operation.

VARICEAL PRESSURE

Pressure in a varix is equal to the pressure necessary to compress it. This may be estimated by a pneumatic pressure gauge fixed at the tip of an endoscope and connected to an electronic manometer [115]. The variceal pressure measured via the endoscope correlates with the wedged hepatic venous pressure and the intrasplenic pressure [43].

Direct puncture of varices at the time of

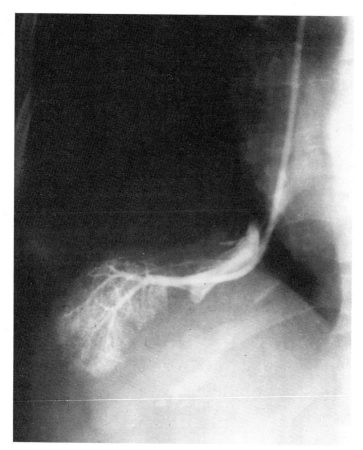

Fig. 10.31. A catheter has been inserted into an hepatic vein via the femoral vein. The wedged position is confirmed by introducing a small amount of contrast which has entered the sinusoidal bed.

sclerotherapy also allows a pressure to be recorded. Values correlate with the endoscopic pressure-gauge method [18]. However, the variceal pressure in cirrhosis (about 15.5 mm Hg) is significantly lower than the main portal pressure (about 18.8 mm Hg) [18].

Estimation of hepatic blood flow

Constant infusion method

Hepatic blood flow may be measured by a constant infusion of the dye bromsulphalein (BSP) and catheterization of the hepatic vein [19].

The formula for calculating flow, by the Fick principle, is as follows:

$$EHBF = \frac{\text{rate of dye removal}}{\text{arterial}-\text{hepatic vein dye conc.}} \times \frac{1}{Hct},$$

where EHBF = estimated hepatic blood flow, Hct = haematocrit.

If arterial level is constant:

rate of infusion = rate of hepatic removal,

e.g.
Q = 5 mg/min,
A = 1.94 mg/100 ml plasma,
H = 1.34 mg/100 ml plasma,

$$EHBF = \frac{5 \times 100}{0.6} = \frac{500}{0.6} = 834 \text{ ml/min.}$$

If haematocrit = 45%

$$EHBF = \frac{834 \times 100}{(100-45)} = 1520 \text{ ml/min.}$$

This method depends on the dye being removed only by the liver at a steady rate, shown by maintenance of constant arterial levels, and on the absence of significant entero-hepatic circulation.

BSP may be replaced by indocyanine green (IG) [26] which has the advantage of being removed only by the liver, and entero-hepatic circulation is minimal. It is not conjugated. Plasma arterial levels are steadier in those with borderline hepatic function. Calculated hepatic flow is lower than for BSP and this is especially so in the cirrhotic.

This method has been used to show a fall in hepatic blood flow in recumbency, fainting [10], heart failure and cirrhosis, and exercise. Fever increases flow and it is unaltered in such high cardiac output states as thyrotoxicosis and pregnancy.

Plasma disappearance method

Hepatic blood flow can be measured after an intravenous injection of indocyanine green, followed by analysis of the disappearance curve in a peripheral artery and hepatic vein.

$$EHBF = K \times \frac{\text{blood volume}}{E},$$

where

K = fraction retained plasma dye disappearing per minute

$$= \frac{0.693}{t_{\frac{1}{2}}}$$

E = percentage extraction by liver

$$= \frac{\text{arterial-hepatic venous conc.}}{\text{arterial conc.}} \times 100.$$

If the extraction of a substance is 100%, i.e. the substance is completely removed in one passage through the liver, then hepatic blood flow could be measured from the peripheral–arterial disappearance curve. A heat-denatured albumin colloidal complex tagged with [131]I ([131]CAI) has minimal extra-hepatic removal and 94% extraction by the liver in man [151]. In normal subjects hepatic blood flow can be determined from the peripheral clearance, without hepatic vein catheterization, by the formula:

$$EHBF = K \times \text{blood volume},$$

where

K = fraction retained plasma colloid disappearing per minute

$$= \frac{0.693}{t_{\frac{1}{2}}}$$

and assuming 100% extraction of colloid by liver.

In patients with cirrhosis up to 20% of the blood perfusing the liver may not go through normal channels and hepatic extraction is reduced. This must be measured by hepatic vein catheterization to obtain estimates of flow in patients with liver disease. Galactose and D-sorbitol have been used in similar fashion to indocyanine green [109].

Electromagnetic flow meters

Flows in exposed vessels may be measured directly using the square-wave electromagnetic flow meter. This enables flow in portal vein and hepatic artery to be measured separately.

Doppler ultrasound

Doppler ultrasound may be used to determine the direction of blood flow, (whether hepato-pedal or hepato-fugal) [116], and the calibre of the portal vein, its branches and the portal–systemic collaterals [133]. The patency of the portal vein and of any surgical portal–systemic shunt can be established. Arterio–portal shunts and portal vein occlusion may be diagnosed.

Oesophageal varices may be predicted by

the demonstration of hepato-fugal flow in an enlarged left gastric vein [123]. Patients with chronic portal systemic encephalopathy have shown hepato-pedal flow in the splenic vein due to large spontaneous spleno—renal shunting [121].

The Doppler method has been used to measure portal blood flow. The average velocity of blood flowing in the portal vein is multiplied by the cross-sectional area of the vessel (fig. 10.32). Measurements are made with the ultrasonic duplex scanner which combines pulsed Doppler with real-time imaging. In a model, results correlate well with those obtained with electromagnetic flow meters [112]. There are however, possible flaws in the technique [24]. The use of a single, highest velocity with a fixed velocity profile [123] is generally inaccurate and a mean velocity using special equipment is preferable [1]. Measurement of the cross-sectional area of the vessel can be difficult. There are technical difficulties in obese individuals. Perhaps the method is most useful in estimating *changes* in flow rather than absolute values.

Using the Doppler technique, the hyperdynamic portal circulation of cirrhosis has been confirmed by finding increased flow in superior mesenteric and splenic arteries [148].

Using Doppler-duplex flow measurements, portal venous pressure measured transhepatically and hepatic venous pressure by catheterization, the portal vascular resistance can be measured and has been shown to be markedly increased in cirrhosis [112].

Variceal blood flow can be assessed during diagnostic endoscopy by a Doppler ultrasound probe passed down the biopsy channel of the standard gastroscope [97].

Estimation of portal—systemic collateral flow

This is a difficult problem. The fraction of portal—systemic shunting may be computed by direct injection of isotope into splenic or mesenteric vein and measurement of the area of an isotope dilution curve recorded in the hepatic vein.

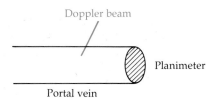

Flow = velocity × cross section vein

Fig. 10.32. The Doppler real-time ultrasound method of measuring portal venous flow.

Trans-hepatic catheterization allows injection of isotopically-labelled materials into splenic or portal vein. Subsequent differential counting over liver and lungs allows calculations of intra- and extra-hepatic shunts. The intra-hepatic shunt indices vary from 1 to 78.4% and the extra-hepatic shunt indices vary from 0 to 50%. These values correlate closely with the size of collaterals opacified by portography.

Azygos blood flow

Most of the blood flowing through gastro-oesophageal varices terminates in the azygos system. Azygos blood flow can be measured using a double thermo-dilution catheter directed under fluoroscopy into the azygos vein (fig. 10.33) [17]. Alcoholic cirrhotic patients who have bled from varices show a flow of about 596 ml/min. Azygos flow is markedly reduced by propranolol [27].

EXPERIMENTAL PORTAL VENOUS
OCCLUSION AND HYPERTENSION

Survival following acute occlusion depends on the development of an adequate collateral circulation. In the rabbit, cat or dog this does not develop and death supervenes rapidly. In the monkey or man, the collateral circulation is adequate and survival is usual [34].

Acute occlusion of one branch of the portal vein is not fatal. The liver cells of the ischaemic lobe atrophy, but bile ducts, Kupffer cells and

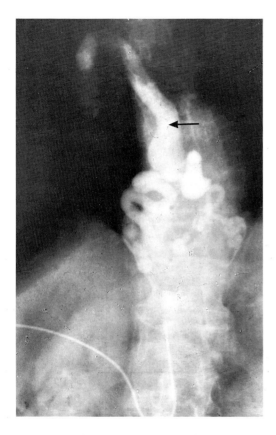

Fig. 10.33. Trans-hepatic catheterization of the azygos vein (arrow) via portal vein and oesophageal collaterals.

connective tissues survive. The unaffected lobe hypertrophies.

Experimentally, portal hypertension can be produced by occluding the portal vein, injecting silica into the portal vein, infecting mice with schistosomiasis, by any experimental type of cirrhosis, or by biliary obstruction. An extensive collateral circulation develops, the spleen enlarges but ascites does not form.

Classification of portal hypertension

Portal hypertension usually follows obstruction to the portal blood flow anywhere along its course. Intrasplenic pressure reflects pressure in the splenic vein. The trans-hepatic route can be used to measure pressure in the main portal vein [162]. The wedged hepatic venous pressure represents sinusoidal pressure. Splenic or portal venography or visceral angiography show the site of obstruction and the nature of the collateral circulation. Liver biopsy helps in localization and diagnosis of the cause of obstruction. Using a selection of these techniques, portal hypertension can be classified into two groups *presinusoidal* (extra-hepatic or intra-hepatic) and a big general group of *hepatic* causes (figs 10.34, 10.35, table 10.3). This distinction is a practical one. The presinusoidal forms, which include obstruction to the sinusoids by Kupffer and other cellular proliferation, are associated with relatively normal hepato-cellular function. Consequently, if patients with this type suffer a haemorrhage from oesophageal varices, liver failure is rarely a consequence. In contrast, the intra-hepatic types are associated with hepato-cellular disease. Patients with this type suffering haemorrhage frequently develop liver failure.

Table 10.2. Methods of visualizing the portal vein

Method	Scanning	Splenic venography	Splanchnic arteriography
Definition of:			
Portal vein	+	+++	++
Splenic vein	±	+++	±
Collaterals	±	+++	+
Hepatic artery	0	0	+++
Estimation of portal pressure	No	Yes	No
Complications	None	Intraperitoneal haemorrhage	Femoral arterial haemorrhage

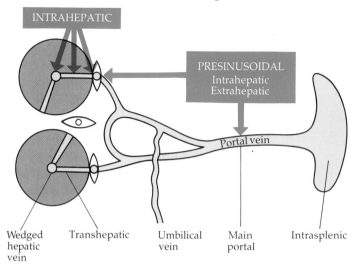

Pressure recordings

INTRAHEPATIC

PRESINUSOIDAL
Intrahepatic
Extrahepatic

Portal vein

Wedged   Transhepatic   Umbilical   Main   Intrasplenic
hepatic   vein   portal
vein

Fig. 10.34. Portal hypertension can be classified into two main groups: presinusoidal and intra-hepatic. The presinusoidal is further divided into extra-hepatic, where the obstruction is the main portal vein, intra-hepatic, where the obstruction is usually in the portal tracts. Pressure recordings allow the anatomical site of the obstruction to be located.

Table 10.3. Classification of portal hypertension

Presinusoidal	
Extra-hepatic	Blocked portal vein
	Increased splenic flow
Intra-hepatic	Portal zone infiltrates
	Toxic
	Hepato-portal sclerosis
Hepatic	
Intra-hepatic	Cirrhosis
Post-sinusoidal	Other nodules
	Blocked hepatic vein

Extra-hepatic portal venous obstruction [119]

This causes extra-hepatic presinusoidal portal hypertension. The obstruction may be at any point in the course of the portal vein. The *venae comitantes* enlarge in an attempt to deliver portal blood to the liver, so assuming a leash-like cavernous appearance [180]. The portal vein, represented by a fibrous strand, is recognized with difficulty in the multitude of small vessels. This cavernous change follows any block in the main vein (fig. 10.25) [156].

AETIOLOGY

Infections, whether septicaemic or intra-abdominal, are the commonest causes. Umbilical infection with or without catheterization of the umbilical vein may be responsible in neonates [175]. The infection spreads along the umbilical vein to the left portal vein and hence to the main portal vein (fig. 10.36). Acute appendicitis and peritonitis are causative in older children.

Portal vein occlusion is particularly common in India accounting for 20–30% of all variceal bleeding. Neonatal dehydration and infections may be responsible.

Ulcerative colitis and Crohn's disease can be complicated by portal vein block. Portal vein obstruction may be secondary to biliary infections due, for instance, to gallstones or primary sclerosing cholangitis.

Post-operative

The portal and splenic veins commonly block after splenectomy, especially when, pre-operatively, the patient had a normal platelet count which, however, rises post-operatively. The thrombosis spreads from the splenic vein

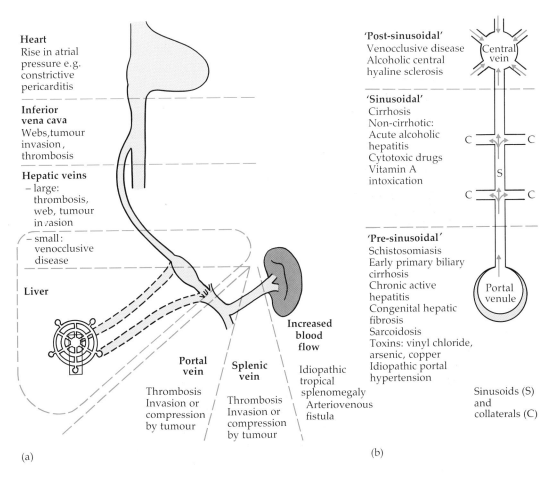

Fig. 10.35. Causes of portal hypertension. (a) Pre- and posthepatic. (b) Intrahepatic. (*NB. Overlap exists; wedge hepatic vein pressure may be high in patients with 'pre-sinusoidal' causes, especially as the disease progresses, indicating sinusoidal and/or collateral involvement. Some 'post-sinusoidal' conditions may also have a sinusoidal component.) (Dick & Dooley, 1987).

into the main portal vein. It is especially likely in patients with myeloid metaplasia [22]. A similar sequence follows occluded surgical portal–systemic shunts. It should be considered where ascites and abdominal pain develop post-operatively.

The portal vein may thrombose as a complication of major, difficult biliary surgery, for instance, repair of a stricture or removal of a choledochal cyst.

Trauma

Portal vein injury usually follows automobile accidents or stabbing and is rare. Laceration of the portal vein carries a mortality of 50% and ligation may be the only method to control the bleeding.

Hypercoagulable state

Enhanced clotting may be a factor, particularly

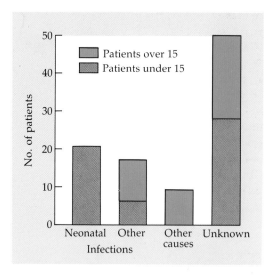

Fig. 10.36. Aetiology of portal vein occlusion in 97 patients over and under 15 years old (Webb & Sherlock 1979).

in the older age group. Myeloproliferative diseases, especially polycythaemia rubra vera are the commonest associations. These must be excluded in all adults with portal vein obstruction.

Invasion and compression

The classic example is hepato-cellular carcinoma. Carcinoma of the pancreas, usually of the body, and of other adjacent organs may lead to portal vein block. Portal and splenic vein thrombosis can complicate chronic pancreatitis, usually in the alcoholic.

Congenital

Congenital obstruction can be produced anywhere along the line of the right and left vitelline veins from which the portal vein develops. The portal vein may be absent with visceral venous return passing to systemic veins particularly the inferior vena cava [111]. Hilar venous collaterals are absent.

Congenital abnormalities of the portal vein are usually associated with congenital defects elsewhere [111, 118, 191].

Cirrhosis

The prevalence of portal vein thrombosis complicating cirrhosis is very low [126]. Invasion by a hepato-cellular carcinoma is the most frequent cause. Post-splenectomy thrombocytosis is another aetiological factor. Mural thrombi found at autopsy are probably terminal [11]. It is easy to overdiagnose thrombosis by finding a non-filled portal vein on imaging. This usually represents 'steal' into massive collaterals or into a large spleen.

Miscellaneous

Portal vein thrombosis has been associated with pregnancy and with oral contraceptives, especially in older women and with long usage [31].

Portal vein block has been associated with general disease of veins and in particular with thrombophlebitis migrans.

Collagen diseases may be related, perhaps due to the lupus anticoagulant.

In retro-peritoneal fibrosis, the portal venous system may be encased by dense fibrous tissue [114].

Unknown

In about half the patients the aetiology, even after the fullest investigation, remains obscure (fig. 10.36). Some of these patients have associated auto-immune disorders such as hypothyroidism, diabetes, pernicious anaemia, dermatomyositis or rheumatoid arthritis [191]. It is difficult to find a link between these conditions and portal venous block. In some instances, the obstruction may have followed undiagnosed intra-abdominal infections such as appendicitis or diverticulitis.

CLINICAL FEATURES

The patient may present with features of the underlying disease, for instance, polycythaemia rubra vera or primary liver cancer.

Bleeding from oesophago-gastric varices is

the commonest mode of presentation. In those of neonatal origin, the first haemorrhage is at about the age of four (fig. 10.37). The frequency increases between 10 and 15 years and decreases after puberty. However, some patients with portal venous block never bleed and in others haemorrhage may be delayed for as long as 12 years. If blood replacement is adequate, recovery usually ensues in a matter of days. Apart from frank bleeds, intermittent minor blood loss is probably common. This is diagnosed only if the patient is having repeated checks for stool blood or if iron deficiency anaemia develops.

Especially in children, haemorrhage may be initiated by a minor, febrile, intercurrent infection. The mechanism is unclear. Aspirin or a similar drug may be the precipitating factor, perhaps by damaging the congested gastric mucosa. Excessive exertion or swallowing a large bolus does not seem to initiate bleeding.

The spleen is always enlarged and symptomless splenomegaly may be a mode of presentation, particularly in children. Peri-umbilical veins are not seen but there may be dilated abdominal wall veins in the left flank.

The liver is normal in size and consistency. Stigmata of hepato-cellular disease, such as jaundice or vascular spiders, are absent. With acute portal venous thrombosis, ascites is early and transient, subsiding as the collateral circulation develops. Ascites is usually related to an additional factor which has depressed hepato-cellular function, such as a haemorrhage or a surgical exploration. It may be seen in the elderly where it is related to the deterioration of liver function and fall in serum albumin with ageing [176].

Hepatic encephalopathy is not uncommon in adults, usually following an additional insult such as haemorrhage, infection or anaesthetic. Chronic encephalopathy may be seen in elderly patients with a particularly large portal–systemic collateral circulation.

Haematology

179 Haemoglobin is normal unless there has been

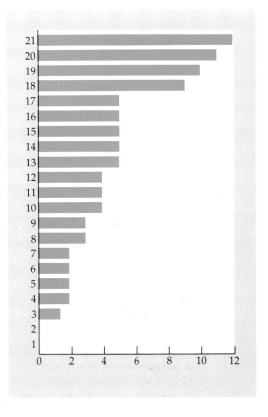

Fig. 10.37. Portal vein occlusion in neonates. Age at time of first haemorrhage in 21 patients in whom the portal vein block occurred in the neonatal period (Webb & Sherlock 1979).

blood loss. Leucopenia and thrombocytopenia are related to the enlarged spleen. Circulating platelets and leucocytes, although in short supply, are adequate and function well.

Hypersplenism is not an indication for splenectomy. Blood coagulation is normal.

Serum biochemistry

All the usual tests of 'liver function' are normal. Elevation of serum globulin may be related to intestinal antigens, particularly *E. coli* bypassing the liver through collaterals. Mild pancreatic hypofunction is presumably related to interruption of the venous drainage of the pancreas (fig. 10.38) [193].

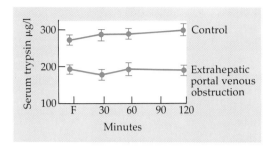

Fig. 10.38. Patients with extra-hepatic portal venous obstruction show lower fasting serum trypsin values and respond less well to a Lundh meal than control subjects (Webb *et al.* 1980).

PROGNOSIS

This depends on the underlying disease. The outlook is much better than for cirrhosis as liver function is normal. The prognosis is surprisingly good in the child and, with careful management of the recurrent bleeding, survival to adult life is to be expected. The number of bleeds seems to get less as time passes. Women may bleed in pregnancy but this is unusual; their babies are normal.

TREATMENT

Any underlying cause must be identified and treated. This may be more important than the portal hypertension. For instance, hepatocellular carcinoma, invading the portal vein, precludes aggressive therapy for bleeding oesophageal varices. If the variceal bleeding is secondary to thrombosis of the portal vein related to polycythaemia rubra vera, reduction of the platelet count by venesection or cytotoxic drugs must precede any surgical therapy; anticoagulants may be needed.

Prophylactic treatment of varices is not indicated. They may never rupture and as time passes collaterals open up.

With acute portal vein thrombosis, anticoagulant therapy is usually too late as the clot will have undergone organization. If diagnosis is early, anticoagulants may prevent spreading thrombosis.

Children should survive haemorrhage with proper management, including transfusion. Care must be taken to give compatible blood and to preserve peripheral veins. Aspirin ingestion should be avoided. Upper respiratory infections should be treated seriously as they seem to precipitate haemorrhage.

Vasopressin infusions may be needed and occasionally the Sengstaken tube.

Endoscopic sclerotherapy is valuable as an emergency procedure. Later endoscopic obliteration of oesophageal varices can be performed but the usually very marked gastric fundal varices are not affected and they may increase after sclerotherapy.

Definitive surgery for reduction of portal pressure is usually impossible as there are no suitable veins for a shunt. Even apparently normal-looking veins seen on venography turn out to be in poor condition, presumably related to extension of the original thrombotic process. In children, veins are very small and difficult to anastomose. Myriads of collateral channels add to the technical difficulties.

Results for all forms of surgery are very unsatisfactory (table 10.4). Splenectomy is the least successful and has the highest complication rate. A shunt (portacaval, mesocaval, or splenorenal) is the most satisfactory treatment but usually proves impossible. However, techniques are improving and in one series of shunts in children with portal vein thrombosis 90% were patent after 3½ years [2].

Surgery is indicated when conservative therapy has failed. When the patient is exsanguinating, despite massive blood transfusion, then an oesophageal transection may have to be performed using the stapling procedure. Here again gastric varices are not treated. Postoperative complications are common.

Splenic vein obstruction

Isolated splenic vein obstruction causes sinistral (left-sided) portal hypertension. It may be due to any of the factors causing portal vein obstruction (table 10.3). Pancreatic disease such as carcinoma (18%), pancreatitis (65%),

Table 10.4. Haemorrhage due to portal vein occlusion (Webb & Sherlock 1979)

Operation	No.	Re-bleed		Operative deaths (within one month of surgery)
		No.	Mean time (years)	
Splenectomy	19	18	1.9	1
Spleno-renal shunt	20	14	3.2	0
Meso− and porta−caval shunt	16	12	2.1	1
Transections and disconnections	52	44	2.7	4

pseudocyst and pancreatectomy are particularly important [103].

If the obstruction is distal to the entry of the left gastric vein, a collateral circulation bypasses the obstructed splenic vein through short gastric veins into the gastric fundus and lower oesophagus, so reaching the left gastric vein and portal vein. This leads to very prominent varices in the fundus of the stomach but few in the lower oesophagus. Thus not all patients develop oesophageal varices or gastro-intestinal bleeding.

Splenic venography with, if necessary, the selective venous phase of an angiogram (fig. 10.39) are diagnostic. Splenectomy, by blocking arterial inflow, is usually curative. Conventional shunt surgery is valueless, although the selective distal splenorenal shunt may be effective.

Hepatic arterial−portal venous fistulae

Portal hypertension results from increased portal venous flow. Increasing intra-hepatic resistance to a rise in portal flow may also be important. The portal zones of the liver show thickening of small portal venous radicles with accompanying mild fibrosis and lymphocyte infiltration. The increased intra-hepatic resistance may persist after obliteration of the fistula so that portal hypertension is not relieved.

These fistulae are usually congenital [75], traumatic or related to adjacent malignant neoplasms. Inferior mesenteric arteriovenous fistulae may be associated with acute ischaemic colitis [29].

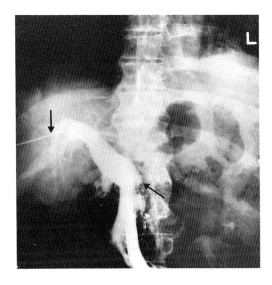

Fig. 10.39. A 64-year-old man with polycythemia rubra vera. Trans-hepatic portal venogram (arrow) shows thrombosed splenic vein marked by black arrow with patent superior mesenteric and portal veins. This patient, after preliminary reduction of red cell and platelet count by radio-active phosphorus, was successfully treated by splenectomy.

With large fistulae, a loud arterial bruit is heard in the right upper abdomen. Pain may be pronounced. Others present with portal hypertension.

Ultrasound and enhanced CT show an enlarged hepatic artery and a dilated intra-hepatic portal vein. The diagnosis is confirmed by angiography.

Selective non-invasive embolization of the fistula is the treatment of choice and has replaced surgery. If portal hypertension persists after obliteration of the fistula, a portal—systemic shunt may be necessary.

Portal—hepatic venous shunts

These are probably congenital and represent persistence of the omphalomesenteric venous system [72]. They may be between the main portal and hepatic veins or between the right or left portal vein and the hepatic veins [33]. They are suggested by ultrasound and confirmed by angiography.

Intra-hepatic presinusoidal and sinusoidal portal hypertension (fig. 10.40)

PORTAL TRACT LESIONS

In *schistosomiasis*, the portal hypertension results from the ova causing a reaction in the minute portal—venous radicles.

In *congenital hepatic fibrosis* the portal hypertension is probably due to a deficiency of terminal branches of the portal vein in the fibrotic portal zones.

The portal hypertension sometimes complicating the *myeloproliferative diseases* results from infiltration of the portal zones with haemopoietic tissue. Portal hypertension has been reported with myelosclerosis, myeloid leukaemia and Hodgkin's disease. Wedged hepatic venous pressure is normal while intrasplenic pressure is increased. Increased hepatic flow is presumably related to the enlarged spleen.

In *systemic mastocytosis*, portal hypertension is related to increased intra-hepatic resistance secondary to mast cell infiltration. Increased splenic flow, perhaps with splenic arteriovenous shunting and with histamine release, may contribute [65].

In *primary biliary cirrhosis*, portal hypertension may be a presenting feature long before the development of the nodular regeneration characteristic of cirrhosis (Chapter 14). The mechanism is uncertain, although portal zone lesions and narrowing of the sinusoids because of cellular infiltration have been incriminated.

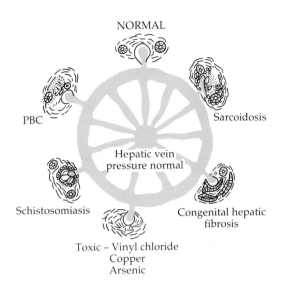

Fig. 10.40. The aetiology of presinusoidal intra-hepatic portal hypertension.

The portal hypertension of *sarcoidosis* may be similar (Chapter 26).

TOXIC CAUSES

The injurious substance is taken up by endothelial cells, mostly lipocytes (Ito cells) in Dissë's space; these are fibrogenic. Minute portal vein radicles are obstructed and intra-hepatic portal hypertension results. *Inorganic arsenic* is a good example. Portal hypertension complicates the treatment of psoriasis with arsenic. Liver disease in vineyard sprayers in Portugal may be related to exposure to copper. Angiosarcoma may be a complication.

Exposure to the vapour of the polymer of *vinyl chloride* leads to sclerosis of portal venules with portal hypertension and angiosarcoma.

Reversible portal hypertension may follow *vitamin A intoxication*—vitamin A being stored in Ito cells [66]. Prolonged use of *cytotoxic drugs*, such as methotrexate, 6-mercaptopurine, and azathioprine can lead to perisinusoidal fibrosis and portal hypertension.

182

IDIOPATHIC PORTAL HYPERTENSION

This has been reported from Japan and is marked by splenomegaly, portal hypertension and relatively mild changes in liver function tests. It affects largely middle-aged women. Intra-hepatic portal veins show occlusive changes. The aetiology is unknown (fig. 10.41).

A very similar condition in India, called *non-cirrhotic portal fibrosis*, largely affects young males. It has been related to arsenic taken in drinking water and in unorthodox medicines. It is more likely due to the effects on the liver of multiple intestinal infections over many years.

Somewhat similar patients have been reported from the United States [107] and the United Kingdom [81].

Hepato—portal sclerosis

This is a confused entity. It has also been termed non-cirrhotic portal fibrosis, non-cirrhotic portal hypertension and idiopathic portal hypertension. Injury to intra-hepatic portal venous radicles and sinusoidal endothelial cells is the common denominator. In every case an increase in intra-hepatic resistance indicates an obstruction to hepatic blood flow. The injury may be infectious, toxic or in many instances unknown.

In childhood, intra-hepatic thrombosis of small portal veins could be the primary disorder [104]. Doppler flow studies suggest increased splenic flow may play a part [124].

Banti's disease, an obsolete term, probably falls into this group.

Liver biopsy shows sclerosis and sometimes obliteration of the intra-hepatic venous bed but the changes, and especially the fibrosis, may be minimal. Large portal veins near the hilum may be thickened and narrow, but this is usually seen only at autopsy. Some of the changes seem to be secondary to partial thrombosis of small portal venous channels with recanalization. Perisinusoidal fibrosis is usually present but may be seen only by electron microscopy.

Portal venography shows small portal vein radicles to be narrowed and sparse. The peripheral branches may be irregular with acute-angle division. Some of the large intra-hepatic portal branches may be non-opacified with

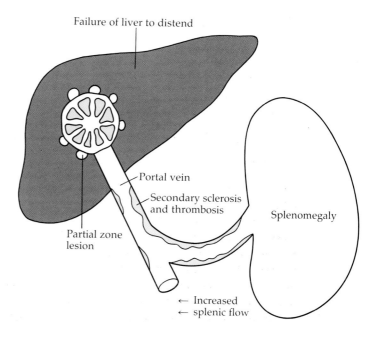

Fig. 10.41. Factors concerned in so-called idiopathic 'primary' portal hypertension.

increase of very fine vasculature around large intra-hepatic portal branches. Hepatic venography confirms the vascular abnormalities and vein-to-vein anastomoses are frequent.

The tropical splenomegaly syndrome

This is marked by residence in a malarial area, splenomegaly, hepatic sinusoidal lymphocytosis and Kupffer cell hyperplasia, raised serum IgM and malarial antibody titres and response to prolonged anti-malarial chemotherapy. Portal hypertension is marked, but variceal bleeding is rare [44].

Congenital intra-hepatic shunting

A three-year-old child has been described with portal hypertension due to an hepatic artery—ductus venosus fistula [106].

An adult with portal—systemic encephalopathy had congenital intra-hepatic shunts between the portal and hepatic veins [139].

This picture was also seen with a shunt through a patent ductus venosus running from the portal vein to the inferior vena cava [120].

Intra-hepatic portal hypertension

CIRRHOSIS [61]

All forms of cirrhosis lead to portal hypertension and the primary event is obstruction to portal blood flow [101]. Portal venous blood is diverted into collateral channels and some bypasses the liver cells and is shunted directly into the hepatic venous radicles in the fibrous septa. These portal—hepatic anastomoses develop from pre-existing sinusoids enclosed in the septa (fig. 10.42) [136]. The hepatic vein is displaced further and further outwards until it lies in a fibrous septum linked with the portal venous radicle by the original sinusoid. The regenerating nodules become divorced from their portal blood supply and are nourished by the hepatic artery. Percutaneous trans-hepatic portography demonstrates even larger portal hepatic venous anastomoses in the cirrhotic liver [122]. About one-third of the total blood flow perfusing the cirrhotic liver may bypass sinusoids, and hence functioning liver tissue, through these channels [151].

The obstruction to portal flow is partially due

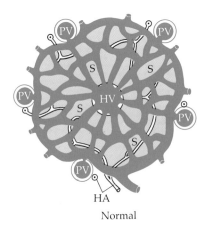
Normal

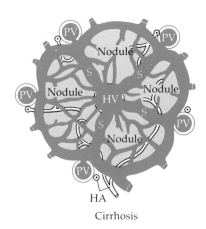
Cirrhosis

Fig. 10.42. Cirrhosis of the liver. The formation of portal venous (PV), hepatic venous (HV) anastomoses or internal Eck fistulae at the site of pre-existing sinusoids (S). Note that the regeneration nodules are supplied by the hepatic artery (HA) (Elias 1952).

to nodules which compress hepatic venous radicles (fig. 10.44) [79]. This would lead to a post-sinusoidal portal hypertension. However, in cirrhosis, the wedged hepatic venous (sinusoidal) and main portal pressures are virtually identical and the stasis must extend to the portal inflow vessels. Sinusoids probably provide the greatest resistance to flow. Changes in Disse's space, particularly collagenization, result in sinusoidal narrowing and this may be particularly important in the alcoholic [128]. Contractile myofibroblasts in the space of Disse could also play a role [6]. Hepatocyte swelling in the alcoholic may also reduce sinusoidal flow [16]. Obstruction is therefore believed to be at all levels from portal zones through the sinusoids to the hepatic venous outflow (fig. 10.43).

The hepatic artery provides the liver with a small volume of blood at a high pressure. The portal vein delivers a large volume at a low pressure (fig. 10.2). The two systems are equilibrated in sinusoids. In normals, the hepatic artery probably plays little part in maintaining portal venous pressure. In the cirrhotic, splenic arterio–portal shunting has been suspected. Hypertrophy of the hepatic artery and relative increase in flow help to maintain sinusoidal perfusion.

NON-CIRRHOTIC NODULES

Various non-cirrhotic nodular conditions of the liver lead to portal hypertension. They are difficult to diagnose, usually being confused with cirrhosis or with 'idiopathic' portal hypertension. A 'normal' needle liver biopsy does not exclude the diagnosis.

Nodular regenerative hyperplasia [40, 186]. Nodules of cells resembling normal hepatocytes and of various sizes involve the liver diffusely. The nodules are not outlined by fibrous tissue. They are probably related to a vasculitis or vascular obstruction of small arteries or portal veins at the level of the acinus [188]. This causes ischaemic atrophy of the involved acinus while adjacent acini, with intact blood supply, undergo compensatory hyperplasia causing micronodularity. They cause marked portal hypertension and there is sometimes haemorrhage into a nodule.

Ultrasound shows hypoechoic or isoechoic masses with anechoic centres with bleeding. CT shows a hypodense pattern with no enhancement on contrast.

The commonest association is with rheumatoid arthritis and Felty's syndrome. Nodules are also seen with monoclonal gammopathy, hyperviscosity syndromes and as a reaction

Fig. 10.43. In patients with cirrhosis the wedged hepatic venous pressure (20 mmHg) is equal to the pressure in the main portal vein (20 mmHg) (measured via umbilical vein). Resistance to flow extends from the central hepatic vein, through the sinusoids to the portal vein. In presinusoidal portal hypertension normal anastomoses exist between small vascular units and prevent the blocking catheter from producing a large area of stasis. Wedged hepatic venous pressure (7 mmHg) is therefore less than the pressure in the main portal vein (20 mmHg) (Reynolds *et al.* 1970).

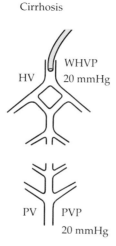

Cirrhosis

HV — WHVP 20 mmHg

PV — PVP 20 mmHg

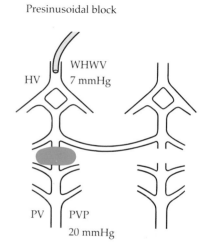

Presinusoidal block

HV — WHWV 7 mmHg

PV — PVP 20 mmHg

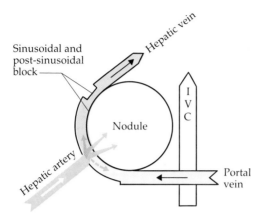

Fig. 10.44. The circulation in hepatic cirrhosis. A nodule obstructs the sinusoids and hepatic veins. The nodule is supplied mainly by the hepatic artery.

to drugs, particularly anabolic steroids and cytotoxics.

Porta—caval shunting for bleeding oesophageal varices is well tolerated as hepato-cellular function is good.

Partial nodular transformation [157] is a very rare disease. The peri-hilar region is replaced by nodules. The periphery of the liver is normal or atrophic (fig. 10.45). Portal hypertension results from obstruction to hepatic blood flow by the nodules. Liver cell function remains good. Fibrosis is inconspicuous, diagnosis is difficult, confirmation often awaits autopsy. The cause is unknown. ·

Focal nodular hyperplasia (Chapter 18).

Veno-occlusive disease (Chapter 11).

Hepatic venous obstruction (Budd—Chiari syndrome (Chapter 11).

Bleeding oesophageal varices

PREDICTING RUPTURE

The prediction of when oesophageal varices will bleed and why is difficult (fig. 10.46). The larger the varices the more likely are they to bleed. Intravariceal pressure is less important although a portal pressure above 12 mmHg appears necessary for varices to form and subsequently bleed [57, 93]. Oesophagitis and

reflux play little, if any, part [135]. Inflammation is not observed histologically in oesophageal rings removed at transection and, in a controlled trial, cimetidine was no better than placebo in preventing recurrent variceal bleeding [100].

Endoscopic appearances of redness and cherry-red spots on the mucosa over the varices may suggest that rupture is imminent. The appearances may be due to intra-epithelial blood-filled channels [167].

Haemorrhage often follows the use of anti-inflammatory drugs. In children, bleeding may follow an upper respiratory infection.

Diagnosis of bleeding

The *clinical features* are those of gastro-intestinal bleeding with the added picture of portal hypertension.

Bleeding may be a slow ooze with melaena, rather than a sudden haematemesis. The intestines may be full of blood before the haemorrhage is recognized and bleeding is liable to continue for days.

Bleeding varices in cirrhosis have injurious effects on the liver cells. These may be due to anaemia diminishing hepatic oxygen supply, or to increased metabolic demands resulting from the protein catabolism following haemorrhage. The fall in blood pressure diminishes hepatic arterial flow, on which the regenerating liver nodules depend, and necrosis may ensue. The increased nitrogen absorption for the intestines often leads to hepatic coma (Chapter 7). Deteriorating liver cell function may precipitate jaundice or ascites.

Non-variceal bleeding is particularly frequent in alcoholic patients in whom duodenal ulcers, gastric erosions and the Mallory—Weiss syndrome are frequent.

Endoscopy is performed routinely to confirm the source of the bleeding (fig. 10.47). Routine ultrasound is used to determine patency of the portal and hepatic veins and to exclude a space-occupying lesion such as a hepato-cellular carcinoma.

Serum biochemical tests are not helpful in

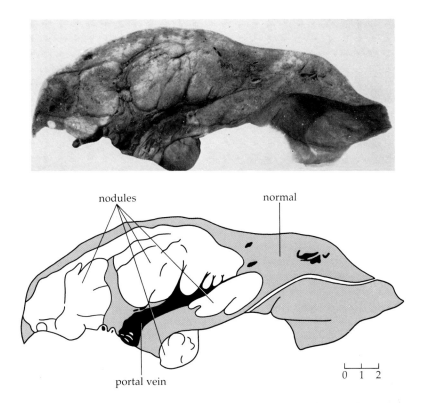

nodules

normal

portal vein

0   1   2

Fig. 10.45. Partial nodular transformation of the liver. Cross-section of liver through the porta hepatis, in which nodules can be seen obstructing the portal vein. The rest of the liver appears normal (Sherlock *et al.* 1960).

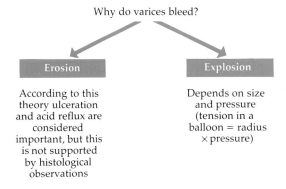

Why do varices bleed?

Erosion

According to this theory ulceration and acid reflux are considered important, but this is not supported by histological observations

Explosion

Depends on size and pressure (tension in a balloon = radius × pressure)

Fig. 10.46. Variceal bleeding.

making the distinction between bleeding varix and bleeding ulcer.

Serial angiography can be used to exclude arterial bleeding and to visualize the portal vein.

Prognosis

In cirrhosis, the mortality of bleeding varices is about 40% with each episode. Recurrence during that hospital admission is 60% and long-term mortality is 60% after two years.

In cirrhosis, the prognosis is determined by the severity of the underlying hepato-cellular disease. The ominous triad of jaundice, ascites and encephalopathy is associated with an 80% mortality. Child classified prognosis into three risk grades: A, B and C (table 10.5) [34]. The one-year survival in good-risk (Child A and B) patients is about 70% and in bad-risk (Child C) about 30% (table 10.6). Alcoholics have a worse prognosis as hepato-cellular disease is greater. Patients with continuing chronic active hepatitis also do poorly. Patients with primary biliary cirrhosis tolerate the haemorrhage reasonably well.

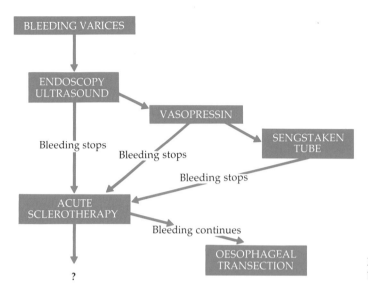

Fig. 10.47. The management of bleeding oesophageal varices.

In portal vein obstruction without cirrhosis, liver failure after haemorrhage is mild and unusual. The prognosis is therefore better. It is determined by availability of peripheral veins and of adequate compatible blood for transfusion.

General measures

The patient should be hospitalized however small the haemorrhage. On admission to hospital, all cirrhotic patients with bleeding oesophageal varices should have their Child's grade recorded in the notes. Bleeding is likely to continue and observation must be close. If possible, the patient should be managed by an intensive care team. A physician and a surgeon must be together in the picture from the start

and subsequent management must be a joint undertaking.

Blood transfusion is a first priority if blood volume is depleted. This may need to be massive. The mean during the first 24 hours is 4 units and the mean total for a hospital admission about 10 units. Saline infusions must be avoided. Over-expansion of the blood volume may initiate re-bleeding. Animal studies suggest this is due to a rise in portal pressure over control levels because of a post-bleeding increase in resistance in portal collaterals [88].

Clotting factors are liable to be deficient and if possible fresh blood or fresh packed red cells or fresh frozen plasma should be used. Platelet transfusions may be necessary. Vitamin K_1 intramuscularly should be routine.

Cimetidine or ranitidine is given. Although

Table 10.5. Child's classification of hepato-cellular function in cirrhosis

Group designation	A	B	C
Serum bilirubin (mg/%)	Below 2.0	2.0−3.0	Over 3.0
Serum albumin (g/%)	Over 3.5	3.0−3.5	Under 3.0
Ascites	None	Easily controlled	Poorly controlled
Neurological disorder	None	Minimal	Advanced coma
Nutrition	Excellent	Good	Poor 'wasting'

there is no controlled evidence of its benefit in patients with severe hepatic failure, stress-induced acute mucosal ulcers are frequent [47].

Sedatives should be avoided and, if essential, oxazepam should be used. Chlordiazepoxide or heminevrin may be useful if the patient is an alcoholic and delirium tremens is a possible development. If the cause of the portal hypertension is presinusoidal and hepato-cellular function is good, hepatic encephalopathy is unlikely and sedation may be liberal.

Routine measures in the cirrhotic patient to prevent hepatic encephalopathy include dietary protein abstention, neomycin 4 g daily, gastric aspiration and enemas, preferably of lactulose, phosphate or lactose (300–500 ml).

If ascites is very tense, intra-abdominal pressure may be reduced by a cautious paracentesis and the use of spironolactone or amiloride.

Endoscopic variceal sclerotherapy is the method of first choice for stopping acute variceal bleeding. However, it is not performed while the patient is actually bleeding as, at this time, injection is difficult and usually fails due to vision being obscured by blood. First, haemorrhage must be controlled by vasopressin (glypressin), followed, if necessary, by the Sengstaken tube.

Vasopressin (Pitressin) [64, 140]

This lowers portal venous pressure by constriction of the splanchnic arteriolar bed, causing an increase in resistance to the inflow of blood to the gut [152]. It controls haemorrhage from oesophageal varices by lowering portal venous pressure [153].

Twenty units of vasopressin in 100 ml 5% dextrose are given intravenously in 10 minutes. Portal pressure falls for 45–60 minutes (fig. 10.48). Alternatively the vasopressin may be given by continuous intravenous infusion (0.4 μ/min.) for a maximum of two hours.

Abdominal colicky discomfort and evacuation of the bowels, together with facial pallor, are usual during the infusion. If these are

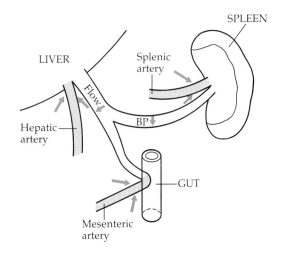

Fig. 10.48. The mode of action of vasopressin on the splanchnic circulation. Hepatic, splenic and mesenteric arteries are shown. Splanchnic blood flow (including hepatic blood flow) and portal venous pressure are reduced by arterial vasoconstriction (arrowed).

absent it may be questioned whether the vasopressin is pharmacologically active. Inert material is the commonest cause of failure.

Vasopressin stimulates smooth muscle and so causes coronary vasoconstriction. A preliminary electrocardiogram should be taken before vasopressin is given.

Cessation of haemorrhage probably results from the temporary drop in portal flow and blood pressure, allowing haemostasis at the bleeding point. The reduction in hepatic arterial blood flow in patients with cirrhosis is undesirable.

Efficacy drops with repeated use. Vasopressin may stop the bleeding but not prolong life. It should be regarded as a preliminary to other forms of treatment.

Despite widespread use there have been very few controlled trials of efficacy and these have given conflicting results [14]. Such trials are difficult to perform while the patient is bleeding and when other therapies are being used. Vasopressin may be less effective during a haemorrhage when endogenous vasopressin is already maximally released [89]. Nevertheless, until proved otherwise vasopressin remains a useful initial, simple, emergency method of controlling variceal bleeding.

Vasopressin may be given with *nitroglycerine* (0.4 mg sublingual). This reduces the cardiac side-effects but does not alter survival or transfusion requirements [58, 179].

Terlipressin (glypressin; tryglycyl lysine vasopressin). This synthetic derivative has the same haemodynamic effect as vasopressin. It is more stable and has a longer action than vasopressin. It is given as a 2 mg bolus 6 hourly. It is more costly than vasopressin and at present it is not clear that it is superior to it [14].

Somatostatin. This drug has similar haemodynamic effects and is as effective as vasopressin but with fewer complications [87]. It is given in a dose of 250 μg per hour after a bolus of 5 μg. However, the drug is costly and probably has little to offer over vasopressin or glypressin.

Long-acting somatostatin is being evaluated. It has no effect on the systemic circulation [51] and is effective in lowering portal pressure [77] in experimental animals. It is extremely costly.

Sengstaken–Blakemore tube (fig. 10.49) [134]

Oesophageal tamponade is done with the Sengstaken–Blakemore tube. The four-lumened tube has an oesophageal and a gastric balloon [134], a tube in the stomach and a fourth lumen for continuous aspiration above the oesophageal balloon. The stomach is emptied. A *new*, tested and lubricated tube is passed through the mouth into the stomach. The gastric balloon is inflated with 250 ml air and doubly clamped. The gastric tube is aspirated continuously. The oesophageal tube is inflated to a pressure of 20–30 mmHg, slightly greater than that expected in the portal vein. Firm traction is exerted using a padded keyhole plywood retainer positioned around the tube at the angle of the mouth and held in position by adhesive tape. Too little traction means that the gastric balloon falls back into the stomach. Too much causes discomfort with retching, and also potentiates gastro-oesophageal ulceration. The position of the tube may be checked radiologically. The gastric balloon should sit well into the fundus

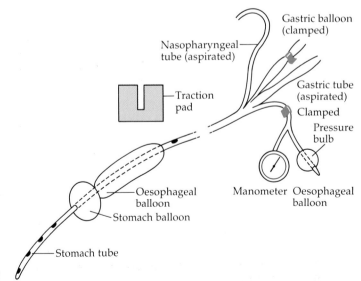

Fig. 10.49. Sengstaken–Blakemore oesophageal compression tube modified by Pitcher (1971). Note fourth oesophageal tube which aspirates the oesophagus above the oesophageal balloon.

Table 10.6. Pugh's (Child's) grading and hospital deaths at index bleed

Grade	No. patients	Hospital deaths (%)
A	65	3 (5%)
B	68	12 (18%)
C	53	36 (68%)
Total	186	51 (27%)

of the stomach. The head of the bed is elevated. A trained attendant is constantly at the bedside and a pair of scissors is available to transect the tube if respiratory distress occurs. Tube traction and oesophageal balloon pressure are checked at 2–4 hour intervals. After 24 hours, traction is released, and the oesophageal balloon deflated leaving the gastric balloon inflated for a further 24 hours. If, during this period, re-bleeding occurs, the traction is re-applied and the oeso-phageal balloon re-inflated for another 24–28 hours or until emergency sclerosis or surgery is performed. Following removal, a soft diet and saltfree liquid antacids are given.

The compression tubes are successful in con-trolling bleeding from oesophageal varices. They do, however, have many complications including obstruction to the pharynx and asphyxia. The gastric balloon may rupture and the tube may migrate into the oesophagus. Ulceration of the lower oesophagus complicates one-third of intubations, particularly if pro-longed or repeated. Aspiration of secretion into the lung is prevented by continuous aspiration of the nasopharynx via the fourth tube.

The *Linton–Nachlas* tube is a single-balloon triple-lumen tube which is more effective for control of gastric variceal haemorrhage but less so for the oesophagus [174].

The modified four-lumen Sengstaken tube is the most certain method for continued control of oesophageal bleeding over hours. Compli-cations are frequent and are in part related to the skill and experience of the operating team [134]. It is unpleasant for the patient. It is useful when patients have to be transferred from one centre to another and when haemorrhage is

torrential. It is a useful preliminary to variceal sclerosis or surgery. The oesophageal tube should not be kept inflated for more than 24 hours.

Endoscopic sclerotherapy [165]

In 1939, injection sclerotherapy for the treat-ment of oesophageal varices was introduced [38]. It did not achieve popularity, but current disenchantment with portal–systemic shunt-ing procedures has led to its re-introduction. The varix is thrombosed by the injection of a sclerosing solution introduced via the endoscope.

TECHNIQUE (table 10.7)

The technique should be as sterile as possible with sterile needles, mouth washes and careful mouth hygiene. A conventional fibre endo-scope is usual with local anaesthesia and sed-ation. The 23-gauge needle protrudes 3–4 mm beyond the catheter sheath (fig. 10.50). Large (3.7 mm channel) or double channel endoscopes allow a clear view and safer injection. They are of particular value to control acute bleeding. The rigid oesophagoscope has been largely abandoned although it provides a more blood-less field of vision.

The sclerosant may be 5% sodium morrhuate, 1% sodium tetradecylsulphate or 5% etha-nolamine oleate. The choice is probably un-important. The injection is made just above the gastro-oesophageal junction and the volume should not exceed 4 ml in any one varix. Gastric

Table 10.7. Royal Free Hospital routine for oesophageal variceal sclerotherapy

1 Sedation (10 mg diazepam I.V.)
2 Local anaesthesia to throat
3 Endoscope (oblique viewing) (Olympus K10)
4 Intravariceal
5 1–4 ml 5% ethanolamine or 5% sodium morrhuate per varix
6 Maximum total sclerosant per session 15 ml
7 Sucralfate (1 g twice daily) for one week

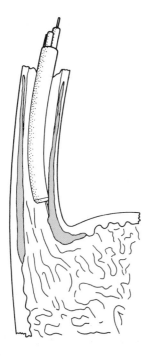

Fig. 10.50. Direct injection with an unmodified fibreoptic endoscope.

varices within 3 cm of the gastro-oesophageal junction may be injected.

The sclerosant may be injected directly into the varix to obliterate the lumen or into the lamina propria to produce inflammation followed by fibrosis. The intra-variceal technique seems more effective in controlling acute haemorrhage and has fewer variceal recurrences [147]. However if methylene-blue is added to the sclerosant it becomes apparent that most injections are both intra- and para-variceal. With acute bleeding, para-variceal and intra-variceal injection may be combined [83]. After sclerosis, a mucosal protective such as sucralfate is given for a few days.

Acute sclerotherapy

Control of acute bleeding is 71 to 96%. Controlled trials have shown significant reduction in re-bleeding [8, 131]. In grade C patients with alcoholic cirrhosis, bleeding was reduced but there was no difference in survival compared with controls [91]. These good results come from experienced groups. The occasional operator should not attempt to deal with bleeding oesophageal varices using the endoscope.

Chronic sclerotherapy

Once bleeding has been controlled the patient usually commences a course of repeated variceal sclerotherapy. The injections are done at weekly intervals until all varices are thrombosed. Each session involves treating three to four varices with 1−2 ml sclerosant. Manometry may be used to assess whether a varix has been sclerosed [73]. Three to five sessions at weekly intervals will probably be needed. In the majority, the procedure should be considered an out-patient one and this considerably reduces the cost [95].

In one uncontrolled trial, the varices were first obliterated by intravariceal injection to be followed by sub-mucosal injections of ethanolamine to cause ulceration and denude the mucosa and sub-mucosa. This would then re-epithelialize with squamous epithelium [83]. This procedure is said to be particularly effective in reducing variceal recurrence.

New varices will undoubtedly develop and the patient has to be followed up endoscopically every six months or so when any new vessel is injected, particularly if it is red. This long-term routine demands much compliance from the patient.

RESULTS

Sclerotherapy is less costly than surgery in treating variceal haemorrhage.

Controlled trials have shown that the frequency of re-bleeding is markedly reduced in the sclerosed group [172, 195]. Any re-bleeding usually takes place before varices have been fully obliterated. Gastric varices remain untreated and indeed may increase with the development of congestive gastropathy and subsequent bleeding. Varices may increase at other sites, for instance the colon. The effect of chronic sclerotherapy on survival is more controversial. Controlled trials from London [195] France [132] and Copenhagen [37] show an improvement of treated over controls, whereas those from South Africa [172] and Los Angeles [86] report no difference. The results of these trials are difficult to compare. Account must be taken of when randomization took place (the later the better) [161], the aetiology of the cirrhosis, the number of grade C patients included, the number treated with acute bleeding as opposed to chronic sclerotherapy, and the number lost to follow-up. One can conclude that variceal bleeding is certainly reduced but survival is much the same, deaths usually being due to hepato-cellular failure (table 10.8).

Prophylactic sclerotherapy

Despite early enthusiastic reports there is now little enthusiasm for this treatment [173]. Indeed it does not significantly reduce the risk of the first variceal bleed [149]. Controlled trials are extremely difficult to construct and continue

Table 10.8. Sclerotherapy of varices

Prophylactic
- Benefit uncertain

Acute
- Skill needed
- Stops bleeding
- ? survival

Chronic
- Less deaths from bleeding
- Complications many
- Compliance
- ? survival unaltered

[26]. One large, multicentre, controlled trial was abandoned because of the high incidence of side-effects in those receiving sclerotherapy [60]. Nevertheless, if, on endoscopy, red varices are seen with weals and cherry-red spots upon them they should probably be sclerosed even if overt haemorrhage has never taken place.

Complications

These depend on the site of injection and are greater with para-variceal than intra-variceal. Other factors include the volume of sclerosant used and the grade of severity of the cirrhosis. Complications are more likely with chronic, repeated sclerotherapy than with acute injection to stop bleeding.

Almost every patient will experience fever, dysphagia and chest pain. This is usually transient.

Bleeding is the most common life-threatening complication. This is not usually from the puncture site but from remaining varices or deep ulcers that have opened on sub-mucosal channels. Re-bleeding is seen in 30% of patients before the varices have been obliterated [166]. If the haemorrhage comes from varices, further sclerotherapy is indicated. If from an ulcer, management should be conservative with sucralfate and transfusion if necessary.

Stricture formation is usually related to underlying inflammatory myonecrosis. Acid clearance from the distal oesophagus is delayed following sclerosis, and swallowing is impaired [164]; these may contribute to stricture formation. Oesophageal dilatation is usually successful but occasionally the strictures are refractory so that surgery becomes necessary [169].

Perforation can follow fibreoptic endoscopic sclerotherapy [154]. Delayed post-necrotic perforation may be followed by broncho-oesophageal fistula.

Pulmonary complications include chest pain, aspiration pneumonia, pleural effusions [4, 5] and mediastinitis. Adult respiratory distress syndrome has been attributed to morrhuate sclerosis [110] although only very little morrhuate reaches the pulmonary endothelium [36].

Pyrexia is frequent and bacteraemia is not uncommon. Prophylactic antibiotics should be given only to those at risk of developing endocarditis [28].

Other recorded complications include cardiac tamponade [168], pericarditis [84] and brain abscess [34].

Trans-hepatic variceal sclerosis (fig. 10.30)

Under local anaesthesia, a catheter can be introduced into the portal vein and the dangerous variceal supply veins selectively catheterized and injected with sclerosant—so obliterating them [96, 163]. The hole in the liver is plugged as the catheter is withdrawn. This is an excellent method of stopping variceal bleeding, particularly in those with severe liver failure. The technique allows fundal and oesophageal varices to be obliterated close to their origin.

Complications include haemorrhage from the liver, biliary peritonitis and, possibly, portal vein thrombosis.

The duration of occlusion is uncertain. The value is as an emergency procedure in poor-risk patients. It demands considerable technical skill and comparison shows it is not so effective as sclerotherapy [170].

Emergency surgery

This should be avoided if at all possible.

A porta−caval shunt performed as an emergency as soon as possible after the bleed virtually eliminates recurrent haemorrhage from varices [127]. The mortality for grade C patients is 50% and for all comers 20%. Alas, only 20% of survivors are alive five years later. Even in mild and moderate cirrhosis, emergency porta−caval shunt has a post-operative encephalopathy rate of 31% [185]. Hospital costs and blood requirements are significantly reduced. Emergency porta−caval shunting has not been universally accepted and it is probable that less experienced surgical groups will not be so successful. It cannot, at present, be recommended.

If bleeding is torrential, and re-bleeding occurs following initial control with vasopressin, sclerotherapy and the Sengstaken tube, an emergency oesophageal transection using the staple gun procedure may be the most suitable operation. An alternative is an emergency meso−caval shunt; this has a high mortality in grade C patients.

Emergency oesophageal transection using the staple gun

Under general anaesthesia, the staple gun is inserted into the lower oesophagus via an anterior gastrotomy (fig. 10.51). A ligature is tied just above the cardia, invaginating a section of oesophageal wall between the two parts of the gun. The stapler is closed and fired, and the oesophageal wall is transected and stapled. The gun with the segment of oesophagus is removed. The gastrotomy and anterior abdominal wall are closed [78]. The stapling transection arrests haemorrhage in every patient. However, a third of the patients die during that hospital admission, usually from hepatic failure. The staple gun procedure has a place in the emergency treatment of bleeding oesophageal varices. Operative time is short, mortality low and complications few. It is not indicated as a prophylactic or elective procedure. Within two

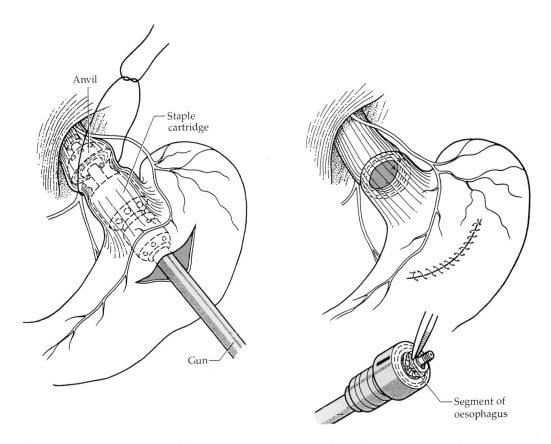

Fig. 10.51. Stapling transection of the lower oesophagus. The staple gun has been introduced into the lower oesophagus via a gastrotomy. A ligature has been tied just above the cardia invaginating a section of oesophageal wall between the two parts of the gun. When the gun is fired, a section of the oesophageal wall will be transected and stapled. (Courtesy K.E.F. Hobbs.)

years, varices have often recurred, enlarged [73] and frequently re-bled.

Surgical portal−systemic shunts
(fig. 10.52)

The aim is to reduce portal venous pressure, maintain total hepatic and, particularly, portal blood flow and, above all, not have a high incidence of complicating hepatic encephalopathy. There is no currently available procedure that fulfils all these criteria satisfactorily. Hepatic reserve determines survival. Hepatocellular function deteriorates after shunting.

Porta−caval

In 1877 Eck [50] first performed a porta−caval shunt in dogs and this remains the most effective way of reducing portal hypertension in man.

The portal vein is joined to the inferior vena cava either end-to-side, with ligation of the portal vein or side-to-side, maintaining its continuity. The portal blood pressure falls, hepatic venous pressure falls and hepatic arterial flow increases.

The end-to-side shunt probably gives a greater fall in portal venous pressure than does

195

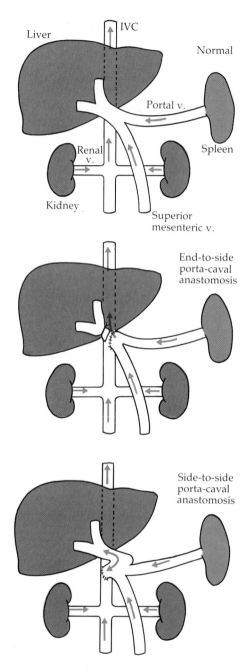

Normal

Liver

IVC

Portal v.

Renal
v.

Spleen

Kidney

Superior
mesenteric v.

End-to-side
porta-caval
anastomosis

Side-to-side
porta-caval
anastomosis

Fig. 10.52. The types of portal—systemic shunt operation performed for the relief of portal hypertension.

the side-to-side procedure, of the order of 10 mmHg. Technically, it is easier to perform. Because of the high incidence of post-shunt

encephalopathy there has been a great reduction in shunt operations. The end-to-side procedure is rarely performed in cirrhotic patients. It is still useful in some patients with early primary biliary cirrhosis, congenital hepatic fibrosis with good hepato-cellular function and with portal vein obstruction at the hilum of the liver.

Patients selected for any shunt should have had a haemorrhage from proven oesophageal varices. Portal hypertension must be established. The portal vein must be good and age preferably less than 50 years. After 40 years, survival is reduced and encephalopathy is twice as common.

The patient should not give a history of hepatic encephalopathy, and should be Child's grade A or B. Serum bilirubin should be less than 2.5 mg/dl in non-biliary cases, serum albumin exceed 3 g/dl and ascites should not be present.

Survival is reduced in chronic active hepatitis where hepato-cellular necrosis continues and increased in primary biliary cirrhosis where hepato-cellular function is maintained. Prognosis in the alcoholic lies between the two and much depends on whether the patient abstains from alcohol.

Meso—caval

This is made between the superior mesenteric vein and the inferior vena cava using a Dacron graft (fig. 10.53) [48]. It is technically easy. The portal vein remains patent but blood flow through it is uncertain. Shunt occlusion is usual with time and is followed by re-bleeding [48].

Selective 'distal' spleno—renal (fig. 10.54)

Veins feeding the dangerous oesophago-gastric collaterals are divided while allowing drainage of portal blood through short gastric—splenic veins through a spleno—renal shunt to the inferior vena cava. Portal blood flow (hepatic perfusion) is maintained.

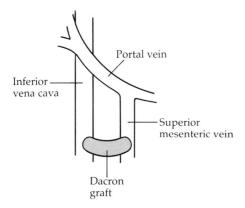

Fig. 10.53. The Drapanas meso-caval shunt using a dacron graft.

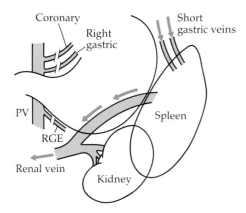

Fig. 10.54. The distal spleno-renal shunt. Veins feeding varices (coronary, right gastric, right gastro-epiploic—RGE) are ligated. A spleno-renal shunt is made, preserving the spleen; retrograde flow in the short gastric veins is possible. Portal blood flow to the liver is preserved. PV = portal vein.

Warren and co-workers [143] report an operative mortality of 4.1%, five year survival was 49%, and the encephalopathy rate 12%, with 30% subclinical encephalopathy; the shunts remained patent. These excellent results may reflect the expertise of this surgical team.

Compared with the standard portal—systemic shunt, the selective one does not improve survival. Some trials report an improved post-operative encephalopathy rate [90, 108] while others do not [35, 69]. These differences

may reflect the type of patient being treated. Re-bleeding may be higher than with a conventional shunt [69].

The selective shunt has not lived up to its original expectations partly due to differences in surgical expertise in various centres. Portal venous perfusion of the liver is not maintained in the long-term. At present, this technically difficult operation should not replace the conventional one except where gastric varices are the main problem.

General results of portal—systemic shunts

Operative mortality in good-risk patients is about 5% with a five year survival of 65—70%. For poor-risk patients, the mortality is 50%.

Shunt closure is often due to operating on a partially thrombosed, diseased portal vein and is often fatal. Hepatic failure is the usual cause of death. Later fibrotic closure of the shunt is unusual.

A patent end-to-side portal—caval anastomosis undoubtedly prevents bleeding from gastro-oesophageal varices, but the advantages have to be weighed against the complications.

After the shunt, abdominal wall collateral veins disappear and spleen size decreases. Endoscopy shows disappearance of varices within six months to one year of the operation.

Portal pressure and hepatic blood flow fall [141] if the shunt is non-selective. The fall in hepatic blood flow accounts for the deterioration in hepatic function while the natural history of the disease also plays a part.

Post-operative jaundice is frequently related to haemolysis and reduction in hepatic function [42].

Oedema of the ankles is due to reduction in portal venous pressure while the serum albumin level remains low. Fluid therefore localizes in dependent parts rather than in the peritoneal cavity. Increased cardiac output with failure may contribute to the oedema.

Shunt patency is confirmed by ultrasound, CT scanning or angiography.

Hepatic encephalopathy may be transient.

Chronic changes develop in 20–40% and personality deterioration in about one-third (Chapter 7). The incidence increases with the size of the shunt. Patients with progressive liver disease are at most risk and particularly so in those with chronic active hepatitis. Encephalopathy is more common in older patients, perhaps due to underlying changes in the ageing brain.

Myelopathy, with paraplegia and a Parkinsonian-cerebellar syndrome are other complications (Chapter 7).

Experimental techniques

Experimental intra-hepatic porta–caval anastomosis. In swine, expandable, stainless-wire Ginturco stents have been introduced via the jugular vein into the inferior vena cava and hence, by liver puncture into the portal vein, identified by trans-hepatic venography [144]. The stent has remained patent at six weeks.

Percutaneous trans-hepatic angioplasty. Extrahepatic portal obstruction has been treated by this technique [181]. This will have a limited application to those patients where part of the intra-hepatic portal venous system is patent.

Percutaneous transluminal angioplasty has been used for stenosis of portal–systemic shunts [146].

Drugs to lower portal pressure
[64, 140]

Theoretically, portal blood pressure (and flow) could be reduced by lowering cardiac output, by reducing inflow by splanchnic vasoconstriction, by splanchnic venodilatation, by reducing intra-hepatic vascular resistance or, of course, by surgical porta–caval shunting (fig. 10.55).

REDUCING CARDIAC OUTPUT

This could be achieved by blocking β_1-receptors in the myocardium. Propranolol acts partially in this way. Metoprolol and atenolol are cardioselective blockers but are less effective than propranolol in reducing portal pressure.

REDUCING PORTAL VENOUS INFLOW

Vasopressin, terlipressin and somatostatin act as splanchnic vasoconstrictors and have already been discussed.

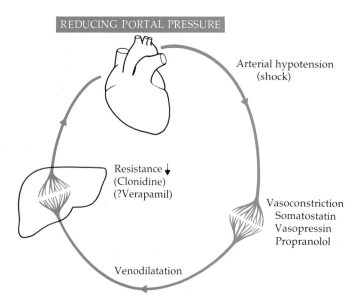

Fig. 10.55. The portal pressure can be reduced by arterial hypotension, splanchnic vasoconstriction, portal venodilation or reduction in intrahepatic resistance.

Table 10.9. Drugs to lower portal pressure

Drug	Oral or intravenous	First pass	Selective β-blocker
Vasopressin	i.v.	–	–
Somatostatin	i.v.	–	–
Propranolol	Oral	Yes	No
Atenolol	Oral	No	Yes
Nitroglycerine	Oral	Yes	–

Propranolol. This non-selective β_1- and β_2-blocker lowers portal venous pressure by reducing cardiac output, but, particularly, by splanchnic vasoconstriction. It is active by mouth, and one dose usually leads to a reduction in portal venous pressure for three to five hours. Azygos blood flow falls even more than portal pressure. There is marked individual variation in the response of the portal blood pressure. Even with large doses, 20 to 50% of patients do not respond [56, 187]. Reduction of the resting pulse rate by 25% measured 12 hours after taking the drug is usually, but not always, a measure of the effect on portal pressure.

Propranolol has been used for the prevention of recurrent variceal bleeding. The first controlled trial in alcoholic, cirrhotic patients with large varices and in good condition showed marked reduction in re-bleeding [94]. Other trials have given conflicting results, some favourable [94, 132], some not so [25, 137, 186] (fig. 10.56). The differences may be related to the type of cirrhosis and, in particular, how many alcoholics were included and how many later abstained. Childs C patients may respond less well than A and B. Compliance may differ from one trial to another.

Blockade may make resuscitation more difficult if the patient re-bleeds. Encephalopathy can also be induced, also a rise in blood ammonia levels. Propranolol is a high 'first pass' rate drug and might be expected to have unpredictable results in patients with advanced cirrhosis where hepatic clearance would be delayed. Propranolol has the advantage of decreasing anxiety. Propranolol whether as prophylaxis or to prevent re-bleeding from varices remains unproven therapy. It should only be given in the context of controlled trials.

PORTAL VASODILATORS

The smooth muscle of the portal vein has α-1-receptors. Portal systemic collaterals are probably already maximally dilated and have a poorly developed smooth muscle layer. They are not likely to respond to vasodilatatory stimuli.

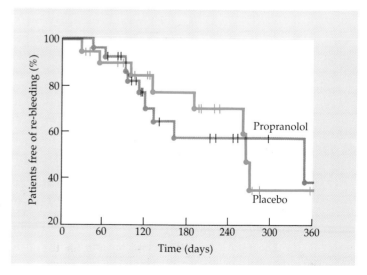

Fig. 10.56. Controlled trial of propranolol for prevention of recurrent variceal haemorrhage in patients with cirrhosis. Percentage of patients in treated and placebo groups free of rebleeding. There is no statistical difference (Burroughs *et al.* 1983).

Nitroglycerin [55] and isosorbide dinitrate [15] probably reduce portal venous pressure as a result of systemic vasodilatation although portal collateral vasodilatation is possible.

Isolated mesenteric veins from portal hypertensive rats are hypersensitive to serotonin. Ketanserin, a 5-HT antagonist, may lower portal blood pressure by dilating the portal venous bed [68].

REDUCING INTRA-HEPATIC VASCULAR RESISTANCE

The increased portal vascular resistance observed in the isolated, perfused, cirrhotic rat liver can be reduced by vasodilators including prostaglandin E1 and isoprenaline [13]. This effect may be on contractile myofibroblasts known to be present in fibrous septa and around sinusoids. The sympathetic is hyperactive in patients with alcoholic cirrhosis [71]. Intravenous clonidine, a centrally acting α-adrenergic agonist, caused a fall in post-sinusoidal hepatic vascular outflow resistance in alcoholic cirrhotic patients [196]. This suggests a labile component of hepatic vascular resistance which is partly under sympathetic control.

Verapamil, a calcium channel antagonist, reduces the hepatic venous pressure gradient and may decrease intra-hepatic resistance [85].

Conclusions

The pharmacology of the portal venous system is difficult to understand. It is uncertain how many results from animal models may be transferred to man where such invasive techniques to study portal blood pressure are impossible.

Interactions between cardiac output, systemic resistance and flow, and portal resistence and flow are difficult to evaluate. A reciprocal relationship exists between the hepatic arterial and portal venous flow, one increasing when the other decreases [92].

The future will hold better agents for the pharmacological control of portal hypertension.

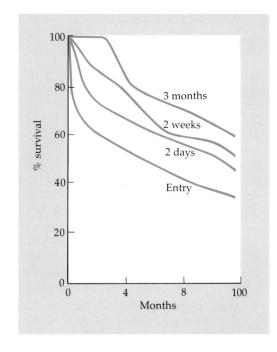

Fig. 10.57. In any trial survival depends on the time elapsed before entry (Smith & Graham, 1982).

These may act on the portal bed or on intra-hepatic resistance. At present, no agent can be recommended for the chronic reduction of portal pressure.

Conclusions

New treatments of gastro-oesophageal varices are usually variants of the old, such as anatomically different shunts or better methods of variceal obliteration. Their proponents are initially enthusiastic, but over the subsequent decade each method takes its place in the background with its forebears. Clinical trials must be interpreted cautiously, the type of patient being entered, the aetiology of the cirrhosis and of the portal hypertension, together with the degree of hepato-cellular failure (how many Child's C grade?) must be noted. The time of randomization is very important. The risk of further haemorrhage and death rapidly diminishes as the patient survives the first few days after a bleed (fig. 10.57) [161]. Endoscopic sclerotherapy, trans-hepatic obliteration or transection oesophageal stapling will stop acute variceal bleeding in 75−100%. Deaths from haemorrhage *per se* should no longer happen. All the procedures have a complication rate, with both procedures the varices may recur and probably bleed again.

The problem of long-term control is a different matter. All the surgical shunting procedures have their drawbacks, particularly encephalopathy. They also have their spectacular individual successes, usually in patients with well compensated hepatic cirrhosis, where the main problem is the height of the portal pressure.

Endoscopic sclerotherapy to obliterate varices gives at least as good results as shunt surgery [143]. Sclerotherapy has a higher re-bleeding rate than the shunt [32, 177, 190] whereas encephalopathy is similar. Survival is better in the endoscopy group provided the patient has a surgical shunt once the sclerotherapy has failed to prevent bleeding [190].

In the group with extra-hepatic portal obstruction, prognosis, even without surgery, is good provided adequate blood transfusion is given.

Medical measures such as bed rest and a good diet may be followed by a fall in portal pressure, especially in alcoholic subjects who lose fat from the liver. This makes assessment of surgical results even more difficult.

References

1 Ackroyd N, Gill R, Griffiths K *et al.* Duplex scanning of the portal vein and porto−systemic shunts. *Surgery* 1986; **99:** 591.
2 Alvarez F, Bernard O, Brunelle E *et al.* Portal obstruction in children. 11 results of surgical porto-systemic shunts. *J. Pediatr.* 1983; **103:** 703.
3 Atkinson M, Sherlock S. Intrasplenic pressure as an index of the portal venous pressure. *Lancet* 1954; **i:** 1325.
4 Bacon BR, Bailey-Newton RS, Connors AF Jr. Pleural effusions after endoscopic variceal sclerotherapy. *Gastroenterology* 1985; **88:** 1910.
5 Bacon BR, Camara DS, Duffy MC. Severe ulceration and delayed perforation of the esophagus after endoscopic variceal sclerotherapy. *Gastrointestin. Endoscopy* 1987; **33:** 311.
6 Balthazar EJ, Megibow A, Naidich D *et al.* Computed tomographic recognition of gastric varices. *Am. J. Roentgenol.* 1984; **142:** 1121.
7 Balthazar EJ, Maidich DP, Megibow AJ *et al.* CT evaluation of esophageal varices. *Am. J. Roentgenol.* 1987; **148:** 131.
8 Barsoum MS, Abdel-Wahab Mooro H, BoLous Fl *et al.* The complications of injection sclerotherapy of bleeding esophageal varices. *Br. J. Surg.* 1982; **69:** 79.
9 Baumgarten P von. Über völlstandiges Offenbleiben der Vena umbilicalis: zugleichein Beitrag zur Frage des Morbus Bantii. *Arb. path. Anat. Inst. Tübingen* 1907; **6:** 93.
10 Bearn AG, Billing B, Edholm OG *et al.* Hepatic blood flow and carbohydrate changes in man during fainting. *J. Physiol.* 1951; **115:** 442.
11 Belli VL, Sansalone CV, Aseni P *et al.* Portal thrombosis in cirrhotics. A retrospective analysis. *Ann. Surg.* 1986; **203:** 286.
12 Bernardino ME, Steinberg HV, Pearson TC *et al.* Shunts for portal hypertension: MR and angiography for determination of patency. *Radiology* 1986; **158:** 57.
13 Bhathal PS, Grossman HJ. Reduction of the increased portal vascular resistance of the isolated perfused cirrhotic rat liver by vasodilators. *J. Hepatol.* 1985; **1:** 325.
14 Blei AT. Vasopressin analogs in portal hypertension: different molecules but similar questions. *Hepatology* 1986; **6:** 146.
15 Blei AT, Gottstein J. Isosorbide dinitrate in experimental portal hypertension: a study of factors that modulate the hemodynamic response. *Hepatology* 1986; **6:** 107.
16 Blendis LM, Orrego H, Crossley IR *et al.* The role of hepatocyte enlargement in hepatic pressure in cirrhotic and non-cirrhotic alcoholic liver disease. *Hepatology* 1982; **2:** 539.
17 Bosch J, Groszmann RJ. Measurement of azygous venous blood flow by a continous thermal dilution technique: an index of blood flow through gastroesophageal collaterals in cirrhosis. *Hepatology* 1984; **4:** 424.
18 Bosch J, Bordas JM, Rigau J *et al.* Non-invasive measurement of the pressure of esophageal varices using an endoscopic gauge: comparison with measurements by variceal puncture in patients undergoing endoscopic sclerotherapy. *Hepatology* 1986; **6:** 667.
19 Bradley SE, Ingelfinger FJ, Bradley GP *et al.* Estimation of hepatic blood flow in man. *J. clin. Invest.* 1945; **24:** 890.
20 Braun SD, Newman GE, Dunnick NR. Digital splenoportography. *Am. J. Roentgenol.* 1985; **144:** 1003.

21 Brazzini A, Hunter DW; Darcy MD *et al.* Safe splenoportography. *Radiology* 1987; **162**: 607.

22 Broe PJ, Conley CL, Cameron JL. Thrombosis of the portal vein following splenectomy for myeloid metaplasia. *Surg. Gynecol. Obstet.* 1981; **152**: 488.

23 Bruix J, Bosch J, Kravetz D *et al.* Effects of prostaglandin inhibition on systemic and hepatic hemodynamics in patients with cirrhosis of the liver. *Gastroenterology* 1985; **88**: 430.

24 Burns P, Taylor K, Blei AT. Doppler flowmetry and portal hypertension. *Gastroenterology* 1987; **92**: 824.

25 Burroughs AK, Jenkins WJ, Sherlock S *et al.* Controlled trial of propanolol for the prevention of recurrent variceal haemorrhage in patients with cirrhosis. *N. Engl. J. Med.* 1983; **309**: 1539.

26 Caesar J, Shaldon S, Chiandussi L *et al.* The use of indocyanine green in the measurement of hepatic blood flow and as a test of hepatic function. *Clin. Sci.* 1961; **21**: 43.

27 Cales P, Braillon A, Jiron MI *et al.* Superior porto-systemic collateral circulations estimated by azygos blood flow in patients with cirrhosis—lack of correlation with oesophageal varices and gastrointestinal bleeding. Effect of propanolol. *J. Hepatol.* 1985; **1**: 37.

28 Camara DS. Bacteremia and injection sclerotherapy. *Arch. int. Med.* 1986; **146**: 458.

29 Capron JP, Gineston J-L, Remond A *et al.* Inferior arteriovenous fistula associated with portal hypertension and acute ischemic colitis. *Gastroenterology* 1984; **86**: 351.

30 Capron JP, Lebrec D, Degott C *et al.* Portal hypertension in systemic mastocytosis. *Gastroenterology* 1978; **74**: 595.

31 Capron JP, LeMay JL, Muir JF *et al.* Portal vein thrombosis and fatal pulmonary thromboembolism associated with oral contraceptive treatment. *J. clin. Gastroenterol.* 1981; **3**: 295.

32 Cello JP, Grendell JH, Crass RA *et al.* Endoscopic sclerotherapy versus porta-caval shunt in patients with severe cirrhosis and acute variceal haemorrhage. *N. Engl. J. Med.* 1987; **316**: 11.

33 Chagnon SF, Vallee CA, Barge J *et al.* Aneurysmal porta hepatic venous fistula: report of two cases. *Radiology* 1986; **159**: 693.

34 Cohen FL, Koerner RS, Taub SJ. Solitary brain abscess following endoscopic injection sclerosis of oesophagal varices. *Gastrointestin. Endoscopy* 1985; **31**: 331.

35 Conn HO, Resnick RH, Grace CE *et al.* Distal splenorenal shunt versus portal-systemic shunt: current status of a controlled trial. *Hepatology* 1981; **1**: 151.

36 Connors AF Jr, Bacon BR, Miron SD. Sodium morrhuate delivery to the lung during endo-

scopic variceal sclerotherapy. *Ann. int. Med.* 1986; **105**: 539.

37 Copenhagen Esophageal Varices Sclerotherapy Project. Sclerotherapy after first variceal hemorrhage in cirrhosis. A randomised multi-center trial. *N. Engl. J. Med.* 1984; **311**: 1594.

38 Crafoord C, Frenckner P. New surgical treatment of varicose veins of the oesophagus. *Acta Otolaryngöl. Stockh.* 1939; **27**: 422.

39 Cruveilhier J. Anatomie pathologique du corps humain. Vol. I. XVI livr. pl. vi- *Maladies du veines* J.B. Ballière. Paris 1829–35.

40 Dachman AH, Ros PR, Goodman ZD *et al.* Nodular regenerative hyperplasia of the liver: clinical and radiologic observations. *Am. J. Roentgenol.* 1987; **148**: 717.

41 Dan SJ, Train JS, Cohen BA *et al.* Common bile duct varices: cholangiographic demonstration of a hazardous porto-systemic communication. *Am. J. Gastroenterol.* 1983; **78**: 42.

42 Da Silva LC, Jamra MA, Maspes V *et al.* Pathogenesis of indirect reacting hyperbilirubinemia after portacaval anastomosis. *Gastroenterology* 1963; **44**: 117.

43 Dawson J, Gertsch P, Mosiman F *et al.* Endoscopic variceal pressure measurements: response to isosorbide dinitrate. *Gut* 1985; **26**: 843.

44 De Cock KM, Awadh S, Raja RS *et al.* Esophagal varices in Nairobi, Kenya: a study of 68 cases. *Am. J. trop. Med. Hyg.* 1982; **31**: 579.

45 Dennis MA, Pretorius D, Manco-Johnson ML *et al.* CT detection of portal venous gas associated with suppurative cholangitis and cholecystitis. *Am. J. Roentgenol.* 1985; **145**: 1017.

46 Dick R, Dooley JS. Suspected portal hypertension in *Imaging in Hepatobiliary Disease.* Dooley JS, Dick R, Viamonte M. *et al.* eds. Blackwell Scientific Publications, Oxford 1987; p. 147.

47 Douglass BE, Baggenstoss AH, Hollinshead WH. Variations in the portal systems of veins. *Proc. Mayo Clin.* 1950; **25**: 26.

48 Dowling JB. Ten years' experience with mesocaval grafts. *Surg. Gynecol. Obstet.* 1979; **149**: 518.

49 Drapanas T. Interposition mesocaval shunt for treatment of portal hypertension. *Ann. Surg.* 1972; **176**: 435.

50 Eck NV. On the question of ligature of the portal vein (trans. title) *Voyenno med. J. (St Petersburg)* 1877; **130**: Sect. 2.1.

51 Eriksson LS, Brundin T, Soderlund C *et al.* Haemodynamic effects of a long-acting somatostatin analogue in patients with liver cirrhosis. *Scand. J. Gastroenterol.* 1987; **22**: 919.

52 Flannigan BD, Gomes AS, Stambuk EC. Intra-arterial digital subtraction angiography: comparison with conventional hepatic arteriography.

Radiology 1983; **148**: 17.

53 Foley WD, Stewart ET, Milbrath JR *et al.* Digital subtraction angiography of the portal venous system. *Am. J. Roentgenol.* 1983; **140**: 497.

54 Freeman JG, Cobden J, Lishman AH *et al.* Controlled trial of terlipressin ('Glypressin') versus vasopressin in the early treatment of oesophagaeal varices. *Lancet* 1982; **ii**: 66.

55 Garcia-Tsao G, Groszmann RJ, Fisher RL *et al.* Portal pressure, presence of gastroesophagaeal varices and varical bleeding. *Hepatology* 1985; **5**: 419.

56 Garcia-Tsao G, Grace ND, Groszmann RJ *et al.* Short-term effects of propanolol on portal venous pressure. *Hepatology* 1986; **6**: 101.

57 Garcia-Tsao G, Groszmann RJ. Portal hemodynamics during nitroglycerin administration in cirrhotic patients. *Hepatology* 1987; **7**: 805.

58 Gimson AES, Westaby D, Hegarty J *et al.* A randomized trial of vasopressin and vasopressin plus nitroglycerin in the control of acute variceal hemorrhage. *Hepatology* 1986; **6**: 410.

59 Goldstein MB, Brandt LJ, Bernstein LH *et al.* Hemorrhage from ileal varices: a delayed complication after total protocolectomy in a patient with ulcerative colitis and cirrhosis. *Am. J. Gastroenterol.* 1983; **78**: 351.

60 Gregory P, Hartigan P, Amodeo D *et al.* Prophylactic sclerotherapy for esophageal varices in alcoholic liver disease: results of a VA cooperative randomized trial. *Gastroenterology* 1987; **92**: 1414.

61 Groszmann RJ, Atterbury CE. The pathophysiology of portal hypertension: a basis for classification. *Semin. Liver Dis.* 1982; **2**: 117.

62 Groszmann RJ, Glickman M, Blei AT *et al.* Wedged and free hepatic venous pressure measured with a balloon catheter. *Gastroenterology* 1979; **76**: 253.

63 Groszmann RJ, Kotelanski B, Cohn J *et al.* Quantitation of porta-systemic shunting from the splenic and mesenteric beds in alcoholic liver disease. *Am. J. Med.* 1972; **53**: 715.

64 Groszmann RJ (ed). Portal hypertension: circulatory and renal abnormalities. *Sem. Liv. Dis.* 1986; **6**: 277.

65 Grundfest A, Cooperman AM, Ferguson R *et al.* Portal hypertension associated with systemic mastocystosis and splenomegaly. *Gastroenterology* 1980; **78**: 370.

66 Guarascio P, Portmann B, Visco G *et al.* Liver damage with reversible portal hypertension from vitamin A intoxication; demonstration of Ito cells. *J. clin. Pathol.* 1983; **36**: 769.

67 Gudjonsson H, Zeiler D, Gamelli RL *et al.* Colonic varices. Report of an unusual case diagnosed by radionuclide scanning, with review of the literature. *Gastroenterology* 1986; **91**: 1543.

68 Hadengue A, Lee SS, Moreau R *et al.* Beneficial hemodynamic effects of ketanserin in patients with cirrhosis: possible role of serotonergic mechanisms in portal hypertension. *Hepatology* 1987; **7**: 644.

69 Harley HAJ, Morgan T. Redecker AG *et al.* Results of a randomized trial of end-to-side portacaval shunt and distal splenorenal shunt in alcoholic liver disease and variceal bleeding. *Gastroenterology* 1986; **91**: 802.

70 Henderson JM, Millikan WJ Jr, Wright-Bacon L *et al.* Hemodynamic differences between alcoholic and nonalcoholic cirrhotics following distal splenorenal shunt—effect on survival? *Ann. Surg.* 1983; **198**: 325.

71 Henriksen JH, Ring-Larsen H, Christensen NJ. Hepatic intestinal uptake and release of catecholamines in alcoholic cirrhosis. Evidence of enhanced hepatic intestinal sympathetic nervous activity. *Gut* 1987; **28**: 1637.

72 Horiguchi Y, Kitano T, Imai H *et al.* Intrahepatic portal—systemic shunt: its etiology and diagnosis. *Gastroenterol. JPN* 1987; **22**: 496.

73 Hosking SW, Johnson AG. What happens to esophagal varices after transection and devascularization? *Surgery* 1987; **101**: 531.

74 Hosking SW, Robinson P, Johnson AG. Usefulness of manometric assessment of varices in maintenance sclerotherapy. A controlled trial. *Gastroenterology* 1987; **93**: 846.

75 Inon AE, D'Agostino D. Portal hypertension secondary to congenital arterioportal fistula. *J. pediat. Gastro. Nutr.* 1987; **6**: 471.

76 Itzchak Y, Glickman MG. Duodenal varices in extrahepatic portal obstruction. *Radiology* 1977; **124**: 619.

77 Jenkins SA, Baxter JN, Corbett WA *et al.* The effects of a somatostatin analogue SM201−995 on hepatic haemodynamics in the cirrhotic rat. *Br. J. Surg.* 1985; **72**: 864.

78 Johnston GW. Six years' experience of oesophageal transection for oesophageal varices using a circular stapling gun. *Gut* 1982; **23**: 770.

79 Kelty RH, Baggenstoss AH, Butt HR. The relation of the regenerated liver nodule to the vascular bed in cirrhosis. *Gastroenterology* 1950; **15**: 285.

80 Kerr DNS, Harrison CV, Sherlock S *et al.* Congenital hepatic fibrosis. *Q. J. Med.* 1961; **30**: 91.

81 Kingham JGC, Levinson DA, Stansfeld AG *et al.* Non-cirrhotic intrahepatic portal hypertension. A long-term follow-up study. *Q. J. Med.* 1981; **50**: 259.

82 Kitano S, Terblanche J, Kahn D *et al.* Venous anatomy of the lower oesophagus in portal hypertension: practical implications. *Br. J. Surg.* 1986; **73**: 525−531.

83 Kitano S, Koyanagi N, Iso Y *et al.* Prevention of recurrence of esophageal varices after endoscopic

injection. Sclerotherapy with ethanolamine oleate. *Hepatology* 1987; **7:** 810.

84 Knauer CM, Fogel MR. Pericarditis: complication of esophageal sclerotherapy. A report of three cases. *Gastroenterology* 1987; **93:** 287.

85 Kong C-W, Lay C-S, Tsai Y-T. The hemodynamic effect of verapamil on portal hypertension in patients with post-necrotic cirrhosis. *Hepatology* 1986; **6:** 423.

86 Korula J, Balart LA, Radvan G *et al.* A prospective, randomized controlled trial of chronic esophageal variceal sclerotherapy. *Hepatology* 1985; **5:** 584.

87 Kravetz D, Bosch J, Teres J *et al.* Comparison of intravenous somatostatin and vasopressin infusions in treatment of acute variceal haemorrhage. *Hepatology* 1984; **4:** 442.

88 Kravetz D, Sikuler E, Groszmann RJ. Splanchnic and systemic haemodynamics in portal hypertensive rats during hemorrhage and blood volume restitution. *Gastroenterology* 1986; **90:** 1232.

89 Kravetz D, Cummings SA, Groszmann RJ. Hyposensitivity to vasopressin in a hemorrhaged-transfused rat model of portal hypertension. *Gastroenterology* 1987; **93:** 170.

90 Langer B, Taylor BR, Mackenzie DR *et al.* Further report of a prospective randomized trial comparing distal splenorenal shunt with end-to-side portacaval shunt. An analysis of encephalopathy, survival and quality of life. *Gastroenterology* 1985; **88:** 424.

91 Larson AW, Cohen H, Zweiban B *et al.* Acute esophageal variceal sclerotherapy. Results of a prospective randomized controlled trial. *J. Am. med. Assoc.* 1986; **255:** 497.

92 Lautt WW. Greenway CV. Conceptual review of the hepatic vascular bed. *Hepatology* 1987; **7:** 952.

93 Lebrec D, de Fleury P. Rueff B. Portal hypertension, size of esophageal varices and risk of gastrointestinal bleeding in alcoholic cirrhosis. *Gastroenterology* 1980; **79:** 1139.

94 Lebrec D, Poynard T, Bernuau J *et al.* A randomized controlled study of propranolol for prevention of recurrent gastro-intestinal bleeding in patients with cirrhosis; a final report. *Hepatology* 1984; **4:** 355.

95 Lewis M. Outpatient esophageal variceal sclerotherapy: it is safe and cost-effective? *Gastrointest. Endosc.* 1986; **32:** 51.

96 Lunderquist A, Vang J. Transhepatic catheterization and obliteration of the coronary vein in patients with portal hypertension and esophageal varices. *N. Engl. J. Med.* 1974; **291:** 646.

97 McCormack T. Martin T, Smallwood RH *et al.* Doppler ultrasound probe for assessment of blood-flow in oesophageal varices. *Lancet* 1983; **i:** 677.

98 McCormack TT, Rose JD, Smith PM *et al.* Perforating veins and blood flow in oesophageal varices. *Lancet* 1983; **ii:** 1442.

99 McCormack TT, Sims J, Eyre-Brook I *et al.* Gastric lesions in portal hypertension: inflammatory gastritis or congestive gastropathy? *Gut* 1985; **26:** 1226.

100 MacDougall BRD, Williams R. A controlled clinical trial of cimetidine in the recurrence of variceal hemorrhage: implication about the pathogenesis of hemorrhage. *Hepatology* 1983; **3:** 69.

101 McIndoe AH. Vascular lesions of portal cirrhosis. *Arch. Path.* 1928; **5:** 23.

102 McMichael J. The pathology of hepatorenal fibrosis. *J. Path. Bact.* 1934; **39:** 481.

103 Madsen MS, Peterson TH, Sommer H. Segmental portal hypertension. *Ann. Surg.* 1986; **204:** 72.

104 Maksoud JG, Mies S, Gayotto LC, Da C. Hepatoportal sclerosis in childhood. *Am. J. Surg.* 1986; **151:** 484.

105 Manenti F, Williams R. Injection of the splenic vasculature in portal hypertension. *Gut* 1966; **7:** 175.

106 Martin LW, Benzing G, Kaplan S. Congenital intrahepatic arteriovenous fistula: report of a successfully treated case. *Ann. Surg.* 1965; **161:** 209.

107 Mikkelsen WP. Extrahepatic portal hypertension in children. *Am. J. Surg.* 1966; **111:** 333.

108 Millikan WJ, Warren WD, Henderson JM *et al.* The Emory prospective randomized trial: selective versus non selective shunt to control variceal bleeding. Ten year follow-up. *Ann. Surg.* 1985; **201:** 712.

109 Molino G, Cavanna A, Avagnina P *et al.* Hepatic clearance of D-sorbitol non-invasive test for evaluating functional liver plasma flow. *Dig. Dis. Sci.* 1987; **32:** 753.

110 Monroe P, Morrow CF Jr, Millen JE *et al.* Acute respiratory failure after sodium morrhuate oesophageal sclerotherapy. *Gastroenterology* 1983; **85:** 693.

111 Morse SS, Taylor KJW, Strauss EB *et al.* Congenital absence of the portal vein in oculoauriculovertebral dysplasia (Goldenhar syndrome). *Pediatr. Radiol.* 1986; **16:** 437.

112 Moriyasu F, Nishida O, Ban N *et al.* Measurement of portal vascular resistance in patients with portal hypertension. *Gastroenterology* 1986; **90:** 710.

113 Moriyasu F, Ban N, Nishida O *et al.* Clinical application of an ultrasonic duplexsystem in the quantitative measurement of portal blood flow. *J. Clin. Ultrasound.* 1986; **14:** 579.

114 Mosimann F, Mange B. Portal hypertension as a complication of idiopathic retroperitoneal fi-

brosis. *Br. J. Surg.* 1980; **67**: 804.

115 Mosimann R. Nonagressive assessment of portal hypertension using endoscopic measurement of variceal pressure. *Am. J. Surg.* 1982; **143**: 212.

116 Nelson RC, Lovett KE, Chezmar JL *et al.* Comparison of pulsed Doppler sonography and angiography in patients with portal hypertension. *Am. J. Roentgenol.* 1987; *149*: 77.

117 North Italian Endoscopic Club for the study and treatment of esophageal varices. Can endoscopy predict the first variceal hemorrhage is cirrhotics? A prospective multicenter study. *Gastroenterology* 1986; **90**: 1752.

118 Odièvre M, Pigé G, Alagille D. Congenital abnormalities associated with extrahepatic portal hypertension. *Arch. Dis. Child.* 1977; **52**: 383.

119 Ohkubo H, Okuda K, Takayasu K *et al.* Cruveilhier-Baumgarten syndrome presenting with precordial murmur and thrill. *Am. J. dig. Dis.* 1978; **23**: 65s.

120 Ohnishi K, Hatano H, Nakayama T *et al.* An unusual portal–systemic shunt, most likely through a patent ductus venous: a case report. *Gastroenterology* 1983; **85**: 962.

121 Ohnishi K, Saito M, Sato S *et al.* Direction of splenic venous flow assessed by pulsed Doppler flowmetry in patients with a large splenorenal shunt. *Gastroenterology* 1985; **89**: 180.

122 Ohnishi K, Chin N, Saito M *et al.* Portographic opacification of hepatic veins and (anomalous) anastomoses between the portal and hepatic veins in cirrhosis—indication of extensive intrahepatic shunts. *Am. J. Gastroenterology.* 1986; **81**: 975.

123 Ohnishi K, Saito S, Sato S *et al.* Clinical utility of pulsed Doppler flowmetry in patients with portal hypertension. *Am. J. Gastroenterol.* 1986; **81**: 1.

124 Ohnishi K, Saito M, Sato S *et al.* Portal haemodynamics in idiopathic portal hypertension (Banti's syndrome). Comparison with chronic persistent hepatitis and normal subjects. *Gastroenterology* 1987; **92**: 751.

125 Okuda K, Kono K, Ohnishi K *et al.* Clinical study of eighty-six cases of idiopathic portal hypertension and comparison with cirrhosis with splenomegaly. *Gastroenterology* 1984; **86**: 600.

126 Okuda K, Ohnishi K, Kimura K *et al.* Incidence of portal vein thrombosis in liver cirrhosis. An angiographic study 708 patients. *Gastroenterology* 1985; **89**: 279.

127 Orloff MJ, Bell RH Jr, Greenburg AG. Prospective randomized trial of emergency portacaval shunt and medical therapy in unselected cirrhotic patients with bleeding varices. *Gastroenterology* 1986; **90**: 1754.

128 Orrego H, Israel Y, Blendis LM. Alcoholic liver

129 Pagani JJ, Thomas JL, Bernardino ME. Computed tomographic manifestations of abdominal and pelvic venous collaterals. *Radiology* 1982; **142**: 415.

130 Papazian A, Braillon A, Dupas JL *et al.* Portal hypertensive gastric mucosa: an endoscopic study. *Gut* 1986; **27**: 1199–1203.

131 Paquet K-J, Feussner H. Endoscopic sclerosis and esophageal balloon tamponade in acute haemorrhage from oesophagogastric varices: a prospective controlled randomized trial. *Hepatology* 1985; **5**: 580.

132 Pascal J-P, Cales P, and a multicenter study group. Propranolol in the prevention of first upper gastrointestinal tract hemorrhage in patients with cirrhosis of the liver and esophageal varices. *N. Engl. J. Med.* 1987; **317**: 856.

133 Patriquin H, Lafortune M, Burns PN *et al.* Duplex doppler examination in portal hypertension. Technique and anatomy. *Am. J. Roentgenol.* 1987; *149*: 71.

134 Pitcher JL. Safety and effectiveness of the modified Sengstaken–Blakemore tube: a prospective study. *Gastroenterology* 1971; **61**: 291.

135 Ponce J, Froufe A, de la Morena E *et al.* Morphometric study of the esophageal mucosa in cirrhotic patients with variceal bleeding. *Hepatology* 1981; **1**: 641.

136 Popper H, Elias H, Petty DE. Vascular pattern of the cirrhotic liver. *Am. J. clin. Path.* 1952; **22**: 717.

137 Queuniet AM, Czernichow P, Lerebours E. *et al.* Étude contrôlée du propranolol dans la prévention des récidives hémoragiques chez les patients cirrhotiques. *Gastroenterol. clin. Biol.* 1987; **11**: 41.

138 Quintero E, Pique JM, Bombi JA *et al.* Gastric mucosal vascular ectasias causing bleeding in cirrhosis. *Gastroenterology* 1987; **93**: 1054.

139 Raskin NH, Price JB, Fishman RA. Portal-systemic encephalopathy due to congenital intrahepatic shunts. *N. Engl. J. Med.* 1964; **270**: 225.

140 Rector WG Jr, Redeker AG. Direct transhepatic assessment of hepatic vein pressure and direction of flow using a thin needle in patients with cirrhosis and Budd–Chiari syndrome. *Gastroenterology* 1984; **86**: 1395.

141 Redeker AG, Geller HM, Reynolds TB. Hepatic wedge pressure, blood flow, vascular resistance and oxygen consumption in cirrhosis before and after end-to-side portacaval shunt. *J. clin. Invest.* 1958; **37**: 606.

142 Reynolds TB, Ito S, Iwatsuki S. Measurement of portal pressure and its clinical application. *Am. J. Med.* 1970; **49**: 649.

143 Rikkers LF, Burnett DA, Valentine GD *et al.*

Shunt surgery *versus* endoscopic sclerotherapy for long-term treatment of variceal bleeding. Early results of a randomized trial. *Ann. Surg.* 1987; **206**: 261.

144 Rösch J, Uchida BT, Putnam JS *et al.* Experimental intrahepatic portacaval anastomosis: use of expandable Gianturco stents. *Radiology* 1987; **162**: 481.

145 Rougier P, Degott C, Rueff B *et al.* Nodular regenerative hyperplasia of the liver. *Gastroenterology* 1978; **75**: 169.

146 Ruff RJ, Chuang VP, Alspaugh JP *et al.* Percutaneous vascular intervention after surgical shunting for portal hypertension. *Radiology* 1987; **164**: 469.

147 Sarin SK, Nanda R, Sachdev G *et al.* Intravariceal versus para-variceal sclerotherapy: a prospective controlled randomized trial. *Gut* 1987; **28**: 657.

148 Sato S, Ohnishi K, Sugita S *et al.* Splenic artery and superior mesenteric artery blood flow: nonsurgical Doppler US measurement in healthy subjects and patients with chronic liver disease. *Radiology* 1987; **164**: 347.

149 Sauerbruch T, Wotzka R, Köpcke W *et al.* Endoscopy sclerotherapy (ST) for prophylaxis of first variceal bleeding in liver cirrhosis: a randomized controlled trial. *J. Hepatol.* 1988; in press.

150 Schuman BM, Beckman JW, Tedesco FJ *et al.* Complications of endoscopic injection sclerotherapy: a review. *Am. J. Gastroent.* 1987; **82**: 823.

151 Shaldon S, Chiandussi L, Guevara L *et al.* The measurement of hepatic blood flow and intrahepatic shunted blood flow by colloid heat denatured human serum albumin labelled with I^{131}. *J. clin. Invest.* 1961; **40**: 1346.

152 Shaldon S, Dollë W, Guevara L *et al.* Effect of pitressin on the splanchnic circulation in man. *Circulation* 1961; **24**: 797.

153 Shaldon S, Sherlock S. The use of vasopressin ('pitpressin') in the control of bleeding from oesophageal varices. *Lancet* 1960; **ii**: 222.

154 Shemesh E. Esophageal perforation after fiberoptic endoscopic injection sclerotherapy for esophageal varices. *Arch. Surg.* 1986; **121**: 243.

155 Sherlock S (ed). Portal hypertension. *Semin. Liver Dis.* 1982; **2**: 17.

156 Sherlock S. Extrahepatic portal venous hypertension in adults. *Clin. Gastroenterol.* 1985; **14**: 1.

157 Sherlock S, Feldman CA, Moran B *et al.* Partial nodular transformation of the liver with portal hypertension. *Am. J. Med.* 1966; **40**: 195.

158 Sibbald WJ, Sweeny JP, Inwood MJ. Portal venous gas (PVG) as an indication for heparinization. *Am. J. Surg.* 1972; **124**: 690.

159 Sivak MV Jr. Endoscopic injection sclerosis of oesophageal varices: A/S/G/E survey (letter). *Gastroint. Endosc.* 1982; **28**: 41.

160 Smallwood RA, Davidson JS. Calcification in the portal system. *Gastroenterology* 1968; **54**: 265.

161 Smith JL, Graham D. Variceal hemorrhage—a critical evaluation of survival analysis. *Gastroenterology* 1982; **82**: 968.

162 Smith-Laing G, Camilo ME, Dick R *et al.* Percutaneous transhepatic portography in the assessment of portal hypertension. *Gastroenterology* 1980; **78**: 197.

163 Smith-Laing G, Scott J, Long RG *et al.* Role of percutaneous transhepatic obliteration in the management of haemorrhage from gastroesophageal varices. *Gastroenterology* 1981; **80**: 1031.

164 Snady H, Korsten MA. Esophageal acid—clearance and motility after endoscopic sclerotherapy of esophageal varices. *Am. J. Gastro.* 1986; **81**: 419.

165 Snady H. The role of sclerotherapy in the treatment of esophageal varices: personal experience and a review of randomized trials. *Am. J. Gastro.* 1987; **82**: 813.

166 Soehendra N, Kempeneers I, Grimm H. Preventions, diagnosis and treatment of complications of sclerotherapy. *Acta Endosc.* 1986; **32**: 4.

167 Spence RAJ, Sloan JM, Johnston GW *et al.* Oesophageal mucosal changes in patients with varices. *Gut* 1983; **24**: 1024.

168 Tabibian N, Alpert E. Refractory sclerotherapy-induced esophageal strictures. *Ann. int. Med.* 1987; **106**: 59.

169 Tabibian N, Schwartz JT, Lacey Smith J *et al.* Cardiac tamponade as a result of endoscopic sclerotherapy: report of a case. *Surgery* 1987; **102**: 546.

170 Terabayashi H, Ohnishi K, Tsunoda T *et al.* Prospective controlled trial of elective endoscopic sclerotherapy in comparison with percutaneous transhepatic obliteration of esophageal varices in patients with nonalcoholic cirrhosis. *Gastroenterology* 1987; **93**: 1205.

171 Terblanche J, Bornman PC, Kahn D *et al.* Failure of repeated injection sclerotherapy to improve long-term survival after oesophageal variceal bleeding. *Lancet* 1983; **ii**: 1328.

172 Terblanche J, Yakoob HI, Bornman PC. Acute bleeding varices: a 5-year prospective evaluation of tamponade and sclerotherapy. *Ann. Surg.* 1981; **194**: 521.

173 Terblanche J. Sclerotherapy for prophylaxis of variceal bleeding. *Lancet* 1986; **i**: 961.

174 Teres J, Cecilia A, Bordas JM *et al.* Esophageal tamponade for bleeding varices. *Gastroenterology* 1978; **75**: 566.

175 Thompson EN, Sherlock S. The aetiology of portal vein thrombosis with particular reference to the role of infection and exchange transfusion. *Q. J. Med.* 1964; n.s. **33**: 465.

176 Thompson EN, Williams R, Sherlock S. Liver function in extra-hepatic portal hypertension. *Lancet* 1964; **ii:** 1352.

177 Torres WE, Gaylord GM, Whitmire L. The correlation between MR and angiography in portal hypertension. *Am. J. Roentgenol.* 1987; **148:** 1109.

178 Triger DR. Extrahepatic portal venous obstruction. *Gut* 1987; **28:** 1193.

179 Tsai Y-E, Lay C-S, Lai K-H *et al.* Controlled trial of vasopressin plus nitroglycerin versus vasopressin alone in the treatment of bleeding esophageal varices. *Hepatology* 1986; **6:** 406.

180 Turner MD, Sherlock S, Steiner RE. Intrasplenic pressure measurement and splenic venography in the clinical investigation of the portal circulation. *Am. J. Med.* 1957; **23:** 846.

181 Uflacker R, Alves MA, Cantisani GG *et al.* Treatment of portal vein obstruction by percutaneous transhepatic angioplasty. *Gastroenterology* 1985; **88:** 176.

182 Valla D, Bercoff E, Menu Y *et al.* Discrepancy between wedged hepatic venous pressure and portal venous pressure after acute propranolol administration in patients with alcoholic cirrhosis. *Gastroenterology* 1984; **86:** 1400.

183 Van Gansbeke D, Avni EF, Delcour C *et al.* Sonographic features of portal vein thrombosis. *Am. J. Roentgenol.* 1985; **144:** 749.

184 Vianna A, Hayes PC, Moscoso G *et al.* Normal venous circulation of the gastroesophageal junction. A route to understanding varices. *Gastroenterology* 1987; **93:** 876.

185 Villeneuve J-P, Pomier-Layrargues G, Infante-Rivard C *et al.* Propranolol for the prevention of recurrent variceal hemorrhage: a controlled trial. *Hepatology* 1986; **6:** 1239.

186 Villeneuve J-P, Pomier-Layrargues G, Duguay L *et al.* Emergency portacaval shunt for variceal hemorrhage. *Ann. Surg.* 1987; **206:** 48.

187 Vorobioff J, Picabea E, Villavicencio R *et al.* Acute and chronic hemodynamic effects of propranolol in unselected cirrhotic patients. *Hepatology* 1987; **7:** 648.

188 Wanless IR, Mawdsley C, Adams R. On the pathogenesis of focal nodular hyperplasia of the liver. *Hepatology* 1985; **5:** 1194.

189 Warren WD, Millikan WJ, Henderson JM *et al.* Ten years' portal hypertensive surgery at Emory. Results and new perspectives. *Ann. Surg.* 1982; **195:** 530.

190 Warren WD, Henderson JM, Millikan WJ *et al.* Distal splenorenal shunt versus endoscopic sclerotherapy for long-term management of variceal bleeding. Preliminary report of a prospective randomized trial. *Ann. Surg.* 1986; **203:** 454.

191 Webb LJ, Sherlock S. The aetiology, presentation and natural history of extrahepatic portal venous obstruction. *Q. J. Med.* 1979; **48:** 627.

192 Webb LJ, Berger LA, Sherlock S. Grey-scale ultrasonography of portal vein. *Lancet* 1977; **ii:** 675.

193 Webb L, Smith-Laing G, Lake-Bakaar G *et al.* Pancreatic hypofunction in extrahepatic portal venous obstruction. *Gut* 1980; **21:** 227.

194 Weinshel E, Chen W, Falkenstein DB *et al.* Hemorrhoids or rectal varices: defining the cause of massive rectal hemorrhage in patients with portal hypertension. *Gastroenterology* 1986; **90:** 744.

195 Westaby D, MacDougall BRD, Williams R. Improved survival following injection sclerotherapy for esophageal varices: final analysis of a controlled trial. *Hepatology* 1985; **5:** 827.

196 Willett IR, Esler M, Jennings G *et al.* Sympathetic tone modulates portal venous pressure in alcoholic cirrhosis. *Lancet* 1986; **ii:** 939.

11 · The Hepatic Artery and Hepatic Veins: the Liver in Circulatory Failure

The hepatic artery

The hepatic artery is a branch of the coeliac axis. It runs along the upper border of the pancreas to the first part of the duodenum where it turns upwards between the layers of the lesser omentum, lying in front of the portal vein and medial to the common bile duct. Reaching the porta hepatis it divides into right and left branches. Its branches include the right gastric artery and the gastroduodenal artery. Aberrant branches are common. Among the many variations, the right hepatic artery may arise from the superior mesenteric, the aorta or the right renal artery. An accessory left hepatic artery may come from the left gastric artery.

Anastomoses occur between the right and left branches, with subcapsular vessels of the liver and with the inferior phrenic artery.

INTRA-HEPATIC ANATOMY

The hepatic artery enters sinusoids adjacent to portal tracts [3, 18]. Direct arterio–portal venous anastamasoses are not seen in man [18].

The hepatic artery forms a capillary plexus around the bile ducts. Interference with this hepatic arterial supply leads to bile duct injury in such conditions as operative trauma, hepatic transplantation and intra-hepatic arterial cytotoxic therapy (fig. 11.1) [15].

The connective tissue in the portal zones is supplied by the hepatic artery.

The *pressure in the hepatic artery* is equal to the general systemic blood pressure; that in the portal vein is much lower. These two pressures are equilibrated within the sinusoids (Chapter 10).

HEPATIC ARTERIAL FLOW

In man, during surgery, the hepatic artery supplies 35% of the hepatic blood flow and 50% of the liver's oxygen supply [16]. The hepatic arterial flow serves to hold total hepatic blood flow constant. It is not regulated by the metabolic demands of the liver, but rather regulates blood levels of nutrients and hormones by maintaining blood flow and thereby hepatic clearance as steady as possible [7].

The proportion of hepatic arterial flow increases greatly in cirrhosis, increasing with the extent of portal–systemic venous shunting. It is the main blood supply to tumours. The proportion varies greatly under different conditions. A drop in systemic blood pressure from haemorrhage or other cause lowers the oxygen content of the portal vein and the liver

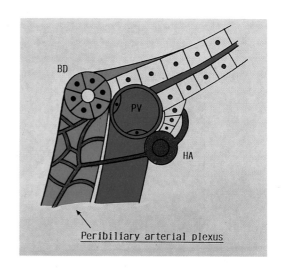

Fig. 11.1. The hepatic artery forms a peribiliary plexus supplying the bile duct.

becomes more and more dependent on the hepatic artery for oxygen. The hepatic artery and the portal vein adapt the volume of blood and of oxygen they supply to the liver according to demand [7].

HEPATIC ARTERIOGRAPHY

The hepatic artery is cannulated via the aorta and coeliac axis. Hepatic arteriography is used for the diagnosis of space-occupying lesions of the liver including cysts, abscesses and benign and malignant tumours (Chapter 28) and vascular lesions such as aneurysms (fig. 11.2) or arterio-venous fistulae. Embolization via the catheter is used for treating tumours, and in the management of hepatic arterial aneurysm or arteriovenous fistulae (figs 11.3, 11.4).

Hepatic arterial pump perfusion of cytotoxic drugs is used to treat patients with hepatic metastases, particularly from colo-rectal cancer (Chapter 28).

HEPATIC ARTERY OCCLUSION

The effects of hepatic artery occlusion depend on the site and on the extent of available collateral circulation. If the division is distal to the origins of the gastric and gastroduodenal arteries the patient may die. Survivors develop a collateral circulation. Slow thrombosis is better than sudden block. Simultaneous occlusion of the portal vein is nearly always fatal.

The size of the infarct depends on the extent of the collateral arterial circulation. It rarely exceeds 8 cm in diameter [13] and has a pale centre with a surrounding congested haemorrhagic band. Liver cells in the infarcted area are jumbled together in irregular masses of eosinophilic, granular cytoplasm without glycogen or nuclei. Subcapsular areas escape because they have an alternative, arterial blood supply.

Hepatic infarction may occur without arterial occlusion in such conditions as shock, cardiac failure [11] or diabetic ketosis [10]. The gallbladder may be infarcted [5]. If sought by scanning, hepatic infarcts are frequent after percutaneous liver biopsy.

AETIOLOGY

Occlusion of the hepatic artery is very rare. Hitherto it was regarded as a fatal condition. However, hepatic angiography has allowed earlier diagnosis and better management, and the prognosis is therefore less serious. Some of the causes are polyarteritis nodosa, giant cell arteritis [12] and embolism in patients with acute bacterial endocarditis. A branch of the artery may be tied during cholecystectomy but recovery is usual. Hepatic arterial dissection

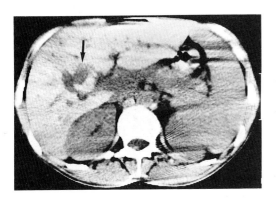 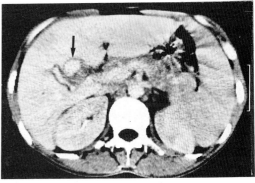

Fig. 11.2. Hepatic artery aneurysm in a patient with subacute bacterial endocarditis. CT scans of the upper abdomen (a) *left*—before and (b) *right*—after contrast enhancement. The aneurysm shows a filling defect (black arrow) with highlights following contrast injection.

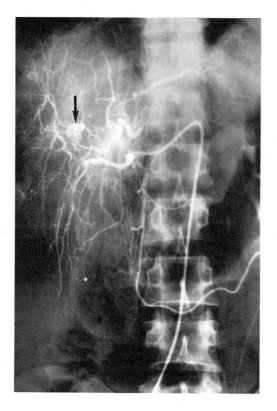

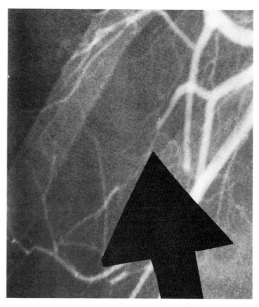

Fig. 11.4. Same patient as Fig. 11.3. Higher magnification of the coeliac angiogram immediately post-embolization showing obliteration of the aneurysm and its feeding vessels (Kibbler *et al*. 1985).

Fig. 11.3. Subacute bacterial endocarditis. Coeliac arteriogram showing a 3 cm false aneurysm of one of the intra-hepatic branches of the right hepatic artery 2.5 cm lateral to its major bifurcation (black arrow).

may follow abdominal trauma or hepatic arterial catheterization.

CLINICAL FEATURES

The condition is rarely diagnosed *ante mortem* and descriptions are meagre. The patient exhibits the features of the cause, such as bacterial endocarditis, or polyarteritis nodosa, or has undergone a difficult upper abdominal operation. Sudden pain in the right upper abdomen is followed by collapse and hypotension. Right upper quadrant tenderness develops and the liver edge is tender. Jaundice deepens rapidly. There is usually fever and leucocytosis and liver function tests show hepato-cellular damage. The prothrombin time rises precipitously and haemorrhages develop.

With major occlusions the patient passes into coma and is dead within ten days.

Hepatic arteriography is essential. The obstruction to the hepatic artery may be shown. Intra-hepatic arterial collaterals develop in the portal zones and subcapsular areas. Extrahepatic collaterals form in the suspensory ligaments and with adjacent structures [2].

Scanning [8]. The infarcts are round or oval, rarely wedge-shaped and are centrally located. Rarely, lesions are hypoechoic on ultrasound and CT shows a poorly demarcated low-density region which does not enhance with contrast. Later lesions are confluent with distinct margins. Bile lakes follow large infarcts and these may contain gas.

Treatment. The causative lesion must be treated. Antibiotics may prevent secondary infection in the anoxic liver. The general management is that of acute hepato-cellular failure. Trauma to the artery is treated by percutaneous arterial embolization [17].

Aneurysms of the hepatic artery

These are rare but make up about one fifth of all visceral aneurysms. The aneurysm may complicate bacterial endocarditis, polyarteritis nodosa or arterio-sclerosis. Trauma is becoming increasingly important including motor vehicle accidents and iatrogenic causes such as biliary tract surgery, liver biopsy, and interventional radiological procedures. Pseudo-aneurysms may complicate chronic pancreatitis with pseudo-cyst formation. The aneurysm may be extra- or intra-hepatic and vary in size from a pin point to a grapefruit. The aneurysm may be recognized by angiography, incidentally at operation or at autopsy.

Clinical presentation is varied. The classical triad of jaundice, abdominal pain and haemobilia is present in only about a third of patients. Abdominal pain is a frequent feature and may last as long as five months before the aneurysm ruptures.

60 to 80% of patients present for the first time with rupture into the peritoneum, biliary tree or gastrointestinal tract with resultant haemoperitoneum, haemobilia or haematemesis.

The *diagnosis* is suggested by sonography and confirmed by hepatic arteriography and a CT scan after enhancement (fig. 11.2) [1, 6]. Real-time plus pulsed Doppler ultrasound may be used to show turbulent flow in the aneurysm [4].

Treatment. Intra-hepatic aneurysms are treated by angiographic embolization (figs 11.3, 11.4). Aneurysms of the common hepatic artery are treated surgically by proximal and distal ligation.

Hepatic arterio—venous shunts

These are usually secondary to blunt trauma, needle liver biopsy or neoplasms, usually primary liver cancer. Multiple shunts may be part of hereditary haemorrhagic telangiectasia; when they can be so extensive that congestive heart failure follows.

Large shunts cause a bruit in the right upper quadrant. The diagnosis is confirmed by hepatic angiography. Embolization with gelfoam is the usual treatment.

References

1 Athey PA, Sax SL, Lamki N *et al.* Sonography in the diagnosis of hepatic artery aneurysms. *Am. J. Roentgenol.* 1986; **147:** 725.

2 Charnsangavej C, Chuang VP, Wallace S *et al.* Angiographic classification of hepatic arterial collaterals. *Radiology* 1982; **144:** 485.

3 Elias H. A re-examination of the structure of the mammalian liver. II. The hepatic lobule and its relation to the vascular and biliary systems. *Am. J. Anat.* 1949; **85:** 379.

4 Falkoff GE, Taylor KJW, Morse S. Hepatic artery pseudoaneurysm: diagnosis with real-time and pulsed Doppler US. *Radiology* 1986; **158:** 55.

5 Henrich WL, Huehnergarth RJ, Rosch J *et al.* Gall bladder and liver infarction occurring as a complication of acute bacterial endocarditis. *Gastroenterology* 1975; **68:** 1602.

6 Kibbler CC, Cohen DL, Cruickshank JK *et al.* Use of CAT scanning in the diagnosis and management of hepatic artery aneurysm. *Gut* 1985; **26:** 752.

7 Lautt WW, Greenaway CV. Conceptual review of the hepatic vascular bed. *Hepatology* 1987; **7:** 952.

8 Lev-Toaff AS, Friedman AC, Cohen LM *et al.* Hepatic infarcts: new observations by CT and sonography. *Am. J. Roentgenol.* 1987; **149:** 87.

9 Lewis DR Jr, Kung JH, Connon JJ. Biliary obstruction secondary to hepatic artery aneurysm: cholangiographic appearance and diagnostic considerations. *Gastroenterology* 1982; **82:** 1446.

10 Ng RCK, Sigmund CJ Jr, Lagos JA *et al.* Hepatic infarction and diabetic ketoacidosis. *Gastroenterology* 1977; **73:** 804.

11 O'Connor PJ, Buhac I, Balint JA. Spontaneous hepatic artery thrombosis with infarction of the liver. *Gastroenterology* 1976; **70:** 599.

12 Oglivie AL, James PD, Toghill PJ. Hepatic artery involvement in polymyalgia arteritica. *J. clin. Pathol.* 1981; **34:** 769.

13 Parker RGF. Arterial infarction of the liver in man. *J. Path. Bact.* 1955; **70:** 521.

14 Pinsky MA, May ES, Taxler MS *et al.* Late manifestations of hepatic artery pseudo aneurysm: case presentation and review. *Am. J. Gastroenterol.* 1987; **82:** 467.

15 Sherlock S. The syndrome of disappearing intrahepatic bile ducts. *Lancet* 1987; **ii:** 493.

16 Tygstrup N, Winkler K, Mellengaard K *et al.* Determination of the hepatic arterial blood flow and

oxygen supply in man by clamping the hepatic artery during surgery. *J. clin. Invest.* 1962; **41**: 447.

17 Wagner WH, Lundell CJ, Donovan AJ. Percutaneous angiographic embolization for hepatic arterial haemorrhage. *Arch. Surg.* 1985; **120**: 1241.

18 Yamamoto K, Sherman I, Phillips MJ *et al.* Three-dimensional observations of the hepatic arterial terminations in rat, hamster and human liver by scanning electron microscopy of micro vascular casts. *Hepatology* 1985; **5**: 452.

19 Zachary K, Geier S, Pellecchia C *et al.* Jaundice secondary to hepatic artery aneurysm: radiological appearance and clinical features. *Am. J. Gastroenterol.* 1986; **81**: 295.

The hepatic veins

The hepatic veins begin as the central veins. These join the sublobular veins and merge into larger hepatic veins, which enter the inferior vena cava while it is still partly embedded in the liver. The number, size and pattern of hepatic veins are very variable. Generally, there are three large veins, one draining the left lobe and the other two emerging from the right lobe. There are variable numbers of small accessory veins particularly from the caudate lobe.

In the normal liver there are no direct anastomoses between portal vein and hepatic vein which are linked only by the sinusoids. In the cirrhotic liver there are anastomoses between portal and hepatic veins so that the blood bypasses the regenerating liver cell nodules (fig. 10.42). There is no evidence, either in the normal or cirrhotic liver, of anastomoses between the hepatic artery and the hepatic vein.

FUNCTIONS

The pressure in the free hepatic vein is approximately 6 mmHg.

The hepatic venous blood is only about 67% saturated with oxygen. The oxygen consumption of the liver (or splanchnic area) can be calculated as 47 ml per square metre body surface per minute.

Dogs have muscular hepatic veins near their caval orifices which form a sluice mechanism. The hepatic veins in man have little muscle.

The hepatic venous blood is usually sterile for the liver is a bacterial filter.

VISUALIZING THE HEPATIC VEIN

Hepatic venography is performed by slow injection of contrast material into a wedged hepatic vein radicle, using a balloon catheter, inserted via the femoral vein. This results in filling of the sinusoidal area draining into the catheter and also in retrograde filling of the portal venous system in that area. The portal radicle then carries the contrast medium to other parts of the liver and so other hepatic vein branches become opacified. Cirrhotic nodules and tumour deposits are surrounded by portal vein−hepatic vein anastomoses and may be outlined. In cirrhosis the sinusoidal pattern is coarsened, beady and tortuous, and gnarled hepatic radicles may be seen. The extent of filling of the main portal vein may indicate the extent to which the portal vein has become the outflow tract of the liver. In the Budd−Chiari syndrome a characteristic lace-like vascular pattern may be seen (fig. 11.8) [6, 32].

The hepatic veins may occasionally be seen after selective coeliac or hepatic arteriography, particularly when hepatic arterial blood flow is increased.

Scanning. The main hepatic veins may also be visualized by ultrasound or by the enhanced CT scan (fig. 11.14).

Experimental hepatic venous obstruction

Individual ligation of all the hepatic veins is impossible. The usual method is to constrict the inferior vena cava by a band placed above the entry of the hepatic veins, and so obstruct the venous return from the liver [2]. Centrizonal (zone 3) haemorrhage and necrosis with fibrosis follow.

The hepatic lymphatics dilate and lymph passes through the capsule of the liver forming ascites with a high protein content.

Budd—Chiari (hepatic venous obstruction) syndrome (fig.11.8) [6, 32]

This condition is usually associated with the names of Budd and Chiari although Budd's description [3] omitted the features and Chiari's paper [5] was not the first to report the clinical picture. The syndrome comprises hepatomegaly, abdominal pain, ascites and hepatic histology showing zone 3 sinusoidal distension and pooling. It may arise from obstruction to hepatic veins at any site from the efferent vein of the lobule to the entry of the inferior vena cava into the right atrium (fig. 11.8). A similar syndrome may be produced by constrictive pericarditis or right heart failure.

Clotting diseases are particularly important in the aetiology. Polycythaemia, both primary and secondary, was believed responsible in 61 of 147 (41%) well-documented cases [34]. The patient is often a young female. Thrombosis is also associated with other myeloproliferative diseases and with essential thrombocythaemia. The erythroid bone-marrow colony test *in vitro* shows that many sufferers, although without peripheral blood changes, have a latent myeloproliferative syndrome [34].

The Budd—Chiari syndrome has been associated with systemic lupus erythematosus [8] and with circulating lupus anticoagulant [18, 21, 37].

Paroxysmal nocturnal haemoglobinuria may be associated with hepatic vein thrombosis, the severity varying from asymptomatic occlusion of hepatic venules to a fatal Budd—Chiari syndrome [36].

Antithrombin-3 deficiency, whether primary or secondary to heavy proteinuria has been associated with hepatic vein thrombosis [7].

There is a 2.37 times increased risk in users of oral contraceptives. This is about the same as for other thrombotic complications such as venous thromboembolism [35]. Oral contraceptives may act synergistically in those predisposed to clotting for some other reason.

Hepatic vein thrombosis has been reported in pregnancy [15].

Trauma (usually of blunt abdominal type)

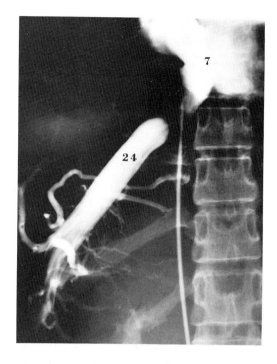

Fig. 11.5. Hepatic venogram in a patient with the Budd—Chiari syndrome due to obstruction of the right main hepatic vein. Right hepatic venous pressure 24 mmHg distal to the obstruction and 7 mmHg proximal to it. (Courtesy D.S. Zimmon.)

due to automobile accidents is an increasingly common association.

Obstruction to the inferior vena cava is usually secondary to thrombosis in malignant disease, for instance an adrenal or renal carcinoma or invasion by a hepato-cellular cancer. Rare tumours include leiomyosarcoma of the hepatic veins [17] and metastatic testicular lesions in the right atrium [9].

In one child with Wilm's tumour, metastases involved the inferior vena cava and hepatic veins. The child survived excision of the primary tumour and of thrombus in the inferior vena cava and hepatic veins. Triple drug therapy was given with a survival of five years [27].

Myxoma of the right atrium has caused hepatic venous obstruction. Invasion of hepatic veins by masses of aspergillosis has been reported in a patient with leukaemia [39].

Membranous obstruction of the suprahepatic

segment of the inferior vena cava is important [24]. The web varies from a thin membrane to a thick fibrotic band. The largest reported series comes from Japan [3]. Webs can also affect children [13]. The web is presumed congenital although the presentation in adults is surprising. A web developed in one patient following hepatic venous thrombosis related to lupus anticoagulant [33]. This suggests that webs can be a consequence of organized thrombosis.

The picture also follows central hepatic vein involvement in the alcoholic and in veno-occlusive disease (Chapter 11).

In many instances the cause remains unknown [6]. The Budd—Chiari syndrome is being diagnosed much more often and in milder forms probably due to the routine use of imaging, especially ultrasound.

PATHOLOGICAL CHANGES

The hepatic veins show thrombosis at various points in their course from the ostia to the smaller radicles. The thrombus may have spread from an occluded inferior vena cava. Thrombus filling the veins may be purulent or may contain malignant cells, depending on the cause. In chronic cases the vein wall is thickened and there may be some recanalization of the lumen. In others it is replaced by a fibrous strand; a fibrous web may be seen.

The liver is enlarged, purplish and smooth. Venous congestion is gross and the cut surface shows a 'nutmeg' change. Hepatic veins beyond the obstruction and, in the acute stage, subcapsular lymphatics, are dilated and prominent.

In the more chronic case, the caudate lobe, which has a separate venous drainage into the cava, is enlarged and compresses the inferior vena cava as it passes posterior to the liver (fig. 11.9). Areas less affected by obstruction form nodules. The spleen may enlarge and a portal—systemic collateral circulation develops. The mesenteric vessels may thrombose.

Histological sections show zone 3 venous dilatation and congestion with haemorrhage and central necrosis of hepatocytes (figs 11.10,

11.11). Blood cells in Dissë's space could represent an extrasinusoidal circulation, attempting to circumvent the venous obstruction. Peri-portal areas are spared. Appearances are indistinguishable from those of any hepatic outflow obstruction, for instance cardiac failure or constrictive pericarditis.

In the later stages, zone 3 fibrosis develops and the picture is that of a cardiac cirrhosis.

CLINICAL FEATURES

These depend on the speed of occlusion and the extent of the hepatic venous involvement. The picture varies all the way from a fulminant course, the patient presenting as encephalopathy and dying within two to three weeks, to presentation as chronic hepato-cellular disease slowly developing and causing confusion with other forms of cirrhosis [22].

In the most *acute form* the picture is of an ill patient, often suffering from some other condition—for instance renal carcinoma, primary cancer of the liver, thrombophlebitis migrans or polycythaemia. The presentation is with abdominal pain, vomiting, liver enlargement, ascites and mild icterus. Watery diarrhoea, following mesenteric venous obstruction, is a terminal, inconstant feature. If the hepatic venous occlusion is total, delirium and coma with hepato-cellular failure and death follow rapidly.

In the more usual *chronic form* the patient presents with pain over an enlarged tender liver and ascites. Jaundice is mild or absent, unless zone 3 necrosis is marked. Pressure over the liver may fail to fill the jugular vein (negative *hepato-jugular reflux*). As portal hypertension increases, the spleen becomes palpable. The enlarged caudate lobe, palpable in the epigastrium, may simulate a tumour.

If the inferior vena cava is blocked, oedema of the legs is gross and veins distend over the abdomen, flanks and back. Albuminuria is found. The condition may develop over months as ascites and wasting.

Biochemical. Serum bilirubin rarely exceeds 2 mg/100 ml. The serum alkaline phosphatase level is raised and the serum albumin value reduced. Serum transaminase values increase and very high concomitant blockage of the portal vein is suggested. The prothrombin time is reduced. Hypoproteinaemia may be due to protein-losing enteropathy.

The protein content of the ascites should, theoretically, be high, but this is not always so.

Needle liver biopsy is essential. Speckled zone 3 areas can be distinguished from the pale portal ones. Histologically, the picture is of zone 3 congestion (figs 11.10, 11.11). Alcoholic hepatitis or phlebitis of the hepatic veins should be noted.

Hepatic venography may fail or show narrow occluded hepatic veins. Adjacent veins show a tortuous, lace-like spider-web pattern (fig. 11.7) [6]. This probably represents abnormal venous collaterals. The catheter cannot be advanced the usual distance along the hepatic vein and wedges 2–12 cm from the diaphragm.

Inferior vena cavography both from above, via the right atrium, or below, via the femoral vein, or both, establishes the patency of the inferior vena cava. The hepatic segment may show side-to-side narrowing due to distortion from the enlarged caudate lobe (fig. 11.12). Pressure measurements should be taken in the inferior vena cava along its length to confirm its patency and to quantify the extent of any membranous or caudate lobe obstruction.

Selective coeliac arteriography. The hepatic artery appears small for the size of the liver and the branches are of fine calibre. They appear stretched and displaced, producing the appearance of multiple space-occupying lesions simulating metastases [14]. The venous phase shows delayed emptying of the portal venous bed.

Ultrasound. This is diagnostic in 87% [23]. It shows hepatic vein abnormalities, caudate lobe hypertrophy with increased reflectivity and compression of the inferior vena cava. The appearances are hypoechogenic in the early stages of acute thrombosis and hyperechogenic with fibrosis in the later stages [1]. Pulsed Doppler ultrasound may show abnormal intra-hepatic channels with blood flowing away from the

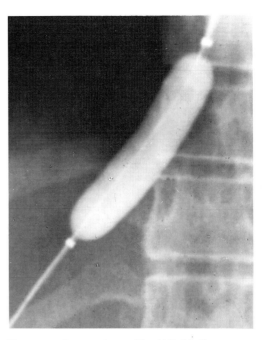

Fig. 11.6a. Same patient as Fig. 11.5. A balloon inflated in the right hepatic vein is dilating the stricture.

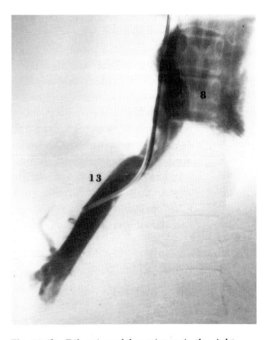

Fig. 11.6b. Dilatation of the stricture in the right hepatic vein has resulted in a fall in distal right hepatic venous pressure to 13 mmHg while the pressure proximally is 8 mmHg.

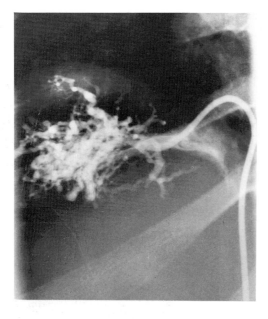

Fig. 11.7. Hepatic venogram in a patient with Budd–Chiari syndrome. Note lace-like spider-web pattern (Clain *et al.* 1967).

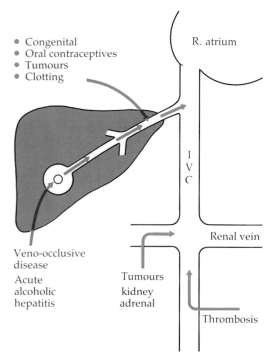

Fig. 11.8. Aetiological factors in the Budd–Chiari syndrome.

site of the hepatic venous ostia [11]. Ascites is confirmed.

CT (fig. 11.14). Shows enlargement of the liver with diffuse hypodensity on plain and patchy enhancement after contrast injection. In subacute or chronic disease peripheral hypodensity is seen. The portal venous blood flow is normal in the enhanced but with inverse flow in atrophic areas [19]. *Hepatic scintiscan* may be useful (fig. 11.13).

Magnetic resonance imaging. This shows reduction in calibre or absence of hepatic veins, intra-hepatic collaterals and any obstruction of the inferior vena cava [30].

DIAGNOSIS

The condition should be suspected if a patient with a tendency to thrombosis or malignant disease in or near the liver or on oral contraceptives develops tender hepatomegaly with gross ascites. Diagnosis, prognosis and correct treatment are only possible if the block is localized by radiological and scanning techniques.

Heart failure and constrictive pericarditis must be distinguished clinically, by echocardiography and by electrocardiography. Tense ascites *per se* can elevate the jugular venous pressure and displace the cardiac apex. Atrial myxoma may cause confusion.

Cirrhosis must be distinguished and the liver biopsy is helpful. The ascitic fluid protein content is usually lower in cirrhosis.

Portal vein thrombosis rarely leads to ascites. Jaundice is absent and the liver is not very large.

Inferior vena caval thrombosis results in distended abdominal wall veins (fig. 10.10) but without ascites. If the renal vein is occluded, albuminuria is gross. Hepatic venous and inferior vena caval thrombosis may, however, co-exist.

Hepatic metastases are distinguished clinically and by the liver biopsy.

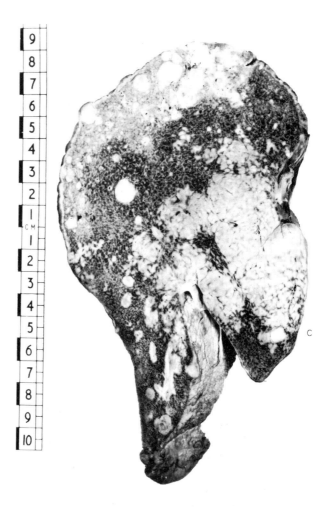

Fig. 11.9. Vertical section of the liver at autopsy in hepatic venous obstruction. The pale areas represent regeneration and the dark areas are congested. Note the marked hypertrophy of the caudate lobe (C).

PROGNOSIS

In the acute form, death in hepatic coma usually results. Thrombosis may spread to the portal and mesenteric veins with infarction of the bowel. In the more chronic and localized instances response to symptomatic therapy may allow prolongation of life for a few years [6].

The demonstration of functioning intrahepatic collaterals improves chances of survival [10].

Prognosis depends on the aetiology, on the extent of the occlusion and whether it can be corrected. Clotting diseases such as polycythaemia are usually found with multiple thrombosis of vessels of varying sizes. The inferior vena cava and portal vein may also be involved.

Haemorrhage from oesophageal varices is usually terminal.

Chronic cases may survive many months or even years and up to 22 years has been recorded.

TREATMENT

If the diagnosis is made early, particularly in those with underlying clotting disorders, anticoagulants and streptokinase may be of value although there is no proof of this. Anticoagulants do not dissolve clots but may prevent extension.

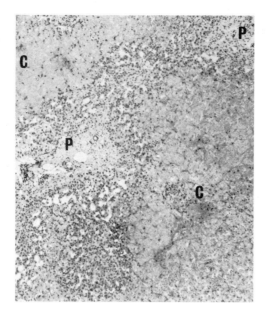

Fig. 11.10. Hepatic venous occlusion (Budd–Chiari syndrome). Hepatic histology shows marked zone 3 haemorrhage (C). The liver cells adjoining the portal zones (P) are spared. (Stained H & E, ×100.)

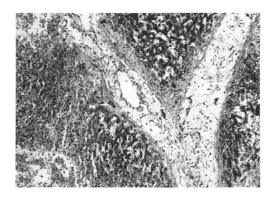

Fig. 11.11. Budd–Chiari syndrome. Longitudinal section of hepatic venules shows fibrosis in lumen, thickening of the wall and surrounding loss of hepatocyte. (Stained chromophobe aniline blue).

In those with polycythaemia or thrombocytosis the haemoglobin and platelet count should be reduced by venesection and cytotoxic drugs.

Ascites is treated with a low sodium diet and diuretics. Severe cases demand ever-increasing

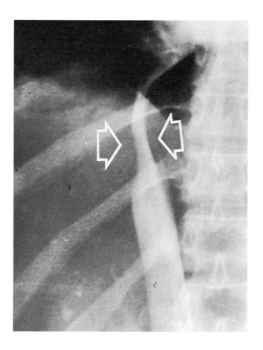

Fig. 11.12. Inferior venacavogram. Antero-posterior view showing side-to-side narrowing and distortion of the inferior vena cava. Extrinsic compression from the left (arrow) is due to an enlarged caudate lobe (Tavill *et al.* 1975).

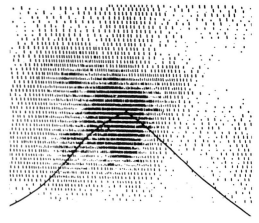

Fig. 11.13. Hepatic scintiscan in hepatic venous obstruction showing maximal uptake of isotope more centrally placed in the liver than normal; this represents the hypertrophied caudate lobe.

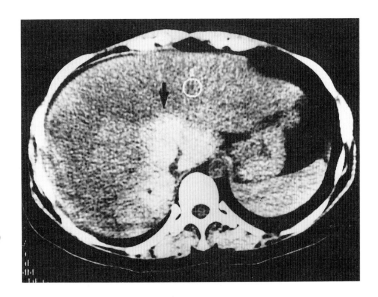

Fig. 11.14. CT scan (unenhanced) shows caudate lobe (arrow) with surrounding underperfused parenchyma.

doses of combinations of potent diuretics and eventually the patient is overtaken by inanition and renal failure. Seventeen of 19 patients treated with diet and diuretics were dead within 3.5 years [32]. Some milder cases, however, respond slowly and require less treatment with time. The peritoneo−jugular (LeVeen) shunt may be useful in some patients, although the shunt often clogs up.

The timing of surgery is difficult. On the one hand, some re-vascularization may continue. On the other, the long-term results of medical therapy are, in general, so poor, that as time passes the patient's chances of surviving major surgery are less.

Surgical portal−systemic shunts

These are considered in patients with symptomatic Budd−Chiari syndrome who have a patent portal vein. The aim is to decompress the congested liver and reverse portal venous flow so allowing the portal vein to serve as an outflow channel.

The underlying clotting defect in many patients increases the likelihood of thrombosis of the portal systemic shunt.

The enlarged caudate lobe increases pressure in the retro-hepatic inferior vena cava so that it

may exceed the portal venous pressure. The anatomic bulk of the caudate lobe makes a technical approach to the portal vein difficult.

Side-to-side porta caval anastomosis. This has proved reliable and effective but may offer technical difficulties [20].

Meso−Caval interposition shunt. This has given good results in some hands but not in all [38].

The shunt may stand a better chance of staying patent if the obstruction from the caudate lobe is first relieved by inserting, preoperatively and percutaneously, an expandable wire spring in the inferior vena cava [12].

Meso−atrial shunt. This is used when the inferior vena cava is obstructed. The shunt is made between the superior mesenteric vein and the right atrium using a prosthetic graft (fig. 11.15) [4, 26].

Trans-atrial membranotomy. Webs may be surgically corrected, either by resection or by fracturing with the finger.

Percutaneous trans-luminal angioplasty [29] or balloon dilatation have been used to dilate webs (fig. 11.6). Re-occlusion may develop when a further angioplasty or balloon dilatation is indicated.

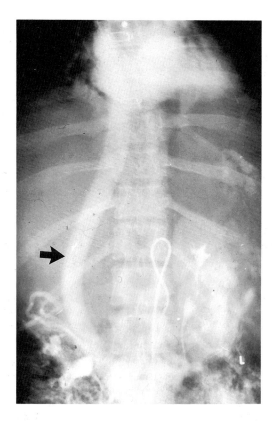

Fig. 11.15. Budd−Chiari syndrome. Surgical relief by meso-atrial stent (arrow).

Hepatic transplantation

This has been used. The major difficulty is the underlying thrombotic condition which favours rethrombosis (see Chapter 35) [28].

Veno-occlusive disease (VOD)
(see Chapter 10)

Spread of disease by the hepatic veins

The hepatic veins link the portal and systemic venous systems. Malignant disease of the liver is spread by the hepatic veins to the lungs and hence to other parts. Liver abscesses can burst into the hepatic vein and metastatic abscesses may result. Parasitic disease, including amoebiasis, hydatid disease and schistosomiasis, is spread by this route. The portal−hepatic venous

anastomoses developing in cirrhosis may allow intestinal organisms to cause septicaemia.

References

1 Becker CD, Scheidegger J, Marincek B. Hepatic vein occlusion: morphologic features on computed tomography and ultrasonography. *Gastrointest. Radiol.* 1986; **11:** 305.

2 Bolton C, Barnard WG. The pathological occurrences in the liver in experimental venous stagnation. *J. Path. Bact.* 1931; **34:** 701.

3 Budd G. *On Diseases of the Liver*, 3rd edn, 1857. Blanchard & Lea, Philadelphia.

4 Cameron JL, Herlong HF, Sanfey H *et al.* The Budd-Chiari syndrome. Treatment by mesenteric-systemic venous shunts. *Ann. Surg.* 1983; **198:** 335.

5 Chiari H. Ueber die selbständige Phlebitis obliterans der Hauptstämme der Venae hepaticae als Todesurache. *Beitr. path. Anat.* 1899; **26:** 1.

6 Clain D, Freston J, Kreel L *et al.* Clinical diagnosis of the Budd-Chiari syndrome. *Am. J. Med.* 1967; **43:** 544.

7 Das M, Carroll SF. Antithrombin III deficiency: an etiology of Budd−Chiari syndrome. *Surgery* 1985; **97:** 242.

8 Disney TF, Sullivan SN, Haddad RG *et al.* Budd−Chiari syndrome with inferior vena cava obstruction associated with systemic lupus erythematosus. *J. clin. Gastroenterol.* 1984; **6:** 253.

9 Feingold ML, Litwak RL, Geller SS *et al.* Budd−Chiari syndrome caused by a right atrial tumor. *Arch. intern. Med.* 1971; **127:** 292.

10 Gupta S, Blumgart LH, Hodgson HJF. Budd−Chiari syndrome: long-term survival and factors affecting mortality. *Q. J. Med.* 1986; **60:** 781.

11 Gupta S, Barter S, Phillips GWL *et al.* Comparison of ultrasonography, computed tomography and ^{99m}Tc liver scan in diagnosis of Budd−Chiari syndrome. *Gut* 1987; **28:** 242.

12 Hobbs KEF, Dick R. Relief of inferior caval obstruction in Budd−Chiari syndrome using a stent (in preparation).

13 Hoffman H du P, Stockland B, von der Heyden U. Membranous obstruction of the inferior vena cava with Budd−Chiari syndrome in children: a report of nine cases. *J. Pediat. Gastroenterol. Nut.* 1987; **6:** 878.

14 Hungerford GD, Hamlyn AN, Lunzer MR *et al.* Pseudo-metastases in the liver: a presentation of the Budd−Chiari syndrome. *Radiology* 1976; **120:** 627.

15 Khuroo MS, Datta DV. Budd−Chiari syndrome following pregnancy. Report of 16 cases with roentgenologic, hemodynamic and histologic

studies of the hepatic outflow tract. *Am. J. Med.* 1980; **68**: 113.

16 Lewis JH, Tice HL, Zimmerman HJ. Budd–Chiari syndrome associated with oral contraceptive steroids. Review of treatment of 47 cases. *Dig. Dis. Sci.* 1983; **28**: 673.

17 McMahon HE, Ball HG III. Leiomyosarcoma of hepatic vein and the Budd–Chiari syndrome. *Gastroenterology* 1971; **61**: 239.

18 Mackworth-Young CG, Melia WM, Harris EN *et al.* The Budd–Chiari syndrome. Possible pathogenetic role of anti-phospholipid antibodies. *J. Hepatol.* 1986; **3**: 83.

19 Mathieu D, Vasile N, Menu Y *et al.* Budd–Chiari syndrome: dynamic CT. *Radiology* 1987; **165**: 409.

20 Pezzuoli G, Spina GP, Opocher E *et al.* Portacaval shunt in the treatment of primary Budd–Chiari syndrome. *Surgery* 1985; **98**: 319.

21 Pomeroy C, Knodell RG, Swaim WR *et al.* Budd–Chiari syndrome in a patient with the lupus anticoagulant. *Gastroenterology* 1984; **86**: 158.

22 Powell-Jackson PR, Ede RJ, Williams R. Budd–Chiari syndrome presenting as fulminant hepatic failure. *Gut* 1986; **27**: 1101.

23 Powell-Jackson PR, Karani J, Ede RJ *et al.* Ultrasound scanning and 99ᵐ TC sulphur colloid scintigraphy in diagnosis of Budd–Chiari syndrome. *Gut* 1986; **27**: 1502.

24 Rector WG, Xu Y, Goldstein L *et al.* Membranous obstruction of the inferior vena cava in the United States. *Medicine* 1985; **64**: 134.

25 Redmond PL, Kadir S, Kaufman SL *et al.* Mesoatrial shunts for Budd–Chiari syndrome and IVC thrombosis: angiographic and hemodynamic evaluations. *Radiology* 1987; **163**: 131.

26 Schaffner F, Gadboys HL, Safran AP *et al.* Budd–Chiari syndrome caused by a web in the inferior vena cava. *Am. J. Med.* 1967; **42**: 838.

27 Schraut WH, Chilcote RR. Metastatic Wilm's tumor causing acute hepatic-vein occlusion (Budd–Chiari syndrome). *Gastroenterology* 1985; **88**: 576.

28 Seltman HJ, Dekker A, van Thiel DH *et al.* Budd–Chiari syndrome recurring in a transplanted liver. *Gastroenterology* 1983; **84**: 640.

29 Sparano J, Chang J, Trasi S *et al.* Treatment of the Budd–Chiari syndrome with percutaneous transluminal angioplasty. Case report and review of the literature. *Am. J. Med.* 1987; **82**: 821.

30 Stark DD, Hahn PF, Trey C *et al.* MRI of the Budd–Chiari syndrome. *Am. J. Roentgenol.* 1986; **146**: 1141.

31 Takeuchi J, Takada A, Hasumura Y *et al.* Budd–Chiari syndrome associated with obstruction of the inferior vena cava. *Am. J. Med.* 1971; **51**: 11.

32 Tavill AS, Wood EJ, Kreel L *et al.* The Budd–Chiari syndrome: correlation between hepatic scintigraphy and the clinical, radiological and pathological findings in nineteen cases of hepatic venous outflow obstruction. *Gastroenterology* 1975; **68**: 509.

33 Terabayashi H, Okuda K, Nomura F *et al.* Transformation of inferior vena caval thrombosis to membranous obstruction in a patient with the lupus anticoagulant. *Gastroenterology* 1986; **91**: 219.

34 Valla D, Casadevall N, Lacombe C *et al.* Primary myeloproliferative disorder and hepatic vein thrombosis: a prospective study of erythroid colony formation *in vitro* in 20 patients with Budd–Chiari syndrome. *Ann. int. Med.* 1985; **103**: 329.

35 Valla D, Le MG, Poynard T *et al.* Risk of hepatic vein thrombosis in relation to recent use of oral contraceptives: a case–control study. *Gastroenterology* 1986; **90**: 807.

36 Valla D, Dhumeaux D, Babany G *et al.* Hepatic vein thrombosis in paroxysmal nocturnal hemoglobinuria. *Gastroenterology* 1987; **93**: 569.

37 Van Steenbergen W, Beyls J, Vermylen J *et al.* "Lupus" anticoagulant and thrombosis of the hepatic veins (Budd–Chiari syndrome). Report of three patients and review of the literature. *J. Hepatol.* 1986; **3**: 87.

38 Vons C, Bourstyn E, Bonnet P *et al.* Results of portal systemic shunts in Budd–Chiari syndrome. *Ann. Surg.* 1986; **203**: 366.

39 Young RC. The Budd–Chiari syndrome caused by *Aspergillus*. *Arch. intern. Med.* 1969; **124**: 754.

Circulatory failure

A rise in pressure in the right atrium is readily transmitted to the hepatic veins. Liver cells are particularly vulnerable to diminished oxygen supply so that a failing heart, lowered blood pressure or reduced hepatic blood flow are reflected in impaired hepatic function. The left lobe of the liver may suffer more than the right.

Hepatic changes in acute heart failure and shock

Hepatic changes are particularly common in acute heart failure and in shock due to trauma, burns, haemorrhage, sepsis, peritonitis or black water fever [2]. Similar ischaemic changes follow cessation of hepatic blood flow during the course of hepatic transplantation or tumour resection [12].

Light microscopy shows congested central areas with local haemorrhage (fig. 11.16). Focal necrosis with eosinophilic hepatocytes, hydropic change and polymorph infiltration is usually centrizonal. Mid-zonal necrosis may be due to tangential section cutting but in some instances is unexplained [8]. The reticulin framework is preserved within the necrotic zone. With recovery, particularly after trauma, mitoses may be prominent [5].

Hepatic calcification can develop in zone 3 areas following shock [30]. This might be related to the disturbance of intracellular Ca^{2+} homeostasis as a result of ischaemic liver injury.

MECHANISM OF THE HEPATIC CHANGES

Changes can be related to the duration of the shock: if longer than 24 hours, hepatic necrosis is almost constant; if less than 10 hours, it is unusual.

The fall in systemic blood pressure leads to a reduction in hepatic blood flow and the oxygen content of the blood is reduced. Hepatic arterial vasoconstriction follows the fall in systemic blood pressure. The cells in zone 3 receive blood at a lower oxygen tension than the peripheral cells and therefore more readily become anoxic and necrotic [11]. Intense selective splanchnic vasoconstriction follows, perhaps in response to endogenous release of angiotensin II [4].

The hepatocyte injury is largely due to oxygen lack. Insufficient substrates and accumulation of metabolites contribute. Energy level is rapidly reduced with, in addition, mitochondrial dysfunction, impaired membrane function, and reduced protein synthesis [12]. Much of the tissue damage develops during reperfusion when there is a large flux of oxygen-derived 'free' radicles [31]. These initiate lipid peroxidation with disruption of membrane integrity.

Lysosomal membranes may be peroxidized with the release of enzymes into the cytoplasm. Attempts are being made to prevent and

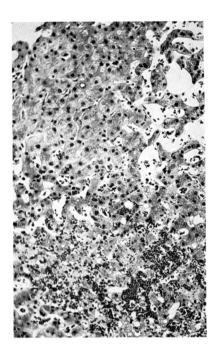

Fig. 11.16. Coronary thrombosis. Serum bilirubin 2.1 mg/100ml. Liver cells have disappeared from zone 3 and are replaced by frank haemorrhage. (Stained H & E, ×120).

treat these effects by hypothermia, methyl prednisolone, ATP and magnesium chloride. 'Free' radicle trapping agents such as vitamin E, glutathione and ascorbic acid are also being evaluated. Allopurinol, a specific inhibitor or xanthine oxidase, the enzyme that generates free radicles from oxygen, may also be useful.

Some patients show mild icterus. Jaundice has been recorded in severely traumatized patients. Serum transaminase levels increase markedly and the prothrombin time rises [2].

Ischaemic hepatitis

This term is applied to acute circulatory failure of the liver [16]. Acute hepatic infarction might be a preferable term [9]. The picture simulates acute virus hepatitis.

The patient usually suffers from cardiac disease, often ischaemic or a cardiomyopathy. He has an acute fall in cardiac output, often due to an arrhythmia or myocardial infarction. Zone 3 necrosis without inflammation results. Clinical evidence of hepatic failure is absent. Congestive cardiac failure is inconspicuous.

Serum bilirubin and alkaline phosphatase values increase slightly but serum transaminases rise rapidly and strikingly to levels 8–10 times normal and these return speedily towards recovery in less than one week. Tests for hepatitis A and B are negative and hepatotoxic drugs cannot be incriminated.

The outcome depends entirely on the cardiovascular status of the patient. The hepatic course is usually benign. However, if the liver has been previously damaged by chronic congestive heart failure, acute circulatory failure may lead to the picture of fulminant hepatic failure [23].

Post-operative jaundice [15]

Jaundice developing *soon* after surgery may have multiple causes [13, 15]. Increased serum bilirubin follows blood transfusion, particularly of stored blood. The haemoglobin in 500 ml blood contains about 250 mg of bilirubin, the normal daily production. Extravasated blood in the tissues gives an additional bilirubin load.

Impaired hepato-cellular function follows operation, anaesthetics and shock. Severe jaundice develops in approximately 2% of patients with shock resulting from major trauma [24]. Hepatic perfusion is reduced. This will be particularly evident if the patient is in incipient circulatory failure and the cardiac output is already reduced. Renal blood flow also falls.

Halothane anaesthetics, especially if multiple, may be followed by a hepatitis-like picture. This is rare less than seven days after a first operation. Other drugs used in the operative period, such as the promazines, must also be considered. Sepsis, *per se*, can produce deep jaundice which may be cholestatic.

Glucose-6-phosphatase dehydrogenase (G6-PD) deficiency affects approximately 10% of United States Blacks. In such patients the administration of the many drugs at the time of surgery may precipitate haemolysis and jaundice.

Rarely, a *cholestatic jaundice* may be noted on the first or second post-operative day. It reaches its height between the fourth and tenth day, and disappears by 14–18 days. Serum biochemical changes are variable. Sometimes, but not always, the alkaline phosphatase and transaminase levels are increased [26]. Serum bilirubin can rise to levels of 23–39 mg/100 ml. The picture simulates extra-hepatic biliary obstruction [10]. Patients have all had an episode of shock, been transfused and suffered heart failure of recent onset. Centrizonal hepatic necrosis, however, is not conspicuous and hepatic histology shows only minor abnormalities. The mechanism of the cholestasis is uncertain. This picture must be recognized [13] and if necessary needle biopsy of the liver performed. Surgical intervention to relieve a non-existent biliary obstruction would be disastrous. The prognosis is good.

Jaundice after cardiac surgery

Jaundice is frequent and develops in 20% of patients having cardio-pulmonary bypass surgery [5, 6]. It carries a bad prognosis. The jaundice is detected by the second post-operative day. Serum bilirubin is conjugated, suggesting failure of canalicular biliary excretion. Serum alkaline phosphatase may be normal or only slightly increased and transaminases are raised, often to very high levels [19]. Patients aged over 50 are particularly at risk. Jaundice is significantly associated with multiple valve replacement, high blood transfusion requirements and a longer bypass time.

Many factors contribute. The patient may have a liver that has already suffered from prolonged heart failure. Operative hypotension, shock and hypothermia contribute. Infections, drugs (including anticoagulants) and anaesthetics must be considered. The serum bilirubin load is increased by blood transfusion and haemolysis. The pump may contribute by decreasing erythrocyte survival, and by adding gaseous micro-emboli and platelet aggregates and debris to the circulation.

Non-A, non-B hepatitis is the commonest cause of post-transfusion hepatitis (see Chapter 16). The acute attack may be virtually asymptomatic and the patient present months or years later with a chronic hepatitis or cirrhosis. Virus B hepatitis is rare since blood for transfusion has been screened. Cytomegalovirus hepatitis may develop after cardiac surgery.

The liver in congestive heart failure

PATHOLOGICAL CHANGES [17]

Hepatic autolysis is particularly rapid in the patient dying in heart failure [28]. Autopsy material is therefore unreliable for the assessment of the effects of cardiac failure on the liver in life.

Macroscopic changes. The liver is usually enlarged, and purplish with rounded edges. Nodularity is inconspicuous but nodular masses of hepatocytes (nodular regenerative hyperplasia) may be seen. The cut surface (fig. 11.17) shows prominent hepatic veins which may be thickened. The liver drips blood. Zone 3 is prominent with alternation of yellow (fatty change) and red areas (haemorrhage) giving a nutmeg-like appearance.

Histological changes. The hepatic venule is always dilated, and the sinusoids entering it are engorged for a variable distance towards the periphery (fig. 11.18). In severe cases, there is frank haemorrhage with focal necrosis of liver cells. The liver cells show a variety of degenerative changes but each portal tract is surrounded by relatively normal cells to a depth that varies inversely with the extent of the zone 3 atrophy. Surviving cells usually retain their glycogen. Biopsy sections show significant fatty change in only about a third. The absence of fat in biopsy material contrasts with the usual post-mortem picture. Cellular infiltration is inconspicuous.

The zone 3 degenerating cells are often packed with brown lipochrome pigment. As they disintegrate, pigment lies free amidst

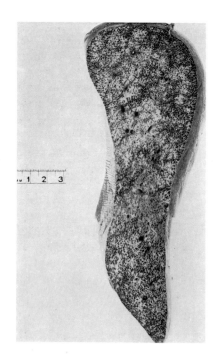

Fig. 11.17. Cut surface of the liver from a patient dying with congestive heart failure. Note dilated hepatic veins. Light areas corresponding to peripheral fatty zones alernate with dark areas corresponding to zone 3 congestion and haemorrhage.

cellular debris. Bile thrombi, particularly periportally, may be seen in deeply jaundiced patients.

Zone 3 reticulin condensation follows loss of liver cells. Then reticulin and collagen increase and the central vein shows phlebosclerosis (fig. 11.19). Cardiac sclerosis consists of eccentric thickening or occlusion of the walls of zone III veins and perivenular scars extending into the lobule [17]. If the heart failure continues or relapses, bridges develop between central veins so that the unaffected portal zone is surrounded by a ring of fibrous tissue (reversed lobulation) (fig. 11.20). Later the portal zones are involved and a complex cirrhosis results. A true cardiac cirrhosis is extremely rare.

Electron microscopy [25] shows atrophy of zone 3 cells, probably related to new fibres in the space of Dissë, which interfere with

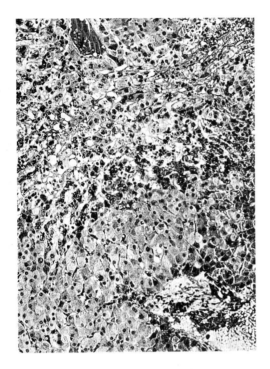

Fig. 11.18. Cor pulmonale. Serum bilirubin 3.4 mg/100ml. Gross zone 3 congestion and liver cell necrosis. Pigment increase is seen in the degenerating liver cells. Liver cells in zone 1 are relatively normal. (Stained H & E, ×120.)

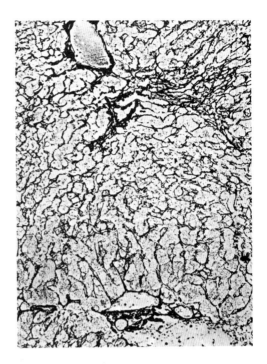

Fig. 11.19. Same section as in Fig. 11.18. Reticulin stains show zone 3 condensation. (Stained H & E, × 120.)

blood—hepatocyte transfer. Canaliculi may dilate and rupture.

MECHANISM (fig. 11.21)

Zone 3 hepatocytes receive blood at a lower oxygen tension than those at the periphery. Hypoxia causes degeneration of the zone 1 liver cells, dilatation of sinusoids [27] and slowing of bile secretion [27]. Endotoxins diffusing through the intestinal wall into the portal blood may augment this effect [29]. The liver attempts to compensate by increasing the oxygen extracted as the blood flows across the sinusoidal bed. Collagenosis of Dissë's space may play a minor role in impairing oxygen diffusion.

Necrosis correlates with a reduced systemic blood pressure and hence with a low cardiac output [1]. The hepatic venous pressure increases in proportion to the rise in central venous pressure and this correlates with zone 3 congestion [1].

CLINICAL FEATURES

Cardiac jaundice

Mild jaundice is common but deeper icterus is rare and associated with chronic congestive failure due, for example, to coronary artery disease or mitral stenosis [22]. In hospital in-patients, cardio-respiratory disease is the commonest cause of a raised serum bilirubin level. Jaundice increases with prolonged and repeated bouts of congestive failure. Oedematous areas escape, for bilirubin is protein-bound and does not enter oedema fluid with a low protein content.

Mechanisms. Jaundice is partly hepatic, for

225

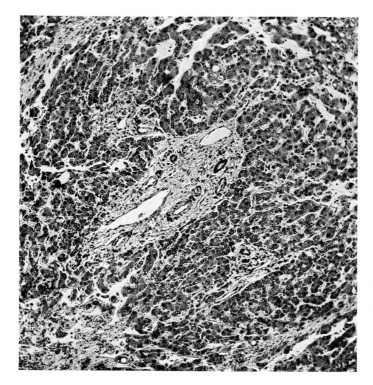

Fig. 11.20. Fibrous tissue bands pass from central vein to central vein. There is 'reversed lobulation' and a fully developed cardiac cirrhosis. Portal tracts show only slight fibrosis. (Stained H & E, × 90.)

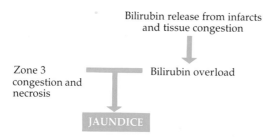

Fig. 11.21. Mechanisms of hepatic jaundice developing in patients with cardiac failure.

the greater the extent of zone 1 necrosis the deeper the icterus (fig. 11.22) [28].

Cholestasis due to bile thrombi or to pressure on bile ducts by distended veins is unlikely.

Bilirubin released from infarcts, whether pulmonary, splenic or renal, or simply from pulmonary congestion, provides an overload on the anoxic liver. Patients in cardiac failure who become jaundiced with minimal hepatocellular damage usually have clear evidence of pulmonary infarction [28]. In keeping with

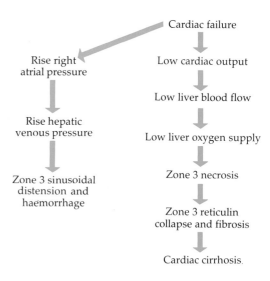

Fig. 11.22. Possible mechanisms of the hepatic histological changes in heart failure.

bilirubin overload the serum shows unconjugated bilirubinaemia and the urine and the faeces show excess of urobilinogen.

The liver

The patient may complain of right abdominal pain probably due to stretching of the nerve endings in the capsule of the enlarged liver. The firm, smooth, tender lower edge may reach the umbilicus.

A rise in right atrial pressure is readily transmitted to the hepatic veins. This is particularly so in tricuspid incompetence when the hepatic vein pressure tracing resembles that obtained from the right atrium. Palpable systolic pulsation of liver can be related to this transmission of pressure. Pre-systolic hepatic pulsation occurs in tricuspid stenosis. The expansion may be felt bimanually with one hand over the liver anteriorly and the other over the right lower ribs posteriorly. This expansibility distinguishes it from the palpable epigastric pulsation due to the aorta or an hypertrophied right ventricle. Correct timing of the pulsation is important.

Hepato-jugular reflux

In heart failure, pressure applied over the liver increases the venous return and the jugular venous pressure rises due to the inability of the failing right heart to handle the increased blood flow.

The reflux is of value for identifying the jugular venous pulse and to establish that venous channels between the hepatic and jugular veins are patent.

The reflux is absent if the hepatic veins are occluded or if the main mediastinal or jugular veins are blocked. It is useful for diagnosing tricuspid regurgitation [21].

Ascites

Ascites is associated with a particularly high venous pressure, a low cardiac output and severe, zone 3 necrosis. This description applies to patients with mitral stenosis and tricuspid incompetence or constrictive pericarditis. In such patients the ascites may be out of proportion to the oedema and symptoms of con-gestive heart failure. The ascitic fluid may have a high protein content similar to that observed in the Budd–Chiari syndrome.

Encephalopathy

Confusion, lethargy and coma are related to cerebral anoxia. Occasionally the whole picture of impending hepatic coma may be seen [22].

Portal hypertension

Splenomegaly is frequent. Other features of portal hypertension are usually absent except in very severe cardiac cirrhosis associated with constrictive pericarditis. However, at autopsy, 6.7% of 74 patients with congestive heart failure showed oesophageal varices, although in only one was there evidence of bleeding.

Cardiac cirrhosis

This should be suspected in patients with prolonged, decompensated mitral valve disease with tricuspid incompetence or in patients with constrictive pericarditis. The prevalence has fallen since both these conditions are relieved surgically.

BIOCHEMICAL CHANGES

In general, the biochemical changes are small and proportional to the severity of the heart failure [14].

In congestive failure the serum bilirubin level usually exceeds 1 mg/dl and in about one-third it is more than 2 mg/dl [28]. The jaundice may be deep, exceeding 5 mg/dl and even up to 26.9 mg. The serum bilirubin level corresponds to the degree of heart failure.

Serum alkaline phosphatase is usually normal or slightly increased. Serum albumin values may be mildly reduced and globulin raised [28]. Protein loss from the intestine may contribute.

Serum transaminases are higher in acute than chronic failure and are proportional to the degree of shock and the extent of zone 3 necrosis. The association of very high values with jaundice may simulate acute viral hepatitis [3].

Urine shows excess urobilinogen and faecal stercobilinogen is increased. Rarely, grey stools accompany deep icterus.

PROGNOSIS

The prognosis of the liver changes is that of the underlying heart disease causing them. Cardiac jaundice, particularly if deep, is always a bad omen.

Cardiac cirrhosis *per se* does not carry a bad prognosis and, if the heart failure responds to treatment, the cirrhosis can be expected to become compensated.

Hepatic dysfunction and cardiovascular abnormalities in paediatric patients

Infants and children with heart failure and cyanotic heart disease show liver dysfunction. Hypoxaemia, systemic venous congestion and a low cardiac output are associated with increased prothrombin time, and serum bilirubin and transaminase values. The most severe changes are found with a low cardiac output. Liver function correlates with cardiac status.

The liver in constrictive pericarditis

The clinical picture and hepatic changes are those of the Budd–Chiari syndrome (page 213).

Cardiac cirrhosis is frequent and marked thickening of the liver capsule simulates sugar icing (*zuckergussleber*). Microscopically the picture is of cardiac cirrhosis.

Jaundice is absent. The liver is enlarged and hard and may pulsate [7]. Ascites is gross.

Diagnosis must be made from ascites due to cirrhosis or to hepatic venous obstruction. This is done by the paradoxical pulse, the venous pulse, the calcified pericardium, the echocardiogram, the electrocardiogram and by cardiac catheterization.

TREATMENT

Treatment is that of the cardiac condition. If pericardectomy is possible, prognosis as regards the liver is good although recovery may be slow. Within six months of a successful operation, liver function tests improve and the liver shrinks. The cardiac cirrhosis cannot be expected to resolve completely, but fibrous bands become narrower and avascular.

References

1 Arcidi JM Jr, Moore GW, Hutchins GM. Hepatic mor-phology in cardiac dysfunction. A clinicopathologic study of 1000 subjects at autopsy. *Am. J. Pathol.* 1981; **104:** 159.
2 Birgens HS, Henriksen J, Matzen P *et al.* The shock liver. *Acta med. Scand.* 1978; **204:** 417.
3 Bloth B, De Faire U, Edhag O. Extreme elevation of transaminase levels in acute heart disease—a problem in differential diagnosis? *Acta med. Scand.* 1976; **200:** 281.
4 Bulkley GB, Oshima A, Bailey RW. Patho-physiology of hepatic ischemia in cardiogenic shock. *Am. J. Surg.* 1986; **151:** 87.
5 Chu C-M, Chang C-H, Liaw Y-F. *et al.* Jaundice after open heart surgery: a prospective study. *Thorax* 1984; **39:** 52.
6 Collins JD, Bassendine MF, Ferner R *et al.* Incidence and prognostic importance of jaundice after cardiopulmonary bypass surgery. *Lancet* 1983; **i:** 1119.
7 Coralli RJ, Crawley IS. Hepatic pulsations in constrictive pericarditis. *Am. J. Cardiol.* 1986; **58:** 370.
8 De La Monte SM, Arcidi JM, Moore GW *et al.* Midzonal necrosis as a pattern of hepatocellular injury after shock. *Gastroenterology* 1984; **86:** 627.
9 Gibson PR, Dudley FJ. Ischemic hepatitis: clinical features, diagnosis and prognosis. *Aust. N.Z. J. Med.* 1984; **14:** 822.
10 Gourley GR, Chesney PJ, Davis JP *et al.* Acute cholestasis in patients with toxic-shock syndrome. *Gastroenterology* 1981; **81:** 928.
11 Gumucio JJ, Miller DL. Functional implications of liver cell heterogeneity. *Gastroenterology* 1981; **80:** 393.
12 Hasselgren P-O. Prevention and treatment of ischemia of the liver. *Surg. Gynec. Obstet.* 1987; **164:** 187.
13 Kantrowitz PA, Jones WA, Greenberger NJ *et al.* Post-operative hyperbilirubinemia simulating obstructive jaundice. *N. Engl. J. Med.* 1967; **276:** 591.

14 Kubo SH, Walter BA, John DHA *et al.* Liver function abnormalities in chronic heart failure. Influence of systemic hemodynamics. *Arch. int. Med.* 1987; **147**: 1227.

15 LaMont JT, Isselbacher KJ. Current concepts: postoperative jaundice. *N. Engl. J. Med.* 1973; **288**: 305.

16 Leading Article. Ischaemic hepatitis. *Lancet* 1985; **i**: 1019.

17 Lefkowitch JH. Bile ductular cholestasis: an ominous histopathologic sign related to sepsis and 'cholangitis lenta'. *Hum. Pathol.* 1982; **13**: 19.

18 Lefkowitch JH, Mendez L. Morphologic features of hepatic injury in cardiac disease and shock. *J. Hepatol.* 1986; **2**: 313.

19 Lockey E, McIntyre N, Ross DN *et al.* Early jaundice after open heart surgery. *Thorax* 1967; **22**: 165.

20 Mace S, Borkat G. Liebman J. Hepatic dysfunction and cardiovascular abnormalities. Occurence in infants, children and young adults. *Am. J. Dis. Child.* 1985; **139**: 60.

21 Maisel AS, Atwood JE, Goldberger AL. Hepatojugular reflux: useful in the bedside diagnosis of tricuspid regurgitation. *Ann. intern. Med.* 1984; **101**: 781.

22 Moussavian SN, Dincsoy HP, Goodman S *et al.* Severe hyperbilirubinemia and coma in chronic congestive heart failure. *Dig. Dis. Sci.* 1982; **27**: 175.

23 Nouel O, Henrion J, Bernuau J *et al.* Fulminant hepatic failure due to transient circulatory failure in patients with chronic heart disease. *Dig. Dis. Sci.* 1980; **25**: 49.

24 Nunes G, Blaisdell FW, Margaretten W. Mechanism of hepatic dysfunction following shock and trauma. *Arch. Surg.* 1970; **100**: 646.

25 Safran AP, Schaffner F. Chronic passive congestion of the liver in man. Electron microscopic study of cell atrophy and intralobular fibrosis. *Am. J. Pathol.* 1967; **50**: 447.

26 Schmid M, Hefti ML, Gattiker R *et al.* Benign post-operative intrahepatic cholestasis. *N. Engl. J. Med.* 1965; **272**: 545.

27 Seneviratne RD. Physiological and pathological responses in the blood-vessels of the liver. *Q. J. exp. Physiol.* 1949; **35**: 77.

28 Sherlock S. The liver in heart failure; relation of anatomical, functional and circulatory changes. *Br. Heart J.* 1951; **13**: 273.

29 Shibayama Y. The role of hepatic venous congestion and endotoxaemia in the production of fulminant hepatic failure secondary to congestive heart failure. *J. Path.* 1987; **151**: 133.

30 Shibuya A, Unuma T, Sugimoto M *et al.* Diffuse hepatic calcification as a sequela to shock liver. *Gastroenterology* 1985; **89**: 196.

31 Weisiger RA. Oxygen radicals and ischemic tissue injury. *Gastroenterology* 1986; **90**: 494.

12 · Jaundice

Bilirubin metabolism [6, 39]

Bilirubin is the end product of haem, coming from haemoglobin and from myoglobin and many respiratory enzymes (fig. 12.1). Approximately 35 g haemoglobin are broken down daily and 300 mg bilirubin are formed. Production takes place in reticulo-endothelial cells.

The enzyme which converts haem to bilirubin is microsomal haem oxygenase which has absolute requirements for oxygen and NADPH. Cleavage of the porphyrin ring occurs selectively at the alpha methane bridge (fig. 12.2). The alpha bridge carbon atom is converted to carbon monoxide and the original bridge function is replaced by two oxygen atoms which are derived from molecular oxygen. The resulting linear tetrapyrrole has the structure of the IX alpha biliverdin. This is further converted to IX alpha bilirubin by an enzyme, biliverdin reductase. Such a linear tetrapyrrole should be water soluble whereas bilirubin is lipid soluble. The lipid solubility is explained by the structure of IX alpha bilirubin which has six intramolecular stable hydrogen bonds (fig. 12.3) [9]. This bonding can be broken by alcohol in the diazo (Van den Bergh) reaction converting unconjugated (indirect) bilirubin to conjugated (direct) reacting bilirubin. *In vivo* the stable hydrogen bonds are altered by esterification of the propionic groups by glucuronic acid.

About 20% of circulating bilirubin is not formed from the haem of mature erythrocytes [5]. A small proportion comes from immature cells in spleen and bone marrow. This component is increased in haemolytic states. The remainder is formed in the liver from haem proteins such as myoglobin, cytochromes and unknown sources. This component is increased in pernicious anaemia, congenital erythropoietic porphyria and the Crigler–Najjar syndrome.

Hepatic transport of bilirubin (figs 12.4, 12.5)

Unconjugated bilirubin is transported in the plasma tightly bound to albumin. A very small amount is dialysable, but this can be increased by substances such as fatty acids and organic anions which compete with bilirubin for albumin binding. This is important in the

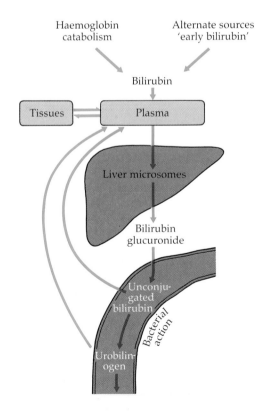

Fig. 12.1. The metabolism of bilirubin.

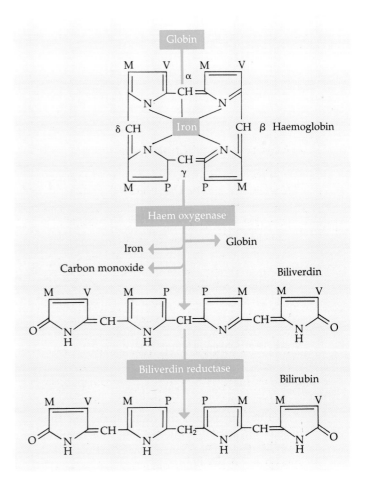

Fig. 12.2. The metabolism of haemoglobin to bilirubin (Billing 1972).

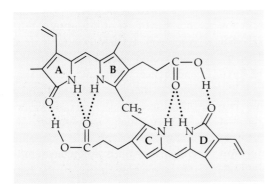

Fig. 12.3. The structure of bilirubin IXα as an involuted hydrogen-bonded structure. The propionic acid groups of pyrrole rings B and C are linked to the nitrogens of the opposite pyrrole rings (broken lines).

231

neonate where such drugs as sulphonamides and salicylates facilitate diffusion of bilirubin into the brain and so increase the risk of kernicterus.

The liver extracts such organic anions as fatty acids, bile acid and non-bile acid cholephils, such as bilirubin, despite tight albumin binding [42]. This results from interaction with the liver cell plasma membrane, perhaps involving a specific albumin receptor. Candidate carrier proteins have been isolated. Binding protein, ligandin, may be concerned with the transport of bilirubin from the plasma membrane to the endoplasmic reticulum.

Unconjugated bilirubin is non-polar (lipid soluble). It is converted to a polar (water

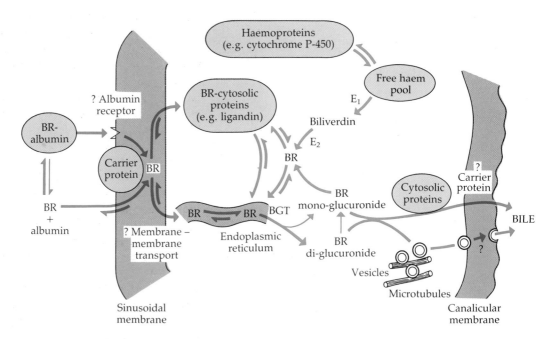

Fig. 12.4. Scheme of bilirubin uptake, metabolism and transport in the hepatocyte. (Courtesy of Gollan 1985.)

soluble) compound by conjugation and this allows its excretion into the bile. This involves an enzyme of the microsomal fraction called bilirubin UDP glucuronyl transferase which converts the unconjugated bilirubin to the conjugated bilirubin monoglucuronide. The process is inducible by such drugs as phenobarbital. Reduced concentrations of the conjugating enzyme are of importance in the neonate and in the Gilbert's and Crigler—Najjar hyperbilirubinaemias. Levels are well maintained in hepato-cellular jaundice and even increased in the cholestatic type [7].

The major bilirubin conjugate in human bile is the diglucuronide. A single microsomal glucuronyl system catalyses both the conversion of bilirubin to the monoglucuronide and also on to the digluronide [31]. With a high bilirubin load, as in haemolysis, monoglucuronide formation is favoured whereas if the bilirubin load is low or following enzyme induction the diglucuronide increases.

Although conjugation as a glucuronide remains the most important mechanism, sulphate, xylose and glucose conjugation also occur to a small extent and may be increased in cholestasis [11].

It has always been unclear why, in the late stages of cholestatic or hepato-cellular jaundice, despite high serum bilirubin levels, none can be detected in the urine. This is apparently due to a third type of bilirubin, a bilirubin monoconjugate, covalently bound to albumin [47]. This would not be filtered by the glomerulus and hence would not reach the urine. This lessens the practical application of urinary bilirubin tests.

Biliary canalicular excretion of bilirubin is thought to be an energy requiring process which transports conjugated bilirubin across the canalicular surface of the hepatocyte into bile against a concentration gradient. Biliary excretion of glucuronide is the rate-limiting factor in the transport of bilirubin from plasma to bile. Secretion of the conjugated pigments involves a carrier-mediated active transport

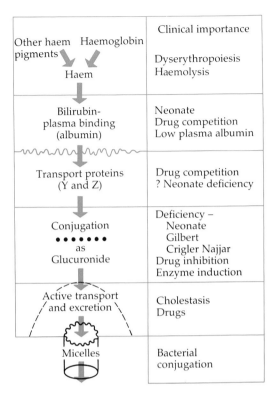

	Clinical importance
Other haem Haemoglobin pigments ↘ ↙ Haem	Dyserythropoiesis Haemolysis
Bilirubin- plasma binding (albumin)	Neonate Drug competition Low plasma albumin
Transport proteins (Y and Z)	Drug competition ? Neonate deficiency
Conjugation •••••• as Glucuronide	Deficiency – Neonate Gilbert Crigler Najjar Drug inhibition Enzyme induction
Active transport and excretion	Cholestasis Drugs
Micelles	Bacterial conjugation

Fig. 12.5. The clinical importance of interference with the stages in the transport of bilirubin, from its production from haem through to its excretion in micellar form into the bile.

small intestine. In the colon, bacterial beta-glucuronidases hydrolyse the conjugated bilirubin, which is then reduced to urobilinogens. In the presence of bacterial cholangitis some hydrolysis of the bilirubin glucuronide is possible and unconjugated bilirubin is precipitated. This may be important in the production of bilirubin gallstones.

Urobilinogen is non-polar and is well absorbed from the small intestine, but only minimally from the colon. The little that is normally absorbed is re-excreted by the liver and kidneys (entero-hepatic circulation). With hepato-cellular dysfunction, re-excretion by the liver is impaired and more is excreted in the urine. This accounts for the urobilinogenuria of alcoholic liver disease, pyrexia, heart failure and in the early stages of viral hepatitis.

Unconjugated bilirubin is tightly bound to albumin and so cannot cross the glomerulus and is not found in normal urine. The bilirubin–glucuronide–albumin complex on the other hand is 1% dialysable and is excreted by glomerular filtration. This unbound conjugated bilirubin is largely reabsorbed in the proximal tubules [20]. Bilirubin is therefore present in the urine in cholestatic jaundice where increases of circulating conjugated bilirubin are found.

system. There are at least two independent mechanisms for biliary secretion of organic anions, one for bile salts and the other for other organic anions, including bilirubin. This is exemplified by the Dubin–Johnson syndrome where there is a defect in the excretion of conjugated bilirubin while bile salt excretion is usually normal. A high proportion of the conjugated bilirubin in bile is incorporated into mixed micelles with cholesterol, phospholipids and bile salts. The role of the Golgi apparatus and of the microfilaments of the cytoskeleton in the intra-hepatic transport of conjugated bilirubin remains to be defined.

Bilirubin diglucuronide in bile is polar (water soluble) and hence is not absorbed from the

Distribution of jaundice in the tissues

Circulating protein-bound bilirubin finds it difficult to enter the protein-low tissue fluids. If the protein is increased, jaundice becomes more evident. Thus exudates tend to be more icteric than transudates.

The cerebrospinal fluid is more likely to be xanthochromic when meningitis is present, the classical example being Weil's disease with both jaundice and meningitis.

The basal ganglia may be stained yellow in the newborn (kernicterus). This is due to the high concentration of circulating, unconjugated bilirubin having an affinity for nervous tissue.

Cerebrospinal fluid from jaundiced subjects contains a small amount of bilirubin, the level being one-tenth to one-hundredth of that found in the serum.

In deep jaundice, the ocular fluids are yellow, and this is considered to explain the extremely rare symptom of xanthopsia (seeing yellow).

Urine, sweat, semen and milk contain bile pigment in the deeply jaundiced patient. Bilirubin is a normal constituent of synovial fluid.

Paralysed parts and oedematous areas tend to remain uncoloured.

Bilirubin is readily bound to elastic tissue. Skin, ocular sclera and blood vessels have a high elastic tissue content, and easily become icteric. This also accounts for the disparity between the depth of skin jaundice and serum bilirubin levels during the stage of recovery.

Factors determining the depth of jaundice

Even after complete bile duct obstruction, the depth of jaundice is very variable. After an initial rapid increase, the serum bilirubin levels off after about three weeks although the obstruction persists. The level of jaundice depends on both bile pigment production and the capacity of the kidney for its excretion. Rates of bilirubin production may vary and products other than bilirubin, which do not give the diazo reaction, may be formed from haem catabolism. The intestinal mucosa may allow the passage of bilirubin, presumably unconjugated, from the blood.

In prolonged cholestasis the skin is greenish, possibly due to biliverdin, which does not give the diazo reaction for bilirubin. Other pigments may play a part.

Conjugated bilirubin, because of its water solubility and penetration of body fluids, produces more jaundice than unconjugated pigment. The extravascular space is greater than the vascular. This accounts for the more intense colour of those with hepato-cellular and cholestatic rather than haemolytic jaundice.

Classification of jaundice (fig. 12.6)

234 Jaundice might arise in four different ways.

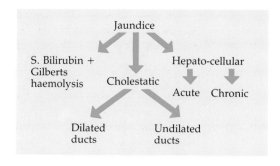

Fig. 12.6. Classification of jaundice.

First, there may be increased bilirubin load on the liver cell. Second, there may be a disturbance in uptake and transport of bilirubin within the hepatocyte. Third, there may be defects in conjugation. Finally, the defect may be in the cell membrane opposite the canaliculus for excretion into the bile or there may be an obstruction to the large bile channels before bilirubin reaches the intestines. A simple classification is into three predominant types, pre-hepatic, hepatic and cholestatic. There is much overlap between them, and particularly between the hepatic and cholestatic varieties.

Pre-hepatic. Total serum bilirubin levels are increased with normal serum transaminases, alkaline phosphatase and proteins. The circulating serum bilirubin is largely unconjugated. Bilirubin cannot be detected in the urine. The cause may be haemolysis or a familial disturbance of bilirubin metabolism.

Hepatic (Chapters 16 and 18). The jaundice usually comes on rapidly and is of an orange tint. Fatigue and malaise are conspicuous. There are varying degrees of liver failure. These may be shown in a mild case as personality change and in the more severe as flapping tremor, confusion and coma. Fluid retention is shown in its mildest form by weight gain and in the more severe by oedema and ascites. The blood pressure is low. Reduced hepatic synthesis of coagulation factors is shown by bruising in relation to venepunctures and also spontaneously. Serum biochemistry shows increases in transaminases. Serum albumin levels are reduced in the long-standing case.

Cholestatic (Chapter 13). This is due to failure of adequate amounts of bile to reach the duodenum. The patient is relatively well, apart from the causative condition, for cholestasis *per se* is compatible with reasonably good health. Pruritus is prominent. With time the patient becomes increasingly pigmented. The serum shows increases in conjugated bilirubin, biliary alkaline phosphatase, total cholesterol and conjugated bile acids. Steatorrhoea is responsible for weight loss and malabsorption of fat-soluble Vitamins A, D, E and K and also of calcium.

Diagnosis of jaundice
(tables 12.1, 12.2)

The importance of a careful history and physical examination with routine biochemical and haematological tests must be stressed. The stool should be inspected and occult blood examination performed. The urine is tested for bilirubin and urobilinogen excess. The place of special tests such as ultrasonic examination, liver biopsy and cholangiography—whether percutaneous or endoscopic—will depend on the category of jaundice.

Clinical history

Occupation of the patient should be noted; particularly any contact with rats carrying Weil's disease, or employment involving alcohol.

Place of origin (Mediterranean, African or Far East) may suggest carriage of hepatitis B.

Family history is important with respect to jaundice, hepatitis, anaemia, splenectomy or cholecystectomy. Positive histories are helpful in diagnosing haemolytic jaundice, congenital hyperbilirubinaemia, hepatitis and gallstones.

Contact with jaundiced persons particularly in nurseries, camps, hospitals and schools is noted. Close contact with patients on renal units or with drug abusers is recorded. Any *injection* in the preceding six months should be recorded. 'Injections' include blood tests, drug abuse, tuberculin testing, dental treatment and tattooing as well as blood or plasma transfusions. The patient is asked about previous *drug treatment* with possible icterogenic agents. Consumption of *shellfish* and previous *travel* to areas where hepatitis is endemic should be noted.

Previous dyspepsia, fat intolerance and biliary colic suggest choledocholithiasis.

Jaundice after biliary tract surgery suggests residual calculus, traumatic stricture of the bile duct or hepatitis. Jaundice following the removal of a malignant growth may be due to hepatic metastases. Post-operative jaundice might be related to multiple administrations of halothane.

Alcoholics usually have associated features such as anorexia, morning nausea, diarrhoea and mild pyrexia. They may complain of pain over the enlarged liver.

Progressive failure of health and weight loss favour an underlying carcinoma.

The onset is extremely important. Preceding nausea, anorexia, in smokers—aversion to smoking, and jaundice, developing in a matter of hours and deepening rapidly—suggest virus hepatitis or drug jaundice. Cholestatic jaundice develops more slowly, often with persistent pruritus. Pyrexia with rigors suggests cholangitis associated with gallstones or biliary stricture.

Table 12.1. First steps in the diagnosis of the jaundiced patient.

Clinical history and examination
Urine, stools
Serum biochemical tests
    Bilirubin
    Transaminase ('AST', 'SGOT')
    Albumin
    Quantitative immunoglobulins
    Alkaline phosphatase
Haematology
    Haemoglobin, WBC, platelets
Blood film
Prothrombin time (before and after i.m. Vitamin K)
X-ray chest
Hepatitis A and B markers

Table 12.2. General features of the common types of acute jaundice

	Gallstones in common bile duct	Carcinoma ampullary region	Acute virus hepatitis	Cholestatic drug jaundice
Antecedent history	Dyspepsia, previous attack	Nil	Contacts, injections, transfusion, or nil	Taking drug
Pain	Constant epigastric, biliary colic, or none	Constant epigastric, back, or none	Ache over liver or none	None
Pruritus	+	+	Transient	+
Rate of development of jaundice	Slow	Slow	Rapid	Rapid
Type of jaundice	Fluctuates or persistent	Usually but not always	Rapid onset, slow fall with recovery	Variable, usually mild
Weight loss	Slight to moderate	Progressive	Slight	Slight
Examination				
Diathesis	Frequently female obese	Over 40 years old	Young usually	Often older female, psychotic
Depth of jaundice	Moderate	Deep	Variable	Variable, rash sometimes
Ascites	0	Rarely with metastases	If severe and prolonged	0
Liver	Enlarged, slightly tender	Enlarged, not tender	Enlarged and tender	Slightly enlarged
Palpable gallbladder	0	+ (sometimes)	0	0
Tender gallbladder area	+	0	0	0
Palpable spleen	0	Occasionally	About 20%	0
Temperature	↑	Not usually	↑ onset only	↑ onset
Laboratory investigations				
Leucocyte count	↑ or normal	↑ or normal	↓	Normal
Differential leucocytes	Polymorphs ↑	—	Lymphocytes ↑	Eosinophilia at onset
Faeces				
Colour	Intermittently pale	Acholic	Variable, light→dark	Pale
Occult blood	0	+	0	0
Urine: urobilin (ogen)	+	Absent + late	− Early + late	− Early
S. bilirubin meq/l	Usually 3−10	Steady rise to 15−30	Varies with severity	Variable

Table 12.2. *cont.*

	Gallstones in common bile duct	Carcinoma ampullary region	Acute virus hepatitis	Cholestatic drug jaundice
S. alkaline phosphatase (times normal)	>3×	>3×	<3×	>3×
S. aspartate transaminase (times normal)	<5×	<5×	>10×	>5×
Radiology				
Plain film abdomen	Gallstones 10%	Hepatomegaly	Hepatomegaly, slight	Hepatomegaly, slight
CT and ultrasound	Gallstones	Dilated ducts	Splenomegaly	Normal

Dark urine and pale stools precede hepato-cellular or cholestatic jaundice by a few days. In haemolytic jaundice the stools are well coloured.

In hepato-cellular jaundice the patient feels ill; in cholestatic jaundice he may be inconvenienced only by the icterus, any symptoms being due to the cause of the obstruction.

Persistent mild jaundice of varying intensity suggests haemolysis. The jaundice of cirrhosis is usually mild and variable and is associated with dark stools, although patients with acute 'alcoholic hepatitis' may be deeply jaundiced and pass pale stools.

Biliary colic may be continuous for hours rather than being intermittent. Back or epigastric pain may be associated with pancreatic carcinoma.

Examination (fig. 12.7)

Age and sex. A parous, middle-aged, obese female may have gallstones. The incidence of type A hepatitis decreases as age advances but no age is exempt from type B and non-A, non-B hepatitis. The probability of cancerous biliary obstruction increases with age. Drug jaundice is very rare in childhood.

General examination. Anaemia may indicate haemolysis, cancer or cirrhosis. Gross weight loss suggests cancer. The patient with haemolytic jaundice is a mild yellow colour, with hepato-cellular jaundice is orange and with prolonged biliary obstruction has a deep greenish hue. A hunched-up position suggests pancreatic carcinoma. In alcoholics, the stigmata of cirrhosis should be noted. Sites to be examined for a primary tumour include breasts, thyroid, stomach, colon, rectum and lung. Lymphadenopathy is noted.

Mental state. Slight intellectual deterioration with minimal personality change may be extremely valuable in suggesting hepato-cellular jaundice. Fetor and 'flapping' tremor indicate impending hepatic coma.

Skin changes. Bruising may indicate a clotting defect. Purpuric spots on forearms, axillae or shins may be related to the thrombocytopenia of cirrhosis. Other cutaneous manifestations of cirrhosis include vascular spiders, palmar erythema, white nails and loss of secondary sexual hair.

In chronic cholestasis, scratch marks, melanin pigmentation, finger clubbing, xanthomas on the eyelids, extensor surfaces and palmar creases, and hyperkeratosis may be found.

Pigmentation of the shins and ulcers may be seen in some forms of congenital haemolytic anaemia.

Malignant nodules should be sought in the skin. Multiple venous thromboses suggest carcinoma of the body of the pancreas. Ankle

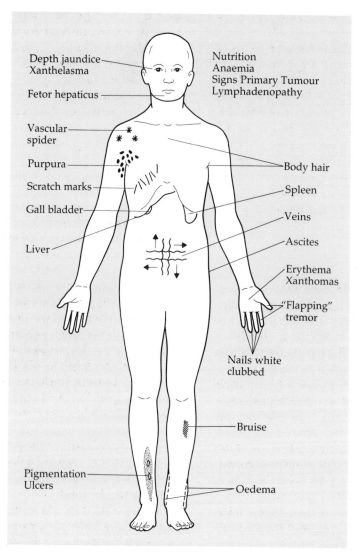

Depth jaundice
Xanthelasma

Nutrition
Anaemia
Signs Primary Tumour
Lymphadenopathy

Fetor hepaticus

Vascular
spider

Purpura

Scratch marks

Gall bladder

Liver

Body hair

Spleen

Veins

Ascites

Erythema
Xanthomas

"Flapping"
tremor

Nails white
clubbed

Bruise

Pigmentation
Ulcers

Oedema

Fig. 12.7. Physical signs in jaundice.

oedema may indicate cirrhosis, or obstruction of the inferior vena cava due to hepatic malignancy.

Abdominal examination. Dilated peri-umbilical veins indicate a portal collateral circulation and cirrhosis. Ascites may be due to cirrhosis or to malignant disease. A very large nodular liver suggests cancer. A small liver may indicate severe hepatitis or cirrhosis, and its presence excludes extra-hepatic cholestasis in which the liver is enlarged and smooth. In an alcoholic, fatty change and cirrhosis may

produce a uniform enlargement of the liver. The edge is tender in hepatitis, in congestive heart failure, with alcoholism, in bacterial cholangitis and occasionally in malignant disease. An arterial murmur over the liver indicates acute alcoholic hepatitis or primary liver cancer.

In choledocholithiasis the gallbladder may be tender and Murphy's sign positive. A pal-pable, and sometimes visibly enlarged, gall-bladder suggests pancreatic cancer.

The abdomen is carefully examined for any

primary tumour. A rectal examination is essential.

Urine and faeces. Bilirubinuria is an early sign of virus hepatitis and drug jaundice. Persistent absence of urobilinogen suggests total obstruction of the common bile duct. Persistent excess of urobilinogen with a negative bilirubin test supports the diagnosis of haemolytic jaundice.

The persistence of acholic stools confirms biliary obstruction. The presence of occult blood favours a diagnosis of ampullary, pancreatic or alimentary carcinoma or of portal hypertension.

Serum biochemical tests

The serum bilirubin level confirms jaundice, indicates depth and is used to follow progress. Serum alkaline phosphatase values more than three times normal strongly suggest biliary obstruction if bone disease is absent; high values may also be found in patients with non-biliary cirrhosis. In doubtful cases the serum γ-glutamyl transpeptidase level is measured when an increase indicates hepato-biliary and not bone disease.

Serum albumin and globulin levels are little changed in jaundice of short duration. In more chronic hepato-cellular icterus the albumin is depressed and globulin increased. Electroph oretic analysis shows raised α_2- and β-globulins in cholestatic jaundice in contrast to γ-globulin elevation in hepato-cellular jaundice.

Serum transaminase increases in hepatitis compared with variable but lower levels in cholestatic jaundice. High values may sometimes be found with cholangitis.

Haematology

A low total leucocyte count with a relative lymphocytosis suggests hepato-cellular jaundice. A polymorph leucocytosis may be found in alcoholic and severe virus hepatitis. Increased leucocyte counts are found with cholestatic jaundice with acute cholangitis or underlying malignant disease. If haemolysis is suspected, investigations should include reticulocyte counts, the examination of blood films, erythrocyte fragility, Coombs' test, and examination of the bone marrow.

If the prothrombin time is prolonged vitamin K_1 10 mg intramuscularly for three days leads to return to normal in cholestatis, whereas patients with hepato-cellular jaundice show little change.

Diagnostic routine

It should now be clear whether the patients' jaundice is pre-hepatic, hepatic or cholestatic. Clinical and biochemical clues are not infallible and consequently neither is clinical evaluation. A small proportion of patients with extra-hepatic biliary obstruction are incorrectly diagnosed as having intra-hepatic cholestatis, whereas a larger proportion of patients with intra-hepatic disease are thought to have extra-hepatic obstruction. Various algorithms are laid down for the investigation of the jaundiced patient. The sequence employed depends on the clinical impression, the facilities available and the risk of each investigation. Cost plays a part.

Computer models have been devised based on clinical history and examination with haematological and biochemical observations made during the first six hours in hospital [36]. These have a performance equalling that of the hepatologist and better than some internists. They predict the most efficient tests selected from 22 that will give the diagnosis. This first special test is usually successful in 69%. Such computer diagnosis may be cost-efficient but so far has not replaced the clinical skill of the internist.

Radiology

A chest film is taken to show primary and secondary tumours and any irregularity and elevation of the right diaphragm due to an enlarged or nodular liver. A barium meal may show oesophageal varices and in patients with hepatomegaly the lesser curve of the stomach may be displaced and even rigid. Distortion and altered motility of the duodenum is seen in carcinoma of the head of the pancreas.

Visualization of the bile ducts

This is indicated if the patient is cholestatic (see Chapter 29). The first procedure in distinguishing hepato-cellular from surgical, main duct 'obstructive' jaundice is ultrasound or CT scanning to show whether or not the intra-hepatic bile ducts are dilated (fig. 12.6). This is followed by percutaneous or endoscopic cholangiography as indicated.

Viral markers

These are indicated for hepatitis A, B cyto-megala and Epstein–Barr infections if viral hepatitis is suspected (Chapter 16).

Needle liver biopsy

Acute jaundice rarely merits liver biopsy and the technique is reserved for the patient who presents diagnostic difficulty and where an intra-hepatic cause is suspected. The method carries extra risk in the jaundiced; the Menghini technique is safest. Mere depth of jaundice is not a contraindication.

Trans-jugular or CT or US guided biopsy with plugging of the puncture site in the liver is useful if clotting defects preclude the 'blind' technique (Chapter 3).

Acute virus hepatitis is usually diagnosed easily. The greatest difficulty arises in the cholestatic group. However, in most instances an experienced histopathologist can distinguish appearances of intra-hepatic cholestasis, for instance due to drugs or to primary biliary cirrhosis, from the appearances of a block to main bile passages. The cause of the cholestasis can be stated with much less certainty.

Laparoscopy

The appearance of a dark green liver with an enormous gallbladder favours extra-hepatic biliary obstruction. Tumour nodules may be seen and needle biopsy may be made under direct vision. A pale yellow-green liver suggests hepatitis and cirrhosis is obvious. The method cannot be relied upon to distinguish extra-hepatic biliary obstruction, especially due to a carcinoma of the main hepatic ducts, from intra-hepatic cholestasis due to drugs.

A photographic record should be taken of the appearances. In the presence of jaundice peritoneoscopy is safer than needle biopsy but, if necessary, the two procedures may be combined.

Prednisolone test

When 30 mg prednisolone daily are given a profound fall in serum bilirubin level in five days indicates hepato-cellular jaundice. Patients with cholestasis show little change. A fall in serum bilirubin level greater than 40% strongly suggests hepatitis [43], but an equivocal change does not exclude it. This test is for the problem case usually when cholestatic viral hepatitis is suspected and hepatitis B has been excluded. It is rarely necessary.

The fate of the bilirubin disappearing from the blood after prednisolone is most obscure. The corticosteroid 'whitewash' cannot be accounted for by changes in erythrocyte survival (reflecting changes in haemoglobin catabolism), faecal or urinary urobilinogen output, or urinary bilirubin [48]. The bilirubin may take an alternative metabolic pathway.

Laparotomy

Jaundice is rarely a surgical emergency (see Chapter 13). If there is any doubt concerning the diagnosis, it is better to investigate further rather than to explore the bile passages of a patient with hepatic jaundice and so run the very real risk of precipitating acute liver failure. The patient rarely suffers from delay.

The familial non-haemolytic hyperbilirubinaemias (table 12.3)

Although the upper limit of serum bilirubin is usually taken to be 0.8 mg/100 ml, in some 5% of healthy blood donors higher values (1—3 mg/100 ml) may be found. When those suffering from haemolysis or from overt liver disease have been excluded there remain the patients with familial abnormalities of bilirubin metabolism. The commonest is Gilbert's syndrome [19]. Other syndromes can also be identified. The prognosis for all these is excellent. Accurate diagnosis, particularly from chronic liver disease, is important for it enables the patient to be reassured. The diagnosis is based on family history, duration, absence of stigmata of hepato-cellular disease and of splenomegaly, and if necessary on the hepatic histology.

Primary hyperbilirubinaemia. This very rare condition is due to increased production of 'early-labelled' bilirubin in the bone marrow. The cause is probably the premature destruction of abnormal red cell precursors (ineffective erythrocyte synthesis). The clinical picture is of compensated haemolysis. Peripheral erythrocyte destruction is normal. The condition is probably familial [1, 22].

Gilbert's syndrome

This is defined as benign, familial, mild, unconjugated hyperbilirubinaemia (serum bilirubin 1—5 mg/dl) not due to haemolysis and with normal routine tests of liver function and hepatic histology. It affects some 2—5% of the population. The number involved in any family is difficult to determine. The serum bilirubin may be only minimally, and inconstantly, elevated. Gilbert's syndrome is probably inherited as an autosomal dominant. Patients are heterozygous for a single mutant gene [33].

It may be diagnosed by chance at a routine medical examination or when the blood is being examined for another reason, for instance to determine completeness of recovery from virus hepatitis. It has an excellent prognosis. Jaundice is mild and intermittent. Deepening may follow an intercurrent infection or fasting and is associated with malaise, nausea and often discomfort over the liver. These symptoms have never been explained but often lead to a mistaken diagnosis of virus hepatitis. There are no other abnormal physical signs; the spleen is not palpable.

The defect in bilirubin metabolism is com-

Table 12.3. Isolated increases in serum bilirubin

Type	Diagnostic points
Unconjugated	
Haemolysis	Splenomegaly. Blood film. Reticulocytosis. Coombs' test
Gilbert's	Familial. S. bilirubin increases with fasting and falls on phenobarbitone. Liver biopsy normal but conjugating enzyme reduced
Crigler—Najjar	
Type 1	No conjugating enzyme in liver. No response to phenobarbitone. Usually die young with kernicterus
Type 2	Absent or deficient conjugating enzyme in liver. Response to phenobarbitone
Conjugated	
Dubin—Johnson	Black liver biopsy. No concentration of cholecystographic media. Secondary rise in BSP test
Rotor	Normal liver biopsy. Cholecystography normal. BSP test no uptake

plex. The conjugating enzyme, UDP glucuronyl transferase, is reduced [7]. Alterations in membrane fluidity might impair the uptake of bilirubin by the liver cell. In spite of reduction of total bilirubin the bile contains increased bilirubin monoglucuronide over the diglucuronide, suggesting a second enzyme defect related to the conversion of monoglucuronide to diglucuronide [18]. Erythrocyte survival may be mildly reduced [33] and dyserythropoiesis may play a part. The bilirubin liberated from the excess erythrocyte breakdown would not be sufficient to account for the jaundice.

Other abnormalities include mild impairment of BSP clearance and of tolbutamide, a drug which does not need conjugation. A variant is marked by defective indocyanine green uptake, but normal BSP metabolism. Peripheral blood cells show abnormalities of the enzymes of biosynthesis. These resemble variegate porphyria and are perhaps due to increased hepato-cellular bilirubin concentrations [27].

The multiplicity of abnormalities suggest that Gilbert's syndrome may not be an entity. The hyperbilirubinaemia may constitute merely the upper end of the normal range [3]. The squirrel monkey provides an animal model for Gilbert's syndrome [32].

Specialist diagnostic tests include the increase in serum bilirubin on fasting (fig. 12.8) [30], the fall on taking phenobarbital which induces the hepatic conjugating enzyme (fig. 12.9) and the increase following intravenous nicotinic acid which raises the osmotic fragility of red blood cells [35].

If unconjugated and conjugated serum bilirubin are measured by high phase liquid chromatography, the level of unconjugated bilirubin is significantly higher in Gilbert's syndrome than in normals, chronic haemolysis or chronic hepatitis; this is diagnostic [41]. The fasting serum bile acids are normal or even low [34, 45]. Low values for bilirubin conjugating enzyme are found in liver biopsies [7]. However, Gilbert's syndrome is usually diagnosed with ease without recourse to these specialist methods [29].

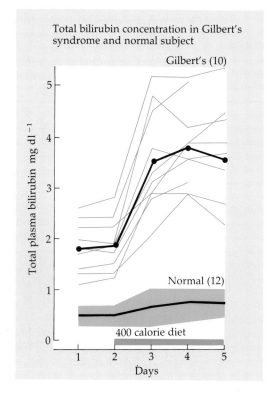

Fig. 12.8. Gilbert's syndrome. The serum unconjugated bilirubin level increases after a 400 calorie diet (Owners & Sherlock 1973).

Gilbert's syndrome has a normal life expectancy and no treatment is needed other than reassurance. Symptoms persist over many years and the serum bilirubin level remains relatively constant.

Serum bilirubin may be reduced by phenobarbital [8] but, as icterus is rarely obvious, few patients will gain cosmetic benefit from this treatment. 'Sufferers' should be warned that jaundice can follow an intercurrent infection, repeated vomiting or missed meals. The 'sufferer' is a normal risk for life insurance.

Crigler−Najjar type

This extreme form of familial non-haemolytic jaundice is associated with very high serum unconjugated bilirubin values [13]. Deficiency

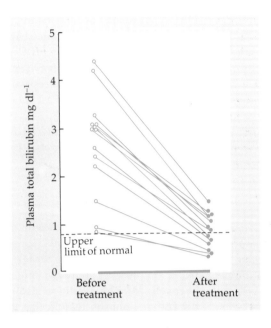

Fig. 12.9. Gilbert's syndrome. The effect of phenobarbital (60 mg, three times a day) on the serum bilirubin level (Black & Sherlock 1970).

of conjugating enzyme can be demonstrated in the liver. Total pigment in bile is minimal [18]. Bilirubin tolerance is impaired but the BSP test gives normal results.

TYPE 1

This is inherited as an autosomal recessive. No bilirubin conjugating enzyme can be detected in the liver. Conjugated bilirubin is absent from the bile. Bilirubin glucuronide is totally absent from serum [28]. As the serum bilirubin levels eventually stabilize, the patient must have some alternative pathway of bilirubin metabolism.

Sufferers usually, but not always, die with kernicterus in the first year of life. There is no response to phenobarbital. Phlebotomy and plasmapheresis have been used to reduce serum bilirubin but with only temporary success. Phototherapy can reduce the serum bilirubin by about 50% and may be carried out at home [17]. Encephalopathy may develop any time in the first or second decade and hepatic transplantation has to be considered; this results in restoration of the serum bilirubin to normal [23].

In the future, clones of the UDP-glucuronyl transferase specific gene might make enzyme replacement possible [25].

TYPE 2

This is inherited as an autosomal dominant. Bilirubin conjugating enzyme is extremely reduced in the liver and although present is undetectable by the usual methods of analysis. The patients respond dramatically to phenobarbital and survive into adult life [21]. Phototherapy lowers the serum bilirubin level.

The *Gunn strain* of congenitally jaundiced rats also lacks the bilirubin glucuronyl transferase enzyme.

Dubin—Johnson type

The Dubin—Johnson type is a chronic, benign, intermittent jaundice with conjugated and some unconjugated hyperbilirubinaemia and with bilirubinuria [14, 15].

The liver, macroscopically, is greenish-black (black-liver jaundice) (figs 12.10, 12.11). In sections the liver cells show a brown pigment which is neither iron nor bile. The pigment may be melanin, which has been found in the urine and spleen of a patient with this syndrome [46]. This seems likely since the pigment in the liver of mutant Corriedale sheep, which have a disorder similar in all respects to the Dubin—Johnson syndrome, appears to be melanin [2]. Electron microscopy shows the pigment in dense bodies related to lysosomes (fig. 12.12).

An unrelated virus hepatitis leads to temporary mobilization of the hepatic pigment [44].

Pruritus is absent and the serum alkaline phosphatase and bile acid levels are normal.

Excretion of organic anions into bile is impaired, hepatic uptake is usually normal. The

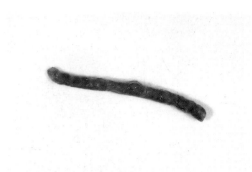

Fig. 12.10. Needle biopsy of patient with Dubin–Johnson syndrome is blackish-brown.

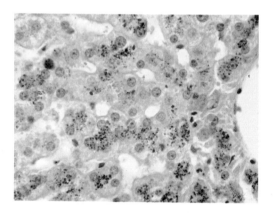

Fig. 12.11. Dubin–Johnson hyperbilirubinaemia. The liver cells and Küpffer cells are packed with a dark pigment which gives the staining reactions of lipofuscin. H & E, ×275.

contrast media used in intravenous cholangiography are not concentrated but ^{99m}Tc-HIDA excretion shows normal liver and gallbladder [4].

In patients a diagnostic pattern is seen in a prolonged BSP test. After an initial fall in serum level the BSP rises so that the value at 120 minutes exceeds that seen at 45 minutes (fig. 12.13) [26].

Urinary coproporphyrins are excreted in normal amounts but there is an increased proportion of coproporphyrin 1.

The condition may present as jaundice during pregnancy or after taking oral contraceptives, both of which reduce hepatic excretory function [12].

Dubin–Johnson syndrome is probably inherited as an autosomal recessive. It is most frequent in the Middle East among Iranian Jews.

There is no correlation between liver pigment and serum bilirubin levels. Prognosis is excellent.

Rotor type

This is a similar form of chronic familial conjugated hyperbilirubinaemia. It resembles the Dubin–Johnson syndrome, the main difference being the absence of brown pigment in the liver cell [38]. The condition also differs from the Dubin–Johnson type in that the gallbladder opacifies on cholecystography and there is no secondary rise in the BSP test. The abnormality causing BSP retention appears to be related to a defect in hepatic uptake rather than excretion as originally demonstrated in the Dubin–Johnson syndrome. ^{99m}Tc-HIDA excretion gives no visualization of the liver, gallbladder or biliary tree.

Total urinary coproporphyrins are raised, as in cholestasis. The proportion of coproporphyrin I in urine is approximately 65% of the total [40]. Electron microscopy may show abnormalities of mitochondria and peroxisomes [16].

Family studies make an autosomal inheritance probable [24]. The Rotor type has an excellent prognosis.

The group of familial non-haemolytic hyperbilirubinaemias

There is much overlap between the various syndromes of congenital hyperbilirubinaemia. Patients are found in the same family with conjugated hyperbilirubinaemia but with or without pigment in the liver cells. Pigmented livers have been found in patients with unconjugated hyperbilirubinaemia [10]. In one large family the propositi had the classic

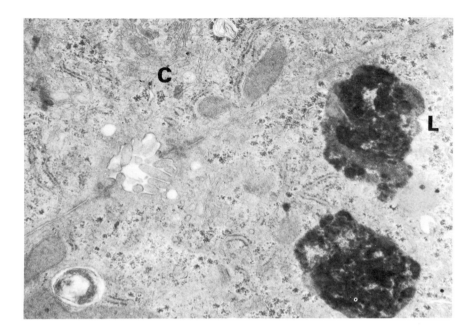

Fig. 12.12. Dubin−Johnson syndrome. Electron microscopy shows normal bile canaliculi with intact microvilli (C). Lysosomes (L) are enlarged, irregularly shaped and contain granular material and often membrane-bound lipid droplets.

Fig. 12.13. Bromsulphalein tolerance test (5 mg/kg i.m.) in a patient with Dubin−Johnson syndrome. At 40 min, the BSP level has almost returned to normal. An increase is then seen at 120, 180 and 240 min. Dye can still be detected in the blood at 48 hours. The indocyanine green test is also shown and is normal at 20 min, but also has a tendency to increase at 30 min.

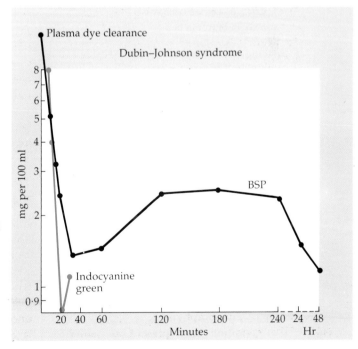

Dubin–Johnson picture, but the commonest abnormality in the family was unconjugated hyperbilirubinaemia [10]. In another family, conjugated and unconjugated hyperbilirubin-aemia alternated in the same patient [37]. Family members of Crigler–Najjar type 2 sufferers may have serum bilirubin levels more typical of Gilbert's syndrome. Such observations add to the confusion in separating the groups and in deciding the mode of inheritance.

References

1 Arias IM. Chronic unconjugated hyperbilirubin-aemia (CUH) with increased production of bile pigment not derived from the hemoglobin of mature, circulating erythrocytes. *J. clin. Invest.* 1962; **41:** 1341.

2 Arias IM, Bernstein L, Toffler R *et al.* Black liver disease in Corriedale sheep: a new mutation affecting excretory function. *J. clin Invest.* 1964; **43:** 1249.

3 Bailey A, Robinson D, Dawson AM. Does Gilbert's disease exist? *Lancet* 1977; **i:** 931.

4 Bar-Meir S, Baron J, Seligson U *et al.* ^{99m}Tc-HIDA cholescintigraphy in Dubin–Johnson and Rotor syndromes. *Radiology* 1982; **142:** 743.

5 Berk PD, Blaschke TF, Scharschmidt BF *et al.* A new approach to quantitation of the various sources of bilirubin in man. *J. lab. clin. Med.* 1976; **87:** 767.

6 Billing BH. Twenty-five years of progress in bilirubin metabolism (1952–1977). *Gut* 1978; **19:** 481.

7 Black M, Billing BH. Hepatic bilirubin UDP-glucuronyl transferase activity in liver disease and Gilbert's syndrome. *N. Engl. J. Med.* 1969; **280:** 1266.

8 Black M, Sherlock S. Treatment of Gilbert's syndrome with phenobarbitone. *Lancet* 1970; **i:** 1359.

9 Bonnett R, Davies JE, Hursthouse MB. Structure of bilirubin. *Nature* 1976; **262:** 326.

10 Butt HR, Anderson VE, Foulk WT *et al.* Studies of chronic idiopathic jaundice (Dubin–Johnson syndrome). II Evaluation of a large family with the trait. *Gastroenterology* 1966; **51:** 619.

11 Chowdhury JR, Chowdhury NR. Conjugation and excretion of bilirubin. *Sem. Liv. Dis.* 1983; **3:** 11.

12 Cohen L, Lewis C, Arias IM. Pregnancy, oral contraceptives and chronic familial jaundice with predominantly conjugated hyperbilirubinaemia (Dubin–Johnson syndrome). *Gastroenterology* 1972; **62:** 1182.

13 Crigler JF Jr, Najjar VA. Congenital familial non-hemolytic jaundice with kernicterus. *Pediatrics* 1952; **10:** 169.

14 Dubin IN. Chronic idiopathic jaundice. A review of fifty cases. *Am. J. Med.* 1958; **24:** 268.

15 Dubin IN, Johnson FB. Chronic idiopathic jaundice with unidentified pigment in the liver cells: a new clinico-pathological entity with a report of twelve cases. *Medicine (Baltimore)* 1954; **33:** 155.

16 Evans J, Lefkowitch J, Lim CK *et al.* Fecal porphyrin abnormalities in a patient with features of Rotor's syndrome. *Gastroenterology* 1981; **81:** 1125.

17 Farrell GC, Gollan JL, Stevens SM *et al.* Crigler–Najjar type 1 syndrome: absence of hepatic bilirubin UDP glucuronyl transferase activity and therapeutic responses to light. *Aust. NZ J. Med.* 1982; **12:** 280.

18 Fevery J, Blanckaert N, Heirweigh KPM *et al.* Unconjugated bilirubin and an increased proportion of bilirubin monoconjugates in the bile of patients with Gilbert's syndrome and Crigler–Najjar disease. *J. clin. Invest.* 1977; **60:** 970.

19 Gilbert A, Leerboullet P. La cholémie simple familiale. *Sem. med. Paris* 1901; **21:** 241.

20 Gollan JL, Dallinger KJC, Billing BH. Excretion of conjugated bilirubin in the isolated perfused rat kidney. *Clin. Sci. molec. Med.* 1978; **54:** 381.

21 Gollan JL, Huang SN, Billing B *et al.* Prolonged survival in three brothers with severe type 2 Crigler–Najjar syndrome. Ultrastructural and metabolic studies. *Gastroenterology* 1975; **68:** 1543.

22 Israels LG, Suderman HJ, Ritzmann SE. Hyper-bilirubinaemia due to an alternate path of bilirubin production. *Am. J. Med.* 1959; **27:** 693.

23 Kaufman SS, Wood RP, Shaw BW Jr *et al.* Orthotopic liver transplantation for type 1 Crigler–Najjar syndrome. *Hepatology* 1986; **6:** 1259.

24 Lima JEP, Utz E, Roisenberg I. Hereditary non hemolytic conjugated hyperbilirubinaemia without abnormal liver cell pigmentation. A family study. *Am. J. Med.* 1966; **40:** 628.

25 Mackenzie PI. Rat liver UDP-glucuronyltransferase. Sequence and expression of a cDNA encoding a phenobarbital-inducible form. *J. biol. Chem.* 1986; **261:** 6119.

26 Mandema E, De Fraiture WH, Nieweg HO *et al.* Familial chronic idiopathic jaundice (Dubin–Sprinz disease) with a note on bromsulphalein metabolism in this disease. *Am. J. Med.* 1960; **28:** 42.

27 McColl KEL, Thompson GG, El Omar E *et al.* Porphyrin metabolism and haem biosynthesis in Gilbert's syndrome. *Gut* 1987; **28:** 125.

28 Muraca M, Fevery J, Blanckaert N. Relationships between serum bilirubins and production and conjugation of bilirubin. Studies in Gilbert's syn-

drome, Crigler—Najjar disease, hemolytic disorders, and rat models. *Gastroenterology* 1987; **92:** 309.

29 Okolicsanyi L, Fevery J, Billing BH *et al.* How should mild, isolated unconjugated hyperbilirubinaemia be investigated? *Semin. Liv. Dis.* 1983; **3:** 36.

30 Owens D, Sherlock S. The diagnosis of Gilbert's syndrome: role of the reduced caloric intake test. *Br. med. J.* 1973; **iii:** 559.

31 Peters WHM, Jansen PLM. Microsomal UDP-glucuronyl-transferase-catalyzed bilirubin diglucuronide formation in human liver. *J. Hepatol.* 1986; **2:** 182.

32 Portman OW, Chowdhury JR, Chowdhury NR *et al.* A nonhuman primate model of Gilbert's syndrome. *Hepatology* 1984; **4:** 175.

33 Powell LW, Hemingway E, Billing BH *et al.* Idiopathic unconjugated hyperbilirubinaemia (Gilbert's syndrome). A study of 42 families. *N. Engl. J. Med.* 1967; **277:** 1108.

34 Roda A, Roda E, Sama C *et al.* Serum primary bile acids in Gilbert's syndrome. *Gastroenterology* 1982; **82:** 77.

35 Röllinghoff W, Paumgartner G, Preisig R. Nicotinic acid test in the diagnosis of Gilbert's syndrome: correlation with bilirubin clearance. *Gut* 1981; **22:** 663.

36 Saint-Marc Girardin M-F, Le Minor M, Alperovitch A *et al.* Computer-aided selection of diagnostic tests in jaundiced patients. *Gut* 1985; **26:** 961.

37 Satler J. Another variant of constitutional familial hepatic dysfunction with permanent jaundice and with alternating serum bilirubin relations. *Acta Hepato-splen.* 1966; **13:** 38.

38 Schiff L, Billing BH, Oikawa Y. Familial non-hemolytic jaundice with conjugated bilirubin in the serum. A case study. *N. Engl. J. Med.* 1959; **260:** 1314.

39 Schmid R. Bilirubin metabolism: state of the art. *Gastroenterology* 1978; **74:** 1307.

40 Shimizu Y, Naruto H, Ida S *et al.* Urinary coproporphyrin isomers in Rotor's syndrome: a study in eight families. *Hepatology* 1981; **1:** 173.

41 Sieg A, Stiehl A, Raedsch R *et al.* Gilbert's syndrome: diagnosis by typical serum bilirubin pattern. *Clin. Chim. Acta* 1986; **154:** 41.

42 Stremmel W, Tavoloni N, Berk PD. Uptake of bilirubin by the liver. *Semin. Liv. Dis.* 1983; **3:** 1.

43 Summerskill WHJ, Clowdus BF II, Bollman JL *et al.* Clinical and experimental studies on the effect of corticotrophin and steroid drugs on bilirubinaemia. *Am. J. med. Sci.* 1961; **241:** 555.

44 Varma RR, Grainger JM, Scheuer PJ. A case of the Dubin—Johnson syndrome complicated by acute hepatitis. *Gut* 1970; **11:** 817.

45 Vierling JM, Berk PD, Hofmann AF *et al.* Normal fasting-state levels of serum cholyl-conjugated bile acids in Gilbert's syndrome: an aid to the diagnosis. *Hepatology* 1982; **2:** 340.

46 Wegmann R, Rangier M, Etévé J *et al.* Mélanose hépato-splénique avec ictère chronique a bilirubine directe: maladie de Dubin—Johnson? Étude clinique et biologique de la maladie. Étude histochimique et spectrographique du pigment anormal. *Semin. Hôp. Paris.* 1960; **36:** 1761.

47 Weiss JS, Gautam A, Lauff JJ *et al.* The clinical importance of a protein-bound fraction of serum bilirubin in patients with hyperbilirubinaemia. *N. Engl. J. Med.* 1983; **309:** 147.

48 Williams R, Billing B. Action of steroid therapy in jaundice. *Lancet* 1961; **ii:** 392.

13 · Cholestasis

Cholestasis is defined as failure of normal amounts of bile to reach the duodenum. The term 'obstructive jaundice' is not used, as in many instances no mechanical block can be shown in the biliary tract.

Biliary cirrhosis follows prolonged cholestasis; the time taken for its development varies from months to years. The transition is not reflected in a sudden change in the clinical picture. The term 'biliary cirrhosis' is reserved for a pathological picture. It is diagnosed when there are features of cirrhosis such as nodule formation, encephalopathy or fluid retention.

Anatomy of the biliary system

Conjugated bilirubin is secreted by the liver cell into the canaliculus. The biliary secretory apparatus comprises the bile canaliculus, the peri-canalicular ectoplasm, lysosomes and Golgi apparatus (fig. 13.1).

The bile canalicular membrane has enzymes as an integral component and some parts of the membrane such as phospholipids are released into the bile. The microvilli increase the surface area.

The tight junctions seal the biliary space from the blood compartment.

The peri-canalicular ectoplasm contains the *cytoskeleton* of the liver cell. Microfilaments provide tone to the canalicular system. Microtubules may be concerned in the arrangement of canalicular membrane proteins and in lecithin and bile acid secretion. The intermediate filaments interconnect with microtubules and microfilaments to maintain the structural organization of the cytoplasm [47]. Peri-canalicular vesicles are probably 'ferry' vesicles conveying substances from sinusoidal to canalicular zones. Lysosomes are involved in biliary excretion.

The role of the Golgi apparatus in biliary secretion is unknown.

The bile canaliculi empty into ductules sometimes called cholangioles or canals of Hering (figs 13.2, 13.3). These are found largely in the portal zones of the liver. The ductule passes into the interlobular bile duct which is the first bile channel to be accompanied by a branch of the hepatic artery and portal vein. These are also found in the portal triad. These channels unite with one another to form septal bile ducts and so on until the two main hepatic ducts emerge from the right and left lobes of the liver at the porta hepatis.

The secretion of bile (figs 13.4, 13.5, 13.6, 13.7)

Bile secretion is relatively independent of perfusion pressure and bile is formed by several different energy dependent transport processes (fig. 13.4) [9, 23].

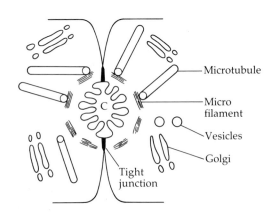

Fig. 13.1. The bile secretory apparatus. A diagram of the ultrastructure of the bile canaliculus (C) and pericanalicular zone of the liver cell.

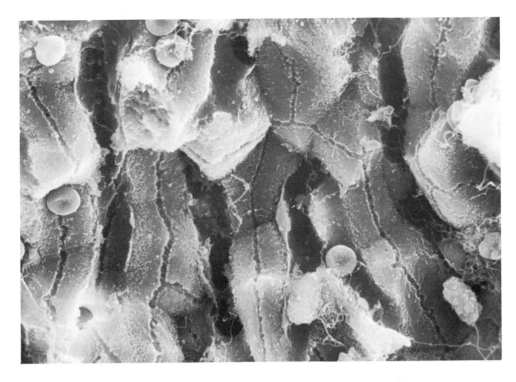

Fig. 13.2. Scanning electron micrograph of the canalicular biliary system (Boyer 1975).

An excellent correlation exists between bile flow and bile salt secretion. Bile salts passing into the biliary canaliculus are the most important factors promoting bile flow. This *bile salt-dependent* active secretion carries with it bile pigments, organic ions and water. The passage of the osmotically active bile salts generates water flow. Changes in osmotic activity may be the regulatory mechanism for the flow of water into the bile.

Bile salt-independent flow is shown by extrapolation of bile salt versus bile flow data to zero bile salt excretion when a positive intercept is shown. This indicates that flow would continue at zero bile salt excretion, presumably by a bile salt-independent method.

The hepatocyte is a polarized secretory epithelial cell with a basolateral (sinusoidal and lateral) and apical (canalicular) membrane. Bile formation requires the uptake of bile acids across the sinusoidal membrane, transport through the hepatocyte and excretion across the canalicular membrane. This is followed by osmotic filtration of water largely along paracellular pathways.

Uptake of bile acids by a specific protein of the basolateral membrane appears to be coupled to sodium uptake (bile acid-sodium co-transport or symport). The energy necessary for this transport against an electrochemical gradient is provided by the sodium gradient (high sodium out, low sodium in) maintained by the Na^+K^+-ATPase on the basolateral membrane. Another important mechanism at the basolateral membrane is a Na^+H^+ exchange (antiport). This system could play a role in regulation of cellular pH and electrolyte transport and is responsible for canalicular bicarbonate secretion. Little is known of the intracellular transport of bile acids.

Transport of bile acids across the canalicular membrane involves binding to a specific protein and is carrier-mediated. Facilitated diffusion is driven by the electrical potential

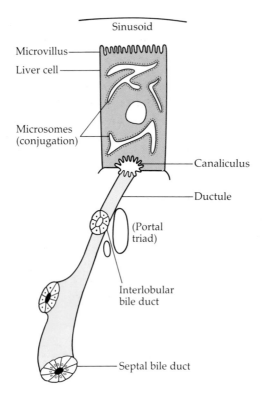

Fig. 13.3. The anatomy of the intra-hepatic biliary system.

difference across the canalicular membrane. Water and inorganic ions (cations, in particular sodium) enter bile by diffusion through the tight junctions which represent negatively charged semi-permeable barriers. Carrier-mediated transport of bile acids as well as other organic acids and electrolytes has been demonstrated in sinusoidal and canalicular lipid plasma membranes [27, 45]. Membrane fluidity refers to the motional freedom of membrane lipids and in particular, cholesterol. Membrane fluidity is known to influence the activity of certain plasma membrane enzymes such as Na^+K^+ ATPase.

The bile canaliculus is limited by tight junctions which may leak in diseased states. Actin microfilaments may help to propel the bile along the canalicular network (fig. 13.6) [58].

Isolated rat hepatocyte couplets, studied in short-term culture, allow the canaliculus to become assessable to standard micropuncture techniques. This will allow the canalicular bile to be studied in great detail.

Ductular bile flow modifies canalicular flow by adding an inorganic electrolyte solution consisting mostly of sodium bicarbonate and sodium chloride. A considerable amount of

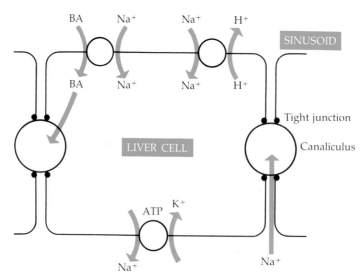

Fig. 13.4. Bile formation and transport systems. Note the Na^+ K^+ ATPase or sodium pump, the $Na^+ -$ bile acid (BA) co-transport (symport) uptake, the Na^+ H^+ exchange (antiport) system and the paracellular pathway for Na^+ and H_2O into the canaliculus.

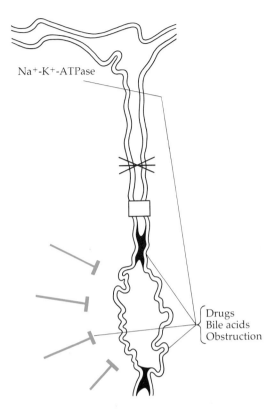

Na$^+$-K$^+$-ATPase

Drugs
Bile acids
Obstruction

Fig. 13.5. Cholestatic drugs or bile acids and biliary obstruction cause cholestasis by interfering with the Na$^+$-K$^+$-ATPase, located on the sinusoidal pole of the hepatocyte, the cytoskeleton, the canalicular membrane and the tight junction between canaliculus and sinusoid.

water and sodium chloride may be absorbed. Ductular flow is largely controlled by secretin. *Gallbladder contraction* is controlled by cholecystokinin. Ductular flow may serve to flush bile salts from the lower end of the common bile duct following gallbladder contraction.

In man, *total bile flow* is about 600 ml per 24 hours of which 225 ml is bile acid-dependent, 225 ml bile acid-independent and 150 ml ductular (fig. 13.8) [49].

The syndrome of cholestasis

Definition. Cholestasis can result from interference with bile flow anywhere from the basolateral membrane of the hepatocyte to the entry of the bile duct into the duodenum.

Morphologically cholestasis is defined as accumulation of bile in liver cells and biliary passages (fig. 13.9).

Clinically cholestasis is the retention in the blood of all substances normally excreted in the bile. Serum bile acid levels are increased.

Functionally cholestasis is defined as a decrease in canalicular bile flow [11, 51]. There is a decreased hepatic secretion of water and/or organic anions (bilirubin−bile acid). The disturbance in bile flow is multi-factorial (fig. 13.7) due to failure of the pumps secreting bile or of the channels into which bile is secreted.

The bile salt-dependent pump fails if inadequate quantities of bile salts reach the canaliculus or leak from it. Failure of the enterohepatic circulation of bile salts may contribute.

Cholestasis may be related to changes in membrane fluidity [9]. Ethinyl oestradiol, for instance, is known to decrease fluidity of the sinusoidal plasma membrane. In rats, this can be prevented by the methyl-donor, S-adenosyl methionine (SAME) which alters membrane fluidity through its protein composition [53]. *E. coli* endotoxin may act in this way [41].

The bile salt-independent sodium− potassium ATPase ion pump may be inhibited. The actin microfilaments around the tight junctions between neighbouring hepatocytes is widened reflecting a defect in the normal depolymerization of the actin−myosin microfilaments. Vesicle transport through the cytoplasm may depend on the cytoskeleton [23]. Phalloiden is a good example where cholestasis is related to depolymerization of actin. Chlorpromazine also affects the polymerization of actin *in vitro*.

The canaliculi may become more rigid, excessively permeable and less contractile (fig. 13.6) [58]. The tight junctions between neighbouring hepatocytes become more permeable and bile salts leak from the liver cell [11].

Ductular abnormalities, such as inflammation and epithelial changes, interfere with bile flow but are probably secondary rather than primary.

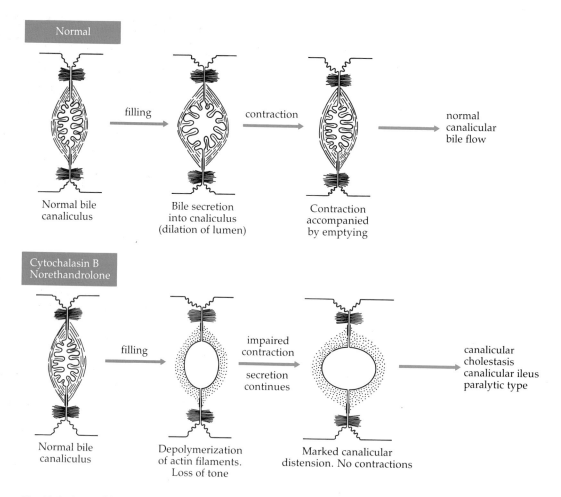

Fig. 13.6. A possible mechanism for intra-hepatic cholestasis. Normal canalicular bile secretion is accompanied by canalicular contraction and canalicular bile flow. Cytochalasin or norethandrolone depolymerizes actin filaments, resulting in loss of tone, canalicular distension and failure to contract, with consequent canalicular ileus and cholestasis. (Courtesy M.J. Phillips.)

The primary event in extra-hepatic chole-stasis is obvious, for instance a gallstone ob-structing the common bile duct. Secondary events are then initiated within the liver cell. In intra-hepatic cholestasis the primary event is particularly obscure, but again secondary changes follow within the liver cell itself. It is often impossible to differentiate the primary events from the secondary ones.

Pathology

All changes depend on duration. The liver is enlarged, green, swollen and with a rounded edge. Nodularity develops late.

Light microscopy [14]. Zone 3 shows marked bilirubin stasis in hepatocytes, Kupffer cells and canaliculi. Hepatocytes may show feathery degeneration, possibly due to retention of bile salts, with foamy cells and surrounding mono

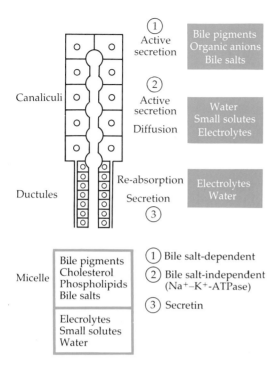

Fig. 13.7. Mechanisms of bile formation.

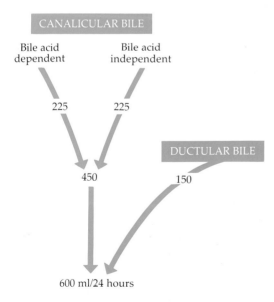

Fig. 13.8. Twenty-four-hour volumes of bile in man (Paumgartner 1977).

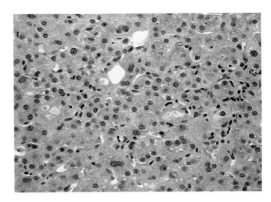

Fig. 13.9. Cholestasis: bile is seen in dilated canaliculi and hepatocytes.

nuclear accumulations. Cellular necrosis, regen eration and nodular hyperplasia are minimal.

Zone 1 shows ductular proliferation due to the mitogenic effect of bile salts. Hepatocytes transform into bile duct cells and form base ment membranes. The peribiliary endothelial cells manufacture γ glutamyl trans-peptidase and alkaline phosphatase. Reabsorption of bile constituents by ductular cells can result in microlith formation.

Fibrosis can be seen in zone 1. This is rever sible if the cholestasis is relieved. The zone 1 fibrosis extends to meet bands from adjacent zones so that eventually zone 3 is enclosed by a ring of connective tissue (figs 13.9, 13.10).

In the early stages, the relationship of hepa tic vein to portal vein is normal and this dis tinguishes the picture from biliary cirrhosis. Continuing periductular fibrosis may lead to disappearance to bile ducts and this is irrever sible.

Zone 1 oedema and inflammation are related to bilio-lymphatic reflux and to leucotrienes. Mallory bodies can accompany the inflamma tion and fibrosis in zone 1. Copper-associated protein, demonstrated by orcein staining, is seen in periportal hepatocytes [32].

Class 2 HLA antigens are displayed on hepa tocyte membranes.

Biliary cirrhosis follows prolonged choles tasis. Fibrous tissue bands in the portal zones coalesce and the lobules are correspondingly

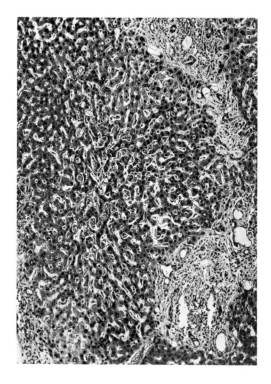

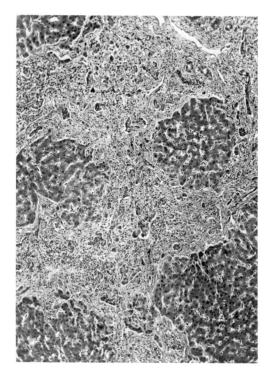

Fig. 13.10. Unrelieved common bile duct obstruction. Bile duct proliferation and fibrosis in the portal tracts which are becoming joined together. Bile pigment accumulations in the centrizonal areas. Hepatic lobular architecture normal. H & E, ×67

Fig. 13.11. Biliary cirrhosis. The normal hepatic architecture is disturbed. The wide intervening fibrous tissue bands show proliferating bile ducts and a heavy infiltration with mononuclear cells. H & E, ×63.

reduced in size. Fibrous bridges join portal and centrizonal areas (fig. 13.11). Nodular regeneration of liver cells follows, but a true cirrhosis rarely follows biliary obstruction. In total biliary obstruction due to cancer of the head of the pancreas death ensues before nodular regeneration has had time to develop. Biliary cirrhosis is associated with partial biliary obstruction due for instance to biliary stricture, primary sclerosing cholangitis or gallstones.

In biliary cirrhosis the liver is larger and greener than in non-biliary cirrhosis. Margins of nodules are clear cut rather than moth-eaten. If the cholestasis is relieved the portal zone fibrosis and bile retention disappear slowly.

Electron microscopy. The biliary canaliculi show changes irrespective of the cause. These include dilatation and oedema, blunting, distortion and sparsity of the microvilli. The Golgi apparatus shows vacuolization. Peri-canalicular bile-containing vesicles appear and these represent the 'feathery' hepatocytes seen on light microscopy. Lysosomes proliferate and contain copper bound as a metalloprotein.

The endoplasmic reticulum is hypertrophied, all these changes are non-specific for the aetiology of the cholestasis.

Changes in other organs

The spleen is enlarged and firm due to reticulo-endothelial hyperplasia and increase in mononuclear cells. Later, cirrhosis results in portal hypertension.

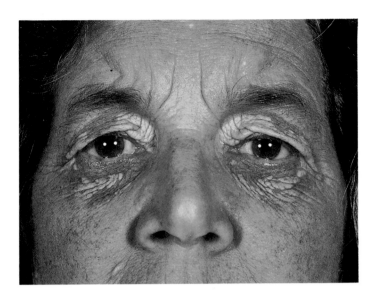

Fig. 13.12. Primary biliary cirrhosis. The patient shows xanthelasma and pigmentation.

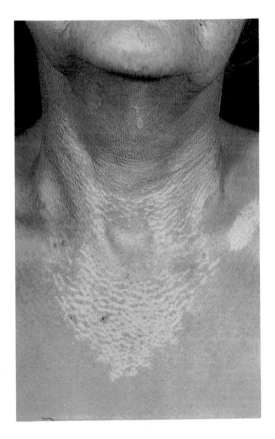

Fig. 13.13. Primary biliary cirrhosis. Xanthomatous skin lesions in the necklace area.

255

The intestinal contents are bulky and greasy; the more complete the cholestasis the paler the stools.

The kidneys are swollen and bile stained. Casts containing bilirubin are found in the distal convoluted tubules and collecting tubules. The casts may be heavily infiltrated with cells and the tubular epithelium is disrupted. The surrounding connective tissue may then show oedema and inflammatory infiltration. Scar formation is absent.

Clinical features

The patient develops jaundice slowly. He feels well and weight loss is slow. This is in contrast to the malaise and physical deterioration of the patient with hepato-cellular disease. Later the skin may become greenish. Skin pigmentation is due to melanin.

Pruritus is often attributed to retained bile acids. However, even with the most sophisticated biochemical methods, pruritus could not be associated with the concentration of any naturally occurring bile acid in serum or on skin [26]. Moreover, in terminal liver failure, when pruritus is lost, serum bile acids may still be increased. The association with cholestasis

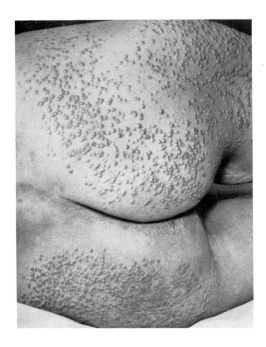

Fig. 13.14. Chronic obstructive jaundice. Xanthomata tuberosa affecting the buttocks.

suggests that pruritus is due to some substance normally excreted in the bile. Relief by the bile salt chelating resin, cholestyramine, also suggests that bile salts are concerned. Disappearance of itching when liver cells fail indicates that the agent responsible is manufactured by the liver.

Xanthomas. The planous varieties (xanthelasma) are flat or slightly raised, yellow and soft. They may also be seen in the palmar creases, below the breast and on the neck (figs 13.12, 13.13), chest or back. The tuberous lesions appear later, and are found on extensor surfaces, especially the wrists, elbows, knees, ankles and buttocks (fig. 13.14), on pressure points and in scars. The xanthomas associated with cholestatic jaundice rarely affect tendon sheaths. They may involve bone (fig. 13.19) or occasionally peripheral nerves [63]. Focal accumulations of xanthoma cells may be found in the liver.

Skin xanthomas develop in proportion to the height of the total serum lipids (fig. 13.21). The serum cholesterol value must be raised to over 450 mg/dl for longer than three months before skin xanthomas appear [36]. Skin xanthomas disappear if serum cholesterol levels fall after cholestasis is relieved or in the late stage of hepato-cellular failure.

The *liver* is usually enlarged with a firm, smooth, non-tender edge. *Splenomegaly* is unusual except in biliary cirrhosis where portal hypertension has developed or if infection is present.

Sinus bradycardia is usual [8].

Faeces

Faecal *colour* gives a good indication whether cholestasis is total, intermittent or decreasing.

Bile salts, deficient in the intestine in cholestasis, are essential for the absorption of dietary fat. Steatorrhoea (fig. 13.15) is proportional to the depth of jaundice. In cholestasis, inadequate bile salts are present in small intestinal contents to achieve micellar solution of lipid (fig. 13.16) [6]. Stools are loose, pale, bulky and offensive. Clubbing of the fingers may be associated.

Steatorrhoea results in failure of proper absorption of calcium and fat-soluble vitamins.

HEPATIC OSTEODYSTROPHY

Bone disease can complicate all forms of chronic cholestasis and hepato-cellular disease especially in the alcoholic [5, 40]. Bone pain is frequent. Serum may show normal or low calcium and phosphate levels and calcium is reduced in the urine. Bone biopsy may reveal either osteomalacia or, more often, osteoporosis. Bone changes cannot be predicted by serum calcium and phosphate values.

In osteomalacia the bone is weakened, osteoblasts multiply and the serum alkaline phosphatase therefore rises; in the presence of cholestasis these values may be enormous. The vertebral bodies become crushed and wedge-shaped (fig. 13.17) and kyphosis is gross. The thoracic cage is decalcified and pseudo-fractures are frequent. Ribbon-like areas of decalcification (Looser's zones) are rare. The hands show rarefaction (fig. 13.18). The lamina

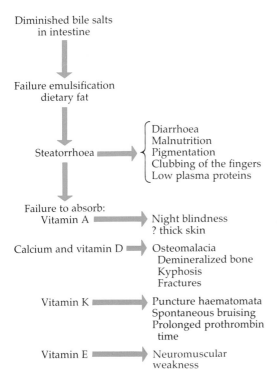

Fig. 13.15. The effects of acholia in chronic cholestatic jaundice.

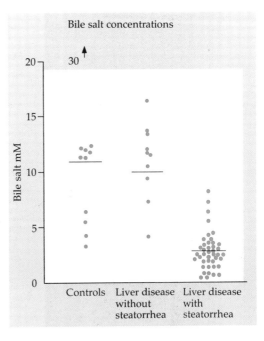

Fig. 13.16. Bile salt concentration of aspirated intestinal contents in patients with non-alcoholic liver disease with or without steatorrhoea (Badley *et al.* 1970).

dura around the teeth disappear and the teeth fall out. Bone biopsy shows wide, uncalcified, osteoid seams surrounding the trabeculae.

Osteoporosis is diagnosed by bone biopsy. It is particularly likely in patients more than 45 years old.

Osteomalacia and osteoporosis are slow to develop and are unlikely unless the cholestasis is deep and has lasted longer than two years. Ill-advised prednisolone therapy hastens their progress.

Painful *osteoarthropathy* may develop in the wrists and ankles (fig. 13.19) [22]. This is non-specific complication of chronic liver disease.

Osteomalacia. Vitamin D_2 (ergo-calciferol) is absorbed from the gut while vitamin D_3 (chol-ecalciferol) is synthesized in the skin (fig. 13.20). In both England and North America, the majority of circulating vitamin D originates from vitamin D_3 rather than vitamin D_2 Both forms are transported in serum by vitamin D binding

globulin which is synthesized by the liver and is usually only 2–5% saturated. 25-hydroxyla-tion of vitamin D takes place in the liver cell and concentrations in the serum roughly corre-late with vitamin D intake. Low serum 25-(OH)D values have been demonstrated in vitamin D-untreated patients with symptomatic primary biliary cirrhosis, alcoholic liver disease, chronic active liver disease and large bile duct obstruc-tion. Such low levels are restored by vitamin D supplements indicating that 25-hydroxylation is not defective [35]. 1, 25-dihydroxy vitamin D is formed normally so that a renal defect in dihydroxy vitamin D synthesis seems unlikely.

The cause is probably multiple. Cholestatic patients fail to go out into the sun or take an adequate diet. Absorption of vitamin D is poor because of steatorrhoea (fig. 13.16). Cholestasis interrupts the enterohepatic circulation of bile salts. Cholestyramine increases steatorrhoea. Jaundiced skin colour may interfere with the

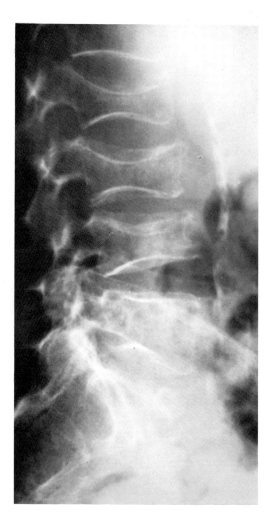

Fig. 13.17. Primary biliary cirrhosis jaundiced for three years. Lumbar spine shows very severe biconcave deformities and vertebral compression.

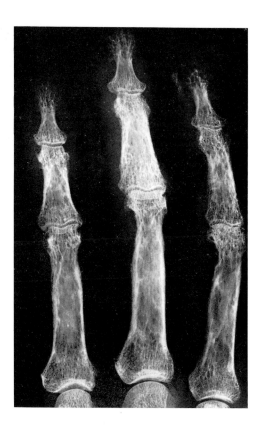

Fig. 13.18. Primary biliary cirrhosis; jaundiced for five years. Many skin xanthomas. Serum cholesterol 2400 mg/dl. X-ray of digits shows gross demineralization. Erosions represent bone xanthomas.

cutaneous synthesis of vitamin D_3. Increased vitamin D metabolites may be lost in the urine.

In practice, osteomalacia is rarely a problem except in the most deeply jaundiced patients, usually elderly, female and with most prolonged cholestasis. In cholestatic patients, vitamin D status can be assessed by measuring serum levels of 25-OH cholecalciferol.

Calcium malabsorption can be related to vitamin D deficiency and the formation of unabsorbable calcium soaps in the intestinal lumen.

Hyperparathyroidism is not a major problem in patients with chronic liver disease.

Osteoporosis. This is the more common component of hepatic osteodystrophy. Cortical and trabecular bone thinning are found and the bone turnover is reduced [13, 61]. The problem is osteoblastic dysfunction rather than excessive bone resorption.

The pathogenesis is probably complex and factors include calcium malabsorption, alcohol, corticosteroid therapy, oestrogen deficiency in post-menopausal women and vitamin D deficiency with secondary parathyroidism. Vertebral crush fractures (fig. 13.17) are the most common clinical complications of osteoporosis.

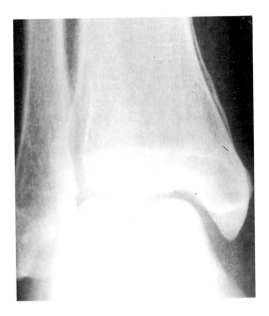

Fig. 13.19. Osteo-arthropathy in chronic cholestasis. New subperiosteal bone is seen at the lower end of the tibia.

FAT SOLUBLE VITAMINS AND COAGULATION FACTORS

Vitamin A. Is fat soluble and plasma levels are low. Hepatic storage is normal and the defects are due to poor absorption [48]. If cholestasis is sufficiently long, hepatic reserves of the vitamin become exhausted and failure of dark adaptation follows (night blindness) [64].

Vitamin K and Factor VII are not absorbed and the *prothrombin time* is prolonged. This is restored to normal by intramuscular vitamin K_1 therapy.

Vitamin E deficiency, related to chronic fat malabsorption, has been reported in children with cholestasis [18, 60]. The picture is of cerebellar ataxia, posterior column dysfunction, peripheral neuropathy and retinal degeneration. If the serum bilirubin level exceeds 6 mg/dl, almost all adult patients with cholestasis will have sub-normal vitamin E levels [33]. However, a specific neurological syndrome does not seem to develop in adults.

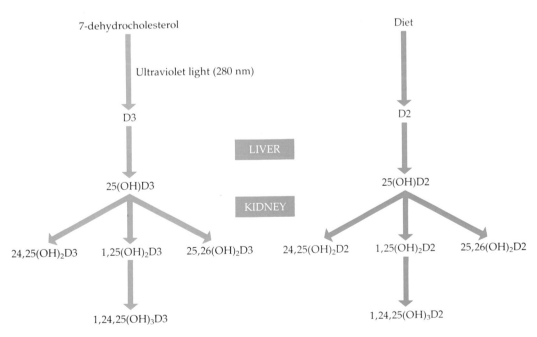

Fig. 13.20. Normal vitamin D metabolic pathway. Vitamin D_3 is formed in the skin. The 25-hydroxylation step of both D_2 and D_3 occurs in the liver; the addition of a second hydroxy group occurs predominantly in the kidney (Long & Sherlock 1979).

CHANGES IN COPPER METABOLISM

Approximately 80% of absorbed copper is normally excreted in the bile and lost in the faeces. In all forms of cholestasis, but particularly if it is chronic (as in primary biliary cirrhosis, biliary atresia or sclerosing cholangitis), copper accumulates in the liver to levels equal to or exceeding those found in Wilson's disease [56]. Pigmented corneal rings resembling the Kayser—Fleischer ring are seen rarely [24].

Hepatic copper may be measured on biopsies or demonstrated histochemically by rhodanine staining [32]. Copper-associated protein may be shown by orcein staining. These methods give circumstantial support to a diagnosis of cholestasis. In cholestasis the retained copper is probably not hepatotoxic [21]. Electron microscopy shows it in electron-dense lysosomes and the characteristic organelle changes associated with cytosolic copper in Wilson's disease are not observed. In cholestasis, the copper is retained within the hepatocyte in a non-toxic form.

HAEMATOLOGICAL CHANGES

These include reduced osmotic fragility of the erythrocytes. Target cells have been related to an accumulation of cholesterol in the red cell membrane. This increases red cell surface area and leads to target formation.

DEVELOPMENT OF HEPATO-CELLULAR FAILURE

This is slow, and it is remarkable how well the liver cells function in the presence of cholestasis. After 3—5 years of chronic jaundice, rapidly deepening jaundice, ascites, oedema and a lowered serum albumin level indicate liver cell failure. Pruritus lessens and the bleeding tendency is not controlled by parenteral vitamin K. Hepatic encephalopathy is terminal.

Microsomal drug oxidation. Patients with intrahepatic cholestasis show a reduction in hepatic cytochrome P^{450} content in proportion to the severity of the cholestasis [34]. This defect is confirmed by an impaired aminopyrine breath test [7].

Biochemistry

All the constituents of the bile show an increased level in the serum. Conjugation of biliary substances is intact but excretion defective.

The *serum ('conjugated', 'ester') bilirubin level* is raised due mainly to conjugated pigment. In unrelieved cholestasis the level rises slowly for the first three weeks and then fluctuates, always tending to increase. When the cholestasis is relieved, serum bilirubin values fall slowly to normal.

The *serum alkaline phosphatase level* is raised, usually to more than three times the upper limit of normal. *Serum γ-glutamyl trans-peptidase levels* are raised. The rises are due to increased synthesis or release of enzymes from liver plasma membranes.

The total *serum cholesterol* increases but not constantly. In chronic cholestasis the total serum lipids are greatly increased (fig. 13.21) and this involves particularly phospholipid and total cholesterol. These changes probably reflect increased hepatic synthesis. Neutral fat is very slightly increased. In spite of the high lipid content, the serum is characteristically clear and not milky. This may be due to the surface-action effect of phospholipid, which keeps the other lipids in solution. Serum cholesterol values fall terminally.

Serum lipoproteins are increased [36], due to a rise in the low density (α_2, β) fraction. The high density lipoproteins are decreased.

The cholestatic liver secretes a variety of unusual lipoproteins and these can be related to low plasma lecithin cholesterol acyl transferase (LCAT) levels [2]. The lipoproteins of cholestasis differ from those found in atherosclerosis. Atheroma is not a complication of prolonged cholestasis. The abnormal lipoproteins appear by electron microscopy as disc-shaped particles.

Lipoprotein-X (LP-X) is a spherical particle, 70 nm in diameter associated with the low density lipoprotein fraction [46]. It is increased

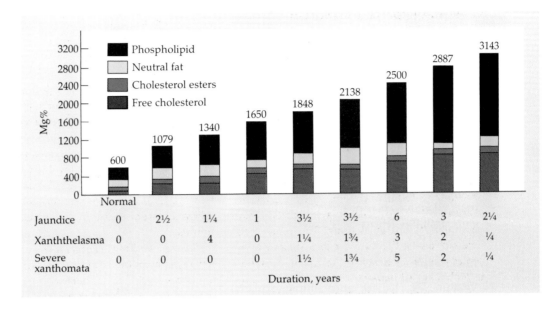

Fig. 13.21. Serum lipid pattern in eight patients with primary biliary cirrhosis (chronic intra-hepatic obstructive jaundice) (Ahrens & Kunkel 1949).

in both intra-hepatic and extra-hepatic cholestasis and is of no practical diagnostic value.

Trihydroxy *bile salts* accumulate in the blood in cholestasis.

Serum albumin and globulin concentrations are normal in acute cholestasis. With the development of biliary cirrhosis the serum albumin tends to fall.

The *serum aspartate trans-aminase* is usually less than 100 i.u./100 ml.

Urine. Conjugated bilirubin is present. Urinary urobilinogen is excreted in proportion to the amount of bile reaching the duodenum.

General treatment

Cholestasis whether of intra-hepatic or extra-hepatic origin should be managed along the same general lines.

NUTRITION (table 13.1)

The problem is essentially that of intestinal bile salt deficiency. Calorie intake should be maintained and protein must be adequate. Neutral

Table 13.1. Management of chronic cholestasis

Dietary fat
Low neutral fat (less than 40 g)
Add medium chain triglyceride, 40 g daily

Intramuscular vitamins
(every four weeks) A   100 000 i.u.
                            D   100 000 i.u.
                            K₁ 10 mg.

Calcium
Extra defatted milk
Calcium
If bone pain, calcium chloride i.v.

Ultraviolet light

fat is poorly tolerated, badly absorbed and reduces calcium absorption. It should be restricted to 40 g daily. Additional fat is supplied by medium chain triglycerides (MCT) which are digested and absorbed quite well in the absence of bile salts into the portal vein as free fatty acids. They can be given as 'Portagen' (Mead–Johnson) or as MCT (coconut) oil for cooking or in salads.

In the chronic case fat soluble vitamins (A, D, K) are necessary and must be given parenterally because they are not absorbed when given by mouth. Patients with night blindness may improve with oral rather than intramuscular vitamin A [64]. Vitamin E is not absorbed [4] and DL tocopherol, as the acetate 10 mg daily, is given by injection to children with chronic cholestasis. Others may take 200 mg daily by mouth.

If there is evidence of bruising or haemorrhage associated with a prolonged prothrombin time, vitamin K_1 may be given intramuscularly daily until the deficiency is corrected.

TREATMENT OF BONE CHANGES

Vitamin D_2 (100 000 units intramuscularly) should be given every four weeks to all patients with chronic cholestasis (fig. 13.22). If possible, treatment should be monitored by measuring serum 25-(OH)D levels. Reduced levels indicate increase of the intramuscular vitamin D_2 supplements or giving oral 25-(OH) vitamin D until the serum 25-(OH)D is normal. In prolonged cholestasis a maintenance oral dose of 6 g calcium gluconate or preferably effervescent calcium (Sandoz) 8 tablets daily, equivalent to 30 g calcium gluconate, should be given. The patient should be encouraged to take extra skimmed (fat-free) milk and expose himself to sunlight or to an ultraviolet lamp.

If the serum phosphate level is low, phosphate supplements must be given. These should be given on alternate days to calcium so that the formation of calcium phosphate complexes in the gut is prevented.

In patients with symptomatic osteomalacia, proven on bone biopsy, oral or parenteral 1,25-dihydroxy-D_3 appears to be the vitamin D metabolite of choice. It is biologically very active and has a short half-life. One could also use 1,alpha vitamin D_3 but full metabolic activity would only follow hepatic 25-hydroxylation.

Severe bone pain may be controlled by intravenous calcium (15 mg calcium per kg body weight as calcium gluconate in 500 ml 5% dextrose) given over four hours daily for about

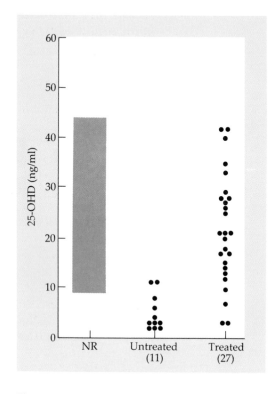

Fig. 13.22. Serum 25-(OH)D values in vitamin D_2-treated (100 000 i.u. in ethyl oleate once monthly i.m.) and untreated patients with primary biliary cirrhosis. The differences are highly significant (Skinner *et al.* 1977).

seven days and repeated as necessary [7].

Hepatic osteodystrophy worsens after liver transplant.

Osteoporosis can be crippling but no treatment is effective. Corticosteroids worsen the process and should be avoided. Oestrogen therapy can be considered in suitable patients. Fluoride is being evaluated.

No specific treatment is available for the periosteal reactions. Simple analgesics may be of use and, if arthropathy is present, physiotherapy may be helpful.

PRURITUS

Biliary drainage. Pruritus can be relieved in patients with biliary obstruction by external biliary drainage. This, presumably, breaks the entero-hepatic circulation of bile salts.

Cholestyramine. This resin binds bile salts in the intestine, so eliminating them in the faeces (fig. 13.23). It will stop itching in 4–7 days in patients with partial biliary obstruction. One sachet should be given before and one after breakfast so that the arrival of the drug in the duodenum coincides with gallbladder contraction. If necessary, a further dose may be taken before the midday and evening meals. The maintenance dose is usually about 12 g per day. The drug causes nausea and reluctance to take it. It is particularly valuable for itching associated with primary biliary cirrhosis, biliary atresia and biliary stricture. Serum bile acid levels fall. Serum cholesterol drops and skin xanthomas diminish or disappear. Cholestyramine increases faecal fat even in normal subjects. The dose should be the smallest that controls pruritus. Hypoprothrombinaemia has developed due to failure to absorb vitamin K. This vitamin must be given by intramuscular injection.

These results suggest that bile salts are responsible for the pruritus. However, the resin might well act in some other way than by removing bile acids.

Cholestyramine may bind calcium, fat soluble vitamins and other drugs having an entero-hepatic circulation, particularly digitoxin. Care must be taken that the cholestyramine and other drugs are given at separate times.

Colestipol is an alternative resin which is equally effective and sometimes better tolerated than cholestyramine.

Anti-histaminics. These are of value only for their sedative action.

Phototherapy. Ultraviolet radiation, 9 to 12 minutes daily, may relieve pruritus and decrease pigmentation.

Plasmapheresis. Has been used to treat intractable pruritus associated with hypercholesterolaemia and xanthomatous neuropathy [12]. 500 to 2000 ml plasma are removed and replaced by 1000 ml 5% glucose with 5% albumin one to

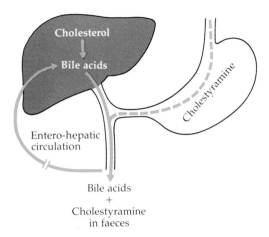

Fig. 13.23. Cholestyramine, a strongly basic anion exchange resin, chelates with bile salts in the intestine and the complex is excreted in the faeces. The enterohepatic circulation is broken.

three times a week. The procedure is temporarily effective but is costly and labour intensive.

Steroids. Glucocorticoids will relieve itching, but at the expense of severe bone thinning particularly in post-menopausal women. Methyltestosterone 25 mg sublingually daily relieves itching within seven days [38] and is appropriate for men. Anabolic steroids such as stanazolol [65] (5 mg daily) are less virilizing and equally effective.

These substances greatly increase jaundice and both can themselves cause an intra-hepatic cholestasis in normal patients (Chapter 18). There are no ill effects on liver function, but these drugs should be given only for intractable pruritus and in the smallest effective dose. They should be used in total biliary obstruction where cholestyramine is not effective.

Ursodeoxycholic acid may be effective by reducing toxic bile salts (see Chapter 14).

Rifampicin (300–450 mg daily) relieves pruritus within seven days [28]. This may be by enzyme induction or by inhibition of bile acid uptake. Potential side-effects include increased risk of gallstone formation, reduction in 25–OH cholecalciferol levels, drug interactions and emergence of resistant organisms. It should be used only short-term.

Hepatic transplantation. May be the only answer for some patients with chronic, really intractable pruritus.

Antibiotics may be indicated for febrile cholangitis but only temporary benefit is given in the presence of continued biliary obstruction.

Terminal hepato-cellular failure or *portal hypertension* are treated along the usual lines.

Classification

Cholestasis is classified into *extra-hepatic*, where there is a mechanical obstruction to the main bile ducts, and *intra-hepatic*, where such an obstructive lesion cannot be demonstrated and the defect is in the hepatocyte or in microscopic bile ducts within the liver. The distinction may be possible by an accurate history and physical examination, with particular attention to pain and pyrexia. This is supplemented by urinary and faecal examination, basic biochemical tests and a prothrombin time. In the cholestatic patient, however, clinical and biochemical evaluation is not infallible. A small proportion of patients with extra-hepatic obstruction are incorrectly diagnosed as having intra-hepatic cholestasis, whereas a larger proportion of patients with intra-hepatic disease are thought to have extra-hepatic obstruction [54]. About 25% of patients with suspected biliary obstruction actually have hepato-cellular disease. Various algorithms are proposed (figs 13.24, 13.25) [54]. The first procedure should be real-time ultrasound, which allows the distinction between cholestasis with dilated bile ducts within the liver and cholestasis where such dilatation cannot be shown. Ultrasound must be followed by direct cholangiography, either endoscopic or percutaneous trans-hepatic. A normal cholangiogram effectively rules out extra-hepatic biliary obstruction, and the site and aetiology are correctly defined in over 90% of patients. The technique chosen should be useful diagnostically and might be helpful therapeutically. Thus, ERCP

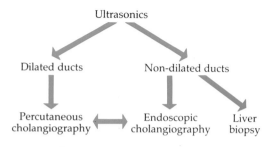

Fig. 13.24. Diagnosis of cholestasis.

might precede endoscopic retrograde sphincterotomy for removal of stones from the common bile duct and percutaneous cholangiography is the choice when stenting is being considered (see Chapter 29).

Extra-hepatic cholestasis

This term implies mechanical obstruction to large bile ducts outside the liver or within the porta hepatis.

Bile is normally secreted at a pressure of about 15–25 cmH$_2$O. A rise to about 35 cm results in suppression of bile flow and so to jaundice.

The liver is enlarged and the intra-hepatic bile ducts are widely dilated. Their contents are at first dark but later so-called *white bile* is the result of the increased pressure in the ducts which suppresses secretion of bile by the liver. White bile is free of bilirubin and bile salts and the cation composition is that of serum [19]. It is found in all forms of extra-hepatic cholestasis. Infection of the bile above the obstruction leads to *cholangitis*; the ducts contain pus and may be surrounded by small abscesses.

Hepatic histology

Bile ducts multiply in the portal zones. They are elongated and tortuous, have a wide lumen and are lined by high cuboidal epithelium (fig. 13.26). With ascending cholangitis histology shows accumulations of polymorphonuclear leucocytes related to bile ducts (fig. 13.26). The sinusoids contain numerous polymorphs.

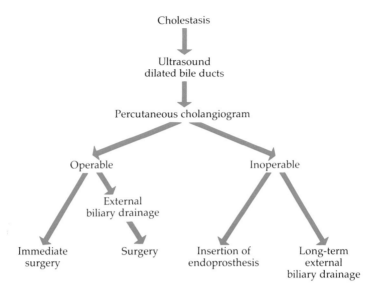

Fig. 13.25. Management of patient with bile duct obstruction (Dooley *et al.* 1979).

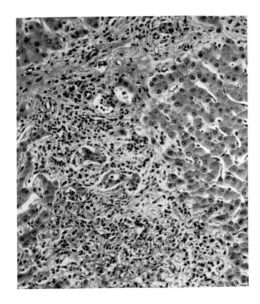

Fig. 13.26. Obstructive jaundice and cholangitis due to choledocholithiasis. The portal tract shows proliferating bile ducts, fibroblasts and an infiltration with polymorphonuclear and round cells. Culture of the biopsy yielded *E. coli*. H & E, ×70.

Bile is toxic and focal necrosis of liver cells, with little surrounding cellularity, is seen early in the mid-zones and later in zone 1.

Bile lakes (fig. 13.27). These represent ruptured interlobular bile ducts.

The hepatic changes develop very rapidly. Cholestasis is seen within 36 hours. Bile duct proliferation is early; portal fibrosis develops later. After about two weeks, duration cannot be related to the extent of hepatic change.

The distinction of *secondary biliary* from other forms of cirrhosis is difficult. In biliary cirrhosis of extra-hepatic origin, bile duct proliferation is more conspicuous; the fibrous bands are more heavily infiltrated with polymorphs. Cholestasis is greater, reflecting the deeper jaundice.

Clinical features

There are additional features to those of general cholestasis. *Pain* varies in type. A fixed right upper quadrant ache is probably due to stretching of the capsule of the liver. The pain of gallbladder disease may be present. Finally, cholestasis of malignant origin may be associated with pain due to the primary tumour.

Fever may indicate ascending cholangitis. When this is due to partial obstruction of the

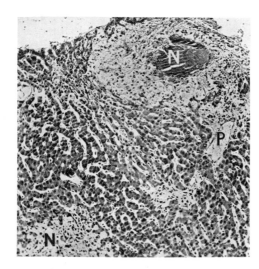

Fig. 13.27. Extra-hepatic obstructive jaundice. Necroses (N) of liver cells are seen in the periportal zones. The larger shows central bile staining. P = branch of portal vein; H = central hepatic vein. H & E, ×70.

common duct by ball-valve calculus or traumatic stricture there may be intermittent high fever with rigors (*Charcot's intermittent biliary fever*).

The liver is enlarged. Nodularity may indicate malignancy; the gallbladder may be palpable or tender.

Other abdominal masses may indicate a primary lesion such as carcinoma of stomach or colon. Endoscopy, rectal examination and sigmoidoscopy may indicate carcinoma.

Haematological changes. Anaemia implies infection, blood loss or malignant disease. A polymorphonuclear leucocytosis suggests some complication such as cholangitis or underlying neoplastic disease.

In the febrile, blood cultures should be performed repeatedly. Septicaemias, especially due to Gram-negative organisms, are common.

Patients with partial biliary obstruction and cholangitis have a very high bacterial population in the bile, rivalling that of the colon [55]. Bacterial contamination of the small bowel leads to some of the features of the blind loop syndrome.

The *mitochondrial antibody test* for primary biliary cirrhosis is consistently negative.

Ultrasound. Dilated bile ducts are most likely if the serum bilirubin level exceeds 10 mg. Gallstones or cancer of the pancreas may be seen.

Cholangiography

Percutaneous techniques are very satisfactory in defining large bile ducts.

Endoscopic techniques are required if bile ducts are not dilated but choledocholithiasis, sclerosing cholangitis or a pancreatic cause is suspected. This specialist method is usually successful in defining main bile and pancreatic ducts.

Intravenous techniques are obsolete.

Liver biopsy

This can be performed safely in patients with cholestatic jaundice, however deep (Chapter 3). However, with the advent of direct cholangiography liver biopsy is rarely needed to diagnose main duct cholestasis.

The portal zones are the most diagnostic areas (fig. 13.26). They show oedema, bile duct reduplication, cubical epithelium and wide lumen, polymorph and mononuclear cells, some fibrosis and a well-defined limiting plate. It is usually possible to diagnose obstruction to main bile ducts (fig. 13.26) from viral hepatitis, alcoholism, drug-associated cholestasis, or primary biliary cirrhosis.

Management

Any laparotomy should be thorough and, if any diagnostic doubt remains, should include operative liver biopsy and direct operative or post-operative cholangiography with biopsy of any suspicious mass or enlarged nodes.

The ideal treatment is relief of the obstruction with removal of the cause. The management therefore differs according to the aetiology.

Important factors associated with increased post-operative morbidity and mortality are an initial haematocrit of 30% or less, a serum bilirubin value exceeding 12 mg/dl, and a malignant obstructive lesion [16]. Anaemia can be corrected. Deep jaundice can be relieved pre-operatively by external biliary drainage [17]. This is a simple technique of value in the very poor risk patient, but with the disadvantages of infections, bacteriaemia, bacterial cholangitis and intra-hepatic abscesses [62]. Fluid and electrolyte balance is difficult to maintain. It is of particular value in the patient with severe obstructive cholangitis [39]. Endoscopic cholangiography with intubation of the common bile duct by the nasal route may be more valuable (see Chapter 31).

Post-operative, acute, renal tubular necrosis (*intrinsic failure*) is a sequel of biliary surgery. The kidney failure is precipitated by a prolonged, difficult operation, hypotension, haemorrhage with diminished renal blood flow, and sepsis such as peritonitis [16]. The diminished renal and hepatic blood flow are contributory. The kidneys of patients with cholestatic jaundice may be particularly susceptible to acute renal tubular necrosis. This may be related to bacterial endotoxins which are increased and which cause renal vasoconstriction and re-distribution of renal blood flow away from the renal cortex. Osmotic diuretics such as mannitol infusions should be given to maintain glomerular infiltration immediately pre-operatively and during the operation in every patient with deep cholestatic jaundice.

Post-operative shock. Patients with cholestasis tend to have arterial hypotension and are susceptible to develop 'shock' after surgery. This seems to be related to a cardio-depressive effect of bile and its constituents causing impaired myocardial contractility. In dogs with obstructive jaundice cardiac function is defective [29]. In rats, common bile duct ligation leads to defective oxygen utilization and ATP synthesis by cardiac mitochondria [31]. Chronic bile duct ligated dogs show vascular instability in response to endogenous or exogenous vasoactive substances, such as noradrenaline and angiotensin 2, and this is associated with evidence of systemic vasodilatation [10].

Intra-hepatic cholestasis

The cause lies within the liver, somewhere distal to the hepato-cellular microsomes and down to the major bile ducts. The general pathological, clinical and biochemical picture and general treatment are the same as for extra-hepatic cholestasis. Febrile cholangitis is absent and there is no pain apart from that associated with the cause. The liver is not necessarily enlarged and is not tender. Bile ducts are not dilated within the liver and, histologically, biliary necrosis and bile duct multiplication are absent.

Cholestasis with undilated intra-hepatic bile ducts (figs 13.28, 13.29) (table 13.2)

HEPATO-CELLULAR

The cholestasis is complex. There is primary injury to intracellular membranes. Leakage of bile salts through defective canaliculi leads to a reduction of bile salt-dependent bile flow. Inhibition of canalicular ATPase interferes with bile salt-independent secretion. Impaired uptake of bile salts by the injured hepatocyte results in loss in the urine. Finally, impaired hydroxylation of cholesterol to bile acids in the endoplasmic reticulum reduces bile salt-dependent flow.

Cholestatic viral hepatitis (Chapter 16). The history of exposure and the nature of the prodromal symptoms may be helpful. The liver biopsy appearances are those of acute viral hepatitis.

Acute alcoholic hepatitis (Chapter 20) can be cholestatic. The history of alcohol abuse, the large tender liver and, often, vascular spiders on the skin are helpful points. Liver biopsy appearances are diagnostic. Chronic pancreatitis may be associated.

SEX HORMONE CANALICULAR MEMBRANE CHANGES

Cholestatic reactions to oral contraceptives (Chapter 18) and in the last trimester of pregnancy (Chapter 25) fall into this group.

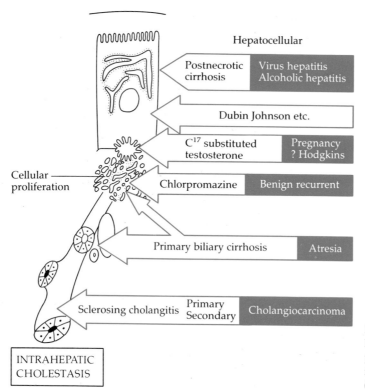

Fig. 13.28. Classification of intrahepatic cholestasis according to possible major sites or involvement of the biliary tree (Sherlock 1966).

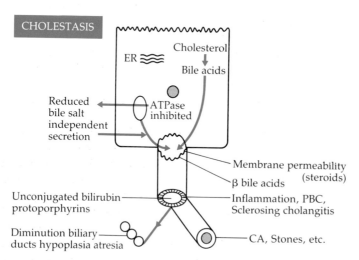

Fig. 13.29. Possible mechanisms of cholestasis. ER = endoplasmic reticulum.

Drugs include the promazine group, long-acting sulphonamides and anti-thyroid drugs (Chapter 18). The history is important and liver biopsy appearances are usually diagnostic.

In some patients with *cryptogenic macronodular cirrhosis* cholestasis may be prominent.

BILE ACIDS

Toxic bile acids have detergent effects on canalicular membranes and are inadequate as micelle formers.

Lithocholic acid is a naturally occurring bile

Table 13.2. Cholestasis with undilated intra-hepatic bile ducts

Type	Diagnostic points
Hepato-cellular	
Viral hepatitis	History. Onset typical. Viral A & B markers
Alcoholic hepatitis	History. Large tender liver. Spiders. Liver biopsy
Drugs	History. Onset six weeks of starting. Liver biopsy
Sex hormones (canalicular)	Hormone therapy. Remit on stopping. Liver biopsy
Bile acids	All rare. Often familial
Biliary	
Intra-hepatic atresia	History. Age. Liver biopsy
Benign recurrent	Repeated. Cholangiography normal. Normal liver between attacks
Primary biliary cirrhosis	Female. Onset pruritus. Positive mitochondrial antibody Raised serum IgM. Liver biopsy
Choledocholithiasis	History. Cholangiography. ERCP
Sclerosing cholangitis	Association ulcerative colitis. ERCP

acid formed in the colon. The human liver probably metabolizes it when it is re-absorbed so preventing its injurious (cholestatic) action. However, it can reduce bile acid-independent flow by inhibiting sodium potassium ATPase and altering the canalicular membrane.

Monohydroxy bile acids, such as 3-beta-hydroxy-5-cholenate, accumulate in canalicular membranes and are cholestatic. They have been found in the bile of infants with established cholestasis, but their role as cause or effect is uncertain.

Coprostanic acid [30]. Two children from two families with cholestasis from birth were found to have this C27 alligator bile acid in bile. They soon died of cirrhosis. An enzyme catalysing C24 hydroxylation may be defective.

Byler's disease. This fatal cholestasis has been reported in Amish kindreds named Byler [15]. Death is usual before the age of eight. Inheritance is autosomal recessive. A defect in the biliary canalicular membrane is postulated. Conjugated bile acids cannot be excreted and this may be related to the cholestasis. Hepatic transplantation has been tried with good results.

Zellweger's syndrome. This is very rare. There is defective formation of hepatic peroxisomes. Side-chain oxidation of bile acids does not occur normally, and C27 bile acids appear in serum and bile. There are other enzymatic defects, and infants die shortly after birth [44].

MISCELLANEOUS

Cholestasis in *severe bacterial infections*, particularly in childhood or post-operatively, is presumably hepato-cellular. It can also be related to the cholestatic effect of endotoxin on Na^+K^+ ATPase [41].

Cholestasis develops with *prolonged parenteral nutrition* especially in neonates (Chapter 24). It may be due to lithocholate formed by bacterial 7 α-dehydroxylation in the intestinal tract.

Hodgkin's disease may be complicated by deep cholestasis. This is not necessarily related to excess haemolysis, hepatic infiltration or invasion of major bile ducts. The cause is unknown (see Chapter 4).

Biliary precipitation of insoluble solutes. Unconjugated bilirubin may precipitate as intra-hepatic pigment stones or as inspissated bile in *cystic fibrosis* or *benoxyprofen toxicity* (Chapter 18).

Protoporphyrins in *erythrocytic protoporphyria* may lead to precipitation in the canalicular ducts.

The cholestasis of *intra-hepatic atresia* (infantile cholangiopathy) (Chapter 24) is probably related to viral injury to intra-hepatic bile ducts.

Benign recurrent intra-hepatic cholestasis (see below).

Primary biliary cirrhosis (see Chapter 14).

Adults with *paucity of intra-hepatic bile ducts* are being increasingly described [67]. The condition may be familial.

LARGE BILE DUCT DISEASE WITH
UNDILATED INTRA-HEPATIC DUCTS

Finally, some diseases which involve main bile ducts do not result in intra-hepatic biliary dilatation. Choledocholithiasis may be found without dilated intra-hepatic ducts if the stone has only recently migrated from the gallbladder, or if it has been present for months so that a secondary bacterial cholangitis has led to sclerosing cholangitis. Primary sclerosing cholangitis involves bile ducts inside and outside the liver. Secondary sclerosing cholangitis can complicate severe biliary infections, sarcoidosis and histiocytosis X (see Chapter 15) [37].

Benign recurrent intra-hepatic cholestasis

Only 70 patients have been recorded with this condition which presents as multiple episodes of cholestatic jaundice [52, 66]. Main bile duct obstruction must be excluded by endoscopic or percutaneous cholangiography. The first patient described has now survived 22 episodes and three laparotomies [66]. Another patient had 27 attacks over 38 years.

The onset is with itching, occasionally an influenza-like illness and vomiting. Serum alkaline phosphatase levels increase but transaminases are virtually normal. Jaundice appears and persists for three to four months.

Hepatic histology shows cholestasis, portal zone expansion, mononuclears and some liver cell degeneration, mainly in zone 1. Hepatic histology and liver function are normal in remission [66].

270 *Aetiology.* In favour of a genetic origin is the

early onset, usually starting before the age of ten, and the familial incidence.

One patient in the anicteric stage showed enhanced bile acid synthesis and abnormal faecal bacteria [20]. Unusual bile acids were found in bile and faeces.

Serum from one patient did not have cholestatic effects on rat liver or isolated rat hepatocytes. Therefore cholestasis is not likely to be mediated by a circulating cholestatic agent, but rather secondary to an intrinsic abnormality in hepatocyte bile salt secretion [42].

Environmental factors are suggested by the allergic diathesis; some patients have rashes. The condition may recur at definite times of the year.

Treatment. The attacks are self-limiting and vary in duration. Corticosteroid treatment is probably of little benefit.

References

1 Adinolfi LE, Utili R, Gaeta GB *et al*. Cholestasis induced by estradiol-17β-D-glucuronide: mechanisms and prevention by sodium taurocholate. *Hepatology* 1984; **4**: 30.
2 Agorastos J, Fox C, Harry DS *et al*. Lecithin-cholesterol acyltransferase and the lipo-protein abnormalities of obstructive jaundice. *Clin. Sci. molec. Med.* 1978; **54**: 369.
3 Ajdukiewicz AB, Agnew JE, Byers PD *et al*. The relief of bone pain in primary biliary cirrhosis with calcium infusions. *Gut* 1974; **15**: 788.
4 Alvarez F, Landrieu P, Laget P *et al*. Nervous and ocular disorders in children with cholestasis and vitamin A and E deficiencies. *Hepatology* 1983; **3**: 410.
5 Atkinson M, Nordin BEC, Sherlock S. Malabsorption and bone disease in prolonged obstructive jaundice. *Q. J. Med.* 1956; **25**: 299.
6 Badley BWD, Murphy GM, Bouchier IAD *et al*. Diminished micellar phase lipid in patients with chronic nonalcoholic liver disease and steatorrhea. *Gastroenterology* 1970; **58**: 781.
7 Baker AL, Krager PS, Kotake AN *et al*. The aminopyrine breath test does not correlate with histologic disease severity in patients with cholestasis. *Hepatology* 1987; **7**: 464.
8 Bashour TT, Antonini C Sr, Fisher J. Severe sinus node dysfunction in obstructive jaundice. *Ann. int. Med.* 1985; **103**: 384.
9 Blitzer B, Boyer JL. Cellular mechanisms of bile formation. *Gastroenterology* 1982; **82**: 346.

10 Bomzon A, Rosenberg M, Gali D *et al.* Systemic hypotension and decreased pressor response in dogs with chronic bile duct ligation. *Hepatology* 1986; **6**: 595.

11 Boyer JL. Tight junctions in normal and cholestatic liver: does the paracellular pathway have functional significance? *Hepatology* 1983; **3**: 614.

12 Cohen LB, Ambinder EP, Wolke AM *et al.* Role of plasmapheresis in primary biliary cirrhosis. *Gut* 1985; **26**: 291.

13 Compston JE. Hepatic osteodystrophy: vitamin D metabolism in patients with liver disease. *Gut* 1986; **27**: 1073.

14 Desmet VJ. Cirrhosis: aetiology and pathogenesis: cholestasis. In *Liver Cirrhosis* eds Boyer JL, Bianchi L. Falk Symposium 44, MTP Press Ltd, Lancaster 1987; p. 101.

15 De Vos R, De Wolf-Peters C, Desmet V *et al.* Progressive intrahepatic cholestasis (Byler's disease): case report. *Gut* 1975; **16**: 943.

16 Dixon JM, Armstrong CP, Duffey SW *et al.* Factors affecting morbidity and mortality after surgery for obstructive jaundice: a review of 373 patients. *Gut* 1983; **24**: 845.

17 Dooley JS, Dick R, George P *et al.* Percutaneous transhepatic endoprosthesis for bile duct obstruction: complications and results. *Gastroenterology* 1984; **86**: 905.

18 Elias E, Muller DPR, Scott J. Association of spino cerebellar disorders with cystic fibrosis or chronic childhood cholestasis and very low serum vitamin E. *Lancet* 1981; **ii**: 1319.

19 Elmslie RG, Thorpe MEC, Colman JVL *et al.* Clinical significance of white bile in the biliary tree. *Gut* 1969; **10**: 530.

20 Endo T, Uchida K, Amuro Y *et al.* Bile acid metabolism in benign recurrent intrahepatic cholestasis: comparative studies on the icteric and anicteric phases of a single case. *Gastroenterology* 1979; **76**: 1002.

21 Epstein O, Arborgh B, Sagiv M *et al.* Is copper hepatotoxic in primary biliary cirrhosis? *J. clin. Pathol.* 1981; **34**: 1071.

22 Epstein O, Dick R, Sherlock S. Prospective study of periostitis and finger clubbing in primary biliary cirrhosis and other forms of chronic liver disease. *Gut* 1981; **22**: 203.

23 Erlinger S. What is cholestasis in 1985? *J. Hepatol.* 1985; **1**: 687.

24 Fleming CR, Dickson ER, Hollenhorst RW *et al.* Pigmented corneal rings in a patient with primary biliary cirrhosis. *Gastroenterology* 1975; **69**: 220.

25 Forker EL, Runyon BA. Canalicular cholestasis. *Gastroenterology* 1978; **75**: 535.

26 Freedman MR, Holzbach RT, Ferguson DR. Pruritus in cholestasis: no direct causative role for bile acid retention. *Am. J. Med.* 1981; **70**: 1011.

27 Gautam A, Oi-Cheng NG, Boyer JL. Isolated rat hepatocyte couplets in short-term culture: structural characteristics and plasma membrane reorganization. *Hepatology* 1987; **7**: 216.

28 Ghent CN, Carruthers SG. Treatment of pruritis in primary biliary cirrhosis with rifampin. Results of a double-blind, crossover, randomized trial. *Gastroenterology* 1988; **94**: 488.

29 Green J, Beyar R, Sideman S *et al.* The 'jaundiced heart': a possible explanation for postoperative shock in obstructive jaundice. *Surgery* 1986; **100**: 14.

30 Hanson RF, Isenberg JN, Williams GC *et al.* The metabolism of 3α, 7α, 12α-trihydroxy-5β-cholestan-26-oic acid in two siblings with cholestasis due to intrahepatic bile duct anomalies: an apparent inborn error of cholic acid synthesis. *J. clin. Invest.* 1975; **56**: 577.

31 Heidenreich S, Brinkema E, Martin A *et al.* The kidney and cardio-vascular system in obstructive jaundice: functional and metabolic studies in conscious rats. *Clin. Sci.* 1987; **73**: 5.

32 Jain S, Scheuer PJ, Archer B *et al.* Histological demonstration of copper and copper-associated protein in chronic liver diseases. *J. clin. Pathol.* 1978; **31**: 784.

33 Jeffrey GP, Muller DPR, Burroughs AK *et al.* Vitamin E deficiency and its clinical significance in adults with primary biliary cirrhosis and other forms of chronic liver disease. *J. Hepatol.* 1987; **4**: 307.

34 Kawata S, Imai Y, Inada M *et al.* Selective reduction of hepatic cytochrome P_{450} content in patients with intrahepatic cholestasis. A mechanism for impairment of microsomal drug oxidation. *Gastroenterology* 1987; **92**: 299.

35 Kehayoglou AK, Holdsworth CD, Agnew JE *et al.* Bone disease and calcium absorption in primary biliary cirrhosis with special reference to vitamin-D therapy. *Lancet* 1968; **i**: 715.

36 Kunkel HG, Ahrens EH Jr. The relationship between serum lipids and the electrophoretic pattern, with particular reference to patients with primary bili-ary cirrhosis. *J. clin. Invest.* 1949; **28**: 1575.

37 Leblanc A, Hadchouel M, Jehan P *et al.* Obstructive jaundice in children with histiocytosis X. *Gastroenterology* 1981; **80**: 134.

38 Lloyd-Thomas HGL, Sherlock S. Testosterone therapy for the pruritus of obstructive jaundice. *Br. med. J.* 1952; **ii**: 1289.

39 Lois JF, Gomes AS, Grace PA *et al.* Risk of percutaneous transhepatic drainage in patients with cholangitis. *Am. J. Roentgenol.* 1987; **148**: 367.

40 Long RG, Meinhard E, Skinner RK *et al.* Clinical, biochemical, and histological studies of osteomalacia, osteoporosis, and para-thyroid function

in chronic liver disease. *Gut* 1978; **19**: 85.

41 Miller DJ, Keeton GR, Webber BL *et al.* Jaundice in severe bacterial infection. *Gastroenterology* 1976; **71**: 94.

42 Minuk GY, Shaffer EA. Benign recurrent intrahepatic cholestasis. Evidence for an intrinsic abnormality in hepatocyte secretion. *Gastroenterology* 1987; **93**: 1187.

43 Morris JS, Gallo GA, Scheuer PJ *et al.* Percutaneous liver biopsy in patients with large bile duct obstruction. *Gastroenterology* 1975; **68**: 750.

44 Moser AE, Singh I, Brown FR *et al.* The cerebrohepatorenal (Zellweger) syndrome. *N. Engl. J. Med.* 1984; **310**: 1141.

45 Moseley RH. Mechanisms of bile formation and cholestasis: clinical significance of recent experimental work. *Amer. J. Gastroenterol.* 1986; **81**: 731.

46 Narayanan S. Biochemistry and clinical relevance of lipoprotein X. *Ann. clin. lab. Sci.* 1984; **14**: 371.

47 Okanoue T, Ohta M, Fushiki S *et al.* Scanning electron microscopy of the liver cell cytoskeleton. *Hepatology* 1985; **5**: 1.

48 Ong DE, Amédée-Manesme O. Liver levels of vitamin A and cellular retinol-binding protein for patients with biliary atresia. *Hepatology* 1987; **7**: 253.

49 Paumgartner G. *Physiology I: Bile Acid-dependent Bile Flow in Liver and Bile*, eds L Bianchi, W Gerok, K Sickinger, Falk Symposium 23, MTP, Lancaster, 1977.

50 Phillips MJ, Oshio C, Miyairi M. Microfilament dysfunction as a mechanism in intrahepatic cholestasis: evidence from time-lapse cinemicrophotography. *Gastroenterology* 1980; **79**: 1120.

51 Popper H. Cholestasis: the future of a past and present riddle. *Hepatology* 1981; **1**: 187.

52 Putterman C, Keidar S, Brook JG. Benign recurrent intrahepatic cholestasism — 25 years of follow-up. *Postgrad. Med. J.* 1987; **63**: 295.

53 Rosario J, Sutherland E, Simon FR. Protection by S-adenosyl-L-methionine against ethinyl estradiol induced cholestasis is not due to alterations in sinusoidal membrane lipids. *Hepatology* 1986; **6**: 1201.

54 Scharschmidt BF, Goldberg HI, Schmid R. Current concepts in diagnosis. Approach to the patient with cholestatic jaundice. *N. Engl. J. Med.* 1983; **308**: 1515.

55 Scott AJ, Khan GA. Origin of bacteria in bileduct bile. *Lancet* 1967; **ii**: 790.

56 Smallwood RA, Williams HA, Rosenoer VM *et al.* Liver-copper levels in liver disease: studies using neutron activation analysis. *Lancet* 1968; **ii**: 1310.

57 Smith DJ, Gordon ER. Membrane fluidity and cholestasis. *J. Hepatol.* 1987; **5**: 362.

58 Smith CR, Oshio C, Miyairi M *et al.* Coordination of the contractile activity of bile canaliculi. Evidence from spontaneous contractions *in vitro*. *Lab. Invest.* 1985; **53**: 270.

59 Sokol RJ, Balistreri WF, Hoofnagle JH *et al.* Vitamin E deficiency during primary biliary cirrhosis. *Hepatology* 1982; **2**: 710.

60 Sokol RJ, Heubi JE, Iannaccone S *et al.* Mechanism causing vitamin E deficiency during chronic childhood cholestasis. *Gastroenterology* 1983; **85**: 1172.

61 Stellon AJ, Webb A, Compston J *et al.* Low bone turnover state in primary biliary cirrhosis. *Hepatology* 1987; **7**: 137.

62 Szabo S, Mendelson MH, Mitty HA *et al.* Infections associated with transhepatic biliary drainage devices. *Am. J. Med.* 1987; **82**: 921.

63 Thomas PK, Walker JG. Xanthomatous neuropathy in primary biliary cirrhosis. *Brain* 1965; **88**: 1079.

64 Walt RP, Kemp CM, Lyness L *et al.* Vitamin A treatment for night blindness in primary biliary cirrhosis. *Br. med. J.* 1984; **288**: 1030.

65 Walt RP, Daneshmend TK, Fellows IW *et al.* Effect of stanozolol on itching in primary biliary cirrhosis. *Brit. med. J.* 1988; **296**: 607.

66 Williams R, Cartter MA, Sherlock S *et al.* Idiopathic recurrent cholestasis: a study of the functional and pathological lesions in four cases. *Q. J. Med.* 1964; **33**: 387.

67 Zafrani ES, Guigui B, Douvin C *et al.* Non-syndromatic paucity of interlobular bile ducts in adults. *J. Hepatol.* 1987; 5, supl.1: s224.

14 · Primary Biliary Cirrhosis

This condition of progressive granulomatous destruction of intra-hepatic bile ducts was first described in 1851 by Addison and Gull [1] and later by Hanot [41]. The association with high serum cholesterol levels and skin xanthomas led to the term 'xanthomatous biliary cirrhosis' [55]. Ahrens and co-workers [2] termed the condition 'primary biliary cirrhosis'. However, in the early stages nodular regeneration is inconspicuous and cirrhosis is not present. The term 'chronic non-suppurative destructive cholangitis' [79] is a better one although too cumbersome to replace the popular 'primary biliary cirrhosis' (PBC) (fig. 14.1).

Aetiology

The aetiology remains unknown but the disease is associated with a profound immunological disturbance and this has been related to the bile duct destruction (table 14.1) [35]. Cytotoxic T-cells have been seen infiltrating the bile duct epithelium [104] as have class 2 restricted T-4 lymphocytes [18]. The final event is an attack by cytotoxic T-cells on biliary epithelium. Suppressor T-cells are reduced in number and function (fig. 14.2). Most patients show increased class 2 HLA histocompatibility antigen expression on bile duct cells [5, 96]. The disease might represent a failure of immuno-regulation, with loss of tolerance to tissues bearing a rich display of histocompatibility antigens. How and why the bile ducts are affected in this way, and the nature of the 'self' antigens presented remains unknown. What triggers off the immunopathological cascade may be a virus or some other neoantigen or simply defective immuno-regulation alone.

In many respects, primary biliary cirrhosis is analogous to the graft-versus-host syndrome, as seen, for instance, after bone marrow transplant and where the immune system has become sensitized to foreign HLA proteins (table 14.2) [28]. Structural changes in the bile ducts are similar. Other ducts with a high concentration of HLA class II antigens on their epithelium such as the lacrimal and pancreatic [24] are involved. The condition can be viewed as a dry gland syndrome. Primary biliary cirrhosis may be regarded as a spontaneous form of chronic liver rejection.

The granulomas might be related to immune complexes and indeed complement has been identified within them [68]. However, they consist predominantly of cytotoxic T-cells, monocytes and macrophages which suggest cell-mediated tissue injury. Patients with many granulomas are usually seen early in the disease where bile duct destruction is not prominent and the prognosis better. Such patients have normal or only slightly decreased concentrations of suppressor cells in the peripheral

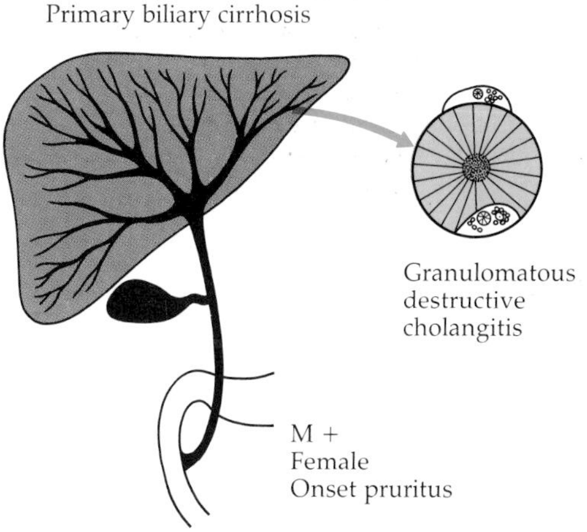

Primary biliary cirrhosis

Granulomatous destructive cholangitis

M +
Female
Onset pruritus

Fig. 14.1. The features of primary biliary cirrhosis (Sherlock 1972).

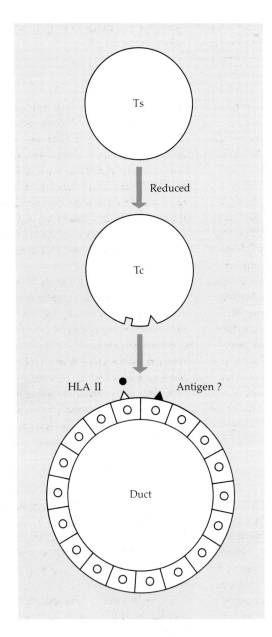

Fig. 14.2. Primary biliary cirrhosis: HLA class 11 antigens and another unknown antigen are displayed on the bile duct. Ts lymphocytes are depressed and there is breach of tolerance to the biliary antigens.

Table 14.1. Immunological changes in primary biliary cirrhosis

Depressed skin energy [47]
Granuloma formation [71]
Circulating immune complexes [53]
Complement activation [39]
Reduction regulator suppressor cells [95]

Table 14.2. Comparison of clinical and immunological aspects of primary biliary cirrhosis and chronic graft-versus-host disease

	PBC	GVH
Clinical		
Cholestatic liver injury (biliary-epithelial damage)	+	+
Sicca complex	+	+
Pancreatic hyposecretion	+	+
Scleroderma-like lesions	+	+
Raynaud's disease	+	+
Immunological		
Chronic inflammatory infiltrate damaging intra-hepatic biliary epithelium	+	+
Granuloma formation	+	+
Macroglobulinaemia	+	+
Failure to convert from IgM to IgG production	+	+
Immune complex formation	+	+
Anergy to DNCB	+	+

Copper is retained in the liver, but in a non-hepatotoxic form [22, 88].

An impaired sulfoxidation pathway has been shown [64]. This is also present with chlorpromazine-induced hepatotoxicity. Significance is uncertain but this may interact with other genetic and immunological factors in the pathogenesis of primary biliary cirrhosis.

Epidemiology and genetics

The disease has been reported from all parts of the world. Asians, Caucasians, Jews, Negroes and Orientals are affected. Death rates are difficult to assess, but are probably of the order of

blood. This might be related to the rarity of diffuse bile duct destruction and the good prognosis [52].

0.6—2% of those dying with cirrhosis. As more patients are diagnosed and subsequently die the figure will undoubtedly change. There is family clustering, and primary biliary cirrhosis has been reported in sisters, twins, mothers and daughters [60, 94]. The prevalence of circulating mitochondrial antibodies is increased in relatives of patients [32, 36]. There is no association with any particular HLA A, B, or DR antigen [7, 46].

Environmental factors are suggested by the development of the disease in a daughter, her mother and an unrelated close friend who nursed the daughter in her terminal illness [21]. A new serum mitochondrial antibody (M_g) on the outer membrane is positive in some sufferers, non blood relatives and technicians handling their blood. This suggests an infective aetiology [10]. In a three-year study (1977 to 1979) of primary biliary cirrhosis in Sheffield, United Kingdom, 90% of patients came from an area that had only 4% of the population and one particular reservoir [95]. No one has so far has matched this experience, and an environmental factor in the water supply could not be identified.

Clinical features

PRESENTATION [85, 86, 88]

Ninety per cent are female usually between the ages of 40 and 59 (range 32—72 years). The reason for the female predominance is unknown. The disease starts insidiously most frequently as pruritus without jaundice. Patients may be referred initially to dermatologists. Jaundice may never develop but in the majority appears within six months to two years of the onset of pruritus. In about a quarter, jaundice and pruritus start simultaneously. Jaundice preceding pruritus is extremely unusual and jaundice without pruritus at any time is very rare. The pruritus can start during pregnancy and be confused with idiopathic cholestatic jaundice of the last trimester.

Examination shows a well-nourished pigmented woman. Jaundice is slight or absent.

The liver is usually enlarged and firm and the spleen palpable.

THE ASYMPTOMATIC PATIENT

Widespread use of automated biochemical screening has resulted in an increasing number of patients being diagnosed when asymptomatic [53]. Liver biopsies performed after finding a positive mitochondrial antibody titre ≥ 1/40 during screening for autoimmune disease are nearly always abnormal and usually show features consistent with primary biliary cirrhosis even if the patient is asymptomatic and the serum alkaline phosphatase is normal [59].

The diagnosis may be made in patients under investigation for a condition known to be associated with primary biliary cirrhosis, such as thyroid or collagen disease, or in the course of family surveys.

Abnormal physical signs may be absent. Mitochondrial antibody is always positive. Serum alkaline phosphatase and bilirubin may be normal or only minimally increased. Serum cholesterol and transaminases can also be normal.

COURSE

Earlier diagnosis in the asymptomatic patient makes the duration seem much longer and these patients usually survive at least ten years (fig. 14.3) [11]. In those with symptomatic disease and jaundice the survival is about seven years [84].

In men, the disease is marked by less common pruritus at diagnosis, less skin pigmentation, less autoimmune features, especially the sickle syndrome. Survival is the same for men and women [54].

Diarrhoea may be due to steatorrhoea. Weight loss is slow. In spite of the jaundice, patients feel surprisingly well and have a good appetite. The course is afebrile and abdominal pain is unusual.

Skin xanthomas develop frequently and sometimes acutely, but many patients remain

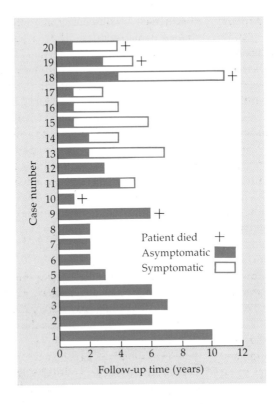

Fig. 14.3. The course of 20 patients with primary biliary cirrhosis diagnosed when asymptomatic. Note that one patient continued asymptomatic for 10 years (Long *et al.* 1977).

in the pre-xanthomatous state throughout their course; terminally xanthomas may disappear.

The skin may be thickened and tough over the fingers, ankles and legs. Pain in the fingers, especially on opening doors, and in the toes may be due to xanthomatous peripheral neuropathy [93]. There may be a butterfly area over the back which is inaccessible and escapes scratching [72].

The bone changes complicating chronic cholestasis are particularly profound in the deeply jaundiced (figs 13.14, 13.15, 13.16). In the late stages the patient complains of backache and pain over the ribs sometimes with pathological fractures. These bone changes are enhanced by prolonged corticosteroid therapy.

Duodenal ulceration and haemorrhage are common.

Bleeding oesophageal varices may be a presenting feature [50, 105], even before nodules have developed in the liver. The portal hypertension is probably presinusoidal. Haemorrhage from varices also accompanies the late cirrhotic stage [84].

Hepato-cellular carcinoma is a very rare termination, perhaps because a true nodular cirrhosis develops so late [51].

ASSOCIATED DISEASES

Non-hepatic disorders are found in 69% [37]. Primary biliary cirrhosis is associated with almost any postulated autoimmune disease. The collagenoses, especially rheumatoid arthritis, dermatomyositis, mixed connective tissue disease [23] and systemic lupus erythematosis [40] are particularly frequent.

Primary biliary cirrhosis may be associated with scleroderma in 4% and with the whole CREST syndrome [73]. The scleroderma is usually limited to sclerodactyly but occasionally involves face, arms and legs. Keratoconjunctivitis may be present [70]. These patients usually have a nuclear centromere antibody [56] and sometimes, circulating immune complexes containing ribonuclear protein AgRo [66]. A sicca complex of dry eyes and mouth, with or without the arthritis completing the Sjögren syndrome, is found in about 75% of patients.

Other associated skin lesions include immune complex capillaritis and lichen planus which is also a feature of graft-versus-host disease [39]. Autoimmune thyroiditis is frequent, affecting about 20% of sufferers [19]. Graves disease has also been reported [63].

Primary biliary cirrhosis and jejunal villous atrophy, resembling coeliac disease, have been reported [8]. Ulcerative colitis is another rare accompaniment [15].

Primary biliary cirrhosis has been associated with autoimmune thrombocytopenia and insulin receptor autoantibodies [82].

Renal complications include IgM associated membranous glomerular nephritis [71].

Renal tubular acidosis is attributed to copper deposits in the distal renal tubule [65]. Hypouricaemia and hyperuricosuria are further expressions of renal tubular damage [43]. Bacteriuria develops in 35% and may be asymptomatic [14]. It is unexplained, but it has been postulated that urinary organisms might be invoked in the pathogenesis of primary biliary cirrhosis.

Primary biliary cirrhosis has been associated with selective immunoglobulin A deficiency in a family [44]. This indicates that the pathogenesis does not require IgA dependent immune mechanisms.

Breast cancer is increased 4.4 times over the rate prevailing in a comparable normal population [38, 103].

Primary biliary cirrhosis has been associated with transverse myelitis due to angiitis and necrotizing myelopathy [80]. Finger clubbing is common, and occasionally there is hypertrophic osteo-arthropathy (fig. 13.19) [26].

Pancreatic insufficiency is secondary to low bile flow [75] and perhaps to immunological damage to the pancreatic duct [24].

Gallstones, usually of pigment type, have been seen by endoscopy in 39%. They are occasionally symptomatic, but rarely migrate to the common bile duct.

Abnormal pulmonary gas-transfer studies are associated with an abnormal chest X-ray showing nodules and interstitial fibrosis. Lung biopsies show interstitial lung disease. Pulmonary interstitial giant cell granulomas have also been described [91]. These patients often have Sjögren's syndrome [98]. Bronchoalveolar lavage shows activated mononuclear cells; similar to those of sarcoidosis.

The CREST syndrome is accompanied by interstitial pneumonitis and pulmonary vascular abnormalities.

A patient with primary biliary cirrhosis and primary pulmonary hypertension had a successful transplantation of liver, heart and lungs [100].

BIOCHEMICAL TESTS

Serum bilirubin values are rarely very high at the onset, usually less than 2 mg/100 ml in symptomatic patients. Serum alkaline phosphatase (gamma-glutamyl transpeptidase) is raised. The total serum cholesterol is increased but not constantly. The serum albumin level is usually normal at presentation and the total serum globulin only moderately increased. Serum immunoglobulin M (IgM) is usually raised and this estimation has been suggested for diagnosis. However, increases are not constant and this method is not reliable for diagnosis, although an increase may add some diagnostic weight.

SERUM MITOCHONDRIAL (M) ANTIBODY TEST

Circulating antibodies against mitochondria are found in virtually 100% of patients with primary biliary cirrhosis [61, 97]. They are non-organ and non-species specific. They are usually detected by an ELISA technique [47] or by dot-immuno-binding [67].

The mitochondrial antibodies represent a heterogenous group of autoantibodies associated with various diseases. They are not confined to primary biliary cirrhosis, being detected in 30% of patients with autoimmune chronic active hepatitis and 3% with connective tissue diseases [97]. They are absent in patients with mechanical obstruction to the bile ducts. They are occasionally present in low titre in patients with primary sclerosing cholangitis.

The mitochondrial antigens can be more clearly defined by separating the outer and inner mitochondrial membranes and the antigens on them (fig. 14.4) [9].

Virtually 100% of patients with primary biliary cirrhosis have serological antibodies against M2, a specific antigen on the inner mitochondrial membrane. A component of this antigen (E2) is part of the pyruvate dehydrogenase of the mitochondrion [105]. This discovery may lead to the development of a specific test. E2 could be related to the unknown antigen believed to exist on biliary epithelium. M2 is produced *in vitro* by peripheral blood mononuclear cells of patients with primary biliary cirrhosis [3]. Two other

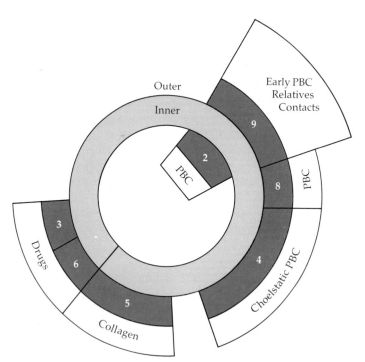

Outer

Inner

Early PBC
Relatives
Contacts

PBC

PBC

Drugs

Choelstatic PBC

Collagen

Fig. 14.4. Mitochondrial (M)
antibodies (after Berg *et al.* 1986).

specific mitochondrial antigens have also been found on the inner membrane and designated P62 and P48 [57, 105].

Anti-M9 is associated with early PBC. It can also be found in 60% of healthy relatives of sufferers and 65% of technicians handling sera from primary biliary cirrhosis patients. Ten to 15% of normal persons are M9 positive.

M8 on the outer mitochondrial membrane is specific for primary biliary cirrhosis and found only in those who are M2 positive. It may be associated with more progressive disease [102].

M3 is associated with drug reactions and the pseudo-lupus syndrome.

M6 is related to iproniazid hepatitis and M6 to collagen vascular diseases.

Mitochondrial antibodies are generally believed to be unrelated to the pathogenesis of primary biliary cirrhosis. However, there are some similarities between bacteria and mammalian mitochondrial components. Persistence of an infectious agent may stimulate mitochondrial autoantigens leading to formation of different types of organ specific and non-specific mitochondrial antibodies in a genetically susceptible individual [10]. Anti-M2 will recognize antigens on some *E. coli*. These observations support the concept that primary biliary cirrhosis may have an infectious origin.

LIVER BIOPSY [79, 81, 85]

The only hepatic lesion diagnostic of primary biliary cirrhosis is the injured septal or inter-lobular bile duct. Such ducts are not often seen in needle biopsy specimens, but are usually well represented in surgical biopsies (fig. 14.5). Histopathological diagnosis is therefore more confident with operative biopsies than with needle ones. Yet the number of such specimens is decreasing with a reduction in laparotomies. Great importance is being placed on the experience of the histopathologist.

The disease begins with damage to the epithelium of small bile ducts. Histometric examinations show that bile ducts less than 70–80 μm in diameter are destroyed and particularly in the early stages [62]. Epithelial cells are

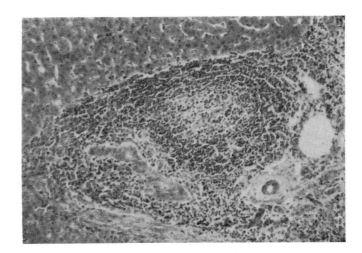

Fig. 14.5. Primary biliary cirrhosis. The portal zone contains a well-formed granuloma. An adjacent bile duct shows damage.

swollen, irregular and more eosinophilic. The bile duct lumen is irregular and the basement membrane is disrupted. The bile duct occasionally ruptures. Surrounding the damaged duct is a cellular reaction which includes lymphocytes, plasma cells, eosinophils and histiocytes. Granulomas commonly form usually in zone 1 (fig. 14.5).

Bile ducts become destroyed. Their sites are marked by aggregates of lymphoid cells and bile ductules begin to proliferate (fig. 14.6). Hepatic arterial branches can be identified in the portal zones but without accompanying bile ducts. Fibrosis extends from the portal tracts and there is a variable degree of piecemeal necrosis. Substantial amounts of copper and copper associated protein can be demonstrated histochemically. The fibrous septa gradually come to distort the architecture of the liver and regeneration nodules form (figs 14.7, 14.8). These are often irregular in distribution and cirrhosis may be seen in one part of a biopsy but not in another. In some areas lobular architecture may be preserved for some time. In the early stages, cholestasis is in zone 1 (portal).

Hepato-cellular hyaline deposits, similar to those of alcoholic disease, are found in hepatocytes in about 25% of cases.

The histological appearances have been divided into four stages: *stage I* florid bile duct lesions; *stage II* ductular proliferation; *stage III* scarring (septal fibrosis and bridging); and *stage*

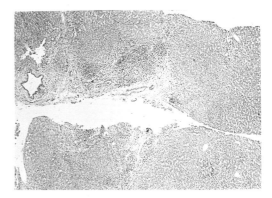

Fig. 14.6. Stage 2 lesion, marked by aggregates of lymphoid cells. Bile ducts begin to proliferate (H & E, ×10).

IV cirrhosis [81]. Such staging is of limited value as the changes in the liver are focal and evolve at different speeds in different parts. Stages overlap. It is particularly difficult to separate stages II and III. The disease has a very variable course and advanced stage III lesions may be seen in the asymptomatic patient. Moreover, serial biopsies have shown that the same stage may persist for many years.

Diagnosis

This is suspected when a middle-aged woman presents with pruritus with or without mild jaundice. It is confirmed by a raised serum

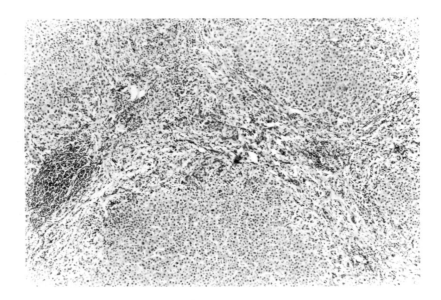

Fig. 14.7. Primary biliary cirrhosis. There is scarring and septa contain lymphoid aggregates. Bile ducts are inconspicuous. Hyperplastic 'regeneration' nodules are beginning to develop. H & E, ×48 (Sherlock & Scheuer 1973).

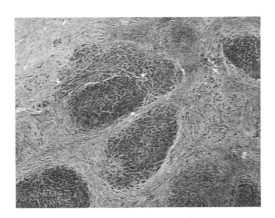

Fig. 14.8. Stage 4: biliary cirrhosis has developed.

alkaline phosphatase level, sometimes a high serum IgM, a positive serum mitochondrial antibody test and diagnostic or compatible hepatic histology on needle biopsy. In the asymptomatic it may be suspected simply by a raised serum alkaline phosphatase level or a positive M test. All biochemical tests may be normal.

Visualization of the bile ducts by endoscopic percutaneous cholangiography may be necessary in atypical patients. These include males and those with a negative serum mitochondrial antibody test, with inconclusive liver biopsy findings or with abdominal pain. Surgical exploration of the bile ducts is not necessary for diagnosis.

Widespread tissue granulomas may suggest sarcoidosis (table 14.3) [6, 31]. In sarcoidosis, however, the Kveim—Siltzbach skin test is positive (75%) and mitochondrial antibody is absent. Liver biopsy shows abundant well-formed granulomas and less bile duct damage than that seen in primary biliary cirrhosis.

The similarities between sarcoidosis and primary biliary cirrhosis are emphasized by the finding of T-lymphocytes (predominantly T-4 positive cells) and activated alveolar macrophages by broncho-alveolar lavage in patients with primary biliary cirrhosis, similar findings to those of sarcoidosis [99].

There are overlaps and occasionally the distinction is impossible.

In later stages, the diagnosis from chronic active hepatitis may be difficult. The pattern of

Table 14.3. Features distinguishing sarcoidosis from symptomatic primary biliary cirrhosis (Stanley *et al.* 1972)

Feature	Sarcoidosis	PBC
Sex (F:M)	Equal	8:1
Erythema nodosum	Yes	No
Uveitis	Yes	No
Pruritus	No	Yes
Xanthomas	No	Yes
Splenomegaly	Yes (in 12%)	Yes (in 50%)
Skin pigmentation	No	Yes
Steatorrhoea	No	Yes
Bilateral hilar lymphadenopathy	Yes	No
Kveim test	Positive (in 75%)	Always negative
Serum angiotensin converting enzyme raised	Yes (in 60%)	Yes (16%)
Depression of delayed-type hypersensitivity	Yes	Yes
Circulating mitochondrial antibodies	No	Yes
Calcium metabolism	Hypercalcaemia (vitamin D sensitivity)	Hypocalcaemia (steatorrhoea)
Alkaline phosphatase raised	Yes (minority)	Yes (majority)
Liver granulomas	Yes	Yes
Corticosteroids	Helpful	Contraindicated
Prognosis	Very good	Progressive disease

biochemical tests of liver function is usually different. Liver biopsy features favouring primary biliary cirrhosis include intact lobules, slight piecemeal necrosis, periseptal cholestasis and lymphoid aggregates.

Primary sclerosing cholangitis may cause diagnostic difficulty, but in this condition the mitochondrial antibody test is always negative or in low titre and cholangiography demonstrates the typical bile duct irregularities.

Chronic drug jaundice, for instance that related to the promazines, may simulate primary biliary cirrhosis. The onset, however, is much more acute, with rapidly deepening jaundice developing 4−6 weeks after the drug is started.

Asymptomatic stage. The diagnosis must be made from other causes of a raised serum alkaline phosphatase such as Paget's disease. The raised serum gamma-glutamyl transpeptidase usually makes the distinction.

Other causes of chronic pruritus have to be considered.

PROGNOSIS

The course of asymptomatic patients is variable and unpredictable and counselling the patient and her family is very difficult. Overall, the life expectancy of these patients does not differ from that of the general population [11, 44]. Only six of 36 asymptomatic patients studied over 6−11.4 years died from liver disease [11].

Serum bilirubin values are the best indicators of prognosis [83]. When values are consistently greater than 6 mg/dl the patient is unlikely to survive more than two years (fig. 14.9) [25]. Other features at diagnosis predicting decreased survival include symptoms, advanced age, hepatosplenomegaly, ascites and hypoalbuminaemia (less than 3 g/dl) [74]. Histologically, piecemeal necrosis, cholestasis, bridging fibrosis and cirrhosis correlate with the worst prognosis. Spread of disease from portal to peri-portal areas implies progression. On the

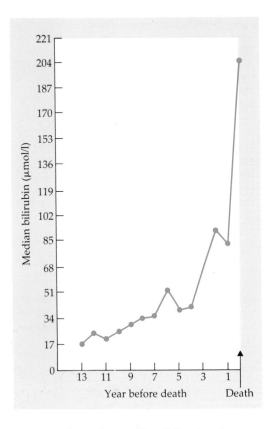

Fig. 14.9. The evolution of liver failure in primary biliary cirrhosis. This nomogram is derived from the medians of pooled serum bilirubin results in patients followed serially from diagnosis to death. Expected survival for any given bilirubin can be extrapolated from this nomogram (Epstein *et al.* 1985).

Bilirubin (μmol/l)	Expected survival (years)
< 34	8–13
35–100	2–7
> 100	< 2
(17 μmol/l=1 mg)	

other hand granulomas seen on an initial biopsy predict a longer survival [52], perhaps because they indicate a less aggressive immune response.

Serum type III procollagen peptide values correlate with the degree of cholestasis and with prognosis [4].

Autoimmune diseases such as thyroiditis,

sicca syndrome or Raynaud's phenomenon correlate with decreased survival [11].

The terminal stages last about one year and are marked by a rapid deepening of jaundice with disappearance of both xanthomas and pruritus. Serum albumin and total cholesterol levels fall. Oedema and ascites develop. The final events include episodes of hepatic encephalopathy with uncontrollable bleeding, usually from the oesophageal varices. An intercurrent infection, sometimes a Gram-negative septicaemia, may be terminal.

Treatment

General measures apply to all patients with cholestasis and include control of itching and the management of steatorrhoea (see Chapter 13). Fat-soluble vitamins A, D and K are given parenterally with oral calcium supplements to all cholestatic patients [60]. Exposure to sunshine should be encouraged. Intractable pruritus and painful neuropathy can be treated by plasmapheresis. This is specialized and costly, but may be considered in the exceptional patient.

Corticosteroids might be expected to be beneficial by reducing inflammation and lessening K-lymphocyte activity. They may also relieve pruritus. In a recent trial, patients treated with prednisolone for one year had less itching and fatigue. Serum alkaline phosphatase, transaminases and procollagen III fell. Liver biopsy improved. However, an increasing development of progressive bone thinning contraindicated this treatment [58].

Azathioprine. In the seventies this drug was used in clinical prospective trials and it was concluded that it did not influence the natural history of the disease. However, in a long-term follow-up of an international trial, it was suggested that azathioprine lowered mortality. 45% of azathioprine-treated patients and 51% of controls died [17]. Although this did not reach statistical significance, the result was deemed significant when a slight imbalance in serum bilirubin between the two groups was 'corrected' by statistical manipulation. The

Table 14.4. Prognostic profiles in PBC (Epstein *et al.* 1985)

	Prognosis		
	Excellent	Intermediate	Poor
Symptoms	No	Yes	Yes
Hepatomegaly	Variable	Variable	Usual
Splenomegaly	Unusual	Variable	Usual
Ascites/ encephalopathy	No	No	Variable
Bilirubin (mg/dl)	1	< 7	> 7
Histology*	1–4	2–4	3–4
Expected survival	Similar to age-matched controls	2–13 years	2 years

* Data of Epstein *et al.* (1985).

conclusion that azathioprine is useful in PBC must be guarded as 63 of the 248 patients were lost to follow-up. Without statistical corrections, it is difficult to see a difference in survival.

D-penicillamine. In two controlled trials, D-penicillamine improved survival and biochemical tests and reduced liver copper content. Biopsies showed reduced inflammation and piecemeal necrosis but hepatic fibrosis progressed [20, 27]. Side-effects were dyspepsia, nausea, taste loss, skin rashes, blood dyscrasias and proteinuria; many patients were withdrawn. More recent trials have failed to confirm the initially good results.

In one, which included 227 patients, there was no difference in mortality over a 10-year follow-up period [20]. The high incidence of side effects were stressed. A further multi-centre trial from Europe showed no difference in mortality between treated and controls. Both trials, however, suggested that the drug may be useful in the early stages. Another trial was terminated due to the severity of adverse effects and continued progression of disease [13]. Further analysis of the Royal Free Hospital trial of 100 patients showed a five-year survival of 70% in the treated and 57% in the placebo group ($P < 0.08$) and to achieve statistical significance 711 patients would be required [29]. This is clearly impractical and no single trial

has been large enough to exclude a type 2 error with confidence. At present, D-penicillamine, particularly in view of its side-effects, cannot be recommended.

Cyclosporin A. In a preliminary study, administration of cyclosporin A to patients with primary biliary cirrhosis was accompanied by improvement in serum biochemistry and the ratio of helper: suppressor/cytotoxic cells fell [78]. Nephrotoxicity was common and the trial was stopped. Use of such a toxic drug is difficult to justify long-term in patients who are symptom-free and with a relatively good life expectancy. Less toxic cyclosporin derivatives are anxiously awaited.

Chlorambucil. In a small trial, after two years this drug reduced serum bilirubin and raised albumin [42]. At two years, hepatic inflammation had decreased although there was no improvement in fibrosis and staging. The long-term toxicity of alkylating agents must be remembered and bone marrow suppression was a complication. Acute leukaemia may develop years later. Its long-term use cannot be recommended.

Colchicine. This alkaloid interferes with collagen synthesis by preventing the assembly of tubulin subunits into microtubules and thereby inhibiting hepatic transport of collagen.

283

CHAPTER 14

Table 14.5. Ursodeoxycholic acid for PBC. 15 patients: 13−15/mg/kg daily (from Poupon *et al.* [69])

	Years		
	0	1	2
% Pruritus	53	27	8
Serum bilirubin mg	2.1	1.4	1.3
Phosphatase (100)	612	287	213
GOT (30)	62	34	28

Colchicine may also degrade collagen by activating hepatic collagenase. Three trials have been undertaken of colchicine in primary biliary cirrhosis. In two trials, biochemical tests of liver function improved [48, 101]. In another trial, there was no change in liver function tests [12]. In all three trials, liver biopsy appearances showed no change. Colchicine is relatively non-toxic, and 0.6 mg twice daily may be given. Side-effects are diarrhoea and granulocytopenia [33]. Long-term benefit is uncertain.

Ursodeoxycholic acid. In primary biliary cirrhosis, bile acids are retained in the liver and systemic circulation and these might contribute to hepatocyte injury. Ursodeoxycholic acid is a hydrophilic and less toxic bile acid and is given to replace the detergent bile acids and to improve liver function. In uncontrolled trials, patients with primary biliary cirrhosis given 13−15 mg/kg body weight ursodeoxy-cholic acid have shown less pruritus, and improved biochemical tests of liver function (table 14.5) [34, 69]. These good results have been confirmed in controlled trials. Liver histology did not improve and this therapy has little effect on the autoimmune process or on histological progression. It should not be used in late-stage disease.

CONCLUSIONS

At present no satisfactory, specific medical treatment can be recommended for primary biliary cirrhosis. Ursodeoxycholic acid looks promising but good results need to be confirmed in large placebo-controlled trials.

Reported trials have usually been too short, too small and poorly controlled. Statistically significant long-term benefits are difficult to establish in a disease with such a long and varied natural history. Any trial must state the numbers of patients included in each grade. The group in the early, asymptomatic, excellent stage require no treatment. The ones with the poor outlook will be too end-stage to respond. It is the intermediate group which should be included in trials. Evaluation of currently available measures should continue only in the context of large controlled clinical trials.

Haemorrhage from oesophageal varices may be early before a true nodular cirrhosis has developed. It is not surprising therefore that porta-caval shunting gives good results in these patients [90]. Hepatic encephalopathy is an unusual complication. These encouraging results apply particularly to good-risk patients (grade A and B), rather than those with poor hepato-cellular function (grade C).

Gallstones should be left *in situ* unless causing severe symptoms or present in the common bile duct. Cholecystectomy is rarely indicated and is badly tolerated.

HEPATIC TRANSPLANTATION

Primary biliary cirrhosis is a disease where the end-stages can be reasonably well predicted (fig. 14.9) (table 14.4). The patient reaches a stage where she is housebound, deeply yellow and itching and life seems scarcely worth living. Once the serum bilirubin level exceeds 6 mg/dl and the patient has been hospitalized with two major complications such as ascites, bleeding varices or encephalopathy, hepatic transplantation must be considered (See chapter 35). The one-year survival is 70% [30] but 25% need a re-transplant. Ninety per cent of those who survive one year will survive three years and probably five. Recurrence of the disease in the transplanted liver is not seen, but the graft-versus-host reaction of chronic rejection may occur [89].

Following liver transplant, mitochondrial antibody titres persist [30]. Sub-types are un-

284

altered. The initial titre does not affect the result of the transplant. Disappearance of mitochondrial antibodies could be due to prednisolone therapy or actual cure by the transplant.

References

1 Addison T, Gull W. On a certain affection of the skin—vitiligoidea—α plana β tuberosa. *Guy's Hosp. Rep.* 1851; **7**: 265.

2 Ahrens EH Jr, Payne MA, Kunkel HG *et al.* Primary biliary cirrhosis. *Medicine (Baltimore)* 1950: **29**: 299.

3 Avigan MI, Adamson G, Hoofnagle JH *et al.* The *in vitro* production of antibodies to mitochondrial antigens by peripheral blood mononuclear cells from patients with primary biliary cirrhosis. *Hepatology* 1986; **6**: 999.

4 Babbs C, Smith A, Hunt LP *et al.* Type III procollagen peptide: a number of disease activity and prognosis in primary biliary cirrhosis. *Lancet* 1988; **i**: 1012.

5 Ballardini G, Mirakian R, Bianchi FB *et al.* Aberrant expression of HLA-DR antigens on bile duct epithelium in primary biliary cirrhosis: relevance to pathogenesis. *Lancet* 1984; **ii**: 1009.

6 Bass NM, Burroughs AK, Scheuer PJ *et al.* Chronic intrahepatic cholestasis due to sarcoidosis. *Gut* 1982; **23**: 417.

7 Bassendine MF, Dewar PJ, James OFW. HLA-DR antigens in primary biliary cirrhosis: lack of association. *Gut* 1985; **26**: 625.

8 Behr W, Barnert J. Adult celiac disease and primary biliary cirrhosis. *Am. J. Gastroenterol.* 1986; **81**: 796.

9 Berg PA, Klein R, Lindenborn-Fotinos J *et al.* ATPase-associated antigen (M2): marker antigen for serological diagnosis of primary biliary cirrhosis. *Lancet* 1982; **ii**: 1423.

10 Berg PA, Klein R, Lindenborn-Fotinos J. Antimitochondrial antibodies in primary biliary cirrhosis. *J. Hepatol.* 1986; **2**: 123.

11 Beswick DR, Klatskin G, Boyer JL. Asymptomatic primary biliary cirrhosis—long term follow-up and natural history. *Gastroenterology* 1985; **89**: 267.

12 Bodenheimer HJ, Schaffner F, Pezzullo J. A randomized double-blind trial of colchicine in primary biliary cirrhosis (Abstr). *Hepatology* 1985; **5**: 968.

13 Bodenheimer HC, Schaffner F, Sternlieb I *et al.* A prospective clinical trial of D-penicillamine in the treatment of primary biliary cirrhosis. *Hepatology* 1985; **5**: 1139.

14 Burroughs AK, Rosenstein IJ, Epstein O *et al.* Bacteriuria and primary biliary cirrhosis. *Gut* 1984; **25**: 133.

15 Bush A, Mitchison H, Walt R *et al.* Primary biliary cirrhosis and ulcerative colitis. *Gastroenterology* 1987; **92**: 2009.

16 Chohan MR. Primary biliary cirrhosis in twin sisters. *Gut* 1973; **14**: 213.

17 Christensen E, Neuberger J, Crowe J *et al.* Beneficial effect of azathioprine and prediction of prognosis in primary biliary cirrhosis: final results of an international trial. *Gastroenterology* 1985; **89**: 1084.

18 Colucci G, Schaffner F, Paronetto F. *In situ* characterization of the cell-surface antigens of the mononuclear cell infiltrate and bile duct epithelium in primary biliary cirrhosis. *Clin. Immunol. Immunopath.* 1986; **41**: 35.

19 Crowe JP, Christensen E, Butler J *et al.* Primary biliary cirrhosis: the prevalence of hypothyroidism and its relationship to thyroid autoantibodies and sicca syndrome. *Gastroenterology* 1980; **78**: 1437.

20 Dickson ER, Wiesner RH, Baldus WP *et al.* D-penicillamine trial for primary biliary cirrhosis. *Gastroenterology* 1984; **86**: 1062A.

21 Douglas JG, Finlayson NDC. Are increased individual susceptibility and environmental factors both necessary for the development of primary biliary cirrhosis? *Br. Med. J.* 1979; **ii**: 419.

22 Epstein O, Arborgh B, Sagiv M *et al.* Is copper hepatotoxic in primary biliary cirrhosis? *J. clin. Pathol.* 1981; **34**: 1071.

23 Epstein O, Burroughs AK, Sherlock S. Polymyositis and acute onset systemic sclerosis in a patient with primary biliary cirrhosis: a clinical syndrome similar to the mixed connective tissue disease. *J.R. Soc. Med.* 1981; **74**: 456.

24 Epstein O, Chapman RWG, Lake-Bakaar G *et al.* The pancreas in primary biliary cirrhosis and primary sclerosing cholangitis. *Gastroenterology* 1982; **83**: 1177.

25 Epstein O, Fraga E, Sherlock S. Importance of clinical staging for prognosis in primary biliary cirrhosis. *Gut* 1985; **26**:A1126.

26 Epstein O, Dick R, Sherlock S. Prospective study of periostitis and finger clubbing in primary biliary cirrhosis and other forms of chronic liver disease. *Gut* 1981; **22**: 203.

27 Epstein O, Jain S, Lee RG *et al.* D-penicillamine treatment improves survival in primary biliary cirrhosis. *Lancet* 1981; **i**: 1257.

28 Epstein O, Thomas HC, Sherlock S. Primary biliary cirrhosis is a 'dry gland' syndrome with features of chronic graft-versus-host disease. *Lancet* 1980; **i**: 1166.

29 Epstein O, Cook DG, Jain S, *et al.* D-penicillamine

in PBC—an untested (and untestable?) treatment. *J. Hepatol.* 1985; **1**: S49.

30 Esquivel CO, Van Thiel DH, Demetris AJ *et al.* Transplantation for primary biliary cirrhosis. *Gastroenterology* 1988; **94**: 1207.

31 Fagan EA, Moore-Gillon JC, Turner-Warwick M. Multiorgan granulomas and mitochondrial antibodies. *N. Engl. J. Med.* 1983; **308**: 572.

32 Feizi T, Naccarato R, Sherlock S *et al.* Mitochondrial and other tissue antibodies in relatives of patients with biliary cirrhosis. *Clin. exp. Immunol.* 1972; **10**: 609.

33 Finklestein M, Goldman L, Grace ND *et al.* Granulocytopenia complicating colchicine therapy for primary biliary cirrhosis. *Gastroenterology* 1987; **93**: 1231.

34 Fisher MM, Paradine ME. Influence of ursodeoxycholic acid (UDCA) on biochemical parameters in cholestatic liver disease. *Gastroenterology* 1986; **90**: 1725.

35 Fox RA, Scheuer PJ, James DG *et al.* Impaired delayed hypersensitivity in primary biliary cirrhosis. *Lancet* 1969; **i**: 959.

36 Galbraith RM, Smith M, Mackenzie RM *et al.* High prevalence of seroimmunologic abnormalities in relatives of patients with active chronic hepatitis or primary biliary cirrhosis. *N. Engl. J. Med.* 1974; **290**: 63.

37 Golding RL, Smith M, Williams R. Multisystem involvement in chronic liver disease: studies on the incidence and pathogenesis. *Am. J. Med.* 1973; **55**: 772.

38 Goudie BM, Burt AD, Boyle P *et al.* Breast cancer in women with primary biliary cirrhosis. *Brit. med. J.* 1985; **291**: 1597.

39 Graham-Brown RAC, Sarkany I, Sherlock S. Lichen planus and primary biliary cirrhosis. *Br. J. Dermatol* 1982; **106**: 699.

40 Hall S, Axelsen PH, Larson DE *et al.* Systemic lupus erythematosus developing in patients with primary biliary cirrhosis. *Ann. intern. Med.* 1984; **100**: 388.

41 Hanot V. *Etude sur une Forme de Cirrhose Hypertrophique de Foie (Cirrhose Hypertrophique avec Ictère Chronique).* JB Bailliere, Paris 1876.

42 Hoofnagle JH, Davis GL, Schafer DF *et al.* Randomized trial of chlorambucil for primary biliary cirrhosis. *Gastroenterology* 1986; **91**: 1327.

43 Izumi N, Hasumura Y, Takeuchi J. Hypouricemia and hyperuricosuria as expressions of renal tubular damage in primary biliary cirrhosis. *Hepatology* 1983; **3**: 719.

44 James O, Macklon AF, Watson AJ. Primary biliary cirrhosis—a revised clinical spectrum. *Lancet* 1981; **i**: 1278.

45 James SP, Jones EA, Schafer DF *et al.* Selective immunoglobulin A deficiency associated with

primary biliary cirrhosis in a family with liver disease. *Gastroenterology* 1986; **90**: 283.

46 Johnston DE, Kaplan MM, Miller KB *et al.* Histocompatability antigens in primary biliary cirrhosis. *Am. J. Gastr.* 1987; **82**: 1127.

47 Kaplan MM, Gandolfo JV, Quaroni EG. An enzyme-linked immunosorbant assay (ELISA) for detecting antimitochondrial antibody. *Hepatology* 1984; **4**: 727.

48 Kaplan MM, Alling DW, Zimmerman HJ *et al.* A prospective trial of colchicine for primary biliary cirrhosis. *N. Engl. J. Med.* 1986; **315**: 1448.

49 Keeffe EB. Sarcoidosis and primary biliary cirrhosis. Literature review and illustrative case. *Am. J. Med.* 1987; **83**: 977.

50 Kew MC, Varma RR, Dos Santos HA *et al.* Portal hypertension in primary biliary cirrhosis. *Gut* 1971; **12**: 830.

51 Krasner N, Johnson PJ, Portman B *et al.* Hepatocellular carcinoma in primary biliary cirrhosis: report of four cases. *Gut* 1979; **20**: 255.

52 Lee RG, Epstein O, Jauregui H *et al.* Granulomas in primary biliary cirrhosis: a prognostic feature. *Gastroenterology* 1981; **81**: 983.

53 Long RG, Scheuer PJ, Sherlock S. Presentation and course of asymptomatic primary biliary cirrhosis. *Gastroenterology* 1977; **72**: 1204.

54 Lucey MR, Neuberger JM, Williams R. Primary biliary cirrhosis in men. *Gut* 1986; **27**: 1373.

55 MacMahon HE, Thannhauser SJ. Xanthomatous biliary cirrhosis (a clinical syndrome). *Ann. intern. Med.* 1949; **30**: 121.

56 Makinen D, Fritzler M, Davis P *et al.* Anticentromere antibodies in primary biliary cirrhosis. *Arthritis Rheum.* 1983; **26**: 9141.

57 Manns M, Gerken G, Kyriatsoulis A *et al.* Two different subtypes of antimitochondrial antibodies are associated with primary biliary cirrhosis: identification and characterization by radioimmunoassay and immunoblotting. *Hepatology* 1987; **7**: 893.

58 Mitchison HC, Bassendine MF, Record CO *et al.* Controlled trial of prednisolone for primary biliary cirrhosis: good for the liver, bad for the bones? *Hepatology* 1986; **6**: 1211 (abstract).

59 Mitchison HC, Bassendine MF, Hendrick A *et al.* Positive antimitochondrial antibody but normal alkaline phosphatase: is this primary biliary cirrhosis? *Hepatology* 1986; **6**: 1279.

60 Mitchison HC, Malcolm AJ, Bassendine MF *et al.* Metabolic bone disease in primary biliary cirrhosis at presentation. *Gastroenterology* 1988; **94**: 463.

61 Munoz LE, Thomas HC, Scheuer PJ *et al.* Is mitochondrial antibody diagnostic of primary biliary cirrhosis? *Gut* 1981; **22**: 136.

62 Nakanuma Y, Ohta G. Histometric and serial

section observations of the intrahepatic bile ducts in primary biliary cirrhosis. *Gastroenterology* 1979; **76**: 1326.

63 Nieri S, Riccardo GG, Salvadori G *et al.* Primary biliary cirrhosis and Graves' disease. *J. clin. Gastroenterol.* 1985; **7**: 434.

64 Olumu AB, Vickers CR, Waring RH *et al.* High incidence of poor sulfoxidation in patients with primary biliary cirrhosis. *N. Engl. J. Med.* 1988; **318**: 1089.

65 Pares A, Rimola A, Bruguera M *et al.* Renal tubular acidosis in primary biliary cirrhosis. *Gastroenterology* 1981; **80**: 681.

66 Penner E. Demonstration of immune complexes containing the ribonucleoprotein antigen R_o in primary biliary cirrhosis. *Gastroenterology* 1986; **90**: 724.

67 Penner E, Goldenberg H, Meryn S *et al.* A dot-immunobinding assay for antimitochondrial antibodies. *Hepatology* 1986; **6**: 381.

68 Potter BJ, Elias E, Thomas HC *et al.* Complement metabolism in chronic liver disease: catabolism of Clq in chronic active liver disease and primary biliary cirrhosis. *Gastroenterology* 1980; **78**: 1034.

69 Poupon R, Chretien Y, Poupon RE *et al.* Is ursodeoxycholic acid an effective treatment for primary biliary cirrhosis? *Lancet* 1987; **i**: 834.

70 Powell FC, Schroeter AL, Dickson ER. Primary biliary cirrhosis and the CREST syndrome. A report of 22 cases. *Q. J. Med.* 1987; **62**: 75.

71 Rai GS, Hamlyn AN, Dahl MGC *et al.* Primary biliary cirrhosis, cutaneous capillaritis and IgM-associated membranous glomerulonephritis. *Br. med. J.* 1977; **i**: 817.

72 Reynolds TB. The 'Butterfly' sign in patients with chronic jaundice and pruritus. *Ann. intern. Med.* 1973; **78**: 545.

73 Reynolds TB, Denison EK, Frankl HD *et al.* Primary biliary cirrhosis with scleroderma, Raynaud's phenomenon and telangiectasia: new syndrome. *Am. J. Med.* 1971; **50**: 302.

74 Roll J, Boyer JL, Barry D *et al.* The prognostic importance of clinical and histologic features in asymptomatic and symptomatic primary biliary cirrhosis. *N. Engl. J. Med.* 1983; **308**: 1.

75 Ros E, Garcia-Puges A, Reixach M *et al.* Fat digestion and exocrine pancreatic function in primary biliary cirrhosis. *Gastroenterology* 1984; **87**: 180.

78 Routhier G, Epstein O, Janossy G *et al.* Effects of cyclosporin A on suppressor and inducer T lymphocytes in primary biliary cirrhosis. *Lancet* 1980; **ii**: 1223.

79 Rubin E, Schaffner F, Popper H. Primary biliary cirrhosis: chronic non-suppurative destructive cholangitis. *Am. J. Pathol.* 1965; **46**: 387.

80 Rutan G, Martinez AJ, Fieshko JT *et al.* Primary

81 Scheuer PJ. Primary biliary cirrhosis. *Proc. R. Soc. Med.* 1967; **60**: 1257.

82 Selinger S, Tsai J, Pulini M *et al.* Autoimmune thrombocytopenia and primary biliary cirrhosis with hypoglycemia and insulin receptor auto-antibodies. *Am. intern. Med.* 1987; **107**: 686.

83 Shapiro JM, Smith H, Schaffner F. Serum bilirubin: a prognostic factor in primary biliary cirrhosis. *Gut* 1979; **20**: 137.

84 Sherlock S. Primary biliary cirrhosis (chronic intrahepatic obstructive jaundice). *Am. J. Gastroenterol.* 1959; **31**: 574.

85 Sherlock S. Primary biliary cirrhosis: critical evaluation and treatment policies. *Scand. J. Gastroenterol.* 1982; Suppl. no. **77**: 63.

86 Sherlock S, Scheuer PJ. The presentation and diagnosis of 100 patients with primary biliary cirrhosis. *N. Engl. J. Med.* 1973; **289**: 674.

87 Sherlock S. The syndrome of disappearing intrahepatic bile ducts. *Lancet* 1987; **ii**: 493.

88 Smallwood RA, Williams HA, Rosenoer VM *et al.* Liver-copper levels in liver disease: studies using neutron activation analysis. *Lancet* 1968; **ii**: 1310.

89 Snover DC, Weisdorf SA, Ramsay NK *et al.* Hepatic graft versus host disease: a study of the predictive value of liver biopsy in diagnosis. *Hepatology* 1984; **4**: 123.

90 Spinsi R, Smith-Laing G, Epstein O *et al.* Results of portal decompression in patients with primary biliary cirrhosis. *Gut* 1981; **22**: 345.

91 Stanley NN, Fox RA, Whimster WF *et al.* Primary biliary cirrhosis or sarcoidosis—or both? *N. Engl. J. Med.* 1972; **287**: 1282.

92 Summerfield JA, Scott J, Berman M *et al.* Benign recurrent intrahepatic cholestasis: studies of bilirubin kinetics, bile acids, and cholangiography. *Gut* 1980; **21**: 154.

93 Thomas PK, Walker JG. Xanthomatous neuropathy in primary biliary cirrhosis. *Brain* 1965; **88**: 1079.

94 Tong MJ, Nies KM, Reynolds TB *et al.* Immunological studies in familial primary biliary cirrhosis. *Gastroenterology* 1976; **71**: 305.

95 Triger DR. Primary biliary cirrhosis: an epidemiological study. *Br. Med. J.* 1980; **281**: 772.

96 Van Den Oord JJ, Sicot R, Desmet VJ. Expression of MHC products by normal and abnormal bile duct epithelium. *J. Hepatol.* 1986; **3**: 310.

97 Walker JG, Doniach D, Roitt IM *et al.* Serological tests in diagnosis of primary biliary cirrhosis. *Lancet* 1965; **i**: 827.

98 Wallace JG Jr, Tong MJ, Ueki BH *et al.* Pulmonary involvement in primary biliary cirrhosis. *J. clin. Gastroenterol.* 1987; **9**: 431.

99 Wallaert B, Bonniere P, Prin L. Primary biliary

cirrhosis. Subclinical inflammatory alveolitis in patients with normal chest roentgenograms. *Chest* 1986; **90:** 842.

100 Wallwork J, Williams R, Calne RY. Transplantation of liyer, heart and lungs for primary biliary cirrhosis and primary pulmonary hypertension. *Lancet* 1987; **2:** 182.

101 Warnes TW, Smith A, Lee FI *et al.* A controlled trial of colchicine in primary biliary cirrhosis. Trial design and preliminary report. *J. Hepatol* 1987; 5:1.

102 Weber P, Brenner J, Stechemesser E *et al.* Characterization and clinical relevance of a new complement-fixing antibody—anti-M8—in patients with primary biliary cirrhosis. *Hepatology* 1986; **6:** 553.

103 Wolke AM, Schaffner F, Kapelman B *et al.* Malignancy in primary biliary cirrhosis. High incidence of breast cancer in affected women. *Am. J. Med.* 1984; **76:** 1075.

104 Yamada G, Hyodo I, Tobe K *et al.* Ultrastructural immunocytochemical analysis of lymphocytes infiltrating bile duct epithelia in primary biliary cirrhosis. *Hepatology* 1986; **6:** 385.

105 Yeaman SJ, Fussey SPM, Danner DJ *et al.* Primary biliary cirrhosis: identification of a major M2 mitochondrial autoantigen. *Lancet* 1988; **i:** 1067.

106 Zeegen R, Stansfeld AG, Dawson AM *et al.* Bleeding oesophageal varices as the presenting feature in primary biliary cirrhosis. *Lancet* 1969: **ii:** 9.

15 · Sclerosing Cholangitis

This is a syndrome which has many causes (table 15.1). The end result is progressive fibrosis and ultimately disappearance of intra- or extra-hepatic ducts or both [49]. In the early stages the impact is on the biliary system and hepatocyte damage is minor; liver failure occurs late. Consequently the prognosis for sclerosing cholangitis is better than for diseases that affect primarily the hepatocyte. Ultimately, biliary cirrhosis and hepato-cellular failure evolve.

Primary sclerosing cholangitis

The condition is of unknown cause. All parts of the biliary tree can be involved in a chronic, fibrosing, inflammatory process which results in obliteration of the biliary tree and ultimately in biliary cirrhosis [7, 24]. The extent of involvement of different parts of the biliary tree varies. The condition may be localized to intra- or extra-hepatic ducts. Eventually interlobular, septal and segmental bile ducts are replaced by fibrous cords. Involvement of very small ducts in the portal (zone 1) areas led to the term *pericholangitis* [59].

Diagnostic criteria are generalized beading and stenosis of the biliary tree on cholangiography with absence of either choledocholithiasis or a history of bile duct surgery [9]. Bile duct cancer must be excluded, usually by prolonged follow-up [60].

AETIOLOGY

About half the patients also suffer from ulcerative colitis and, very rarely, from regional ileitis. The cholangitis may even precede colitis [53] by as much as three years.

Copper is retained in the liver as with all types of cholestasis, but is probably non-toxic.

There is a familial occurrence of primary sclerosing cholangitis and ulcerative colitis [40]. Three sets of siblings from three families have been reported with primary sclerosing cholangitis and ulcerative colitis [40].

The histocompatibility antigen HLA-B8 is associated with ulcerative colitis and with many diseases in which autoantibodies are found. There is an increased prevalence of HLA-B8 in patients with primary sclerosing cholangitis with or without ulcerative colitis [8]. Circulating antibodies to some antigen in obstructed portal tracts are found, especially in those with the HLA-B8 phenotype [9]. Nevertheless, it is difficult to fit primary sclerosing cholangitis into the immunological pattern seen in such diseases as primary biliary cirrhosis or auto-immune chronic active hepatitis which are

Table 15.1. Sclerosing cholangitis

Primary

Associated with immunodeficiency
  Genetic
  AIDS
  Graft-versus-host disease

Infective
  Bacterial with biliary obstruction
  Parasitic (*Clonorchis sinesis*)
  Opportunistic

Vascular
  Trauma
  Allograft rejection
  Hepatic arterial chemotherapy
  Clotting diseases

Drug-related
  Hydatid caustics
  Thiabendazole

Histiocytosis X

associated with an increased prevalence of HLA-B8 among patients [49]. In primary sclerosing cholangitis, circulating antibodies to tissue components such as nuclei, actin or mitochondria are absent or present in low titre. However, enhanced autoreactivity of T-lymphocytes has been shown in the blood [26]. Primary sclerosing cholangitis has also been associated with several immunodeficiency syndromes. These may reduce host defences allowing intestinal bacteria to overgrow and so cause ascending cholangitis. The association may be analogous to that seen with ulcerative colitis, i.e. sclerosing cholangitis could well be infectious rather than immunological.

Serum immune-complex activity is higher in patients with ulcerative colitis and primary sclerosing cholangitis than in those with ulcerative colitis alone [5]. Moreover, Fc receptor-mediated systemic clearance of immune-complex-like material is impaired in patients with ulcerative colitis and chronic liver disease [35]. Finally, concentrations of biliary immune complexes are increased in patients with primary sclerosing cholangitis [2]. It is uncertain whether all these changes are simply secondary to biliary damage or whether they indicate primary immune-complex injury.

When toxic pro-inflammatory bacterial peptides are introduced into the colon of rats with experimental colitis, an increased biliary excretion is found [20]. The liver shows pericholangitis. This is a link between ulcerative colitis and sclerosing cholangitis.

It is difficult to fit all these genetic and immunological observations together with the association with ulcerative colitis. An infective agent operating on a genetically and immunologically susceptible individual remains a possibility.

CLINICAL FEATURES (table 15.2) [7, 24]

Males are twice as commonly affected as females, usually between the ages of 25 and 45, but primary sclerosing cholangitis can affect children as young as two (mean age 5) usually

Table 15.2. Symptoms at presentation in 29 patients with primary sclerosing cholangitis (Chapman *et al.* 1980). n=number of patients

Symptoms	n	%
Jaundice	21	72
Pruritus	20	69
Weight loss	23	79
Right upper quadrant pain	21	72
Acute cholangitis	13	45
Bleeding oesophageal varices	4	14
Malaise	1	3
Asymptomatic	2	7
Total	29	

with associated chronic ulcerative colitis [17, 51].

The patient presents with weight loss, fatigue, right upper quadrant abdominal pain and pruritus, and with intermittent jaundice. The patient can present with an established cirrhosis and portal hypertension usually presinusoidal without prior symptoms and signs of cholangitis or cholestasis. The patient may have been treated for cryptogenic cirrhosis for many years.

An increasing number are being diagnosed when asymptomatic and without any abnormal physical signs. This may be when a persistently raised serum alkaline phosphatase is found incidentally in screening patients with ulcerative colitis. About 4% of such patients will have sclerosing cholangitis if cholangiography is performed [48]. These patients may remain well over many years without any evidence of deterioration in laboratory findings or despite, in some cases, progressive cholangiographic changes. It can be present on a cholangiogram even if biochemical tests, including serum alkaline phosphatase, are normal [10]. Ulcerative colitis (but rarely Crohn's disease) should be sought by barium enema, sigmoidoscopy and rectal biopsy, even if there are no features of colonic disease. The colitis is usually chronic, diffuse and mild to moderate. The activity of the cholangitis is inversely related to that of the colitis. There are prolonged remissions. The primary sclerosing cholangitis may be diagnosed before or after the colitis. The course does not differ whether or not there is associated ulcerative colitis [24].

Perfusion studies of bile ducts in livers removed at the time of transplantation show intra-hepatic tubular and saccular cholangiectasia with transformation of bile ducts into fibrous cords and eventually complete loss of ducts [27].

LABORATORY INVESTIGATIONS

Serum biochemical tests usually show cholestasis with alkaline phosphatase three times above normal. Serum bilirubin values are variable. They can exceed 10 mg/dl, but this is unusual. Serum copper, ceruloplasmin and liver copper contents are increased as in all patients with cholestasis.

The serum mitochondrial antibody is always absent.

Eosinophilia is a rare finding.

LIVER BIOPSY (table 15.3) [7, 25]

The portal zones are infiltrated with small and large lymphocytes, polymorphs and occasional macrophages and eosinophils (fig. 15.1). The interlobular ductules show a periductular inflammation with occasional epithelial desquamation. Intralobular inflammatory cell

Table 15.3. Histological findings in 29 patients with primary sclerosing cholangitis (Chapman *et al.* 1980)

	−	+	++
Portal changes			
Inflammation	0	17	12
Bile duct diminution	12	10	7
Periductal fibrosis	18	9	2
Bile ductular proliferation	4	7	18
Lobular changes			
Piecemeal necrosis	10	8	11
Focal necrosis	11	18	0
Focal inflammation	12	17	0
Kupffer cell hyperplasia	5	11	13

accumulations may be noted and the Kupffer cells are swollen and prominent. Cholestasis is inconspicuous unless jaundice is deep.

As the disease continues fibrosis develops in the portal tracts until the small ducts are surrounded by a cuff of fibrous tissue (fig. 15.3). The portal zones adopt a stellate appearance (fig. 15.2).

The appearances are not diagnostic, but the association of reduced numbers of bile ducts, ductular proliferation and substantial copper deposition with piecemeal necrosis is very suggestive of primary sclerosing cholangitis and indicates the need for cholangiography [7].

Histology of the common bile ducts shows non-diagnostic fibrosis and inflammation (figs 15.3, 15.4).

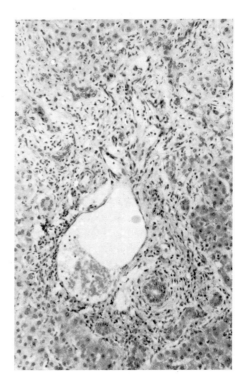

Fig. 15.1. Sclerosing cholangitis and pericholangitis. The portal zone is oedematous and expanded with proliferated bile ducts and an inflammatory cell infiltrate. H & E, ×160.

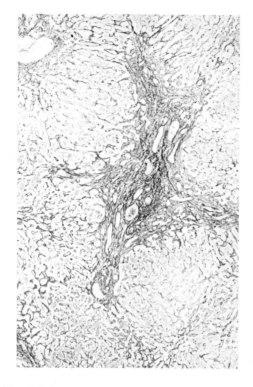

Fig. 15.2. Reticulin preparation of liver biopsy shows stellate expansion of portal zones (Thorpe *et al.* 1967).

CHOLANGIOGRAPHY [7, 28]

ERCP is the most successful technique, although percutaneous trans-hepatic cholangiography may be successful. The appearances are diagnostic with areas of irregular stricturing and dilatation (beading) of the intra- and extra-hepatic biliary tree (fig. 15.5).

The strictures are short (1 to 2 cm long) and angular with intervening segments of apparently normal or slightly dilated ducts. Diverticulum-like output pouchings may be seen along the common bile duct [27].

Cholangiograms may show involvement of the intra-hepatic ducts alone, the extra-hepatic ducts alone or even one hepatic duct.

IMAGING

Ultrasound shows thickening of the bile ducts

[58]. CT shows focal discontinuous minimal biliary dilatation, mimicked only by rare, diffuse cholangiocarcinoma [41].

^{99m}Technetium-labelled iminodiacetic acid planar and single photon emission CT scintigraphy has been used for diagnosis. The half-life may be useful in assessing the course [43].

DIAGNOSIS

The cholangiographic appearances and the negative mitochondrial antibody test distinguish primary sclerosing cholangitis from primary biliary cirrhosis (table 15.4).

Primary sclerosing cholangitis can present as a cryptogenic cirrhosis. The increased serum alkaline phosphatase provides the clue to the diagnosis and indicates cholangiography.

Bile duct carcinoma may complicate large or small duct (pericholangiitis) primary sclerosing cholangitis, usually in those with ulcerative colitis (fig. 15.6) [60]. The prevalence rate is 0.5% and the mean survival 11.8 months [36]. It should be suspected if the patient becomes progressively jaundiced. Suggestive cholangiographic features are biliary dilatation, progressive biliary stricture and intra-duct polyps [28]. If biliary stents are being introduced every attempt should be made to obtain early confirmation by brushings, cytology and needle biopsy.

The differentiation from secondary sclerosing cholangitis due to such conditions as post-operative biliary stricture or choledocholithiasis depends on the history of previous surgery or the demonstration of gallstones.

Histiocytosis X may simulate primary sclerosing cholangitis and is diagnosed by the clinical features and biopsy of affected tissues [56].

PROGNOSIS

The main complications are recurrent acute cholangitis bleeding from oesophageal varices, and cholangiocarcinoma. The course is very variable. Some patients remain asymptomatic for many years, while others develop deep jaundice and liver failure and are dead in a few

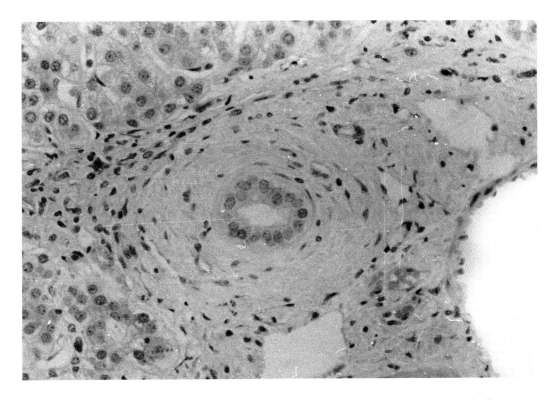

Fig. 15.3. Intra-hepatic bile duct shows abnormal epithelium and concentric periductal whorls of collagen.

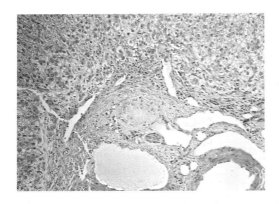

Fig. 15.4. A heavily fibrosed portal zone contains a ring representing an obliterated bile duct.

months. In one series, the mean duration in eleven patients from onset of symptoms to death was seven years [7]. In another series of 53 patients, 75% were alive nine years after diagnosis [18]. Involvement of extrahepatic ducts is worse than intrahepatic alone (fig. 15.7) [19].

Because of portal hypertension, peristomal varies may bleed after proctocolectomy [61].

TREATMENT

There is no specific treatment. Systemic corticosteroids have not proven of value although controlled trials have not been conducted.

D-penicillamine is of little benefit.

Colectomy does not affect the course of primary sclerosing cholangitis associated with ulcerative colitis. Diagnostic surgery is not required except, occasionally, when there is difficulty in excluding bile duct carcinoma.

Attempts at complete surgical relief of the biliary obstruction are clearly impractical as the entire biliary tract is involved. Local strictures in major bile ducts may be amenable to the

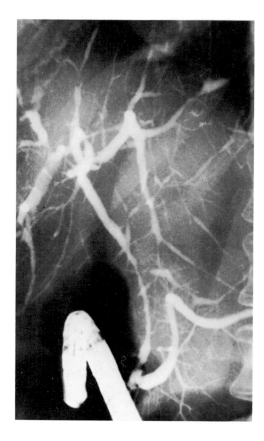

Fig. 15.5. ERCP in primary sclerosing cholangitis shows an irregular common bile duct and beading irregularities in the intra-hepatic bile ducts.

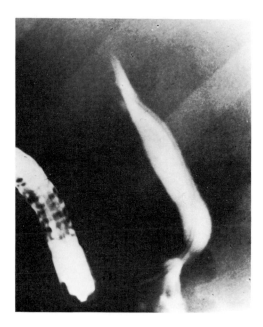

Fig. 15.6. ERCP in bile duct carcinoma shows the common bile duct terminating in a nipple-like deformity.

trans-hepatic introduction of stents, or temporarily to balloon dilatation via the trans-hepatic or endoscopic route [33]. More aggressive surgery is said to be beneficial in the deeply jaundiced patient with hilar or common bile duct biliary obstruction. These may increase cholangitis and have never been subjected to controlled trials.

Primary sclerosing cholangitis is the third most common indication for *liver transplantation* in adults. About 70% of those transplanted survive one year with a five-year survival of 57% (table 15.5) [32]. The decision to transplant should not be postponed too long. Previous palliative surgery on bile ducts should be avoided as it makes the transplant more difficult, it takes longer and greater

quantities of blood transfusion are required. In 5 of 50 patients in one series, a cholangiocarcinoma was diagnosed from the removed liver [32]. In two of these the tumour has already returned.

In post-transplant patients the ulcerative colitis becomes active in about a third but this is usually mild and responds to medical treatment.

Sclerosing cholangitis associated with immunodeficiency

Genetic

Immunodeficiency may reduce host defences, allowing intestinal bacteria to overgrow and so cause ascending cholangitis. The clinical picture, liver biopsy and cholangiographic appearances are indistinguishable from primary sclerosing cholangitis.

Associated immunodeficiency syndromes ,include familial combined immunodeficiency [42, 55], hyperimmunoglobulin M immunodeficiency [15], angioimmunoblastic lymphadenopathy

Table 15.4. Primary sclerosing cholangitis (PSC) and primary biliary cirrhosis (PBC)

	PSC	PBC
Sex	66% male	90% female
Presentation	Fatigue, jaundice, pruritus, cholangitis, weight loss, RUQ pain	Pruritus Jaundice
Serum mitochondrial antibody	−ve or low titre	+ve
Cholangiography (bile ducts)	Beaded, irregular	Pruned
Liver biopsy		
Bile duct lesions	+	+
Granulomas	−	+
Copper	+	+
Associated diseases	Ulcerative colitis Retro-orbital and retro-peritoneal fibrosis Immunodeficiency Cholangiocarcinoma	Arthritis Sicca syndrome Autoimmune diseases Thyroiditis

Table 15.5. Hepatic transplantation in primary sclerosing cholangitis (Marsh *et al.* 1988)

Number	Survived (%)		Incidental cholangiocarcinoma
	1 year	5 years	
55	71	57	5

[3], X-linked immunodeficiency [38] and immunodeficiency with transient T-cell abnormalities [12]. Sclerosing cholangitis in childhood is often associated with immuno-deficiency.

AIDS

In patients with AIDS, opportunist infections can lead to secondary sclerosing cholangitis [44, 47].

In immunosuppressed patients, *crypto-sporidium*, a protozoa, can cause sclerosing cholangitis and biliary strictures [12, 31]. Cytomegalovirus infection can cause progressive

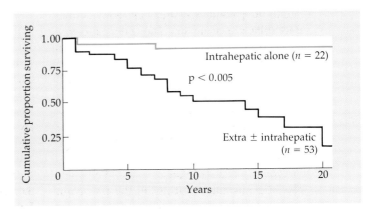

Fig. 15.7. Cumulative survival of patients with primary sclerosing cholangitis according to distribution of cholangiographic changes (Herrmann *et al.* 1988).

mucosal irregularities of the intra and extra-hepatic bile ducts, with ultimate bile duct destruction [1].

The infection may be a mixed one and in one patient with transfusion-related AIDS, sclerosing cholangitis was related to *Cryptococcus*, *Candida albicans* and *Klebsiella pneumoniae* [11].

Primary sclerosing cholangitis and AIDS cholangitis are different. In sclerosing cholangitis the inflammatory infiltration surrounding diseased bile ducts is rich in T-4 lymphocytes, the sub-population specifically depleted in AIDS patients [45].

Graft-versus-host disease

Aberrant expression of HLA class 2 antigen on bile ducts is seen in the transplanted human liver undergoing rejection and in patients with graft-versus-host disease following allogenic bone marrow transplantation (fig. 15.8) [14, 34]. Rejection is marked by progressive non-suppurative cholangitis culminating in disappearance of interlobular bile ducts [57]. The bile duct epithelium is penetrated by mononuclear cells with focal necrosis and rupture of the epithelium. Similar lesions are found in graft-versus-host disease following allogenic bone marrow transplantation [52]. In one such patient, marked cholestatic jaundice lasted 10 years, and serial liver biopsies confirmed progressive biliary-type fibrosis and cirrhosis [23]. She ultimately died in liver failure progressing rapidly during the last year of life. This course strongly resembles that of primary biliary cirrhosis.

Vanishing bile ducts after human liver transplantation may be related to donor/recipient HLA class 1 mismatch with class 1 antigen expression on bile duct epithelium and also to an immunological reaction at the level of HLA class 2 antigens [16].

Infective cholangitis

Bacterial cholangitis is rare in the absence of mechanical biliary obstruction. The infection

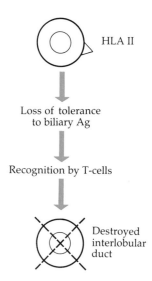

Fig. 15.8. Hepatic rejection (graft-versus-host disease). HLA class antigens are displayed on the bile duct. There is loss of tolerance to biliary antigens which are recognized by cytotoxic T-cells and the interlobular ducts are destroyed.

presumably ascends from the gut. The presence of a biliary stricture results in overgrowth of enteric organisms in the upper small intestine.

The damaged ducts show infiltration of their walls with polymorphs and destruction of the epithelium. Ultimately, the bile duct is replaced by a fibrous cord, the appearances resembling those of primary sclerosing cholangitis. The causes include choledocholithiasis, biliary strictures and stenosis of biliary-enteric anastomoses. The bile duct loss is irreversible and a point comes when, even if the cause of the biliary obstruction can be removed, for instance gallstones, the bile duct destruction with biliary cirrhosis persists.

If the common bile or hepatic duct is surgically anastomosed to a stagnant loop of duodenum, continued access of the biliary system to gut organisms can result in bacterial cholangitis without biliary obstruction (fig. 15.9). A similar sequence may follow sphincteroplasty.

The sclerosing cholangitis associated with infection by the Chinese liver fluke (*Clonorchis sinensis*) is related to secondary infection,

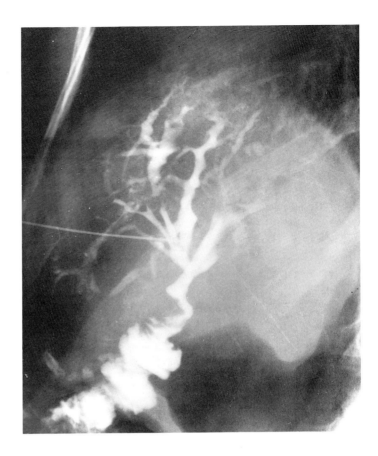

Fig. 15.9. Percutaneous cholangiography following choledochojejunostomy. There is no obstruction to flow of contrast into the jejunum but an intrahepatic sclerosing cholangitis, marked by strictures and beading has developed.

usually with *E. coli*, following biliary obstruction by the fluke.

Vascular cholangitis

The bile ducts have a rich blood supply from the hepatic artery (see Chapter 11). Interference leads to ischaemic necrosis of the bile ducts, both extra- and intra-hepatic, and to their ultimate disappearance.

The hepatic arterial supply of the bile ducts between the confluence of the right and left hepatic duct and the first part of the duodenum is essentially axial, and largely from below [39]. Injury to this supply, for instance during cholecystectomy, leads to ischaemia of the duct wall and damage to the ductal mucosa so allowing bile to enter the duct causing fibrosis and stricture [54]. A similar sequence can complicate hepatic transplantation [62] particularly if the segment of recipient duct is too short so depriving it of its arterial supply.

Biliary ischaemia secondary to intimal thickening of hepatic arterioles is a rare feature of chronic allograft rejection in man [57].

Chronic infusion of 5-fluorodeoxyuridine (5-FUDR) into the hepatic artery though an implantable pump can be used to treat hepatic mestastases from colo-rectal adenocarcinoma. This therapy may be followed by biliary sclerosis in 8–21% of cases resembling primary sclerosing cholangitis [6, 21]. Ducts in zone 1 (portal) are involved as these depend mainly on hepatic arterial supply. The stricturing of main bile ducts can be so severe that treatment by the insertion of an endoscopic biliary stent may be necessary [50]. Severe portal hypertension can result [13].

Bile duct necrosis has also followed hepatic arterial embolization for malignant liver tumours [29]. Lupus anticoagulant, a spontaneously acquired immuno-globulin that interferes with phospholipid-dependent coagulation, has been reported in association with primary sclerosing cholangitis [22]. This is possibly related to hepatic arterial microthrombi. The association of primary sclerosing cholangitis with immune complexes might have a similar mechanism.

Drug-related cholangitis

Hydatid cysts often communicate with the biliary tree and sclerosing cholangitis has followed the injection of a scolicidal solution (2% formaldehyde, 20% sodium chloride or alcohol) [4, 37, 46]. Within months, the strictures result in jaundice, biliary cirrhosis and portal hypertension. Only a part of the biliary tree is usually involved. Similar lesions have been produced in animals by injecting formaldehyde or 20% sodium chloride into the biliary tree.

Thiabendazole therapy has been associated with the cholangiographic appearances of sclerosing cholangitis [30].

Histiocytosis X

A cholangiographic picture identical with that of primary sclerosing cholangitis may complicate histiocytosis X [56]. The biliary lesions progress from a hyperplastic to a granulomatous, xanthomatous and, finally, a fibrotic stage. Clinically, the picture resembles primary sclerosing cholangitis.

References

1 Agha FP, Nostrant TT, Abrams GD *et al.* Cytomegalovirus cholangitis in a homosexual man with acquired immune deficiency syndrome. *Am. J. Gastroenterol.* 1986; **81**: 1068.

2 Alberti-Flor JJ, De Medina M, Jeffers L *et al.* Elevated levels of immunoglobulins and immune complexes in the bile of patients with primary sclerosing cholangitis. *Am. J. Gastroenterol.* 1986; **81**: 325.

3 Bass NM, Chapman RW, O'Reilly A *et al.* Primary sclerosing cholangitis associated with angioim-munoblastic lymphadenopathy. *Gastroenterology* 1983; **85**: 420.

4 Belghiti J, Beuhamou J-P, Heuly S *et al.* Caustic sclerosing cholangitis. A complication of the surgical treatment of hydatid disease of the liver. *Arch. Surg.* 1986; **121**: 1162.

5 Bodenheimer HC, LaRusso NF, Thayer WR *et al.* Elevated circulating immune complexes in primary sclerosing cholangitis. *Hepatology* 1983; **3**: 150.

6 Chang AE, Schneider PD, Sugarbaker PH *et al.* A prospective randomized trial of regional versus systemic continuous 5-fluorodeoxyuridine chemotherapy in the treatment of colorectal liver metastases. *Ann. Surg.* 1987; **206**: 685.

7 Chapman RWG, Arborgh BAM, Rhodes JM *et al.* Primary sclerosing cholangitis—a review of its clinical features, cholangiography and hepatic histology. *Gut* 1980; **21**: 870.

8 Chapman RW, Varghese Z, Gaul R *et al.* Association of primary sclerosing cholangitis with HLA-B8. *Gut* 1983; **24**: 38.

9 Chapman RW, Cottone M, Selby WS *et al.* Serum autoantibodies, ulcerative colitis and primary sclerosing cholangitis. *Gut* 1986; **27**: 86.

10 Clements D, Rhodes JM, Elias E. Severe bile duct lesions without biochemical evidence of cholestasis in a case of sclerosing cholangitis. *J. Hepatol* 1986; **3**: 72.

11 Cockerill FR, Hurley DV, Malagelada JR *et al.* Polymicrobial cholangitis and Kaposi's sarcoma in blood product transfusion-related acquired immune deficiency syndrome. *Am. J. Med.* 1986; **80**: 1237.

12 Davis JJ, Heyman MB, Ferrell L *et al.* Sclerosing cholangitis associated with chronic cryptosporidiosis in child with a congenital immunodeficiency disorder. *Am. J. Gastroenterol.* 1987; **82**: 1196.

13 Dikengil A, Siskind BN, Morse SS *et al.* Sclerosing cholangitis from intra-arterial floxuridine. *J. clin. Gastroenterol.* 1986; **8**: 690.

14 Dilly SA, Sloane JP. An immunohistological study of human hepatic graft-versus-host disease. *Clin. exp. Immunol.* 1985; **62**: 545.

15 Di Palma JA, Strobel CT, Farrow JG. Primary sclerosing cholangitis associated with hyperimmunoglobulin M immuno-deficiency (dysgammaglobulinemia). *Gastroenterology* 1986: **91**: 464.

16 Donaldson PT, Alexander GJM, O'Grady J *et al.* Evidence for an immune response to HLA class 1 antigens in the vanishing-bile duct syndrome after liver transplantation. *Lancet* 1987; **i**: 945.

17 El-Shabrawi M, Wilkinson ML, Portmann B *et al.* Primary sclerosing cholangitis in childhood. *Gastroenterology* 1987; **92**: 1226.

18 Helzberg JH, Petersen JM, Boyer JL. Improved survival with primary sclerosing cholangitis. A

review of clinicopathologic features and comparison of symptomatic and asymptomatic patients. *Gastroenterology* 1987; **92**: 1869.

19 Herrmann R, Dooley J S, Sherlock S. *et al*. Natural history and mortality in primary sclerosing cholangitis. Gut 1988; in press.

20 Hobson CH, Butt TJ, Ferry DM *et al*. Enterohepatic circulation of bacterial chemotactic peptide in rats with experimental colitis. *Gastroenterology* 1988; **94**: 1006.

21 Kemeny MM, Battifora H, Blayney DW *et al*. Sclerosing cholangitis after continuous hepatic artery infusion of FUDR. *Ann. Surg.* 1985; **202**: 176.

22 Kirby DF, Blei AT, Rosen ST *et al*. Primary sclerosing cholangitis in the presence of a lupus anticoagulant. *Amer. J. Med.* 1986; **81**: 1077.

23 Knapp AB, Crawford JM, Rappeport JM *et al*. Cirrhosis as a consequence of graft-versus-host disease. *Gastroenterology* 1987; **92**: 513.

24 LaRusso NF, Wiesner RH, Ludwig J *et al*. Primary sclerosing cholangitis. *N. Engl. J. Med.* 1984; **310**: 899.

25 Lefkowitch JH. Primary sclerosing cholangitis. *Arch. intern. Med.* 1982; **142**: 1157.

26 Lindor KD, Wiesner RH, LaRusso NF *et al*. Enhanced autoreactivity of T-lymphocytes in primary sclerosing cholangitis. *Hepatology* 1987; **7**: 884.

27 Ludwig J, MacCarty RL, LaRusso NF. Intrahepatic cholangiectases and large duct obliteration in primary sclerosing cholangitis. *Hepatology* 1986; **6**; 560.

28 MacCarty RL, LaRusso NF, Wiesner RH *et al*. Primary sclerosing cholangitis: findings on cholangiography and pancreatography. *Radiology* 1983; **149**: 39.

29 Makuuchi M, Sukigara M, Mori T *et al*. Bile duct necrosis: complication of transcatheter hepatic arterial embolization. *Radiology* 1985; **156**: 331.

30 Manivel JC, Bloomer JR, Snover DC. Progressive bile duct injury after thiabendazole administration. *Gastroenterology* 1987; **93**: 245.

31 Margulis SJ, Honig CL, Soave R *et al*. Biliary tract obstruction in the acquired immuno-deficiency syndrome. *Ann. int. Med.* 1986; **105**: 207.

32 Marsh JW Jr, Iwatsuki S. Makowka L *et al*. Orthotopic liver transplantation for primary sclerosing cholangitis. *Ann. Surg.* 1988; **207**: 21.

33 May GR, Bender CE, LaRusso NF *et al*. Nonoperative dilatation of dominant strictures in primary sclerosing cholangitis. *Am. J. Roent.* 1985; **145**: 1061.

34 Miglio M, Pignatelli M, Mazzeo V *et al*. Expression of major histocompatibility complex class II antigens on bile duct epithelium in patients with hepatic graft-versus-host disease after bone marrow trans-plantation. *J. Hepatol.* 1987; **5**; 182.

35 Minuk GY, Hershfield NB, Lee WY *et al*. Reticulo-endothelial system Fc receptor-mediated clearance of IgG-tagged erythrocytes from the circulation of patients with idiopathic ulcerative colitis and chronic liver disease. *Hepatology* 1986; **6**: 1.

36 Mir-Madjlessi SH, Farmer RG, Sivak MV. Bile duct carcinoma in patients with ulcerative colitis. Relationship to sclerosing cholangitis: report of six cases and re-view of the literature. *Dig. Dis. Sci.* 1987; **32**: 145.

37 Mirouze D, Bories P, Pommier-Layrargues G *et al*. Cholangite sclérosante secondaire à une formolisation accidentelle des voies biliares chez 5 malades porteurs d'un kystehydratique du foie (re production expérimentale) (Abstract). *Gastroenterol. clin. Biol.* 1983; **7**: 200.

38 Naveh Y, Mendelsohn H, Spira G *et al*. Primary sclerosing cholangitis associated with immuno-dificiency. *Am. J. Dis. Child.* 1983; **137**: 114.

39 Northover JMA, Terblanche J. A new look at the arterial supply of the bile duct in man and its surgical implications. *Br. J. Surg.* 1979; **66**: 379.

40 Quigley EMM, LaRusso NF, Ludwig J *et al*. Familial occurrence of primary sclerosing cholangitis and ulcerative colitis. *Gastroenterology* 1983; **85**: 1160.

41 Rahn RH III, Koehler RE, Weyman PJ *et al*. CT appearance of sclerosing cholangitis. *Am. J. Roentgenol.* 1983; **141**: 549.

42 Record CO, Eddleston ALWF, Shilkin KB *et al*. Intrahepatic sclerosing cholangitis associated with a familial immunodeficiency syndrome. *Lancet* 1973; **ii**: 18.

43 Rodman CA, Keeffe EB, Lieberman DA *et al*. Diagnosis of sclerosing cholangitis with technetium 99m-labelled iminodiacetic acid planar and single photon emission computed tomographic scintigraphy. *Gastroenterology* 1987; **92**: 777.

44 Romano AJ, Van Sonnenberg E, Casola G *et al*. Gall bladder and bile duct abnormalities in AIDS. Sonographic findings in 8 patients. *Am. J. Roent.* 1988; **150**: 123.

45 Roulot D, Valla D, Brun-Vezinet F *et al*. Cholangitis in the acquired immuno-deficiency syndrome: report of two cases and review of the literature. *Gut* 1987; **28**: 1653.

46 Russo A, Giannone G, Virgilio C. Sclerosing cholangitis following removal of an echinococcus cyst. *Endoscopy* 1987; **19**: 178.

47 Schneiderman DJ, Cello JP, Laing FC. Papillary stenosis and sclerosing cholangitis in the acquired immunodeficiency syndrome. *Ann. int. Med.* 1987; **106**: 546.

48 Shepherd HA, Selby WS, Chapman RWG *et al*. Ulcerative colitis and persistent liver dysfunction. *Q. J. Med.* 1983; **52**: 503.

49 Sherlock S. The syndrome of disappearing intra-

hepatic bile ducts. *Lancet* 1987; **ii:** 493.

50 Siegel JH, Ramsey WH. Endoscopic biliary stent placement for bile duct stricture after hepatic artery infusion of 5FUDR. *J. Clin. Gastroenterol.* 1986; **8:** 673.

51 Sisto A, Feldman P, Garel L *et al.* Primary sclerosing cholangitis in children: study of five cases and review of the literature. *Pediatrics* 1987; **80:** 918.

52 Sloane JP, Farthing MJG, Powles RL. Histopathological changes in the liver after allogeneic bone marrow transplantation. *J. clin. Path.* 1980; **33:** 344.

53 Steckman M, Drossman DA, Lesesne HR. Hepatobiliary disease that precedes ulcerative colitis. *J. clin. Gastroenterol.* 1984; **6:** 425.

54 Terblanche J, Allison HF, Northover JMA. An ischemic basis for biliary strictures. *Surgery* 1983; **94:** 52.

55 Thomas IT, Ochs HD, Wedgwood RJ. Liver disease and immunodeficiency syndromes. *Lancet* 1974; **i:** 311.

56 Thompson HH, Pitt HA, Lewin KJ *et al.* Sclerosing cholangitis and histocytosis X. *Gut* 1984: **25:** 526.

57 Vierling JM, Fennell RH Jr. Histopathology of early and late human hepatic allograft rejection: evidence of progressive destruction of interlobular bile ducts. *Hepatology* 1985; **5:** 1076.

58 Vrla RF, Gore RM, Schachter H *et al.* Ultrasound demonstration of bile duct thickening in primary sclerosing cholangitis. *J. clin. Gastroenterol.* 1986; **8:** 213.

59 Wee A, Ludwig J. Pericholangitis in chronic ulcerative colitis: primary sclerosing cholangitis of the small bile ducts? *Ann. int. Med.* 1985; **102:** 581.

60 Wee A, Ludwig J. Coffy RJ Jr *et al.* Hepatobiliary carcinoma associated with primary sclerosing cholangitis and chronic ulcerative colitis. *Human Path.* 1985; **16:** 719.

61 Wiesner RH, LaRusso NF, Dozois RR *et al.* Peristomal varices after proctocolectomy in patients with primary sclerosing cholangitis. *Gastroenterology* 1986; **90:** 316.

62 Zajko AB, Campbell WL, Logsdon GA *et al.* Cholangiographic findings in hepatic artery occlusion after liver transplantation. *Am. J. Roent.* 1987; **149:** 485.

16 · Virus Hepatitis

The first reference to epidemic jaundice has been ascribed to Hippocrates. The earliest record in Western Europe is in a letter written in 751 AD by Pope Zacharias to St Boniface, Archbishop of Mainz. Since then there have been numerous accounts of epidemics, particularly during wars. Hepatitis was a problem in the Franco−Prussian War, the American Civil War and World War I. In World War II huge epidemics occurred, particularly in the Middle East and Italy [144].

There are three main varieties [137]. Hepatitis A is a self-limited, faecal-spread disease. Hepatitis B is a parenterally transmitted disease that often becomes chronic. Non-A, non-B hepatitis is ill-defined. It contains many types, some faecally, others parenterally transmitted. It has a high chronicity rate.

Hepatic pathology

The basic pathology of virus A, B and non-A, non-B hepatitis is virtually identical [32, 59].

The essential lesion is an acute inflammation of the entire liver [32]. Hepatic cell necrosis is associated with leucocytic and histiocytic re-action and infiltration. Zone 3 shows the necrosis most markedly and the portal tracts the greatest cellularity (figs 16.1, 16.2 16.3). The sinusoids show cellular infiltration, poly-morphs and eosinophils. Surviving liver cells retain their glycogen. Fatty change is rare. Zone 3 liver cells may show eosinophilic change (*acidophil bodies*), ballooning pleomorphism and hyalinization, and giant multi-nucleated cells may be present. Mitoses are sometimes prominent. Zone 3 cholestasis may be found. Focal 'spotty' necrosis may be seen. Bile duct proliferation is usual and damage is an occasional feature [98]. Hepatitis is found even before the development of jaundice.

The reticulin framework is usually well preserved even in the midst of extreme disorganization. This framework provides a scaffolding when the liver cells regenerate. Inflammatory cells disappear gradually from the portal zones, and some new portal connective tissue can often be found for many months (fig. 16.4). During recovery reticulo-endothelial activity increases throughout, apparently a 'scavenger' phenomenon. A slight increase in stainable fat is seen. The Kupffer cells contain lipofusein pigment and iron.

Occasionally the necrosis may be *confluent* (sub-massive), affecting substantial groups of adjacent liver cells, usually zone 3.

In massive fulminant necrosis the whole acinus is involved. Macroscopically the liver is reduced in size, being smallest in those who die the soonest. It is flaccid and shrunken and the left lobe may be disproportionately atrophied. Nodular regeneration is seen in those surviving for more than two weeks (fig. 16.5). The cut surface shows a 'nutmeg' appearance, red areas of haemorrhage alternating with

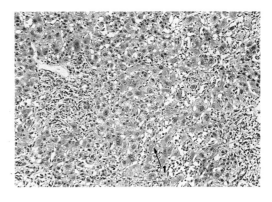

Fig. 16.1. Virus hepatitis: zone 3 (central) (arrow) shows marked loss of liver cells. Zone 1 (portal) shows expansion with cellular infiltration and bile ductular proliferation. (H & E ×40.)

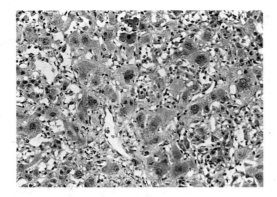

Fig. 16.2. Virus hepatitis: zone 3 shows swollen cells, mitoses and acidophilic bodies. (H & E × 80.)

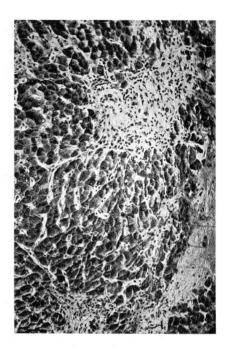

Fig. 16.4. Residual portal zone scarring seen 33 days after the onset of jaundice. (Best's carmine ×100) (Sherlock, 1946).

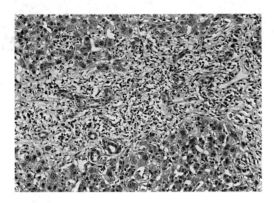

Fig. 16.3. Virus hepatitis: zone 1 (portal tract) shows an acute inflammatory reaction with ductular proliferation. (H & E ×50.)

Electron microscopy

This shows non-specific changes. The rough endoplasmic reticulum is disrupted into vesicles and adherent ribosomes become detached. Large and irregular lysosomes develop which form autophagic vacuoles. The light cells represent ballooned cells and dark cells the eosinophilic bodies and dehydrated remnants of hepatocytes. Mitochondria are clumped, forming hyaloplasmic blebs. Macrophages have approached the sinusoidal cell surface.

During healing, the many polyribosomes form new profiles of endoplasmic reticulum and the smooth endoplasmic reticulum hypertrophies.

Changes in other organs

Regional lymph nodes are large. Splenomegaly is related to cellular proliferation and venous congestion. The bone marrow is moderately hypoplastic, but maturation is usually normal.

yellow patches of necrosis. Necrosis in life is always less than that seen in autopsy material as autolysis proceeds particularly rapidly in the presence of acute hepatitis.

If the confluent necrosis extends from zone 3 to zone 1 the reticulum collapses leaving connective tissue septa. This is termed *bridging* (fig. 16.6). Such bridging may be followed by the development of active fibrous septa nodules and cirrhosis. More usually it is followed by scar formation (*post-necrotic scarring*) (fig. 16.7).

Acute viral hepatitis may be followed by chronic persistent or chronic active hepatitis (Chapter 17).

302

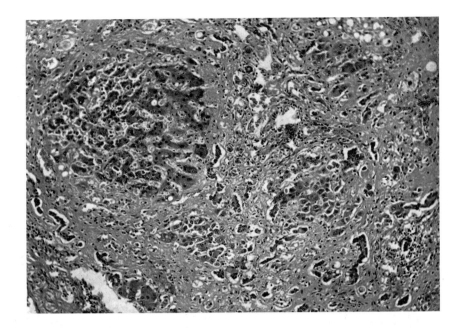

Fig. 16.5. Acute virus hepatitis. Sub-acute massive necrosis with nodular regeneration. (H & E ×120.)

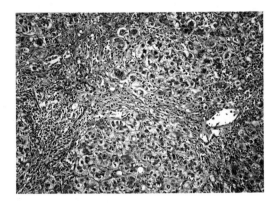

Fig. 16.6. Acute virus hepatitis. A passive septum (bridge) (arrow) has formed between zones 1 and 2. (H & E ×40.)

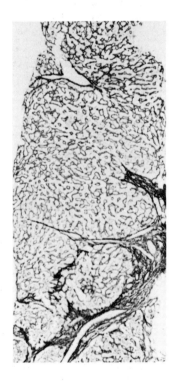

Fig. 16.7. Post-necrotic scarring. The liver biopsy specimen shows scarring, involving and extending from portal tracts. (Reticulin ×34.)

Fatal marrow aplasia has, however, been reported [54]. The pathogenesis is obscure. In about 15% of fatal cases there is ulceration of the gastrointestinal tract—particularly caecal.

The brain shows an acute non-specific degeneration of ganglion cells. Because of the short duration, the cerebral lesions of hepatic coma (Chapter 7) are rarely evident. Occasionally acute pancreatitis and myocarditis have

303

been noted. Haemorrhages are found in most organs.

Virus hepatitis is a multi-system infection involving many organs.

Clinical types

ACUTE HEPATITIS

Note is taken of ethnic origin, jaundiced contacts, recent travel, injections, tattooing, dental treatment, transfusions, homosexuality or ingestion of shellfish. All drugs taken in the previous two months are listed.

The picture varies widely, ranging from anicteric with only slight malaise to a severe and fatal disease culminating in hepatic coma.

In general, type A, type B and non-A, non-B hepatitis run the same clinical course. Type B and non-A, non-B tend to be more severe and may be associated with a serum sickness-like syndrome.

The mildest attack is without symptoms and marked only by a rise in serum transaminase levels. Alternatively, the patient may still be anicteric but suffer gastrointestinal and influenza-like symptoms. Such patients are likely to remain undiagnosed unless there is a clear history of exposure or the patient is being followed up after a blood transfusion. Increasing grades of severity are then encountered ranging from the icteric, from which recovery is usual, through to fulminant, fatal viral hepatitis.

The usual icteric attack in the adult is marked by a prodromal period, usually about three or four days, even up to two or three weeks, during which the patient feels generally unwell, suffers digestive symptoms, particularly anorexia and nausea, and may, in the later stages, have a mild pyrexia. Rigors are unusual. An ache develops in the right upper abdomen. This is increased by jolting movements. There is loss of desire to smoke or to drink alcohol. Malaise is profound and increases towards evening; the patient feels wretched.

Occasionally headache may be severe and, in children, its association with neck rigidity may suggest meningitis. Protein and lymphocytes in the CSF may be raised.

The prodromal period is followed by darkening of the urine and lightening of the faeces. This heralds the development of jaundice and symptoms decrease. The temperature returns to normal and there may be bradycardia. Appetite returns and abdominal discomfort and vomiting cease. Pruritus may appear transiently for a few days.

The liver is palpable with a smooth, tender edge in 70%. Heavy percussion over the right lower ribs posteriorly causes sickening discomfort. The spleen is palpable in about 20% of patients.

The adult loses about 4 kg weight. A few vascular spiders may appear transiently.

After an icteric period of about 1–4 weeks the adult patient usually makes an uninterrupted recovery. In children, improvement is particularly rapid and jaundice mild or absent. The stools regain their colour. The appetite returns. After apparent recovery lassitude and fatigue persist for some weeks. Clinical and biochemical recovery is usual within six months of onset. However, chronic hepatitis may follow types B and non-A, non-B.

Neurological complications, including the Guillain–Barré syndrome, can complicate all forms of viral hepatitis [127].

PROLONGED CHOLESTASIS

Occasionally, prolonged jaundice is of cholestatic type. Onset is acute, jaundice appears and deepens but, within three weeks, the patient starts to itch. After the first few weeks the patient feels well, gains weight and there are no physical signs apart from icterus and slight hepatomegaly. Jaundice persists for 8–29 weeks and recovery is then complete [115]. It is particularly associated with hepatitis A (fig. 16.8) [48].

Liver biopsy shows conspicuous cholestasis which tends to mask the definite, usually mild, hepatitis that is also present.

This type must be differentiated from surgical obstructive jaundice [48]. The acute onset

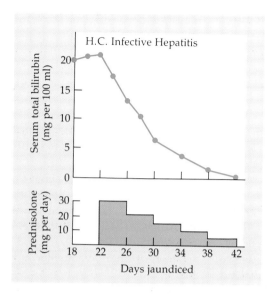

Fig. 16.8. Cholestatic, type A virus hepatitis. Prednisolone therapy was associated with a fall in serum bilirubin values.

and only moderately enlarged liver are the most helpful points. Cholestatic drug jaundice is excluded by the history.

If doubt remains needle biopsy is helpful. Surgical exploration is to be avoided as it may precipitate hepato-cellular failure.

The prognosis is usually excellent with complete clinical recovery and restitution of a normal liver [115].

RELAPSES

These occur in 1.8−15%. In some the original attack is duplicated, usually in milder form. More often, the relapse is simply shown by an increase in serum transaminases and sometimes bilirubin. The relapse may be precipitated by premature activity or by taking large amounts of alcohol. Multiple episodes may occur. Recovery after relapses is usually complete. In some patients relapses may indicate progression to chronic hepatitis.

FULMINANT HEPATITIS (see Chapter 8)

This rare form of the disease usually overwhelms the patient within 10 days. It may develop so rapidly that jaundice is inconspicuous and the disease is confused with an acute psychosis or meningo-encephalitis. Alternatively, the patient, after a typical acute onset, becomes deeply jaundiced. Ominous signs are repeated vomiting, fetor hepaticus, confusion and drowsiness. The 'flapping' tremor may be only transient, but rigidity is usual. Coma supervenes rapidly and the picture becomes that of acute liver failure. Temperature rises, jaundice deepens and the liver shrinks. Widespread haemorrhages may develop.

Leucocytosis may be found in contrast to the usual leucopenia of virus hepatitis. The biochemical changes are those of acute liver failure (Chapter 8). The height of the serum bilirubin and transaminase are poor indicators of prognosis. Transaminase levels may actually fall as the patient's clinical condition worsens. Blood coagulation is grossly deranged and a test of prothrombin is the best indicator of prognosis.

The time relationships and the course depend on whether the cause is A, B or non-A, non-B (table 16.1) [47].

The frequency of the fulminant course in the various types of viral hepatitis depends on the type of patient and the prevalence of hepatitis B carriage. In the United Kingdom and California [86], the non-A, non-B type is more frequent, whereas in Denmark and Greece, hepatitis B predominates [86, 93].

There are clinical differences in the fulminant course of the three types [47]. Pyrexia is most frequent with hepatitis A. The duration of illness before encephalopathy is longer with non-A, non-B. The prothrombin time is greatest with hepatitis B. The bad prognosis in those with a longer duration from onset of illness to encephalopathy is probably related to the greater number of non-A, non-B patients in that group (table 16.1).

POST-HEPATITIS SYNDROME

Adult patients feel below par for variable periods after acute hepatitis. Usually this is a matter of weeks but it may extend to months. This is termed the post-hepatitis s

[117]. It is particularly common in the intelligent, perhaps because of their knowledge of the possible sequelae of hepatitis. Features are anxiety, fatigue, failure to regain weight, anorexia and alcohol intolerance, and right upper abdominal discomfort. The liver edge may be palpable and tender.

Serum transaminases may be raised up to three times normal. Too much attention should not be focused on them and they should not be repeated frequently. This exacerbates the anxiety and a 'transaminitis' is engendered. Serum globulin levels are normal.

Hepatic histology shows only mild, residual, portal zone cellularity and fibrosis with perhaps some fatty change in the liver cells. These features do not differ from those found in patients recovering normally who are now symptom-free. They rarely persist for longer than one year after the acute attack. In general, liver biopsy should not be performed too soon after acute hepatitis, certainly not less than six months, because of the difficulty in distinguishing the usual residual changes from a developing chronic hepatitis.

Treatment consists of reassurance after full investigation. If the acute attack has been type A, chronicity is excluded.

Investigations

URINE AND FAECES

Bilirubin appears in the urine before jaundice. The urinary threshold for bilirubin varies. It is found before the serum level is raised: later it disappears although serum levels remain elevated.

Urobilinogenuria is found in the late pre-icteric phase. At the height of the jaundice, very little bilirubin reaches the intestine, so urobilinogen disappears. Its reappearance indicates commencing recovery. It persists in excess in gradually diminishing amounts until final recovery.

The onset of jaundice is marked by lightening of the faeces. There is moderate steator-rhoea. Reappearance of stool colour denotes impending recovery.

BLOOD CHANGES

Total serum bilirubin levels range widely. Deep jaundice generally implies a prolonged clinical course. An increase in conjugated pigment is early, even when the total bilirubin level is still normal.

Serum alkaline phosphatase level is usually less than three times the upper limit of normal. Serum albumin and globulin are quantitatively unchanged. The serum iron level is raised.

Serum immunoglobulins G and M are raised in about one-third of patients during the acute phase.

Serum transaminase estimations are useful in early diagnosis, in detecting the anicteric case, and for detection of inapparent cases in epidemics. The peak level is found one or two days before or after onset of jaundice. Later in the course the level falls, even if the clinical condition is worsening. The estimation cannot be used prognostically. Values may remain elevated for six months in those who are recovering uneventfully.

In both type A and type B hepatitis antibody against smooth muscle is present, usually in low titre. Mitochondrial antibody is absent.

HAEMATOLOGICAL CHANGES

The pre-icteric stage is marked by leucopenia, lymphopenia and neutropenia. These revert towards normal as jaundice appears. Some 5−28% show atypical lymphocytes (virucytes), resembling those seen in infectious mononucleosis. Acute Coombs' test positive haemolytic anaemia is a rare complication. Haemolysis is commonly precipitated in patients with glucose-6PD deficiency [21].

Aplastic anaemia is very rare [54]. It appears weeks or months after the acute episode and is particularly severe and irreversible. It is not usually associated with A or B infection and may be due to a hitherto unidentified non-A, non-B type. It has been treated by bone marrow transplantation.

The *prothrombin time* is lengthened in the more severe cases and does not return completely to normal with vitamin K therapy.

The *sedimentation rate* of the red cells (ESR) is high in the pre-icteric phase, falls to normal with jaundice, and rises again when the jaundice subsides. It returns to normal with complete recovery.

NEEDLE LIVER BIOPSY

This is rarely indicated in the acute stage. It may ocasionally be needed in older patients to differentiate from extra-hepatic or other forms of intra-hepatic cholestasis and from drug jaundice. It may be used to diagnose the presence and type of chronic complications but should not be performed less than six months after the acute episode else the distinction between the picture of normal recovery and chronic hepatitis may be impossible.

Differential diagnosis

In the *pre-icteric stage*, hepatitis can be confused with other acute infectious diseases, with acute surgical abdomen, especially acute appendicitis, and with acute gastroenteritis. Bile in the urine, tender enlargement of the liver and a rise in serum transaminase values are the most helpful points. The distinction from infectious mononucleosis is outlined in table 16.10. Viral markers are essential.

In the *icteric stage*, the diagnosis must be made from surgical cholestasis. This is outlined in Chapter 12.

The diagnosis of acute virus hepatitis from the drug-related disease depends largely on the history.

Needle liver biopsy is valuable in the problem case. Attempts at a surgical diagnosis are disastrous.

The distinction from Weil's disease is discussed in Chapter 27.

In the *post-icteric stage*, the diagnosis of

organic from non-organic complications necessitates routine investigations for the diagnosis of chronic hepatitis, and these may include needle biopsy.

Prognosis (table 16.1)

Type B infection is said to have the highest mortality. In a survey of 1675 cases in a group of Boston hospitals, one in eight sufferers from transfusion hepatitis (B and non-A, non-B) succumbed whereas only one in 200 died with the type A disease. As many non-icteric cases are not included in the statistics the overall mortality rate is undoubtedly very much lower. In the United Kingdom, non-A, non-B hepatitis had the poorest survival [47].

Those who are elderly or in poor general health clearly have a poor prognosis. Fulminant hepatitis is rare in those less than 15 years old. The non-A, non-B patients tend to be more than 45. Survival rate is the same for males as for females.

Treatment

Prevention

Compulsory notification leads to earlier detection and hence identification of methods of infection, for instance food or water contamination, sexual spread or carriage by blood donors.

Treatment of the acute attack

Treatment has little effect in altering the course. At the outset this is unpredictable and it is wise to treat all attacks as potentially fatal and to insist upon bed rest with bathroom privileges. Traditionally this is enforced until the patient is free of jaundice. A less strict regime may be possible if the patients are young and previously healthy. They can be allowed up when they feel well, regardless of the degree of jaundice. They rest after each meal. If symptoms return, the patient is immediately returned to bed rest. Selected patients treated along these

Table 16.1. Fulminant virus hepatitis in the United Kingdom: aetiology, duration from onset to fulminant and survival (Gimson *et al.* 1983)

	A	B	Non-A, non-B
Frequency (%)	31.5	24.7	43.8
Duration from onset (days)	10	7	21
Survival (%)	43.4	16.6	9.3

liberal lines do not show an increased incidence of later complications.

Convalescence is not allowed until the patient is symptom-free, the liver no longer tender, and the serum bilirubin is less than 1.5 mg/100 ml. The period of convalescence should be twice the period spent in hospital or in bed at home.

The traditional low-fat, high-carbohydrate diet is popular because it has proved the most palatable to the anorexic patient. Apart from this, no benefit accrues from the rigid insistence upon a low-fat diet.

When the appetite returns, high protein intake may hasten recovery. Excess protein, however, is harmful to the severely ill patient in impending hepatic coma. The usual diet in hepatitis is composed of the food most appetizing to the patient. Supplementary vitamins, amino acids and lipotrophic agents are not necessary.

Corticosteroids do not alter the degree of liver necrosis, accelerate the rate of healing or assist in immunity in virus hepatitis. Hepatitis tends towards spontaneous recovery and any benefit is not sufficient to justify the use of this treatment. The drug must be continued into convalescence, for premature withdrawal leads to relapse. A usual course is 30, 20, 15, 10 and 5 mg prednisolone, each dose being given for five days (duration of course 25 days). It should be reserved only for the patient with prolonged cholestasis (fig. 16.8) or the non-B patient who seems to be passing into a subacute stage with persistent jaundice, high serum globulin and transaminase values. The steroid 'whitewash'

improves the morale of both patient and physician but probably has little effect on the healing of the liver [115].

Patients showing signs of acute hepatocellular failure with pre-coma require more active measures and the regime described in Chapter 8 must be instituted.

FOLLOW-UP

The patient should be seen 3–4 weeks after discharge, and if necessary at monthly intervals for the next three months. Special attention should be paid to recurrence of jaundice and to the size of the liver and spleen. Tests should include serum bilirubin, globulin and transaminase levels and hepatitis B markers if originally positive.

The patient should not be questioned too closely about symptoms and feelings of weakness, for the 'post-hepatitis syndrome' can readily be induced by the physician. Exercise must be undertaken and within the limits of fatigue. Alcohol must be denied for six months and preferably one year afterwards. The patient often has little inclination for it and excessive consumption leads to relapses. Diet can be unrestricted.

Virus A (HAV) hepatitis

Hepatitis A accounts for 20–25% of clinical hepatitis in the developed world [79]. It is due to a small 27 nm, cubically symmetrical RNA picorna virus (type 72) (figs 16.9, 16.10) [41].

Like other picorna viruses (small RNA viruses) it has four capsid polypeptides, virus protein (VP 1–4) [131]. Only a single serotype has been identified. However, the genome has been cloned and characterized and a number of minor differences have been identified among isolates from different parts of the world.

The virus has been transmitted to marmosets and chimpanzees and cultivated *in vitro*. It is noncytopathic and grows in a variety of epithelial cell lines. DNA complementary to genomic hepatitis A virus RNA has been cloned in *E. coli*. The mode of elimination of the virus

Table 16.2. Serological viral hepatitis markers and their significance

Marker	Significance
Hepatitis A	
IgM anti-HAV	Acute hepatitis A
IgG anti-HAV	Immune to hepatitis A
Hepatitis B	
HBsAg	Acute or chronic hepatitis B carriage
IgM anti-HBe	Acute hepatitis B (high titre) Chronic hepatitis B (low titre)
IgG anti-HBc	Past exposure to hepatitis B (with negative HBsAg) Chronic hepatitis B (with positive HBsAg)
Anti-HBs	Immune to hepatitis B
HBeAg	Acute hepatitis B. Persistence means continued infectious state
Anti-HBe	Convalescence or continued infectious state
HBV DNA	Continued infectious state
Delta	Acute or chronic infection with delta agent
IgM anti-delta	Chronic delta infection (high titre with + ve IgM anti-delta)
IgG anti-delta	Past delta infection (low titre with − ve IgM anti-delta)

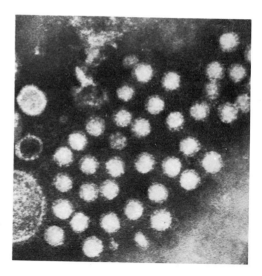

Fig. 16.9. Electron microscopy of hepatitis A antigen particles in faeces. These are shown as 22 nm spheres. (×250 000.)

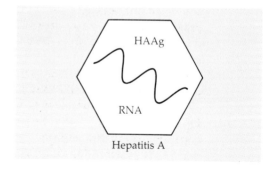

Fig. 16.10. Diagram of the hepatitis A virus shown as a hexagonal body containing single stranded RNA.

from the liver is unknown, but cytolytic T-cells probably play a part [134].

A serum antibody (anti-HAV) appears as the stool becomes negative for virus, reaches a maximum in several months and is detectable for many years (fig. 16.10). IgG anti-HAV probably gives immunity from further infection with hepatitis A. The appearance of serum IgM anti-HAV is more helpful diagnostically and implies a recent infection. This antibody persists for only 2−6 months (figs 16.11, 16.12) and rarely, in low titre, up to one year [64].

Chronic carriers have not been identified.

Epidemiology

The disease occurs sporadically or in epidemic form and has an incubation time of 15−50 days. It is usually spread by the faecal−oral route. Parenteral transmission is extremely rare, but can follow transfusion of blood from a donor who is in the incubation stage of the disease [56].

Age 5−14 is the group most affected and adults are often infected by spread from children.

Spread is related to overcrowding, poor hygiene and poor sanitation. With an improved standard of living the prevalence is decreasing world-wide. In urban areas, 29% (Switzerland)

Table 16.3. Type A, type B and transfusion-related non-A, non-B hepatitis contrasted

	A	B	Transfusion-related non-A, non-B
Virus	RNA	DNA	
Incubation (days)	15–20	50–60	42–56
Spread			
Blood	No	Yes	Yes
Faeces	Yes	No	No
Saliva	Yes	Yes	?
Vertical	No	Yes	?No
Intra-family	Yes	Yes	?No
Acute attack	Depends on age	Mild or severe	Usually mild
Rash	Yes	Yes	Yes
Serum diagnosis	IgM anti-HAV	IgM anti-HBc. HBsAg	Awaited
Peak SGPT (ALT)	800–1000	1000–1500	300–800
Waxing and waning	No	No	Yes
Treatment	Symptomatic	Symptomatic ? Anti-virals	Symptomatic
Prevention	Vaccine Immunoglobulin	Vaccine Immunoglobulin	None
Antibody prevalence	40–60% (urban areas)	10–80% (geographic variations)	?
Chronic hepatitis	No	10%	60%
Liver cancer	No	Yes	Rare

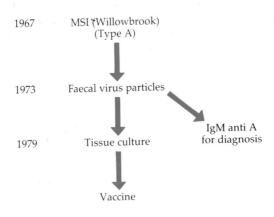

1967	MSI (Willowbrook) (Type A)	
1973	Faecal virus particles	IgM anti A for diagnosis
1979	Tissue culture	
	Vaccine	

Fig. 16.11. Landmarks in hepatitis A (Sherlock, 1984).

to 96.9% (Yugoslavia) of adults show circulating IgG anti-HAV. In underdeveloped countries, 90% of children have the antibody by the age of 10. Young people not previously exposed, and visiting endemic areas, are increasingly becoming affected. Medical staff in developed countries are at risk. A large outbreak among nurses and mothers in a nursery spread from acute hepatitis A in a neonate with an ileostomy [3].

Most sporadic cases follow person-to-person contact. Children in day-care centres and promiscuous homosexuals are at risk.

Explosive water-borne and food-borne epidemics are described. Use of human sewage for soil fertilization can result in frozen fruit-related epidemics.

Ingestion of raw clams and oysters from polluted waters is known to have caused four epidemics. Steaming the clams may not kill the virus, for the temperature achieved inside the clams is not sufficiently high.

Contamination during preparation has resulted in transmission via other foods, including sandwiches, orange juice, potato salad and meat.

Clinical course

The hepatitis is usually mild, particularly in children where it is frequently subclinical or passed off as gastroenteritis. The disease is more serious and prolonged in adults.

ⴟ The rare fulminant course may be related to the dose of virus or impaired antibody responsiveness.

Needle liver biopsy in patients with acute type A hepatitis shows a particularly florid portal zone lesion with expansion, marked cellular infiltration and erosion of the limiting plate [129]. Cholestasis is marked. It is therefore surprising that hepatitis A infection never leads to ongoing chronic hepatitis or cirrhosis.

Cholestatic hepatitis A affects adults [48]. The jaundice lasts 42 to 110 days and itching is severe. Serum IgM anti-HAV is positive. The prognosis is excellent. A case can be made for cutting short the jaundice and relieving the itching by a short course of prednisolone 30 mg reducing to zero over about three weeks (fig. 16.8).

Relapsing hepatitis A. Occasionally after 30 to 90 days the patient relapses. The serum transaminase levels have never returned to normal.

The relapse resembles the original attack clinically and biochemically and virus A is found in the stools [122]. The relapse may last several months but recovery eventually ensues.

Rarely, the relapse can be associated with arthritis, vasculitis and cryoglobulinaemia [58].

PROGNOSIS

This is excellent, and recovery is usually full. Mortality in large epidemics is less than 1 per 1000 and virus A accounts for less than 1% of cases of fulminant viral hepatitis. The average adult with icteric hepatitis can anticipate six weeks illness and this will rarely exceed three months.

Chronicity does not develop. Follow-ups of large epidemics in World War I [26] showed no long-term sequelae. Viral carriage is transient in faeces. Antibodies develop and the patient becomes immune.

Prevention

The virus is excreted in the faeces for as long as two weeks before the appearance of jaundice. The anicteric patient may excrete the virus for a similar period. Virus is therefore disseminated before the diagnosis is made. For this reason, isolation of patients and contacts cannot be expected to influence significantly the spread of hepatitis.

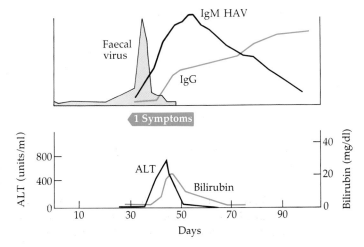

Fig. 16.12. The course of acute hepatitis A. ALT is alanine transferase (GPT) HAV is hepatitis A virus.

Virus A is relatively resistant to inactivation by heat, ether or acid, but is inactivated by formalin 1 in 4000 at 37°C for 72 hours and chlorine 1 ppm for 30 minutes.

IMMUNE SERUM GLOBULIN (ISG)
PROPHYLAXIS (table 16.6)

If possible, any candidate for ISG should be tested for anti-HAV. If present, the ISG is not necessary.

Efficacy depends on the antibody content and hence the source of the plasma.

ISG should be given to close personal contacts of sufferers. Casual contacts in office and work do not need ISG. Routine prophylaxis of hospital staff is not indicated but sound hygiene should be insisted upon.

When a common source of infection is identified, for instance food or water, ISG should be given to all those exposed. This particularly applies to epidemics in schools, hospitals, prisons and other institutions.

HEPATITIS A VACCINES

These are under development (fig. 16.13). A live attenuated vaccine has been prepared from hepatitis A growing in fetal monkey kidney cell cultures and human lung cell cultures [100]. It is effective in human volunteers but doubt remains concerning its safety and there is difficulty in getting fully attenuated strains.

Inactivated vaccines have been prepared from cultures of virus A adapted on human fibroblasts [10, 43, 99]. These will be costly and duration of protection is uncertain.

A recombinant vaccine has been prepared

using the viral protein (VP1) of the virus. Finally, a synthetic vaccine is being considered.

Where available, hepatitis A vaccines will replace immune globulin for travellers and for the military proceeding abroad. Children in nursery schools, homosexuals and workers handling faeces will also be candidates.

Type B (HBV) hepatitis

In 1965, Blumberg and colleagues in Philadelphia found an antibody in two multiply-transfused haemophiliac patients which reacted with an antigen in a single serum in their panel which came from an Australian Aborigine (fig. 16.14) [11]. Later the antigen was found in patients with viral hepatitis. Because of its discovery in an aboriginal serum the antigen was called Australia antigen. In 1977, Blumberg was awarded the Nobel prize for his discovery. Australia antigen is now known to be the surface of the hepatitis B virion and is termed hepatitis B surface antigen (HBsAg).

Three types of particle can be seen in hepatitis B serum: small 20 nm spheres, tubules 20 nm in diameter and 100 nm long, and the more complex 42 nm Dane particles (fig. 16.15) [27]. The Dane particle is the complete hepatitis B virus

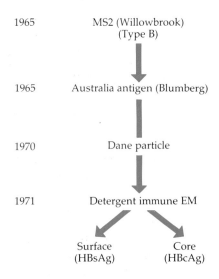

1965	MS2 (Willowbrook) (Type B)
1965	Australia antigen (Blumberg)
1970	Dane particle
1971	Detergent immune EM
	Surface (HBsAg) — Core (HBcAg)

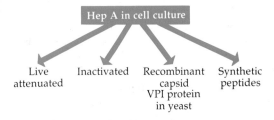

Hep A in cell culture

Live attenuated — Inactivated — Recombinant capsid VPI protein in yeast — Synthetic peptides

312 Fig. 16.13. Possible vaccines against hepatitis A.

Fig. 16.14. Landmarks in hepatitis B (Sherlock, 1984).

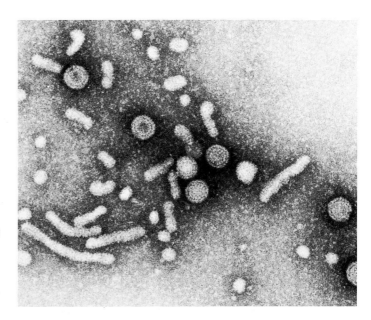

Fig. 16.15. Electron microscopy of hepatitis B antigen particles in blood. These are shown as spherical and tubular forms and the large Dane particles. ×250 000. (Courtesy J.D. Almeida.)

(HBV), whereas the small spheres and tubules are excess viral protein (HBsAg) (fig. 16.16).

The core of the Dane particle is formed by the hepatocyte nucleus whereas the smaller, surface particles are produced in the cytoplasm.

The core of the virus particle contains a DNA polymerase and the DNA has a molecular weight of $1.8 - 2.3 \times 10^6$. The DNA structure has been characterized and shown to be double stranded and circular. It is approximately 3200 nucleotides in length and has a single stranded gap of 600—2100 nucleotides. The DNA polymerase reaction appears to repair the gap. The core contains a core antigen and another antigen, called little 'e', is a protein sub-unit of the core.

DNA recombinant technology has allowed cloning and sequencing of the double-stranded DNA genome of HBV. The open reading frames coding for putative proteins have been identified (fig. 16.17). The genome contains four major polypeptide reading frames. The S-gene codes for an HBsAg polypeptide. The C-gene codes for viral core polypeptide (HBcAg). The third, the putative DNA polymerase 'P-gene', overlaps the S-gene and the fourth reading frame is designated X. The pre-S (S1 and S2) region is a nucleic acid sequence preceding the

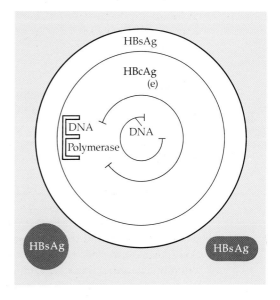

Fig. 16.16. Diagram of the virion of hepatitis B (HBV: Dane particle). The core contains DNA polymerase, double-stranded DNA, core antigen and e antigen. The surface consists of HbsAg. Spheres and tubules of HbsAg are free in serum.

gene coding for the major hepatitis B surface antigen polypeptide [88]. It may be concerned with the ability of the hepatitis B virus to interact with the host hepatocyte.

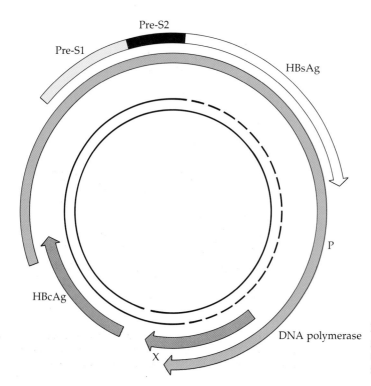

Fig. 16.17. Organization of the genome of the hepatitis B virus showing the four open reading frames, P, HBsAg, HBcAg and X.

A similar disease affects woodchucks, ground squirrels and Peking ducks, and these animals have been extensively used for research [92, 97]. The whole group of agents have been termed *hepadna viruses*.

SUB-TYPES OF HBsAg

HBsAg particles have surfaces that are antigenically complex and this had led to the recognition of antigenic determinants [76]. A common determinant is *a*. The other subdeterminants are designated *d*, *y*, *w* and *r*. The four major determinants are therefore *adw*, *adr*, and *ayr*. They breed true and are very helpful epidemiologically.

SEROLOGICAL DIAGNOSIS (table 16.2)

HBsAg appears in the blood about six weeks after infection and has disappeared by three months (fig. 16.18). Persistence for more than six months implies a carrier state.

Anti-HBs appears late, some three months after the onset, and persists. Anti-HBs levels are rarely high and 10–15% of patients with acute type B hepatitis never develop the antibody. Anti-HBs accounts for recovery and immunity. In the past, HBsAg and HBsAb were believed to be mutually exclusive. However, as many as one-third of carriers of HBsAg also have HBsAb. The mechanism is uncertain, but it has been attributed to simultaneous infection with different sub-types.

HBeAg correlates with ongoing viral synthesis and with infectivity. It is transiently present during the acute attack. It is present for a shorter time than HBsAg. Persistence for more than ten weeks strongly suggests the development of chronicity (Chapter 17).

Anti-HBe is a marker of relatively low infectivity. The appearance of anti-HBe is strong evidence that the patient will recover completely.

HBcAg cannot be detected in circulating blood, but its antibody (anti-HBc) can. High

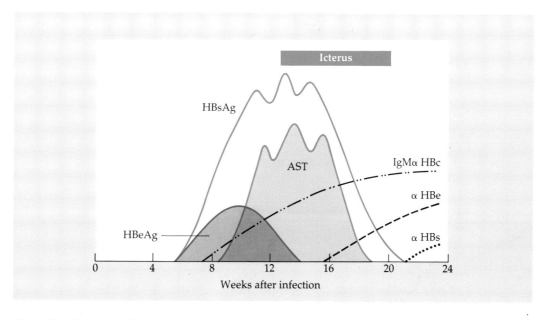

Fig. 16.18. The course of acute type B hepatitis. HBsAg = hepatitis B surface antigen, HBeAg = hepatitis Be antigen, AST = aspartate transaminase, IgMαHBc = IgM antibody against hepatitis B core antigen, αHBe = antibody against hepatitis e antigen, αHBs = antibody against hepatitis B surface antigen.

titres of IgM anti-HBc mark present acute virus hepatitis [22]. This antibody is detected after HBsAg has been cleared from the serum. This is true of 5−6% of cases with acute hepatitis B and is encountered particularly in fulminant hepatitis [120]. It is also useful in determining whether an acute attack of hepatitis is due to virus B or to superinfection with another virus. Persistence of *IgM anti-HBc* implies ongoing virus B-related chronic disease, usually chronic active hepatitis. Lower titres of *IgG anti-HBc* with anti-HBs mark hepatitis B infection in the remote past. Higher titres of IgG anti-HBc without anti-HBs indicate persistence of viral infection.

HBV DNA is the most sensitive index of viral replication. This can now be assessed by molecular hybridization using the Southern blot technique [83, 112]. It can be present in anti-HBe positive sera when it indicates severe ongoing disease [12]. Routine testing for serum HBV DNA will undoubtedly replace tests for HBeAg.

Hepatitis B markers in hepatocytes

HBsAg may be stained orange with orcein (fig. 16.19) in the hepatocytes of carriers and chronic hepatitis patients, but not in those in the acute stage [18]. Electron microscopy and immune histochemistry demonstrate the HBcAg to be in nuclei and the HBsAg in the membranes of liver cells [34]. Core markers are not found in the liver in the acute stage.

INFECTIVITY OF BODY FLUIDS

HBV-containing blood or any body fluid contaminated with blood is infectious. Mere positivity of a fluid for HBsAg is not synonymous with infectivity. However, concentrated samples of saliva, urine and seminal fluid from HBeAg-positive males have shown the presence of HBV-DNA by molecular hybridization [65]. HBV-DNA has also been found in monocytes and leucocytes [51, 96]. The hepatitis B virus probably replicates in extra-hepatic sites.

315

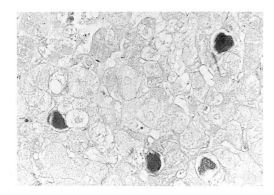

Fig. 16.19. Orcein staining shows liver cells containing HBsAg (brown).

Bone marrow cells have been infected by HBV [142] and light microscopy has shown hepatitis B viral antigens in the human pancreas [121].

Epidemiology (tables 16.3, 16.4 16.5)

The disease is transmitted parenterally or by intimate, often sexual, contact.

Epidemiological methods have proved particularly important in identifying hepatitis B virus infection, indicating its relationship to hepato-cellular carcinoma and in evaluating the effect of vaccine [84].

The carrier rate of HBsAg varies worldwide from 0.1 to 0.2% in Britain, United States and Scandinavia to more than 3% in Greece and Southern Italy and even up to 10 to 15% in Africa and the Far East. If anti-HBs is measured the rate of exposure to hepatitis B in any community is much higher [75]. Carriage of HBsAg is even higher in some isolated communities, 45% in Alaskan Eskimos [87], and 85% in Australian Aborigines.

In high carriage-rate areas infection is probably acquired by passage from the mother to the neonate. The infection is usually not via the umbilical vein but from the mother at the time of birth and during close contact afterwards. The chance of transmission increases as term approaches and is greater with acute than chronic carriers. The mother is HBsAg positive

Table 16.4. Approximate percentage carrier rate or HBsAg (by **RIA**) in 'healthy' blood donors

Scandinavia	0.1
United Kingdom	0.1
United States	0.1
Holland	0.2
Switzerland	0.2
Belgium	0.5
France	0.5
Spain	2.0
Southern Italy	3.0
Japan	3.0
Greece	5.0
South Africa	11.3
Taiwan	15.0
Singapore	15.0
Hong Kong	15.0

Table 16.5. Groups in which acute and chronic type-B hepatitis should be suspected

Immigrants from Mediterranean countries, Africa or the Far East
Drug abusers
Homosexuals
Neonates of HBsAg positive mothers
Hospital staff
Patients with:
    Renal failure
    Reticuloses
    Cancer
    Organ transplants
Staff and patients of hospitals for mentally retarded
Post-transfusion

and also usually, but not always, HBeAg positive. Antigenaemia develops in the baby within two months of birth and tends to persist.

In other areas the peak incidence is in childhood rather than in neonates. In such areas, including Africa [13], Greece and Hong Kong intra-family spread seems particularly important. This may be by close contact such as kissing. Shared utensils, toothbrushes and razors may also be important. In the family group the sexual contacts of carriers are at risk.

Homosexuals are at risk of contracting type B hepatitis. In one multi-centred trial, conducted in the United States, 61% of 3816 'gay' men had markers of hepatitis B (6% HBsAg, 52% HBsAb, and 3% HBcAb) [111]. Infection was related to duration of homosexual activity, number of sexual contacts and anal contact.

Blood-sucking arthropods such as mosquitoes or bed bugs may be important vectors, particularly in the tropics. However, there is no evidence that the virus replicates in the arthropod.

Blood transfusion continues to cause hepatitis B in countries where donor blood is not screened for HBsAg by radioimmunoassay. Transmission is more likely with blood from paid donors than when volunteer blood is transfused.

Opportunities for parenteral infection include the use of unsterile instruments for dental treatment, ear piercing and manicures, neurological examination, prophylactic inoculations, subcutaneous injections, acupuncture, and tattooing (fig. 16.20).

Parenteral drug abusers develop hepatitis from using shared, unsterile equipment. The mortality may be very high in this group. Multiple attacks are seen and chronicity is frequent. Liver biopsy may show, in addition to acute or chronic hepatitis, foreign material, such as chalk, injected with the illicit drug.

Hospital staff in contact with patients, and especially patient's blood, usually have a higher carrier rate than the general community. This applies particularly to staff on renal dialysis or oncology units. Patients are immunosuppressed and, on contracting the disease, become chronic carriers [67]. Danger to the patient's attendant comes from contact with blood parenterally, such as from pricking or through skin abrasions. Surgeons and dentists are particularly at risk in operating on HBsAg-positive patients with a positive HBeAg (fig. 16.20). Holes in gloves and cuts on hands are common. Wire sutures may be a particular hazard in penetrating the skin. Four surgeons developed hepatitis 80–105 days after performing proctocolectomy (with wire sutures) on a patient who developed a positive HBsAg [106]. Checks of 75 additional medical personnel who cared for the patient revealed no other cases of hepatitis. Other methods of casual contact in hospital are much less likely causes of infection.

Using standard cleansing procedures there is no evidence that HBV infection is spread by endoscopes [136].

Special care must be taken in transporting and handling *all* blood samples, but especially those coming from patients with hepatitis.

Institutionalized mentally retarded children (especially with Down's syndrome) and their attendants have a high carrier rate [73].

Clinical course

The course may be anicteric. The high carriage rate of serum markers in those who give no

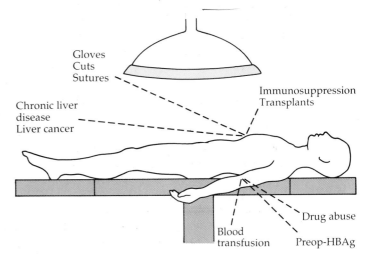

Fig. 16.20. The hepatitis hazard for hospital workers and particularly surgeons. This comes from skin lacerations and pricks when handling blood from a patient with a positive hepatitis B antigen test, especially those with chronic liver disease or cancer, those on immuno-suppression or having organ transplantation or abusing drugs. Care in handling all blood specimens is emphasized.

history of an acute hepatitis B attack suggests that subclinical episodes must be extremely frequent. The non-icteric case is more liable to become chronic than the icteric one.

The usual clinical attack diagnosed in the adult tends to be more severe than for virus A or non-A, non-B infections. The overall picture is, however, similar. The self-limited, benign icteric disease usually lasts less than four months. Jaundice rarely exceeds four weeks. Occasionally, a prolonged benign course is marked by increased serum transaminase values for more than 100 days. Relapses are rare. Cholestatic hepatitis with prolonged deep jaundice is unusual.

There may be features suggesting immune complex disease. This is shown in the prodromal period by a *serum sickness-like* syndrome. This develops about a week before the onset of jaundice. It can be associated with an icteric or an anicteric attack. The syndrome has also been described with chronic hepatitis B [138]. Fever is usual. The skin lesion is urticarial, and rarely, in children, a papular acrodermatitis may be seen. [45].

The arthropathy is symmetrical, non-migratory and affects small joints. Serum rheumatoid factor is negative. It is usually transitory but can persist.

These events can be related to circulating immune complexes containing HBsAg, anti-HBs and complement [130]. Serum complement levels are reduced. Immunoglobulins, complement and HBsAg can be shown in vessel walls.

A fulminant course of hepatitis B in the first four weeks may be related to an enhanced immune response. There is more rapid clearing of virus. Antibodies to surface and 'c' antigen increase, and multiplication of virus ceases [15]. In fulminant hepatitis B, the surface antigen may be in low titre or undetectable and hepatitis Bs antigen is less frequently found. The diagnosis may be made only by finding serum IgM anticore titres.

Another viral hepatitis, superimposed on the symptomless hepatitis B carrier, may precipitate a fulminant course. The new agent may be A [95] or delta; non-A, non-B has also been postulated [93].

Subacute hepatic necrosis is marked by increasing severe disease evolving over one to three months.

Chronic hepatitis can develop insidiously (see Chapter 17).

Extra-hepatic associations

These conditions are often associated with circulating immune complexes containing HBsAg. The accompanying liver disease is usually mild, at the most a chronic persistent hepatitis. The liver disease itself is not due to immune complex injury. Turnover of the C_3 component of complement is not increased in acute type B hepatitis, and is less in chronic active than chronic persistent hepatitis [130]. Acute and chronic type B hepatitis can develop in patients with agammaglobulinaemia.

Polyarteritis (systemic necrotizing vasculitis). This multi-system disease affects the gastrointestinal tract, peripheral and central nervous system. The course is similar to other types of polyarteritis, 31 to 54% have mononeuritis multiplex [127].

Immune complexes containing HBsAg, IgG and complement have been found in the vascular lesions [89]. The presence of circulating complexes correlates with disease activity. As the lesions become less active, evidences of viral infection disappear [89].

The importance of hepatitis B virus in the whole picture of polyarteritis is probably low, perhaps representing some 10% of cases.

Glomerulonephritis. Membranous or membrano-proliferative glomerulonephritis has been found either isolated or as part of a generalized vasculitis [17]. The association is a rare one. Circulating HBcAg antigen—antibody complexes are found in the capillaries [128].

The patient usually has no clinical features of acute or chronic liver disease [74]. The course is indolent but relentlessly progressive.

Polymyalgia rheumatica has been connected with hepatitis B infection [4].

Essential mixed cryoglobulinaemia. A patient

with peripheral neuropathy and cryoglobu-linaemia showed a cryoprecipitate with a high concentration of HBsAg. However, anti-HBsAg and complement were not found [82]. The relationship of hepatitis B to this condition has not been proved [35].

The *Guillain–Barré syndrome* has been reported with HBsAg-containing immune complexes in serum and cerebrospinal fluid [94].

Myocarditis may have an immune complex basis [133].

Hepatitis B carriers

There are an estimated 300 million hepatitis B carriers in the world.

Approximately 10% of patients contracting hepatitis B as an adult and 90% of those infected as neonates will not clear HBsAg from the serum within six months (fig. 16.21). Such patients become carriers and this is likely to persist. Reversion to a negative HBsAg is rare but may develop in old age. Males are six times more likely to become carriers than females.

The dilemma of a person, such as a hospital worker, carrying the antigen and coming from an area where it is prevalent is a very difficult one. The HBsAg carrier of today must not replace the leper of yesterday. Hospital staff who develop HBsAg-positive hepatitis and clear the antigen from the blood are immune to type B hepatitis. If they become carriers, the position is difficult. The extent of the infectivity of surgeons, dentists or indeed any hospital worker to patients and casual contacts has not been established but cannot be very great.

'Healthy' carriers may show changes on liver biopsy ranging from non-specific minimal abnormalities through to chronic active hepatitis and cirrhosis [103]. The extent of the changes is not reflected by serum biochemical tests and may only be revealed by liver biopsy. The carrier presenting by chance is likely to have minor hepatic changes compared to the patient presenting to a gastroenterology department where more serious liver disease is likely. In a survey of patients found to be HBsAg positive at blood donation, 95% had near normal liver

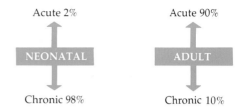

Acute 2%   Acute 90%

NEONATAL   ADULT

Chronic 98%   Chronic 10%

Fig. 16.21. The course of acute hepatitis B in the neonate and adult.

biopsies and only 1.6% proceeded to chronic active hepatitis or cirrhosis [37]. Ninety per cent were serum HBeAg negative and anti-HBe positive.

In a carrier, a positive serum HBV-DNA and HBeAg indicate infectivity and ongoing disease. Mechanisms of chronicity are discussed in Chapter 17.

Chronic organic sequelae

Exposure to HBV can have different results (fig. 16.22). Some are immune and have no clinical attack; they presumably have anti-HBV. In others, an acute attack develops varying from anicteric to fulminant. Previously normal persons usually clear the antigen from the serum within about 4–6 weeks from the onset of symptoms. Chronic liver disease is associated with persistent antigenaemia. In general, the more florid and acute the original attack, the less likely are chronic sequelae.

If the patient survives a fulminant attack of viral hepatitis, ultimate recovery is complete without the development of chronic residuals. Chronicity is more likely after the mildly icteric, anicteric or relapsing episode and in those with immunological incompetence such as neonates, homosexuals, sufferers from AIDS, leukaemia and cancer, renal failure or those receiving immunosuppressive treatment (see Chapter 17) [39].

Prevention

HEPATITIS B IMMUNOGLOBULIN (HBIG)

HBIG is a special hyperimmune serum globulin

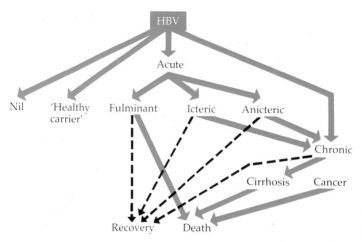

Fig. 16.22. The effect of exposure to hepatitis B virus (HBV).

with a high antibody titre. It is effective for passive immunization against hepatitis B if given prophylactically or within hours of infection [113]. If hepatitis vaccine is available it should always be given with the HBIG, particularly if the subject is at risk of re-infection. It is indicated for sexual contacts of acute sufferers, babies born to HBsAg-positive mothers [8, 141], and victims of parenteral exposure (needle stick) to HBsAg-positive blood (tables 16.6, 16.7, 16.8).

Pre-exposure HBIG, for instance before a blood transfusion, is of possible value.

HEPATITIS B VACCINES

Vaccines are prepared from the uninfectious outer surface of the virus (HBsAg) (fig. 16.23).

The *plasma-derived vaccine* comes from plasma of hepatitis B carriers. It is highly effective in preventing hepatitis B in high risk groups. It is completely safe and no evidence of AIDS has occurred in over one million vaccinees at low risk of exposure to AIDS. The only side-effects are an occasional sore arm and pyrexia, probably due to the alum preservative. Recombinant DNA technology has been used to express HBsAg in yeast cells. The resultant *recombinant yeast vaccine* is free of human plasma. It is safe and as effective as the plasma derived one [16, 125].

Hepatitis B vaccines have been shown to be effective in preventing hepatitis B in promiscuous homosexuals [126], haemodialysis patients [31], Down's syndrome and other mentally retarded patients [55], health care workers [36],

Table 16.6. Immunoprophylaxis of virus hepatitis A and B

Type	Immunoglobulin	Indication	Regime
A	Conventional	Close exposure to virus	3 ml within 14 days
		Travel to 'dirty areas'	6 ml every six months
B (adults)	HBIG	Exposure to HBsAg +ve blood	
		Sexual consorts	0.06 ml/kg as soon as possible combined first dose of vaccine*
Neonates	HBIG	HBsAg +ve mother	0.5 ml as soon as possible combined first dose of vaccine†

* Full course of vaccine given if subject is anti-HBc negative.
† Full course of vaccine given.

Table 16.7. Indications for hepatitis vaccination

Surgical and dental staff including medical students
Hospital and laboratory staff in contact with blood
Patients and staff in departments of oncology and
 haematology, kidney, mental subnormality and
 liver disease
Mental subnormality
Accidental exposure to HBsAg + ve blood
Close family and sexual contacts of HBsAg + ve
 carriers
Babies born to HBsAg +ve mothers
Children in high risk populations
Drug abusers
Homosexually active men
Travellers to high risk areas

Table 16.8. Prophylaxis of persons accidentally
exposed to possibly infectious blood

Check donor blood for HbsAg; victim's blood for
HBsAg and HbcAb
Give at once 0.06 ml/kg HBIG plus first dose hepatitis
B vaccine

	HbsAg	HBcAb	Further action to victim
Victim	+ve	+ve	None: immune
Donor	+ve		Continue vaccine course
	−ve		None or continue vaccine course if victim is at risk of further hepatitis B exposure

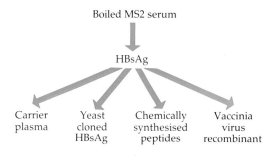

Boiled MS2 serum

HBsAg

| Carrier plasma | Yeast cloned HBsAg | Chemically synthesised peptides | Vaccinia virus recombinant |

Fig. 16.23. The stages of hepatitis B vaccine
production.

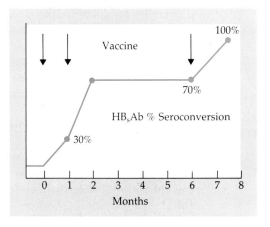

Fig. 16.24. The use of hepatitis B vaccine. Three
injections result in about 93% seroconversion at
eight months in young healthy subjects.

babies born to HBsAg-positive mothers [8, 141],
in children in Africa [24] and susceptibles in
Alaska [87].

In healthy individuals the recombinant vaccine is given in a dose of 10 µg (1 ml) intramuscularly at 0, 1 month and a booster at 6 months
(fig. 16.24). This induces sufficient antibody
response in 94%. The reason for the failure of
some healthy individuals to respond is uncertain. These persons should be given a further
booster of 20 µg before failure is admitted.
Older patients, renal dialysis patients or those
who are immuno-suppressed for any reason
may have a reduced antibody response and the
larger dose of 20 µg intramuscularly should be
given.

The vaccine is usually given intramuscularly into the arm. Intradermal administration is effective although antibody titres are
not so high as with the intramuscular route
[143].

Pre-testing. Vaccination is unnecessary if the
person has a positive HBsAb or HBcAb.

The cost-effectiveness of pre-testing to save
vaccine depends on the prevalence of serum B
markers in a community.

The finding of an isolated serum anti-HBs
does not mean immunity to hepatitis B. A
positive serum anti-HBc is preferable as this
detects infected as well as immune persons.

This test is done in high-risk populations such as homosexuals, drug abusers and spouses of chronic carriers. In low-risk groups, such as health-care workers, it is unnecessary to perform preliminary tests.

Antibody response

The long-term protection depends on the antibody response which is 85–95% in healthy young subjects. Anti-HBs should be measured one to three months after completion of the basic course of vaccine.

Non-responders have peak anti-HBs levels of ⩽ 10 IU/l and lack of protection.

Low responders have peak anti-HBs levels of 10–100 IU/l and generally lack detectable anti-HBs levels within about 5–7 years. They may respond to a further booster of double the dose of vaccine.

Good responders have peak anti-HBs ⩾ 100 IU/l and usually have long-term immunity.

Failure to develop adequate antibodies may be related to freezing the vaccine or giving it into the buttocks rather than the deltoid region [20].

A poor antibody response is seen in the aged and in the immuno-compromised. These should be given doses of 20 µg.

Approximately 5–10% of normal persons have absent or poor antibody responses. Some may respond to a booster [25].

Duration of protection. This remains unknown. Immunity may persist even after anti-HBs has declined to undetectable levels [53]. Until more data are available, one might consider revaccinating individuals once again, five to seven years after the initial course. Immuno-compromised individuals should be re-vaccinated more frequently.

Indications (table 16.7)

The need for vaccination depends on the chance of that person being exposed to hepatitis B. Vaccination is mandatory for health care staff in close contact with hepatitis B patients, particularly those working on renal dialysis units, liver units, haemophilia and oncology units, genitourinary departments treating homosexuals or those working in homes for the mentally retarded. Surgeons and dentists and their assistants, medical students and laboratory workers regularly exposed to infected blood are also candidates. The vaccine should be given to medical personnel proceeding overseas to areas where the prevalence of hepatitis B is high and where they will be directly involved in patient care.

Acute sufferers from hepatitis B are highly infectious and their sexual contacts should be vaccinated and given hyperimmuneglobulin. Sexual and family contacts of hepatitis B carriers should also, if at all possible, be vaccinated after their antibody status has been determined.

Promiscuous homosexuals requesting vaccine should be screened for HBsAg and HBcAb and, if they are not carrying the virus and are not immune, should be vaccinated. The same rules apply to drug abusers.

Babies born to HBsAg-positive, and particularly HB 'e' antigen-positive mothers should be vaccinated and given immune globulin at birth (table 16.7). In countries with a high carrier rate it may be cost-effective to vaccinate all babies without the expense of testing the mothers for HBsAg.

Even in countries with a low carrier rate, it is essential to screen *all* pregnant women for HBsAg and not only those with a high risk of being carriers [63].

The problem of the health care worker, accidentally exposed parenterally to blood which may be infectious, demands special consideration (table 16.8).

The possibility of eliminating hepatitis B and its attendant chronic liver disease and hepato-cellular cancer depends on mass vaccination, particularly of neonates and children in the high carrier areas of the third world. This is turn depends on supplies of an inexpensive vaccine.

OTHER VACCINES

The most simple is derived from *heat-inactivated plasma containing HBsAg* and is based on the original observation of Krugman who boiled infectious hepatitis B-positive serum and showed it protected against hepatitis B [31]. This vaccine is relatively crude and highly immunogenic. It has proved effective in neonates in Hong Kong [141], and in dialysis patients [31].

The cost could be reduced to as little as one dollar per dose.

Polypeptide vaccines are composed of specific immunogenic antigenic determinants of HBsAg. So far they have not proved potent antibody stimulants and are uneconomical to produce.

Hybrid virus vaccines. The coding sequence for HBsAg has been inserted into the vaccinia virus genome and a live vaccine against hepatitis B produced. This has protected chimpanzees against hepatitis B [91]. Vaccinia is clearly not the most satisfactory choice. Other recombinant viruses, such as adenoviruses, are under investigation.

Hepatitis B core antigen [60]. Hepatitis B virus clearance from infected hepatocytes may well require the activity of cytotoxic T-lymphocytes specifically reactive against HBcAg. In chimpanzees, protection against hepatitis B can be induced by immunization with hepatitis B core antigen in adjuvant. This may be useful in the design of further vaccines.

The pre-S region. The hepatitis B virus has a second surface antigen which is coded for by the pre-S region of the HBV-genome (fig. 16.17). Pre-S is important for immunological clearance of hepatitis B viral particles [18]. Recombinant yeast vaccines are now under investigation which will contain pre-S (pre-S1 and pre-S2) [69]. It remains to be determined whether they will be more effective.

Delta virus (hepatitis D virus, HDV)

In 1977, Rizzetto and colleagues, working in Turin, recognized a new antigen—antibody system in the hepatocyte nuclei of HBsAg-positive patients and called it 'delta' [104]. Delta agent is a very small RNA particle coated with HBsAg (figs 16.25, 16.26). It is not able to replicate on its own, but is capable of infection only when activated by the presence of hepatitis B virus. It resembles satellite viruses of plants which cannot replicate without another specific virus. The interaction between the two viruses is very complex. Synthesis of delta may depress the appearance of hepatitis B viral markers in infected cells and even lead to elimination of active hepatitis B viral replication [72].

Delta virus is a single-stranded circular anti-sense RNA of 1.7 kilobases [70, 139]. It is highly infectious and can induce hepatitis in a HBsAg positive host. It has been transmitted to chimpanzees carrying hepatitis B [42].

Hepatitis B and delta infection may be simultaneous (*co-infection*) or delta may infect a chronic HBsAg carrier (*super-infection*).

EPIDEMIOLOGY

Delta virus infection is not a new disease. Prospective analysis of stored blood shows it among the American army in 1947, in Los Angeles since 1967 [28], and in liver specimens from Brazil in the 1930s.

Delta infection is strongly associated with intravenous drug abuse, but can affect all groups at risk of acquiring hepatitis B infection including homosexuals [124], health care workers, transfusion recipients [80, 107],

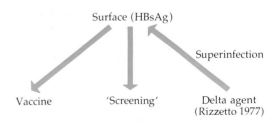

Fig. 16.25. Hepatitis B surface antigen (HBsAg) is the source of the hepatitis B vaccine. It is used for screening for hepatitis B and is superinfected with the delta agent.

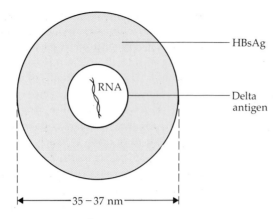

Fig. 16.26. Delta antigen is a small RNA particle coated by HBsAg.

Table 16.9. Diagnosis of delta hepatitis

	Acute	Chronic
Delta antigen		
Serum	+ (transient)	−
Liver	+	+
IgG anti-delta	+ (rising titre)	+ (high titre)
IgM anti-delta	+	+
Delta RNA	+	+

haemophiliacs, immigrants [119] and institutionalized patients. Delta can be spread heterosexually [80]. Intra-family spread with clustering has been noted in Southern Italy [12]. Children can be affected [40]. Delta infection may be reactivated if the sufferer develops HIV infection [116].

Delta infection is world-wide, but particularly in Southern Europe, the Balkans, Middle East [132], South India, and parts of Africa [118]. In general, it is rare in the Far East (including Japan), Brazil, Chile, and Argentina. However, epidemics of delta infection have been reported from the Amazon Basin, Brazil (Labrea fever) [9], Colombia (Santa Marta hepatitis) [19], Venezuela [52] and Equatorial Africa. In these areas children of the indigent population are affected and mortality is high.

DIAGNOSIS (table 16.9)

Serum delta antigenaemia is present only for the first few days of illness.

Co-infection is diagnosed by the finding of serum IgM anti-delta in the presence of high titre IgM anti-HBc. These markers appear at one week, and IgM anti-delta is gone by five to six weeks but may last up to twelve weeks [1]. When serum IgM anti-delta disappears, serum IgG anti-delta is found. There may be a window period between the disappearance of one and

the detection of another. Loss of IgM anti-HDV confirms resolution of delta infection, persistence predicts chronicity.

HBsAg is positive, but often in low titre and may seem negative. Serum IgM anti-HBc is also suppressed by acute delta infection. Unless delta markers are sought, the patient may be misdiagnosed as acute non-A, non-B hepatitis.

Superinfection of a hepatitis B carrier with delta virus is marked by the early presence of serum IgM anti-delta, usually at the same time as early IgG anti-delta and both antibodies persist. These patients are usually IgM anti-HBc negative, but may have low titres of this antibody. Sufferers of chronic delta infection with chronic active hepatitis and active cirrhosis usually have a positive serum IgM anti-delta.

Serum and liver HDV-RNA are found in IgM anti-delta positive patients with acute and chronic delta infection [123].

CLINICAL FEATURES (figs 16.27, 16.28)

With *co-infection*, the acute delta hepatitis is usually self-limited as the delta cannot outlive the transient HBs antigenaemia. The clinical picture is usually indistinguishable from hepatitis due to hepatitis B alone. However, a biphasic rise in aspartate transaminase may be noted, the second rise due to the acute effects of delta [50].

The attack may be fulminant and about a third of fulminant hepatitis B is related to coincidental delta infection. There are marked geographic differences in severity [118].

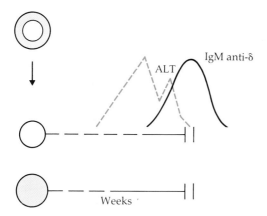

Fig. 16.27. Simultaneous infection with hepatitis B and delta results in acute hepatitis B with rise in ALT (alanine transaminase). Delta infection follows with a second peak of ALT and the appearances of IgM anti-delta in the blood. Clearing of HbsAg is associated with clearing of delta (Rizzetto 1983).

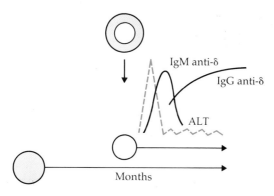

Fig. 16.28. Delta infection in an HBsAg carrier results in an attack of acute hepatitis with the appearance of IgM anti-delta followed by IgG anti-delta in the blood (Rizzetto 1983).

With *super-infection*, the acute attack may be severe and even fulminant, or may be marked only by a rise in serum transaminase levels. Delta infection should always be considered in any hepatitis B carrier, often clinically stable, who has a relapse.

Delta infection reduces active hepatitis B viral synthesis and patients are usually HBeAg and HBV-DNA negative. Two to 10% lose HBsAg. However, chronic delta hepatitis is usual and this results in acceleration towards cirrhosis [140].

Hepato-cellular cancer seems less common in HBsAg carriers with delta. Whether this represents inhibition by the delta virus or such rapid progression of the liver disease that death occurs before cancer can develop remains uncertain. However, when delta is found with late stage chronic liver disease it does not seem to influence survival and hepato-cellular cancer may be a complication in these patients [132].

Delta super-infection modifies the course of healthy B carriers rendering the liver disease more severe.

HEPATIC HISTOLOGY

There may be difficulty in distinguishing the effects of delta virus from those of hepatitis B [135]. However, there is increased histological severity in delta positive patients compared with the usual hepatitis B carriers. Inflammatory activity is greater being particularly marked in intra-lobular portal and peri-portal zones. Focal confluent and bridging necrosis may be seen. Eosinophilic change is noted in the hepatocytes with the formation of acidophilic bodies.

The South American and Equatorial African epidemics are marked by microvesicular fat in hepatocytes, intense eosinophilic necrosis and large amounts of delta antigen within the liver [19]. These changes have also been noted in a New York drug abuser with delta infection [78]. Morula (plant-like) cells may be seen.

Using immunoperoxidase-linked anti-delta serum, delta antigen may be shown in the hepatocyte nuclei. This is reduced in acute delta hepatitis but increases with chronic active liver disease and becomes low in the late stage of cirrhosis (fig. 16.29).

Immune electron microscopy shows nuclear delta as irregular granular structures with aggregates of 20—30 nm similar to those described for non-A, non-B hepatitis [68].

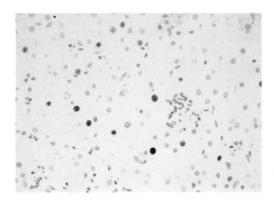

Fig. 16.29. Delta virus hepatitis: immuno peroxidase staining shows delta in hepatocyte nuclei (×100).

PREVENTION

Vaccination against hepatitis B, by rendering the recipient immune to hepatitis B virus infection, protects against delta virus infection. Patients likely to contract delta infection should be encouraged to have hepatitis B vaccine.

Hepatitis B carriers must be educated concerning the risks of acquiring delta by continued drug abuse. A vaccine against delta virus infection is urgently needed.

TREATMENT

This is unsatisfactory. Delta virus infection is unaffected by immunosuppressive therapy. Clinical trials with interferon show inhibition of delta replication with clearance or reduction of serum HBV-RNA and a fall in serum transaminases. Unfortunately delta usually returns to the liver and serum transaminases increase again. More clinical trials are needed, perhaps with larger doses and for a longer time.

Hepatic transplantation of delta infected patients has given disappointing results as delta virus usually returns to the transplanted liver [105].

Non-A, non-B hepatitis

In 1977, on the basis of multiple episodes of viral hepatitis it was suggested that a third variety of acute virus hepatitis existed and this was called non-A, non-B [90]. Diagnosis is made after exclusion of infection with known hepatitis viruses including A, B, cytomegalo- and Epstein—Barr [33, 34]. Non-A, non-B hepatitis has been transmitted to chimpanzees immune to both hepatitis A and B, so confirming a carrier state.

There seem to be two main types, *a bloodborne variety* associated with blood transfusion and drug abuse and an *enteric type* that may be epidemic or sporadic [61]. A possible third type is associated with the administration of blood products such as factor VIII.

PARENTERAL

The causative agent(s) has not hitherto been identified. Under electron microscopy, particles have been seen in the hepatocytes of both chimpanzees and man; their significance is uncertain. Filtration studies give the size of the agent as between 27 and 31 nm [14].

A *viral genomic clone* has been isolated from infected plasma and liver. This encodes the antigen associated with non-A, non-B viral hepatitis in man and chimpanzees [57]. The antibody to it can be measured by radioimmunoassay and has been shown in blood donors and acute and chronic sufferers from parenteral non-A, non-B hepatitis. This opens the prospect of diagnosing chronic non-A, non-B hepatitis and of detecting blood donors carrying the disease.

Hepatic pathology [109]

Various features are suggestive but not diagnostic of non-A, non-B hepatitis. They include sinusoidal cell infiltration, eosinophilic granulomas with acidophilic bodies, giant cells and microvesicular fat. Portal and peri-portal lesions and mild. Bile duct lesions, if present, suggest non-A, non-B hepatitis. Lymphoid follicles may be seen (fig. 16.30).

Epidemiology

The incubation period is about seven weeks.

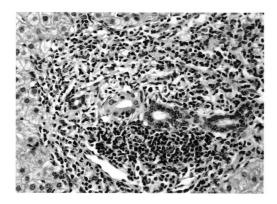

Fig. 16.30. Non-A, non-B hepatitis. Zone 1 (portal) shows cellular infiltration, bile ducts with damaged epithelium and a lymphoid follicle. (H & E ×100.)

Non-A, non-B hepatitis accounts for over 90% of post-transfusion hepatitis in areas where donor blood is screened for hepatitis B. In the United States, it is estimated that 1.6% of volunteer donor blood and 6% of commercial blood carry the virus. In other countries the carrier rate may even be higher, up to an estimated 15% in Brazil.

Recipients of blood products such as Factor VIII and IX are at risk of contracting non-A, non-B hepatitis. In these patients the incubation period may be markedly shortened to 3–21 days. This type may be due to a different virus or to a difference in the infectious dose. Cross-challenge experiments in non-human primates suggest at least two distinct non-A, non-B viruses. The disease has been spread by intravenous immunoglobulin given to agammaglobulinaemics [81].

Non-A, non-B hepatitis also affects dialysis and renal transplant patients and drug abusers. Intra-familial spread is unusual. There is no evidence of heterosexual or homosexual transmission. The high carrier rate in those who give no history of blood transfusion implies that there must be various modes of spread.

Clinical picture

This rather resembles hepatitis B infection. In 73% the patient is completely asymptomatic [23]. In 25%, the picture is that of any other acute virus hepatitis. There may be serum sickness-like prodromata. Rarely the hepatitis is severe and even fulminant (table 16.1).

Serum transaminase values are only moderately elevated, with the peak serum alanine transaminase being about 15 times the upper limit of normal [23]. 60% of patients will have raised serum transaminases one year later. In 68% the disease becomes chronic and in 20% cirrhosis develops [10%] (see Chapter 17).

Hepato-cellular carcinoma, often of clear cell type, is a rare complication [46, 77]. Marrow aplasia may be fatal [7].

Prevention

The use of volunteer instead of commercial blood donors reduces the prevalence. Blood transfusions should be used only when absolutely necessary and blood substitutes are often adequate. The use of free, donated blood will further reduce the risk.

Surrogate tests are being used to identify the donor carrying non-A non-B hepatitis. If blood with an alanine transaminase level exceeding 50 is discarded 30% of non-A, non-B hepatitis would be prevented with a donor loss of 1–3%. The usual cause of the raised transaminase is obesity or alcohol abuse and only 20% are presumptive carriers of non-A, non-B [44]. Serum hepatitis B core antibody can also be used for screening [71]. Those exposed to B are likely to have been exposed to non-A, non-B. This test would reduce post-transfusion hepatitis by 37% with a donor loss of 4–8%.

Factor VIII may be rendered non-infectious by heat inactivation [110]. The risk of factor VIII transmission will disappear when factor VIII is prepared by genetic engineering.

The use of prophylactic immune-globulin before a blood transfusion is given has given good results [108].

A radioimmunoassay test which will diagnose, and hopefully prevent, at least one type of transfusion-related non-A, non-B hepatitis will shortly be available [57].

Treatment of chronic non-A, non-B virus hepatitis (see Chapter 17)

EPIDEMIC (ENTERIC) [101]

In general, this resembles hepatitis A. It affects young adults and has a self-limited course. The mortality is very high in women in the last trimester of pregnancy. The course can be cholestatic, hepatic histology showing marked cholestasis. Epidemic non-A, non-B hepatitis has been reported from India, Pakistan [66], Mexico, Central and South East Asia, North Africa and in travellers returning from these areas [29, 85].

Virology

The disease has been transmitted to Macaque monkeys with recovery of 27–34 nm virus-like particles from the faeces [2]. 27 nm virus particles have been found in the stools of human sufferers and these are aggregated by antibody in acute and convalescent sera from epidemic, but not sporadic, enteric non-A, non-B hepatitis [2]. It is an RNA virus of the calissi group.

Prevention

This depends on improved hygiene and the provision of a clean water supply.

Immunoprophylaxis may be possible using immunoglobulin prepared from donors from countries with a high prevalence of the disease. This may be especially valuable in pregnant women.

SPORADIC (ENTERIC)

This occurs in the general population in the absence of identifiable modes of transmission. Non-A, non-B hepatitis accounts for about 20–30% of acute hepatitis in the Western World [5]. A non-parenteral route of infection, perhaps involving an agent resembling that of epidemic non-A, non-B hepatitis remains possible.

It has a predominance in young men. It is a commoner cause of fulminant hepatitis than either virus A or virus B (table 16.1). The fulminant disease is of slow onset.

Chronicity is uncertain, but is not frequent.

References

1 Aragona M, Macagno S, Caredda F *et al.* Serological response to the hepatitis delta virus in hepatitis D. *Lancet* 1987; **1**: 478.

2 Arankalle VA, Ticehurst J, Sreenivasan MA *et al.* Aetiological association of a virus-like particle with enterically transmitted non-A, non-B hepatitis. *Lancet* 1988; **i**: 550.

3 Azimi PH, Roberto RR, Guralnik J *et al.* Transfusion acquired hepatitis A in a premature infant with secondary nosocomial spread in an intensive care nursery. *Am. J. Dis. Child.* 1986; **140**: 23.

4 Bacon PA, Doherty SM, Zuckerman AJ. Hepatitis B antibody in polymyalgia rheumatica. *Lancet* 1975; **ii**: 476.

5 Bamber M, Murray A, Arborgh BAM *et al.* Short incubation non-A, non-B hepatitis transmitted by factor VIII concentrates in patients with congenital coagulation disorders. *Gut* 1981; **22**: 854.

6 Bamber M, Thomas HC, Bannister B *et al.* Acute type A, B, and non-A, non-B hepatitis in a hospital population in London: clinical and epidemiological features *Gut* 1983; **24**: 561.

7 Bannister P, Miloszewski K, Barnard D *et al.* Fatal marrow aplasia associated with non-A, non-B hepatitis. *Br. med. J.* 1983; **286**: 1314.

8 Beasley RP, Hwang LY, Lee GCY *et al.* Prevention of perinatally transmitted hepatitis B virus infections with hepatitis B immune globulin and hepatitis B vaccine. *Lancet* 1983; **ii**: 1099.

9 Bensabath G, Hadler SC, Soares MCP *et al.* Hepatitis delta virus infection and labrea hepatitis. Prevalence and role in fulminant hepatitis in the Amazon Basin. *J. Am. med. Ass.* 1987; **258**: 479.

10 Binn LN, Bancroft WH, Lemon SM *et al.* Preparation of a prototype inactivated hepatitis A virus vaccine from infected cell cultures. *J. Infect. Dis.* 1986; **153**: 749.

11 Blumberg BS, Alter HJ, Visnich S. A 'new' antigen in leukemia sera. *J. Am. med. Assoc.* 1965; **191**: 541.

12 Bonino F, Caporaso N, Dentico P *et al.* Familiar clustering and spreading of hepatitis delta virus infection. *J. Hepatol.* 1985; **1**: 221.

13 Botha JF, Ritchie MJJ, Dusheiko GM *et al.* Hepatitis B virus carrier state in black children in Ovamboland: role of perinatal and horizontal infection. *Lancet* 1984; **i**: 1210.

14 Bradley DW, Krawczynski K, Cook EHJ *et al.* Enterically transmitted non-A, non-B hepatitis:

serial passage of disease in cynomolgus macaques and tamarins and recovery of disease-associated 27–34 nm virus-like particles. *Proc. Nat. Acad. Sci.* 1987; **84:** 6277.

15 Brechot C, Bernuau J, Thiers V *et al.* Multiplication of hepatitis B virus in fulminant hepatitis. *Br. med. J.* 1984; **288:** 270.

16 Brown SE, Stanley C, Howard CR *et al.* Antibody responses to recombinant and plasma derived hepatitis B vaccines. *Brit. med. J.* 1986; **292:** 159.

17 Brzosko WJ, Krawczynski K, Nazarewicz T *et al.* Glomerulonephritis associated with hepatitis-B surface antigen immune complexes in children. *Lancet* 1974; **ii:** 477.

18 Budkowska A, Dubreuil P, Capel F *et al.* Hepatitis B virus pre-S gene-encoded antigenic specificity and anti-pre-S antibody: relationship between anti-pre-S response and recovery. *Hepatology* 1986; **6:** 360.

19 Buitrago B, Popper H, Hadler SC *et al.* Specific histologic features of Santa Marta hepatitis: a severe form of hepatitis delta-virus infection in Northern South America. *Hepatology* 1986; **6:** 1285.

20 Centers For Disease Control. Update on hepatitis B prevention. Recommendations of the immunization practices advisory committee. *Ann. int. Med.* 1987; **107:** 353.

21 Chan TK, Todd D. Haemolysis complicating viral hepatitis in patients with glucose-6-phosphate dehydrogenase deficiency. *Br. med. J.* 1975; **i:** 131.

22 Chau KH, Hargie MP, Decker RH *et al.* Serodiagnosis of recent hepatitis B infection by IgM class anti-HBC. *Hepatology* 1983; **3:** 142.

23 Colombo M, Oldani S, Donato MF *et al.* A multicenter, prospective study of posttransfusion hepatitis in Milan. *Hepatology* 1987; **7:** 709.

24 Coursaget P, Yvonnet B, Chotard J *et al.* Seven-year study of hepatitis B vaccine efficacy in infants from an endemic area (Senegal). *Lancet* 1986; **2:** 1143.

25 Craven DE, Awdeh ZL, Kunches LM *et al.* Non-responsiveness to hepatitis B vaccine in health care workers. *Ann. int. Med.* 1986; **105:** 356.

26 Cullinan ER, King RC, Rivers JS. The prognosis of infective hepatitis. A preliminary account of a long-term follow-up. *Br. med. J.* 1958; **i:** 1315.

27 Dane DS, Cameron CH, Briggs M. Virus-like particles in serum of patients with Australia-antigen-associated hepatitis. *Lancet* 1970; **i:** 695.

28 De Cock KM, Govindarajan S, Chin KP *et al.* Delta hepatitis in the Los Angeles Area: a report of 126 cases. *Ann. int. Med.* 1986; **105:** 108.

29 De Cock KM, Bradley DW, Sandford NL *et al.* Epidemic non-A, non-B hepatitis in patients from Pakistan. *Ann. int. Med.* 1987; **106:** 227.

30 Deodhar KP, Tapp E, Scheuer PJ, Orcein staining of hepatitis B antigen in paraffin sections of liver biopsies. *J. clin. Pathol.* 1975; **28:** 66.

31 Desmyter J, Colaert J, De Groote G *et al.* Efficacy of heat-inactivated hepatitis B vaccine in haemodialysis patients and staff: double-blind placebo-controlled trial. *Lancet* 1983; **ii:** 1323.

32 Dible JH, McMichael J, Sherlock SPV. Pathology of acute hepatitis. Aspiration biopsy studies of epidemic, arsenotherapy and serum jaundice. *Lancet* 1943; **ii:** 402.

33 Dienstag JL. Non-A, non-B hepatitis. I. Recognition, epidemiology, and clinical features. *Gastroenterology* 1983; **85:** 439.

34 Dienstag JL, Non-A, non-B hepatitis. II. Experimental transmission, putative virus agents and markers, and prevention. *Gastroenterology* 1983; **83:** 741.

35 Dienstag JL, Wands JR, Isselbacher KJ. Hepatitis B and essential mixed cryoglobulinemia. *N. Engl. J. Med.* 1977; **297:** 946.

36 Dienstag JL, Werner BG, Polk BF *et al.* Hepatitis B vaccine in health care personnel: safety, immunogenicity, and indicators of efficacy. *Ann. intern. Med.* 1984; **101:** 34.

37 Dragosics B, Ferenci P, Hitchman E, *et al.* Long-term follow-up study of asymptomatic HBsAg-positive voluntary blood donors in Austria: a clinical and histologic evaluation of 242 cases. *Hepatology* 1987; **7:** 302.

38 Dreesman GR, Sanchez Y, Ionescu-Matui I *et al.* Antibody to hepatitis B surface antigen after a single inoculation of uncoupled synthetic HBsAg peptides. *Nature* 1982; **295:** 158.

39 Dudley FJ, Scheuer PJ, Sherlock S. Natural history of hepatitis-associated antigen-positive chronic liver disease. *Lancet* 1972; **ii:** 1388.

40 Farci P, Barbera C, Navone C *et al.* Infection with the delta agent in children. *Gut* 1985; **26:** 4.

41 Feinstone SM, Kapikian AZ, Purcell RH. Hepatitis A: detection by immune electron microscopy of a virus-like antigen associated with acute illness. *Science* 1973; **182:** 1026.

42 Fields HA, Govindarajan S, Margolis HS *et al.* Experimental transmission of the delta virus to a hepatitis B chronic carrier chimpanzee with the development of persistent delta carriage. *Am. J. Pathol.* 1986; **122:** 308.

43 Flehmig B, Haage A, Pfisterer M. Immunogenicity of a hepatitis A virus vaccine. *J. med. Virol.* 1987; **22:** 7.

44 Friedman LS, Dienstag JL, Watkins E *et al.* Evaluation of blood donors with elevated alanine aminotransferase levels. *Ann. intern. Med.* 1987; **107:** 137.

45 Gianotti F. Papular acrodermatitis of childhood: an Australian antigen disease. *Arch. Dis. Childh.* 1973; **48:** 794.

46 Gilliam JH III, Geisinger KR, Richter JE. Primary hepatocellular carcinoma after chronic non-A, non-B post-transfusion hepatitis. *Ann. intern. Med.* 1984; **101**: 794.

47 Gimson AES, White YS, Eddleston ALWF *et al.* Clinical and prognostic differences in fulminant hepatitis type A, B, and non-A, non-B. *Gut* 1983; **24**: 1194.

48 Gordon SG, Reddy KR, Schiff L *et al.* Prolonged intra-hepatic cholestasis secondary to acute hepatitis A. *Ann. intern. Med.* 1984; **101**: 635.

49 Govindarajan S, Valinluck B, Peters RL. Relapse of acute B viral hepatitis—role of delta agent. *Gut* 1986; **27**: 19.

50 Govindarajan S, De Cock KM, Redeker AG. Natural course of delta superinfection in chronic hepatitis B virus-infected patients: histopathologic study with multiple liver biopsies. *Hepatology* 1986; **6**: 640.

51 Gu J-R, Chen Y-C, Jiang H-Q *et al.* State of hepatitis B virus DNA in leucocytes of hepatitis B patients. *J. Med. Virol.* 1985; **17**: 73.

52 Hadler SC, De Monzon M, Ponzetto A *et al.* Delta virus infection and severe hepatitis: an epidemic in the Yupca Indians of Venzuela. *Ann. intern. Med.* 1984; **100**: 339.

53 Hadler SC, Francis DP, Maynard JE. *et al.* Long-term immunogenicity and efficacy of hepatitis B vaccine in homosexual men. *N. Engl. J. Med.* 1986; **315**: 209.

54 Haglar L, Pastore RA, Bergin JJ *et al.* Aplastic anemia following viral hepatitis. *Medicine (Baltimore)* 1975; **54**: 139.

55 Heijtink RA, De Jong P, Schalm SW *et al.* Hepatitis B vaccination in Down's syndrome and other mentally retarded patients. *Hepatology* 1984; **4**: 611.

56 Hollinger FB, Khan NC, Oefinger PE. Post-transfusion hepatitis type A. *J. Am. med. Assoc.* 1983; **250**: 2313.

57 Houghton M *et al.* Parenteral non-A, non-B hepatitis: molecular isolation and immunity. In press 1989.

58 Inman RD, Hodge M, Johnston MEA. *et al.* Arthritis, vasculitis and cryoglobulinemia associated with relapsing hepatitis A virus infection. *Ann. intern. Med.* 1986; **105**: 700.

59 International Group. Morphological criteria in viral hepatitis. *Lancet* 1971; **i**: 333.

60 Iwarson S, Tabor E, Thomas HC *et al.* Protection against hepatitis B virus infection by immunization with hepatitis B core antigen. *Gastroenterology* 1985; **88**: 763.

61 Iwarson SA, Non-A, non-B hepatitis: dead ends or new horizons? *Br. Med. J.* 1987; **295**: 946.

62 Jacobson IM, Dienstag JL, Zachoval R *et al.* Lack of effect of hepatitis B vaccine on T-cell phenotypes. *N. Engl. J. Med.* 1984; **311**: 1030.

63 Jonas MM, Schiff ER, O'Sullivan MJ *et al.* Failure of centers for disease control criteria to identify hepatitis B infection in a large municipal obstetrical population. *Ann. intern. Med.* 1987; **107**: 335.

64 Kao HW, Ashcavai M, Redeker AG. The persistence of hepatitis A IgM antibody after acute clinical hepatitis A. *Hepatology* 1984; **4**: 933.

65 Karayiannis P, Novick DM, Lok ASF *et al.* Hepatitis B virus DNA in saliva, urine and seminal fluid of carriers of hepatitis B antigen. *Br. Med. J.* 1985; **290**: 1853.

66 Khuroo MS. Study of an epidemic of non-A, non-B hepatitis: possibility of another human hepatitis virus distinct from post-transfusion non-A, non-B type *Am. J. Med.* 1980; **68**: 818.

67 Knight AH, Fox RA, Baillod RA *et al.* Hepatitis associated antigen and antibody in haemodialysis patients and staff. *Br. Med. J.* 1970; **ii**: 603.

68 Kojima T, Callea F, Desmyter J *et al.* Immune electron microscopy of hepatitis delta-antigen in hepatocytes. *Lab. Invest.* 1986; **55**: 217.

69 Konriskern PJ, Hagopian A, Burke P *et al.* A candi-date vaccine for hepatitis B containing the complete viral surface protein. *Hepatology* 1988; **8**: 82.

70 Kos A, Dijkema R, Arnberg AC *et al.* The hepatitis delta (δ) virus possesses a circular RNA. *Nature* 1986; **323**: 558.

71 Koziol DE, Holland PV, Alling DW *et al.* Antibody to hepatitis B core antigen as a paradoxical marker for non-A, non-B hepatitis agents in donated blood. *Ann. intern. Med.* 1986; **104**: 488.

72 Krogsgaard K, Kryger P, Aldershvile J *et al.* δ-infection and suppression of hepatitis B virus replication in chronic HBsAg carriers. *Hepatology* 1987; **7**: 42.

73 Krugman S, Overby LR, Mushahwar IK *et al.* Viral hepatitis type B: studies on natural history and prevention re-examined. *N. Engl. J. Med.* 1979; **300**: 101.

74 Lai KN, Lai FM, Wai Chan K *et al.* The clinicopathologic features of hepatitis B virus-associated glomerulonephritis. *Quart. J. Med.* 1987; **63**: 323.

75 Lander JJ, Holland PV, Alter HJ *et al.* Antibody to hepatitis-associated antigen. Frequency and pattern of response as detected by radioimmunoprecipitation. *J. Am. med. Assoc.* 1972; **220**: 1079.

76 Le Bouvier GL, Subtypes of hepatitis B antigen: clinical relevance? *Ann. intern. Med.* 1973; **99**: 894.

77 Lefkowitch JH, Apfelbaum TF, Liver cell dysplasia and hepatocellular carcinoma in non-A, non-B hepatitis. *Arch. Path. lab. Med.* 1987; **111**: 170.

78 Lefkowitch JH, Goldstein H, Yatto R *et al.* Cytopathic liver injury in acute delta virus hepatitis. *Gastroenterology* 1987; **92**: 1262.

79 Lemon SM. Type A viral hepatitis: new developments in an old disease. *N. Engl. J. Med.* 1985; **313:** 1059.

80 Lettau LA, McCarthy JG, Smith MH *et al.* Outbreak of severe hepatitis due to delta and hepatitis B viruses in parenteral drug abusers and their contacts. *N. Engl. J. Med.* 1987; **317:** 1256.

81 Lever AML, Webster ADB, Brown D *et al.* Non-A, non-B hepatitis occurring in agammaglobulinaemic patients after intravenous immunoglobulin. *Lancet* 1984; **ii:** 1062.

82 Levo Y, Gorevic PD, Kassab HJ *et al.* Association between hepatitis B virus and essential mixed cryoglobulinemia. *N. Engl. J. Med.* 1977; **296:** 1501.

83 Lieberman HM, La Brecque DR, Kew MC *et al.* Detection of hepatitis B virus DNA directly in human serum by a simplified molecular hybridization test: comparison to HBeAg anti-HBe status in HBsAg carriers. *Hepatology* 1983; **3:** 285.

84 London WT, Blumberg BS. Comments on the role of epidemiology in the investigation of hepatitis B virus. *Epidemiologic reviews* 1985; **7:** 59.

85 Margulies A, Bernuau J, Balayan MS *et al.* Non-A, non-B fulminant viral hepatitis in France in returnees from Asia and Africa. *Dig. Dis. Sci.* 1987; **32:** 1151.

86 Mathiesen LR. The Copenhagen Hepatitis Acute Programme. Immunofluorescence studies for Hepatitis A virus and Hepatitis B surface antigen and core antigen in liver biopsies from patients with acute viral hepatitis. *Gastroenterology* 1979: **77:** 623.

87 McMahon BJ, Rhoades ER, Heyward WL *et al.* A comprehensive programme to reduce the incidence of hepatitis B virus infection and its seqelae in Alaskan natives. *Lancet* 1987; **ii:** 1134.

88 Meyer zum Büschenfelde K-H, Gerken G, Hess G *et al.* The significance of the pre-S region of the hepatitis B virus. *J. Hepatol* 1986; **3:** 273.

89 Michalak T. Immune complexes of hepatitis B surface antigen in the pathogenesis of periarteritis nodosa: study of seven necropsy cases. *Am. J. Pathol.* 1978; **90:** 619.

90 Moseley JW, Redeker AG, Feinstone SM *et al.* Multiple hepatitis viruses in multiple attacks of acute viral hepatitis. *N. Engl. J. Med.* 1977; **296:** 75.

91 Moss B, Smith GL, Gerin JL *et al.* Live recombinant vaccinia virus protects chimpanzees against hepatitis B. *Nature* 1984; **311:** 67.

92 Omata M, Uchiumi K, Ito Y *et al.* Duck hepatitis B virus and liver diseases. *Gastroenterology* 1983; **85:** 260.

93 Papaevangelou G, Tassopoulous N, Roumeliotou-Karayannis A *et al.* Etiology of fulminant viral hepatitis in Greece. *Hepatology* 1984; **4:** 369.

94 Penner E, Maida E, Mamoli B *et al.* Serum and cerebrospinal fluid immune complexes containing hepatitis B surface antigen in Guillain–Barré syndrome. *Gastroenterology* 1982; **82:** 576.

95 Piazza M, Guadagnino V, Orlando R *et al.* Acute B viral hepatitis becomes fulminant after infection with hepatitis A virus. *Br. Med. J.* 1982; **284:** 1913.

96 Pontisso P, Poon MC, Tiollais P *et al.* Detection of hepatitis B virus DNA in mononuclear blood cells. *Br. med. J.* 1984; **288:** 1563.

97 Popper H, Shih J W-K, Gerin JL *et al.* Woodchuck hepatitis and hepatocellular carcinoma: correlation of histologic with virologic observations. *Hepatology* 1981; **1:** 91.

98 Poulsen H, Christoffersen P. Abnormal bile duct epithelium in liver biopsies with histological signs of viral hepatitis. *Acta Path. microbiol. Scand.* 1969; **76:** 383.

99 Provost PJ, Bishop RP, Gerety RJ *et al.* New findings in live, attenuated hepatitis A vaccine development. *J. med. Virol.* 1986; **20:** 165.

100 Provost PJ, Hughes JV, Miller WJ *et al.* An inactivated hepatitis A viral vaccine of cell culture origin. *J. med. Virol.* 1986; **19:** 23.

101 Ramalingaswami V, Purcell RH. Waterborne non-A, non-B hepatitis. *Lancet* 1988; **1:** 571.

102 Realdi G, Alberti A, Rugge M *et al.* Long-term follow-up of acute and chronic non-A, non-B post-transfusion hepatitis: evidence of progression to liver cirrhosis. *Gut* 1982; **23:** 270.

103 Reincke V, Dybkjaer E, Poulsen H *et al.* A study of Australia-antigen-positive blood donors and their recipients, with special reference to liver histology. *N. Engl. J. Med.* 1972; **286:** 867.

104 Rizzetto M. The delta agent. *Hepatology* 1983; **3:** 729.

105 Rizzetto M, Macagno S, Chiaberge E *et al.* Liver transplantation in hepatitis delta virus disease. *Lancet* 1987; **ii:** 469.

106 Rosenberg JL, Jones DP, Lipitz LR *et al.* Viral hepatitis: an occupational hazard to surgeons. *J. Am. med. Assoc.* 1973; **223:** 395.

107 Rosina F, Saracco G, Rizzetto M. Risk of post-transfusion infection with the hepatitis delta virus: a multicenter study. *N. Engl. J. Med.* 1985; **312:** 1488.

108 Sanchez-Quijano A, Pineda JA, Lissen E **et al**. Prevention of post-transfusion non-A, non-B hepatitis by non-specific immunoglobulin in heart surgery patients. *Lancet* 1988; **i:** 1245.

109 Scheuer PJ, Texeira MR, Weller IVD *et al.* Pathology of acute hepatitis A, B and non-A, non-B. *J. Pathol.* 1981; **134:** 323.

110 Schimpf K, Mannucci PM, Kreutz W *et al.* Absence of hepatitis after treatment with a pasteurized factor VIII concentrate in patients with hemophilia and no previous transfusions. *N. Engl. J.*

Med. 1987; **316**: 918.

111 Schreeder MT, Thompson SE, Hadler SC *et al.* Hepatitis B in homosexual men: prevalence of infection and factors related to transmission. *J. Infect. Dis.* 1982; **146:** 7.

112 Scotto J, Hadchouel M, Hery C *et al.* Detection of hepatitis B virus DNA in serum by a single spot hybridization technique: comparison with results for other viral markers. *Hepatology* 1983; **3**: 279.

113 Seeff LB, Koff RS. Passive and active immuno-prophylaxis of hepatitis B. *Gastroenterology* 1984; **86:** 958.

114 Seeff LB, Zimmerman HJ, Wright EC *et al.* A randomised, double-blind controlled trial of the efficacy of immune serum globulin for the prevention of post-transfusion hepatitis: a veterans administration cooperative study. 1977; **72:** 111.

115 Shaldon S, Sherlock S. Virus hepatitis with features of prolonged bile retention. *Br. med. J.* 1957; **ii:** 734.

116 Shattock AG, Finlay H, Hillary IB. Possible reactivation of hepatitis D with chronic delta antigenaemia by human immunodeficiency virus. *Br. Med. J.* 1987; **294:** 1656.

117 Sherlock S, Walshe VM. The post-hepatitis syndrome, *Lancet* 1946; **ii:** 482.

118 Sherlock S, Thomas HC. Conference Report: delta virus hepatitis. *J. Hepatol.* 1986; **3**: 419.

119 Shiels MT, Czaja AJ, Taswell HF *et al.* Frequency and significance of delta antibody in acute and chronic hepatitis B. A United States experience. *Gastroenterology* 1985; **89:** 1230.

120 Shimizu M, Ohyama M, Takahashi Y *et al.* Immunoglobulin M antibody against hepatitis B core antigen for the diagnosis of fulminant type B hepatitis. *Gastroenterology* 1983; **84:** 604.

121 Shimoda T, Shikata T, Karasawa T *et al.* Light microscopic localization of hepatitis B virus antigens in the human pancreas. *Gastroenterology* 1981; **81:** 998.

122 Sjogren MH, Tanno H, Fay O *et al.* Hepatitis A virus in stool during clinical relapse. *Ann. intern. Med.* 1987; **106:** 221.

123 Smedile A, Rizzetto M, Denniston K *et al.* Type D hepatitis: the clinical significance of hepatitis D virus RNA in serum as detected by a hybridisa tion-based assay. *Hepatology* 1986; **6**: 1297.

124 Solomon RE, Kaslow RA, Phair JP *et al.* Human immuno-deficiency virus and hepatitis delta virus in homosexual men. A study of four cohorts. *Ann. intern. Med.* 1988; **108:** 51.

125 Stevens CE, Taylor PE, Tong MJ *et al.* Yeast-recombinant hepatitis B vaccine. Efficacy with hepatitis B immune globulin in prevention of perinatal hepatitis B virus transmission. *J. Am. med. Ass.* 1987; **257:** 2612.

126 Szmuness W, Stevens CE, Harley EJ *et al.* Hepatitis B vaccine: demonstration of efficacy in a controlled trial in a high-risk population in the United States. *N. Engl. J. Med.* 1980; **303**: 833.

127 Tabor E. Guillain−Barré syndrome and other neurologic syndromes in hepatitis A, B, non-A, non-B. *J. Med. Virol.* 1987; **21:** 207.

128 Takeda S, Kida H, Katagiri M *et al.* Characteristics of glomerular lesions in hepatitis B virus infection: *Am. J. Kidney Dis.* 1988; **11:** 57.

129 Texeira MR Jr, Weller IVD, Murray A *et al.* The pathology of hepatitis A in man. *Liver* 1982; **2:** 53.

130 Thomas HC, Potter BJ, Elias E *et al.* Metabolism of the third component of complement in acute type B hepatitis, HB_s antigen positive glomerulonephritis, polyarteritis nodosum and HB_s antigen positive and negative chronic active liver disease. *Gastroenterology* 1979; **76:** 673.

131 Ticehurst JR, Hepatitis A virus: clones, cultures, and vaccines. *Semin. Liver Dis.* 1986; **6**: 46.

132 Toukan AU, Abu-El-Rub OA, Abu-Laban SA. The epidemiology and clinical outcome of hepatitis D virus (Delta) infection in Jordan. *Hepatology* 1987; **7**: 1340.

133 Ursell PC, Habib A, Sharma P *et al.* Hepatitis B virus and myocarditis. *Hum. Pathol.* 1984; **15:** 481.

134 Vallbracht A, Gabriel P, Maier K *et al.* Cell-mediated cytotoxicity in hepatitis A virus infection. *Hepatology* 1986; **6:** 1308.

135 Verme G, Amoroso P, Lettieri G *et al.* A histological study of hepatitis delta virus liver disease. *Hepatology* 1986; **6:** 1303.

136 Villa E, Pasquinelli C, Rigo G *et al.* Gastrointestinal endoscopy and HBV infection: no evidence for a causal relationship. *Gastrointest. Endosc.* 1984; **30:** 15.

137 Vyas GN, Dienstag JL, Hoofnagle JH (eds). *Viral Hepatitis and Liver Disease.* Grune & Stratton, New York. 1984.

138 Wands JR, Alpert E, Isselbacher KJ. Arthritis associated with chronic active hepatitis. Complement activation and characterization of circulating immune complexes. *Gastroenterology* 1975; **69:** 1286.

139 Wang K-S, Choo Q-L, Weiner AJ *et al.* Structure sequence and expression of the hepatitis delta (δ) viral genome. *Nature* 1986; **323:** 508.

140 Weller IVD, Karayiannis P, Lok ASF *et al.* Significance of delta agent infection in chronic hepatitis B virus infection: a study in British carriers. *Gut* 1983; **24:** 1061.

141 Wong VCW, Ip HMH, Reesink HW *et al.* Prevention of the HBsAg carrier state in newborn infants

of mothers who are chronic carriers of HBsAg and HBeAg by administration of hepatitis-B vaccine and hepatitis-B immunoglobulin. *Lancet.* 1984; **i**: 921.

142 Zeldis JB, Mugishima H, Steinberg HN *et al. In vitro* hepatitis B virus infection of human bone marrow cells. *J. Clin. Invest.* 1986; **78**: 411.

143 Zoulek G, Lorbeer B, Jilg W *et al.* Evaluation of a reduced dose of hepatitis B vaccine administered intradermally. *J. med. Virol* 1984; **14**: 27.

144 Zuckerman AJ. The chronicle of viral hepatitis. *Bull. Hyg. trop. Dis.* 1977; **54**: 113.

Yellow fever

This acute infection is due to a group B arbovirus transmitted to man by the bite of infected mosquitoes. The virus cycle is a direct human one in urban yellow fever, or may involve wild monkeys of the jungle variety.

The two endemic regions are South America and equatorial Africa.

PATHOLOGY

In man, the liver histology shows predominantly mid-zonal acidophilic hepato-cellular necroses (Councilman bodies). Ceroid is abundant and inflammation scanty. Under electron microscopy viral particles are absent. The acidophilic bodies are composed of round or elliptical cytoplasmic masses, surrounded by a cellular membrane and densely packed with organelles, fat vacuoles, ceroid pigment and residual bodies [1, 2]. These changes are not seen in acidophilic bodies found in other liver diseases.

With recovery, regeneration is complete and chronicity does not result.

The *spleen* is enlarged with reticulo-endothelial proliferation; the *kidneys* show tubular necrosis; the *stomach* contains altered blood; and the *heart* is pale and flabby.

CLINICAL FEATURES

Following an incubation period of 3—6 days, the disease has a sudden onset with fever, chills, headache, backache, prostration and vomiting, often of altered blood. The blood pressure falls, haemorrhages become widespread, jaundice and albuminuria are conspicuous and there is a relative bradycardia. Delirium proceeds to coma and death within nine days. If there is recovery the temperature becomes normal within this time and convalescence progresses rapidly and completely. There are no sequelae and life-long immunity follows. Apart from the classical course described, the majority of infections are probably milder, with no detectable jaundice and only a few constitutional symptoms.

Diagnosis [3]. Serum within the first three days of the illness is injected intracerebrally into mice and the encephalitis noted. Acute-phase and convalescent sera should be obtained for the demonstration of protective antibodies in mice. Prothrombin deficiency parallels the severity of the liver lesion. The serum cholesterol level falls in the fatal case. Serum transaminases are increased relative to severity.

TREATMENT

There is no specific treatment. Death results principally from renal damage. The hepatic lesion is self-limited and of short duration and does not demand special treatment.

Prevention consists of vaccination and control of mosquitoes. It is necessary to be vaccinated at least ten days before arrival in endemic areas.

References

1 Soper FL, Rickard ER, Crawford PJ. The routine post-mortem removal of liver tissue from rapidly fatal fever cases for the discovery of silent yellow fever foci. *Am. J. Hyg.* 1934; **19**: 549.

2 Vieira WT, Gayotto LC, De Lima CP. *et al.* Histopathology of the human liver in yellow fever with special emphasis on the diagnostic role of the Councilman body. *Histopathology* 1983; **7**: 195.

3 World Health Organisation Arboviruses and human disease. *WHO tech. Report Series*, 1967, 369.

Infectious mononucleosis

This virus infection is due to human herpes virus IV (Epstein–Barr) (EBV) which excites a generalized reticulo-endothelial reaction [5]. It largely affects adolescents and young adults and may mimic type A, type B, or non-A, non-B viral hepatitis.

Presentation, particularly in adults, may be as fever with right upper quadrant abdominal discomfort [1, 3]. Pharyngitis and lymphadenopathy may be absent.

HEPATIC HISTOLOGY (fig. 16.31)

The changes are seen within five days of the onset and reach their peak between the tenth and thirtieth days.

The sinusoids and portal tracts are infiltrated with large, mononuclear cells. Polymorphonuclear leucocytes and lymphocytes increase, and the Kupffer cells proliferate. The appearances may resemble those of leukaemia. The portal tract lesions resemble those of early A, B, or non-A, non-B viral hepatitis. The architecture of the liver is preserved.

Zone 3 necrosis is absent, although focal necroses may be randomly distributed. The necroses are not bile stained and there is no surrounding cellular reaction.

In later biopsies, binucleate liver cells and mitoses are conspicuous. The evidences of regeneration are out of proportion to cell necrosis. After clinical recovery, abnormal cells disappear although this may take as long as eight months. Chronic hepatitis and cirrhosis are not sequelae.

CLINICAL FEATURES

Occasionally jaundice can be deep [2]. Large glands in the porta hepatis do not compress the common bile duct.

Fatal acute hepatic necrosis is a rare complication [4].

Persistent infection is a cause of chronic ill health.

Immune responses determine the clinical and pathological expression. Using monoclonal antibodies direct hepatic viral infection has been shown.

DIAGNOSIS

The total serum albumin level may be slightly decreased and the serum globulin value slightly elevated.

Hyperbilirubinaemia is present in about one-half of patients. Serum transaminase values are raised to about 20 times the normal in 80% of patients. Values are usually less than those found in the early stages of an acute virus

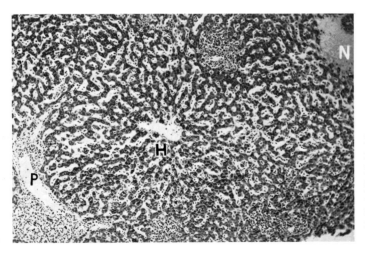

Fig. 16.31. Infectious mononucleosis. The sinusoids and portal tracts (P) are filled with mononuclear cells. H is a central hepatic vein. One small local necrosis (N) is seen in the upper right-hand corner. Best's carmine, ×70.

hepatitis. In about one-third the serum alkaline phosphatase value is increased, often more than the bilirubin.

Alkaline phosphatase and transaminase levels are found in those with severe, mononuclear round-cell infiltration in the hepatic sinusoids.

The 'monospot' reaction is usually but not always positive. The disease is diagnosed conclusively by an increase in serum IgM antibodies against Epstein−Barr capsid antigens.

DISTINCTION FROM VIRUS HEPATITIS (table 16.10)

Although the diagnosis of virus hepatitis from infectious mononucleosis is usually easy, in an occasional instance of mild anicteric hepa-titis or severe mononucleosis this may be impossible.

References

1 Horwitz CA, Henle W, Hewle G *et al.* Infectious mononucleosis in patients aged 40 to 72 years, including 3 without heterphile-antibody, 13 responses. *Medicine (Baltimore)* 1983; **62:** 256.
2 Fuhrman SA, Gill R, Horwitz CA *et al.* Marked hyper-bilirubinemia in infectious mononucleosis. *Arch. intern. Med.* 1987; **147:** 850.
3 Jacobson IM, Gang DL, Schapiro RH. Epstein Barr viral hepatitis: an unusual case and review of the literature. *Am. J. Gastroenterol.* 1984; **79:** 628.
4 Markin RS, Linder J, Zuerlein K *et al.* Hepatitis in fatal infectious mononucleosis. *Gastroenterology* 1987; **93:** 1210.
5 White NJ, Juel-Jensen BE. Infectious mononucleosis hepatitis. *Semin. Liv. Dis.* 1984; **4:** 301.

Other viruses

All viruses may affect the liver in common with other organs. The histological changes are

Table 16.10. Comparison of infectious mononucleosis and virus hepatitis

	Infectious mononucleosis	Virus hepatitis
Epidemic history	Suggestive	Suggestive
Onset		
Fever	+	+
Anorexia	−	+
Sore throat	+	−
Rash	+	Rare
Pruritus	−	+
Physical signs		
Lymphadenopathy	++	±
Jaundice	Mild, transient	Well-developed, persisting
Liver	Enlarged; not usually tender	Enlarged and tender
Spleen	Enlarged and tender	Enlarged but not tender
Pale stools	−	+
Dark urine	±	++
Peripheral blood		
Leucocytes	Usually increased. Characteristic cells	Decreased, with relative lymphocytosis
Monospot	+ve	−ve
IgM EB	Present	Absent
HBsAg	−ve	+ve, type B
IgM anti hep A	−ve	+ve, type A
Liver biopsy	Diffuse mononuclear infiltration. Focal necroses	Zone 3 'spotty' necrosis. Mononuclear infiltration

usually non-specific, consisting of fatty change, or focal necrosis and lymphocytic infiltration of the portal zones. Biochemical tests are usually unchanged or show mild rises in transaminases. Occasionally the patient may be frankly icteric when the picture of type A, B, or non-A, non-B hepatitis is closely simulated.

The upsurge of AIDS has increased the prevalence of hepatitis due to various, unusual viruses. These frequently prove fatal (Chapter 27). They are also important in those receiving large doses of immunosuppression such as liver and bone marrow recipients, or patients with reticulosis. They are seen in neonates (Chapter 24) and may follow a blood transfusion.

Cytomegalovirus

In neonates it is usually inapparent. Confirmed disease in early infancy is rare. Sometimes, however, in association with the respiratory distress syndrome, cytomegalovirus may cause a devastating fatal pneumonitis [3]. In adults, the clinical picture can be very diverse.

Cytomegalovirus can cause a disease strongly resembling EBV-related mononucleosis [10]. Patients usually lack pharyngitis and posterior cervical lymphadenopathy. Serum transaminase and alkaline phosphatase levels are increased and atypical lymphocytes are found in the peripheral blood. The monospot test is usually negative.

The picture may simulate type A, type B or non-A, non-B hepatitis, having a similar onset but with failure of the pyrexia to subside with the onset of jaundice. Icterus lasts two to three weeks and even up to three months.

Occasionally, massive hepatic necrosis may be fatal.

Granulomatous hepatitis can develop in a previously normal adult with prolonged unexplained fever and without lymphadenopathy [4]. In these patients, liver biopsy shows non-caseating granulomas. The immunosuppressed show characteristic inclusions.

Cholangitis, papillary stenosis and sclerosing cholangitis can accompany cytomegaloinfections in AIDS patients (see Chapter 15) [12, 17].

Cytomegalovirus infection is an important cause of post-transfusion hepatitis.

Cytomegalovirus may cause disseminated disease, of which hepatitis is only a part, in the immuno-suppressed, such as the leukaemic or renal or hepatic transplant recipient. This probably represents a reaction to endogenous virus.

Diagnosis is by isolation of virus from urine or saliva. Complement fixing antibodies rise and CMV IgM antibodies can be found. The virus cannot usually be shown in liver biopsy but direct hepatic involvement has been confirmed by demonstrating nuclear and cytoplasmic inclusions in hepatocytes by monoclonal antibodies, immunoperoxidase and immunofluorescent techniques [19].

Herpes simplex

Human herpes virus types I and II affect all humans at some time during their lives.

In *infants* herpes hepatitis may be part of generalized herpetic disease.

In *adults*, disseminated herpes simplex is very rare. It can affect those with underlying diseases e.g. ulcerative colitis [20], with AIDS, receiving immunosuppressive treatment and having organ transplants. Fulminant hepatic failure can also affect the previously normal and immunocompetent [9]. It may complicate genital herpes [18].

Herpetic mucocutaneous lesions are usually absent. The onset is with fever, prostration, marked elevation of transaminases and leucopenia [13]. Jaundice is absent. Fulminant liver failure with fatal coagulopathy can develop.

Liver biopsy shows patchy areas of coagulative necrosis with surrounding hepatocytes containing viral inclusions [9]. The virus can be shown by electron microscopy. It can be cultured from the liver and, using immunoperoxidase staining, may be shown in affected hepatocytes [13].

OTHER VIRUSES

Coxsackie virus B may cause hepatitis in the adult. Coxsackie virus, group A, type IV, has been isolated from the plasma of a child with hepatitis, and complement fixing antibodies appeared in the serum during convalescence.

Adenovirus has caused fulminant hepatitis in a young immuno-suppressed adult [3]. Intranuclear inclusions were confined to the liver.

Varicella and varicella-zoster may be complicated by hepatitis in both normal and immunologically compromised individuals [16]. In children the picture must be distinguished from Reye's syndrome [16].

Measles is affecting an older age group. Eighty per cent of adult sufferers have liver involvement—5% becoming jaundiced [7]. It is most frequent in the seriously ill. Resolution is complete. A similar picture is seen with the atypical measles syndrome [6].

Rubella can be associated with serum transaminase elevations and may be mistakenly diagnosed as non-A, non-B hepatitis [22].

Hepatitis due to exotic viruses

This term is applied to very dangerous, newly identified and unusual viruses where the liver appears to be the primary target [11]. They include Marburg, Lassa and Ebola viruses. They are becoming increasingly important as man encroaches into underdeveloped areas, as ecology changes and as a source of infection to medical or laboratory staff dealing with patients or their blood.

Lassa fever is due to an arena virus transmitted from rodents to man or from man to man. It is largely found in West Africa. The case fatality rate is 36–67%. It has been successfully treated with ribavirin [15].

The liver shows eosinophilic necrosis of individual hepatocytes with little inflammation. Bridging necrosis is usual.

Marburg virus disease is due to an RNA virus transmitted by Vervet monkeys. In 1967, an outbreak of this disease occurred in persons in contact with monkeys in experimental institutes in Germany [16]. Further patients have been reported from South Africa [8] and Kenya [21].

After an incubation of 4–7 days the patients present with headache, pyrexia, vomiting, a characteristic rash, a haemorrhagic diathesis and central nervous system involvement. Serum transaminase levels are very high.

Liver pathology [2] shows single-cell acidophilic necrosis and Kupffer cell hyperactivity. This is followed by eccentric and radial extension of the necrosis, cytoplasmic inclusions and portal zone cellularity. A steatosis is noted in the severely affected. Virus can persist in the body for 2–3 months after initial infection [8].

Ebola virus infection resembles Marburg in clinical course, hepatic histology and electron microscopy [5]. It has been reported from Zaïre and Sudan and has been transmitted to biologists working with it.

TREATMENT

There is no specific treatment for these exotic virus infections. Symptomatic measures are used and very strict precautions are necessary to avoid spread to contacts.

References

1 Ballard RA, Drew L, Hoofnagle KG *et al.* Acquired cytomegalovirus infection in preterm infants. *Am. J. Dis. Child.* 1979; **133**: 482.

2 Bechtelsheimer H, Korb G, Gedigk P. The morphology and pathogenesis of 'Marburg-virus' hepatitis. *Hum. Pathol.* 1972; **3**: 255.8

3 Carmichael GP, Zarhadnik JM, Moyer GH *et al.* Adenovirus hepatitis in an immunosuppressed adult patient. *Am. J. clin. Pathol.* 1979; **71**: 352.

4 Clarke J, Craig RM, Saffro R *et al.* Cytomegalovirus granulomatous hepatitis. *Am. J. Med.* 1979; **66**: 264.

5 Ellis DS, Simpson DIH, Francis DP *et al.* Ultrastructure of Ebola virus particles in human liver. *J. clin. Pathol.* 1978; **31**: 201.

6 Frey HM, Krugman S. Case report. Atypical measles syndrome: unusual hepatic, pulmonary, and immunologic aspects. *Am. J. med. Sci.* 1981; *281*: 51.

7 Gavish D, Kleinman Y, Morag A *et al.* Hepatitis

and jaundice associated with measles in young adults. *Arch. intern. Med.* 1983; **13**: 674.

8 Gear JSS, Cassell GA, Gear AJ *et al.* Outbreak of Marburg virus disease in Johannesburg. *Br. Med. J.* 1975; **iv**: 489.

9 Goodman ZD, Ishak KG, Sesterhenn IA *et al.* Herpes simplex hepatitis in apparently immuno-competent adults. *Am. J. Clin. Path.* 1986; **85**: 694.

10 Horwitz CA, Henle W, Henle G *et al.* Clinical and laboratory evaluation of cytomegalovirus-induced mononucleosis in previously healthy individuals. *Medicine (Baltimore)* 1986; **65**: 124.

11 Howard CR, Ellis DS, Simpson DIH. Exotic viruses and the liver. *Semin. Liv. Dis.* 1984; **4**: 361.

12 Jacobson MA, Cello JP, Sande MA. Cholestasis and disseminated cytomegalovirus disease in patients with the acquired immunodeficiency syndrome. *Am. J. Med.* 1988; **84**: 218.

13 Marrie TJ, McDonald ATJ, Conen PE *et al.* Herpes simplex hepatitis—use of immunoperoxidase to demonstrate the viral antigen in hepatocytes. *Gastroenterology* 1982; **82**: 71.

14 Martini GA, Knauff HG, Schmidt HA **et al**. Uber eine bisher unbekannte von Affen eingeschleppte Infektionskrankheit: Marburg-Virus-Krankheit. *Dtsch. med. Wschr.* 1968; **57**: 559.

15 McCormick JB, King IJ, Webb PA *et al.* Lassa fever. Effective therapy with ribavirin. *N. Engl. J. Med.* 1986; **314**: 20.

16 Myers MG. Hepatic cellular injury during varicella. *Arch. Dis. Child.* 1982; **57**: 317.

17 Roulot D, Walla D, Brun-Vezinet F *et al.* Cholangitis in the acquired immunodeficiency syndrome: report of two cases and review of the literature. *Gut* 1987; **28**: 1653.

18 Rubin MH, Ward DM, Painter J. Fulminant hepatic failure caused by genital herpes in a healthy person. *J. Am. med. Ass.* 1985; **253**: 1299.

19 Sacks SL, Freeman HJ. Cytomegalovirus hepatitis: evidence for direct hepatic viral infection using monoclonal antibodies. *Gastroenterology* 1984; **86**: 346.

20 Shlien RD, Meyers S, Lee JA *et al.* Fulminant herpes simplex hepatitis in a patient with ulcerative colitis. *Gut* 1988; **29**: 257.

21 Smith DH, Johnson BK, Isaacson M. Marburg-virus disease in Kenya. *Lancet* 1982; **i**: 816.

22 Zeldis JB, Miller JG, Dienstag JL. Hepatitis in an adult with rubella. *Am. J. Med.* 1985; **79**: 515.

17 · Chronic Hepatitis

A spectrum of chronic inflammatory diseases of the liver extends from acute hepatitis to chronic hepatitis and finally to cirrhosis. Whatever the type of chronic hepatitis, the same basic underlying liver histology is seen. Superimposed are histological features relative to the aetiology. However, before needle liver biopsy can be recommended, the physician must be aware of the mode of presentation and of the associated laboratory findings which suggest the diagnosis (table 17.1) [84].

Classification

Chronic hepatitis is defined as a chronic inflammatory reaction in the liver continuing without improvement for at least six months [81].

Cirrhosis is defined as widespread fibrosis with nodule formation (Chapter 19). The normal zonal architecture of the liver cannot be recognized.

Chronic hepatitis was originally classified into two types—chronic persistent and chronic active (aggressive) [21]. This has proved to be an over-simplification of the problem; a further type, chronic lobular hepatitis, has been introduced and the chronic active form has been subdivided into a mild and severe type (figs 17.1, 17.2) [46].

Chronic persistent hepatitis (fig. 17.3) is marked by expansion of the portal zone by mononuclear cells and some fibrosis. The limiting plate of liver cells between portal zones and liver cell columns is intact. Piecemeal necrosis of liver cells is not seen.

Chronic lobular hepatitis is sometimes termed prolonged or unresolved acute hepatitis. Many of the histological features resemble acute viral hepatitis, but the duration is greater than three months. The picture is predominantly that of

Table 17.1. The investigation of suspected chronic hepatitis

Presentation
Fatigue: generally unwell
Following blood donation—positive hepatitis B test
Following acute hepatitis—failure of recovery, whether clinical or biochemical or both
Abnormal liver function tests or positive hepatitis B antigen test at routine check-up
Abnormal physical findings—hepatomegaly ± splenomegaly
Jaundice
Blood transfusions in the past

Careful history and physical examination

Routine laboratory tests
Liver function tests
  Bilirubin
  Aspartate transaminase (SGOT)
  Gamma-globulin
  Albumin
  Alkaline phosphatase
Haematology
  Haemoglobin
  White cell count
  Platelet count
  Prothrombin time
Hepatitis B surface antigen

Special tests
Serum antibodies
  Nuclear
  Smooth muscle
  Mitochondrial
Serum ceruloplasmin and copper
Slit lamp cornea
'e' antigen
'e' antibody
Alpha-fetoprotein

Needle liver biopsy
Haematoxylin and eosin and connective tissue stains
Skilled interpreter

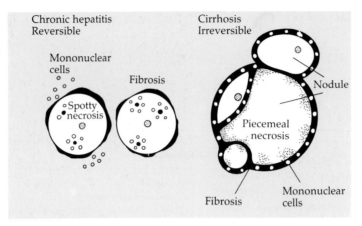

Fig. 17.1. In chronic hepatitis the zonal architecture of the liver is preserved. In cirrhosis, nodular regeneration leads to loss of the essential hepatic architecture. Chronic hepatitis is essentially reversible, cirrhosis is not.

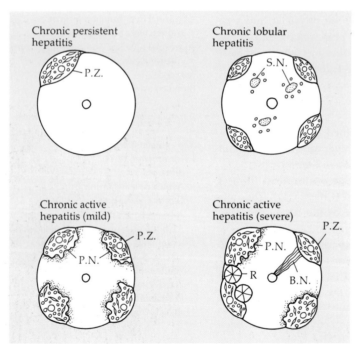

Fig. 17.2. Chronic hepatitis may be divided into three types. Chronic persistent has a good prognosis. Chronic active is divided into a mild and a severe form. Chronic lobular hepatitis usually has a good prognosis. P.Z. = portal zone; S.N. = spotty necrosis; P.N. = piecemeal necrosis; B.N. = bridging necrosis. R = rosettes.

intralobular inflammation and necrosis. Piecemeal necrosis and bridging necrosis are not seen.

Chronic active hepatitis is marked by the presence of an inflammatory infiltrate, primarily of lymphocytes and plasma cells, which greatly expands the portal areas. This inflammatory infiltrate extends into the liver lobule, causing erosion of the limiting plate and piecemeal necrosis.

The *severe form* is marked by fibrous septa extending into the liver cell columns with isolation of groups of liver cells in the form of rosettes (figs 17.4, 17.5, 17.7). Intra-hepatic 'bridging', either portal–central (fig. 17.7) or portal–portal, is seen.

The *milder form* (fig. 17.6) of chronic active hepatitis shows only slight erosion of the limiting plate with some piecemeal necrosis but without bridging or rosette formation.

340

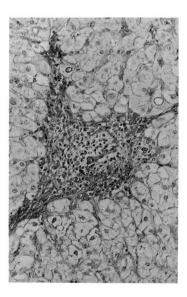

Fig. 17.3. Persistent hepatitis. Part of the liver biopsy shows an inflammed expanded portal zone but a well defined limiting plate and no piecemeal necrosis. (Stained H & E ×100.)

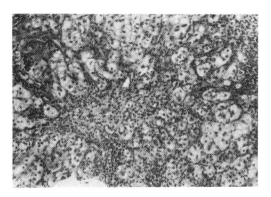

Fig. 17.4. Chronic active liver disease. The lobular architecture is completely disturbed. Isolated groups of liver cells, which often assume a rosette-like appearance, are separated by the septa of connective tissue. Remaining cells are large with clear cytoplasm. Lymphocytic and plasma cell infiltration is conspicuous. H & E, ×40 (Sherlock, 1962).

This classification of chronic hepatitis is important in terms of prognosis. The chronic persistent and chronic lobular types do not usually progress. Mild chronic active hepatitis may occasionally progress to cirrhosis but this is unusual. The severe chronic active hepatitis does progress and indeed cirrhosis may already be present, co-existing with the chronic active hepatitis.

Difficulties in liver biopsy interpretation [80]

Accurate categorization of the type of chronic hepatitis is clearly important because of the prognostic implications.

The liver lesion may vary in severity from place to place and this accounts for sampling errors which are particularly likely if the liver biopsy is small.

It can be difficult to distinguish peri-portal piecemeal necrosis from simple spill-over of inflammatory cells into the lobule, as in acute hepatitis.

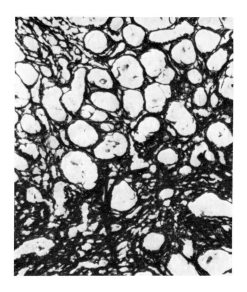

Fig. 17.5. Same case as Fig. 17.4. Reticulin stains confirm the isolation of liver cells by bands of fibrous tissue, ×120 (Sherlock, 1962).

If the patient is on corticosteroid therapy, the inflammatory reaction is reduced and a falsely optimistic interpretation may be made.

In diseases with cholestasis, hepatocytes near the portal zones may swell and become

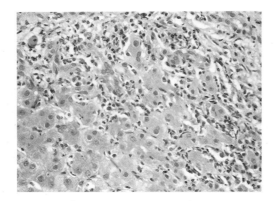

Fig. 17.6. Chronic active hepatitis. Part of a liver biopsy specimen, showing piecemeal necrosis of the limiting plate in the portal zone. (Stained H & E ×100.)

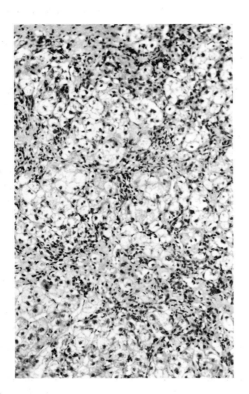

Fig. 17.7. Severe chronic active hepatitis with a positive hepatitis B antigen test. Shown are isolation of cell groups, fibrosis, and many plasma cells. The appearance is indistinguishable from active chronic hepatitis in patients not showing a positive hepatitis B antigen test. H & E, ×40.

necrotic. However, lymphocytes are relatively sparse, neutrophils prominent and hepatocellular copper is often increased.

Difficulties in diagnosing cirrhosis on small samples [83] are discussed in Chapter 19.

A skilled, experienced histopathologist is required to interpret these small samples.

Chronic persistent hepatitis

Aetiology and presentation

In many instances the aetiology is *unknown*. The patient presents with fatigue or when 'check-up' biochemical tests are found to be abnormal. Unexplained mild hepatomegaly is another mode of presentation. Patients are often males in the fourth or fifth decade.

Association with hepatitis B. These patients may come from geographic areas where carriage of hepatitis B is frequent or may be hospital workers in contact with blood. They may present as asymptomatic blood donors, found to be HBsAg positive.

Diagnosis may follow an acute attack of hepatitis with failure of HBsAg to be cleared from the blood. These patients are usually also anti-HBc positive. Others may simply show anti-HBs alone. HBe is usually negative. HBsAg can be demonstrated in the liver.

Hepatitis non-A, non-B. This, at present ill-defined, condition can proceed to chronic persistent hepatitis. It is diagnosed by exclusion of other known causes of chronic persistent hepatitis and by its relation to blood transfusion or exposure to blood products possibly contaminated with virus.

Alcohol. After recovery from an acute attack of alcoholic hepatitis the portal zones may show inflammation persisting for some months.

Inflammatory bowel disease. Chronic persistent hepatitis may complicate long-standing chronic colonic disease, for instance ulcerative colitis, regional ileitis or infection with *E. histolytica* or *Salmonella*. Chronic persistent hepatitis may accompany infection with *Schistosoma mansoni* but here residua of ova are usually seen in the portal veins.

Clinical features

The patient may be asymptomatic. He may complain of fatigue, poor appetite, fat and alcohol intolerance and discomfort over the liver. These symptoms may only develop after the patient has been told he has chronic hepatitis.

Clinical examination may be normal or the liver edge may be tender. Physical signs of chronic liver disease, such as vascular spiders and splenomegaly, are absent.

Investigations

The serum bilirubin level is normal or slightly increased. Serum transaminase values may be elevated and values may continue to fluctuate up to about four times the normal limit for many years.

Serum alkaline phosphatase is usually normal.

Serum total globulin is usually within normal limits and the serum immunoglobulin G (IgG) is but slightly increased. This is a point of distinction from the active forms of chronic hepatitis.

Tests for serum hepatitis B antigen (HbsAg) and, if positive, for HBc antibody should be performed.

In those with opportunities of contracting *Schistosoma mansoni* infection, evidence of this must be sought.

Needle liver biopsy

This is an invaluable method of confirming the diagnosis and particularly of distinguishing the persistent from the more serious forms of chronic hepatitis. The histological appearances may be difficult to distinguish from those of an acute attack of virus hepatitis which is recovering normally and which will not be persistent. If there is any difficulty in interpreting the first biopsy it may be prudent to wait six months and perform a second one.

Differential diagnosis

Chronic active hepatitis is distinguished by the physical signs of chronic liver disease and by the hyperglobulinaemia. Needle biopsy appearances are helpful although mildly aggressive appearances in one portal zone with persistent hepatitis appearances in others can be extremely difficult to interpret. A longer period of follow-up with repeated needle biopsies of the liver may give a clear differentiation between the benign and the serious forms of chronic hepatitis.

Sclerosing cholangitis should be considered if the serum alkaline phosphatase is elevated. Endoscopic cholangiography is diagnostic.

Alcoholic liver disease is distinguished by the history of alcohol excess and by the physical stigmata of chronic alcoholism, including a large tender liver. Histologically, the biopsy may show the features of alcoholic liver disease. However, if the patient has abstained from alcohol for some time, such acute appearances may have vanished and the picture can be indistinguishable from other forms of chronic persistent hepatitis.

Gilbert's syndrome must be considered, for both conditions can present after a hepatitis-like illness. Patients with Gilbert's syndrome show unconjugated hyperbilirubinaemia with normal serum transaminases and liver histology.

Treatment

This is by reassurance of the patient after the fullest possible investigations which may have to include needle biopsy of the liver.

Corticosteroid or immunosuppressant treatment, such as with azathioprine, should not be given.

No specific dietary regime is indicated. In particular, there is no scientific justification for a low-fat diet, with avoidance of eggs and butter. Additional vitamins and 'liver tonics' are not necessary.

Alcohol can be permitted within reason provided it is believed that excess is unlikely in

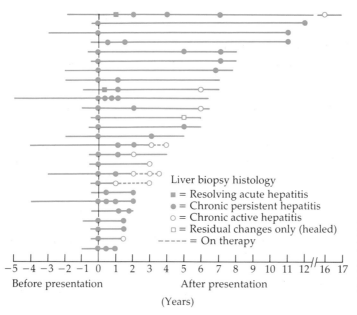

Fig. 17.8. Chronic persistent hepatitis. Liver biopsies and length of observation in 26 patients. Mild chronic active hepatitis was seen histologically in nine. Cirrhosis did not develop (Chadwick *et al.* 1979).

Liver biopsy histology
■ = Resolving acute hepatitis
● = Chronic persistent hepatitis
○ = Chronic active hepatitis
□ = Residual changes only (healed)
- - - - - = On therapy

−5 −4 −3 −2 −1 0 1 2 3 4 5 6 7 8 9 10 11 12 16 17

Before presentation   After presentation

(Years)

that individual and that the persistent hepatitis has not followed alcoholism.

Prognosis

Twenty-six untreated patients were followed for 1−17 years (mean 5.6 years) (fig. 17.8) [9]. These patients did not develop any clinical features of chronic liver disease. Serial liver biopsies showed that nine patients progressed to a very mild chronic active hepatitis but none developed cirrhosis. In no case was there clinical or biochemical deterioration. Those who developed mild chronic active hepatitis were usually HBsAg positive and often 'e' antigen positive.

Chronic lobular hepatitis

This rare condition presents in much the same way as chronic persistent hepatitis. Patients, usually males, are diagnosed after an acute viral hepatitis-like illness [101]. Most may be due to non-A, non-B hepatitis. HbsAg is negative. The course is of remissions and relapses which are marked by elevations of serum transaminases. Serum autoantibodies (smooth

muscle and mitochondrial) may be weakly positive.

Chronic lobular hepatitis may develop during the acute exacerbation accompanying seroconversion from hepatitis B e antigen positive to hepatitis B e antibody positive.

The differential diagnosis from other forms of chronic hepatitis can only be made by liver biopsy.

Chronic active hepatitis

All types of chronic active hepatitis obey certain clinical, biochemical and histological criteria.

Clinically symptoms range from none to incapacitating exhaustion. Fluctuating hepatocellular jaundice is usual. Features of clinically diagnosable and symptomatic portal hypertension (ascites, bleeding oesophageal varices) are late.

Biochemical tests show a variably elevated serum bilirubin level. Serum transaminase values are usually increased and the gamma-globulin concentration is also elevated.

Hepatic histology shows the features of chronic active hepatitis.

Aetiology

A common clinical, biochemical and hepatic histological picture has been associated with more than one aetiological agent (fig. 17.9) [56]. Three main types have been identified (tables 17.2, 17.3, 17.4). One is associated with persistence of hepatitis B infection. Another is associated with a negative result for hepatitis B, but has been termed 'lupoid' or autoimmune because of the association with positive serum autoantibodies. The third, non-A, non-B hepatitis can be followed by a chronic active hepatitis. In the neonate, and occasionally in the immunosuppressed patient, other viral infections such as cytomegalovirus may lead to chronic active hepatitis. Identical clinical, functional and morphological features may be found associated with some drug reactions, among them to methyl dopa and to isoniazid (Chapter 18). α_1-antitrypsin deficiency may lead to a chronic hepatitis but more often presents as cholestasis in the neonate (Chapter 23). A liver biopsy in the alcoholic occasionally shows the picture of chronic active hepatitis (Chapter 20).

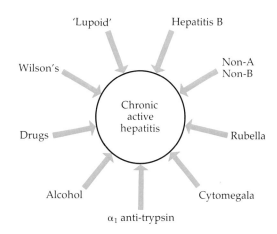

Fig. 17.9. The aetiology of chronic active hepatitis.

Immunological mechanisms of hepato-toxicity

Chronic active hepatitis is the liver disease *par excellence* where immunological factors are invoked in the perpetuation of the liver cell injury.

Liver histology shows heavy infiltration by lymphocytes and plasma cells with peri-portal

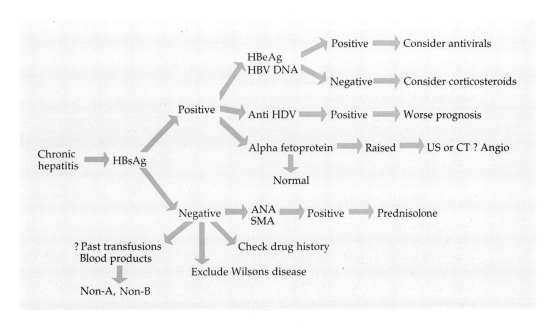

Fig. 17.10. The management of chronic hepatitis.

Table 17.2. Classification of chronic hepatitis (Sherlock, 1984)

Aetiology	Sex predominance	Age predominance	Associations	Diagnostic tests	Histological features
Hepatitis B and delta	M	All	Immigrants from Orient, Africa and Mediterranean, health care workers, homosexuals, drug abusers, immunosuppressed	HBsAG HBeAG anti-HBe HBV-DNA anti HDV	Usually mild, ground glass cells. Orcein positive. Delta antigen in hepatocyte nuclei
Hepatitis non-A, non-B	Equal	All ages	Blood transfusion, Blood products, drug abuse	None	Fat, lobular component
Autoimmune	F	14−25 and post-menopausal	Multi-system (diabetes, arthralgia, haemolytic anaemia, nephritis)	Anti-nuclear antibody + ve 70% Smooth muscle antibody + ve 70% Serum gamma-globulin high, 'florid' liver histology	Rosettes, plasma cell infiltrates bridging
Drug	F	Middle-aged and elderly	INAH, methyl dopa, furantoin, dantrolene antithyroid drugs, etc.	History, liver histology	Eosinophils, fat, granulomas
Wilson's	Equal	10−30	Family history, haemolysis, neurological signs	Kayser−Fleischer rings. Serum copper, ceruloplasmin, urinary copper, liver copper	Ballooned hepatocytes, glycogenic nuclei, fat

piecemeal necrosis, suggesting a type IV hypersensitivity reaction. Hyperglobulinaemia and circulating tissue antibodies are often present. In chronic active hepatitis, it is postulated that an immunological reaction is mounted against membrane constituents of the hepatocyte which serve as antigens. A self-perpetuating antigen−antibody reaction follows with resultant chronic liver disease [28]. Cell-mediated immunity to liver cell antigens has been demonstrated in chronic hepatitis and this process is mediated by sensitized

Table 17.3. Chronic hepatitis: prognosis and treatment (Sherlock, 1984)

Aetiology	Prognosis	Treated	Treatment
Hepatitis B	10–20% remission (HBeAg + →anti-HBe+), develop cirrhosis & primary liver cancer	?	?antivirals (occasionally corticosteroids)
Non-A, non-B	Mild disease. May remit completely or develop cirrhosis	?	?antivirals
Autoimmune	60% dead in 5 years	15% dead in 5 years	Prednisolone
Drugs	Excellent		Withdraw drug

Table 17.4. Chronic hepatitis: bad prognostic signs (Sherlock, 1984)

Aetiology	Bad signs
Hepatitis B	Decompensated cirrhosis Primary liver cancer Super-added delta infection HBeAg positive 'Active' liver histology
Non-A, non-B hepatitis	Sustained elevation of serum transaminases for more than one year Decompensated cirrhosis
Autoimmune	Poor response to prednisolone Decompensated cirrhosis
Drugs	Failure to diagnose with development of acute and sub-acute hepatic necrosis

lymphocytes and mononuclear cells. In both HBsAg positive and negative chronic active hepatitis a candidate membrane protein antigen has been termed liver specific protein (LSP). This is also found in acute hepatitis A and probably reflects only hepato-cellular necrosis [60].

In the case of non-B chronic active hepatitis a liver membrane protein (LMP) is the postulated antigen. In this group a membrane-fixed IgG has been shown on hepatocytes [90] and continuing necrosis of liver cells is seen in patients with this antibody. It is not found in HBsAg positive patients. These results support the

existence of different pathogenetic mechanisms for chronic active hepatitis in the autoimmune type and in the hepatitis virus B-induced type [60]. Cell-mediated immunity to both membrane proteins has been shown in chronic active hepatitis. It is, of course, possible that chronic hepatitis may not be an immunologically perpetuated disease. The separation of primary events from immunological changes secondary to liver damage *per se* is almost impossible. Chronic active hepatitis is more a mode of progression than a disease identity.

Presentation

The patient comes to the clinician through general circumstances, symptoms, physical signs or abnormal serum biochemical tests. The most important general symptom is fatigue. Physical signs include jaundice, rarely vascular spiders, a large or small liver and splenomegaly. Suggestive abnormal biochemical tests are a modestly raised serum bilirubin level, increased transaminases and gamma-globulin values, with a moderately raised serum alkaline phosphatase. The next step is to test for serum hepatitis B surface antigen (HBsAg). Management depends on whether this is positive or negative (fig. 17.10, table 17.3).

SUGGESTIVE CLINICAL PROFILES (table 17.2)

Chronic hepatitis B is suggested by the ethnic origin of the patient, homosexuality, drug abuse or a likely contact with blood of patients carrying hepatitis B. The patient may present because of fatigue. Serum transaminases may be found at a routine medical check or by biochemical screening for some unrelated condition. Hepatitis B may be diagnosed at the time of blood donation.

In a known hepatitis B carrier, a relapse with high transaminase values may indicate super-added infection with Delta virus.

The history of receiving a blood transfusion or blood products, however distant, suggests non-A, non-B hepatitis. The patient may bring a chart recording up and down serum transaminase levels over many months or years.

THE ROLE OF LIVER BIOPSY

Liver biopsy is essential to confirm the diagnosis, assess activity, show the presence or absence of cirrhosis, to indicate a possible aetiology and to follow treatment.

Chronic autoimmune 'lupoid' hepatitis

In 1950, Waldenström [97] drew attention to a chronic hepatitis occurring predominantly in young people, especially women. The syndrome has since been given various titles [3, 102]. None of the names is satisfactory and rather than dogmatize concerning aetiology, sex, age or pathology, all of which may vary, the term 'chronic active autoimmune (lupoid) hepatitis' has been used. The frequency of the condition seems to be decreasing, but this may be simply due to more accurate diagnosis of other causes of chronic active hepatitis, for instance drug-related or hepatitis B.

Aetiology

The aetiology is unknown. Immunological changes are conspicuous. Serum gamma-globulin levels are grossly elevated. The finding of a positive LE cell test in about 15% led to the term 'lupoid hepatitis'. Tissue antibodies are found in a high proportion of patients.

Chronic active (lupoid) hepatitis is not the same as classical systemic lupus erythematosus [36, 39] for the liver rarely shows any lesions in classical lupus. Moreover, the smooth muscle antibody and the mitochondrial antibody are not present in the blood of patients with systemic lupus erythematosus.

Table 17.5. Chronic active hepatitis: comparison of types negative and positive for hepatitis B surface antigen

	Autoimmune (HBsAg − ve)	Type B (HBsAg + ve)
Sex predominance	Female	Male
Age preference	15−25	Older
	Menopause	Neonates
Serum HBsAg	Absent	Present
Autoimmune disease	Frequent	Rare
Serum gamma-globulin increase	Marked	Moderate
Smooth muscle antibody and ANF	High titre (70%)	Low or absent titre
LE cells	15%	Absent
Increased titre viral and bacterial antibodies	Yes	No
Liver membrane antibody	Present	Absent
Risk of primary liver cancer	Low	High
Response to corticosteroids	Good	Uncertain
Liver biopsy		
Shikata stain for HBsAg	−	+
'Ground glass' cells	−	+
Residual acute hepatitis	0	Frequent

Chronic non-A, non-B hepatitis seems unlikely, for in this condition circulating autoantibodies are not detected.

Immunology

Auto-immune chronic active hepatitis is a disease of disordered immunoregulation marked by a defect in suppressor T-cells. This results in production of autoantibodies against hepatocyte surface antigens (fig. 17.11) [91]. It is uncertain whether the defect in the immune regulatory apparatus is primary or secondary to an acquired change in the antigenicity of the tissues.

The nature of the target antigen on the hepatocyte membrane remains to be determined. One candidate, liver membrane protein (LMP) [100], is found in the sera of patients with auto-immune chronic active hepatitis and with primary biliary cirrhosis. It seems to be largely related to piecemeal necrosis. Using monoclonal antibodies, attempts are being made to map out the various epitopes contained within the liver membrane antigens so that the immunogenic defect may be studied in more detail.

The mononuclear infiltrate in the portal zones consists of B lymphocytes and helper T-cells with relatively fewer cytotoxic/suppressor cells [62]. This is consistent with the view that antibody-dependent cytotoxicity is the main effector mechanism (fig. 17.11).

Patients have persistent high titres of circulating measles antibodies. This can be related to persistence of part of the measles virus genome in the lymphocytes [76]. The relation of this to pathogenesis is unknown.

Genetics [55]

The female sex predominance (8:1) is similar to other autoimmune diseases. Humoral immune responsiveness is generally increased in females.

There is a strong association with HLA-B8, and DR3, also with the immunoglobulin allotype Gma + × +. This suggests an HLA-linked aberration in regulation of immune

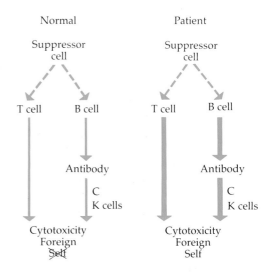

Fig. 17.11. The mechanism of immunological hepatocyte injury in auto-immune 'lupoid' chronic active hepatitis in the patient, related to a defect in T suppressor cells, cytotoxicity is directed not only against foreign antigens but against self (Thomas & Lok 1984).

responses. HLA-DR3 may be linked with a regulator gene for suppressor cells.

HLA-B8 positive patients show an improved response to corticosteroid therapy [48].

A genetically determined low serum C_4 has been found in patients with autoimmune hepatitis and in their families [95]. C_4 plays a key role in virus neutralization and the low value might support viral persistence as an important aetiologic factor.

Hepatic pathology

The lesion is a severe chronic active hepatitis. Activity is variable from place to place and some areas may be near normal.

Cellular infiltrates, largely lymphocytes and plasma cells, are seen in zone 1 and infiltrating between the liver cells. Aggressive septum formation isolates groups of liver cells as rosettes. Fatty change is inconspicuous. Areas of collapse may be seen. The connective tissue encroaches on the parenchyma. Cirrhosis develops rapidly and is usually of the macro-nodular type. The chronic hepatitis and the cirrhosis seem to develop almost simultaneously.

As time passes the activity subsides, the cellularity decreases, the piecemeal necrosis lessens and the fibrous tissue becomes denser. At necropsy in the long-standing case, the lesion is an inactive cirrhosis. In most cases, however, careful search will reveal areas of piecemeal necrosis and rosette formation remaining at the periphery of a nodule.

Although inflammation and necrosis may subside completely during remissions, and the disease remain inactive for a variable interval, regeneration appears inadequate as the peri-lobular architecture is not restored to normal and the pattern of injury remains detectable late in the disease.

Cirrhosis is present in only one-third early in the disease but is usually present two years after the onset [70]. Repeated episodes of necrosis with further stromal collapse and fi-brosis lead to a more severe cirrhosis. Event-ually the liver becomes small and grossly cirrhotic.

Clinical features

The condition is predominantly but not ex-clusively one of young people: half the patients present between 10 and 20 years old. A further peak of incidence is seen about the menopause. Three-quarters are female.

The onset is usually insidious, the patient feels generally unwell and is noticed to be jaundiced. In about a quarter, the disease seems to present as a typical attack of acute viral hepatitis [61]. It is only when the jaundice persists that the physician is alerted to the possibility of a more chronic liver disorder. It is unclear whether the disease can be initiated by acute viral hepatitis, or whether this is simply an intercurrent infection in a patient with long-standing chronic active hepatitis.

In most instances, the hepatic lesion on pres-entation does not agree with the stated duration of symptoms. Chronic active hepatitis must remain asymptomatic for some months or possibly years before jaundice becomes overt and the diagnosis is made. Patients may be recognized sooner if a routine medical examin-ation reveals stigmata of liver disease or if biochemical tests of liver function are per-formed and found to be abnormal.

Although the serum bilirubin level is usually increased, some are anicteric [61]. Frank jaun-dice is often episodic. Rarely, deep cholestatic jaundice is seen.

Amenorrhoea is usual and regular menses is a good sign. However, if a period does occur it may be associated with increase of symptoms and deepening of jaundice. Epistaxis, bleeding gums and bruising with minimal trauma are other complaints.

Examination shows a tall girl, often above normal stature, well built and generally looking healthy (fig. 17.12). Spider naevi are virtually constant on face, necklace area or arms. They tend to be small and to come and go with changes in the activity of the disease. Livid cutaneous striae may sometimes be found on thighs, lateral aspect of the abdominal wall, and also, in severe cases, on upper arms, breasts and back (fig. 17.13). The face may be rounded even before administration of corticosteroids. Acne is prominent and hirsuties may be seen. The skin may show bruises.

Abdominal examination in the early stages shows a firm liver edge some 4 cm below the right costal margin. The left lobe may be dis-proportionately enlarged in the epigastrium; nodules are rarely palpable. In the later stages the liver shrinks and becomes impalpable. The spleen is almost universally enlarged. Ascites, oedema and hepatic encephalopathy are late features.

Recurrent episodes of active liver disease punctuate the course.

Associated conditions

Chronic autoimmune active hepatitis is not a condition confined to the liver (table 17.6). The association with diseases such as Hashimoto's thyroiditis or Coombs'-positive haemolytic

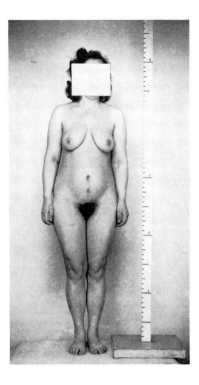

Fig. 17.12. Active juvenile cirrhosis. Well developed girl with good nutrition.

Table 17.6. Associated lesions in 81 cases of autoimmune chronic active hepatitis (Read *et al.* 1963)

Purpura	2
Erythemas	4
Arthralgia	9
Lymphadenopathy	2
Pulmonary infiltrates	7
Pleurisy	2
Rheumatic heart disease	4
Ulcerative colitis	5
Diabetes	3
Hashimoto's thyroiditis	2
Renal tubular defects	3
Lupus kidney	3
Haemolytic anaemia	1

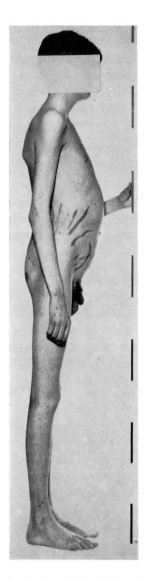

Fig. 17.13. Active chronic 'lupoid' hepatitis. Note tall boy with ascites and striae on abdominal wall and upper arms.

LE cells, there may be sustained pyrexia [70]. Such patients may also have an acute, recurrent, non-deforming migrating polyarthritis of large joints. In most cases pain and stiffness are present without marked swelling. The changes usually resolve completely.

Associated skin conditions include allergic capillaritis, acne, erythema, LE type changes and purpura.

anaemia, has been partly responsible for the view that chronic active hepatitis represents an example of auto-aggression.

In those particularly ill, usually with positive

351

Splenomegaly may be present without portal hypertension, often with generalized lymphadenopathy, presumably part of the same process of lymphoid hyperplasia.

Renal biopsy often shows mild glomerulitis [87]. Nodular deposits of immunoglobulins and complement have been found in the glomeruli. Complexes containing small nuclear ribonucleoprotein and IgG are restricted to those with kidney disease [66]. Glomerular antibodies are present in about half the patients, but do not seem to relate to the extent of renal damage.

Pulmonary changes, including pleurisy and transitory pulmonary infiltrations and collapse, are found when the disease is active. The mottled chest radiograph may be related to dilated precapillary blood vessels. The high cardiac output of chronic liver disease would add to the pulmonary vascular plethora. Multiple pulmonary arteriovenous anastomoses are also found (Chapter 6). Fibrosing alveolitis is another possibility.

Primary pulmonary hypertension has been described in one patient with multi-system involvement [8].

Endocrine changes include the Cushingoid appearance, acne, hirsuties and cutaneous striae. Boys may develop gynaecomastia. Amenorrhoea is virtually constant. Hashimoto's thyroiditis may be seen [70] and other thyroid abnormalities include myxoedema and thyrotoxicosis. Patients develop diabetes mellitus, before and after diagnosis of the chronic hepatitis [70].

Mild anaemia, leucopenia and thrombocytopenia are associated with the enlarged spleen ('hypersplenism'). A positive Coombs' test with haemolytic anaemia is another rare complication [70]. Rarely, a hypereosinophilic syndrome is associated [14].

Ulcerative colitis tends to present with the chronic active hepatitis or to follow it.

Hepato-cellular cancer is reported but is very rare [8, 47].

Biochemistry

The picture is of very active disease. Apart from the hyperbilirubinaemia of about 2–10 mg/dl, the serum gamma-globulin levels are very high (fig. 17.14). Electrophoresis shows a polyclonal gammopathy and, rarely, monoclonal. Serum albumin is maintained until the later stages of clinical liver failure. Serum transaminases are very high. During the course, transaminases and gamma-globulin levels fall spontaneously.

Serum antibodies (table 17.7)

Antinuclear factor. This is present in about 80% of patients. The titres correlate with the serum gamma-globulin levels.

Double-stranded DNA is increased in all types of chronic hepatitis with highest titres in the autoimmune group where it disappears after corticosteroid therapy [103]. It is a non-specific manifestation of inflammatory activity.

Smooth muscle antibody. This is detected in about 70% of patients with autoimmune chronic active hepatitis. It is found in about 50% of patients with primary biliary cirrhosis. It is also present in low titre in patients with acute type A or B viral hepatitis or with infectious mononucleosis [29]. Titres exceeding 1 in

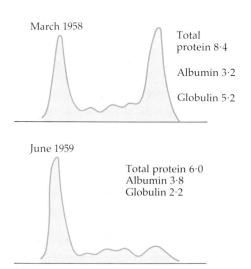

March 1958

Total protein 8·4

Albumin 3·2

Globulin 5·2

June 1959

Total protein 6·0
Albumin 3·8
Globulin 2·2

Fig. 17.14. Chronic active 'lupoid' hepatitis. Effect of corticosteroid treatment on the plasma proteins.

Table 17.7. Serum antibodies

	Antibody				
Type	Smooth muscle	Nuclear	Soluble liver	LKM	Mitochondrial
Classic 'lupoid'	+	+	−	−	−
LKM*	−	−	−	+	−
Soluble liver	±	−	+	−	−
Primary biliary cirrhosis	−	−	−	−	+

*LKM—Liver−kidney-microsomal.

40 are rare except in autoimmune chronic active hepatitis. The antibody is of IgM type. The antigen is related to the S actin of smooth and skeletal muscle. This is also present in cell membranes and in the contractile elements (cytoskeleton) of the liver cell. Smooth muscle antibody can be regarded therefore as a result of liver cell injury.

Soluble liver antigen-antibodies [58]. Non-organ specific autoantibodies against a soluble liver antigen are found in one sub-group, usually in young women. Antibodies against nuclei and liver kidney microsomes are absent. These patients respond well to corticosteroid treatment.

A liver-kidney microsomal antibody (LKM) may be found in high titre particularly in female children and young people [7, 65, 74]. Other serological autoantibodies are usually absent. This microsomal antibody seems to be against endoplasmic reticulum [22]. There are no histocompatibility antigen associations. Insulin-dependent diabetes vitiligo and thyroiditis may be found. The disease is severe but corticosteroids are usually effective therapy [41].

Mitochondrial antibody. This antibody is present in 30% of patients.

Serum α-fetoprotein levels may be increased to greater than 15 ng/ml in about a third of patients. This frequently resolves after corticosteroid therapy.

Haematology

Thrombocytopenia and leucopenia are frequent even before the late stage of portal hypertension and very large spleen. A mild normochromic normocytic anaemia is also usual. The survival of erythrocytes is reduced, presumably related to splenic hyperfunction. Prothrombin time is often prolonged even in the early stages when hepato-cellular function seems preserved.

Needle biopsy of the liver

This is very valuable, but may prove impossible to perform because of the coagulation defect. If biopsy is possible, the classical chronic active hepatitis is seen.

Differential diagnosis

Needle liver biopsy may be required to determine whether *cirrhosis* is also present.

The distinction from *hepatitis B-positive chronic active hepatitis* is made by testing for hepatitis B markers.

The distinction from *Wilson's disease* is vital. A family history of liver disease is important. Presentation is often with haemolysis and ascites. Slit lamp examination of the cornea should be performed to look for Kayser−

Fleischer rings. This should be done in all patients under the age of 30 with HBsAg-negative chronic active hepatitis. Confirmation of the diagnosis of Wilson's disease is made by finding a reduced serum copper and ceruloplasmin and increased urinary copper values. Liver copper is increased.

Ingestion of *drugs*, such as nitrofurantoin, methyl dopa or isoniazid, must be excluded.

Chronic active hepatitis may co-exist with *ulcerative colitis*. Distinction must be made between the combination and *sclerosing cholangitis* where serum alkaline phosphatase values are usually increased and serum smooth muscle antibodies absent. ERCP is diagnostic.

Alcoholic liver disease. The history, stigmata of chronic alcoholism and large tender liver are helpful diagnostic points. Liver histology shows fat (a rare association of chronic active hepatitis) alcoholic hyaline of Mallory, focal polymorph infiltration and maximally centrizonal liver damage.

The distinction from *non-A, non-B chronic hepatitis* is important and difficult. Liver biopsy appearances may be helpful. Non-A, non-B hepatitis can only be excluded when all tissue antibodies including LKMA and the soluble liver antigen have been estimated.

Treatment

Three prospective controlled clinical trials have shown that corticosteroid treatment prolongs life in severe chronic active hepatitis [13, 63, 88], although all the trials have imperfections (table 17.8). Benefit was particularly seen in the first two years (figs 17.15, 17.16) [49]. Well-being is increased, appetite improves, fever and arthralgias are controlled. Biochemical changes are less constant, although serum bilirubin, transaminase and gamma-globulin levels usually fall. Serum albumin concentrations rise.

The effect on hepatic histology is variable and unconvincing. Certainly progression from the stage of chronic hepatitis to cirrhosis does not seem to be prevented.

If the patient is symptomatic, has very high serum transaminase and gamma-globulin levels and there is severe chronic active hepatitis on liver biopsy, the decision to start is easy. If symptoms are mild or absent and biochemical tests are only modestly impaired, but liver biopsy shows a definite chronic active hepatitis, the decision is less easy. Clinical judgement—a vague term—must be invoked. Liver biopsy must precede the commencement of therapy. If coagulation defects prohibit this procedure the biopsy must be done as soon as possible after a remission has been induced by corticosteroids.

The usual dose is 30 mg prednisolone for one week, reducing to a maintenance dose of 10–15 mg daily (table 17.9). The initial course lasts six months. This small maintenance dose may be adequate because patients with reduced liver function have impaired metabolism of prednisolone [73]. If a remission has ensued, judged clinically, biochemically and if possible by a further liver biopsy, the drug should be tapered off slowly over a period of about two months. In general, prednisolone therapy extends over

Table 17.8. Significance between the difference in mortality in corticosteroid and control patients with chronic active hepatitis (Cook *et al.* 1971)

Group	Total no. patients	Deaths from liver failure	Deaths from other causes	Total deaths
Corticosteroid	22	3	0	3
Control	27	13	2	15
Significance		5.09		7.45
(Xu21 with Yates' correction)		($P<0.05$)		($P<0.01$)

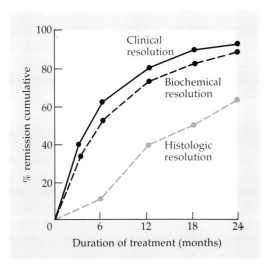

Fig. 17.15. The effect of prednisolone treatment in severe chronic active hepatitis (Summerskill *et al.* 1975).

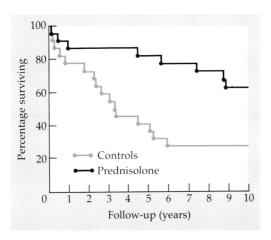

Fig. 17.16. Later results of the Royal Free Hospital trial of prednisolone in chronic active hepatitis. Note the improved survival in the treated group (Kirk *et al.* 1980).

Table 17.9. Prednisolone in autoimmune chronic active hepatitis

First week
10 mg prednisolone three times a day (30 mg/day)

Second and third weeks
Reduce prednisolone to maintenance dose (10−15 mg/day)

Every month
Clinical check—liver tests

At six months
Full check—clinical and biochemical
Liver biopsy

Full remission
Withdraw prednisolone slowly
Re-start if relapse

No remission
Continue maintenance dose for six more months, consider adding azathioprine (50−100 mg/day)
Maximum dose—20 mg prednisolone with 100 mg azathioprine

Table 17.10. Autoimmune chronic active hepatitis: duration of prednisolone treatment

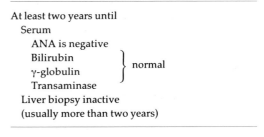

At least two years until
  Serum
    ANA is negative
    Bilirubin
    γ-globulin   } normal
    Transaminase
  Liver biopsy inactive
  (usually more than two years)

2−3 years and usually longer, sometimes for life (table 17.10) [40]. Premature withdrawal leads to relapse. Although control is usually re-established within 1−2 months, there are occasional fatalities. It is indeed difficult to decide when to withdraw therapy. Long-term low-dose prednisolone maintenance is probably preferable.

Prednisolone rather than prednisone should be given. Before it exerts its glucocorticoid effect prednisone has to be converted by 11-hydroxylation to prednisolone. This takes place largely in the liver. Blood levels are more predictable after prednisolone than prednisone and there may be a difficulty in the conversion with severely impaired liver function [57]. Alternate-day prednisolone treatment is not recommended as the incidence of serious complications is higher and histological remission less frequent.

Complications of treatment include facial mooning, acne, obesity, hirsuties and striae. These are particularly unwanted by female patients. More serious complications include growth retardation in those younger than 10 years, diabetes and serious infections.

Bone loss is found even with only 10 mg prednisolone daily and is related to duration of therapy [89]. Calcium and vitamin D must be given.

Side effects are rare if the dose of prednisolone is not more than 15 mg daily. If this is exceeded or serious complications have arisen, alternative measures must be considered.

If 20 mg prednisolone daily has not produced a remission, azathioprine 50−100 mg daily may be added. It is not given as a routine. Continual use of such a drug over many months or even years has obvious disadvantages. Other indications for azathioprine include gross Cushingoid features, associated diseases such as diabetes and other side-effects at doses required to induce remission. Azathioprine should never be given alone as controlled trials have shown the results are no better than with placebo. Azathioprine should not be given to candidates for pregnancy.

Cyclosporin has been used in a patient resistant to corticosteroid therapy [44]. This toxic drug should not be given except as a last resort when conventional therapy has failed.

When the target antigens of the abnormal immune response have been identified on the hepatocyte it is possible that, using either anti-idiotypic or clonal deletion, more specific immunological therapy may be possible [91].

The later picture of cirrhosis is managed along the usual lines (Chapters 6, 7, 9, 10). The incidence of hepatic encephalopathy after porta−caval anastomosis is high. This may be related to the continuing activity of the disease; portal hypertension is relieved by the shunt, but the hepato-cellular necrosis continues. Injection sclerotherapy is probably the best available treatment.

In the later stages, hepatic transplantation must be considered. This is technically difficult because of portal hypertension and a small cirrhotic liver. There is also a chance of recurrence of the autoimmune chronic active hepatitis.

Course and prognosis

This is extremely variable. The course is a fluctuant one marked by episodes of deterioration when jaundice and malaise are enhanced. The ultimate effect of this continuing chronic active hepatitis is inevitably cirrhosis with very few exceptions.

The ten-year survival is 63% [49]. After an initial remission following two years of corticosteroid therapy, a third achieve a five-year remission while two-thirds relapse and have to be retreated [15, 16]. Further corticosteroids have more side-effects. The mean survival is 12.2 years. Mortality is greatest during the first two years when the disease is most active. Sustained remission is more likely if the patient is diagnosed early and if immunosuppression is adequate. Corticosteroid therapy prolongs life, but most patients eventually reach the end stage of cirrhosis.

Oesophageal varices are an uncommon initial finding. Nevertheless bleeding from oesophageal varices and hepato-cellular failure are the usual causes of death.

Pregnancy in patients with chronic active hepatitis is discussed later (Chapter 25).

Chronic hepatitis B virus infection

In the majority, chronic liver disease is not preceded by a recognizable acute attack of hepatitis B (fig. 17.17). In others, the acute episode progresses directly to chronicity. In others, again, although the clinical picture at the apparent onset is of an acute illness, chronic hepatitis already exists. About 10% of adult patients suffering acute type B hepatitis fail to clear HBsAg from the blood in twelve weeks and become chronic carriers. Neonates acquiring hepatitis B have a 90% chance of becoming

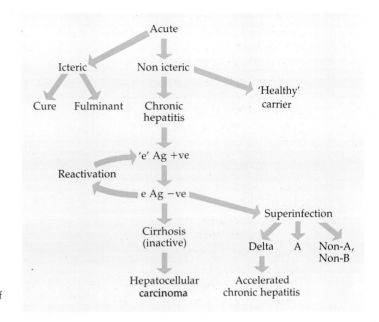

Fig. 17.17. The natural history of hepatitis B virus infection.

chronic carriers (fig. 17.19). The clinical course is not related to any particular hepatitis B subtype. Males are particularly affected.

Mechanisms of chronicity

Progression depends on a combination of continuing viral replication in the liver and the background of the patient (particularly his immunological status). The virus is not directly cytopathic and lysis of infected hepatocytes with progression to chronicity depends on the immune response of the host [28].

Those developing chronic hepatitis show a poor cell-mediated immune response to the virus [28]. If the response is particularly poor, little or no liver damage ensues and the virus continues to proliferate in the presence of normal liver function. Such a patient would be an apparently healthy carrier. The livers of such patients have been shown to contain enormous amounts of HBsAg in the absence of hepatocellular necrosis [37]. Serum levels of HBsAg are also high. Patients with a slightly better cell-mediated immune response show continuing hepato-cellular necrosis, but the response

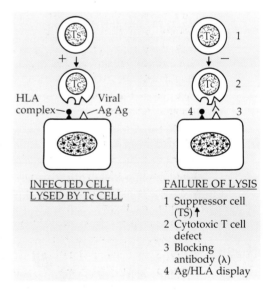

INFECTED CELL LYSED BY Tc CELL

FAILURE OF LYSIS

1 Suppressor cell (TS) ↑
2 Cytotoxic T cell defect
3 Blocking antibody (λ)
4 Ag/HLA display

Fig. 17.18. T lymphocyte lysis of infected hepatocytes and mechanisms of failure of lysis in chronic hepatitis. Ts = suppressor cell, Tc = cytotoxic cell (Thomas 1980).

is insufficient to clear the virus and a chronic hepatitis results [28].

Impairment of humoral and cell-based im-

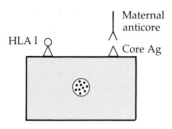

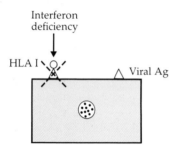

Fig. 17.19. Neonatal hepatitis B may become chronic because maternal anticore blocks expression of viral antigens on the hepatocyte membrane.

Fig. 17.20. Hepatitis B infection in the adult may become chronic because of interferon deficiency resulting in defective expression of HLA class 1 antigens on the hepatocyte membrane.

munity thus determines the outcome in type B hepatitis. When this is defective, viral replication continues and a carrier state with or without chronic hepatitis results. This is particularly important in patients with leukaemia, renal failure or organ transplants, and in those receiving immuno-suppressive therapy, in homosexuals, sufferers from AIDS and neonates.

Failure of lysis of virally infected hepatocytes has various mechanisms (fig. 17.18) [91]. It could be due to increased suppressor T-cell function, to a defect in cytotoxic (K) lymphocytes, or to blocking antibodies on the cell membrane.

Cytotoxic T-cells recognize viral antigen on the infected hepatocyte only in the context of class 1 HLA antigens [10]. Failure of lysis could be due to failure of HLA class 1 antigen display or of viral antigen display.

In the neonatally acquired disease, perpetuation may be related to maternal anticore blocking expression of viral core antigens on the hepatocyte membrane (fig. 17.19).

Some patients with adult acquired chronic hepatitis B show a reduced capacity to produce alpha- and gamma-interferons with resultant defective expression of HLA class 1 antigens on the hepatocyte membrane (fig. 17.20) [45].

STAGES OF HEPATITIS B

There are two phases of hepatitis B (HBV) infection, the replicative and the integrated (fig. 17.21) (table 17.11).

REPLICATIVE

During the phase of active viral replication, the patient's serum is positive for HBeAg and HBV-DNA. The peri-portal mononuclear cells are largely OKT3 (all T-cells) and T-8 (cytotoxic suppressor) cells [62]. Hepatitis B core antigen, and possibly other viral antigens are displayed on the hepatocyte membrane. HBV-DNA is detected in the hepatocyte in episomal form. During the period of HBeAgaemia, the patient is highly infectious and there is rapid progression of hepatic inflammation.

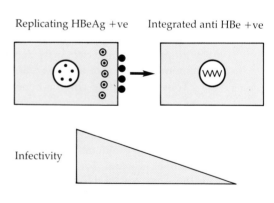

Fig. 17.21. The stages of hepatitis B viral infection. In the early replicative stages, the patient is HBeAg positive, core antigen is exposed on the hepatocyte membrane. With time, infectivity lessens and the patient becomes 'e' antibody positive. The viral nuclear DNA has integrated with the host DNA.

Table 17.11. The stages of infection with hepatitis B

	Replicating	Integrated
Infectivity	High	Low
Serum		
HBeAg	+ve	−ve
Anti-HBe	−ve	+ve
HBV DNA	+ve	−ve
Hepatocyte		
Viral DNA	Unintegrated	Integrated
Histology	Active	Inactive
	CAH.C	CPH.C.HCC
Portal zone		
Suppressors	Increased	Normal
Inducers	Reduced	Reduced
Treatment	?Antivirals	?Immuno-suppression

CAH = Chronic active hepatitis
C   = Cirrhosis
CPH = Chronic persistent hepatitis
HCC = Hepato-cellular carcinoma

INTEGRATED

After a variable period, often of several years, HBe antigen disappears from the blood and HBe antibody is detected.

At some stage of hepatitis B infection, the viral genome has become an integral part of the patient's genome so that viral genes are transcribed along with those of the host (fig. 17.22). The hepatocytes secrete HBsAg but core markers are not produced. Clones of these integrated cells form the basis of malignant transformation and in particular to hepato-cellular carcinoma [69].

The patient now shows serum e antibody which reflects low or absent HBV replication and presumably low activity. However, in some patients who are anti-HBe, some viral replication is undoubtedly continuing as shown by serum HBV-DNA [5] and/or core antigen (HbcAg) in hepatocyte nuclei. HBV-DNA can be detected in the hepatocyte nuclei in integrated form [43].

In the integrated (HBeAb) stage, the inflammatory infiltrate is similar to that found in autoimmune chronic active hepatitis with more helper T-cells and more B-cells being present. The actual membrane antigen is unknown.

HEPATITIS B MARKERS IN THE LIVER

Immunoperoxidase stains allow identification of hepatitis B antigens in liver biopsies [38]. The HBsAg is usually found in largest amounts in the healthy carrier. In the replicative stage, HBcAg is invariably present in liver. It may be

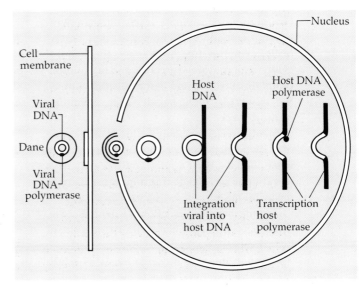

Fig. 17.22. The hepatitis B virion enters the hepatocyte and the core reaches the nucleus. At first the virus replicates using its own viral DNA. Then the viral DNA integrates with host DNA and the host DNA polymerase transcribes for the virus.

diffuse in asymptomatic carriers, the inactive and the immunosuppressed and focal in those with much hepatic inflammation or with later disease [38].

More sophisticated techniques involving molecular hybridization allow identification of the state of HBV-DNA in liver whether episomal or integrated, this is the best indication of the replicative and integrated stages.

Clinical features

The very young and the very old are at particular risk. Chronic hepatitis B is found predominantly in males.

Features suggesting an association of chronic hepatitis with virus B include ethnic origin from a high carrier rate country, work in contact with human blood, patients having transplants or immuno-suppressive treatment, drug abusers and homosexuals. Neonates born to an HBsAg carrier mother may develop chronic hepatitis. There may be none of these associations.

The condition may follow an unresolved acute hepatitis B. The acute attack is usually mild and of 'grumbling' type. The patient having an explosive onset and deep jaundice usually recovers completely. Similarly survivors of fulminant virus hepatitis seldom, if ever, develop progressive disease. Following the attack, serum transaminase levels fluctuate with intermittent jaundice. The patient may be virtually symptom-free with only biochemical evidence of continued activity, and may simply complain of fatigue and being generally unwell the diagnosis being made after a routine medical check.

The diagnosis may only be made at the time of a blood donation or routine blood screen when the HBsAg of a symptom-free patient is found to be positive and serum transaminases modestly raised.

Chronic hepatitis is often a silent disease. Symptoms do not correlate with the severity of liver damage.

In about one-half, presentation is as established chronic liver disease with jaundice, ascites or portal hypertension. Encephalopathy is unusual at presentation. The patient usually gives no history of a previous acute attack of hepatitis. Some present as primary liver carcinoma.

CLINICAL RELAPSE

An apparently stable patient with chronic liver disease due to hepatitis B may have a clinical relapse. This is marked by increasing fatigue and usually rises in serum transaminase values.

Relapse may be related to seroconversion from an HBe Ag positive state to an HBe Ag negative one (fig. 17.23). Liver biopsy shows an acute lobular type hepatitis which ultimately subsides and the serum transaminase values fall. Seroconversion may be spontaneous in 10–15% of patients per annum [96] or it may follow antiviral therapy (see on). HBV-DNA can remain positive even when anti-HBe has developed [33].

Spontaneous reactivation from HBe Ag negative to HBe Ag positive has also been described [17]. The liver disease becomes more active [94] and the picture is that of an acute viral hepatitis which may be fatal [18, 19]. Reactivation may be marked serologically simply by finding a positive IgM anti-HBc and this is useful in making the diagnosis from a superadded virus non-A, non-B, or A infection [50]. Reactivation can follow cancer chemotherapy, organ transplantation [20, 31] or administration of immunosuppressants to HBeAg positive patients [99].

The patient may be superinfected with delta virus (see Chapter 16) [35, 85]. This leads to a

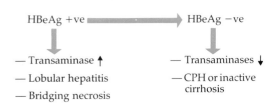

Fig. 17.23. Changes in a patient with chronic hepatitis B on conversion from HBeAg positive to HBeAg negative.

marked acceleration in the progress of chronic active hepatitis.

Finally, any deterioration in a hepatitis B carrier should raise the possibility of hepatocellular carcinoma (fig. 17.25).

Laboratory tests

Serum bilirubin, aspartate transaminase and gamma-globulin are only moderately increased (fig. 17.24). Serum albumin is usually normal. At time of presentation evidences of hepatocellular disease are usually mild.

Smooth muscle antibody, if present, is in low titre [29]. Serum mitochondrial antibody is negative.

Serum HbsAg is present, the titre being inversely proportional to the severity of the chronic hepatitis. In the later stages, HbsAg may be detected with difficulty in the blood yet HBcAb is usually present. HBe antigen or antibody and HBV-DNA are variably detected.

Needle liver biopsy. This establishes the diagnosis and categorizes the type of chronic hepatitis. Hepatic histology varies widely and includes chronic persistent and active cirrhosis and primary liver carcinoma. There are no constant diagnostic features for distinguishing this from other forms of chronic active or persistent hepatitis unless HBsAg is demonstrated as ground glass cells or by the orcein method [23, 37]. Cirrhosis is less frequent at presentation than in the autoimmune type.

Clinical and biochemical features and the presence or absence of HBeAg correlate poorly with hepatic histology and biopsy is particularly important in assessing severity.

The focal necroses may represent lysis of susceptible infected hepatocytes during the replicative stage. The peri-portal piecemeal necrosis may represent an immune attack on non-infected hepatocytes and hence an autoimmune component.

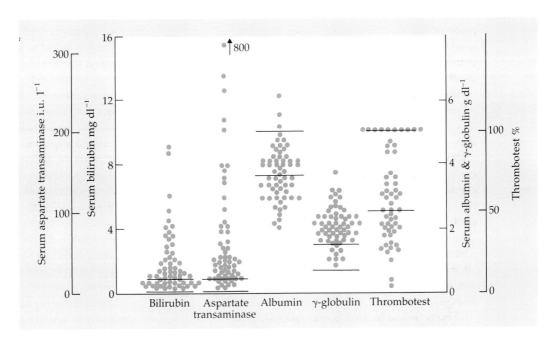

Fig. 17.24. Liver function tests of 59 hepatitis B antigen-positive patients when first seen at the Royal Free Hospital. Note that serum bilirubin, transaminase and gamma-globulin values are not particularly high and serum albumin is well maintained (Dudley *et al.* 1972).

Treatment

The patient must be counselled concerning personal infectivity. This is particularly important if he is HBeAg positive. Close family and sexual contacts should be checked for HBsAb, HbcAb and, if negative, hepatitis B vaccination should be offered.

Bed rest is not helpful. Physical fitness is encouraged by graduated exercises. Diet is normal. Alcohol excess should be avoided as this enhances the effects of HBsAg carriage. However, one or two glasses of wine or beer a day are allowed if this is part of the patient's lifestyle.

The majority of patients with chronic hepatitis B lead normal lives. Strong reassurance from the physician will avoid introspection by the patient.

The patient's problem should be considered whether largely of infectivity, of symptoms or of liver failure. Needle biopsy is essential before therapy is instituted. The presence of a severe, chronic active hepatitis with cirrhosis will obviously make treatment more urgent. The patient in the infectious, replicating stage must be distinguished from the relatively non-infectious patient in the integrated stage. Knowledge of HBe antigen and HBe Ab status is mandatory.

THE HBe ANTIGEN POSITIVE PATIENT

Clearance of hepatocytes containing replicating or integrated non-replicating HBV-DNA is necessary for effective treatment. This can be achieved with antiviral drugs although the effects may not persist. The stage of viral integration with the host is uncertain but this is likely to increase with time. Early treatment before stable clones of integrated HBV-DNA are established might lead to complete eradication of the virus. Antiviral treatment should therefore be early. This might reduce the development of cirrhosis and, despite viral integration with the host, lessen the changes of a subsequent hepato-cellular cancer.

Antiviral treatment aims at converting the

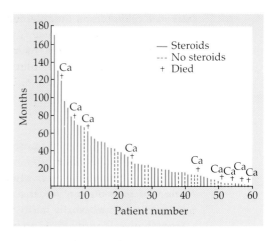

Fig. 17.25. Hepatitis B antigen chronic liver disease. Duration of disease in months after onset of symptoms. Ca = carcinoma. Note that most of the early deaths were related to hepato-cellular carcinoma. Thirty-three patients have been followed up for an average of two years without clinical or biochemical deterioration (Dudley *et al.* 1972).

patient from the replicative (serum HBeAg and HBV-DNA positive) to the integrated (serum HBeAb positive and HBV-DNA negative) (fig. 17.23). Infectivity will fall. This conversion is marked at eight to twelve weeks by an increase of serum transaminases as infected cells undergo immune lysis. HBsAg very rarely disappears [1]. Hepatic histology changes from a chronic active hepatitis with a marked lobular inflammation to an inactive chronic hepatitis. Loss of HBeAg is usually associated with the presence of integrated HBV-DNA in liver biopsy specimens [24].

Antiviral treatment should be considered if the patient is likely to be a serious source of infection to others (table 17.12). Candidates include health care workers (surgeons, dentists, nurses, medical students, technicians) and the sexually promiscuous.

Adenine arabinoside monophosphate (ARA-MP) has a wide spectrum of activity against DNA viruses. Patients show inhibition of HBV-DNA but only a third show long-term disappearance of HBV-DNA with conversion of e antigen to anti-HBe; HBsAg persists. Serum transaminases later fall. Side-effects include fever, malaise and a muscular pain syndrome. These preclude larger doses and longer courses. It has largely been replaced by the interferons, but is valuable in treating hepatitis B-related polyarteritis.

Interferons

Interferons inhibit viral protein synthesis and are also immunostimulatory. Interferon deficiency may predispose to the chronic carrier state in patients with HBV infection [45]. Interferons enhance display of HLA class 1 proteins and may increase interleukin-2 activity and so enhance destruction of diseased hepatocytes.

Results are equal whether lymphoblastoid interferon (a mixture of α-1 interferons) or recombinant α-2 interferon is used. 10 mega units per m² interferon are given intramuscularly three times a week for three months (fig.

17.26). Side-effects include malaise and fever on the day of treatment and the interferon is best given at night. Platelets and white cell count may fall slightly. Side-effects are less if the drug is given three times a week rather than daily.

Results. The ideal candidate should have a 70% chance of converting from serum HBeAg positive to anti-HBe (table 17.12).

The most important factor in determining the result is the time when the infection was acquired. Those infected in early childhood are likely to be well on the way to viral DNA integration before antiviral treatment is given and so do not respond. This may explain why the Oriental and Southern European peoples, who have a high infection rate in early life, do poorly with antiviral therapy [52]. Northern Europeans, developing disease later and treated earlier, achieve better results [86]. If the patient has a deficiency in cell-mediated immunity,

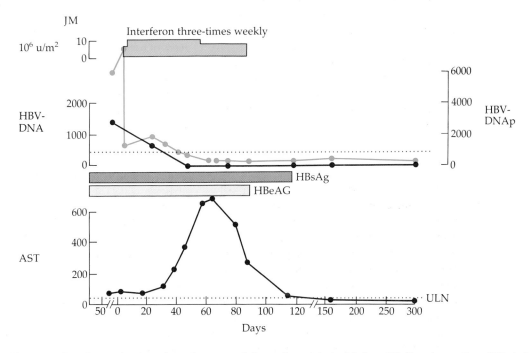

Fig. 17.26. Interferon was given three times a week for twelve weeks to this hepatitis B surface antigen (HBsAg) and hepatitis 'e' antigen (HBeAg) positive patient with chronic hepatitis. HBV DNA and HBV DNAp fell to undetectable levels as did HBsAg and HBeAg. There was a rise in serum aspartate transaminase (AST, GOT) which then fell to below the upper limit of normal (ULN). This result can be expected in 60-70% of treated patients although it is rare for HBsAg to become undetectable (Thomas & Scully, 1986).

Table 17.12. Chronic hepatitis B: ideal candidate for antiviral treatment (Sherlock, 1988)

Hepatitis 'e' antigen-positive
Recently acquired infection
Caucasian (i.e., not from high carrier area)
Heterosexual
Human immunodeficiency virus (HIV) negative
No other diseases
High serum transaminase level
Hepatic histology: lobular and peri-portal activity marked
Low serum HBV-DNA level
No evidence of delta virus infection

results will be poor. Hence, homosexuals respond poorly to therapy particularly if they have the AIDS antibody.

Patients are more likely to respond if the underlying disease is active as shown by liver biopsy and high transaminases. Superadded delta virus infection reduces the response.

Corticosteroids followed by antivirals

Corticosteroid therapy in HBeAg positive patients enhances viral replication. Withdrawal results in 'rebound immune stimulation' with a fall of viral markers including HBV-DNA. Immunocompetence is restored and cells expressing target viral antigens are destroyed [64]. Antiviral therapy is given after the prednisolone withdrawal.

Prednisone is started in a dose of 40 mg daily and is reduced over the next six weeks. After two weeks free of corticosteroid a three-month course of interferon, 5 million units daily, is given [67]. This routine may result not only in HBeAg conversion, but loss of HBsAg. However, it can be dangerous; enhancing the immune response by corticosteroids followed by withdrawal may lead to hepato-cellular failure. This therapy therefore should not be used for ill patients with severe liver disease evidenced by such features as jaundice or ascites.

Acyclovir (acycloguanosine) inhibits herpes simplex virus *in vitro* and *in vivo*, its action being dependent on phosphorylation by a

virus-coded thymidine kinase. In a limited trial acyclovir inhibited DNAp and HNV-DNA [79]. More work is needed using this agent for longer periods. It has the disadvantage of intravenous administration.

Levamisole

This is a potent immunostimulant particularly of T-cells. In limited studies it has improved hepatic histology and resulted in conversion of HBeAg positive to HBeAb positive with serum DNA becoming negative [32]. It may be useful combined with antivirals.

THE ANTI-HBe AND HBV-DNA POSITIVE PATIENT

Patients who fall into this group tend to be older and have more advanced liver disease. If they are asymptomatic or with only mild symptoms, conservative measures are all that should be offered. Advanced age, concomitant disease such as diabetes or a history of many years of non-progressive liver disease also contraindicate treatment. Such patients should have six-monthly clinical and biochemical checks with liver biopsies as indicated to assess progress.

Prednisolone therapy must be considered for those who are symptomatic HBeAg and HBV-DNA negative and where liver biopsy shows chronic active hepatitis, with or without cirrhosis [77]. There is some evidence in the anti-HBe patient that perpetuation of the chronic hepatitis may be immunologically mediated. Prednisolone therapy is started in a dose of 30 mg for one week and reduced to a maintenance of 10−15 mg daily which is continued for three months. If there is no clinical or biochemical evidence of benefit, the drug is stopped. It cannot be dis-counted that prednisolone may increase the chances of developing hepato-cellular carci-noma. Such therapy must in no sense be regarded as desirable. Indeed, it is indicated only if the disease is rapidly progressive and/or other available therapy has failed.

Course and prognosis

Some 300 million carriers of hepatitis B are said to exist in the world. With these large numbers it is clear that the disease must, in most patients, be mild and only occasionally progressive, and that slowly.

The clinical course varies considerably (figs 17.17, 17.25). Many patients remain in a stable, com-pensated state. This is particularly so in the asymptomatic and where hepatic histology shows only a mild, chronic active hepatitis. Such patients, with or without therapy, may go into remission, the histological picture being that of chronic persistent hepatitis.

The prognosis is proportional to the severity of the underlying liver disease [98]. Follow-up of 379 patients showed the five-year survival was 97% for chronic persistent hepatitis, 86% for chronic active hepatitis and 55% for chronic active hepatitis with cirrhosis. Women had less severe disease. Aged greater than 40, ascites and vascular spiders were bad signs.

Clinical deterioration in a previously stable hepatitis B carrier can have varying explanations. The patient may be converting from a replicative to an integrated state. This is usually followed by a remission [71] which may be permanent, serum enzyme levels falling into the normal range and liver histology improving; 10−20% per year may follow this course.

Seven-year follow-up of patients with chronic hepatitis due to hepatitis B showed that one-third had improved, one-third were unchanged and one-third were worse.

Super-infection of a chronic HBV carrier with delta may lead to fulminant disease. The resultant chronic hepatitis is accelerated (see Chapter 16).

Patients who are HBsAg positive with chronic hepatitis or cirrhosis, especially if male and more than 45 years old, should be screened regularly so that hepato-cellular carcinoma may be diagnosed early when surgical resection may prove possible. It is suggested that serum alpha-fetoprotein be measured and ultrasound examination performed at six-monthly intervals (see Chapter 28).

Chronic non-A, non-B hepatitis

Acute non-A, non-B hepatitis is frequently followed by a carrier state (see Chapter 16). In the United States, this may be about 3% after a single unit blood transfusion and in other countries it can be considerably higher. It is not surprising, therefore, that chronic liver disease has been related to the non-A, non-B viruses [26, 27]. Chronic liver disease can follow blood transfusion [72] or blood product-related acute disease (fig. 17.27). 60% of sufferers from parenterally transmitted acute non-A, non-B hepatitis will develop chronic hepatitis, and 20% will proceed to cirrhosis, usually after many years. This progression applies to symptomatic, asymptomatic and non-icteric acute attacks.

Many patients with chronic non-A, non-B hepatitis give no history of a previous possible aetiological event such as transfusion or drug abuse and the diagnosis can be made only by exclusion. The route of infection in these sporadic cases is unknown. Possible parenteral spread by the instruments of barbers and beauticians must be considered. In many instances, the disease develops insidiously and the acute episode would not be recognized if the patient were not under medical observation, for instance after a blood transfusion.

The hepatitis non-A, non-B viruses are probably more important than hepatitis B virus as a world-wide cause of chronic liver disease and cirrhosis.

The mechanism of the liver injury is unknown, but it may be mediated by cytotoxic T-cells which are lymphokine activated. Hepatocellular carcinoma is an extremely rare complication.

Liver histology [25, 80] shows the general features of chronic hepatitis, usually of persistent or mild, chronic active type. However, chronic lobular lesions and cirrhosis may be seen [72]. Histological features suggesting non-A, non-B hepatitis include fatty change, lymphoid aggregates and a disproportionate degree of sinusoidal cellular infiltration. Evidence of mild bile duct damage may be noted.

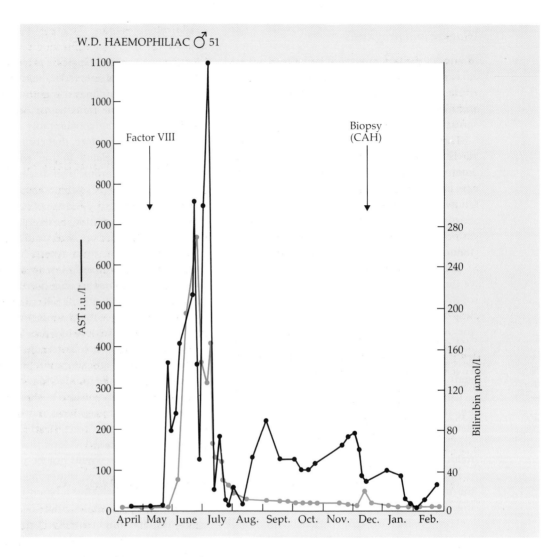

Fig. 17.27. W.D. haemophiliac patient developed acute hepatitis three weeks after a factor VIII concentrate known to cause non-A, non-B hepatitis. Serum HbsAg and hepatitis A IgM antibody were absent. Note very high serum bilirubin and aspartate (AST) levels. Serum bilirubin returned to normal, but aspartate transaminase fluctuated over the next seven months. Liver biopsy showed that a mild chronic active hepatitis (CAH) had developed. Normal AST = 5–15 i.u./l; normal bilirubin = 5–17 μmol/l.

Clinical features

The most characteristic feature is the fluctuating serum transaminase values extending over many months or years. A normal value is rarely recorded. Introspective patients keep charts of their blood test results and these soon cover many pages.

Serum γ-globulin is usually less than 2.5 g/dl

and serum bilirubin and albumin values are well preserved.

The patient may be symptom-free. The most frequent complaint is fatigue and of always feeling below par. This varies from time to time. Clinical symptoms do not always parallel the serum transaminase values.

Serum autoantibodies (ANF, smooth muscle and mitochondrial) are not detected.

Diagnosis

In view of the lack of a specific marker in blood or liver, diagnosis can never be precise. Any known type of chronic hepatitis must be excluded.

All possible *hepatotoxic drugs* must be sought.

Markers of present *hepatitis B* must be absent. However, some patients with chronic hepatitis due to B virus do get misdiagnosed as non-A, non-B when titres of HBsAg and HBV DNA are too low to be detected.

Autoimmune chronic active hepatitis is suggested by very high serum transaminase and gamma-globulin levels combined with high titres of autoantibodies.

Prognosis

This is very variable. In some, the diseases are benign with spontaneous biochemical improvement over one to three years. In others, chronic persistent hepatitis and chronic active hepatitis can convert to more serious disease and even go on to cirrhosis.

In general, however, in spite of biochemical disease, the patient is asymptomatic and the development of hepatic failure is rare [12, 50].

Hepato-cellular cancer has been recorded but is exceedingly rare [34, 53].

Treatment

There is no benefit from rest, diet or vitamin supplements.

Interferon treatment is giving promising results in patients with post-transfusion non-A, non-B chronic hepatitis but reported trials are limited. Serum transaminases fall and hepatic histology becomes less active [42, 93]. The course is 3 million units interferon intramuscularly three times a week for six months with one million units three times a week continued probably indefinitely as transaminases rise again when interferon is stopped.

More severe symptoms, biochemical abnormalities and hepatic histology may indicate

prednisolone therapy. This can be tried in a dose of 10−15 mg prednisolone daily and the biochemical and histological responses noted after six months' therapy. The use of corticosteroids is not on a sound scientific basis, as controlled clinical trials have not proved possible.

Drug-related chronic active hepatitis

The whole picture of chronic active hepatitis can be related to drug reactions (Chapter 18). Such drugs include oxyphenisatin, methyl dopa, isoniazid, ketoconazole and nitrofurantoin. Older females are affected most frequently. Clinical features include jaundice and hepatomegaly. Serum transaminase and globulin levels are raised and LE cells may be found in the blood. Liver biopsy shows chronic active hepatitis and even cirrhosis. Bridging hepatic necrosis is not so serious in this group.

Clinical and biochemical improvement follows drug withdrawal. Exacerbations of hepatitis follow re-exposure to the drug. Drug reactions must be considered in the aetiology of any patient with the clinical syndrome of chronic active hepatitis.

Hepatic transplantation

Clearly, transplantation should not be considered at the stage of chronic hepatitis but only when the stage of advanced cirrhosis is reached. Age, psychosocial status, economics, infections and previous upper abdominal surgery are among the pre-operative considerations (see Chapter 35).

Transplant of the cirrhotic liver is difficult because of portal hypertension and poor blood clotting. Removal of a small cirrhotic liver may be difficult. Recurrence of the original disease is likely with hepatitis B and Delta virus infections. The position of recurrence of non-A, non-B hepatitis is uncertain. Patients with autoimmune chronic active hepatitis and cirrhosis rarely show a return of their disease.

References

1 Alexander GJM, Brahm J, Fagan EA *et al.* Loss of HBsAg with interferon in chronic hepatitis B virus infection. *Lancet* 1987; **ii:** 66.

2 Bamber M, Murray A, Arborgh BAM *et al.* Short incubation non-A, non-B hepatitis transmitted by factor VIII concentrates in patients with congenital coagulation disorders. *Gut* 1981; **22:** 854.

3 Bearn AG, Kunkel HG, Slater RJ. The problem of chronic liver disease in young women. *Am. J. Med.* 1956; **21:** 3.

4 Berman M, Alter HJ, Ishak KG *et al.* The chronic sequelae of non-A, non-B hepatitis. *Ann. intern. Med.* 1979; **91:** 1.

5 Bonino F, Rosina F, Rizzetto M *et al.* Chronic hepatitis in HBsAg carriers with serum HBV-DNA and anti-HBe. *Gastroenterology* 1986; **90:** 1268.

6 Bradley DW, Krawcyznski K, Cook EHJ *et al.* Enterically transmitted non-A, non-B hepatitis: serial passage of disease in cynomolgus macaques and tamarins and recovery of disease-associated 27–34-nm virus-like particles. *Proc. Nat. Acad. Sci.* 1987; **84:** 6277.

7 Buffet C, Homberg J-C, Pelletier G *et al.* Chronic active hepatitis associated with liver-kidney microsomal antibody of an autoimmune type: two familial cases. *Dig. Dis. Sci.* 1986; **31:** 1273.

8 Burroughs AK, Bassendine MF, Thomas HC *et al.* Primary liver cell cancer in autoimmune chronic liver disease. *Br. med. J.* 1981; **282:** 273.

9 Chadwick RG, Galizzi J, Heathcote J *et al.* Chronic persistent hepatitis: hepatitis B virus markers and histological follow-up. *Gut* 1979; **20:** 372.

10 Chu C-M. Shyu W-C, Kuo R-W *et al.* HLA class 1 antigen display on hepatocyte membrane in chronic hepatitis B virus infection: its role in the pathogenesis of chronic type B hepatitis. *Hepatology* 1987; **7:** 1311.

11 Cohen N, Mendelow H. Concurrent 'active juvenile cirrhosis' and 'primary pulmonary hypertension'. *Am. J. Med.* 1965; **39:** 127.

12 Colombo M, Oldani S, Donato MF *et al.* A multi-center, prospective study of post-transfusion hepatitis in Milan. *Hepatology* 1987; **7:** 709.

13 Cook GC, Mulligan R, Sherlock S. Controlled prospective trial of corticosteroid therapy in active chronic hepatitis. *Q. J. Med.* 1971; **40:** 159.

14 Croffy B, Kopelman R, Kaplan M. Hypereosinophilic syndrome. Association with chronic active hepatitis. *Dig. Dis. Sci.* 1988; **33:** 233.

15 Czaja AJ, Beaver SJ, Shiels MT. Sustained remission after corticosteroid therapy of severe hepatitis B surface antigen-negative chronic active hepatitis. *Gastroenterology* 1987; **92:** 215.

16 Czaja AJ, Beaver SJ, Wood JR *et al.* Frequency and significance of serum alpha-fetoprotein elevation in severe hepatitis B surface antigen-negative chronic active hepatitis. *Gastroenterology* 1987; **93:** 687.

17 Davis GL, Hoofnagle JH, Waggoner JG. Spontaneous reactivation of chronic hepatitis B virus infection. *Gastroenterology* 1984; **86:** 203.

18 De Cock KM, Govindarajan S, Sandford N *et al.* Fatal reactivation of chronic hepatitis B *J. Am. med. Ass.* 1986; **256:** 1329.

19 De Cock KM, Bradley DW, Sandford NL *et al.* Epidemic non-A, non-B hepatitis in patients from Pakistan. *Ann. intern. Med.* 1987; **106:** 227.

20 Degos F, Lugassy C, Degott C *et al.* Hepatitis B virus and hepatitis B-related viral infection in renal transplant recipients. A prospective study of 90 patients. *Gastroenterology* 1988; **94:** 151.

21 De Groote J, Desmet VJ, Gedigk P *et al.* A classification of chronic hepatitis. *Lancet* 1968; **ii:** 626.

22 De Lemos-Chiarandini C, Alvarez F, Bernard O *et al.* Anti-liver kidney microsome antibody is a marker for the rat hepatocyte endoplasmic reticulum. *Hepatology* 1987; **7:** 468.

23 Deodhar KP, Tapp E, Scheuer PJ. Orcein staining of hepatitis B antigen in paraffin sections of liver biopsies. *J. clin. Pathol.* 1975; **28:** 66.

24 Di Bisceglie AM, Waggoner JG, Hoofnagle JH. Hepatitis B virus deoxyribonucleic acid in liver of chronic carriers. Correlation with serum markers and changes associated with loss of hepatitis Be antigen after antiviral therapy *Gastroenterology* 1987; **93:** 1236.

25 Dienes HP, Popper H, Arnold W *et al.* Histologic observations in human hepatitis non-A, non-B. *Hepatology* 1982; **2:** 562.

26 Dienstag JL. Non-A, non-B hepatitis. I. Recognition, epidemiology and clinical features. *Gastroenterology* 1983; **85:** 439.

27 Dienstag JL. Non-A, non-B hepatitis. II. Experimental transmission, putative virus agents and markers, and prevention. *Gastroenterology* 1983; **85:** 743.

28 Dudley FJ, Fox RA, Sherlock S. Cellular immunity and hepatitis associated (Australia) antigen liver disease. *Lancet* 1972; **i:** 743.

29 Dudley FJ, O'Shea MJ, Ajdukiewicz A *et al.* Serum autoantibodies and immunoglobulins in hepatitis-associated antigen (HAA)-positive and -negative liver disease. *Gut* 1973; **14:** 360.

30 Dudley FJ, Scheuer PJ, Sherlock S. Natural history of hepatitis-associated antigen-positive chronic liver disease. *Lancet* 1972; **ii:** 1388.

31 Dusheiko G, Song E, Bowyer S *et al.* Natural history of hepatitis B virus infection in renal transplant recipients—a fifteen-year follow-up. *Hepatology* 1983; **3:** 330.

32 Fattovich G, Brollo L, Pontisso P *et al.* Levamisole therapy in chronic type B hepatitis. Results of a double-blind randomized trial. *Gastroenterology* 1986; **91**: 692.

33 Fattovich G, Rugge M, Brollo L *et al.* Clinical, virologic and histologic outcome following seroconversion from HBeAg to anti-Hbe in chronic hepatitis type B. *Hepatology* 1986; **6**: 167.

34 Gilliam JH III, Geisinger KR, Richter JE. Primary hepato-cellular carcinoma after chronic non-A, non-B post-transfusion hepatitis. *Ann. intern. Med.* 1984; **101**: 794.

35 Govindarajan S, De Cock KM, Redeker AG. Natural course of delta superinfection in chronic hepatitis B virus-infected patients: histopathologic study with multiple liver biopsies. *Hepatology* 1986; **6**: 640.

36 Gurian LE, Rogoff TM, Ware AJ *et al.* The immunologic diagnosis of chronic active 'autoimmune' hepatitis: distinction from systemic lupus erythematosus. *Hepatology* 1985; **5**: 397.

37 Hadziyannis S, Vissoulis C, Moussouros A *et al.* Cytoplasmic localisation of Australia antigen in the liver. *Lancet* 1972; **i**: 976.

38 Hadziyannis SJ, Lieberman HM, Karvountzis GG *et al.* Analysis of liver disease, nuclear HBcAg, viral replication, and hepatitis B virus DNA in liver and serum of HBeAg versus anti-HBe positive carriers of hepatitis B virus. *Hepatology* 1983; **3**: 656.

39 Hall S, Czaja AJ, Kaufman DK *et al.* How lupoid is lupoid hepatitis? *J. Rheumatol.* 1986; **13**: 95.

40 Hegarty JE, Nouri Aria KT, Portmann B *et al.* Relapse following treatment withdrawal in patients with autoimmune chronic active hepatitis. *Hepatology* 1983; **3**: 685.

41 Homberg J-C, Abuaf N, Bernard O *et al.* Chronic active hepatitis associated with antiliver-kidney microsome antibody type 1: a second type of 'autoimmune' hepatitis. *Hepatology* 1987; **7**: 1333.

42 Hoofnagle JH, Mullen KD, Jones DB *et al.* Treatment of chronic non-A, non-B, hepatitis with recombinant alpha interferon. *N. Engl. J. Med.* 1986; **315**: 1575.

43 Hoofnagle JH, Sharfitz DA, Popper H. Chronic type B hepatitis and the 'healthy' HBsAg carrier state. *Hepatology* 1987; **7**: 758.

44 Hyams JS, Ballow M, Leichtner AM. Cyclosporine treatment of autoimmune chronic active hepatitis. *Gastroenterology* 1987; **93**: 890.

45 Ikeda T, Lever AML, Thomas HC. Evidence for a deficiency of interferon production in patients with chronic hepatitis B virus infection acquired in adult life. *Hepatology* 1986; **6**: 962.

46 International Group. Acute and chronic hepatitis revisited. *Lancet* 1977; **ii**: 914.

47 Jakobovits AW, Gibson PR, Dudley FJ. Primary liver cell carcinoma complicating auto-immune chronic acute hepatitis. *Dig. Dis. Sci.* 1981; **26**: 694.

48 Kilby AE, Albertini RJ, Krawitt EL. HLA typing and autoantibodies in hepatitis B surface antigen-negative chronic active hepatitis. *Tissue Antigens* 1986; **28**: 214.

49 Kirk AP, Jain S, Pocock S *et al.* Late results of Royal Free Hospital controlled trial of prednisolone therapy in hepatitis B surface antigen-negative chronic active hepatitis. *Gut* 1980; **21**: 78.

50 Koike K, Iino S, Kurai K *et al.* IgM anti-HBc in anti-HBe positive chronic type B hepatitis with acute exacerbations. *Hepatology* 1987; **7**: 573.

51 Koretz RL, Stone O, Mousa M *et al.* Non-A, non-B post-transfusion hepatitis—a decade later. *Gastroenterology* 1985; **88**: 1251.

52 Lai C-L, Lok A S-F, Lin H-J *et al.* Placebo-controlled trial of recombinant alpha 2 interferon in Chinese HBsAg-carrier children. *Lancet* 1987; **ii**: 877.

53 Lefkowitch JH, Apfelbaum TF. Liver cell dysplasia and hepato-cellular carcinoma in non-A, non-B hepatitis. *Arch. Path. lab. Med.* 1987; **111**: 170.

54 Lok ASF, Weller IVD, Karayiannis P *et al.* Thrice weekly lymphoblastoid interferon is effective in inhibiting hepatitis B virus replication. *Liver* 1984; **4**: 45.

55 Mackay IR. Genetic aspects of immunologically mediated liver disease. *Semin. Liver Dis.* 1984; **4**: 13.

56 Maddrey WC. Subdivisions of idiopathic autoimmune chronic active hepatitis. *Hepatology* 1987; **7**: 1372.

57 Madscad S, Bjerregaard B, Henricksen JH *et al.* Impaired conversion of prednisone to prednisolone in patients with liver cirrhosis. *Gut* 1980; **21**: 52.

58 Manns M, Gerken G, Kyriatsoulis A *et al.* Characterization of a new subgroup of autoimmune chronic active hepatitis by autoantibodies against a soluble liver antigen. *Lancet* 1987; **i**: 292.

59 Margulies A, Bernuau J, Balayan MS *et al.* Non-A, non-B fulminant hepatitis in France in returnees from Asia and Africa. *Dig. Dis. Sci.* 1987; **32**: 1151.

60 Meyer zum Büschenfelde K-H, Manns M, Hütteroth TH *et al.* LM Ag and LSP—two different target antigens involved in the immuno-pathogenesis of chronic active hepatitis? *Clin. exp. Immunol* 1979; **37**: 205.

61 Mistilis SP, Blackburn CRB. Active chronic hepatitis. *Am J. Med.* 1970; **48**: 484.

62 Montano L, Aranguibel F, Boffill M *et al.* An analysis of the composition of the inflammatory

infiltrate in autoimmune and hepatitis B virus-induced chronic liver disease. *Hepatology* 1983; **3:** 292.

63 Murray-Lyon IM, Stern RB, Williams R. Controlled trial of prednisone and azathioprine in active chronic hepatitis. *Lancet* 1973; **i:** 735.

64 Nair PV, Tong MJ, Stevenson D *et al.* A pilot study on the effects of prednisone withdrawal on serum HBV DNA and HBeAg in chronic active hepatitis B. *Hepatology* 1986; **6:** 1319.

65 Odièvre M, Maggiore G, Homberg JC *et al.* Seroimmunologic classification of chronic active hepatitis in 57 children. *Hepatology* 1983; **3:** 407.

66 Penner E. Nature of immune complexes in autoimmune chronic active hepatitis. *Gastroenterology* 1987; **92:** 304.

67 Perrillo RP, Regenstein FG. Corticosteroid therapy for chronic active hepatitis B: Is a little too much? *Hepatology* 1986; **6:** 1416.

68 Perrillo R P, Regenstein F G, Peters M G. *et al.* Prednisone withdrawal followed by recombinant alpha interferon in the treatment of chronic type B hepatitis. A randomized, controlled trial. *Ann. int. Med.* 1988; **109:** 95.

69 Popper H, Shafritz DA, Hoofnagle JH. Relation of the hepatitis B virus carrier state to hepatocellular carcinoma. *Hepatology* 1987; **7:** 764.

70 Read AE, Harrison CV, Sherlock S. 'Juvenile cirrhosis'; part of a system disease. The effect of corticosteroid therapy. *Gut* 1963; **4:** 378.

71 Realdi G, Alberti A, Rugge M *et al.* Seroconversion from hepatitis Be antigen to anti-HBe in chronic hepatitis B virus infection. *Gastroenterology* 1980 **79:** 195.

72 Realdi G, Alberti A, Rugge M. *et al.* Long-term follow-up of acute and chronic non-A, non-B post-transfusion hepatitis: evidence of progression to liver cirrhosis. *Gut* 1982; **23:** 270.

73 Renner E, Horber FF, Jost G *et al.* Effect of liver function on the metabolism of prednisone and prednisolone in humans. *Gastroenterology* 1986; **90:** 819.

74 Rizzetto M, Swana G, Doniach D. Microsomal antibodies in active chronic hepatitis and other disorders. *Clin. exp. Immunol* 1973; **15:** 331.

75 Rizzetto M, Macagno S, Chiaberge E *et al.* Liver transplantation in hepatitis Delta virus disease. *Lancet* 1987; **ii:** 469.

76 Robertson DAF, Zhang SL, Guy EG *et al.* Persistent measles virus genome in auto-immune chronic active hepatitis. *Lancet* 1987; **ii:** 9.

77 Sagnelli E, Piccinino F, Manzillo G *et al.* Effect of immunosuppressive therapy on HBsAg-positive chronic active hepatitis in relation to presence or absence of HBeAg and anti-HBe. *Hepatology* 1983, **3:** 690.

78 Schalm SW, Summerskill WHJ, Gitnick GL *et al.*

Contrasting features and responses to treatment of severe chronic active liver disease with and without hepatitis B$_s$ antigen. *Gut* 1976; **17:** 781.

79 Schalm SW, Heytink RA, Van Buuren HR *et al.* Acyclovir enhances the antiviral effect of interferon in chronic hepatitis B. *Lancet* 1985; **ii:** 358.

80 Scheuer PJ, Texeira MR, Weller IVD *et al.* Pathology of acute hepatitis A, B and non-A, non-B. *J Pathol.* 1981; **134:** 323.

81 Scheuer PJ. Changing views on chronic hepatitis. *Histopathology* 1986: **10:** 1.

82 Scheuer PJ. Chronic hepatitis. In *Liver Biopsy Interpretation*, 4th edn. London, Baillière Tindall, 1988.

83 Schlichting P, Holund B, Poulson H. Liver biopsy in chronic aggressive hepatitis. Diagnostic reproducibility in relation to size of specimen. *Scand. J. Gastroenterol.* 1983; **18:** 27.

84 Sherlock S. Chronic hepatitis and cirrhosis. *Hepatology* 1984; **4:** 25S.

85 Sherlock S, Thomas HC. Conference Report: delta virus hepatitis. *J. Hepatol.* 1987; **3:** 419.

86 Sherlock S. Treatment of chronic viral hepatitis. *J. Hepatol.* 1988; **6:** 113.

87 Silva H, Hall E, Hill KR *et al.* Renal involvement in active 'juvenile' cirrhosis. *J. clin. Pathol.* 1965; **18:** 157.

88 Soloway RD, Summerskill WH, Baggenstoss AH *et al.* Clinical, biochemical, and histological remission of severe chronic active liver disease: a controlled study of treatments and early prognosis. *Gastroenterology* 1972; **63:** 820.

89 Stellon AJ, Davies A, Compston J. *et al.* Bone loss in autoimmune chronic active hepatitis on maintenance corticosteroid therapy. *Gastroenterology* 1985; **89:** 1078.

90 Tage-Jensen U, Arnold W, Dietrichson O *et al.* Liver cell membrane autoantibody specific for inflammatory liver diseases. *Br. med. J.* 1977; **i:** 206.

91 Thomas HC, Lok ASF. The immuno-pathology of autoimmune and hepatitis B virus-induced chronic hepatitis. *Semin. Liver Dis.* 1984; **4:** 36.

92 Thomas HC, Scully LJ. Antiviral therapy in hepatitis B infection. *Br. med. Bull.* 1985; **41:** 374.

93 Thomson BJ, Doran M, Lever AML *et al.* Alpha-interferon therapy for non-A, non-B hepatitis transmitted by gammaglobulin replacement therapy. *Lancet* 1987; **1:** 539.

94 Tong MJ, Sampliner RE, Govindarajan S *et al.* Spontaneous reactivation of hepatitis B in Chinese patients with HBsAg-positive chronic active hepatitis. *Hepatology* 1987; **7:** 713.

95 Vergani D, Wells L, Larcher VF *et al.* Genetically determined low C4: a predisposing factor to autoimmune chronic active hepatitis. *Lancet* 1985; **ii:** 294.

96 Viola LA, Barrison IG, Coleman JC *et al*. Natural history of liver disease in chronic hepatitis B surface antigen carriers. *Lancet* 1981; **ii:** 1156.

97 Waldenström J. *Leber, Blutproteine und Nahrungsweiss Stoffwechs Krh.*, Sonderband: XV, p 8. Tagung, Bad Kissingen 1950.

98 Weissberg JI, Andres LL, Smith CI *et al*. Survival in chronic hepatitis B: an analysis of 379 patients. *Ann. intern. Med.* 1984; **101:** 613.

99 Weller IVD, Bassendine MF, Murray A *et al*. The effects of prednisolone/azathioprine in chronic hepatitis B viral infection. *Gut* 1982; **23:** 650.

100 Wiedmann KH, Bartholemew TC, Brown DJC *et al*. Liver membrane antibodies detected by immunoradiometric assay in acute and chronic virus-induced and autoimmune liver disease. *Hepatology* 1984; **4:** 199.

101 Wilkinson SP, Portmann B, Cochrane AMG *et al*. Clinical course of chronic lobular hepatitis. *Q. J. Med.* 1978; **47:** 421.

102 Willock RG, Isselbacher KJ. Chronic liver disease in young people. Clinical features and course in thirty-three patients. *Am. J. Med.* 1961; **30:** 185.

103 Wood JR, Czaja AJ, Beaver SJ *et al*. Frequency and significance of antibody to double-stranded DNA in chronic active hepatitis. *Hepatology* 1986; **6:** 976.

18 · Drugs and the Liver

The liver is particularly concerned with drug metabolism, and especially of drugs given orally (fig. 18.1). These must be lipid-soluble to have passed the membrane of the intestinal cell. They must then be presented to the liver and converted to water-soluble (more polar) compounds for excretion via the urine or bile.

PHARMACOKINETICS [84]

The hepatic clearance of drugs given by mouth (CLH) depends on the efficiency of the drug metabolizing enzymes, the intrinsic clearance, (CLint), the liver blood flow (HBS) and the extent of plasma protein binding (fb) (fig. 18.2). Drugs vary in their pharmacological effects according to the relative importance of these different pharmacokinetic factors (table 18.1).

Drugs which are avidly taken up by the liver (high intrinsic clearance) are said to have a high *first-pass metabolism*. The rate-limiting factor in their hepatic uptake is liver blood flow and indeed their clearance can be used to measure liver blood flow. Indocyanine green is one such drug. These drugs are usually highly lipid soluble. If liver blood flow falls, for instance, due to cirrhosis or heart failure, the systemic effect of the high first-pass rate drug will be enhanced. Administration of drugs such as propranolol or cimetidine which lower hepatic blood flow will have a similar effect [43].

Because of its high first-pass rate, a drug such as glyceryl trinitrate has to be given sublingually to avoid entry into the portal vein. Similarly, lignocaine has to be given intravenously.

Drugs with a low intrinsic clearance, such as theophylline, depend on enzyme function and changes in hepatic blood flow have little effect.

Plasma protein binding limits the presentation of the drug to hepatic enzymes. This will be affected by changes in the synthesis and degradation of plasma proteins.

HEPATIC DRUG METABOLISM

Phase 1. The main drug-metabolizing system resides in the microsomal fraction of the liver

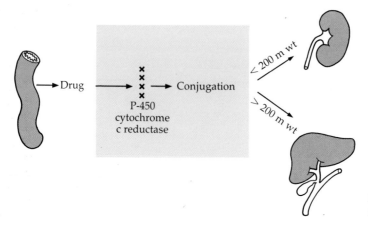

Fig. 18.1. Hepatic drug metabolism (Sherlock, 1979).

$$CLH = QH \left[\frac{CLint.fb}{QU + CLint.fb} \right]$$

Fig. 18.2. Formula for calculating clearance (CLH) of a drug by the liver. QH = liver blood flow, CLint = intrinsic clearance, fb = plasma protein binding.

cell (smooth endoplasmic reticulum). The enzymes concerned are mixed function mono-oxygenases, cytochrome C-reductase and cytochrome P450. Reduced NADPH in the cell sap is a co-factor. The drug is rendered more polar by hydroxylation or oxidation. Alternative phase 1 drug metabolizing reactions include the conversion of alcohol to acetaldehyde by alcohol dehydrogenases found mainly in the cytosolic fraction.

The drug metabolizing enzyme system may be induced non-specifically, so increasing drug oxidation, by many lipid-soluble substances. Inducing agents increase drug metabolizing enzyme activity by genomal de-repression of

Table 18.1. Classification of drugs based on pharmacokinetic parameters obtained in normal subjects (Larrey & Branch 1983)

	Hepatic extraction	Protein binding	Effect of shunting on systemic availability	Examples
Enzyme limited, binding insensitive	Low	High	0	Antipyrine Amobarbital Caffeine Theophylline Aminopyrine
Enzyme limited, binding sensitive	Low	High	0	Chlordiazepoxide Diazepam Diphenylhydantoin Indomethacin Phenylbutazone Rifampicin Tolbutamide Warfarin
Flow and enzyme sensitive	Medium	Medium	+	Acetaminophen Chlorpromazine Isoniazid Merperidine Metoprolol Nortriptyline Quinidine
Flow limited	High	Medium	+++	Galactose Indocyanine green Labetalol Lidocaine Morphine Pentazocine Propoxyphene Propranolol Verapamil

protein synthesis that results in enhanced production of the specific drug metabolizing enzyme. Enzyme inducers include barbiturates, alcohol, anaesthetics, hypoglycaemic and anticonvulsant agents, griseofulvin, rifampicin, glutethimide, phenylbutazone and meprobamate. Enlargement of the liver following the introduction of drug therapy can be related to enzyme induction. Inhibitors of the enzyme system include para-amino-salicylic acid. Two active drugs competing for an enzyme-binding site may lead to the drug with a lower affinity being metabolized more slowly and thus having a more prolonged action.

Phase 2. These biotransformations involve conjugation of the drug or drug metabolite with a small endogenous molecule. The enzymes concerned are usually not confined to the liver, but are present there in high concentration.

Active transport. This system is located at the biliary pole of the hepatocyte. The mechanism is energy dependent and can be saturated.

Biliary and urinary excretion. Factors determining whether the metabolized drug will be excreted ultimately in bile or urine are multiple and many are unclear. Highly polar substances are excreted unaltered in the bile and also those which become more polar after conjugation. Those with a molecular weight exceeding 200 tend to be excreted in the bile. As the molecular weight gets smaller, the urinary route becomes more important.

Risk factors for hepatic drug injury

Liver disease. The impaired metabolism is proportional to the extent of hepato-cellular failure and is greatest in cirrhosis. A correlation exists between the half-life of a drug and the prothrombin time, serum albumin level, hepatic encephalopathy and ascites [40].

The causes of the impaired drug metabolism are multiple. Reduced hepatic blood flow leads to impaired metabolism particularly of high first-pass drugs. Impaired oxidative metabolism is seen particularly with barbiturates such as hexobarbital, phenobarbital and also with

chlordiazepoxide. Glucuronidation is preserved so that morphine, which is a high-clearance drug normally inactivated in this way, is eliminated normally.

Reduced plasma protein binding follows failure of hepatic albumin synthesis. Benzodiazepines, for instance, are eliminated almost solely by hepatic biotransformation, highly protein bound and this is restrictive in their elimination. In hepato-cellular disease there is a decrease in drug clearance from plasma, and an increase in its volume of distribution accounted for by decreased drug binding.

There is evidence of increased cerebral sensitivity, particularly to sedatives, and increased cerebral receptors in liver disease may increase this effect. Oxazepam seems to be the most satisfactory sedative for patients with liver disease.

Chronic drug ingestion can induce drug-metabolizing enzymes and so shorten the half-life of a drug in a patient with cirrhosis (fig. 18.3) [92].

Age and sex. Hepatic drug reactions are rare in children, apart from accidental overdose. They even may be resistant, as children with paracetamol overdose have much less liver damage than an adult with an equivalent paracetamol serum concentration [97]. Valproate hepatotoxicity, however, does affect children and rarely halothane [73]. The ageing liver may be more at risk [67]. Hepatic drug reactions are more frequent in the female sex.

Genetics. Genetic polymorphism arises from the occurrence of mutant alleles that influence the structure or amount of an enzyme synthesized. This leads to certain individuals having a genetic inability to perform a particular biotransformation. A good example is the fast and slow acetylation of isoniazid. Debrisoquine, a antihypertensive drug, exhibits genetic polymorphism. Individuals showing impaired debrisoquine oxidation also fail to metabolize the drug perhexiline and can develop liver injury [113].

Sensitivity to electrophilic attack may be an inherited autosomal dominant in sufferers from halothane hepatitis [41].

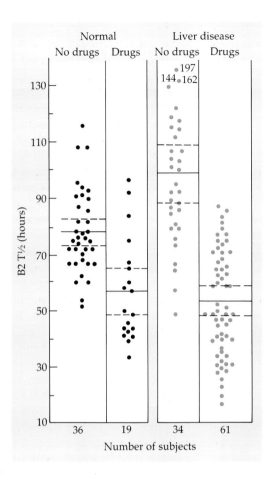

Fig. 18.3. The effect of preliminary treatment with drugs on the half-life of phenylbutazone. In those who were not pre-treated with drugs, the group of cirrhotics has a longer half-life than the controls. After pre-treatment there is no statistical difference in the half-life (Levi *et al.* 1968).

Such genetic defects may apparently explain idiosyncratic hepatic drug reactions where only a small number of patients receiving the drug are affected. The identification of those susceptible is important in prevention.

Drugs causing interference with bilirubin metabolism

Drugs can affect bilirubin metabolism at any **375** stage from its production from haem to its

canalicular excretion. The effects can be investigated in man, and methods used in animals are usually applicable. The reactions are predictable, reversible and not serious in the adult. In the neonate, however, a rise in unconjugated bilirubin in the brain is very important (fig. 18.4) as this potentiates bilirubin encephalopathy (kernicterus). In the adult, those with an underlying tendency to, or actual, hyperbilirubinaemia will have the jaundice enhanced by a drug which interferes with bilirubin metabolism. This applies to such conditions as Gilbert's syndrome, chronic active hepatitis or primary biliary cirrhosis. Organic anions such as salicylates or sulphonamides compete with unconjugated bilirubin for albumin binding and lead to its detachment (fig. 18.4).

Haemolytic reactions increase the bilirubin load on the liver cell. This is rare as a single defect and is usually combined with a hypersensitivity reaction which decreases hepatocellular function. Sulphonamides, phenacetin or quinine can cause such reactions. Such drugs may also precipitate haemolysis in those with a congenitally determined defect—for instance,

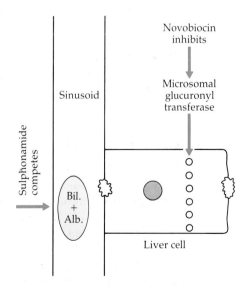

Fig. 18.4. Drugs given to neonates may compete with unconjugated bilirubin for serum albumin binding or may inhibit the microsomal conjugating enzymes.

glucose 6PD deficiency. In the Far East, glucose 6PD deficiency is a common cause of neonatal jaundice. The offending drug may be transmitted in the mother's milk. The toxic effects of synthetic Vitamin K preparations given to neonates may partially be due to increased haemolysis.

Certain drugs interfere with the uptake and transport of bilirubin in the hepatocyte. They include cholecystographic media and rifampicin. Transport proteins may be decreased in neonates making them susceptible to drugs that compete with bilirubin for transport. These drugs would potentiate kernicterus.

The antibiotic, novobiocin, inhibits bilirubin conjugation and the resultant hyperbilirubinaemia is particularly important in neonates (fig. 18.4).

Cholestasis follows interference of drugs such as sex hormones with bilirubin canalicular excretion.

Hepatotoxicity due to drugs

Drugs in common use can cause toxic effects on the liver which can mimic almost every naturally occurring liver disease affecting man (table 18.2). About 2% of all cases of jaundice in hospitalized patients are drug-induced. About a quarter of cases of fulminant hepatic failure in the United States are thought to be drug-related.

In every patient with liver disease it is essential to record all medicaments which have been taken over the last three months. The physician may have to take on the role of a detective to identify them all. History must include dose, route of administration, duration and any concomitant drugs [201]. Other causes of a hepatic reaction, such as hepatitis A or B, must be excluded.

Early suspicion of a drug-related hepatic reaction, and, if possible, diagnosis of the cause, are essential. Severity is greatly increased if the drug is continued after symptoms develop or after serum transaminases rise. This action provides grounds for negligence claims.

Hepato-cellular zone 3 necrosis

Hepato-cellular injury seems to be the primary event. This is rarely due to the drug itself and a toxic metabolite is usually responsible (fig. 18.5) The drug-metabolizing enzymes activate chemically stable drugs to produce electrophilic metabolites. These potent alkylating, arylating or acylating agents bind covalently to liver molecules which are essential to the life of the hepatocyte and necrosis ensues (fig. 18.6). This follows exhaustion of intra-cellular substances such as glutathione which are capable of preferentially conjugating with the toxic metabolite. In addition, metabolites with an unpaired electron are produced by oxidative reactions of cytochrome P450. These *free radicals* can also bind covalently to proteins and to unsaturated fatty acids of cell membranes. This results in *lipid peroxidation* and membrane damage. The end result is hepatocyte death related to failure to pump calcium from the cytosol and to depressed mitochondrial function (fig. 18.6) [69]. Necrosis is greatest in zone 3, where drug metabolizing enzymes are found in highest concentration and where the oxygen tension is lowest in sinusoidal blood [25]. Fatty change is also seen with little inflammatory reaction.

The hepatic necrosis is dose-dependent. Animal models exist. Other organs also suffer and renal damage is often the most important. In mild cases, jaundice may be mild, slight and transient. Serum biochemical tests show marked rises in transaminases. Prothrombin time increases rapidly. Light microscopy shows clear-cut zone 3 necrosis, with scattered fatty change and little inflammatory reaction (fig. 18.7). Peri-portal fibrosis may sometimes be marked. Paracetamol (acetaminophen) is a good example of this type.

Some drugs cause zone 3 hepatic necrosis, but in only a small proportion of those exposed. The mechanism cannot be straightforward dose-dependent toxicity, and metabolic idiosyncrasy is postulated. Halothane occasionally causes confluent zonal or massive necrosis as well as hepatitic reaction [11]. The products of reductive metabolism are reactive as are the

Table 18.2. Classification of hepatic drug reactions

Type	Features	Examples
Zone 3 necrosis	Dose dependent, multi-organ failure	Carbon tetrachloride Paracetamol Halothane
Microvesicular fat	Affects children Reyes's-like syndrome Cirrhosis	Valproate
'Alcoholic hepatitis	Long half-life Cirrhosis	Perhexiline Amiodarone
Fibrosis	Portal hypertension Cirrhosis	Methotrexate Vinyl chloride Vitamin A
Vascular Veno-occlusive disease	Dose dependent	Irradiation Cytotoxics
Sinusoidal dilatation and peliosis		Azathioprine Sex hormones
Hepatic vein obstruction	Thrombotic effect	Sex hormones
Acute hepatitis	Bridging necrosis Short term, acute Long term, chronic active hepatitis	Methyl dopa Isoniazid Halothane Ketoconazole
General hyper-sensitivity	Often with granulomas	Sulphonamides Quinidine Allopurinol
Cholestasis Canalicular	Dose dependent, reversible	Sex hormones
Hepato-canalicular	Reversible surgical 'obstructive' jaundice	Chlorpromazine Erythromycin Nitrofurantoin Azathioprine
Ductular	Age related, renal failure	Benoxaprofen
Sclerosing cholangitis	Cholestasis	FUDR (intra-arterial)
Neoplastic Focal nodular hyperplasia	Benign. Presents space occupying lesion	Sex hormones
Adenoma	May rupture. Usually regress	Sex hormones
Hepato-cellular carcinoma	Very rare. Relatively benign	Sex hormones

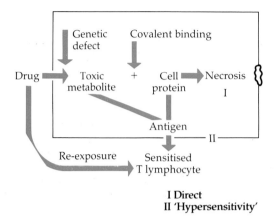

Fig. 18.5. The mechanisms of hepatotoxicity, direct, metabolic related and immunological hypersensitivity.

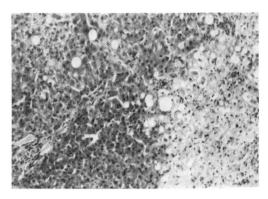

Fig. 18.7. Accidental carbon tetrachloride poisoning. To the right of the section liver cells are necrotic and show hydropic degeneration and fatty change. Surviving liver cells to the left of the section show occasional fatty change. The portal zones are unaffected.

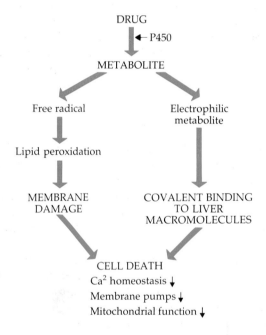

Fig. 18.6. The mechanism of metabolite-related direct hepato-cellular necrosis.

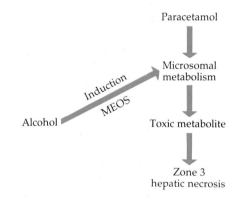

Fig. 18.8. Alcohol, as an enzyme inducing agent, increases the production of toxic metabolites of paracetamol, so potentiating hepatic necrosis (Sherlock 1986). MEOS = microsomal enzyme oxidizing system.

oxidative ones. The metabolites produced by either mechanism could bind to cellular macromolecules and cause lipid peroxidation and inactivation of drug-metabolizing and other enzymes [31]. The idiosyncrasy might be explained by inherited sensitivity to electrophilic attack. Ketoconazole may have a similar hepatotoxic mechanism [12, 94].

Effects of enzyme induction and inhibition. Induction of the P450 drug metabolizing enzymes enhances the production of toxic drug metabolites. Thus rats pre-treated with phenobarbital show increased zone 3 necrosis following carbon tetrachloride. Halothane toxicity may be greater in patients who have been receiving previous anticonvulsant therapy [123].

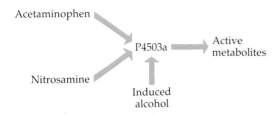

Fig. 18.9. Alcohol, by inducing P 450 3a (P450 11E1) drug-metabolizing enzymes enhances the toxicity of paracetamol and the carcinogen nitrosamine (Sherlock 1986).

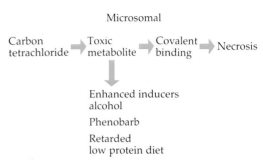

Fig. 18.10. Carbon tetrachloride liver injury mediated by a toxic metabolite (Sherlock 1979).

Alcohol ingestion considerably enhances paracetamol toxicity so that as little as 4 to 8 g can cause serious liver damage (fig. 18.8) [160]. This is apparently due to the induction by alcohol of a distinct liver cytochrome, P450 3a (P450 11E1) which is important in generating toxic metabolites. It is also concerned in oxygenation of nitrosamines at the alpha-carbon (fig. 18.9) [197]. Theoretically, this could increase the risk of cancer in alcoholics. Cimetidine inhibits P-450 mixed-function oxidase activities and modifies the hepatotoxic effects of paracetamol [89]. Omeprazole acts similarly [54]. Ranitidine in high doses reduces metabolic activation of paracetamol but at low doses it potentiates hepatotoxicity [91]. Isoniazid is much more hepatotoxic when combined with rifampycin (an enzyme inducer) than with para-amino salicylate (an enzyme inhibitor). Interferon inhibits theophylline metabolism [192].

The administration of drugs which induce microsomal enzymes, for instance phenytoin, results in increases in serum gamma-glutamyl-transpeptidase [72].

Carbon tetrachloride

This may be taken accidentally or suicidally. It may be inhaled, for instance in dry-cleaning or in filling fire extinguishers, or mixed in drinks.

The liver injury is induced by a toxic metabolite which combines covalently with cell proteins and induces necrosis (fig. 18.10) [108]. The effect is enhanced by enzyme inducers such as alcohol and barbiturates and reduced by protein malnutrition which depresses drug metabolizing enzymes. This may explain the apparent resistance of those in underdeveloped countries to the hepatotoxic effects of carbon tetrachloride and similar compounds when used to treat helminth infestation.

CLINICAL FEATURES

Vomiting, abdominal pain and diarrhoea are followed within 48 hours by jaundice. The liver may be enlarged and tender. Spontaneous haemorrhages reflect the profound hypoprothrombinaemia. Serum transaminase values are very high (fig. 18.11); the serum albumin level falls.

In severe cases acute renal failure overshadows hepatic destruction. Acute haemorrhagic gastritis is prominent. Since carbon tetrachloride is an anaesthetic the patient becomes increasingly drowsy.

PATHOLOGY

Zone 3 cells show hydropic degeneration marked by clear cytoplasm and pyknotic nuclei (fig. 18.7). Fatty change varies from a few droplets to diffuse involvement of liver cells. Polymorphonuclear infiltration of the portal zones is slight, fibrosis is uncommon. With recovery the liver pattern returns to normal.

379

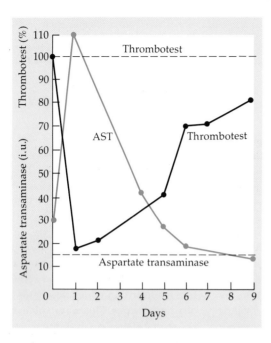

Fig. 18.11. Suicidal inhalation of carbon tetrachloride in a young male. Note the rapid fall in thrombotest with rise in transaminase values. At six days they have virtually resumed normal levels.

PROGNOSIS

Death in the acute stage is due to kidney failure. If the patient survives the acute episode there are no late hepatic sequelae. In rats one oral dose of carbon tetrachloride causes acute hepatic injury followed by complete recovery, but repeated administration leads to cirrhosis. This sequence is not seen in man. Liver cells may even be more resistant with prolonged exposure. Carbon tetrachloride is not an aetiological factor in hepatic cirrhosis in man.

TREATMENT

Screening tests in workers should include routine examination for liver enlargement and tenderness, urine testing for urobilinogen and serum transaminase estimation.

Acute poisoning is treated by a high calorie, high carbohydrate diet and along the usual lines for acute hepato-renal failure including

dialysis. Prompt treatment with acetyl cysteine may minimize hepatorenal damage [151].

RELATED COMPOUNDS

Other chlorinated hydrocarbons and benzol derivatives may act similarly. Teenagers sniffing cleaning fluid which contains trichlorethylene [34] or glue containing toluene [125] suffer jaundice with liver necrosis and renal failure.

Benzene derivatives include trinitrotoluene (TNT), dinitrophenol and toluene. The maximum effect is on the bone-marrow with aplasia. The liver may be involved acutely, but chronic sequelae are rare.

Chronic industrial exposure to organic solvents can lead to abnormal transaminase values with minor changes on liver biopsy [34]. Such effects of occupational exposure to toxic materials are probably of little clinical importance but further research is needed to be certain.

Occupational exposure to 2-nitropropane may be fatal [57].

Muscarine

Acute liver failure follows ingestion of various *Amanita* mushrooms, including *A. phalloides* and *A. verna*. Three stages of illness can be recognized. The first, starting 8—12 hours after ingestion, consists of nausea, cramping abdominal pain and rice-water diarrhoea and lasts for 3—4 days. The second phase is characterized by apparent improvement. The third stage includes hepato-renal and central nervous system degeneration with massive cell destruction. The liver shows zone 3 necrosis without much inflammation. Fatty change is seen in fatal cases [190]. The condition is life-threatening although recovery can occur. The mushroom toxins, phalloidin and phalloin, are extremely lethal to liver cells.

Supportive measures are all that can be offered. Haemodialysis may be helpful. Hepatic transplantation has been successfully employed.

Paracetamol (acetaminophen)

Paracetamol is used as a suicidal agent [12]. About 10 g produces hepatic necrosis, but the dose actually ingested is difficult to assess because of early vomiting and unreliable histories. Alcohol, by its enzyme-inducing effect, enhances the hepatotoxicity of paracetamol [160]. As little as 10 g paracetamol per day may produce significant hepatotoxicity in an alcoholic and even less if there is underlying liver disease.

The electrophilic metabolite of paracetamol preferentially conjugates with hepatic glutathione. When the glutathione is exhausted, the paracetamol metabolite arylates essential nucleophilic macromolecules, so producing hepatic necrosis (fig. 18.12) [109].

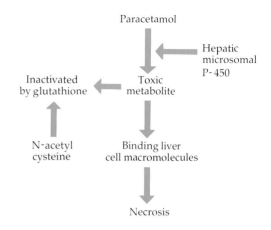

Fig. 18.12. The mechanism of paracetamol (acetaminophen) liver injury and of *N*-acetyl cysteine treatment (Sherlock 1979).

CLINICAL FEATURES

Within a few hours of ingestion, the patient becomes nauseated and vomits. Consciousness is preserved. After about 48 hours recovery seems in progress; then about the third or fourth day the patient deteriorates and becomes jaundiced when the liver is tender. Serum transaminase and prothrombin levels are enormous. In the more seriously affected, deterioration is then rapid with the signs of acute hepatic necrosis (Chapter 8). Myocardial and renal damage and hypoglycaemia are prominent.

Hepatic histology shows zone 3 necrosis, some fatty change and very little inflammation [137]. Reticulin collapse may be confluent and massive, but cirrhosis is not a sequel.

Chronic hepatitis. Long-term (about one year) exposure to paracetamol (within the therapeutic upper limit of 4 g daily) is said to lead to chronic hepatitis [20]. Underlying liver disease may potentiate the effect [12]. Chronic disease is potentiated by alcoholism.

PROGNOSIS

The overall mortality for 201 patients admitted to a general hospital was 3.5%. A prothrombin ratio of 20% and hepatic coma are unfavourable prognostic signs. Severity can also be assessed by the paracetamol blood levels which should always be determined. If the plasma level four hours after the overdose exceeds 300 µg/ml there is 100% incidence of hepatic toxicity, and if less than 120 µg/ml there is no danger. If the paracetamol level 12 hours after administration exceeds 50 µg/ml hepatic toxicity is likely, and if less than 50 µg/ml there is no danger [137].

TREATMENT

The stomach is washed out. The patient is admitted to hospital. Evidences of hepatic necrosis are delayed and early improvement should not give a sense of false security.

Forced diuresis and renal dialysis do not increase the excretion of paracetamol or its metabolites already bound to tissues. The treatment of acute liver failure is outlined in Chapter 7.

Treatment is aimed at replenishing the glutathione reserves of the liver cell. Unfortunately the penetration of glutathione itself into liver cells is poor. Precursors of glutathione and glutathione-like substances have therefore been employed. They are necessary only when hepatic damage is likely. This is assessed by plasma levels. The patient's value is plotted against a line joining 200 µg/ml at four hours, and 60 µg/ml at 12 hours on a semi-log graph of concentration versus time [137]. If the patient's concentration is below this line, liver damage will be clinically insignificant and treatment can be stopped.

Cysteamine and methionine have been replaced by intravenous acetyl cysteine (Mucomist, Parvolex) [136]. This is rapidly hydrolysed to cysteine *in vivo*. It has fewer side-effects than cysteamine. It is very effective in preventing severe liver damage if administered up to eight hours after an overdose and is worth giving even after 20 hours. Treatment after 15 hours is ineffective. The dose is 150 mg/kg in 200 ml 5% glucose over 15 minutes, followed by 50 mg/kg in 500 ml 5% dextrose over four hours and 100 mg/kg in one litre 5% dextrose over the next 16 hours (total dose 300 mg/kg in 20 hours).

Salicylates

Patients on salicylate therapy for acute rheumatic fever, juvenile and adult rheumatoid arthritis, and systemic lupus erythematosus, may develop acute hepatic injury and even chronic active hepatitis. This may develop even with serum salicylate levels below 25 mg/100 ml [126].

Piroxicam

Causes zone 3 hepato-cellular necrosis [90].

Mineral oil

Chronic ingestion of mineral oils can lead to hepatic inflammation and scarring related to deposits in portal triads [17].

Hyperthermia [75, 150]

Heat stroke is accompanied by hepato-cellular damage. In 10% of cases it is severe and may contribute to death. Pathologically it is marked by microvesicular fat, congestion, cholestasis (some-times ductal), haemosiderosis and

sinusoidal infiltration with primitive cells [150]. Dilatation of portal venules is prominent in fatal cases. Biochemically there may be jaundice, increased transaminases and a fall in prothrombin and albumin levels. The damage is due to hypoxia and to direct thermal injury. Some of the changes resemble those of the toxic shock syndrome and may be related also to endotoxaemia. Obesity is a risk factor.

Hypothermia

Although the changes in experimental animals are impressive, in man they are inconspicuous. The effect of low temperatures on the liver is unlikely to be of serious consequence.

Burns

Within 36–48 hours of burning, the liver shows changes very similar to those seen in carbon tetrachloride poisoning. These are reflected in minor changes in liver function tests.

Hepato-cellular zone 1 necrosis

This type of injury resembles that of zone 3 but is maximal in zone 1 (peri-portal) areas.

Ferrous sulphate

Accidental ingestion of large quantities of ferrous sulphate is followed by zone 1 coagulative degeneration with nuclear pyknosis and karyorrhexis with little or no inflammation.

Cocaine

The active hepatotoxic metabolite is norcaine nitroxide produced by oxidative metabolism and catalysed by P450. Free radicals are generated causing lipid peroxidation [52]. The liver in man shows zone 1 (peri-portal) inflammation and necrosis with mild fatty change [128].

Phosphorus

The red form is relatively non-toxic but the

yellow is extremely lethal, as little as 60 mg being fatal. It is usually taken accidentally or suicidally as rat poison or in fire crackers [107].

Poisoning causes acute gastric irritation. Phosphorus may be found by gastric lavage. The patient's breath has a characteristic garlic odour and the faeces are frequently phosphorescent. Jaundice appears on the third or fourth day. The course may be fulminating with coma and death within 24 hours or, more usually, within the first four days.

The liver biopsy shows zone 1 necrosis with macro and medium sized fat droplets. Inflammation is minimal.

About one-half recover and ultimate recovery will probably be complete. There is no specific treatment.

Microvesicular fat

The picture is that of a microvesicular fat disease with vomiting and apathy prominent (Chapter 23).

Sodium valproate

Asymptomatic rises in serum transaminases, which subside on withdrawing the drug or reducing the dose, are reported in about 11% of patients receiving valproate. However, a more severe, even fatal, hepatic reaction may develop [135]. The patients are usually young, between 2½ months and 34 years with 69% being 10 years old or less. Males are particularly affected. Presentation is usually within one to two months of starting the drug and is not seen after 6 to 12 months therapy. Vomiting and disturbed consciousness are seen with hypoglycaemia and clotting defects. Other features of the microvesicular fat syndrome are also found.

Liver biopsy shows microvesicular fat mainly in zone 1 where, in rats, valproate has been shown to depress ketogenesis to a greater extent than in zone 3 hepatocytes [127]. Variable hepatocellular necrosis is seen in zone 3. Electron microscopy shows obvious mitochondrial changes.

The mechanism is probably interference with mitochondrial function and fatty acid oxidation by valproate or one of its metabolites, particularly 2-propyl-pentenoic acid [202]. Polypharmacy, presumably by enzyme induction, may be a risk factor for fatal hepatotoxicity in young children [35]. In both Reye's syndrome and valproate toxicity, blood ammonia levels rise, indicating inhibition of mitochondrial urea-cycle enzymes. Even in healthy subjects valproate induces inhibition of urea synthesis with hyperammonaemia [61]. It is possible that patients having severe reactions to valproate have an inborn deficiency of urea-cycle enzymes, but this has never been proved, although one patient with inherited carbamoyl transferase deficiency died when receiving valproate therapy [61].

Tetracyclines

Chlortetracycline and oxychlortetracycline interfere with protein synthesis. In 1963, six women in the last trimester of pregnancy were given large doses (3.5–6 g per day intravenously) of tetracycline for the treatment of pyelonephritis. Death followed in hepato-renal failure [157]. Autopsy showed a markedly fatty liver. Tetracyclines have been associated with fatty liver of pregnancy although the condition is also common without drug administration. Tetracycline may be inhibitory to protein synthesis particularly affecting the transport lipoproteins which remove triglyceride from the liver. It should be avoided during pregnancy, although large doses intravenously are probably necessary for significant hepatotoxicity.

'Alcoholic hepatitis' (Phospholipidosis)

The reaction histologically resembles acute alcoholic hepatitis with sometimes in addition electron microscopical evidence of lysosomal phospholipidosis. Mallory's hyaline is found in zone 3 in distinction to true alcoholic hepatitis.

Perhexiline maleate

Perhexiline maleate, an anti-anginal drug now withdrawn, has been associated with hepatic histology resembling acute alcoholic hepatitis [129]. Patients with this reaction lack a gene concerned with the oxidation of the antihypertensive drug, debrisoquine [113]. The genetic defect leads to a deficiency of a monoxygenase reaction in liver microsomes [59].

Amiodarone

This is an effective drug for the management of cardiac arrhythmias. It has however been associated with toxic damage particularly to lung, cornea, thyroid, peripheral nerves and liver. Abnormal biochemical tests of liver function are found in 15 to 55% of patients receiving the drug [146].

Hepatic toxicity usually develops more than a year after the start of therapy but can occur within one month. It is marked by hepatomegaly, a rise in serum transaminases and rarely by jaundice. Symptoms may be absent and toxicity detected only by routine monitoring and hepatomegaly is not constant [145]. Fatal cirrhosis can develop. Children can be affected [195].

Amiodarone has a very large volume of distribution and a very long half-life, so that blood levels may remain raised for many months after withdrawal of therapy (fig. 18.13). Amiodarone and its major metabolite N-desethyl-amiodarone are present in the liver for several months after stopping the drug [168]. The incidence and severity of side-effects correlates with the serum concentration and the daily dose must be kept between 200 and 600 mg daily.

Amiodarone is an iodinated compound and accumulation in the liver results in an increased density on a CT scan [50].

Hepatic histology shows an acute alcoholic hepatitis-like picture with fibrosis and sometimes, pronounced bile-ductular proliferation. Fatal cirrhosis can develop. Electron microscopy shows phospholipid-laden lysosomal lamellar

bodies containing myelin figures (fig. 18.14) [135]. In animal experiments a number of amphiphilic compounds have produced similar ultrastructural changes in the liver [102]. Swollen granular zone 3 macrophages, presumably iodine-laden lysosomal bodies, may be an early marker of amiodarone hepatotoxicity [163].

Either the drug itself or its main metabolite, desethyl-amiodarone, probably inhibits lysosomal phospholipases responsible for catabolizing phospholipids [58].

Synthetic oestrogens

A picture of 'alcoholic hepatitis' has been associated with massive doses of synthetic oestrogen used to treat prostatic cancer [161].

Amodiaquine

This drug is used for malaria prophylaxis and treatment. It may lead to a hepatic reaction of variable severity 4 to 15 weeks after starting

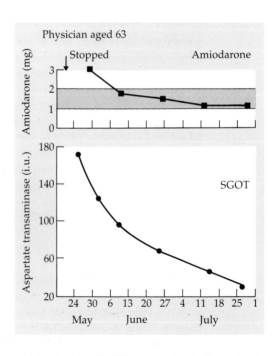

Fig. 18.13. AST (SGOT) and blood amiodarone levels in a 63-year-old physician.

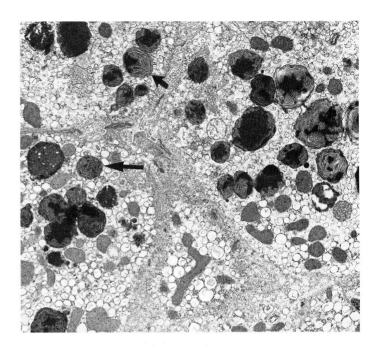

Fig. 18.14. Amiodarone hepatotoxicity: electron microscopy of the liver shows lysosomal lamellar bodies containing myelin figures.

[85] and after a total dose exceeding 1.5 g. Agranulocytosis may be associated [119]. Amodiaquine inhibits protein synthesis in cultured mammalian cells and a toxic effect on both bone marrow and liver is possible.

Cyanamide

This aldehyde dehydrogenase inhibitor is used for alcohol aversion therapy. Liver biopsy from asymptomatic recipients shows ground glass hepatocytes in zone 3 resembling those of hepatitis B surface antigen carriers but negative to orcein and positive to PAS staining [23]. The cells disappear when the drug is stopped.

Fibrosis

Fibrosis forms part of most drug reactions, but in some it may be the predominant feature. The fibrous tissue is deposited in the Dissë space, where it obstructs sinusoidal blood flow, causing non-cirrhotic portal hypertension and hepato-cellular dysfunction. The lesion is related to toxic drug metabolites and is usually in

zone 3, an exception being methotrexate where the damage is in zone 1.

Methotrexate

Methotrexate is first metabolized to 6-mercaptopurine. Hepato-toxicity results from a toxic metabolite of microsomal origin which induces fibrosis and ultimately cirrhosis (fig. 18.15) [3]. Primary liver cancer can develop [152]. Electron microscopy shows membrane whorls, lipid droplets and autophagic vacuoles. This complication is likely to follow long-term therapy, usually for psoriasis [27] rheumatoid arthritis or leukaemia. A cumulative dose exceeding 2 g is especially dangerous. When given in three 5-mg doses at twelve-hour intervals each week (i.e., 15-mg a week) it seems safe [83]. Increased alcohol intake adds to the risk. Serum transaminases and needle biopsy should be performed before starting and at regular intervals afterwards. Normal serum transaminases do not exclude the development of hepatic fibrosis. Repeated liver biopsies are necessary to follow the course. Ultrasound may

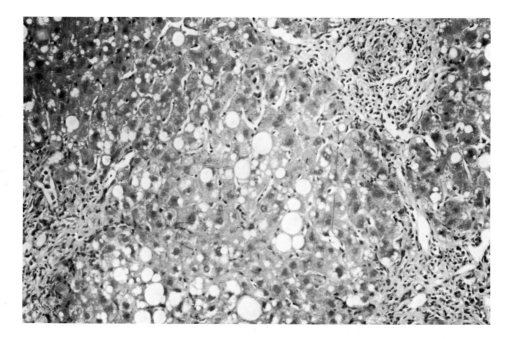

Fig. 18.15. Methotrexate liver injury. Zonal architecture is maintained. The portal zones are expanded with fibrous tissue and mononuclear cells. The hepatocytes show fatty change. H & E, ×65.

be useful in detecting fibrosis and indicating cessation of therapy [111].

Other cytotoxic drugs

These have a wide-range of hepatotoxicity [174]. The liver, however, is surprisingly resistant to injury by cytotoxic drugs, perhaps due to its low proliferative rate and extensive detoxifying capabilities.

Cytotoxic drugs cause rises in serum transaminases if large amounts are given. Drugs such as methotrexate, azathioprine and cyclophosphamide cause zone 3 necrosis, fibrosis and cirrhosis. Veno-occlusive disease is associated with cyclophosphamide, busulphan and irradiation. Cholestasis may be dose-related due to such drugs as cytosine arabinoside or hepato-canalicular due to such drugs as azathioprine. Sinusoidal dilatation, peliosis and tumours are associated with sex and anabolic hormone therapy. One drug may enhance the toxicity of another, for instance 6-mercaptopurine effects are worsened by doxorubicin.

Long-term use of cytotoxic agents in recipients of renal transplants or in children with acute lymphatic leukaemia leads to chronic hepatitis, fibrosis and portal hypertension [118].

Arsenic

The organic, trivalent compounds are particularly poisonous. Arsenic trioxide 1% (Fowler's solution) given for long periods for the treatment of psoriasis has resulted in presinusoidal intra-hepatic portal hypertension [114]. Arsenic in drinking water and native drugs in India may be related to 'idiopathic' portal hypertension. The liver shows portal tract fibrosis and sclerosis of the portal vein branches. Angiosarcoma is a complication [147].

Vinyl chloride

Workmen exposed to vinyl chloride monomer

over many years may develop hepato-toxicity (fig. 18.16). The earliest change is a sclerosis of portal venules in zone 1 of the liver with the clinical changes of splenomegaly and portal hypertension. Later associations include angiosarcoma of the liver and peliosis hepatis [131]. Early histological alterations indicative of vinyl monomer exposure are focal hepato-cellular hyperplasia and focal mixed (hepato-cytes and sinusoidal cells) hyperplasia. This is followed by subcapsular portal and perisinus-oidal fibrosis [176].

Vitamin A

Chronic ingestion results in hepatomegaly, abnormal biochemical tests and portal hyper-tension (64). Ascites, either exudate or tran-sudate, may develop.

Electron microscopy shows perisinusoidal, lipid-filled Ito cells which store the vitamin [124].

Vitamin A is slowly metabolized from hepatic stores and may be identified in the liver, months after stopping treatment.

Hepar lobatum

This is coarse lobulation caused by extensive fibrosis and has been reported in patients with metastatic breast carcinoma treated by combi-nation chemotherapy [26, 138].

Vascular

Sinusoidal dilatation

Focal dilatation of zone 1 sinusoids may com-plicate contraceptive or anabolic steroid ther-apy [193] This can cause hepatomegaly and abdominal pain with rises in serum enzymes. Hepatic arteriography shows stretched, attenu-ated branches of the hepatic artery with a patchy parenchymal pattern where areas of contrast alternate with areas not well filled.

The condition regresses on stopping the hormone.

387   A similar change may complicate azathioprine

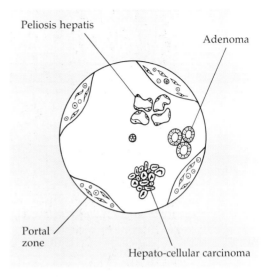

Fig. 18.16. Toxic effects of vinyl chloride, arsenic and thorotrast on the liver.

given after renal transplantation and this may be followed one to three years later by fibrosis and cirrhosis [49].

Peliosis hepatis

This consists of large blood-filled cavities which may or may not be lined with sinusoidal cells (figs 18.17, 18.26). They are distributed ran-domly, the diameter varying from 1 mm to several cm [200]. Electron microscopy shows passage of red blood cells through the endo-thelial barrier and perisinusoidal fibrosis may develop. These alterations might constitute the primary event [198].

Peliosis has been described in patients taking oral contraceptives, in men having androgenic and anabolic steroids, and in a woman receiv-ing tamoxifen for breast cancer [99]. Peliosis has been reported in recipients of renal trans-plants, perhaps due to azathioprine blocking blood flow from the sinusoids (30).

It has complicated Danazol therapy [120]

Veno-occlusion

Small zone 3 hepatic veins are particularly

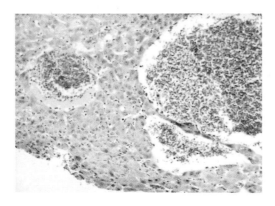

Fig. 18.17. Peliosis hepatis. A dilated blood space is seen with no clear cut wall.

sensitive to toxic damage reacting by subendo-thelial oedema and subsequent collagenization.

Veno-occlusive disease (VOD): this disease was originally described from Jamaica due to toxic injury to the minute hepatic veins by pyrrolizidine alkaloids taken as senecio in medicinal bush teas [173]. It has since been described from India [177], Israel, Egypt and even Arizona [146]. It has been related to contamination of wheat [112, 177].

The disease is marked by an acute stage with painful hepatomegaly, ascites and inconspicuous jaundice. The patient may recover, die or pass into a subacute stage of hepatomegaly and recurrent ascites. The chronic type re-sembles any other cirrhosis. Diagnosis is made by liver biopsy.

Veno-occlusion may follow any *cytotoxic therapy* but especially with alkylating agents such as cyclophosphamide or busulphan, azathioprine [70], fluxidine and decarbazone. It can be part of the graft-versus-host reaction in patients having bone marrow transplantation [148]. Zone 1 hepatic veins are also character-istically affected in acute alcoholic hepatitis.

Hepatic irradiation leads to veno-occlusion. The liver has a low tolerance to radiotherapy. Radiation hepatitis increases when doses reach or exceed 3500 rads to the whole organ delivered as 1000 rads a week. The hepatitis appears one to three months after completion of treatment as an enlarged liver, ascites and jaundice. The

condition may be transient or death may ensue from liver failure. Histologically, haemorrhage and congestion are seen with minimal hepato-cellular damage. Zone 1 hepatic veins show fibrosis and obliterate. Combination with vincristin may lead to fulminant hepatic necrosis [55].

Vasculopathic hepatotoxicity has followed treatment with E-ferol, a preparation containing dl-alpha-tocopherol acetate given to low birth weight infants. The liver shows sinusoidal veno-occlusion, fibrosis and cholestasis [21].

Hepatic vein occlusion (Budd–Chiari syndrome) has been reported following oral contraceptives (see Chapter 11) [182].

Acute hepatitis

Only a very small proportion of patients taking the drug will have the reaction. There is usually no method of selecting who will be susceptible. The reaction is unrelated to dose but is commoner after multiple exposures to the drug. The onset is delayed about one week after exposure.

The pre-icteric period of gastrointestinal symptoms resembles acute hepatitis and is followed by jaundice associated with pale stools and dark urine and an enlarged tender liver. Biochemical tests indicate hepato-cellular damage. Serum gamma-globulins are increased.

In those patients who recover, maximum serum bilirubin levels are reached after 2–3 weeks. The more seriously affected show a shrinking liver and die of hepatic failure. The mortality is high for those that are clinically recognized, higher than for sporadic virus hepatitis. If hepatic pre-coma or coma is reached the mortality is 70%.

Hepatic histology shows a picture virtually indistinguishable from that of acute virus hepatitis [65]. Milder cases show spotty necrosis becoming more extensive and reaching a stage of diffuse liver injury and collapse, bridging is frequent; inflammatory infiltration is marked. Chronic active hepatitis may sometimes be a sequel.

The drugs causing this type of reaction may

do so by the production of toxic metabolites injurious to the liver *per se* or the metabolite may act as a hapten with cell protein, so inducing immunological liver injury (fig. 18.5). These mechanisms may apply to such drugs as isoniazid, methyl dopa, halothane and chlorpromazine.

An enormous number of drugs cause this hepatic reaction and it is impossible to describe them all. They may emerge only after the drug has been released on the general market. Specialist text books should be consulted for individual drugs [151, 171].

An individual drug may cause more than one type of reaction. There may be an overlap between acute hepatitic, cholestatic and hypersensitivity reactions. Halothane, for instance, which can cause zone 3 necrosis may also produce an acute hepatitis picture. The promazines provide an overlap between the hepatitic and the cholestatic types. Methyl dopa can cause acute or chronic hepatitis, cirrhosis, hepatic granulomas or cholestasis.

The reactions tend to be severe, and often fatal, particularly if the drug is continued after liver damage has started. Patients with acute, fulminant drug-related liver failure must be considered for hepatic transplantation (see Chapter 8). Corticosteroids are of doubtful benefit.

Older women are at particular risk for hepatitic drug reactions, these are unusual in children.

Isoniazid

This hydrazine weak amine-oxidase inhibitor has been associated with severe hepato-toxicity. This followed its use alone in asymptomatic persons with positive tuberculin skin tests. In one serious outbreak, 19 of 2231 government employees in Washington devel-oped clinical signs of liver disease within six months of starting isoniazid [48]. Thirteen sub-jects were jaundiced and two died.

The liver injury is metabolite-related (fig. 18.18). After acetylation the isoniazid is converted to a hydrazine which is changed by

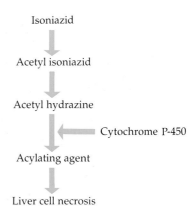

Fig. 18.18. The possible mechanism of isoniazid liver injury (Sherlock 1979).

drug-metabolizing enzymes to a potent acylating agent which produces liver necrosis [110].

Combination of the isoniazid with an enzyme inducer such as rifampicin increases the risk. Anaesthetic drugs and alcohol may also enhance isoniazid toxicity. Para-amino salicylate, on the other hand, is an enzyme retarder, and this may account for the relative safety of the para-amino salicylate—isoniazid combination formerly used in the treatment of tuberculosis.

The relation to acetylator status is uncertain although in Japanese patients fast acetylators are more susceptible [196].

The possibility of immunological liver injury cannot be excluded. However, 'allergic' manifestations are absent and the incidence of 12—20% developing sub-clinical liver injury is very high.

Elevated serum transaminase values are frequently seen during the first eight weeks of therapy. There are usually no symptoms and the transaminases subside despite continuing isoniazid. Nevertheless, transaminases should be monitored before treatment is started and four weeks later. If increases are found they should be repeated at weekly intervals. Rising levels indicate stopping therapy.

CLINICAL FEATURES

Serious reactions commonly affect those more than 50 years old, usually female. After treatment for about 2–3 months, non-specific symptoms develop, including anorexia and weight loss. These continue for 1–4 weeks before the onset of jaundice. There is a discrepancy between a well-looking patient and hepatic histological appearances.

The hepatitis usually resolves rapidly on stopping the drug, but if jaundice develops there is a 10% mortality [13].

Severity is greatly increased if the drug is continued after symptoms develop or serum transaminases rise. The reactions are more serious if the patient presents after more than two months on the drug [13].

The *liver biopsy* may show spotty necrosis or extensive bridging necrosis and fibrosis. Continued administration leads to chronic active hepatitis [104]. This is probably non-progressive if the drug is withdrawn.

Rifampicin

In the majority of patients reporting with rifampicin hepatotoxicity, isoniazid has also been given. Rifampicin on its own may cause a mild hepatitis, but this is usually in the context of a general hypersensitivity reaction.

Methyl dopa

Asymptomatic increases in serum transaminases, which generally subside despite continued drug administration, are reported in 5% of those taking methyl dopa. This may be metabolite-related, for human microsomes can convert methyl dopa to a potent arylating agent.

Methyl dopa hepatotoxicity may also be immunological related to metabolic activation and the production of a drug-associated antigen [121].

The patient is often post-menopausal and has been on methyl dopa for 1–4 weeks. The reaction usually appears within the first three months. Prodromata include pyrexia and are

short. The reaction is much more severe in those continuing the drug. Liver biopsy shows bridging and multilobular necrosis. Death may occur in the acute state, but clinical improvement usually follows stopping the drug.

Halothane

The frequency of halothane-associated liver damage is estimated to be between 1 in 7000 and 1 in 30 000. It seems of two types, mild, evidenced by raised serum transaminase and fulminant in a few patients who have usually been previously exposed to halothane.

MECHANISMS

Toxic products of reductive metabolism have been demonstrated and these are particularly hepatotoxic in the presence of hypoxaemia [31]. The oxidative metabolites are also reactive. Active metabolites produced by either mechanism could cause lipid peroxidation and inactivation of drug metabolising enzymes [121].

Metabolites are stored in adipose tissue and may be released slowly; obesity is frequently associated with halothane hepatitis.

The association with multiple exposures (fig. 18.19), the pattern of fever and the occasional eosinophilia and skin rash would suggest immunological mediation. 80% of patients treated for halothane hepatitis have antibodies that react with halothane-altered liver cell membranes [122, 192]. Lymphocytes from patients with halothane hepatitis, but not those from controls or from patients not sensitive to halothane, have shown an increased cytotoxicity in an *in vitro* test to determine cell damage from electrophilic drug metabolites [42]. The abnormality persisted for up to 13 months and was found in family members of halothane-sensitive patients. The extreme rarity of the fulminant reaction implies an unusual pathway for drug biotransformation in susceptible patients and/ or abnormal tissue responses to electrophilic halothane metabolites.

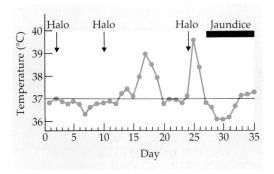

Fig. 18.19. Hepatitis associated with multiple exposures to halothane. Note the febrile response to the halothane anaesthetics. The patient became jaundiced after the third anaesthetic and rapidly became pre-comatose, developing deep coma on the fourth day and dying on the seventh day.

CLINICAL FEATURES [115]

Halothane hepatitis is much more frequent after multiple anaesthetics. Obese, elderly females seem particularly at risk [115]. Children can be affected [73].

The first abnormal event is fever, usually with rigors, developing more than seven days (range 8−13) after the first operation and usually accompanied by malaise and non-specific gastro-intestinal symptoms, including right upper abdominal pain. After several exposures the temperature is noted 1−11 days post-operatively (fig. 18.19). Jaundice appears rapidly after the pyrexia, about 10−28 days after a *single* exposure and 3−17 days after *multiple* anaesthetics. This delay before jaundice, usually of about a week, is helpful in excluding other causes of post-operative icterus.

The total white cell count is usually normal, but there may be an eosinophilia. Serum bilirubin levels may be very high, particularly in fatal cases, but are under 10 mg in 40%. The condition may be anicteric. Serum transaminases are in the range found in viral hepatitis. An occasionally high serum alkaline phosphatase level may be seen. If the patient becomes icteric the mortality is very high. Altogether 139 of 310 patients in one series

died (46%). If coma ensues and the one stage prothrombin time rises markedly in spite of intramuscular vitamin K therapy, the condition is virtually hopeless. The mortality is obviously less in the anicteric cases.

HEPATIC CHANGES

These may be virtually indistinguishable from those of acute viral hepatitis (fig. 18.20). Leucocytic infiltration in the sinusoids, granulomas and fatty change may suggest a drug aetiology. Necrosis may be sub-massive and confluent or massive [10].

Alternatively, the picture in the first week may be that of direct metabolite-related liver injury with zone 3 massive necrosis involving two thirds or more of each lobule (fig. 18.21)

CONCLUSIONS

Halothane administration should not be repeated if there is the slightest suspicion of

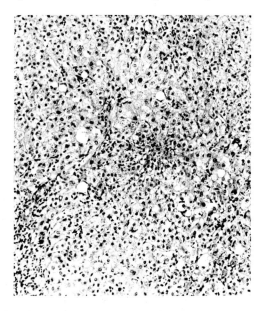

Fig. 18.20. Halothane-associated hepatitis. Hepatic histology shows cellular infiltration largely with mononuclear cells. Centrizonal areas show necrosis and cell swelling. Liver cell columns are disorganized. The appearances are virtually identical with those of acute virus hepatitis. H & E, ×96.

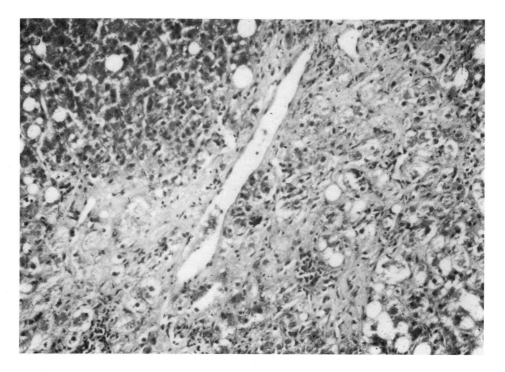

Fig. 18.21. Halothane liver injury. Centrizonal area shows well-defined necrosis without inflammatory reaction. Hepatocytes show fatty change. H & E, ×220.

even a mild reaction after the first anaesthetic. All case records should be scrutinized carefully before *any* second anaesthetic is given. There is no increased likelihood of an adverse reaction if the patient has underlying liver disease. Those requiring multiple anaesthetics during a short period should not be given halothane. A second anaesthetic with halothane should not be repeated within six months of the first. Obese females, especially with a history of allergy, should be assessed with particular care.

Enflurane and *isoflurane* are metabolized much less than halothane and low gas solubilities ensure rapid expiration from the body. Consequently, less toxic metabolites are produced. Used under similar conditions to halothane, isoflurane did not lead to demonstrable impairment of hepato-cellular integrity [2]. Although a few cases of liver damage have been reported after enflurane [95] they are exceedingly rare. Despite increased cost,

enflurane or preferably isoflurane should replace halothane.

Ketoconazole

A hepatic reaction causing symptoms is very rare, about 1:1500 exposed individuals. However, reversible increases in serum transaminases are seen in 5 to 10% of those taking the drug.

The reaction usually affects older people (mean age 57.9), and often women. The patient has usually taken the drug for at least four weeks (mean 6 to 7 weeks) and not for less than 10 days. A course of up to six weeks with hepatotoxicity has been reported [94]. Seventy-five cases have been reported in the United Kingdom, 16 probable, 48 possible and 11 unlikely [82]. Cholestasis was often a histological feature. There were three deaths. A positive challenge has been reported [184].

The reaction is idiosyncratic but does not seem immunological as fever, rash eosinophilia and granulomas are rare [11]. Two fatal cases showed massive, predominantly zone 3 hepatic necrosis. Paracetamol is one metabolite of ketoconazole in the dog but the amount generated by normal therapeutic doses is unlikely to be significant. It is also suggested that ketoconazole might interfere with the synthesis of DNA [82].

Glafenine

This analgesic has been associated with a hepatitic reaction in 39 patients usually between two weeks and four months of starting. The picture resembles that described for cincophen. Five of 12 patients died [172].

Chlorzoxazone

This muscle relaxant derived from zoxazolamine has been related to an acute hepatitic reaction which is sometimes fatal [133].

Disulfiram

This drug, used for the treatment of chronic alcoholism has been associated with an acute hepatitis picture, sometimes fatal [6].

Verapamil

This drug is said to cause an acute hepatitis-like reaction [53].

Chronic active hepatitis

The picture strikingly resembles 'autoimmune' chronic active hepatitis in clinical, biochemical, serological and histological features. The patients usually recover when the drug is withdrawn. Anti-organelle antibodies have been found in a number of patients [62, 103].

Chronic hepatitis was first described following the laxative oxyphenisatin and this has now been withdrawn from most parts of the world [143]. Chronic active hepatitis can develop insidiously after many years of methyl dopa therapy and without an acute episode. Improvement follows withdrawal of the drug [104].

Nitrofurantoin has rarely been related to chronic active hepatitis developing insidiously, usually in women, four weeks to 11 years after starting the drug [14, 162].

Other causes [62] include clometacin, fenofibrate, isoniazid and papaverine.

General hypersensitivity

A large number of drugs cause hepatic reactions of 'hypersensitivity' type of variable severity and with or without jaundice [101]. Other features such as rash, arthritis, haemolytic anaemia and eosinophilia may be present. Sometimes the picture resembles infectious mononucleosis. The reaction usually appears within four weeks of starting therapy and is most frequent with multiple exposures. Challenge is usually positive. There is considerable overlap with the acute hepatitic and hepato-canalicular groups. Liver histology shows focal, spotty necrosis of liver cells, with a mononuclear and sometimes eosinophilic reaction in the portal zones. Granulomas are sometimes found (fig. 18.22).

Sulphonamides and derivatives

A spectrum of pathological changes in the liver have been associated with sulphonamides. Widespread granulomas may be found.

Sulfasalazine. The hepatic reaction is usually part of a systemic hypersensitivity reaction. A serum sickness picture may be present. The patient has usually been taking the drug for less than one month. Re-challenge is positive [44]. There is an association with HLA-B8- DR3. The reaction can be fatal [144].

Cotrimoxazole (Septrin). The reaction tends to be cholestatic [180] and may be fatal [141].

Pyremethamine—sulfadoxine (Fansidar). This reaction is associated with severe cutaneous reactions and transient liver damage. Occasionally the reaction may be fatal [203]. The sulfadoxine is the likely hepatotoxin.

Non-steroidal anti-inflammatory drugs

These can all cause occasional rises in serum transaminases and alkaline phosphatase values. They include clinoril [194], feldene, naprosyn and salicylates.

Salicylates. Cross hepatotoxicity may develop between derivatives of proprionic acid such as naproxen and fenoprofen [4].

Phenylbutazone. Is associated with a high instance of general hypersensitivity reactions. Hepatitis is rather uncommon and is usually found with evidence of a general reaction. Sometimes cholestasis may develop. A granulomatous reaction simulating sarcoidosis has been reported [66].

Diclofenac. This can cause a hypersensitivity or acute hepatitis-like reaction which may be fatal [22]. Drug challenge is positive [36].

Allopurinol. Can be associated with a hepatic reaction which can include granulomas of fibrin type similar to those of Q fever [183]. *Pirprofen* [28] can cause an acute hepatic reaction which may be fatal.

Anti-thyroid drugs

Propylthiouracil has been implicated in hypersensitivity hepatic injury [56, 98].

Carbimazole has induced cholestasis [18].

Quinidine [77] and Quinine

This reaction is marked by rash and fever 6 to 12 days after starting treatment. Liver biopsy shows inflammatory infiltrates and granu-lomas. Prompt withdrawal leads to resolution, continued use may cause chronic liver damage.

Diltiazem

This calcium channel-blocking agent has been associated with fevers, headache and abnormal transaminases within 18 days of starting. Liver

biopsy shows many well-defined granulomas [154].

Anti-convulsants

Diphenylhydantoin [1]. The reaction usually affects adults two to four weeks after starting the drug. The picture closely resembles infectious mononucleosis. Eosinophilia is usual.

Mortality is 50% in those who develop jaundice usually due to streptococcal skin infections. Sufferers may have a genetic lack of epoxide hydroxylase so allowing accumulation of a toxic metabolite, arene oxide. Corticosteroids may be of value therapeutically.

Dantrolene is a phenytoin derivative used to treat spasticity. In one study, 19 (1.8%) of 1044 patients taking the drug for more than 60 days developed abnormal biochemical tests. Six became jaundiced and three died [181]. Challenge is positive [181]. Hepatic histology showed acute hepatitis and massive hepatic necrosis. A cholangitic picture has also been seen. Chronic active hepatitis and cirrhosis may follow its prolonged use. There is a disparity between clinical severity and the hepatic histological picture.

Carbamazepine. This drug, used for seizures and trigeminal neuralgia, has a wide spectrum of hepatic side-effects, the most usual being hepato-cellular necrosis with granulomas (fig. 18.22) [192]. Sometimes however, itching, fever and right upper quadrant pain may suggest cholangitis and hepatic histology may show marked cholestasis [86].

Canalicular cholestasis [169, 187]

Sex hormones contained in all oral contraceptives are potentially cholestatic. The oestrogen is the important agent although the progestin may augment the effect.

Bile salt-independent bile flow is consistently reduced by oestrogens probably through suppression of Na^+-K^+-ATPase activity. Liver sinusoidal membranes become less fluid. This may be modulated by s-adenosyl-L-methionine [19]. Paracellular permeability (tight junctions)

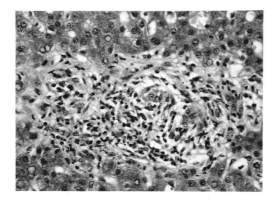

Fig. 18.22. Carbamazepine granulomatous hepatitis.

may be increased. The cytoskeleton of the liver cell is affected, with failure of the pericanalicular microfilaments to contract [130].

The hormone concerned is usually, but not always, a C17-alkylated testosterone. The reaction is dose-dependent and reversible even if large doses have been taken over many years [100]. The hormones are often taken in oral contraceptive pills. However, the reaction is rare in relation to the millions of users and is decreasing as the hormone content is reduced. Patients with a genetic predisposition to cholestasis of pregnancy remain at risk (see Chapter 25). This type of cholestasis is also seen with norethandrolone, methyltestosterone 1g-norandrostenolone and stanozolol [38].

CLINICAL FEATURES

Itching occurs during the first or second cycle and rarely after the third. Bilirubinaemia is variable but often exceeds 10 mg/dl. Serum alkaline phosphatase levels are raised. Serum transaminase values are variable but may exceed five times normal in about one-third of cases.

The effects are enhanced in those with a tendency to cholestasis such as sufferers from the Dubin–Johnson syndrome or presymptomatic primary biliary cirrhosis.

Theoretically, patients with acute hepatitis who continue to take oral contraceptives should develop deep jaundice and pruritus. This is not always so, for in a controlled trial, women taking oral contraceptives during the course of acute hepatitis had an illness of similar severity to matched controls [159]. A woman convalescent from viral hepatitis may resume use of 'the Pill' as soon as she wishes.

Liver biopsy shows normal architecture and central cholestasis with surrounding reaction. Electron microscopy shows cholestasis and mild hepato-cellular damage.

Prognosis is excellent. Rarely jaundice is severe and prolonged [96]. The patient recovers when the drug is stopped. Recurrence is liable to follow resumption. The patient may develop cholestasis in a subsequent pregnancy.

Hepato-canalicular cholestasis

Here the reaction is predominantly cholestatic but, in addition, hepato-cellular features are present. In many, immunological liver injury is suggested.

Chlorpromazine

Only 1–2% of those taking the drug develop cholestasis. The reaction is unrelated to dose and in 80–90% the onset is in the first four weeks. There may be associated hypersensitivity. Excess eosinophils may be found in the liver (fig. 18.23). This suggests idiosyncracy.

Chlorpromazine is also directly hepatotoxic. Histologically, damage to liver cells is virtually constant.

Chlorpromazine is a cationic detergent, highly concentrated in bile and with a significant entero-hepatic circulation. The parent compound and some of its metabolites decrease membrane fluidity and inhibit NaK ATPase [153, 169]. This would reduce biliary flow. They can intercalate into membranes and alter the lipid bilayer structure. Direct hepatotoxicity also may be related to the production of free chlorpromazine radicals [153]. The liver cell has two inbuilt safeguards; first the production of more stable chlorpromazine sulphoxide, and second, the protective action of hepatic glutathione (fig. 18.24).

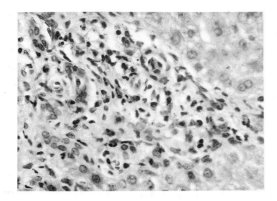

Fig. 18.23. Chlorpromazine hepatitis shows a portal zone reaction with eosinophils prominent.

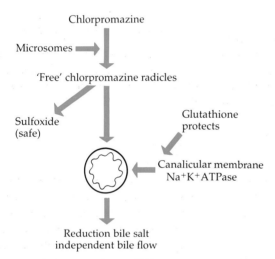

Fig. 18.24. The possible mechanisms of chlorpromazine cholestasis (after Samuels & Carey 1978) (Sherlock 1979).

Genetically determined differences in the biotransformation of chlorpromazine could, theoretically lead to the selective accumulation of cholestatic metabolites.

The delay in onset of jaundice, the extra-hepatic manifestations and the lack of a dose relationship remains unexplained.

CLINICAL PICTURE

The onset may simulate viral hepatitis, prodromata lasting some 4–5 days. Anorexia is

rarely so absolute and prostration is never so great. Cholestatic jaundice appears concurrently or within a week of the systemic reaction and lasts 1–4 weeks. Pruritus may precede jaundice. Recovery is usually complete.

Serum biochemistry shows the features of cholestatic jaundice. A sustained rise in alkaline phosphatase values may be the only change.

An eosinophilia may be seen in the peripheral blood in the very early stages.

HEPATIC CHANGES

Light microscopy shows cholestasis and, in the portal zones, a marked cellular reaction with mononuclear cells and eosinophils prominent (fig. 18.23). The reaction is not merely a cholestatic one. Even in the uncomplicated case a certain amount of damage to liver cells can be noted. 'Feathery' degeneration of liver cells, focal cell necrosis with cellular reaction, mild fatty change, anisocytosis and mitoses are all seen. Ballooned liver cells, peripheral vacuolation and hyaline deposits may also be noted [142]. Damage to the liver is greater than that observed with simple obstruction to main bile ducts. Granulomas may be present.

PROGNOSIS AND TREATMENT

Jaundice of the chlorpromazine type rarely proves fatal.

Occasionally jaundice is more prolonged, lasting more than three months and even up to three years [142]. The clinical picture is of prolonged cholestatic jaundice with steatorrhoea and weight loss. The biochemical changes include the early appearance of very high serum alkaline phosphatase and cholesterol levels. The clinical picture simulates primary biliary cirrhosis. The onset is, however, much more explosive and, in contrast to primary biliary cirrhosis, which is inevitably progressive, recovery always ensues. However, in two patients biliary cirrhosis is said to have developed six years and four years after the onset.

The diagnosis is not easy in these chronic cases for hepatic histology may be difficult to interpret. Cholangiography may be necessary. The mitochondrial antibody test for primary biliary cirrhosis is negative or in low titre.

In the usual case of chlorpromazine jaundice no active treatment is required and recovery is complete. Corticosteroids do not affect the course.

OTHER PROMAZINES

An essentially similar picture can complicate therapy with other phenothiazine derivatives such as promazine, prochlorperazine, mepazine or trifluoperazine [79].

Erythromycin

Hepatic reactions are usually associated with the estolate, but the proprionate and ethylsuccinate have also been incriminated [5, 199].

Two patients reacting to the estolate had a further cholestatic reaction when given the ethylsuccinate 12 and 15 years later [71].

The effect of the drug-metabolite on mixed drug oxidation is very complex.

The onset is 1–4 weeks after starting therapy with right upper quadrant pain, which may be severe, simulating biliary disease, fever, itching and jaundice. The blood may show eosinophilia and atypical lymphocytes.

Liver biopsy shows cholestasis, hepatocellular injury and acidophil bodies. Portal zones show the bile duct wall to be infiltrated with leucocytes and eosinophils and the bile duct cells may show mitoses. At autopsy the gallbladder has been shown to be inflamed.

A challenge is positive within hours [5].

Nitrofurantoin

This drug has been associated with cholestatic jaundice and chronic active hepatitis four weeks to 11 years after starting the drug [162].

The serum albumin is reduced while gamma-globulin is increased. Serum nuclear antibodies and smooth muscle antibodies are positive.

Patients usually improve when the drug is stopped. Cirrhosis, however, can develop and patients may die with fatal progressive liver failure. The mechanism may be direct cytotoxicity to the parent compound or to a metabolite. Association with a lupus-like syndrome with positive lymphocyte transformation [137] suggests that an immunological mechanism may also be concerned.

Haloperidol

This drug may rarely cause a cholestatic reaction resembling that related to chlorpromazine. It may become chronic [33].

Cimetidine and ranitidine [158, 185]

Very rarely, cimetidine or ranitidine can cause a mild, non-fatal cholestatic jaundice usually developing within four weeks of starting the drug.

Imipramine

In general, the triclyclic anti-depressants are very free from hepatotoxic effects. A promazine-type jaundice, however, has been reported following imipramine, which is not surprising in view of the structural resemblance of imipramine to the phenothiazines. Cross-hepato-toxicity may occur between tricyclic anti-depressants [85].

Oral hypoglycaemics

Cholestasis has been related to chlorpropamide [156], tolazamide [117] and glyburide [51].

Other causes

Cholestasis can complicate therapy with oxacillin [178], flucloxacillin, cloxacillin [80], and dicloxacillin [76]. Prolonged cholestasis can follow cyproheptadine (an appetite suppressant) [87], triacetyloleandomycin [86] and flucloxacillin [186].

Cholestasis has also been associated with

gold [55], tamoxifen [16], azathioprine [32], hydralazine [116] and captopril [139].

Dextropropoxyphene

This analgesic can induce a reaction with recurrent jaundice, upper abdominal pain and rigors, mimicking biliary tract disease [7].

Ductular cholestasis

The bile ducts and canaliculae are filled with dense, inspissated bile casts without any surrounding inflammatory reaction. The plugs contain bilirubin, probably in combination with a drug metabolite. The picture has been particularly associated with benoxyprofen, which has a half-life of 30 hours in the young, but 111 hours in the elderly [175]. It accumulates if given daily to old people. Indeed five elderly patients, given the recommended doses of benoxyprofen, died with jaundice and renal failure. The cause of death was not established, but generalized poisoning by the drug and its metabolites seems likely. Benoxyprofen has now been withdrawn.

Sclerosing cholangitis (see Chapter 15)

Causes include hepatic arterial infusion of cytotoxic drugs such as 5-flurouridine [81], thiabendazole [105], caustics introduced into hydatid cysts [9] and the Spanish toxic oil syndrome [170].

Hepatic tumours

The association of hepatic adenoma, a hitherto very rare benign tumour, with oral contraceptives was first suggested in 1973 [8]. The association is rare, believed to be about 3–4 per 100 000 long-term users of oral contraceptives in the United States [136]. About 400 patients a year are reported. The association with oral contraceptive use is statistically significant [60]. The risk increases dramatically with duration of use, particularly after 48 months [37].

The risk is five-hundred-fold greater for women taking oral contraceptives for longer than seven years than in controls. The use of pills with a high hormone content and in women over the age of 30 may increase the risk of adenoma [149].

Familial adenomas have been described, the sufferers never having taken oral contraceptives [46].

Adenomas have been induced by norethisterone in patients on renal dialysis [68].

MECHANISMS

The mechanism of tumour formation is complex (fig. 18.25). Oestrogens promote hepatic neoplasia [189]. Hepatic adenoma lacks oestrogen receptors [132]. Oral contraceptives, as enzyme inducers, might potentiate the carcinogenesis of certain compounds by increasing their rate of conversion to toxic (?carcinogenic) metabolites. Cholestatic properties of steroids might enhance the potentially carcinogenic action of substances normally excreted in the bile. Concomitant drugs might act as additional enzyme inducers. The vascular changes probably represent part of the general vasodilatation associated with sex hormones and are analogous both to the vascular spiders developing in the skin and to the endometrial arterial hypertrophy found in pregnancy.

TYPES OF TUMOUR

Adenomas. These smooth, encapsulated tumours are usually single but may be multiple. They are about 8–10 cm in diameter, usually subcapsular and sometimes pedunculated (fig. 18.26). They are most frequent in the right lobe. Microscopically the tumour consists of sheets of near-normal liver cells without portal tracts or central veins. Bile ducts are conspicuously absent (fig. 18.27). Granulomas may be associated [106].

Focal nodular hyperplasia (figs 18.28, 18.29). This well-circumscribed, unencapsulated lesion presents as a nodular mass in an otherwise normal liver. The lesion is commonly subcap-

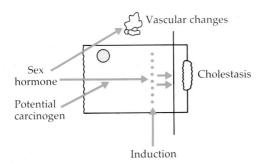

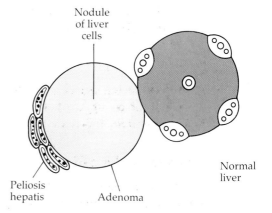

Fig. 18.25. Possible mechanisms of hepatic tumour production by sex hormones (Sherlock 1979).

Fig. 18.26. Structure of hepatic adenoma and peliosis hepatis compared with normal liver.

sular but can be pedunculated and can occur in either lobe. The lesions vary in size between 1 and 15 cm and may be multiple.

On cut section, a stellate, central scar containing an artery in seen from which septa radiate, subdividing the mass into nodules which simulate cirrhosis.

Histologically, the central core consists of fibrous tissue and proliferating bile ducts. The hepatocytes are normal.

Focal nodular hyperplasia does not have such

a strong association with oral contraceptives as adenoma [47]. It affects both sexes, including children, and women who have never taken contraceptives. The lesion is larger and more vascular than adenoma. This would explain the regression when the oral contraceptives are stopped.

The lesion is supplied by a central artery,

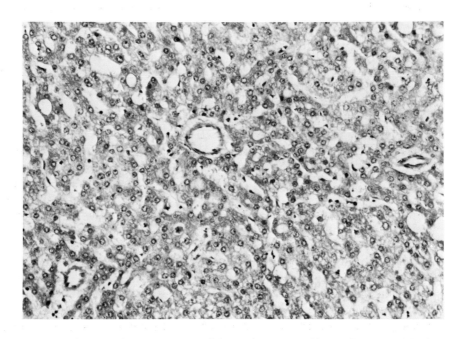

Fig. 18.27. Hepatic adenoma. The appearance is of sheets of near normal liver cells without portal tracts. H & E, ×185.

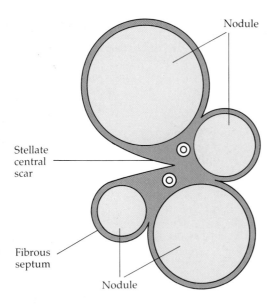

Nodule

Stellate central scar

Fibrous septum

Nodule

Fig. 18.28. The structure of focal nodular hyperplasia.

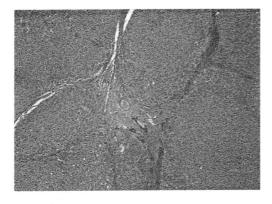

Fig. 18.29. Focal nodular hyperplasia. Note stellate central scar containing an artery.

and may represent a vascular anomaly [188]. This is supported by the association with other vascular lesions such as haemangioma [188].

Hepato-cellular carcinoma. There is a low, although probably increased, risk of hepato-cellular carcinoma in women receiving oral contraceptives for eight years or more [45, 122]. The tumour develops in a non-cirrhotic liver, metastases rarely, and does not infiltrate [60].

The features of hepato-cellular carcinoma in young women with or without exposure to oral contraceptives have been compared [63]. Those taking oral contraceptives tended to survive longer, had fewer symptoms and lower serum alpha-fetoprotein levels. The tumours were more vascular and haemoperitoneum was more common.

Hepato-cellular carcinoma has developed in an area of the liver where a contraceptive steroid-induced adenoma had previously regressed.

Hepato-cellular carcinoma has been associated with *danazol*.

Vascular lesions may accompany adenoma or focal nodular hyperplasia. Large arteries and veins are present in excess, sinusoids may be focally dilated and peliosis may be present.

CLINICAL FEATURES [74, 78]

The tumour may be symptomless and discovered incidentally at autopsy or at the time of surgery or hepatic scanning for another condition. This presentation is particularly true for focal nodular hyperplasia.

The patient may present with a right upper quadrant mass.

Haemorrhage into the tumour, or infarction, leads to abdominal pain and the tumour is tender.

Rupture is associated with the symptoms and signs of acute intraperitoneal bleeding.

Serum biochemical tests may be normal. Necrosis and rupture are associated with increase in transaminases and alkaline phosphatase. Serum alpha-fetoprotein is not increased.

Needle liver biopsy is contraindicated because of the vascular nature of the tumour.

LOCALIZATION

Ultrasound is useful. Technetium scans usually demonstrate the filling defect. However, both this method and a *CT scan*, enhanced by contrast, may fail to demonstrate the tumour when it closely resembles normal liver.

Arteriography (figs 18.30, 18.31) shows

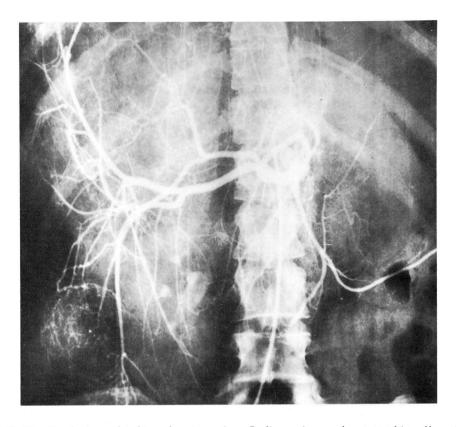

Fig. 18.30. Hepatic adenoma related to oral contraceptives. Coeliac angiogram shows stretching of branches of the hepatic artery around a relatively avascular lesion in the upper part of the right lobe of the liver.

stretching of the feeding arteries around the mass with branches penetrating the tumour from the periphery. Irregular vessels course through the lesion. Areas of haemorrhage may be demonstrated. There is a marked capillary blush.

Focal nodular hyperplasia shows a spokes-of-a-wheel appearance on arteriography.

Combined angiography and liver scan may be helpful in distinguishing between focal nodular hyperplasia, which is hypervascular and exhibits normal uptake on the scan, and liver cell adenoma, which is hypovascular and cold on a scan [78].

MANAGEMENT

Women who take oral contraceptives, particularly for many years, should be warned of the possibility of tumours developing and encouraged to examine their abdomens regularly.

The temptation to operate on space-filling lesions in the liver is almost overwhelming to some surgeons. However, in most uncomplicated cases it is advisable to be conservative. If, when operating for intraperitoneal haemorrhage, multiple tumours are found, all cannot be removed. If the tumour is diagnosed but there are no complications, it should be left *in situ* and sex hormones stopped. Tumours may regress [24, 140] although this is not always the case [107]. Women must be warned of the possibility of rupture and the significance of any unexplained right upper quadrant pain or swelling in the abdomen. Rupture becomes more likely in pregnancy. Liver ultrasound or scans should be repeated initially every six months and then yearly. A yearly serum alka-

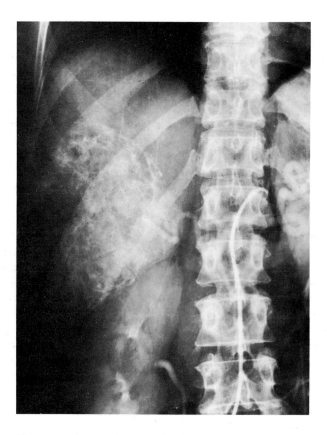
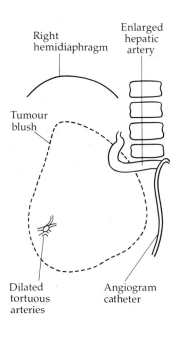

Right hemidiaphragm

Enlarged hepatic artery

Tumour blush

Dilated tortuous arteries

Angiogram catheter

Fig. 18.31. Hepatic adenoma related to oral contraceptives. Late stage of coeliac angiogram shows abnormal vascularity in the tumour in the lower part of the right lobe of the liver.

line phosphatase value should be performed in all women taking the pill for longer than three years.

Surgery may be needed for complications, particularly intraperitoneal or intratumour bleeding with severe abdominal pain and anaemia. Hepatic arteriography is particularly valuable in planning surgery. Local resection of the tumour is advised in amounts sufficient to control haemorrhage. In some instances hepatic lobectomy may be needed.

Even if present, lymph node metastases may regress [179].

Androgenic hormones

Adenoma, peliosis and particularly hepato-cellular carcinoma may complicate long-term use of C_{17} substituted testosterones. Angiosarcoma has also been associated [39]. These hormones may be given for the treatment of aplastic anaemia [41], hypopituitarism, eunuchoidism, impotency, in female transsexuals [191] and in athletes to increase muscle mass.

Hepato-cellular cancer of a rather benign type is much more frequent with male than with female hormone therapy, perhaps due to the much larger doses needed. The incidence of hepatic abnormality is particularly high; in one series, 19 of 60 patients given methyl testosterone showed abnormal liver function tests [191].

Other tumours

Angiosarcoma may follow androgenic–anabolic steroids [39], vinyl chloride [176], thorotrast and inorganic arsenic [147].

Epithelioid haemangioendothelioma. This rare malignant vascular tumour has been related to oral contraceptive use [29].

Conclusions

Before marketing a new drug testing must always be done on both an acute and chronic basis and on more than one species or strain. Both the drug and its known metabolites must be used. The albumin-binding properties of the drug must be noted. The role of the drug as a hepatic enzyme inducer must be studied. Clinical trials must include regular pre- and post-treatment estimations of serum bilirubin and transaminase levels. A needle liver biopsy, after informed consent, is particularly helpful in establishing the relation between a drug and liver injury and in determining the type of injury. An experienced histopathologist is essential for correct interpretation.

The serum transaminases may rise during the first four weeks of therapy only to subside although the drug is continued. When a hepatic reaction is possible, as with isoniazid, it is wise to check serum transaminases three and four weeks after commencing treatment. If more than three times increased the drug should be stopped. If less, a further value is taken one week later when an increase is an indication for stopping the drug. Continuence of therapy once a hepatic reaction has commenced is the commonest cause of a fatal outcome.

The safety of a drug which causes transient rises in transaminases and apparently no other hepatic effects remains obscure. Many valuable drugs in widespread use fall into this category. In many instances, challenge is the only method of linking a drug with a hepatic reaction, but if its consequence is likely to be serious, this is ethically impossible. However, reporting agencies and drug manufacturers should pay particular attention to the results of inadvertent challenge and to the effects of withdrawing the drug (dechallenge).

Intake of a drug, such as paracetamol, within the therapeutic range may cause liver injury if the patient is ingesting another drug such as alcohol which by enzyme induction increases the production of hepatotoxic metabolites.

An iatrogenic cause must be considered in any patient presenting with any clinical pattern of hepato-biliary disease. This is particularly so with a picture suggesting viral hepatitis in a middle aged or elderly patient, especially a woman. In the absence of a factor supporting genuine viral hepatitis, such as a recent blood transfusion, the cause is very frequently drug-related.

Widespread recognition of the relation between a drug and a hepatic reaction would follow increased reporting to agencies such as the Committee for Safety of Medicines in the United Kingdom, or the Washington Registry for Drug-Induced Liver Injury (telephone (202) 745−8123) in the United States.

Some catastrophies would be avoided if clinical trials included subjects of all ages from children to old people and those with liver disease.

References

1 Aaron JS, Bank S, Ackert G. Diphenylhy-dantoin — induced hepatotoxicity. *Am. J. Gastroenterol.* 1985; **80**: 200.
2 Allan LG, Hussey AJ, Howie J *et al* Hepatic glutathine. S-transferase release after halothane anaesthesia: open randomized comparison with isoflurane. *Lancet* 1987; **i**: 771.
3 Almeyda J, Barnardo D, Backer H *et al.* Structural and functional abnormalities of the liver before and during methotrexate therapy. *Br. J. Dermatol.* 1972; **87**: 623.
4 Andrejak M, Davion T, Gineston JL *et al.* Cross hepatotoxicity between non-steroidal anti-inflammatory drugs. *Br. med. J.* 1987; **295**: 180.
5 Bachman BA, Boyd WP Jr, Brady PG. Erythro-mycin ethylsuccinate-induced cholestasis. *Am. J. Gastroenterol.* 1982; **77**: 397.
6 Bartle WR, Fisher MM, Kerenyi N. Disulfiram-induced hepatitis. Report of two cases and review of the literature. *Dig. Dis. Sci.* 1985; **30**: 834.
7 Bassendine MF, Woodhouse KW, Bennett M *et al.* Dextropropoxyphene induced hepatotoxicity mimicking biliary tract disease. *Gut* 1986; **27**: 444.
8 Baum JK, Bookstein JJ, Holtz F *et al.* Possible association between benign hepatomas and oral contraceptives. *Lancet* 1973; **ii**: 926.

403

9 Belghiti J, Benhamou J-P, Houry S et al. Caustic sclerosing cholangitis. A complication of the surgical treatment of hydatid disease of the liver. *Arch. Surg.* 1986; **121:** 1162.

10 Benjamin SB, Goodman ZD, Ishak KG et al. The morphologic spectrum of halothane-induced hepatic injury. Analysis of 77 cases. *Hepatology* 1985; **5:** 1163.

11 Benson GD, Anderson PK, Combes B, et al. Prolonged jaundice following ketoconazole-induced hepatic injury. *Dig. Dis. Sci.* 1988; **33:** 240.

12 Black M. Acetaminophen hepatotoxicity. *Gastroenterology* 1980; **78:** 382.

13 Black M, Mitchell JR, Zimmerman HJ et al. Isoniazid-associated hepatitis in 114 patients. *Gastroenterology* 1975; **69:** 289.

14 Black M, Rabin L, Schatz N. Nitro-furantoin-induced chronic active hepatitis. *Ann. intern. Med.* 1980; **92:** 62.

15 Black M, Scott WE Jr, Kanter R. Possible ranitidine hepatotoxicity. *Ann. Intern. Med.* 1984; **101:** 208.

16 Blackburn AM, Amiel SA, Millis RR et al. Tamoxifen and liver damage. *Br. med. J.* 1984; **289:** 288.

17 Blewitt RW, Bradbury K, Greenall MJ et al. Hepatic damage associated with mineral oil deposits. *Gut* 1977; **18:** 476.

18 Blom H, Stolk J, Schreuder HB et al. A case of carbimazole-induced intrahepatic cholestasis. An immune-mediated reaction? *Arch. intern. Med.* 1985; **145:** 1513.

19 Boelsterli UA, Rakhit G, Balazs T. Modulation by S-adenosyl-L-methionine of hepatic Na$^+$, K$^+$-ATPase, membrane fluidity, and bile flow in rats with ethinyl estradiol-induced cholestasis. *Hepatology* 1983; **3:** 12.

20 Bonkowsky HL, Mudge GH, McMurtry RJ. Chronic hepatic inflammation and fibrosis due to low doses of paracetamol. *Lancet* 1978; **i:** 1016.

21 Bove KE, Kosmetatos N, Wedig KE et al. Vasculopathic hepatotoxicity associated with E-Ferol syndrome in low birth-weight infants. *J. Am. Med. Ass.* 1985; **254:** 2422.

22 Breen EG, McNicholl J, Cosgrove E et al. Fatal hepatitis associated with diclofenac. *Gut* 1986; **27:** 1390.

23 Bruguera M, Pares A, Heredia D et al. Cyanamide hepatotoxicity. Incidence and clinicopathological features. *Liver* 1987; **7:** 216.

24 Buhler H, Pirovino M, Akovbiantz A et al. Regression of liver cell adenoma: a follow-up study of three consecutive patients after discontinuation oral contraceptive use. *Gastroenterology* 1982; **82:** 775.

25 Chianale J, Dvorak C, May M et al. Heterogeneous expression of phenobarbital inducible cytochrome P-450 genes within the hepatic acinus in the rat. *Hepatology* 1986; **6:** 945.

26 Chin NW, Chapman I, Jimenez FA. Complete chemotherapeutic regression of hepatic metastases with resultant hepar lobatum. *Am. J. Gastroenterol.* 1987; **82:** 149.

27 Dahl MGC, Gregory MM, Scheuer PJ. Liver damage due to methotrexate in patients with psoriasis. *Br. med. J.* 1971; **i:** 625.

28 Davan G, Bernuau J, Moullot X et al. Amitriptyline-induced fulminant hepatitis. *Digestion* 1984; **30:** 179.

29 Dean PJ, Haggitt RC, O'Hara CJ. Malignant epithelioid hemangioendothelioma of the liver in young women: relationship to oral contraceptive use. *Am. J. Surg. Pathol.* 1985; **9:** 695.

30 Degott C, Rueff B, Kreis H et al. Peliosis hepatitis in recipients of renal transplants. *Gut* 1978; **19:** 748.

31 De Groot H, Noll T. Halothane hepatotoxicity: relation between metabolic activation, hypoxia, covalent binding, lipid peroxidation and liver cell damage. *Hepatology* 1983; **3:** 601.

32 DePinho RA, Goldberg CS, Lefkowitch JH. Azathioprine and the liver: evidence favoring idiosyncratic, mixed cholestatic-hepatocellular injury in humans. *Gastroenterology* 1984; **86:** 162.

33 Dincsoy HP, Saelinger DA. Haloperidol-induced chronic cholestatic liver disease. *Gastroenterology* 1982; **83:** 694.

34 Døssing M, Arlien-Søborg P, Milling Peterson L et al. Liver damage associated with occupational exposure to organic solvents in house painters. *Eur. J. clin. Invest.* 1983; **13:** 151.

35 Dreifuss FE, Santilli N. Valproic acid hepatic fatalities. Analysis of US cases. *Neurology* 1986; **36:** (Suppl. 1) 175.

36 Dunk AA, Walt RP, Jenkins WJ et al. Diclofenac hepatitis. *Br med. J.* 1982; **284;** 1605.

37 Edmondson HA, Henderson B, Benton B. Liver-cell adenomas associated with the use of oral contraceptives. *N. Engl. J. Med.* 1976; **294:** 470.

38 Evely RS, Triger DR, Milnes JP et al. Severe cholestasis associated with stanozolol. *Br. med. J.* 1987; **294:** 612.

39 Falk H, Thomas LB, Popper H et al. Hepatic angiosarcoma associated with androgenic-anabolic steroids. *Lancet* 1979; **ii:** 1120.

40 Farrell GC, Cooksley WGE, Hart P et al. Drug metabolism in liver disease: identification of patients with impaired hepatic drug metabolism. *Gastroenterology* 1978; **75:** 580.

41 Farrell G, Prendergast D. Halothane hepatitis: detection of individual susceptability by an *in vitro* test. *Hepatology* 1984; **4:** 1013.

42 Farrell G, Prendergast D, Murray M. Halothane hepatitis: detection of a constitutional susceptability factor. *N. Engl. J. Med.* 1985; **313:** 1310.

43 Feely J, Wilkinson GR, Wood AJ. Reduction of liver blood flow and propranolol metabolism by cimetidine. *N. Engl. J. Med.* 1981; **304:** 692.

44 Fich A, Schwartz J, Braverman D *et al.* Sulfasalazine hepatotoxicity. *Am. J. Gastroenterol* 1984; **79:** 401.

45 Forman D, Vincent TJ, Doll R. Cancer of the liver and the use of oral contraceptives. *Br. med. J.* 1986; **292:** 1357.

46 Foster JH, Donohue TA, Berman MM. Familial liver-cell adenoma and diabetes mellitus. *N. Engl. J. Med.* 1978; **299:** 239.

47 Friedman LS, Gang DL, Hedberg SE *et al.* Simultaneous occurrence of hepatic adenoma and focal nodular hyperplasia: report of a case and review of the literature. *Hepatology* 1984; **4:** 536.

48 Garibaldi RA, Drusin RE, Ferebee SH *et al.* Isoniazid-associated hepatitis: report of an outbreak. *Am. Rev. respir. Dis.* 1972; **106:** 357.

49 Gerlag PGG, Lobatto S, Driessen WMM *et al.* Hepatic sinusoidal dilatation with portal hypertension during azathioprine treatment after kidney transplantation. *J. Hepatol.* 1985; **1:** 339.

50 Goldman IS, Winkler ML, Raper SE *et al.* Increased hepatic density and phospholipidosis due to amiodarone. *Am. J. Roentgenol.* 1985; **144:** 541.

51 Goodman RC, Dean PJ, Radparvar A *et al.* Glyburide-induced hepatitis. *Ann. intern. Med.* 1987; **106:** 837.

52 Gottfreid MR, Kloss MW, Graham D *et al.* Ultrastructure of experimental cocaine hepatoxicity. *Hepatology* 1986; **6:** 299.

53 Guarascio P, D'Amato C, Sette P *et al.* Liver damage from verapamil. *Br. med. J.* 1984; **288:** 362.

54 Gugler R, Jensen JC. Omeprazole inhibits oxidative drug metabolism. Studies with diazepam and phenytoin *in vivo* and 7-ethoxycoumarin *in vitro. Gastroenterology* 1985; **89:** 1235.

55 Hansen MM, Ranek L, Walbom S *et al.* Fatal hepatitis following irradiation and vincristine. *Acta med. Scand.* 1982; **212:** 171.

56 Hanson JS. Propylthioracil and hepatitis. *Arch. intern. Med.* 1984; **144:** 994.

57 Harrison R, Letz G, Pasternak G *et al.* Fulminant hepatic failure after occupational exposure to 2-nitropropane. *Ann. intern. Med.* 1987; **107:** 466.

58 Heath MF, Costa-Jussa FR, Jacobs JM *et al* The induction of pulmonary phospolipidosis and the inhibition of lysosomal phospholipases by amiodarone. *Br. J. exp. Pathol.* 1985; **66:** 391.

59 Heier PJ, Mueller HK, Dick B *et al.* Hepatic monooxygenase activities in subjects with a genetic defect in drug oxidation. *Gastroenterology* 1983; **85:** 682.

60 Henderson BE, Preston-Martin S, Edmondson HA *et al.* Hepatocellular carcinoma and oral contraceptives. *Br. J. Cancer.* 1983; **48:** 437.

61 Hjelm M, de Silva LVK, Seakins JWT *et al.* Oberholzer VG. Evidence of inherited urea cycle defect in a case of fatal valproate toxicity. *Br. med. J.* 1986; **292:** 23.

63 Hromas RA, Srigley J, Murray JL. Clinical and pathological comparison of young adult women with hepatocellular carcinoma with and without exposure to oral contraceptives. *Am. J. Gastroenterol.* 1985; **80:** 479.

64 Inkeles SB, Connor WE, Illingworth DR. Hepatic and dermatologic manifestations of chronic hypervitaminosis A in adults: report of two cases. *Am. J. Med.* 1986; **80:** 491.

65 International Group, Guidelines for diagnosis of therapeutic drug-induced liver injury in liver biopsies. *Lancet* 1974; **i:** 854.

66 Ishak KG, Kirchner JP, Dhar JK. Granulomas and cholestatic-hepatocellular injury associated with phenylbutazone. *Am. J. dig. Dis.* 1977; **22:** 611.

67 James OFW. Drugs and the ageing liver. *J. Hepatol.* 1985; **1:** 431.

68 Kalra PA, Guthrie JA, Dibble JB *et al.* Hepatic adenomas induced by norethisterone in patients receiving renal dialysis. *Br. med. J.* 1987; **294:** 808.

69 Kaplowitz N. Drug-induced hepatotoxicity. *Ann. intern. Med.* 1986; **104:** 826.

70 Katzka DA, Saul SH, Jorkasky D *et al.* Azathioprine and hepatic venoocclusive disease in renal transplant patients. *Gastroenterology* 1986; **90:** 446.

71 Keeffe EB, Reis TC, Berland JE. Hepatotoxicity to both erythromycin estolate and erythromycin ethylsuccinate. *Dig. Dis. Sci.* 1982; **27:** 701.

72 Keeffe EB, Sunderland M, Gabourel JD. Serum gamma-glutamyl transpeptidase activity in patients receiving chronic phenytoin therapy. *Dig. Dis. Sci.* 1986; **31:** 1056.

73 Kenna JG, Neuberger J, Mieli-Vergani G *et al.* Halothane hepatitis in children. *Br. med. J.* 1987; **294:** 1209.

74 Kerlin P, Davis GL, McGill DB *et al.* Hepatic adenoma and focal nodular hyperplasia: clinical, pathologic, and radiologic features. *Gastroenterology* 1983; **84:** 994.

75 Kew M, Bersohn I, Seftel H *et al.* Liver damage in heatstroke. *Am. J. Med.* 1970; **49:** 192.

76 Kleinman MS, Presberg JE. Cholestatic hepatitis after dicloxacillin-sodium therapy. *J. Clin. Gastroenterol.* 1986; **8:** 77.

77 Knobler H, Levij IS, Gavish D *et al.* Quinidine-induced hepatitis. A common and reversible hypersensitivity reaction. *Arch. intern. Med.* 1986; **146:** 526.

78 Knowles DM, Casarella WJ, Johnson PM *et al.* The clinical, radiologic and pathologic characterization of benign hepatic neoplasms. *Medicine (Baltimore)* 1978; **75:** 223.

79 Kohn N, Myerson RM. Cholestatic hepatitis associated with trifluoperazine. *N. Engl. J. Med.* 1961; **264**: 549.

80 Konikoff F, Alcalay J, Halevy J. Cloxacillin-induced cholestatic jaundice. *Am. J. Gastroenterol* 1986; **81**: 1082.

81 Lafon PC, Reed K, Rosenthal D. Acute cholecystitis associated with hepatic arterial infusion of floxuridine. *Am. J. Surg.* 1985; **150**: 687.

82 Lake-Bakaar G, Scheuer PJ, Sherlock S. Hepatic reactions associated with ketoconazole in the United Kingdom. *Br. med. J.* 1987; **294**: 419.

83 Lanse SB, Arnold GL, Gowans JDC *et al.* Low incidence of hepatotoxicity associated with long-term, low-dose oral methotrexate in treatment of refractory psoriasis, psoriatic arthritis and rheumatoid arthritis. An acceptable risk/benefit ratio *Dig. Dis. Sci.* 1985; **30**: 104.

84 Larrey D, Branch RA. Clearance by the liver: current concepts in understanding the hepatic disposition of drugs. *Semin. Liver Dis.* 1983; **3**: 285.

85 Larrey D, Castot A, Pessayre D *et al.* Amodiaquine-induced hepatitis. A report of seven cases. *Ann. intern. Med.* 1986; **104**: 801.

86 Larrey D, Geneve J, Pessayre D *et al.* Prolonged cholestasis after cyproheptadine-induced acute hepatitis. *J. clin. Gastroenterol.* 1987; **9**: 102.

87 Larrey D, Amouyal G, Danan G *et al.* Prolonged cholestasis after trioleandomycin-induced acute hepatitis. *J. Hepatol.* 1987; **4**: 327.

88 Larrey D, Hadengue A, Pessayre D *et al.* Carbamazepine-induced acute cholangitis. *Dig. Dis. Sci.* 1987; **32**: 554.

89 Lauterburg BH, Todd EL, Smith CV *et al.* Cimetidine inhibits the formation of the reactive, toxic metabolite of isoniazid in rats but not in man. *Hepatology* 1985; **5**: 607.

90 Lee SM, O'Brien CJ, Williams R *et al.* Subacute hepatic necrosis induced by piroxicam. *Br. med. J.* 1986; **293**: 540.

91 Leonard TB, Morgan DG, Dent JG. Ranitidine: acetaminophen interaction effects on acetaminophen-induced hepatotoxicity in Fischer 344 rats. *Hepatology* 1985; **5**: 480.

92 Levi AJ, Sherlock S, Walker D. Phenylbutazone and isoniazid metabolism in patients with liver disease in relation to previous drug therapy. *Lancet* 1968; **i**: 1275.

93 Lewis JH, Tice HL, Zimmerman HJ. Budd–Chiari syndrome associated with oral contraceptive steroids: review of treatment of 47 cases. *Dig. Dis. Sci.* 1983; **28**: 673.

94 Lewis JH, Zimmerman HH, Benson GD *et al.* Hepatic injury associated with ketoconazole therapy: analysis of 33 cases. *Gastroenterology* 1984; **86**: 503.

95 Lewis JH, Zimmerman HJ, Ishak KG *et al.* Enflurane hepatotoxicity: a clinicopathologic study of 24 cases. *Ann intern. Med.* 1983; **98**: 984.

96 Lieberman DA, Keeffe EB, Stenzel P. Severe and prolonged oral contraceptive jaundice. *J. Clin. Gastroenterol.* 1984; **6**: 145.

97 Lieh-Lai MW, Sarnaik AP, Newton JF *et al.* Metabolism and pharmacokinetics of acetaminophen in a severely poisoned young child. *J. Pediat.* 1984; **105**: 125.

98 Limaye A, Ruffolo PR. Propylthiouracil-induced fatal hepatic necrosis. *Am. J. Gastroenterol.* 1987; **82**: 152.

99 Loomus GN, Aneja P, Bota RA. A case of peliosis hepatitis in association with tamoxifen therapy. *Am. J. clin. Pathol.* 1983; **80**: 881.

100 Lowdell CP, Murray-Lyon IM. Reversal of liver damage due to long term methyltestosterone and safety of non 17α alkylated androgens. *Br. med. J.* 1985; **291**: 637.

101 Ludwig J, Axelsen R. Drug effects on the liver. An updated tabular compilation of drugs and drug-related hepatic diseases. *Dig. Dis. Sci.* 1983; **28**: 651.

102 Lüllman H, Lüllman-Rauch R, Wassermann O. Drug-induced phospholipidoses. II Tissue distribution of the amphiphilic drug chlorphentermine. *CRC Crit. Rev. Toxicol.* 1975; **4**: 185.

103 Mackay IR. Induction by drugs of hepatitis and autoantibodies to cell organelles: significance and interpretation. *Hepatology* 1985; **5**: 904.

104 Maddrey WC, Boitnott JK. Drug-induced chronic liver disease. *Gastroenterology* 1977; **72**: 1348.

105 Manivel JC, Bloomer JR, Snover DC. Progressive bile duct injury after thiobendazole administration. *Gastroenterology* 1987; **93**: 245.

106 Malatjalian DA, Graham CH. Liver adenoma with granulomas. *Arch. pathol. lab. Med.* 1982; **106**: 244.

107 Mariani AF, Livingstone AS, Pereiras RV Jr *et al.* Progressive enlargement of an hepatic cell adenoma. *Gastroenterology* 1979; **77**: 1319.

108 McLean AEM, McLean EK. Diet and toxicity. *Br. med. Bull.* 1969; **25**: 278.

109 Mitchell JR, Jollow DJ. Metabolite activation of drugs to toxic substances. *Gastroenterology* 1975; **68**: 392.

110 Mitchell JR *et al.* Isoniazid liver injury: clinical spectrum, pathology and probable pathogenesis. *Ann. intern. Med.* 1976; **84**: 181.

111 Miller JA, Dodd H, Rustin MHA *et al.* Ultrasound as a screening procedure for methotrexate-induced hepatic damage in severe psoriasis. *Br. J. Dermatol.* 1985; **113**: 699.

112 Mohabbat O, Younos MS, Merzad AA *et al.* An attack of hepatic veno-occlusive disease in

North-Western Afghanistan. *Lancet* 1976; **ii**: 269.

113 Morgan MY, Reshef R, Shah RR *et al* Impaired oxidation of debrisoquine in patients with perhexiline liver injury. *Gut* 1984; **25**: 1057.

114 Morris JS, Schmid M, Newman S *et al*. Arsenic and non-cirrhotic portal hypertension. *Gastroenterology* 1974; **66**: 86.

115 Moult PJA, Sherlock S. Halothane-related hepatitis. A clinical study of twenty six cases. *Q. J. Med.* 1975; **44**: 99.

116 Myers JL, Augur NA Jr. Hydralazine-induced cholangitis. *Gastroenterology* 1984; **87**: 1185.

117 Nakao NL, Gelb AM, Stenger RJ *et al*. A case of chronic liver disease due to tolazamide. *Gastroenterology* 1985; **89**: 192.

118 Nataf C, Feltmann G, Lebrec D *et al*. Idiopathic portal hypertension (perisinusoidal fibrosis) after renal transplantation. *Gut* 1979; **20**: 531.

119 Neftel KA, Woodtly W, Schmid M *et al*. Amodiaquine-induced agranulocytosis and liver damage. *Br. med. J.* 1986; **292**: 721.

120 Nesher G, Dollberg L, Zimran A *et al*. Hepatosplenic peliosis after danazol and glucocorticoids for ITP. *N. Engl. J. Med.* 1985; **312**: 242.

121 Neuberger J, Williams R. Halothane anaesthesia and liver damage. *Br. med. J.* 1984; **289**: 1136.

122 Neuberger J, Kenna JG, Nouri Aria K *et al*. Antibody mediated hepatocyte injury in methyldopa induced hepatotoxicity. *Gut* 1985; **26**: 1233

123 Nomura F, Hatano H, Ohnishi K *et al*. Effects of anticonvulsant agents on halothane-induced liver injury in human subjects and experimental animals. *Hepatology* 1986; **6**: 952.

124 Noseda A, Borsch G, Muller K-M *et al*. Methimazole-associated cholestatic liver injury: case report and brief literative review. *Hepato-Gastroenterol.* 1986; **33**: 244.

125 O'Brien ET, Yeoman WB, Hobby JAE, Hepatorenal damage from toluene in a 'glue sniffer'. *Br. med. J.* 1971; **ii**: 29.

126 O'Gorman T, Koff RS. Salicylate hepatitis. *Gastroenterology* 1977; **72**: 726.

127 Olson MJ, Handler JA, Thurman RG. Mechanism of zone-specific hepatic steatosis caused by valproate: inhibition of ketogenesis in periportal regions of the liver lobule. *Molec. Pharm.* 1986; **30**: 520.

128 Perino LE, Warren GH, Levine JS. Cocaine-induced hepatotoxicity in humans. *Gastroenterology* 1987; **93**: 176.

129 Pessayre D, Bichara M, Feldmann G *et al*. Perhexiline maleate-induced cirrhosis. *Gastroenterology* 1979; **76**: 170.

130 Phillips MJ, Oda M, Mak E *et al*. Microfilament dysfunction as a possible cause of intrahepatic cholestasis. *Gastroenterology* 1975; **69**: 48.

131 Popper H, Thomas LB, Telles NC *et al*. Development of hepatic angiosarcoma in man induced by vinyl chloride, thorotrast and arsenic. *Am. J. Pathol.* 1978; **92**: 349.

132 Poncin E, Silvain C, Touchard G *et al*. Papaverine-induced chronic liver disease. *Gastroenterology* 1986; **90**: 1051.

133 Porter LE, Elm MS, Van Thiel DH *et al*. Characterization and quantitation of human hepatic estrogen receptor. *Gastroenterology* 1983; **84**: 704.

134 Poucell S, Ireton J, Valencia-Mayoral P *et al*. Amiodarone-associated phospholipidosis and fibrosis of the liver: light, immunohistochemical and electron microscropic studies. *Gastroenterology* 1984; **86**: 926.

135 Powell-Jackson PR, Tredger JM, Williams R. Progress report, hepatotoxicity to valproate: a review. *Gut* 1984; **25**: 673.

136 Prescott LF, Illingworth RN, Critchley JAJH *et al*. Intravenous N-acetylcysteine: the treatment of choice for paracetamol poisoning. *Br. med. J.* 1979; **ii**: 1097.

137 Prescott LF, Wright N, Roscoe P, *et al*. Plasma paracetamol half-life and hepatic necrosis in patients with paracetamol overdosage. *Lancet* 1971; **i**: 591.

138 Qizilbash A, Kontozoglou T, Sianos J *et al*. Hepar lobatum associated with chemotherapy and metastatic breast cancer. *Arch. Pathol. lab. Med.* 1987; **111**: 58.

139 Rahmat J, Gelfand RL, Gelfand MC *et al*. Captopril-associated cholestatic jaundice. *Ann. intern. Med.* 1985; **102**: 56.

140 Ramseur WL, Cooper R. Asymptomatic liver cell adenomas. Another case of resolution after discontinuation of oral contraceptive use. *J. Am. med. Assoc.* 1978; **239**: 1647.

141 Ransohoff DF, Jacobs G, Terminal hepatic failure following a small dose of sulfamethoxazole-trimethoprim. *Gastroenterology* 1981; **80**: 816.

142 Read AE, Harrison CV, Sherlock S. Chronic chlorpromazine jaundice: with particular reference to its relationship to primary biliary cirrhosis. *Am. J. Med.* 1961; **31**: 249.

143 Reynolds TB, Lapin AC, Peters RL *et al*. Puzzling jaundice. Probable relationship to laxative ingestion. *J. Am. med. Assoc.* 1970; **211**: 86.

144 Ribe J, Benkov KJ, Thung SN *et al*. Fatal massive hepatic necrosis: a probable hypersensitivity reaction to sulfasalazine. *Am. J. Gastroenterol.* 1986; **81**: 205.

145 Rigas B, Rosenfeld LE, Barwick KW. Amiodarone hepatotoxicity: a clinicopathologic study of five patients. *Ann. intern. Med.* 1986; **104**: 348.

146 Rinder HM, Love JC, Wexler R. Amiodarone hepatotoxicity. *N. Engl. J. Med.* 1986; **314**: 318.

147 Roat JW, Wald A, Mendelow H *et al*. Hepatic

angiosarcoma associated with short-term arsenic ingestion. *Am. J. Med.* 1982; **73**: 933.

148 Rollins BJ. Hepatic veno-occlusive disease. *Am. J. Med.* 1986; **81**: 297.

149 Rooks JB, Ory HW, Ishak KG *et al.* Epidemiology of hepatocellular adenoma. The role of oral contraceptive use. *J. Am. med. Assoc.* 1979; **242**: 644.

150 Rubel LR, Ishak KG. The liver in fatal exertional heatstroke. *Liver* 1983; **3**: 249.

151 Ruprah M, Mant TGK, Flanagan RJ. Acute carbon tetrachloride poisoning in 19 patients: implications for diagnosis and treatment. *Lancet* 1985; **i**: 1027.

152 Ruymann FB, Mosijczuk A, Sayers RJ. Hepatoma in a child with methotrexate-induced hepatic fibrosis. *J. Am. med. Assoc.* 1977; **238**: 2631.

153 Samuels AM, Carey MC. Effects of chlorpromazine hydrochloride and its metabolites on Mg^{2+} and Na^+K^+-ATPase activities of canicular-enriched rat liver plasma membranes. *Gastroenterology* 1978; **74**: 1183.

154 Sarachek NS, London RL, Matulewicz TJ. Diltiazem and granulomatous hepatitis. *Gastroenterology* 1985; **88**: 1260.

155 Schenker S, Olson KN, Dunn D *et al.* Intra-hepatic cholestasis due to therapy of rheumatoid arthritis. *Gastroenterology* 1973; **64**: 622.

156 Schneider HL, Horbach KD, Kniaz JL *et al.* Chlorpropamide hepatotoxicity: a report of a case and review of the literature. *Am. J. Gastroenterol.* 1984; **79**: 721.

157 Schultz JC, Adamson JS Jr, Workman WW *et al.* Fatal liver disease after intravenous administration of tetracycline in high dosage. *N. Engl. J. Med.* 1963; **269**: 999.

158 Schwartz JT, Gyorkey F, Graham DY. Cimetidine hepatitis. *J. clin. Gastroenterol.* 1986; **8**: 681.

159 Schweitzer IL, Weiner JM, McPeak CM *et al.* Oral contraceptives in acute viral hepatitis. *J. Am. med. Assoc.* 1975; **233**: 979.

160 Seeff LB, Cuccherini BA, Zimmerman HJ *et al.* Acetaminophen hepatotoxicity in alcoholics: a therapeutic misadventure. *Ann. intern. Med.* 1986; **104**: 399.

161 Seki K, Minami Y, Nishikawa M *et al.* 'Nonalcoholic steatohepatitis' induced by massive doses of synthetic estrogen. *Gastroenterol. Jpn.* 1983; **18**: 197.

162 Sharp JR, Ishak KG, Zimmerman HJ. Chronic active hepatitis and severe hepatic necrosis associated with nitrofurantoin. *Ann. intern. Med.* 1980; **92**: 14.

163 Sheperd NA, Dawson AM, Crocker PR *et al.* Granular cells as a marker of early amiodarone hepatotoxicity: a pathological and analytical study. *J. Clin. Path.* 1987; **40**: 418.

164 Sherlock S. Hepatic reactions to drugs. *Gut* 1979;
20: 634.

165 Sherlock S. The spectrum of hepatotoxicity due to drugs. *Lancet* 1986; **ii**: 440.

166 Sherlock S. Needle biopsy of the liver: a review. *J. clin. Path.* 1962; **15**: 291.

167 Sherlock S, Acute fatty liver of pregnancy and the microvesicular fat diseases. *Gut* 1983; **24**: 265.

168 Simon JB, Manley PN, Brien JF *et al* Amiodarone hepatotoxicity simulating alcoholic liver disease *N. Engl. J. Med.* 1984; **311**: 167.

169 Simon FR, Pathogenesis of drug-induced cholestasis. In Kaplowitz N, *Drug-induced Hepatotoxicity. Ann. intern. Med.* 1986; **104**: 826.

170 Solis-Herruzo JA, Castellano G, Colina F *et al.* Hepatic injury in the toxic epidemic syndrome caused by ingestion of adulterated cooking oil (Spain 1981). *Hepatology* 1984; **4**: 131.

171 Stricker BHC, Spoelstra P. *Drug-induced Hepatic Injury.* Amsterdam, Elsevier, 1985.

172 Stricker BHC, Blok APR, Bronkhorst FB Glafenine-associated hepatic injury. Analysis of 38 cases and review of the literature. *Liver* 1986; **6**: 63.

173 Stuart KL, Bras G. Veno-occlusive disease of the liver. *Q. J. Med.* 1957; **26**: 291.

174 Sznol M, Ohnuma T, Holland JF. Hepatic toxicity of drugs used for hematologic neoplasia. *Semin. Liv. Dis.* 1987; **7**: 237.

175 Taggart HMcA, Alderdice JM. Fatal cholestatic jaundice in elderly persons taking benoxaprofen. *Br. med. J.* 1982; **284**: 1372.

176 Tamburro CH, Makk L, Popper H. Early hepatic histologic alterations among chemical (vinyl monomer) workers. *Hepatology* 1984; **4**: 413.

177 Tandon BN, Tandon RK, Tandon HD *et al.* An epidemic of veno-occlusive disease of liver in central India. *Lancet* 1976; **ii**: 271.

178 Tauris P, Jørgensen NF, Petersen CM *et al.* Prolonged severe cholestasis induced by oxacillin derivatives. A report on two cases. *Acta Med. Scand.* 1985; **217**: 567.

179 Terpstra OT, Ten Kate FJW, Van Urk H. Long-term survival after resection of a hepatocellular carcinoma with lymph node metastasis and discontinuation of oral contraceptives. *Am. J. Gastroenterol.* 1984; **79**: 474.

180 Thies PW, Dull WL. Trimethoprin-sulfamethoxazole-induced cholestatic hepatitis—inadvertent rechallenge. *Arch. intern. Med.* 1984; **144**: 1691.

181 Utili R, Boitnott JK, Zimmerman HJ. Dantrolene-associated hepatic injury. *Gastroenterology* 1977; **72**: 610.

182 Valla D, Le MG, Poynard T *et al.* Risk of hepatic vein thrombosis in relation to recent use of oral contraceptives: a case-control study. *Gastroenterology* 1986; **90**: 807.

183 Vanderstigel M, Zafrani ES, Lajonc JL *et al.* Allopurinol hypersensitivity syndrome as a cause of hepatic fibrin-ring granulomas. *Gastroenterology* 1986; **90**: 188.

184 Van Parys G, Evenepoel C, van Damme B *et al.* Ketoconazole-induced hepatitis: a case with a definite cause-effect relationship. *Liver* 1987; **7**: 27.

185 Van Steenbergen W, Vanstapel MJ, Desmet V *et al.* Cimetidine-induced liver injury. Report of three cases. *J. Hepatol.* 1985; **1**: 359.

186 Victorino RMM, Maria VA, Pinto Correia AP *et al.* Floxacillin-induced cholestatic hepatitis with evidence of lymphocyte sensitisation. *Arch. intern. Med.* 1987; **147**: 987.

187 Vore M. Estrogen cholestasis. Membranes metabolites, or receptors? *Gastroenterology* 1987; **93**: 643.

188 Wanless IR, Mawdsley C, Adams R. On the pathogenesis of focal nodular hyperplasia of the liver. *Hepatology* 1985; **5**: 1194.

189 Wanless IR, Medline A. Role of estrogens as promoters of hepatic neoplasia. *Lab. Invest.* 1982; **46**: 313.

190 Wepler W, Opitz K. Histologic changes in the liver biopsy in *Amanita phalloides* intoxication. *Hum. Pathol.* 1972; **3**: 249.

191 Westaby D, Ogle SJ, Paradinas FJ *et al.* Liver damage from long term methyltestosterone. *Lancet* 1977; **ii**: 261.

192 Williams SJ, Baird-Lambert JA, Farrell GC. Inhibition of theophylline metabolism by interferon. *Lancet* 1987; **ii**: 939.

193 Winkler K, Poulsen H. Liver disease with peri-portal sinusoidal dilatation. A possible complication to contraceptive steroids. *Scand. J. Gastroenterol.* 1975; **10**: 699.

194 Wood LJ, Searle J, Mundo F *et al.* Sulindac hepatotoxicity: effects of acute and chronic exposure. *Aust. NZ J. Med.* 1985; **15**: 397.

195 Yagupsky P, Gazala E, Sofer S *et al.* Fatal hepatic failure and encephalopathy associated with amiodarone therapy. *J. Pediat.* 1985; **107**: 967.

196 Yamamoto T, Suou T, Hirayama C. Elevated serum aminotransferase induced by isoniazid in relation to isoniazid acetylator phenotype. *Hepatology* 1986; **6**: 295.

197 Yang CS, Tu YY, Koop DR *et al.* Metabolism of nitrosamines by purified rabbit liver cytochrome P-450 isozymes. *Cancer Res.* 1985; **45**: 1140.

198 Zafrani ES, Cazier A, Baudelot A-M *et al.* Ultrastructural lesions of the liver in human peliosis: a report of 12 cases. *Am. J. Pathol.* 1984; *114*: 349.

199 Zafrani ES, Ishak KG, Rudzki C. Cholestatic and hepatocellular injury associated with erythromycin esters. *Dig. Dis. Sci.* 1979; **24**: 385.

200 Zafrani ES, Pinaudeau Y, Dhumeaux D. Drug-induced vascular lesions of the liver. *Arch. intern. Med.* 1983; **143**: 495.

201 Zimmerman HJ. *Hepatotoxicity. The Adverse Effects of Drugs and Other Chemicals on the Liver.* Appleton-Century-Crofts, New York, 1979.

202 Zimmerman HJ, Ishak KG. Valproate-induced hepatic injury: analyses of 23 fatal cases. *Hepatology* 1982; **2**: 591.

203 Zitelli BJ, Alexander J, Taylor S *et al.* Fatal hepatic necrosis due to pyrimethamine-sulfadoxine (fansidar). *Ann. intern. Med.* 1987; **106**: 393.

19 · Hepatic Cirrhosis

Definition

Cirrhosis is defined anatomically as a diffuse process with fibrosis and nodule formation [2]. It has followed hepato-cellular necrosis. Although the causes are many, the end result is the same.

Fibrosis is not synonymous with cirrhosis. Fibrosis may be in zone 3 in heart failure, or in zone 1 in bile duct obstruction and congenital hepatic fibrosis (fig. 19.1) or interlobular in granulomatous liver disease, but without a true cirrhosis.

Nodule formation without fibrosis, as in Felty's syndrome, or partial nodular transformation (fig. 19.1), is not cirrhosis.

The relation of chronic active hepatitis to cirrhosis is discussed in Chapter 17.

Production of cirrhosis

The responses of the liver to necrosis are strictly limited; the most important are collapse of hepatic lobules, formation of diffuse fibrous septa and nodular regrowth of liver cells. Thus, irrespective of the aetiology, the ultimate histological pattern of the liver is the same, or nearly the same. Necrosis may no longer be apparent by the time the cirrhotic liver is examined.

Fibrosis follows hepato-cellular necrosis (figs 19.2, 19.3). This may be piecemeal in Rappaport's zone 1 leading to portal–portal fibrous bridges [8]. Confluent necrosis in zone 3 leads to centro–portal bridging and fibrosis. Spotty necrosis is followed by focal fibrosis. The necrosis is followed by nodules which disturb the hepatic architecture and a full cirrhosis has developed.

Sinusoids persist at the periphery of the regenerating nodules at the site of the portal–central bridges. Portal blood is diverted past functioning liver tissue leading to vascular insufficiency at the centre of the nodules (zone 3) and even to persistence of the cirrhosis after the initial causative injury has been controlled. Basement membranes form in the Dissë space, so impeding metabolic exchange with the liver cells.

New fibroblasts form round necrotic liver cells and proliferated ductules. The fibrosis (collagen) progresses from a reversible to an irreversible state where acellular permanent septa have developed in zone 1 and hepatic parenchyma. The distribution of the fibrous septa varies with the causative agent.

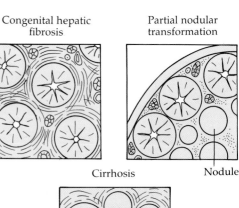

Congenital hepatic fibrosis

Partial nodular transformation

Cirrhosis

Nodule

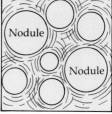

Fig. 19.1. Cirrhosis is defined as widespread fibrosis and nodule formation. Congenital hepatic fibrosis consists of fibrosis without nodules. Partial nodular transformation consists of nodules without fibrosis.

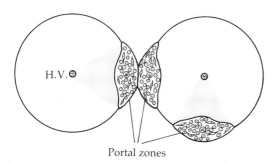

Fig. 19.2. Bridging necrosis and fibrosis is often precirrhotic and the site of internal portal—systemic shunts.

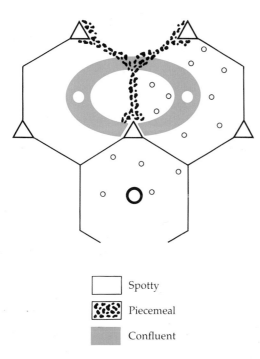

Fig. 19.3. Spotty, piecemeal and confluent necrosis and their relationship to portal—portal and portal—central fibrosis. (Courtesy L. Bianchi.)

In haemochromatosis, the iron excites portal zone fibrosis. In alcoholism, the fibrosis is predominantly in zone 3.

Fibrogenesis

Collagen is a heterogeneous class of extracellular proteins characterized by a unique amino acid composition (about 30% glycine, 20% proline + hydroxyproline and a variable content of hyroxylysine). There are four distinct types (table 19.1). The cirrhotic liver shows an increase in all collagen types irrespective of aetiology. The ratio of type I to type III increases with the quantity of collagen formed. This may reflect duration of chronicity: type III is abundant in fetal tissue, whereas type I increases during ageing. The increased collagen is harmful by disrupting the hepatic architecture and by converting sinusoids to capillaries, so impeding metabolic exchange through basement membranes between liver cells and the blood and causing portal hypertension.

In cirrhosis, synthesis of collagen is increased due both to a greater collagen synthesis per fibroblast and to an increase in the number of collagen-producing cells.

Typical *fibroblasts* are found only in portal tracts.

Ito cells are the resting precursor fibroblasts of the parenchyma. Myofibroblasts in Dissë space may similarly produce collagen.

Pathological fibrosis represents excessive or disordered production of hepatic extracellular matrix which contains collagen and also large glycoproteins and proteoglycans [3]. In normal human liver, hepatocytes, fat storing cells and endothelial cells produce components of the extracellular matrix. In fibrosis, hepatocytes which normally do not synthesize types III and types IV collagen may produce them [14].

Fibronectin is a cell surface glycoprotein serving the attachment of collagen fibrils and proteoglycans to hepatocytes. It is formed by

Table 19.1. The types of collagen

Type	Site	Stained by
I	Portal zones, central zones, broad scars	Van Giesen
II	Sinusoids (elastic tissue)	Elastin
III	Reticulin fibres (sinusoids, portal zones)	Silver
IV	Basement membranes	Periodic-acid Schiff (PAS)

411

endothelial cells in the space of Dissë [41]. Together with collagen, it is deposited in areas of liver cell damage as early as one hour after the injury. It stimulates fibroplasia and its breakdown products are chemotactic for fibroblasts. It also moderates cell differentiation and function, particularly during the healing response. Fibronectin is found around all hepatocytes but not in portal tracts.

Laminin is a large, rigid glycoprotein produced in normal rat liver by lipocytes. It is present in the presinusoidal matrix and forms a continuous distribution round hepatic sinusoids adjacent to hepatocytes and sinusoidal lining cells [32]. It is also present in basement membranes of ducts, ductules and capillaries. It forms a basement membrane round hepatocytes when regenerating or injured.

Mediators of fibrosis. Hepato-cellular necrosis is the stimulus for collagen formation. Necrotic cells could produce stimulating factors or there might be a pre-formed inactive precursor in plasma. In monolayer culture, the rat hepatocyte can secrete collagen—raising the possibility that the hepatocyte may elaborate its own matrix and play a role in fibrogenesis.

The nature of the stimulant is unknown. Candidates include gamma-interferon but in fact interleukin 1-α is a more potent stimulator of fibroblast-produced collagen. In chronic hepatitis B infection, interleukin 1 production from mononuclear cells is markedly increased and correlates with the severity of fibrosis. Lymphokines and monokines are produced by specifically T-lymphocytes and macrophages and can be formed in the absence of necrosis and inflammation so raising the possibility that fibrosis can develop without an intervening stage of chronic active hepatitis and cell necrosis. The mediators may differ in different types of liver disease.

MONITORING FIBROGENESIS [24]

The proteins and metabolites of connective tissue metabolism which are secreted by the cell spill-over into the plasma where they can be measured. Unfortunately, results reflect fibrosis generally and do not give information on localization and specifically about hepatic fibrosis.

Aminoterminal *procollagen type III peptide* is cleaved off the procollagen molecule in the synthesis of a collagen type III fibril. It can be measured in serum by radio-immunoassay. Values are not of practical *diagnostic* value. They are useful in *monitoring* liver fibrosis, particularly in the alcoholic [18, 37]. However, increased levels may reflect inflammation and necrosis rather than fibrosis in chronic liver disease [35, 47], primary biliary cirrhosis [4] and haemochromatosis [43]. Increased values are found in children, the pregnant or in patients with renal failure.

Collagen type 1 deposition may be studied by immunofluorescence on liver biopsies using a monoclonal antibody [33]. Active production of collagen type 1 by hepatocytes could become a useful marker of progressive liver disease.

Levels of *fibronectin* and *laminin* have also been used to mark increased connective tissue metabolism.

These estimations are of largely experimental interest, but it will clearly not be too long before a satisfactory estimate of hepatic fibrosis becomes available.

Classification

Morphological

Three anatomical types are recognized: micronodular, macronodular and mixed, the liver showing both micro- and macronodular features.

Micronodular is characterized by thick, regular septa, by regenerating small nodules varying little in size and by involvement of every lobule (figs 19.4, 19.6). The micronodular liver may represent impaired capacity for regrowth as in alcoholism, malnutrition, old age or anaemia.

Macronodular is characterized by septa and nodules of variable sizes and by normal lobules in the larger nodules (figs 19.5, 19.7). Previous

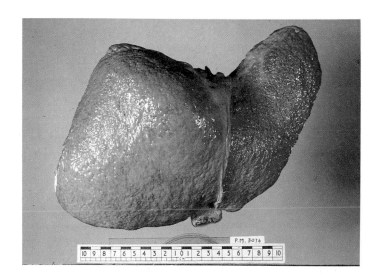

Fig. 19.4. The small finely nodular liver of micronodular cirrhosis.

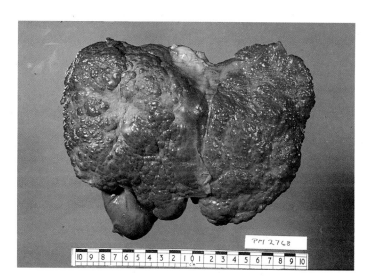

Fig. 19.5. The grossly distorted coarsely nodular liver of macronodular cirrhosis.

collapse is shown by juxtaposition in the fibrous scars of three or more portal tracts. Regeneration is reflected by large cells with large nuclei and by cells plates of varying thicknesses.

Regeneration in a micronodular cirrhosis results in a macronodular or mixed appearance. With time, micronodular cirrhosis often converts to macronodular [17].

Aetiology (table 19.2)

The following are usually accepted.

1 Viral hepatitis types B; ± Delta; non-A, non-B.
2 Alcohol.
3 Metabolic, e.g. haemochromatosis, Wilson's disease, α_1-antitrypsin deficiency, diabetes mellitus, type IV glycogenosis, galactosaemia, congenital tyrosinosis.

413

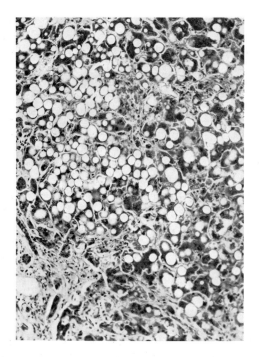

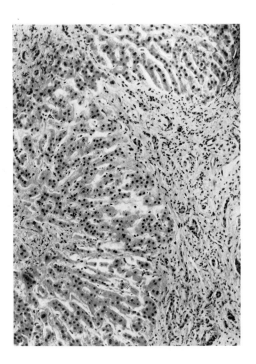

Fig. 19.6. Micronodular cirrhosis. Gross fatty change. The liver cells are often necrotic. Fibrous septa dissect the liver. H & E, ×135.

Fig. 19.7. Macronodular cirrhosis. Nodules of regenerating liver cells of different sizes are intersected by fibrous bands of various widths containing proliferating bile ducts. Fatty change is not seen. H & E, ×135.

Table 19.2. Aetiology and definitive treatment of cirrhosis

Aetiology	Treatment
Virus hepatitis (B and non-A, non-B)	?Antivirals
Alcohol	Abstention
Metabolic	
Iron overload	Venesection. Desferrioxamine
Copper overload (Wilson's disease)	Penicillamine
α_1-antitrypsin deficiency	?Transplant
Type IV glycogenosis	?Transplant
Galactosaemia	Withdraw milk and milk products
Tyrosinaemia	Withdraw dietary tyrosine. ?Transplant
Cholestasis (biliary)	Relieve biliary obstruction
Hepatic venous outflow block	
Budd–Chiari syndrome	Relieve main vein block
Heart failure	Treat cardiac cause
Immunological ('Lupoid' hepatitis)	Prednisolone
Toxins and drugs, e.g. methotrexate, amiodarone	Identify and stop
Indian childhood	?Penicillamine
Cryptogenic	—

4 Prolonged cholestasis intra- and extra-hepatic.

5 Hepatic-venous outflow obstruction, e.g. veno-occlusive disease, Budd—Chiari syndrome, constrictive pericarditis.

6 Disturbed immunity 'lupoid' hepatitis.

7 Toxins and therapeutic agents, e.g. methotrexate, amiodarone.

8 Intestinal bypass.

9 Indian childhood cirrhosis.

Other possible factors to be considered include:

Malnutrition (Chapter 23).

Infections. Malarial parasites do not cause cirrhosis. The co-existence of malaria and cirrhosis probably reflects malnutrition, virus hepatitis and toxic factors in the community.

Syphilis causes cirrhosis in neonates but not in adults.

In schistosomiasis, the ova excite a fibrous tissue reaction in the portal zones. The association with cirrhosis in certain countries is probably related to other aetiological factors.

Granulomatous lesions. Focal granuloma in such conditions as brucellosis, tuberculosis and sarcoidosis heal with fibrosis, but the liver dose not show nodular regrowth.

Cryptogenic cirrhosis. The aetiology is unknown and this is clearly a heterogeneous group. Frequency varies in different parts of the world; in the United Kingdom it is about 30% whereas in other areas such as France or in urban parts of the United States where alcoholism is prevalent the level drops. As specific diagnostic criteria appear, so the percentage falls. The advent of HBsAg transferred many previously designated cryptogenic cirrhotics to the post-hepatitic group. Estimations of serum smooth muscle and mitochondrial antibodies and better interpretation of liver histology separate others into the chronic active hepatitis—primary biliary cirrhosis category. Some of the remainder may be alcoholics who deny alcoholism or have forgotten that they ever consumed alcohol. There remains a hard core of patients in whom the cirrhosis remains cryptogenic. Aetiological diagnosis in these awaits further specific criteria and particularly tests for non-A, non-B viral hepatitis.

Mechanisms are discussed in individual chapters. The clinical and pathological picture may be that of 'chronic active hepatitis' which has proceeded to cirrhosis (Chapter 17).

Anatomical diagnosis

The diagnosis of cirrhosis depends on the demonstration of widespread nodules in the liver combined with fibrosis. This may be done by *direct visualization*, for instance at laparotomy or at laparoscopy. However laparatomy should never be used to diagnose cirrhosis, because it may precipitate liver failure even in those with apparently very well-compensated disease.

Laparoscopy visualizes the nodular liver and allows directed liver biopsy (fig. 19.8). It has some advantages in the presence of a coarsely nodular liver where a 'blind' liver biopsy can extract virtually normal liver tissue from a large nodule.

Radio-isotope scanning gives suggestive evidence of cirrhosis such as generalized decrease in hepatic uptake of isotope, an irregular pattern and uptake of isotope by the spleen and bone marrow. Nodules are not identified.

Using *ultrasound*, cirrhosis is suggested by dense reflective areas of irregular distribution and increased attenuation. The caudate lobe is enlarged relative to the right lobe [20]. However, ultrasound is not reliable for the diagnosis of cirrhosis unless ascites is present. Frequency demodulation may be useful in following hepatic fibrosis [25]. *CT scan* is cost-effective for the diagnosis and its complications (fig. 19.9). Liver size can be assessed and the irregular nodular surface seen. Fatty change, increased density due to iron and a space-occupying lesion can be recognized. After intravenous contrast, the portal vein and hepatic vein can be identified in the liver, and a collateral circulation with splenomegaly may give confirmation to the diagnosis of portal hypertension. Large collateral vessels, usually perisplenic or paraoesophageal, may add confirmation to a clinical diagnosis of chronic portal—systemic encephalopathy. Ascites can be seen. Gallstones may be noted in the gallbladder or common bile duct. The CT provides

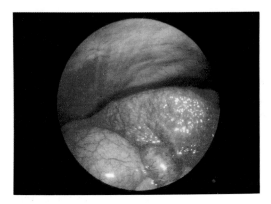

Fig. 19.8. Laparoscopy shows the nodular liver of cirrhosis. Note gall bladder to the left.

an objective record useful for following the course. Directed biopsy of a selected area can be performed safely.

Biopsy diagnosis of cirrhosis may be difficult, especially when Menghini-type needles are used, and the Trucut method may be preferable. The soft parenchyma may be aspirated leaving fibrous tissue behind. Reticulin and collagen stains are essential for demonstration of a rim of fibrosis around the nodule (fig. 19.10).

Helpful diagnostic points include absence of portal tracts, abnormal vascular arrangements, hepatic arterioles not accompanied by portal veins, the presence of nodules with fibrous septa, variability in liver cell size and appearance in different areas and thickened liver cell plates [45].

Functional

An assessment of hepatic function should always be attempted.

Liver failure is estimated by such features as jaundice, ascites (Chapter 9), encephalopathy (Chapter 7), low serum albumin, raised transaminase levels and a prothrombin deficiency not corrected by Vitamin K.

Portal hypertension (Chapter 10) is shown by splenomegaly, oesophageal varices and by the newer methods of measuring portal pressure.

Evolution is assessed by serial clinical, biochemical and histological observations, and classified whether progressing, regressing or stationary.

Examples of classification

In every patient, diagnosis must be in terms of aetiology, morphology and hepatic function. Examples of such complete diagnoses are:
1 Macronodular cirrhosis following type B

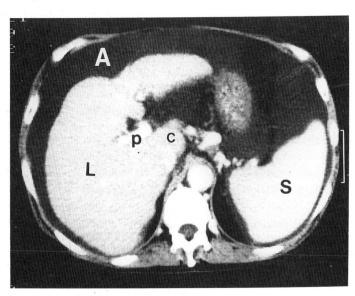

Fig. 19.9. CT, after intravenous contrast, in cirrhosis shows ascites (A). Small liver with irregular surface (L), enlarged caudate lobe (c), splenomegaly (S), patent portal vein (p).

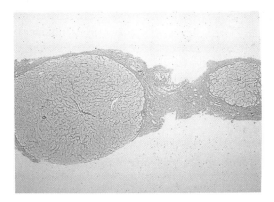

Fig. 19.10. Liver biopsy in cirrhosis: the specimen is small but nodules are shown outlined by reticulin. Stained reticulin ×40.

hepatitis with liver cell failure and portal hypertension. Progressing.

2 Micronodular cirrhosis in an alcoholic with liver cell failure and minimal portal hypertension. Regressing.

3 Mixed micronodular and macronodular cirrhosis following bile duct stricture with minimal liver cell failure and portal hypertension. Progressing.

Clinical cirrhosis

Cirrhosis, apart from other features peculiar to the cause, results in two major events, hepatocellular failure (Chapters 6, 7, 8, 9) and portal hypertension (Chapter 10). Prognosis and treatment depend on the magnitude of these two factors. In clinical terms, the types are either 'latent and well compensated' or 'active and decompensated'. In addition, cirrhosis, whatever its type, has certain clinicopathological associations.

It is difficult to associate the clinical picture with the underlying pathology although there are certain similarities. In Europe and the United States, post-hepatitic cirrhosis, cirrhosis of the alcoholic, chronic active hepatitis and cryptogenic cirrhosis account for the majority. The age and sex distribution of the various types differ.

Table 19.3. General investigations in the patient with cirrhosis (see also table 10.1)

Occupation, age, sex, domicile

Clinical history
  Fatigue and weight loss
  Anorexia and flatulent dyspepsia
  Abdominal pain
  Jaundice. Colour of urine and faeces
  Swelling of legs or abdomen
  Haemorrhage—nose, gums, skin, alimentary tract
  Loss of libido
  Past health: jaundice, hepatitis, drugs ingested, blood transfusion
  Social
  Hereditary. Alcohol consumption

Examination
  Nutrition, fever, fetor hepaticus, jaundice, pigmentation, purpura, finger clubbing, white nails, vascular spiders, palmar erythema, gynaecomastia, testicular atrophy, distribution of body hair. Parotid enlargement. Dupuytren's contracture. Blood pressure
  Abdomen: ascites, abdominal wall veins, liver, spleen
  Peripheral oedema
  Neurological changes: mental functions, stupor, tremor

Special investigations
Biochemical:
  Serum—bilirubin concentration
            alkaline phosphatase concentration
            albumin and globulin concentration
            immunoglobulins
            transaminase concentration
If ascites present:
  serum sodium potassium, bicarbonate, chloride and urea levels
  Weigh daily
  24-hour urine volume and sodium excretion
Serum immunological:
  Smooth muscle, mitochondrial and nuclear antibodies
  Hepatitis-B antigen (HBsAg) (other markers of hepatitis, Chapter 16)
  α_1-fetoprotein
Haematology:
  Haemoglobin, absolute values, leucocyte and platelet count, prothrombin time
Endoscopy
Needle liver biopsy if blood coagulation permits
EEG. If neuropsychiatric changes
Hepatic scan or ultrasound

The terminal stages of the various types may be identical and differences must not be stressed. The aetiological distinction, however, is important both for prognosis and for specific treatment such as alcohol withdrawal, venesection in haemochromatosis or prednisolone in autoimmune chronic active hepatitis (table 19.2). Finally, comparison of cirrhosis in different parts of the world must allow for different aetiologies, although the basic pattern of liver cell failure and portal hypertension may be similar. Results of treatment of one type cannot be compared with those for another.

Clinical and pathological associations

1 Splenomegaly and abdominal wall venous collaterals usually indicate *portal hypertension*.
2 Chronic relapsing *pancreatitis* and pancreatic calcification are often associated with alcoholic liver disease [40].
3 *Gastrointestinal*. Varices may collapse and be overlooked at autopsy. Peptic ulcer is frequent with cirrhosis of alcoholics. Intestinal absorption of glucose and protein loss into the gastrointestinal tract are normal [27]. Taste and smell acuity may be reduced [11].
4 *Steatorrhoea* is frequent even in the absence of pancreatitis or alcoholism. It can be related to reduced hepatic bile salt secretion.
5 *Abdominal herniae* are common with ascites. They should not be repaired unless endangering life or unless the cirrhosis is very well compensated.
6 *Primary liver cancer* is frequent with all forms of cirrhosis except the biliary and cardiac types. *Metastatic cancer* is said to be rare, due to the reduced frequency of extrahepatic carcinoma in cirrhosis [21, 44]. However, when groups of patients with cancer with and without cirrhosis were compared the incidence of hepatic metastases was the same in each group.
7 *Gallstones*. At autopsy, gallstones were found in 29.4% of cirrhotic patients (irrespective of the type) and 12.8% of the non-cirrhotic population [9]. Gallstones are usually of pigment type and hence not related to lithogenic (low-cholesterol holding) bile (see Chapter 31).

When discovered, surgical intervention should be avoided unless life-saving, for the patient is potentially a poor operative risk.
8 *Digital clubbing* and *hypertrophic osteoarthropathy* may complicate cirrhosis, especially biliary [16].
9 *Parotid gland enlargement* and *Dupuytren's contracture* are seen in some alcoholic patients with cirrhosis.
10 *Renal*. Changes in intrarenal circulation, and particularly a redistribution of blood flow away from the cortex, are found in all forms of cirrhosis. This predisposes to the *hepatorenal syndrome*. Intrinsic renal failure follows periods of hypotension and shock.

Glomerular changes include a thickening of the mesangial stalk and to a lesser degree of the capillary walls (cirrhotic glomerular sclerosis) [6]. Deposits of IgA are most frequent. These are usually found with alcoholic liver disease. The changes are usually latent, but occasionally associated with proliferative changes and the clinical manifestations of glomerular involvement.
11 *Infections*. Reticulo-endothelial system phagocytic activity is impaired [42], largely related to intra-hepatic portal—systemic shunting. Bacterial infections, often of intestinal origin, are common, affecting 4.5% cirrhotic patients per year [22].

Septicaemias are frequent in end-stage cirrhosis and should always be suspected in patients with unexplained pyrexia or deterioration. The diagnosis is often missed. Spontaneous bacterial peritonitis must always be considered (Chapter 10).

Tuberculosis has, in general, decreased, but tuberculous peritonitis is still encountered and is often unsuspected [10]. Respiratory infections have also lessened in severity.
12 *Cardiovascular*. Cirrhotics are less liable to coronary and aortic atheroma than the rest of the population [38]. At autopsy, the incidence of myocardial infarction is about a quarter of that among total cases examined without cirrhosis [26]. Patients with compensated or decompensated cirrhosis have a lower arterial blood pressure than healthy controls [36].

13 *Eye signs.* Lid retraction and lid lag is significantly increased in patients with cirrhosis compared with a control population [46].

There is no evidence of thyroid disease. Serum-free thyroxin is not increased.

Histocompatibility antigens (HLA)

Sixty per-cent of patients with HBsAg negative chronic active hepatitis are HLA-B8 positive. The patients who are positive tend to be female, less than 40 years old, have a remission with corticosteroid therapy and show positive non-specific serum antibody tests and high serum gamma-globulins. This association does not apply to HBsAg positive chronic active hepatitis. The D locus antigen DW3 may show an even stronger association with non-B chronic active hepatitis than does locus B8.

In alcoholic liver disease there are geographic differences in the HLA association but no consistent pattern (Chapter 20).

In idiopathic haemochromatosis, there is an association with HLA-B3,-B7 and -14 (Chapter 21). This observation may be useful in detecting family members at risk of developing the disease.

In primary biliary cirrhosis, there is no association with HLA-B8, nor indeed with any particular histocompatibility antigen.

In general, detection of HLA types are not of practical importance in the investigation of patients with liver disease. They may be useful in family studies and in detection of relatives at risk of developing genetically related diseases.

Hyperglobulinaemia

Elevation of the total serum globulin, and particularly gamma level is a well-known accompaniment of most forms of chronic liver disease. Electrophoresis of the serum proteins shows a polyclonal gamma response, but rarely a monoclonal picture may be seen . The increased gamma-globulin values may be related in part to increased tissue autoantibodies, such as smooth muscle antibody. However, the major factor seems to be failure of the damaged liver to clear intestinal antigen (fig. 19.11). Patients with cirrhosis show increased serum antibodies to gastrointestinal tract antigens, particularly *E. coli* [3,49]. Such antigens bypass the liver through portal—systemic channels or through the internal shunts developing round the cirrhotic nodule. Once in the systemic circulation these intestinal antigens provoke an increased antibody response from such organs as the spleen. Systemic endotoxaemia may arise similarly. Polymeric IgA and IgA-antigen complexes of gut origin can also reach the systemic circulation [30]. Suppressor T-lymphocyte function is depressed in chronic liver disease and this would reduce the suppression of B-lymphocytes and so favour antibody production [48].

Clinically latent cirrhosis

The disease may be discovered at a routine examination or biochemical screen or at operation undertaken for some other condition (fig. 19.12). Cirrhosis may be suspected if the patient has mild pyrexia, vascular spiders, palmar erythema, or unexplained epistaxis or oedema of the ankles. Firm enlargement of the liver and splenomegaly are helpful diagnostic signs. Vague morning indigestion and flatulent dyspepsia may be early features in the alcoholic cirrhotic. Confirmation should be sought by biochemical tests and, if necessary, by aspiration liver biopsy.

Biochemical tests may be quite normal in this group. The most frequent changes are a slight increase in the serum transaminase or gamma-GT level.

Diagnosis is confirmed by *needle liver biopsy*.

These patients may remain compensated until they die from another cause. Some proceed, in a period from months to years, to the stage of hepato-cellular failure. In others the problem is of portal hypertension with oesophageal bleeding. Portal hypertension may present even with normal liver function tests. The course in the individual patient is very difficult to predict.

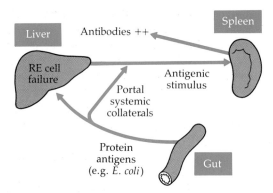

Fig. 19.11. A possible mechanism for the increased serum antibody (and globulin) levels in cirrhosis. Protein antigens from the gut bypass reticulo-endothelial (RE. Kupffer) cells in the liver and produce an antigenic stimulus to other organs, particularly the spleen, so increasing serum antibodies.

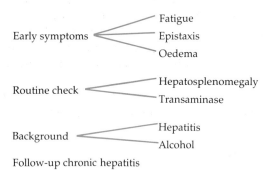

Follow-up chronic hepatitis

Fig. 19.12. Presentation of 'compensated' hepatic cirrhosis.

Decompensated cirrhosis

The patient usually seeks medical advice because of ascites and/or jaundice. General health fails with weakness, muscle wasting and weight loss. Continuous mild fever (37.5–38°C) is often due to Gram-negative bacteriaemia, to continuing hepatic cell necrosis or to a complicating liver cell carcinoma. Fetor hepaticus may be present. Cirrhosis is the commonest cause of hepatic encephalopathy.

Jaundice implies that liver cell destruction exceeds the capacity for regeneration and is always serious. The deeper the jaundice the greater the inadequacy of the liver cell function.

The skin may be pigmented, due to increased amounts of melanin. Clubbing of the fingers is occasionally seen. Purpura over the arms, shoulders and shins may be associated with a low platelet count. Spontaneous bruising and epistaxes reflect a prothrombin deficiency. The circulation is over-active. The blood pressure is low. Sparse body hair, vascular spiders, palmar erythema, white nails and gonadal atrophy are common.

Ascites is usually preceded by abdominal distension. Oedema of the legs is frequently associated.

The liver may be enlarged, with a firm regular edge, or contracted and impalpable. The spleen may be palpable.

The differential diagnosis of ascites, hepatic encephalopathy and jaundice are described in Chapters 7, 9, 12.

Laboratory findings

Urine. Urobilinogen is present in excess; bilirubin is also present if the patient is jaundiced. The urinary sodium excretion is diminished in the presence of ascites, and in a severe case less than 4 mEq are passed daily.

Serum biochemical changes. In addition to the raised serum bilirubin level, albumin is depressed and gamma-globulin raised. The percentage of esterified cholesterol is depressed. The serum alkaline phosphatase is usually raised to about twice normal; very high readings are occasionally found particularly with alcoholic cirrhosis. Serum transaminase values may be increased.

Haematology. There is usually a mild normocytic, normochromic anaemia; it is occasionally macrocytic. Gastrointestinal bleeding leads to hypochromic anaemia. The leucocyte and platelet counts are reduced ('hypersplenism'). The prothrombin time is prolonged and does not return to normal with vitamin K therapy. The bone-marrow is macronormablastic. Plasma cells are increased in proportion to the hyperglobulinaemia.

Needle biopsy diagnosis (table 19.4)
[2, 45]

If there are no contraindications, such as ascites or a coagulation defect, this may give a clue to aetiology and to activity. Serial biopsies are useful in assessing progress.

In cirrhosis, directed biopsies, using ultrasound or CT, are particularly helpful in obtaining adequate samples and avoiding other viscera especially the gallbladder.

Prognosis

Cirrhosis is usually believed to be irreversible, but fibrosis may regress as seen in treated haemochromatosis or Wilson's disease and the concept of irreversibility is not proven.

Cirrhosis need not be a progressive disease. With therapy the downhill progress may be checked.

Improved results for liver transplantation have emphasized the need for making an accurate prognosis in cirrhotic patients so that surgery may be performed at the best time.

Child's classification (Grades A, B, C)—which depends on jaundice, ascites, encephalopathy, serum albumin concentration and nutrition—gives a good short-term prognostic guide [28]. Cox's regression model using proportional hazards has been applied to cirrhosis and the prognostic index formulated [13]. Poor prognosis is associated with a low prothrombin index, marked ascites, GI bleeding, advanced age, high daily alcohol consumption, high serum bilirubin and alkaline phosphatase and low albumin values, little liver connective tissue inflammation and poor nutrition.

In a very large series of cirrhotic patients from Southern Italy, those originally compensated became decompensated at the rate of 10% per year. Ascites was the usual first sign and the six-year survival was 54%. Decompensated patients had a 21% six-year survival. Significant indicators of death risk were advanced age, male sex, encephalopathy, haemorrhage, varices, prothrombin time, HBsAg positivity and, of course, hepato-cellular carcinoma [15].

Specialist tests of hepatocyte function are not particularly helpful prognostically although the

Table 19.4. Histopathology and aetiology of cirrhosis

Aetiology	Morphological pattern	Fat	Chole-stasis	Iron	Copper	Acido-philic bodies	PAS-positive globules	Mallory's hyatin	Ground-glass hepato-cytes
Viral hepatitis B	Macro- or micronodular	−	−	−	−	+	−	−	+
Alcoholism	Micro- or macronodular	+	±	±	−	±	−	+	−
Haemochromatosis	Micronodular	±	−	+	−	−	−	−	−
Wilson's disease	Macronodular	±	±	−	+	+	−	+	−
α_1-antitrypsin deficiency	Micro- or macronodular	±	± +	−	±	±	+	±	−
Primary biliary	Biliary	−		−	+	−	−	±	−
Venous outflow obstruction	Reversed	−	−	−	−	−	−	−	−
Intestinal bypass operation	Micronodular	+	−	−	−	±	−	±	−
Indian childhood	Micronodular	−	±	−	+	−	−	+	−

− usually absent; ± may be present; + usually present.

serum bile acid concentration gives comparable results to Child's classification [34].

The following points are useful prognostically:

1 *Aetiology.* Alcoholic cirrhotics, if they abstain, respond better than those with 'cryptogenic' cirrhosis.

2 If decompensation has followed haemorrhage, infection or alcoholism, the prognosis is better than if it is spontaneous, because the *precipitating factor* is correctable.

3 The *response to therapy.* If the patient has failed to improve within one month of starting hospital treatment, the outlook is poor.

4 *Jaundice*, especially if persistent, is a serious sign.

5 *Neurological complications.* The significance depends on their mode of production. Those developing in the course of progressive hepato-cellular failure carry a bad prognosis, whereas those developing chronically and associated with an extensive portal−systemic collateral circulation respond well to dietary protein restriction.

6 *Ascites* worsens the prognosis, particularly if large doses of diuretics are needed for control.

7 *Liver size.* A large liver carries a better prognosis than a small one because it is likely to contain more functioning cells.

8 *Haemorrhage from oesophageal varices.* Portal hypertension must be considered together with the state of the liver cells. If function is good, haemorrhage may be tolerated: if poor, hepatic coma and death are probable.

9 *Biochemical tests.* If the serum albumin is less than 2.5 g the outlook is poor. Hyponatraemia (serum sodium < 120 mEq/l), if unrelated to diuretic therapy, is grave.

Serum transaminase and globulin levels give no guide to prognosis.

When the ratio of the total serum bilirubin (μmol/l) to the gamma glutamyl transpeptidase (i.u./1) exceeds one, the prognosis is very poor. Only 12% of 129 largely alcoholic cirrhotic patients with this ratio survived one year [39].

10 Persistent *hypoprothrombinaemia* with spontaneous bruising is serious.

11 Persistent hypotension (systolic BP < 100 mmHg) is serious.

12 *Hepatic histological changes.* Sections are useful in evaluating the extent of necrosis and of inflammatory infiltration. A fatty liver responds well to treatment.

CONCLUSIONS

The prognosis is determined by the extent of hepato-cellular failure. Jaundice, spontaneous bruising and ascites resistant to treatment are grave signs. If specific treatment is available the outlook is better.

Treatment

The management of the *well-compensated* cirrhotic is that of the early detection of hepato-cellular failure. The principles of an adequate mixed diet and avoidance of alcohol should be explained.

A diet of 1 g protein/kg body weight is adequate unless the patient is obviously malnourished. Additional choline or methionine or various 'hepato-protectives' are unnecessary. Avoidance of butter and other fats, eggs, coffee or chocolate is not of any therapeutic value.

The onset of hepato-cellular failure with oedema and ascites demands sodium restriction and diuretics (Chapter 9); complicating encephalopathy is an indication for a lowered protein intake (Chapter 7).

Portal hypertension may demand special treatment (Chapter 10).

Anti-fibrotic drugs

The therapy of cirrhosis may reside in switching off collagen synthesis [12].

Penicillamine inhibits the formation of cross-links in collagen. Its use in cirrhosis remains uncertain and toxic effects are numerous.

Pro-collagen secretion requires the polymerization of microtubules, a process which can be inhibited by micro-tubular disruptive drugs such as *colchicine*. One long-term clinical trial reported that colchicine improved survival in cirrhotic patients [29]. However, collagen production in cell and tissue cultures treated with colchicine is unchanged and this suggests that any beneficial effect in liver fibrosis is mediated by other mechanisms including anti-inflammatory and stimulation of collagenase secretion. Evidence is not sufficiently strong to recommend the use of colchicine long-term for patients with cirrhosis. It is however, relatively harmless, the only sideeffect being diarrhoea.

Corticosteroids are anti-inflammatory and inhibit the activity of prolyl hydroxylase. They inhibit collagen synthesis but also inhibit procollagenase. Corticosteroids also suppress the formation of collagen by cultured rat hepatocytes [23].

Other promising drugs for the treatment of hepatic fibrosis exist, such as *γ-interferon*, *2-oxoglutarate analogues* and *prostaglandins*. They have not been subjected to clinical trial.

Other therapeutic strategies for the future include the augmentation of the activity of extracellular proteases responsible for degrading collagen. The possibility of directly blocking the synthesis of connective tissue proteins by somatic gene therapy remains for the future.

SURGICAL PROCEDURES

All operations in cirrhotic patients carry a high risk and a high mortality. Surgery in non-bleeding cirrhotic patients has an operative mortality of 30% and an additional morbidity rate of 30% [19]. These are related to Child's grades—mortality being 10% in A, 31% in B, and 76% in grade C patients. Operations on the biliary tract, for peptic ulcer disease or for colon resection have a particularly bad prognosis. Poor predictive features include a low serum albumin, the presence of infection and a prolonged prothrombin time. Surgical procedures should be undertaken in cirrhotic patients only when there are clear indications and where they are life saving.

Using modern segmental surgery, small hepato-cellular carcinomas arising in a cirrhotic liver can be successfully resected [7].

423

References

1 Anastassakos C, Alexander GJM, Wolstencroft RA et al. Interleukin-1 and interleukin-2 activity in chronic hepatitis B virus infection. *Gastroenterology* 1988; **94**: 999.

2 Anthony PP, Ishak KG, Nayak NC et al. The morphology of cirrhosis; definition, nomenclature and classification. *Bull. WHO* 1977; **55**: 521.

3 Arenson DM, Bissell DM. Glycosaminoglycan, proteoglycan and hepatic fibrosis. *Gastroenterology* 1987; **92**: 536.

4 Babbs C, Smith A, Hunt LP et al. Type III procollagen peptide: a marker of disease activity and prognosis in primary biliary cirrhosis. *Lancet* 1988; **i**: 1021.

5 Badley BWD, Murphy GM, Bouchier IAD et al. The role of bile salts in the steatorrhoea of chronic liver disease. *Gastroenterology* 1969; **56**: 1136.

6 Berger J, Yaneva H, Nabarra B. Glomerular changes in patients with cirrhosis of the liver. *Adv. Nephrology* 1977−8; **7**: 3.

7 Bismuth H, Houssin D, Ornowski J et al. Liver resections in cirrhotic patients: a Western experience. *World J. Surg.* 1986; **10**: 311.

8 Bjørneboe M, Prytz H, Orskov F. Antibodies to intestinal microbes in serum of patients with cirrhosis of the liver. *Lancet* 1972; **i**: 58.

9 Bouchier IAD. Postmortem study of the frequency of gallstones in patients with cirrhosis of the liver. *Gut* 1969; **10**: 705.

10 Burack WR, Hollister RM. Tuberculous peritonitis: a study of forty-seven proved cases encountered by a general medical unit in twenty-five years. *Am. J. Med.* 1960; **28**: 510.

11 Burch RE, Sackin DA, Ursick JA et al. Decreased taste and smell acuity in cirrhosis. *Arch. intern. Med.* 1978; **138**: 743.

12 Chojkier M, Brenner DA. Therapeutic strategies for hepatic fibrosis. *Hepatology* 1988; **8**: 176.

13 Christensen E, Schlichting P, Anderson PK et al. Updating prognosis and therapeutic evaluation in cirrhosis with Cox's multiple regression model for time-dependent variables. *Scand. J. Gastroenterol.* 1986; **21**: 163.

14 Clement B, Grimaud J-A, Campion J-P et al. Cell types involved in collagen and fibronectin production in normal and fibrotic human liver. *Hepatology* 1986; **6**: 225.

15 D'Amico G, Morabito A, Pagliaro L et al. Survival and prognostic indicators in compensated and decompensated cirrhosis. *Dig. Dis. Sci.* 1986; **31**: 468.

16 Epstein O, Ajdukiewicz AB, Dick R et al. Hypertrophic hepatic osteoarthropathy. *Am. J. Med.* 1979; **67**: 88.

17 Fauerholdt L, Schlichting P, Christensen E et al.

Conversion of micronodular cirrhosis into macronodular cirrhosis. *Hepatology* 1983; **3**: 928.

18 Frei A, Zimmermann A, Weigand K. The N-terminal propeptide of collagen type III in serum reflects activity and degree of fibrosis in patients with chronic liver disease. *Hepatol.* 1984; **4**: 830.

19 Garrison RN, Cryer HM, Howard DA *et al.* Clarification of risk factors for abdominal operations in patients with hepatic cirrhosis. *Ann. Surg.* 1984; **199**: 648.

20 Giorgio A, Amoroso P, Lettieri G *et al.* Cirrhosis: value of caudate to right lobe ratio in diagnosis with US. *Radiology* 1986; **161**: 443.

21 Goldstein MJ, Franle WJ, Sherlock P. Hepatic metastases and portal cirrhosis. *Am. J. med. Sci.* 1966; **252**: 26.

22 Graudal N, Milman N, Kirkegaard E *et al.* Bacteremia in cirrhosis of the liver. *Liver* 1986; **6**: 297.

23 Guzelian PS, Lindblad WJ, Diegelmann RF. Glucocorticoids suppress formation of collagen by the hepatocyte: studies in primary monolayer cultures of parenchymal cells prepared from adult rat liver. *Gastroenterology* 1984; **86**: 897.

24 Hahn EG. Blood analysis for liver fibrosis. *J. Hepatol.* 1984; **1**: 67.

25 Hoefs JC, Aufrichtig D, Lottenberg S *et al.* Noninvasive evaluation of hepatic fibrosis using frequency demodulation of ultra-sound signals. *Dig. dis. Sci.* 1986; **31**: 1046.

26 Howel WL, Manion WC. The low incidence of myocardial infarction in patients with portal cirrhosis of the liver: a review of 639 cases of cirrhosis of the liver from 17,731 autopsies. *Am. heart J.* 1960; **60**: 341.

27 Iber FL. Protein loss into the gastrointestinal tract in cirrhosis of the liver. *Am. J. clin. Nutr.* 1967; **19**: 219.

28 Infante-Rivard C, Esnaola S, Villeneuve J-P *et al.* Clinical and statistical validity of conventional prognostic factors in predicting short-term survival among cirrhotics. *Hepatology* 1987; **7**: 660.

29 Kershenobich HD, Vargas F, Garcia-Tsao G *et al.* Effectiveness of colchicine in patients with cirrhosis (Abstract). *Hepatology* 1987; **7**: 1104.

30 Kleinman RE, Harmatz PR, Walker WA. The liver: an integral part of the enteric mucosal immune system. *Hepatology* 1982; **2**: 379.

31 MacSween RNM, Anthony PP, Scheuer PJ. *Pathology of the Liver*, 2nd edn. Churchill Livingstone, Edinburgh 1987.

32 Maher JJ, Friedman SL, Roll FJ *et al.* Immuno-localisation of laminin in normal rat liver and biosyntheses of laminin by hepatic lipocytes in primary culture. *Gastroenterology* 1988; **94**: 1053.

33 Malizia G, Giannuoli G, Caltagirone M *et al.* Procollagen type 1 production by hepatocytes: a marker of progressive liver disease? *Lancet* 1987; **ii**: 1055.

34 Mannes GA, Thieme C, Stellaard F *et al.* Prognostic significance of serum bile acids in cirrhosis. *Hepatology* 1986; **6**: 50.

35 McCullough AJ, Stassen WN, Wiesner RH *et al.* Serum type III procollagen peptide concentrations in severe chronic active hepatitis: relationship to cirrhosis and disease activity. *Hepatol.* 1987; **7**: 49.

36 Minuk GY, MacCannell KL. Is the hypotension of cirrhosis a GABA-mediated process? *Hepatology* 1988; **8**: 73.

37 Niemela O, Risteli L, Sotaniemi EA *et al.* Aminoterminal propeptide of type III procollagen in serum in alcoholic liver disease. *Gastroenterology* 1983; **85**: 254.

38 Platt D, Kie FE, Luboeinski HP. Der Einfluss des Atters auf die negative Syntropie zwischen malignen Tumören, Lebercirrhöse und arterioskleorischen Umbaurorgangen der Aortawand Coronar und Cerebral. *Arterien Klin. Wschr.* 1973; **51**: 176.

39 Poynard T, Zouvabichvili O, Hilpert G *et al.* Prognostic value of total serum bilirubin/gamma-glutamyl transpeptidase ratio in cirrhotic patients. *Hepatology* 1984; **4**: 324.

40 Renner IG, Savage WT III, Stace NH *et al.* Pancreatitis associated with alcoholic liver disease: a review of 1022 autopsy cases. *Dig. Dis. Sci.* 1984; **29**: 593.

41 Rieder H, Ramadori G, Dienes H−P *et al.* Sinusoidal endothelial cells from guinea pig liver synthesize and secrete cellular fibronectin *in vitro*. *Hepatology* 1987; **7**: 856.

42 Rimola A, Soto R, Bory F *et al.* Reticuloendothelial system phagocytic activity in cirrhosis and its relation to bacterial infections and prognosis. *Hepatology* 1984; **4**: 53.

43 Roberts FD, Sandford NL, Bradbear RA *et al.* Serum procollagen-III-peptide: failure to reflect the extent of hepatic fibrosis. *J. Gastro. Hepatol.* 1986; **1**: 27.

44 Ruebner BH, Green R, Miyai K *et al.* The rarity of intrahepatic metastasis in cirrhosis of the liver. *Am. J. Pathol.* 1961; **39**: 739.

45 Scheuer PJ. *Liver Biopsy Interpretation*, 4th edn. Ballière Tindall, London. 1988.

46 Summerskill WHJ, Molnar GD. Eye signs in hepatic cirrhosis. *N. Engl. J. Med.* 1962; **266**: 1244.

47 Surrenti C, Casini A, Milani S *et al.* Is determination of serum N-terminal procollagen type III peptide (s PIII P) a marker of hepatic fibrosis? *Dig. Dis. Sci.* 1987; **32**: 705.

48 Thomas HC, Ryan CJ, Benjamin IS *et al.* The immune response in cirrhotic rats: the induction of tolerance to orally administered protein antigens. *Gastroenterology* 1976; **71**: 114.

49 Triger DR, Wright R. Hyperglobulinaemia in liver disease. *Lancet* 1973; **i**: 1494.

20 · Alcohol and the Liver

The association of alcohol with cirrhosis was recognized by Matthew Baillie in 1793. Over the last 20 years alcohol consumption has correlated with deaths from cirrhosis (fig. 20.1). At the Royal Free Hospital, London, between 1959 and 1965 alcoholism accounted for only 4.3% of patients with cirrhosis, compared with 25% between 1978 and 1983 [58]. In the United States, cirrhosis is the fourth commonest cause of death in adults.

The prevalence of alcoholic liver disease in various countries depends largely on religious and other customs and on the relation between the cost of alcohol and earnings—the lower the cost of alcohol, the more are lower socio-economic groups affected (fig. 20.2).

France is one of the few countries where alcohol consumption has decreased over the past 20 years (fig. 20.3). This can be related to government propaganda against alcoholism.

Risk factors for alcoholic liver diseases

Not all those who abuse alcohol develop liver damage and the incidence of cirrhosis among alcoholics at autopsy is about 10−15% (fig. 20.4) [76]. The explanation of the apparent predisposition of certain people to develop alcoholic cirrhosis is unknown.

DRINKING PATTERNS

The average intake of alcohol in a large group of male alcoholic cirrhotics was 160 g/day for

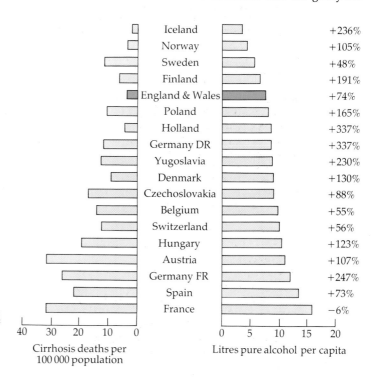

Fig. 20.1. Cirrhosis deaths related to litres pure alcohol drunk per year in various European countries.

Iceland +236%
Norway +105%
Sweden +48%
Finland +191%
England & Wales +74%
Poland +165%
Holland +337%
Germany DR +337%
Yugoslavia +230%
Denmark +130%
Czechoslovakia +88%
Belgium +55%
Switzerland +56%
Hungary +123%
Austria +107%
Germany FR +247%
Spain +73%
France −6%

Cirrhosis deaths per 100 000 population

Litres pure alcohol per capita

SMR All groups =100

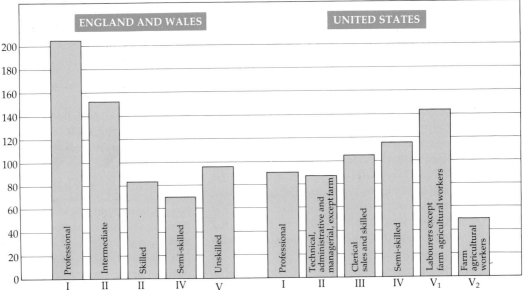

Fig. 20.2. Cirrhosis of the liver, standardized mortality ratios (SMR), men aged 20–64, by occupational level and social class; United States 1950, England and Wales 1949–53 (Office of Home Economics).

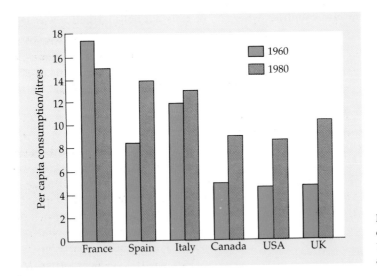

Fig. 20.3. Changing alcohol consumption per person between 1960 and 1980. Only France shows a decrease.

eight years [38]. Alcoholic hepatitis, a precirrhotic lesion, was noted in 14% of those who drank less than 160 g a day. For most individuals the danger dose is greater than 80 g alcohol daily (table 20.1). Duration is important. Neither cirrhosis nor alcoholic hepatitis

was seen in patients who consumed an average of 160 g of ethanol per day for less than five years, whereas 50% of 50 patients consuming high levels of alcohol for an average of 21 years developed cirrhosis.

The liver injury is unrelated to the type of

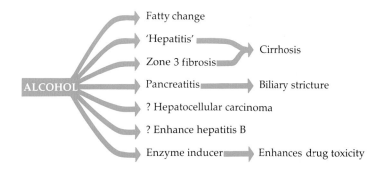

Fig. 20.4. The hepato-biliary effects of alcohol abuse. 80–90% of abusers have no liver disease.

Table 20.1. Alcohol equivalents

Whisky	30 ml	10 g
Wine	100 ml	10 g
Beer	250 ml	10 g

?80 g daily safe.

Table 20.2. Alcoholic liver disease—males:females (Morgan & Sherlock 1977)

Females suspected	38%
Males suspected	77%
Continued to abuse alcohol	
Males	71%
Females	91%

beverage consumed; it is related only to its alcohol content. The non-alcoholic constituents of the drink—congeners—are not particularly hepato-toxic.

Continued daily imbibing is more dangerous than intermittent when the liver is given a chance to recover. It is recommended that for at least two days in the week a person should not drink alcohol.

Those who develop alcoholic liver damage are only mildly dependent on alcohol [102]. They escape the florid symptoms of alcohol dependence, such as withdrawal symptoms, and are at greater risk of developing liver damage because they are able to maintain a high consumption over many years.

SEX

Alcoholism is increasing among women, being related to lesser social stigmata attached to drinking and to the ready availability of alcohol in supermarkets. Women are less likely to be suspected of alcohol abuse; they present at a later stage, are more susceptible to hepatic damage and are more likely to relapse after treatment (table 20.2) [59]. Women develop

higher blood ethanol values following a standard dose of ethanol, possibly because of a smaller mean apparent volume of distribution of alcohol [43]. Women are more likely to progress from alcoholic hepatitis to cirrhosis even if they stop drinking [74].

GENETICS

Patterns of alcohol drinking behaviour are inherited, but no single genetic marker has been shown to be associated with susceptibility to alcoholic liver damage. However, the rates of alcohol elimination vary as much as three-fold among individuals. Twin studies show that about one half of this variability is genetic.

Various HLA histocompatibility types have been associated with susceptibility to alcohol liver injury. In Britain HLA-B8 has been linked to florid alcoholic hepatitis, and to shorter drinking time and lower cumulative alcohol consumption [60], but in Norway the association is with B40 and in Chile with B13. In France, a significant increase in B15 and DR4 with a decrease in B13 has been noted [20]. All these results are very inconsistent and relatively crude.

Different rates of alcohol elimination may be related to genetic polymorphism of two enzyme systems (MEOS and ADH) which metabolize alcohol. Genetic polymorphism for alcohol dehydrogenase (ADH) has been found at two gene loci [8]. Differences account for different rates of ethanol oxidation and acetaldehyde generation. Genotyping can now be performed and this opens up the possibility of identifying the person deficient in metabolizing alcohol through the ADH reaction. Its practical application unfortunately is a long way away. The embarrassing acetaldehyde flush reaction seen in about 50% of Orientals when they consume alcohol is explained by the mitochondrial form of acetaldehyde dehydrogenase in the liver being inactive. This obviously inhibits Orientals taking alcohol and is a negative risk for the development of alcoholic liver damage.

Hepatitis B is another possible co-factor, there being an increased tendency to alcoholic liver damage in alcohol abusers who have hepatitis B virus markers [101].

Alcoholics have higher than normal blood acetaldehyde levels after alcohol. This might be secondary to chronic alcohol abuse, but could be a primary genetic abnormality.

NUTRITION

The role of malnutrition is controversial. Much depends on the population of alcoholics being studied, whether of low socio-economic status where protein-calorie malnutrition often precedes liver injury [51], or in the socially adequate where diet is good and damage cannot be related to nutrition [91].

Alcohol given to rats does not produce liver damage unless accompanied by a diet deficient in essential nutrients, particularly choline. Baboons apparently develop cirrhosis when given alcohol even if the diet is good [40], whereas in rhesus monkeys, the liver damage induced by alcohol could be prevented by increasing dietary protein and choline [85]. Certainly patients with decompensated liver disease, given a third of their calories as alcohol together with a nutritious diet, improve steadily [84], whereas liver function does not improve with alcohol abstinence if dietary protein remains low [80]. Severe alcoholics, imbibing for a mean of 23.8 years, are usually protein-calorie malnourished and this can precede clinical evidence of liver dysfunction [52]. The role of nutrition in the perpetuation or initiation of alcoholic liver disease cannot be discounted [79]. Both nutrition and hepatotoxicity may act synergistically. Alcohol may increase the minimum daily requirements of choline, folic acid and other nutrients. Nutritional deficiencies, particularly of protein, may promote the toxic effects of alcohol by depleting hepatic amino acids and enzymes.

It seems likely that both alcohol and nutrition play a part in alcoholic hepato-toxicity, alcohol being the more important. There may be a range of alcohol intake that is tolerated without liver damage under optimal dietary conditions. However, it is also likely that there is a threshold of alcohol toxicity beyond which no protection is afforded by dietary manipulation [75].

Metabolism of alcohol (figs 20.5, 20.6) [96]

Alcohol cannot be stored and obligatory oxidation must take place, predominantly in the liver. The healthy individual cannot metabolize more than 160–180 g per day. Alcohol induces enzymes used in its catabolism, and the alcoholic, at least while his liver is relatively unaffected, may be able to metabolize more. One gram of alcohol gives seven calories, and alcoholics literally run on spirit. One litre of wine provides 670 calories and a half a litre of spirits 1200 calories. These empty calories make no contribution to nutrition other than to give energy.

The major route of ethanol oxidation is by initial conversion to acetaldehyde catabolized by the enzyme alcohol dehydrogenase (ADH) (fig. 20.6). This takes place in the cytosol. Acetaldehyde in mitochondria and cytosol may be

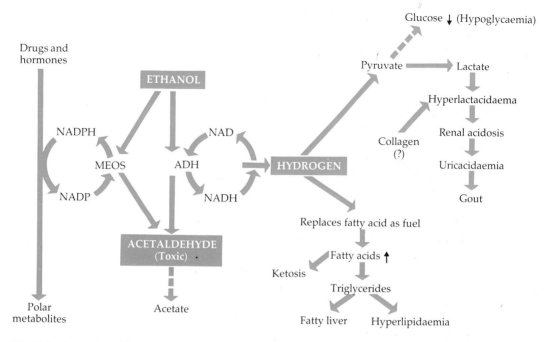

Fig. 20.5. Oxidation of alcohol in the hepatocyte. The production of acetaldehyde (toxic) is enhanced and conversion to acetate reduced. The hydrogen produced replaces fatty acid as a fuel so that fatty acids accumulate with consequent ketosis, triglyceridaemia, fatty liver and hyperlipidaemia. Unwanted hydrogen is used to convert pyruvate to lactate, which is produced in excess. Hyperlactacidaemia leads to renal acidosis, a rise in serum uric acid and gout. Collagen synthesis may be stimulated. Reduction of the pyruvate to glucose pathway results in hypoglycaemia.

Stimulation of the MEOS drug metabolizing system leads to drug and alcohol tolerance, and increased testosterone metabolism may be related to feminization and to infertility.

Broken lines indicate depressed pathways.

H = excess hydrogen equivalents; ADH = alcohol dehydrogenase; MEOS = microsomal ethanol oxidizing system; NAD = nicotinamide adenine dinucleotide; NADP = nicotinamide adenine dinucleotide phosphate (after Lieber 1978).

Ethanol $\xrightarrow{\text{ADH}}$ acetaldehyde $\xrightarrow{\text{ALDH}}$ acetate

Fig. 20.6. Alcohol metabolism in the liver. ADH = alcohol dehydrogenase; ALDH = acetaldehyde dehydrogenase.

injurious, causing membrane damage and cell necrosis. The acetaldehyde is converted to acetyl CoA with acetaldehyde dehydrogenase acting as a co-enzyme (fig. 20.5). This can be further broken down to acetate, which may be oxidized to carbon dioxide and water, or converted by the citric acid cycle to other biochemically important compounds including fatty acids. NAD is a co-factor and hydrogen acceptor when alcohol is converted to acetaldehyde and further to acetyl CoA. The NADH generated shuttles into the mitochondria and changes the NADH: NAD ratio and the redox state of the liver. The hydrogen generated replaces fatty acid as a fuel and is followed by triglyceride accumulation and fatty liver. The redox state of the liver changes, protein synthesis is inhibited and lipid peroxidation increases.

Alcohol dehydrogenase made by the stomach may play a role in metabolizing some alcohol and the gastric atrophy of the alcoholic may reduce this process.

The activity of the citric acid cycle is reduced, and this may be responsible for decreased fatty acid oxidation. Lipoprotein synthesis is increased by alcohol. The NADH may serve as the hydrogen barrier for the conversion of pyruvate to lactate and blood lactate and uric acid levels rise after alcohol. Post-alcoholic hypoglycaemia and gout after alcohol ingestion may be explained by this mechanism. The conversion of alcohol to acetaldehyde also leads to inhibition of protein synthesis.

Alcohol is also metabolized by a microsomal ethanol oxidizing system (MEOS). This is inducible by alcohol and microsomal P-450 increases after alcohol. A specific form of P-450, 11 E1, has a high affinity for alcohol and for some drugs such as paracetamol (acetaminophen) and carcinogens [42]. This accounts for the susceptibility of the alcoholic to drugs such as paracetamol which are hepatotoxic on account of metabolites and when given in recognized therapeutic doses can cause serious liver injury (Chapter 18).

Enhanced metabolism of toxic substances to carcinogens may increase the risk of cancer [42].

Mechanisms of liver injury [40, 42]

Relation to alcohol and its metabolites

Only a fatty liver is produced by alcohol in rodents. Rats, however, cannot match the quantities of alcohol consumed by the human alcoholic who may take 50% of total calories as alcohol. This level can be achieved in the baboon, who after 2−5 years of alcoholism, develops cirrhosis [40]. However, in another study, baboons receiving 70% of their calories as alcohol with an adequate diet for 30 months failed to produce significant liver damage [1]. Evidence for the direct hepato-toxic affect of alcohol, apart from nutritional changes, comes from human volunteers, both normal and alcoholic who, after 10−20 ounces (300−600 dl) of 86% proof alcohol daily for 8−10 days, develop fatty change and EM abnormalities on liver biopsy [40].

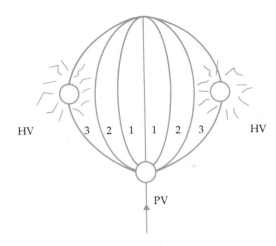

Fig. 20.7. Zone 3 collagenosis HV hepatic venule PV portal venule.

Acetaldehyde [78]

Acetaldehyde, is the major product of hepatic ethanol oxidation. It is oxidized by the liver. The enzyme responsible is an NAD^+-linked acetaldehyde dehydrogenase (fig. 20.6). In the rat this enzyme is mitochondrial but in man cytosolic acetaldehyde dehydrogenase may be important [33]. Blood acetaldehyde levels in alcoholics are increased after chronic ethanol consumption, but only very small amounts of acetaldehyde leave the liver. Acetaldehyde is metabolically extremely reactive and toxic (table 20.3). It binds to phospholipids, amino acid residues and sulphydryl groups. Acetaldehyde reacts with serotonin, dopamine and noradrenaline, yielding pharmacologically active compounds. It affects the plasma membranes by depolymerizing proteins and producing altered surface antigens. It forms stable protein−acetaldehyde adducts which may stimulate antibody formation. It may stimulate collagen synthesis [30].

Changes in the intracellular redox potential

The marked increase in the NADH:NAD ratio in hepatocytes actively oxidizing produces profound metabolic consequences. Thus the redox ratio of lactate to pyruvate is markedly

Table 20.3. The possible hepatotoxic effects of acetaldehyde

1 Increases lipid peroxidation
2 Binds plasma membranes
3 Interferes mitochondrial electron-transport chain
4 Inhibits nuclear repair
5 Interferes with microtubule function
6 Forms adducts with proteins
7 Activates complement
8 Stimulates superoxide formation by neutrophils
9 Increases collagen synthesis

increased, leading to lactic acidosis. This acidosis, in conjunction with ketosis, impairs urate excretion and leads to gout. The altered redox potential has also been implicated in the pathogenesis of fatty liver, collagen formation, altered steroid metabolism and impaired gluconeogenesis [40].

In man, in contrast to the rat, the entire pathway from ethanol to acetate is in the cytosol, so that these unfavourable redox changes are unlikely to be particularly striking. This may underlie the greater susceptibility of man to alcoholic liver diseases compared with many experimental animals.

Mitochondria. Morphological changes in mitochrondria are a feature of alcoholic liver injury [10]. Functionally the mitochondria are probably abnormal, certainly in the baboon model. This may be due to damage by acetaldehyde. However, in early alcoholic liver disease in man, mitochondrial enzymes are normal [33], although later functional abnormalities undoubtedly do develop.

Liver cell water and protein retention

Using rat liver slices, alcohol inhibits secretion of newly synthesized glycoprotein and albumin by the hepatocyte [5]. This may be due to acetaldehyde binding to tubulin so impairing the microtubules of the cytoskeleton on which protein secretion from the cell depends [5, 99]. In rats fed alcohol, fatty acid binding protein increases and this accounts for some of the total rise in cytosolic protein [81].

Water is retained in proportion to the protein and the resultant hepatocyte swelling is the major cause of hepatomegaly in alcoholics.

Hypermetabolic state

Chronic alcohol ingestion results in an increased consumption of oxygen. This seems largely to be due to the increased mitochondrial re-oxidation of NADH. The hypermetabolic state has been confirmed in hepatocytes isolated from alcohol-fed animals, and this is directly related to cell viability. The increased oxygen requirement in the liver following chronic alcohol consumption results in a steeper oxygen gradient along the sinusoidal length so that cell necrosis in hepatitis is in zone 3 (centrizonal). It is conceivable that necrosis in this area may be hypoxic [70].

Enzymes metabolizing alcohol to acetaldehyde are found in greatest concentration in zone 3 where the redox changes are also most marked.

Increased liver fat

Increased amounts of fat can be of exogenous (dietary) origin, can come from adipose tissue being transported to the liver as free fatty acids, or can come from lipids synthesized in the liver itself. The origin depends upon the dose of ethanol ingested and the lipid content of the diet. After an acute isolated ingestion of a large dose of ethanol the fatty acids found in the liver originate from adipose tissue, whereas following chronic ingestion, there is an increased synthesis and decreased degradation of fatty acids in the liver.

Immunological liver damage

Occasional progression of hepatic injury, despite cessation of alcohol intake, has been attributed to immunological mechanisms. In some patients, the histological appearances resemble those of other types of chronic active hepatitis with mononuclear cell accumulations, piecemeal necrosis and rosette formation [26, 67].

In alcohol-related liver disease, cell-mediated immunity is impaired, as judged by *in vitro* tests of suppressor cell function and helper/ suppressor cell ratios [2], but such abnormalities probably reflect no more than systemic illness.

There is increased prevalence of non-organ specific antibodies with alcoholic liver injury. Liver specific autoantibodies (anti-LSP and anti-LMA) may circulate. Patients with alcoholic hepatitis may have antibodies reacting with ethanol-altered rabbit liver cell membrane antigens (3, 68). Circulating lymphocytes from patients with alcoholic hepatitis are directly cytotoxic to different target cells. However, peripheral lymphocytes may not be important and may not reflect what is actually happening in the liver. All these immunological reactions are difficult to interpret and may be consequences of the liver injury rather than causal.

Mallory's alcoholic hyaline has been invoked as a possible neoantigen [35], but there are doubts concerning the purity of the material and the results have not been confirmed.

Immunological mechanisms may be concerned in the perpetuation of liver damage in a limited number of alcoholics, who show liver damage and abnormal immunological response.

Fibrosis

In the alcoholic baboon and in man, cirrhosis can develop from fibrosis without an intervening acute alcoholic hepatitis [82]. The mechanism of the fibrosis is uncertain. Lactic acid, which increases fibrogenesis, seems to be related to any severe liver disease [90].

The fibrosis is due to transformation of fat-storing Ito cells to fibroblasts and myofibroblasts. Type III procollagen is found in these presinusoidal collagen deposits (fig. 20.7) [54, 57]. Alcohol dehydrogenase can be found in the Ito cells of rat liver [104].

Although cell necrosis is the major stimulus to collagen formation there are other possibilities. Centrizonal (zone 3) anoxia might be the stimulus. Increased intracellular pressure due to hepatocyte enlargement is another possible fibrogenic stimulus [6].

The inflammatory response

Leucotrienes might be produced by the hepatocyte as it metabolizes alcohol or could be related to impairment of hepatocyte uptake and metabolism. Although leucotrienes are undoubtedly important mediators of inflammatory liver disease, their relation to alcoholic damage remains unclear [37].

The macrophages, lymphocytes and polymorphs infiltrating the alcohol damaged liver might release cytokines which could increase fibrosis [105].

It is known that hepatocyte membranes altered by acetaldehyde can increase free radical production by polymorphoneutrophils.

A neutrophil chemotactic factor inactivator is increased in patients with alcoholic liver disease and this may contribute to the predisposition to infection.

Morphological changes

The changes are usually classified into fatty liver, alcoholic hepatitis and cirrhosis [23, 31].

FATTY LIVER (steatosis) (fig. 20.11)

The fat accumulates in zones 3 and 2 (centrizonal and mid-zonal). In the more severely affected, the fatty change is diffuse. The fat may be present as macrovesicular, large droplet form. Less often it is in micro-vesicular (small droplet) form.

Large fat droplets appear in hepatocytes within three to seven days of excess alcohol ingestion.

Microvesicular, small-droplet, fat represents more active lipid synthesis by the hepatocyte.

ALCOHOLIC HEPATITIS

Acute and chronic inflammation of the liver

develops in response to alcohol-induced hepato-cellular damage. It may occur separately or be combined with an established cirrhosis. Hepatocytes are swollen, and the cytoplasm is granular, film-like and often dispersed into fine strands. The nucleus is small and hyperchromatic.

Mallory's alcoholic hyaline bodies are seen as intracytoplasmic inclusions within swollen hepatocytes; they usually stain a purplish red with haematoxylin and eosin, but are more readily seen with connective tissue stains like Masson's trichrome or chromotrope aniline blue (figs 20.10, 20.11). They are found in centrizonal areas and they may persist for as long as six months after alcohol withdrawal. They consist of intermediate filaments of varying thickness which are randomly orientated [22]. They are apparently connected to plasma membrane vesicles and the nucleus. They may result from failure of microtubules which leads to intermediate filament increase within the hepatocyte. The polymorph reaction is related to necrotic and Mallory-containing hepatocytes, polymorphs being arrayed around them in satellite fashion. Polymorphs can also be seen within the injured hepatocytes.

Giant mitochondria form globular intracytoplasmic inclusions, sometimes surrounded by a distinct halo.

Pericellular fibrosis is in zone 3 (fig. 20.8). Collagen fibres are perisinusoidal and enclose normal or ballooned hepatocytes. The picture produced is like lattice or chicken wire and has also been termed 'creeping collagenosis' [21].

Collagenization of the space of Dissë can be shown by electron microscopy (fig. 20.9). Eventually a continuous membrane forms under the sinusoidal endothelium [88]. This change may impede interchange between blood and hepatocytes and so contribute to reduction in hepatocyte function [70] and to portal hypertension. Venous lesions include lymphocytic phlebitis in terminal hepatic venules and sublobular veins, perivenular scarring with gradual obliteration of the lumen of terminal hepatic venules and veno-occlusive lesions consisting of intimal proliferation, fibrosis and narrowing of the lumen of terminal hepatic venules and occasionally portal veins [27].

Portal zone changes are inconspicuous with mild to moderate chronic inflammatory infiltrate in the advanced case. Marked portal zone fibrosis suggests a complicating chronic pancreatitis (fig. 20.15) [62].

Occasionally the histological picture is of chronic active hepatitis [26] but this is very rare.

The histological patterns form a spectrum from minimal alcoholic hepatitis to an

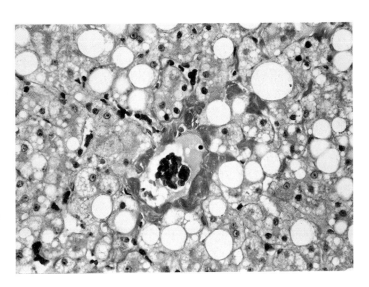

Fig. 20.8. Perivenular (zone 3) and phlebosclerosis fibrosis with adjacent fatty change. (Chromophobe aniline blue ×100).

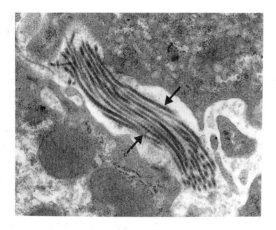

Fig. 20.9. Electron micrograph of liver in patient with alcoholic liver disease. Note deposition of collagen fibrils in Dissë's space (arrowed). This could interfere with oxygen and metabolite exchange between blood and hepatocyte.

advanced, probably irreversible, picture, where necrosis is more extensive and fibrotic scars form [31]. Alcoholic hepatitis can be regarded as a precursor of cirrhosis.

Hyperplastic nodules develop in those who reduce their oxygen consumption [25]. This suggests that alcohol inhibits hepato-cellular proliferation.

CIRRHOSIS

Classically, cirrhosis of the alcoholic is of micro-nodular type (fig. 20.13). No normal lobular architecture can be identified, and zone 3 venules are difficult to find. The formation of regenerative nodules is often slow because of a presumed inhibitory effect of alcohol on hepatic regeneration. The amount of fat is variable and acute alcoholic hepatitis may or may not co-exist. With continuing necrosis and replacement fibrosis, the cirrhosis may progress from a micro- to a macronodular pattern, but this is usually accompanied by a reduction in steatosis. When this end-stage picture is reached, an alcoholic aetiology is difficult to confirm on histological grounds.

Cirrhosis may follow pericellular fibrosis without apparent hepatic necrosis and inflammation [23]. Zone 3 myofibroblastic proliferation and collagen deposition may be the first

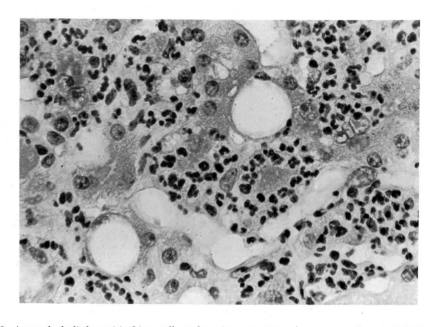

Fig. 20.10. Acute alcoholic hepatitis. Liver cells undergoing necrosis and containing clumps of Mallory's hyaline are surrounded by cuffs of polymorphonuclear cells. There is fatty change. H & E, ×120.

apparent lesions in the sequence of events leading to alcoholic cirrhosis.

Increased hepatic iron can be related to increased iron absorption, the iron content of beverages (especially wines), haemolysis and porta−caval shunting. Body iron stores are only moderately increased [32].

Early recognition

This depends on a high index of suspicion on the part of the physician. A patient may present with non-specific digestive symptoms such as anorexia, morning nausea with dry retching, diarrhoea, vague right upper abdominal pain and tenderness or pyrexia.

The patient may seek medical advice because of the effects of alcoholism such as social disruption, poor work performance, accidents, violent behaviour, fits, tremulousness or depression.

The diagnosis may be made when hepatomegaly, a raised serum transaminase or gamma-glutamyl transpeptidase level or macrocytosis are discovered at a routine examination, for instance at a life insurance checkup or during investigation of another condition.

Physical signs may be non-contributory, although tender hepatomegaly, prominent vascular spiders and associated features of alcoholism may be helpful. The clinical features do not reflect the hepatic histology and biochemical tests of liver function may be normal.

BIOCHEMICAL TESTS

Serum transaminase levels are only modestly increased. SGOT (AST), which is derived from alcoholic damage to mitochondria or smooth muscle generally, is more increased than the SGPT (ALT) which is confined to the liver. The relatively low serum aspartate transaminase levels and the high SGOT:SGPT ratio are also reflected by changes in the liver activities of these enzymes [50]. Pyridoxal 5-phosphate, the biologically active form of vitamin B_6, is necessary for the activity of both transaminases.

In alcoholics, pyridoxal 5-phosphate depletion is partially responsible for the high SGOT:SGPT ratio. In alcoholic liver disease, this ratio usually exceeds 2.

The serum gamma-glutamyl transpeptidase (GGTP) is a widely used screening test for alcohol abuse. The rise results mainly from hepatic induction of the enzyme, although hepatocellular damage and cholestasis may contribute. There are many false positives due to factors other than alcohol, such as drugs, other diseases and the patient having a value at the upper limit of the normal range.

Serum alkaline phosphatase may be markedly increased (greater than four times normal) especially in those with severe cholestasis and alcoholic hepatitis [77]. Serum IgA values may be very high.

Various combinations of haematological and biochemical tests have been advocated. Using quadratic multiple discriminant analysis of 25 commonly ordered laboratory tests, 100% of non-alcoholics without overt liver disease, 98% of alcoholism treatment programme patients with mild liver involvement, 96% of alcoholics with liver disease and 89% of non-alcoholics with liver disease were correctly classified [86].

Blood alcohol levels can be used in the clinic to refute the individual who has a high blood alcohol level but denies imbibing.

Non-specific serum changes in acute and chronic alcoholism include elevations in uric acid, lactate, triglyceride and reductions in glucose, phosphate and magnesium. Low serum tri-iodothyronine (T3) levels presumably reflect decreased hepatic conversion of T3 to T4. Levels correlate inversely with the severity of alcoholic liver disease.

Serum procollagen type 111 peptides are under study [87].

Other serum tests are markers of chronic alcohol intake rather than alcoholic liver damage. They include serum glutamate dehydrogenase [34], the mitochondrial isoenzyme of aspartate transaminase [43, 64] and desialylated transferrin [94, 97].

Even sensitive biochemical methods may fail

to reveal alcoholic liver damage, and liver biopsy is necessary in cases of doubt.

HAEMATOLOGICAL CHANGES

Macrocytosis (MCV) greater than 95 μm is very useful for screening. It is presumably due to a direct effect of alcohol on bone marrow. Deficiencies of folate and vitamin B_{12} contribute in the malnourished.

LIVER BIOPSY

This confirms the presence of liver disease and identifies alcohol abuse as the likely cause. The dangers of the liver damage can be emphasized more forcibly to the patient.

Liver biopsy is important prognostically. Fatty change alone is not nearly so serious as perivenular sclerosis, which is a precursor of cirrhosis [92]. An established cirrhosis can be confirmed.

Diagnostic difficulties may arise when the histological picture of alcoholic liver disease is shown in a patient who denies alcohol abuse. Other causes are Indian childhood cirrhosis, gross obesity, jejuno-ileal bypass operation, Wilson's disease, diabetes, prolonged parenteral nutrition and drugs such as perihexilene or amiodarone (table 20.4).

PORTAL HYPERTENSION

Splenomegaly is not prominent. Portal hypertension and gastrointestinal bleeding, however, are frequent at all stages. Bleeding comes not only from oesophageal varices but from duodenal ulcers, gastritis and Mallory—Weiss lower oesophageal tears following repeated vomiting.

The portal hypertension may be related to cirrhosis. Fatty change and zone 3 collagenosis (perivenular sclerosis) lead to a presinusoidal portal hypertension [27]. Collagenization of the space of Disse decreases sinusoidal diameter, increases resistance to sinusoidal blood flow and raises portal pressure [70]. An increase in hepatocyte volume may also be a factor [6].

Table 20.4. Differential diagnosis of the hepatic histological picture of alcoholic hepatitis in the non-alcoholic

Condition	Diagnostic points
Diabetes and prediabetes	Fasting blood glucose
Obesity	Body weight
Jejuno—ileal bypass	History
Prolonged parenteral nutrition	History—cholestasis
Wilson's disease	Kayser—Fleischer ring Copper metabolism
Drugs: Amiodarone	History
Indian childhood cirrhosis	Age—clinical picture Excess liver copper

SCANNING

With severe acute alcoholic hepatitis or advanced cirrhosis isotopes, such as technetium, are hardly taken up by the liver because the blood shunts past the reticulo-endothelial cells.

Ultrasound will not detect minimal change, fat or fibrosis. However, in more advanced alcoholic liver disease, the liver is diffusely abnormal and the changes correlate with those seen on liver biopsy.

CT scanning is very useful in demonstrating fatty liver (low attenuation), irregular liver surface, splenomegaly, portal collateral circulation, ascites and pancreatitis (fig. 19.9).

Clinical syndromes

FATTY LIVER

The patients are usually asymptomatic, diagnosis being made when an enlarged, smooth, firm liver is discovered. In these patients liver function tests may be normal or the transaminases and alkaline phosphatase slightly increased. If the alcoholic fatty liver is sufficiently severe to merit admission to hospital the patient has usually been drinking heavily for some time and has lost his appetite. There may be nausea and vomiting with periumbilical, epigastric or right upper quadrant pain. Clinically, the fatty liver patient cannot be separated from one with mild alcoholic hepatitis. Needle liver biopsy is essential to diagnose alcoholic hepatitis.

ACUTE HEPATITIS

The clinical picture is variable, from a mild syndrome resembling fatty liver through to severe, life-threatening liver decompensation.

In the milder form the symptoms are fatigue, anorexia and weight loss, with a large, tender liver.

In the more severe, the patient has usually been drinking particularly heavily. The severe hepatic decompensation may be precipitated by vomiting, diarrhoea, an intercurrent infection such as pneumonia or an infection of the urinary tract, or by prolonged anorexia. Otherwise unexplained pyrexia is usual.

The patient may be obese, but some features of malnutrition are present in 90% of patients. The blood pressure is usually low, with a hyperdynamic circulation. Signs of associated vitamin deficiencies, such as beri beri, scurvy or a raw, red tongue, are usual in the malnourished ('skid row') type of alcoholic. The liver is very large, smooth, firm and tender. An arterial bruit may be heard over the liver, causing confusion with the diagnosis of primary liver cancer. The spleen is not palpable unless there is a concomitant cirrhosis. Ascites often develops rapidly. Diarrhoea with steatorrhoea can be related to decreased biliary excretion of bile salts, to pancreatic insufficiency and to a direct, toxic effect of alcohol on the intestinal mucosa.

Patients with acute fatty liver may die suddenly in shock, attributable to pulmonary fat emboli. Sudden deaths have also been reported in hypoglycaemia.

Gastrointestinal haemorrhage is frequently from a local gastric or dudodenal lesion, and is secondary to the general bleeding tendency, rather than related to portal hypertension.

Acute alcoholic hepatitis may be confused with acute virus hepatitis. Helpful diagnostic points are the florid vascular spiders, the very large liver and the leucocytosis.

Laboratory tests. The serum aspartate transaminase is only mildly increased, usually less than 100 IU/ml. The SGOT:SGPT ratio is greater than two. Serum alkaline phosphatase levels are usually increased.

The severity is best correlated with the serum bilirubin level and prothrombin time after Vitamin K administration [44]. Serum IgA is markedly increased with IgG and IgM raised to a much lesser extent, and serum IgG falls with improvement. The serum albumin level is decreased, increasing as the patient improves. Serum cholesterol levels are usually increased.

The serum potassium value is particularly low, largely due to the low dietary protein intake, to diarrhoea, and to secondary hyperaldosteronism if fluid retention is present. Albumin-bound serum zinc is decreased, and this is related to a low liver zinc concentration, not found in patients with non-alcoholic liver disease. The blood urea and creatinine values increase and these reflect severity. They predict the development of the hepato-renal syndrome.

Alcoholic liver disease is associated with severely decreased hepatic vitamin A levels, even when liver injury is moderate (fatty liver) and when blood levels of vitamin A and prealbumin are still unaffected [39].

A polymorph leucocytosis of about $15-20 \times 10^9$ is found in about a third of patients in proportion to the severity of the alcoholic hepatitis.

Platelet function is depressed even in the absence of thrombocytopenia or of alcohol in the blood [55]. The changes reverse on abstention.

HEPATIC CIRRHOSIS

Established cirrhosis can present without a stage of acute alcoholic hepatitis having been recognized clinically or histologically and the picture can resemble any end-stage liver disease. The points suggesting an alcoholic aetiology include the history of alcohol abuse (which may be forgotten), the hepatomegaly

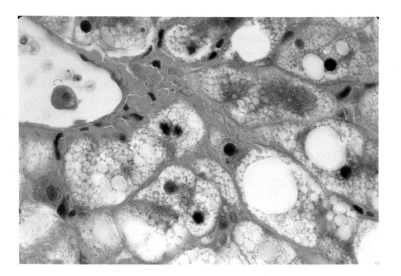

Fig. 20.11. Acute alcoholic hepatitis: hepatocytes are ballooned and contain micro- and macro-vesicular fat and clumps of purplish-red Mallory's alcoholic hyaline. (Chromophobe aniline blue ×100).

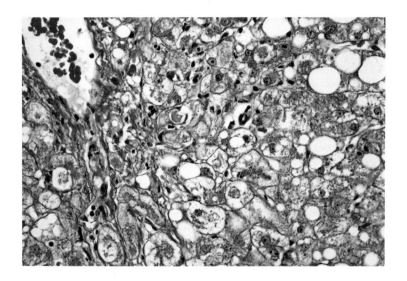

Fig. 20.12. Advanced zone 3 collagenosis with fatty change. Thickened hepatic vein is upper left. (Chromophobe aniline blue ×100).

and the associated features of alcoholism. Splenomegaly is a late feature.

Liver biopsy findings supporting an alcoholic aetiology include a micronodular cirrhosis, perivenular sclerosis and paucity of hepatic veins. In many instances, however, it is impossible on histological grounds to determine an alcoholic cause [31].

CHOLESTATIC SYNDROMES

Occasionally, the patient may present with deep jaundice, hepatomegaly and an increase in serum alkaline phosphatase, transaminases and cholesterol [48, 98]. Functional renal failure is usual. This is usually the first episode of decompensation.

Liver biopsy shows massive accumulation of microvesicular fat (fig. 20.11) with cholestasis in centrizonal areas. Inflammation is inconspicuous and there is little or no hyaline. Electron microscopy shows extensive disorganization of the organelles in affected hepatocytes. The condition has been termed *alcoholic foamy degeneration* [98] Prognosis is very variable.

Cholestasis may also be due to compression of the intra-hepatic portion of the common bile duct by chronic pancreatitis (89). ERCP confirms the diagnosis (figs 20.15, 20.16)

RELATIONSHIP OF ALCOHOLIC LIVER
DISEASE TO HEPATITIS B

Markers of past or current hepatitis B are commoner in patients with alcoholic liver disease than in the general population [29]. There is, however, considerable doubt as to which is the cart and which is the horse for, when liver biopsies are performed, the underlying changes are not those of alcoholism, suggesting that hepatitis B or another aetiological agent is the primary event. Alcohol may enhance the liver damage caused by hepatitis B and carriers should be advised to abstain from alcohol or take very small amounts [101].

Hepato-cellular cancer occasionally develops in the alcoholic cirrhotic liver, usually after a period of abstention when a macronodular cirrhosis has developed (Chapter 28) [41].

There is a strong association between hepatitis B and cancer developing in an alcoholic. Integrated hepatitis B sequences are frequently found in the livers of alcoholic patients with primary liver cancer.

Associated features

The occasional, bilaterally enlarged parotids may be analogous to those seen with other types of malnutrition. Gynaecomastia often appears after treatment and is a frequent complication of spironolactone therapy. The testes atrophy and infertility may be a feature. Muscle mass wastes.

Dupuytren's contracture of the palmar fascia

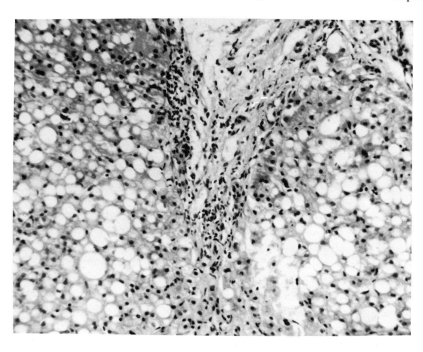

Fig. 20.13. Cirrhosis of the alcoholic. Fibrous bands divide the liver into small regular nodules. Fatty change is conspicuous. H & E, ×120.

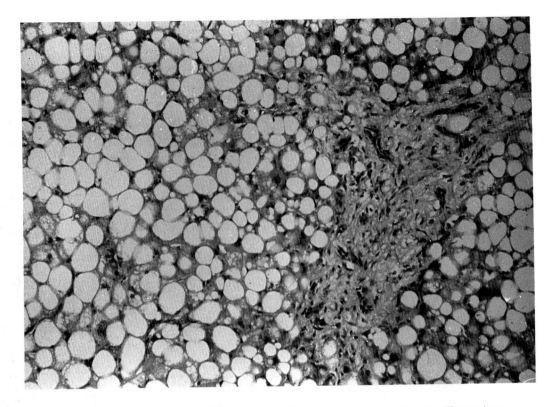

Fig. 20.14. Portal zone (zone 1) with marked fibrosis and fatty change in the hepatocytes. This patient suffered from chronic alcoholic pancreatitis with partial biliary obstruction (H & E, ×120).

is related to the alcoholism and not to the cirrhosis [9].

Loss of memory and concentration, insomnia, irritability, hallucinations, convulsions, 'rum-fits' and tremor may be the stigmata of alcoholism. These must be distinguished from early hepatic pre-coma.

Hepato-renal syndrome seems particularly common in alcoholics.

Serum IgA is increased and deposits are found along the sinusoids. They are probably related to local stimulation of the secretory immune system [100]. They are probably unrelated to liver damage.

Renal glomerular abnormalities, in particular mesangial expansion with deposits of IgA, are frequently found in patients showing glomerulo-nephritis and renal failure [57]. Other constituents of the deposits are Mallory-body antigen and complement [12].

Impaired renal acidification in alcoholic liver disease may be a sign of liver cell failure [73].

Prognosis

The prognosis in alcoholics is much better than with other forms of cirrhosis. Everything depends on whether the alcoholic can overcome his addiction. This in turn is related to family support, financial resources and socio-economic state. In a large group of working-class, often 'skid row' type, alcoholic cirrhotics studied in Boston, the mean life expectancy for men was 33 months, compared with 16 months for a non-alcoholic group of cirrhotics [24]. In a study at Yale, the patients of a higher socio-economic class, with cirrhosis complicated by ascites, jaundice and haematemesis, showed an overall 5-year survival of 50%. If they persisted in alcoholism, this fell to 40%, whereas if

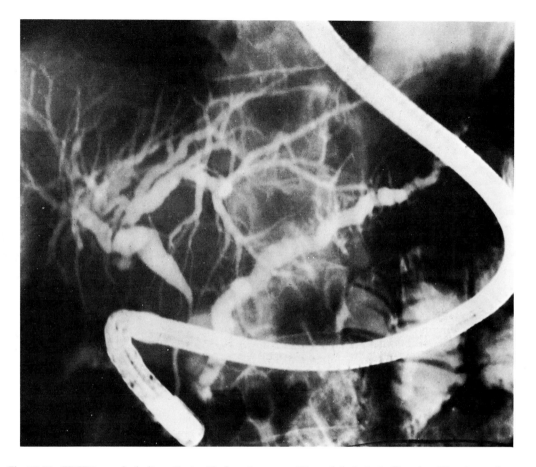

Fig. 20.15. ERCP in an alcoholic patient with chronic pancreatitis and cholestasis. Showing dilatation and irregularity of the pancreatic duct and smooth constriction of the common bile duct as it passes behind the inflamed pancreas (Scott *et al.* 1977).

they abstained it was 60% [83]. Very similar figures come from the United Kingdom (fig. 20.17) [11]. It is generally agreed that continued heavy drinking is associated with poor survival for alcoholic cirrhotics [7].

Women with alcoholic cirrhosis survive a shorter time than men (fig. 20.18).

Liver biopsy appearances give the best indication of prognosis. Zone 3 fibrosis and perivenular sclerosis are very unfavourable features [48, 103]. At present this lesion can only be detected by liver biopsy with appropriate connective tissue staining.

In one study, 50% of patients with alcoholic hepatitis developed cirrhosis after 10 to 13 years [73]. In another study, 23% of patients with

alcoholic liver disease but without cirrhosis developed it after an average of 8.1 years [48]. Fatty change is probably not a risk factor. Over a given threshold of 40 to 50 g of alcohol daily, the risk of developing cirrhosis is unrelated to average daily alcohol consumption.

Patients with fibrosis and nodules *per se* but without hepatitis have the same prognosis as those with non-cirrhotic liver disease without hepatitis and usually with fatty liver [71].

Features with independent but bad prognostic significance seem to be encephalopathy, low serum albumin, increased prothrombin time and low haemoglobin level [69]. Pre-coma, persistent jaundice and azotaemia are bad signs and patients with these features are very liable

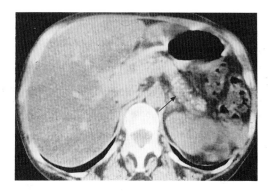

Fig. 20.16. CT scan showing an enlarged fatty liver with a chronic calcific pancreatitis (arrowed).

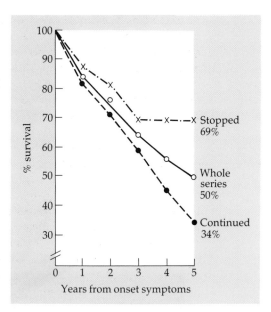

Fig. 20.17. The probability of survival of patients with established alcoholic liver disease: 50% survived five years, 69% of those who abstained from alcohol were alive at five years, but only 34% of those who continued to imbibe (Brunt *et al.* 1974).

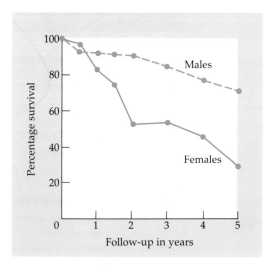

Fig. 20.18. The percentage survival of males and females with cirrhosis of the alcoholic.

to develop the hepato-renal syndrome.

The patient with decompensated cirrhosis improves slowly. Overt jaundice and ascites after three months carry a grave prognosis. Even total abstention may not improve the prognosis when portal hypertension is prominent. In the very late, irreversible stage, abstinence from alcohol cannot be expected to affect the prognosis. The damage has been done and there is no turning back. The highest mortality for patients with either cirrhosis or alcoholic hepatitis or both is in the first year of follow-up [71].

Megamitochondria on liver biopsy categorize a mild illness with a good long-term survival [15].

Patients with acute alcoholic hepatitis often deteriorate during the first few weeks in hospital. It may take 1−6 months for resolution, and 20−50% die. Those with a markedly prolonged prothrombin time, unresponsive to intramuscular vitamin K and with a serum bilirubin level greater than 20 mg, have a particularly bad outlook [44]. Alcoholic hepatitis is slow to resolve even in those who abstain [23].

Treatment

The most important measure is to ensure total and immediate abstinence from alcohol. Patients with severe physical ailments are more likely to abstain than those who present

psychological problems. In a long-term follow-up of men attending a liver clinic, severe medical illness was critical in the decision to stop drinking [75]. Continued medical care is also essential. The development of a with-drawal syndrome (delirium tremens) should be anticipated by the administration of chlormethiazole or chlordiazepoxide [13]. Improvement following abstinence and bed rest may be so striking that it is virtually diagnostic of previous alcoholism.

During 'drying out' or recovery from hepatic decompensation, the alcoholic requires dietary supplements of protein and vitamins. Dietary protein should be 0.5 g per kg initially, increasing to 1 g per kg as soon as possible. Encephalopathy may restrict protein intake. Potassium stores are usually low and supplements of potassium chloride together with magnesium and zinc are usually given to patients with decompensated alcoholic liver disease. Vitamins, especially the B complex, C and K are given in large doses, if necessary intravenously.

· Stable middle-class alcoholics should, of course, be advised to abstain completely particularly if the liver biopsy shows zone 3 fibrosis. If they fail they should be encouraged to take at least 2000 calories daily of a well-balanced diet containing 1 g protein per kg body weight. Modest vitamin supplements are advisable (table 20.5) [91].

Acute alcoholic hepatitis

The measures recommended for encephalopathy should be started. Ascites is treated cautiously as functional renal failure is a likely development.

The results of therapy with corticosteroids have been extremely conflicting. They seem to depend on the type of patient, the severity and on associated features such as presence or absence of cirrhosis, encephalopathy or renal failure. If liver biopsy is a necessary criterion for entry into any clinical trial, then the patients will inevitably be less seriously ill than those in whom impaired clotting prevents biopsy. In seven clinical trials of corticosteroid therapy in mild or moderately ill patients with acute alcoholic hepatitis, there seemed to be no effect on the rate of clinical recovery, improvement in

Table 20.5. Minimum daily requirements for an alcoholic (Sherlock 1984)

Item	Amounts	Remarks
Protein	1 g/kg body weight	Eggs, lean meat, cheese, chicken, liver
Calories	2000	Mixed foods with fruit and vegetables
Vitamins		
A	} One multivitamin tablet	or one carrot
B complex		or yeast
C		or one orange
		Sunlight
D		Good mixed diet
Folate		Good mixed diet
K_1		

biochemical tests or rate of histological progression [18]. In another study, methylprednisolone [1 g daily for three days) failed to affect mortality [95].

A further multi-centre trial showed that methylprednisolone improved short-term survival in patients with severe, alcoholic hepatitis [46], and in these desperate cases, corticosteroids may be tried. In most instances they are unnecessary [52].

Testosterone or anabolic-androgenic steroids have been used to treat alcoholic hepatitis and cirrhosis again with conflicting results [45]. In one study, oxandrolone given long-term (the patients had to survive 30 days) to those with moderately severe disease decreased mortality [52]. In another, oral testosterone apparently increased mortality [17]. These agents are not of proven value.

Severe protein malnutrition can favour immuno-incompetence and infections and exacerbate hypoalbuminaemia and ascites. Controlled trials of intravenous *amino acid supplementation* have given conflicting results. In one, 70 to 85 g daily lowered mortality and improved serum bilirubin and albumin concentrations [65]. In another, benefit was transient and not significant [19]. In yet another, sepsis and fluid retention were enhanced in the treated group, although serum bilirubin level was reduced [66]. Trials of branched-chain amino acid-enriched enteral diets have showed no effect on mortality [14, 53]. Oral or intravenous amino acid supplementation should be reserved for the very few jaundiced and obviously malnourished patients. Most patients can take adequate natural protein by mouth.

In a small controlled trial, the hepatotrophic factors insulin and glucagon were given with some benefit [4]. However, patients with hepato-cellular disease already have high plasma insulin and glucagon levels and further treatment with insulin may be dangerous.

Cirrhosis

Cirrhosis is irreversible and therapy has to be directed at the complications. These include portal hypertension, encephalopathy and ascites. Drug metabolism is impaired and particular care must be taken, especially with sedatives. Oxazepam seems to be the safest.

Porta−caval shunting in alcoholics is associated with a reduction of bleeding from varices, but a 30% incidence of hepatic encephalopathy and a marginal increase in survival. Results with the selective spleno−renal shunt are less good in alcoholic than in non-alcoholic patients. In general, alcoholics are not good candidates for surgical procedures, especially if they continue to imbibe.

Other measures

Hepatic transplantation is rarely done for alcoholic cirrhosis. It may be considered if the patient has taken no alcohol for six months, is psycho-socially stable and has no other alcohol-related disease [93].

In animals, chronic feeding of alcohol leads to a hypermetabolic state, with increased hepatic oxygen consumption abolished by pre-treatment with *propyl thiouracil*. This drug has been used in the short-term in patients with active alcoholic liver disease and improvement was enhanced [70]. A further double-blind

controlled trial of propyl thiouracil in severe alcoholic hepatitis showed no effect on survival or in the frequency or incidence of complications [28]. In yet another controlled trial of thiouracil (300 mg daily), the long-term mortality was reduced by half in the treated group and particularly in those who continued to drink modestly [72]. Drop-outs were equal in treated and placebo groups but, in fact, 104 of 157 patients failed to complete the trial; this must affect the significance of the results. It is uncertain whether a hepatic hypermetabolic state exists in human alcoholics and persists in those with severe alcoholic hepatitis, and this treatment has not been accepted [36, 77].

Colchicine inhibits microtubule-mediated transcellular movement of collagen. It has been used to treat alcoholic cirrhotics (see Chapter 19).

Cyanidanol-3 (catechin) is a bioflavonoid with free radical scavenger and anti-oxidant actions. In a randomized double-blind controlled trial over three months, the course of patients with pre-cirrhotic alcohol-related liver disease was not changed [16]. The treated patients consumed more alcohol.

References

1 Ainley C, Senapati A, Brown IMH *et al.* Is alcohol hepatotoxic in the baboon? *J. Hepatol.* 1988; **7**: 85.
2 Alexander GJM, Nouri-Aria K-T, Eddleston ALWF *et al.* Contrasting relations between suppressor-cell function and suppressor-cell number in chronic liver disease. *Lancet* 1983; **i:** 1291.
3 Anthony RS, Farquharson M, MacSween RNM. Liver membrane antibodies in alcoholic liver disease. II. Antibodies to ethanol-altered hepatocytes. *J. clin. Pathol.* 1983; **36**: 1302.
4 Baker AL, Jaspan JB, Haines NW *et al.* A randomized clinical trial of insulin and glucagon infusion for treatment of alcoholic hepatitis: progress report on 50 patients. *Gastroenterology* 1981; **80**: 1410.
5 Baraona E, Leo MA, Borowsky SA *et al.* Pathogenesis of alcohol-induced accumulation of protein in the liver. *J. clin. Invest.* 1977; **60**: 546.
6 Blendis LM, Orrego H, Crossley IR *et al.* The role of hepatocyte enlargement in hepatic pressure in cirrhotic and noncirrhotic alcoholic liver disease.

Hepatology 1982; **2**: 539.

7 Borowsky SA, Strome S, Lott E. Continued heavy drinking and survival in alcoholic cirrhosis. *Gastroenterology* 1981; **80**: 1405.

8 Bosron WF, Li T-K. Genetic polymorphism of human liver alcohol and aldehyde dehydrogenases, and their relation to alcohol metabolism and alcoholism. *Hepatology* 1986; **6**: 502.

9 Bradlow A, Mowat AG. Dupuytren's contracture and alcohol. *Ann. Rheum. Dis.* 1986; **45**: 304.

10 Bruguera M, Bertran A, Bombi JA *et al.* Giant mitochondria in hepatocytes. A diagnostic hint for alcoholic liver disease. *Gastroenterology* 1977; **73**: 1383.

11 Brunt PW, Kew MC, Scheuer PJ *et al.* Studies in alcoholic liver disease in Britain. I. Clinical and pathological patterns related to natural history. *Gut* 1974; **15**: 52.

12 Burns J, D'Ardenne AJ, Morton AJ *et al.* Immune complex nephritis in alcoholic cirrhosis: detection of Mallory body antigen in complexes by means of monoclonal antibodies to Mallory bodies. *J. clin. Path.* 1983; **36**: 751.

13 Burroughs AK, Morgan MY, Sherlock S. Double-blind controlled trial of bromocriptine, chlordiazepoxide and chlormethiazole for alcohol withdrawal symptoms. *Alcohol & Alcoholism* 1985; **20**: 263.

14 Calvey H, Davis M, Williams R. Controlled trial of nutritional supplementation, with and without branched chain amino acid enrichment, in treatment of acute alcoholic hepatitis. *J. Hepatol.* 1985; **1**: 141.

15 Chedid A, Mendenhall CL, Tosch T *et al.* Significance of megamitochondria in alcoholic liver disease. *Gastroenterology* 1986; **90**: 1858.

16 Colman JC, Morgan MY, Scheuer PJ *et al.* Treatment of alcohol-related liver disease with (+)-cyanidanol3: a randomised double-blind trial. *Gut* 1980; **21**: 965.

17 Copenhagen Study Group for Liver Disease. Testosterone treatment of men with alcoholic cirrhosis: a double-blind study. *Hepatology* 1986; **6**: 807.

18 Depew W, Boyer T, Omata M *et al.* Double-blind controlled trial of prednisolone therapy in patients with severe acute alcoholic hepatitis and spontaneous encephalopathy. *Gastroenterology* 1980; **78**: 524.

19 Diehl AM, Boitnott JK, Herlong HF *et al.* Effect of parenteral amino acid supplementation in alcoholic hepatitis. *Hepatology* 1985; **5**: 57.

20 Doffoel M, Tongio MM, Gut J-P *et al.* Relationships between 34 HLA-A, HLA-B and HLA-DR antigens and three serological markers of viral infections in alcoholic cirrhosis. *Hepatology* 1986; **6**: 457.

21 Edmondson HA, Peters RL, Reynolds TB *et al.* Sclerosing hyaline necrosis of the liver in the chronic alcoholic. A recognizable clinical syndrome. *Ann. intern. Med.* 1963; **59**: 646.

22 French SW. The Mallory body: structure, composition, and pathogenesis. *Hepatology* 1981; **1**: 76.

23 Galambos JT. Natural history of alcoholic hepatitis. III. Histological changes. *Gastroenterology* 1972; **63**: 1026.

24 Garceau AJ & The Boston Inter-Hospital Liver Group. The natural history of cirrhosis. II. The influence of alcohol and prior hepatitis on pathology and prognosis. *N. Engl. J. Med.* 1964; **271**: 1173.

25 Gluud C, Christoffersen P, Eriksen J *et al.* Influence of ethanol on development of hyperplastic nodules in alcoholic men with micronodular cirrhosis. *Gastroenterology* 1987; **93**: 256.

26 Goldberg SJ, Mendenhall CL, Connell AM *et al.* 'Non-alcoholic' chronic hepatitis in the alcoholic. *Gastroenterology* 1977; **72**: 598.

27 Goodman ZD, Ishak KG. Occlusive venous lesions in alcoholic liver disease. *Gastroenterology* 1982; **83**: 786.

28 Halle P, Pare P, Kaptein E *et al.* Double-blind, controlled trial of propylthiouracil in patients with severe acute alcoholic hepatitis. *Gastroenterology* 1982; **82**: 925.

29 Hislop WS, Follett EA, Bouchier IAD *et al.* Serological markers of hepatitis B in patients with alcoholic liver disease: a multi-centre survey. *J. clin. Pathol.* 1981; **34**: 1017.

30 Holt K, Bennett M, Chojkier M. Acetaldehyde stimulates collagen and noncollagen protein production by human fibroblasts. *Hepatology* 1984; **4**: 843.

31 International Group. Alcoholic liver disease: morphological manifestations. *Lancet* 1981; **i**: 707.

32 Jakobovits AW, Morgan MY, Sherlock S. Hepatic siderosis in alcoholics. *Dig. Dis. Sci.* 1979; **24**: 305.

33 Jenkins WJ, Peters TJ. Mitochondrial enzyme activities in liver biopsies from patients with alcoholic liver disease. *Gut* 1978; **19**: 341.

34 Jenkins WJ, Rosalki SB, Foo Y *et al.* Serum glutamate dehydrogenase is not a reliable marker of liver cell necrosis in alcoholics. *J. clin. Pathol.* 1982; **35**: 207.

35 Kanagasundaram N, Kakumu S, Chen T *et al.* Alcoholic hyaline antigen (AHAg) and antibody (AHAb) in alcoholic hepatitis. *Gastroenterology* 1977; **73**: 1368.

36 Kaplowitz N. Propylthiouracil treatment for alcoholic hepatitis: should it and does it work? *Gastroenterology* 1982; **82**: 1468.

37 Keppler D. Inflammatory mediation of alcoholic liver injury. *Molecular aspects of medicine 1988,*

Pergamon Press (in press).

38 Lelbach WK. Cirrhosis in the alcoholic and the relation to the volume of alcohol abuse. *Ann. NY Acad. Sci.* 1975; **252:** 85.

39 Leo MA, Sato M, Lieber CS. Effect of hepatic vitamin A depletion on the liver in humans and rats. *Gastroenterology* 1983; **84:** 562.

40 Lieber CS. *Medical disorders of alcoholism: pathogenesis and treatment.* WB Saunders, Philadelphia 1982.

41 Lieber CS, Garro A, Leo MA *et al.* Alcohol and cancer. *Hepatology* 1986; **5:** 1005.

42 Lieber CS. Biochemical and molecular basis of alcohol-induced injury to liver and other tissues. *New Engl. J. Med.* 1988; **319:** 1639.

43 Lumeng L. New diagnostic markers of alcohol abuse. *Hepatology* 1986; **4:** 742.

44 Maddrey WC, Boitnott JK, Bedine MS *et al.* Corticosteroid therapy of alcoholic hepatitis. *Gastroenterology* 1978; **75:** 193.

45 Maddrey WC. Is therapy with testosterone or anabolic-androgenic steroids useful in the treatment of alcoholic liver disease? *Hepatology* 1986; **6:** 1033.

46 Maddrey WC, Carithers RL Jr, Herlong HF *et al.* Prednisolone therapy in patients with severe alcoholic hepatitis: results of a multicenter trial. *Hepatology* 1986; **6:** 1202 Abst.

47 Maddrey WC. Hepatic effects of acetaminophen. Enhanced toxicity in alcoholics. *J. clin. Gastroenterol.* 1987; **9:** 180.

48 Marbet UA, Bianchi L, Meury U *et al.* Long-term histological evaluation of the natural history and prognostic factors of alcoholic liver disease. *J. Hepatol.* 1987; **4:** 364.

49 Marshall AW, Kingstone D, Boss M *et al.* Ethanol elimination in males and females: relationship to menstrual cycle and body composition. *Hepatology* 1983; **3:** 701.

50 Matloff DS, Selinger MJ, Kaplan MM. Hepatic transaminase activity in alcoholic liver disease. *Gastroenterology* 1980; **78:** 1389.

51 Mendenhall CL, Anderson S, Weesner RE *et al.* Protein calorie malnutrition associated with alcoholic hepatitis. Veterans Administration Cooperative Study Group on alcoholic hepatitis. *Am. J. Med.* 1984; **76:** 211.

52 Mendenhall CL, Anderson S, Garcia-Pont P *et al.* Short-term and long-term survival in patients with alcoholic hepatitis treated with oxandrolone and prednisolone. *N. Engl. J. Med.* 1984; **311:** 1464.

53 Mendenhall C, Bongiovanni G, Goldberg S *et al.* VA cooperative study on alcoholic hepatitis III: changes in protein calorie malnutrition associated with 30 days of hospitalization with and without enteral nutritional therapy. *J. parenter.*

enteral Nutr. 1985; **9:** 590.

54 Mezey E, Potter JJ, Maddrey WC. Hepatic collagen proline hydroxylase activity in alcoholic liver disease. *Clin. Clim. Acta.* 1976; **68:** 313.

55 Mikhailidis DP, Jenkins WJ, Barradas MA, Jeremy JY *et al.* Platelet function defects in chronic alcoholism. *Br. med. J.* 1986; **293:** 715.

56 Mills PR, Spooner RJ, Russell RI *et al.* Serum glutamate dehydrogenase as a marker of hepatocyte necrosis in alcoholic liver disease. *Br. med. J.* 1981; **283:** 754.

57 Minato Y, Hasumura Y, Takeuchi J. The role of fat-storing cells in Dissë space fibrogenesis in alcoholic liver disease. *Hepatology* 1983; **3:** 559.

58 Morgan MY. The epidemiology of alcoholic liver disease in the United Kingdom. In *Alcoholic Liver Disease* ed. P Hall, p 193. Edward Arnold, London 1985.

59 Morgan MY, Sherlock S. Sex-related differences among 100 patients with alcoholic liver disease. *Br. med. J.* 1977; **i:** 939.

60 Morgan MY, Ross MGR, Ng CM *et al.* HLA-B8 immunoglobulins and antibody responses in alcohol-related liver disease. *J. clin. Pathol.* 1980; **33:** 488.

61 Morgan MY, Sherlock S, Scheuer PJ. Acute cholestasis, hepatic failure and fatty liver in the alcoholic. *Scand. J. Gastroenterol.* 1978; **13:** 299.

62 Morgan MY, Sherlock S, Scheuer PJ. Portal fibrosis in the livers of alcoholic patients. *Gut* 1978; **19:** 1015.

63 Nakamoto MY, Iida H, Kobayashi K *et al.* Hepatic glomerulonephritis: characteristics of hepatic glomerulonephritis as the major part. *Virchow's Arch. [A]* 1981; **392:** 45.

64 Nalpas B, Vassault A, Charpin S *et al.* Serum mitochondrial aspartate aminotransferase as a marker of chronic alcoholism: diagnostic value and interpretation in a Liver Unit. *Hepatology* 1986; **4:** 608.

65 Nasrallah SM, Galambos JT. Aminoacid therapy of alcoholic hepatitis. *Lancet* 1980; **ii:** 1276.

66 Naveau S, Pelletier G, Poynard T *et al.* A randomized clinical trial of supplementary parenteral nutrition in jaundiced alcoholic cirrhotic patients. *Hepatology* 1986; **6:** 270.

67 Nei J, Matsuda Y, Takada A. Chronic hepatitis induced by alcohol. *Dig. Dis. Sci.* 1983; **28:** 207.

68 Neuberger J, Crossley IR, Saunders JB *et al.* Antibodies to alcohol-altered liver cell determinants in patients with alcoholic liver disease. *Gut* 1984; **25:** 300.

69 Orrego H, Israel Y, Blake JE *et al.* Assessment of prognostic factors in alcoholic liver disease: toward a global quantitative expression of severity. *Hepatology* 1983; **3:** 896.

70 Orrego H, Israel Y, Blendis LM. Alcoholic liver

disease: information in search of knowledge? *Hepatology* 1981; **1**: 267.

71 Orrego H, Blake JE, Blendis LM *et al.* Medline A. Prognosis of alcoholic cirrhosis in the presence and absence of alcoholic hepatitis. *Gastroenterology* 1987; **92**: 208.

72 Orrego H, Blake JE, Blendis LM *et al.* Long-term treatment of alcoholic liver disease with propylthiouracil. *N. Engl. J. Med.* 1987; **317**: 1421.

73 Pare P, Reynolds TB. Impaired renal acidification in alcoholic liver disease. *Arch. intern. Med.* 1984; **144**: 941.

74 Pares A, Caballeria J, Bruguera M *et al.* Histological course of alcoholic hepatitis. Influence of abstinence, sex and extent of hepatic damage. *J. Hepatol.* 1986; **2**: 33.

75 Patek AJ Jr, Hermos JA. Recovery from alcoholism in cirrhotic patients: a study of 45 cases. *Am. J. Med.* 1981; **70**: 782.

76 Pequignot G, Cyrulnik F. Chronic disease due to overconsumption of alcoholic drinks (excepting neuropsychiatric pathology). In *International Encyclopaedia of Pharmacology and Therapeutics*, Vol. II, Chapter 14, pp. 375–412. Pergamon Press, Oxford 1970.

77 Perrillo RP, Griffin R, De Schryver-Kecskemeti K *et al.* Alcoholic liver disease presenting with marked elevation of serum alkaline phosphatase. A combined clinical and pathological study. *Am. J. dig. Dis.* 1978; **23**: 1061.

78 Peters TJ, Ward RJ. Role of acetaldehyde in the pathogenesis of alcoholic liver disease. *Molecular Aspects of Medicine* 1988; **10**: 179

79 Phillips GB. Acute hepatic insufficiency of the chronic alcoholic revisited. *Am. J. Med.* 1983; **75**: 1.

80 Phillips GB, Gabuzda GJ Jr, Davidson CS. Comparative effects of a purified and an adequate diet on the course of fatty cirrhosis in the alcoholic. *J. clin. Invest.* 1952; **31**: 351.

81 Pignon J-P, Bailey NC, Baraona E *et al.* Fatty acid-binding protein: a major contributor to the ethanol-induced increase in liver cytosolic proteins in the rat. *Hepatology* 1987; **7**: 865.

82 Popper H, Lieber CS. Histogenesis of alcoholic fibrosis and cirrhosis in the baboon. *Am. J. Pathol.* 1980; **98**: 695.

83 Powell WJ Jr, Klatskin G. Duration of survival in patients with Laennec's cirrhosis. *Am. J. Med.* 1968; **44**: 406.

84 Reynolds TB, Redeker AG, Kuzma OT. Role of alcohol in pathogenesis of alcoholic cirrhosis. In *Therapeutic Agents and the Liver* p. 131, eds N McIntyre & S Sherlock. Blackwell Scientific Publications, Oxford. 1965.

85 Rogers AE, Fox JG, Whitney K *et al.* Acute and chronic effects of ethanol in non human primates. In *Primates in nutritional research* p. 249,

ed K C Hayes. Academic Press, New York. 1979.

86 Ryback RS, Eckardt MJ, Felsher B *et al.* Biochemical and hematologic correlates of alcoholism and liver disease. *J. Am. med. Assoc.* 1982; **248**: 2261.

87 Sato S, Nouchi T, Worner TM *et al.* Liver fibrosis in alcoholics: detection by Fab radio-immunoassay of serum procollagen III peptides. *J. Am. med. Assoc.* 1986; **256**: 1471.

88 Schaffner F, Popper H. Capillarization of hepatic sinusoids in man. *Gastroenterology* 1973; **44**: 239.

89 Scott J, Summerfield JA, Elias E *et al.* Chronic pancreatitis: a cause of cholestasis. *Gut* 1977; **18**: 196.

90 Shaw S, Worner TM, Lieber CS. Frequency of hyperprolinemia in alcoholic liver cirrhosis: relationship to blood lactate. *Hepatology* 1984; **4**: 295.

91 Sherlock S. Nutrition and the alcoholic. *Lancet* 1984; **i**: 436.

92 Sorensen TIA, Orholm M, Bentsen KD *et al.* Prospective evaluation of alcohol abuse and alcoholic liver injury in men as predictors of development of cirrhosis. *Lancet* 1984; **ii**: 241.

93 Starzl TL, van Thiel D, Tzakis AG. Orthotopic liver transplantation for alcoholic cirrhosis. *J. Am. med. Assoc.* 1988; **260**: 2542.

94 Storey E, Anderson GJ, Mack U *et al.* Desialylated transferrin as a serological marker of chronic excessive alcohol ingestion. *Lancet* 1987; **i**: 1292.

95 Theodossi A, Eddleston ALWE, Williams R. Controlled trial of methylprednisolone therapy in severe acute alcoholic hepatitis. *Gut* 1982; **23**: 75.

96 Thompson RPH. Measuring the damage—ethanol and the liver. *Gut* 1986; **27**: 751.

97 Torres-Salinas M, Pares A, Caballeria J *et al.* Serum procollagen type III peptide as a marker of hepatic fibrogenesis in alcoholic hepatitis. *Gastroenterology* 1986; **90**: 1241.

98 Uchida T, Kao H, Quispe-Sjogren M *et al.* Alcoholic foamy degeneration—a pattern of acute alcoholic injury of the liver. *Gastroenterology* 1983; **84**: 683.

99 Volentine GD, Ogden KA, Kortje DK *et al.* Role of acetaldehyde in the ethanol-induced impairment of hepatic glycoprotein secretion in the rat in vivo. *Hepatology* 1987; **7**: 490.

100 Van de Weil A, Delacroix DL, van Hattum J *et al.* Characteristics of serum IgA and liver IgA deposits in alcoholic liver disease. *Hepatology* 1987; **7**: 95.

101 Villa E, Rubbiani L, Barchi T *et al.* Susceptibility of chronic symptomless HBsAg carriers to ethanol-induced hepatic damage. *Lancet* 1982; **ii**: 1243.

102 Wodak AD, Saunders JB, Ewuis-Mensah I *et al.* Severity of alcohol dependence in patients with alcoholic liver disease. *Br. med. J.* 1983; **287**: 1420.

103 Worner TM, Lieber CS. Perivenular fibrosis as precursor lesion of cirrhosis. *J. Am med. Assoc.* 1985; **253:** 627.

104 Yamauchi M, Potter JJ, Mezey E. Characteristics of alcohol dehydrogenase in fat-storing (Ito) cells of rat liver. *Gastroenterology* 1988; **94:** 163.

105 Zama MA. Collagen gene expression in alcoholic liver disease. *Molecular Aspects of Medicine.* Pergamon Press, 1988 (in press).

Normal iron metabolism

Dietary iron is absorbed from the intestine in ferrous form to the extent of 1–1.5 mg daily. The amount depends on body stores, more being absorbed the greater the need. In the intestinal cell the iron links to a glycoprotein called *transferrin* by which it is carried in serum. Transferrin is largely synthesized by the hepatocyte and this process is reduced in alcoholic cirrhosis [40]. The serum iron binding capacity (transferrin) is about 250 µg/100 ml and is one-half to one-third saturated with iron. The absorptive process is active, capable of transporting iron against a gradient.

The morning fasting serum iron is about 125 µg/100 ml. The normal total body content of iron is about 4 g, of which 3 g are present in haemoglobin, myoglobin, catalase and other respiratory pigments or enzymes. Storage iron comprises 0.5 g; of this 0.3 g is in the liver but is not revealed by the usual histological stains for iron. The liver is the predominant site for storage of iron absorbed from the gut. When its capacity is exceeded, iron is deposited in other parenchymal tissues, including the acinar cells of the pancreas, the adrenals, and other secreting tissues throughout the body. The liver, however, contains the bulk of storage iron. The reticulo-endothelial system plays only a limited part in iron storage unless the iron is given intravenously, when it becomes a preferential site for deposition. Iron from erythrocyte breakdown is concentrated in the spleen.

When excess iron is deposited, three pigments may be found in the liver—ferritin, haemosiderin and lipofuscin.

Ferritin is a combination of the protein apoferritin and iron and appears under electron microscopy as particles 50 Å in diameter lying free in the cytoplasm.

Aggregates of ferritin molecules make up *haemosiderin* which stains as blue granules with ferrocyanide. Under the electron microscope the ferritin takes the form of paracrystalline aggregates. The iron-containing nucleus of the molecule consists of six sub-units arranged at the apices of a regular octahedron.

Lipofuscin, or wear and tear pigment, is yellow-brown in colour and does not contain iron. These granules may form the organic basis for iron deposition.

Iron contained in depots as ferritin or haemosiderin is available for mobilization and haemoglobin formation should the demand arise.

Iron overload and liver damage

Fibrosis and hepato-cellular damage are directly related to the iron content of the liver cell. The pattern of damage is similar irrespective of the aetiology: for instance, whether the overload is due to idiopathic haemochromatosis or to multiple transfusions. The severity of fibrosis is maximal in peri-portal areas where iron is particularly deposited. Cirrhosis has been produced in dogs by massive iron overload [31].

When iron deposition is low it is stored as ferritin. As the load increases more is present as haemosiderin [60].

Removal of iron by venesections or chelation leads to clinical and biochemical improvement with reduction or prevention of hepatic fibrosis [15].

Iron damages the hepatocyte by two possible mechanisms. Haemosiderin is deposited in peribiliary lysomes where release of iron leads to membrane fragility and disruption so allowing hydrolytic enzymes to reach the cytosol

[37, 48, 49]. The second, but not exclusive, theory invokes microsomal and mitochondrial lipid peroxidation with consequent functional disturbances in mitochondria and microsomes [3, 54].

Idiopathic (genetic) haemochromatosis

This is a genetically determined metabolic disorder with increased iron absorption over many years [21]. It is a rare disease described in 1886 as *bronzed diabetes* [23]. The tissues contain enormous quantities of iron, of the order of 20–60 g. If 10 mg dietary iron were retained by the tissues daily it would take about 14 years for 50 g to accumulate.

Pathology

A fibrous tissue reaction is found wherever the iron is deposited.

The *liver* in the early stages may show only portal zone fibrosis with deposition of iron in the peri-portal liver cells and, to a lesser extent, in the Kupffer cells. Fibrous septa then surround groups of lobules and irregularly shaped nodules (*holly-leaf appearance*). There is partial preservation of the architecture, although ultimately a macronodular cirrhosis develops (fig.

21.1). Fatty change is unusual and the glycogen content of the liver cells is normal.

The *pancreas* shows fibrosis and parenchymal degeneration with iron deposition in acinar cells, macrophages, islets of Langerhans and fibrous tissue.

Iron is found in the enlarged *spleen*, in *gastric* and *intestinal* epithelium and to a lesser extent in the kidneys.

Heart muscle is heavily involved, muscle fibres being replaced by a mass of iron pigment within the sheath. Degeneration of the fibres is rare. Coronary sclerosis, however, is common.

Brain and nervous tissue are usually free of iron.

Epidermal atrophy may reduce the *skin* to a flattened sheet. Hair follicles and sebaceous glands are inconspicuous. Characteristically, pigment is increased in the melanin content of the basal layer. Iron is usually absent from the epidermis but can often be seen deeper, especially in the basal layer.

Endocrine glands, including adrenal cortex, anterior lobe of pituitary and thyroid, show varying amounts of iron and fibrosis.

The testes are small and soft with atrophy of the germinal epithelium without iron overload. There is interstitial fibrosis and iron is found in the walls of capillaries.

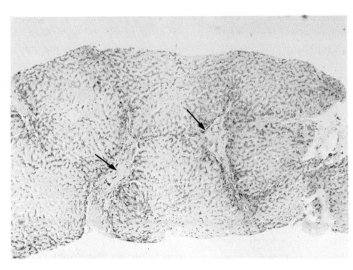

Fig. 21.1. The liver in idiopathic haemochromatosis. Cirrhosis is seen, the liver cells being filled with blue-staining iron pigment. Fibrous tissue is also infiltrated with iron. (Stained Perls, ×13.)

Aetiology

Increased, inappropriate, intestinal absorption of iron dates from birth. Absorption only becomes normal when storage iron reaches injurious levels and then increases again after iron stores have been reduced by venesection [58].

Control of iron absorption is at the level of the mucosal cell. Under normal circumstances only a proportion of the iron taken up by the mucosal cell is retained; the rest is stored and lost as the intestinal epithelium is exfoliated. In patients with idiopathic haemochromatosis, much more of the absorbed iron is retained in spite of increased body stores.

The primary abnormality in iron metabolism is unknown. A defect in the intestinal mucosal cell is possible. Absorption may follow the binding of iron to specific, intracellular, binding proteins such as mucosal transferrin or ferritin. However, transferrin receptors in the human gastrointestinal tract are not increased in haemochromatosis and transferrin is unlikely to be a mediator of mucosal iron absorption [4]. A specific microvillous membrane protein with a high affinity binding capacity for iron has been identified and is compatible with a membrane-associated iron uptake mechanism [53]. This might be abnormal in haemochromatosis. Another possibility is an abnormality in the process by which the hepatocyte binds iron transferrin. Adult hepatocytes in culture show transferrin-bound iron to be taken up by a non-saturable process, possibly fluid-phase or non-specific absorptive endocytosis, and a saturable phase involving transferrin receptors. Hepatic iron uptake from transferrin is known to be abnormal in treated haemochromatosis [12], but the exact defect is not known.

Genetics

Sheldon [50], in his classical monograph, described idiopathic haemochromatosis as an inborn error of metabolism. Family studies have shown first degree relatives with raised serum iron levels and/or variable degrees of excess iron in the liver [57]. A heterozygote state exists in 8–10% and a homozygous state in 0.3% of the Caucasian population [20]. Overt disease is unusual in two generations. Increased hepatic iron has been shown in siblings, even when serum iron values are normal [57].

There is a genetic linkage with the histocompatibility antigen A3 which is found in 72% of sufferers compared with 28% of the general population. The genotype varies in different countries; in France it is HLA3-B14 [51], and in Australia, HLA3-B7 [8]. The haemochromatosis gene is located on the short arm of chromosome 6, close to the HLA3 locus. The gene has not yet been cloned or sequenced.

Inheritance is autosomal recessive [7]. The heterozygote shows intermediate increase in transferrin saturation and in hepatic iron, but has no clinical manifestations. However, heterozygotes are at risk if they are alcoholic, take oral iron or excess ascorbic acid or suffer from another disturbance in iron metabolism such as haemolytic anaemia [35].

RELATION TO ALCOHOLISM AND NUTRITION

Alcoholism is frequent in patients with clinical haemochromatosis, but low among asymptomatic relatives with disordered iron metabolism [57]. Abuse of alcohol may accelerate the accumulation of iron in a subject genetically disposed to the disease. High dietary iron intake or liver or pancreatic damage from any other cause may act similarly.

The picture of haemochromatosis has been repeatedly described in abstainers from alcohol and the well nourished and also in children and in young relatives of sufferers. Genetic haemochromatosis is regarded as a definite entity independent of alcohol excess.

Clinical features

The classical picture (fig. 21.2) is of a lethargic, middle-aged man with pigmentation, hepatomegaly, diminished sexual activity and loss of

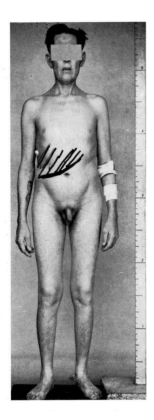

Fig. 21.2. Pigmented man showing loss of secondary sexual hair, gonadal atrophy and hepatomegaly.

body hair; diabetes is common.

Diagnosis depends on a high degree of suspicion and should be considered in any male with symptomless hepatomegaly and virtually normal biochemical tests of liver function. In view of the high heterozygote frequency in the community, the condition must be considerably more frequent than is recognized.

Haemochromatosis is ten times as frequent in males as females [21, 50]. Women are spared by iron loss with menstruation and pregnancy. Female patients with haemochromatosis, usually, but not always [32], have absent or scanty menstruation, have had a hysterectomy, or are many years post-menopausal. Families have been reported including two generations of women, two of whom were menstruating [32]. Familial juvenile haemochromatosis is described [29, 38]. The symptoms appear earlier in males than in females.

Haemochromatosis is rarely diagnosed before the age of 20, and the peak incidence is between 40 and 60. Children developing the disease show a more acute course [20], presenting with skin pigmentation, endocrine changes and cardiac disease [38].

Profound psychic disturbances are often shown by depression or suicidal tendencies.

The grey-slatey pigmentation is maximal in the the axillae, groins, genitalia, old scars and exposed parts. It can occur in the mouth. The colour, due to increased melanin in the basal layer, appears through the atrophied, superficial epidermis. The skin is shiny, thin and dry, like that of eunuchs.

HEPATIC CHANGES

The liver is enlarged and firm. Abdominal pain, usually a dull ache with hepatic tenderness, is noted in 37% [21]. The pain may be so severe that an acute abdominal emergency is simulated [34]. Circulatory collapse and sudden death can occur. The mechanism is obscure, although release of ferritin, a vasoactive substance, from the liver has been postulated.

Signs of hepato-cellular failure are usually absent and ascites rare. The signs of portal hypertension are also inconspicuous. The spleen is palpable but rarely large. Bleeding from oesophageal varices is rare.

Primary liver cancer develops in about 14% [21]. It may be a method of presentation, particularly in the elderly. It should be suspected if the patient shows clinical deterioration with rapid liver enlargement, abdominal pain and ascites. Erythrocytosis can be associated [44]. The serum iron may fall. Serum alpha-fetoprotein may be increased.

ENDOCRINE CHANGES

Clinical diabetes is present in about two-thirds [19]. This may be complicated by nephropathy, neuropathy, peripheral vascular disease and proliferative retinopathy [19]. The diabetes may be easy to control or may be resistant to large doses of insulin. It could be related to a family history of diabetes, to cirrhosis of the liver which impairs glucose tolerance or to direct damage to the pancreas by iron deposition.

Pituitary function is impaired to a variable extent in about two-thirds of patients. This can be related to iron deposition in the anterior pituitary, and not to severity of liver disease or to the degree of abnormality of iron metabolism. Gonadotrophin producing cells are selectively affected. Basal serum prolactin and luteinizing hormone levels are low with impaired response to thyroid or luteinizing releasing hormones [56] or to clomiphene. Hypogonadotrophic testicular failure is shown by impotence, loss of libido, testicular atrophy, skin atrophy and loss of secondary sexual hair. Plasma testosterone levels are subnormal. Urinary oestrogens increase following administration of gonadotrophins suggesting that the testes are capable of responding.

Pan-hypopituitarism with hypothyroidism and adrenal cortico-deficiency are rarer.

CARDIAC CHANGES

Although only 15% of patients with haemochromatosis present with heart failure, about a third subsequently develop cardiac symptoms. They are particularly frequent in the younger subject. The picture is of progressive right-sided heart failure sometimes with sudden death. Constrictive pericarditis or cardiomyopathy may be simulated. The 'iron heart' is a weak one. The heart is globular in shape. Arrhythmias are also seen.

Cardiac complications are presumably related to iron deposits in the myocardium and conducting system.

ARTHROPATHY

In about two-thirds of patients a specific arthropathy starts in the metacarpo-phalangeal joints and also involves larger ones. It may be a presenting feature [2]. It is related to an acute crystal synovitis with calcium pyrophosphate. Radiologically, chondrocalcinosis is seen in menisci and articular cartilage (fig. 21.4).

Special investigations

Biochemical tests show surprisingly little disturbance. Later the changes are those of cirrhosis of the liver.

The *serum iron* is raised to about 220 µg/dl compared with the normal of about 125 µg/dl. The *serum transferrin* is about 90% saturated compared with 30% in the normal.

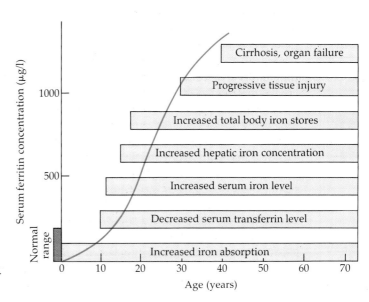

Fig. 21.3. Natural history of idiopathic haemochromatosis, progression of events leading to the clinical syndrome (Powell *et al.* 1978).

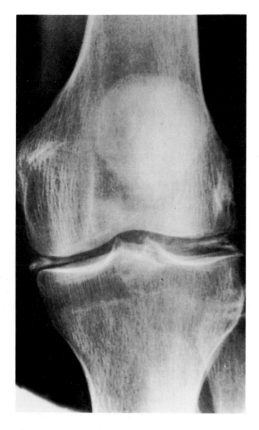

Fig. 21.4. Idiopathic haemochromatosis. Radiograph of the knee joint shows chondrocalcinosis in menisci and articular cartilage. (Courtesy M. Barry.)

Serum ferritin

Ferritin is the major cellular iron-storage protein present in normal serum. Its function there is uncertain. The concentration is proportional to body iron stores. It is of value in assessing uncomplicated iron overload [43], but can be unreliable in early diagnosis of the pre-cirrhotic stage [20]; it is useful in following treatment. A normal value does not exclude iron storage disease [11, 43].

With severe hepato-cellular necrosis, serum ferritin levels increase as it is released from liver cells [43]. Increases are also seen with some cancers.

Needle liver biopsy

This is the best method of confirming the diagnosis. The tough, fibrous liver may cause technical difficulties, but, if a sample is obtained, this shows the characteristic pigmentary cirrhosis (fig. 21.1).

The amount of iron in the specimen correlates well with total body storage of iron [6]. If the liver iron is less than 1.5% dry weight in a cirrhotic liver, the condition is unlikely to be genetic haemochromatosis. In the homozygote, hepatic iron correlates with age [10]. Fibrosis and cirrhosis develop only when the liver iron concentration is at least 2.2% dry weight (4500 μg/g wet weight) in the liver. Needle liver biopsy is a useful method of following treatment.

Imaging

Using single energy *CT scanning*, hepatic density correlates with serum ferritin [46]. If serum ferritin is elevated, an increased hepatic CT density confirms iron overload without the need for liver biopsy [26]. The accuracy is greatly improved if dual-energy CT scanning is available.

Magnetic resonance imaging (MRI) is particularly important as iron is a naturally occurring paramagnetic contrast agent. In overload states, marked decreases in P2 relaxation time are shown [52]. MRI may be of particular value in following therapy.

Differential diagnosis

Haemochromatosis may be confused with other forms of cirrhosis, especially in the alcoholic. The association of diabetes mellitus and cirrhosis is not uncommon, and patients with cirrhosis may become impotent, hairless and develop skin pigmentation. Hepato-cellular failure is usually minimal in haemochromatosis. Liver biopsy resolves any doubt, although moderate increases in iron may be found in cirrhosis, especially in alcoholics. Although hepatic siderosis is frequent in alcoholics (57%), significant siderosis is rare (7%) and hepatic iron concentration is lower than in hereditary haemochromatosis.

The serum iron level in cirrhosis may be raised but the iron-binding protein is not saturated. The distinction from other forms of *secondary haemosiderosis* is discussed later.

Prognosis

Much depends on early diagnosis and treatment. Those diagnosed in the pre-cirrhotic stage have a normal life expectancy [36]. Cardiac failure worsens the outlook and such patients rarely survive longer than one year without treatment. Hepatic failure or bleeding oesophageal varices are rare terminal features.

The outlook is better than for cirrhosis in alcoholics who stop drinking (fig. 21.5) [41]. However, the patient with haemochromatosis who also abuses alcohol does worse than the abstinent patient.

The risk of developing hepatocellular carcinoma is increased about 200 times [16].

Treatment

Iron can be removed by venesection and can be mobilized from tissue stores at rates as high as 130 mg/day [33]. Blood regeneration is extraordinarily rapid, haemoglobin production increasing to six or seven times normal. Large quantities of blood must be removed, for 500 ml removes only 250 mg of iron, whereas the tissues contain up to 200 times this amount. Depending on the initial iron stores, the amount necessary to reduce them effectively varies from 7 to 45 g. Venesections of 500 ml are carried out weekly, or even twice weekly in particularly co-operative patients, and continued for about two years until the haemoglobin and serum iron levels fall. Liver biopsy is a good check that de-ironing is complete. Comparison of a venesection-treated with an untreated group showed a survival of 8.2 compared with 4.9 years and a five-year mortality of 11% compared with 67% [42, 58]. Venesection treatment results in increased well-being and gain in weight. Pigmentation and hepa-

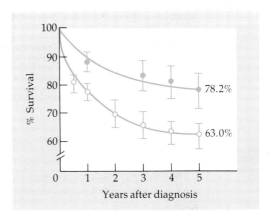

Fig. 21.5. Cumulative survival after diagnosis in 51 patients with haemochromatosis (solid line) compared with that reported by Powell & Klastskin (1968) for 93 patients with alcoholic cirrhosis who had stopped drinking (interrupted line). The vertical lines at each time interval represent plus or minus one standard error and the differences between the two curves are statistically significant at the fifth year ($P < 0.001$). Both curves were constructed by the same life-table (Powell 1970).

tosplenomegaly decrease. Liver function tests improve. Control of diabetes improves in some patients [15]. The arthropathy is unaffected. Cardiac failure may decrease [45]. Hypogonadism may lessen [27]. In two patients, serial hepatic biopsies showed apparent reversal of established cirrhosis [42]. This would agree with the type of fibrosis seen in haemochromatosis, architecture is preserved so making reversibility possible.

Rates of iron accumulation vary between 1.4 and 4.8 mg daily [15] and after de-ironing a 500 ml venesection every three months should prevent iron accumulation.

Primary liver cancer is not prevented by adequate venesection therapy [15].

Siblings with significant iron depositions should also be treated by venesection until liver biopsy shows absence of stainable iron [57].

A low iron diet is impossible to achieve. An alternative is to prescribe large doses of phosphate which prevent iron absorption by forming a precipitate and so increase faecal excretion of dietary iron.

Gonadal atrophy may be treated by substitution therapy with an intramuscular, depot testosterone. Human chorionic gonadotrophin (HCG) injections will increase testicular volume and sperm counts.

Diabetes should be treated by diet and if necessary, insulin. Resistant cases may be encountered.

The *cardiac complications* respond poorly to the usual measures but can be reversible with venesection [45].

DETECTION OF EARLY HAEMOCHROMATOSIS IN RELATIVES

First degree relatives, particularly male siblings should be screened so that treatment may be started before tissue damage has ensued. Pigmentation and hepatomegaly are helpful, but they may not be early signs. If serum iron, percentage transferrin saturation and serum ferritin are normal, significantly increased iron stores are very unlikely. The combination of an increased transferrin saturation (greater than 50%) with an elevated serum ferritin concentration (greater than 200 µg/l in men or 150 µg/l in women) is 94% sensitive and 86% specific for genetic haemochromatosis in younger homozygotes [9]. If any test is abnormal, liver biopsy, with measurement of hepatic iron, is indicated.

Relatives may be classified as homozygous, heterozygous or normal by comparing their HLA phenotype with that of the proband. Any relative whose phenotype is the same is at particular risk of developing homozygous haemochromatosis. Progressive iron overload rarely develops in heterozygotes and they can be reassured and reassessed at yearly intervals.

If significant iron deposition is shown the relative even if symptom-free should be venesected.

Other iron storage diseases

TRANSFERRIN DEFICIENCY

Absence of this binding protein has been found in a child with haemochromatosis [24]. The haematological picture was of severe iron deficiency although the tissues were loaded with iron. The parents were heterozygotes and the patient a homozygote.

CANCER INDUCING IRON OVERLOAD

A primary bronchial carcinoma produced an abnormal ferritin that was thought to cause excess iron deposition in the liver and spleen [30].

PORPHYRIA CUTANEA TARDA (Chapter 23)

Increased hepatic iron has been related to additional heterozygosity for the haemochromatosis gene [28] although this is uncertain [13]. Results may depend on the population studied.

ERYTHROPOIETIC SIDEROSIS

Siderosis is associated with extremely high rates of erythropoiesis. The hyperplastic bone-marrow may in some way direct the intestinal mucosa to take in excessive quantities of iron. This continues even in the presence of anaemia and of large iron stores. The iron is deposited first in the macrophages of the reticulo-endothelial system and later in parenchymal cells of liver, pancreas and other organs.

Siderosis can therefore be expected in chronic haemolytic states, especially beta thalassaemia sickle cell disease, congenital spherocytosis [5] and hereditary dyserythropoietic anaemia. Patients with chronic aplastic anaemia may also be at risk. Iron overload may develop in mild sideroblastic anaemia without severe anaemia or transfusions [39].

The siderosis is enhanced by blood transfusions as the iron given with the blood cannot be utilized. More than 100 units must have been transfused before siderosis is clinically recognizable. Misdirected iron therapy enhances the siderosis.

The siderosis is recognized clinically by increasing skin pigmentation and by hepatomegaly. Children fail to grow and to develop secondary sexual characteristics. Liver failure and frank portal hypertension are rare. The fasting blood glucose is raised, but clinical diabetes is excessively rare.

Although the amount of iron deposited in the heart is relatively small myocardial damage is a major factor determining prognosis, especially in younger children [47]. In children, symptoms arise when body iron reaches 20 g (100 units blood transfused); death from heart failure is likely when 60 g is reached.

Treatment is difficult. Splenectomy may reduce transfusion needs. A well-balanced low-iron diet is virtually impossible. Twelve-hour overnight subcutaneous infusion of of 2−4 g desferrioxamine given with a small syringe pump into the anterior abdominal wall is effective [25]. Such measures can only be available to a very few children with haemoglobinopathies: the cost is prohibitive.

Serum ferritin is reduced relative to iron stores and this can be raised by oral ascorbic acid [17].

BANTU SIDEROSIS

This condition is seen in South African Blacks whose diet consists of porridge fermented in iron pots at an acid pH. Absorption is facilitated by the acid diet and by malnutrition. Traditional beer brewed in steel drums continues to cause iron overload in rural sub-Saharan Africa [22].

CIRRHOSIS OF THE ALCOHOLIC

Multiple factors contribute to increased hepatic iron deposition. Protein deficiency is frequent. Increased iron absorption is found in cirrhotic patients irrespective of aetiology [59]. Cirrhotic patients with a large portal−systemic collateral circulation may absorb somewhat more.

Alcoholic beverages, particularly wine, have a high iron content (table 21.1). Chronic pancreatitis seems to increase iron absorption. Iron medications and haemolysis add to the load of iron, whereas intestinal blood loss diminishes it.

Iron deposition is rarely as great as in genetic haemochromatosis. Iron deficiency soon follows multiple venesections and body iron stores are only moderately increased. Hepatic histology shows the features of alcoholism as well as iron deposition. The chemical measurement of hepatic iron concentration, when corrected for the age of the subject, will distinguish early haemochromatosis from alcoholic siderosis [10]. Some alcoholic patients with hepatic cirrhosis may be heterozygotes for genetic haemochromatosis but this is not likely unless hepatic iron levels are very greatly increased. Diagnostic difficulties arise when a homozygote is also a heavy drinker.

SIDEROSIS AFTER PORTA−CAVAL SHUNTING

Iron may accumulate rapidly in the liver with surgical or spontaneous portal−systemic shunts [18, 59]. In general, siderosis is slight and clinically insignificant. It is probably an exaggeration of that frequently observed in cirrhosis.

HAEMODIALYSIS

Massive overload in liver and spleen reflect transfusion and haemolysis [1].

Table 21.1. Average alcohol and iron content of common beverages (Jakobovits et al. 1979)

Beverage	Alcohol (g/100 ml)	Iron (mg/100 ml)
Beers	2.2−6.6	0.01−0.05
Ciders	3.8−10.5	0.3−0.5
Wines—heavy ports, sherry	15.6−16.1	0.3−0.5
Table wines—white	8.8−10.2	0.5−1.2
—red	8.9−10.1	0.65−1.3
Spirits—70% proof	31.5	Trace

RELATION OF THE PANCREAS TO IRON
METABOLISM

Increased iron absorption and storage have
been found in experimental pancreatic damage
and also in patients with calcific pancreatitis
and with cystic fibrosis where absorption of
inorganic iron but not haemoglobin iron was
increased [55]. This suggests that some factor
in the exocrine secretion of the pancreas can
increase iron absorption.

NEONATAL HAEMOCHROMATOSIS

This very rare and fatal disorder must be related
to abnormal trans-placental passage of iron
[14].

References

1 Ali M, Fayemi AO, Rigolisi R *et al.* Hemosiderosis
in hemodialysis patients. *J. Am. med. Assoc.* 1980;
244: 343.

2 Askari AD, Muir WA, Rosner IA *et al.* Arthritis of
haemochromatosis. Clinical spectrum, relation to
histocompatibility antigens and effectiveness of
early phlebotomy. *Am. J. Med.* 1983; **75;** 957.

3 Bacon BR, Healey JF, Brittenham GM *et al.* Hepatic
microsomal function in rats with chronic dietary
iron overload. *Gastroenterology* 1986; **90:** 1844.

4 Banerjee D, Flanagan PR, Cluett J *et al.* Transferrin
receptors in the human gastrointestinal tract. Relationship to body iron stores. *Gastroenterology*
1986; **91:** 861.

5 Barry M, Scheuer PJ, Sherlock S *et al.* Hereditary
spherocytosis with secondary haemochromatosis.
Lancet 1968; ii: 481.

6 Barry M, Sherlock S. Measurement of liver iron
concentration in needle biopsy specimens. *Lancet*
1971; i: 100.

7 Bassett ML, Doran TJ, Halliday JW *et al.*
Idiopathic haemochromatosis: demonstration of
homozygous-heterozygous mating by HLA
typing in families. *Human Genet.* 1982; **60:** 352.

8 Bassett ML, Halliday JW, Powell LW. HLA typing
in idiopathic hemochromatosis: distinction between homozygotes and heterozygotes with biochemical expression. *Hepatology.* 1981; **1:** 120.

9 Bassett ML, Halliday JW, Ferris RA *et al.* Diagnosis
of hemochromatosis in young subjects: predictive
accuracy of biochemical screening tests. *Gastroenterology* 1984; **87:** 628.

10 Bassett ML, Halliday JW, Powell LW. Value of
hepatic iron measurements in early hemochromatosis and determination of the critical iron level
associated with fibrosis. *Hepatology* 1986; **6:** 24.

11 Batey RG, Hussein S, Sherlock S *et al.* The role of
serum ferritin in the management of idiopathic
haemochromatosis. *Scand. J. Gastroenterol.* 1978;
13: 953.

12 Batey RG, Pettit JE, Nicholas AW *et al.* Hepatic
iron clearance from serum in treated hemochromatosis. *Gastroenterology* 1978; **75:** 856.

13 Beaumont C, Fauchet R, Phung LN *et al.* Porphyria
cutanea tarda and HLA-linked hemachromatosis:
evidence against a systematic association. *Gastroenterology* 1987; **92:** 1833.

14 Blisard KS, Bartow SA. Neonatal hemochromatosis. *Hum. Path.* 1986; **17:** 376.

15 Bomford A, Williams R. Long term results of
venesection therapy in idiopathic haemochromatosis. *Q. J. Med.* 1976; **45:** 611.

16 Bradbear RA, Bain C, Siskind V *et al.* Cohort
study of internal malignancy in genetic haemochromatosis and other chronic non alcoholic liver
diseases. *J. Natl. Cancer Inst.* 1985; **75:** 81.

17 Chapman RWG, Hussain MAM, Gorman A *et al.*
Effect of ascorbic acid deficiency on serum ferritin
concentration in patients with beta-thalassaemia
major and iron overload. *J. clin. Pathol.* 1982; **35:**
487.

18 Conn HO. Portacaval anastomosis and hepatic
haemosiderin disposition: a prospective controlled investigation. *Gastroenterology.* 1972; **62:**
61.

19 Dymock IW, Cassar J, Pyke DA *et al.* Observations
on the pathogenesis, complications and treatment
of diabetes in 115 cases of haemochromatosis.
Am. J. Med. 1972; **52:** 203.

20 Edwards CQ, Griffen LM, Goldgar D *et al.* Prevalence of hemochromatosis among 11,068 presumably healthy blood donors. *N. Engl. J. Med.* 1988;
318: 1355.

21 Finch SC, Finch CA. Idiopathic hemochromatosis.
Medicine (Baltimore) 1955; **34:** 381.

22 Gordeuk VR, Boyd RD, Brittenham GM. Dietary
iron overload persists in rural sub-Saharan Africa.
Lancet 1986; i: 1310.

23 Hanot V, Schachmann M. Sur le cirrhose pigmen-
taire dans le diabète sucré. *Arch. Physiol. norm.
path.* 1886; **7:** 50.

24 Heilmeyer L, Keller W, Vivell O *et al.* Congenital
transferrin deficiency in a seven-year-old girl.
Germ. med. Mth. 1961; **6:** 385.

25 Hoffbrand AV, Gorman A, Laulicht M *et al.* Improvement in iron status and liver function in
patients with transfusional iron overload with
long-term subcutaneous desferrioxamine. *Lancet*
1979; i: 947.

26 Howard JM, Ghent CN, Carey LS *et al.* Diagnostic
efficacy of hepatic computed tomography in the
detection of body iron overload. *Gastroenterology*

1983; **84:** 209.

27 Kelly TM, Edwards CO, Meikle AW *et al.* Hypogonadism in hemochromatosis: reversal with iron depletion. *Ann. intern. med.* 1984; **101:** 629.

28 Kushner JP, Edwards CQ, Dadone MM *et al.* Heterozygosity for HLA-linked hemochromatosis as a likely cause of the hepatic siderosis associated with sporadic porphyria cutanea tarda. *Gastroenterology* 1985; **88:** 1232.

29 Lamon JM, Marynick SP, Rosenblatt R *et al.* Idiopathic hemochromatosis in a young female. A case study and review of the syndrome in young people. *Gastroenterology* 1979; **76:** 178.

30 Li AKC, Batey RG. A tumour inducing iron overload. *Br. med J.* 1977; **ii:** 1327.

31 Lisboa PE. Experimental hepatic cirrhosis in dogs caused by chronic massive iron overload. *Gut* 1971; **12:** 363.

32 Lloyd HM, Powell LW, Thomas MJ. Idiopathic haemochromatosis in menstruating women. *Lancet* 1964; **ii:** 555.

34 McAllen PM, Coghill NF, Lubran M. The treatment of haemochromatosis with particular reference to the removal of iron from the body by repeated venesection. *Q. J. Med.* 1957; **26:** 251.

35 Mohler DN, Wheby MS. Case report: hemochromatosis heterozygotes may have significant iron overload when they also have hereditary spherocytosis. *Am. J. med. Sci.* 1986; **29:** 320.

36 Niederau C, Fischer R, Sonnenberg A *et al.* Survival and causes of death in cirrhotic and non cirrhotic patients with primary hemochromatosis. *N. Engl. J. Med.* 1985; **313:** 1256.

37 O'Connell MJ, Ward RJ, Baum H *et al.* Role of iron in ferritin and haemosiderin mediated lipid peroxidation in lipsomes. *Biochem. J.* 1985; **229:** 135.

38 Perkins KW, McInnes IWS, Blackburn CRB *et al.* Idiopathic haemochromatosis in children. *Am. J. Med.* 1965; **39:** 118.

39 Peto TEA, Pippard MJ, Weatherall DJ. Iron overload in mild sideroblastic anaemias. *Lancet* 1983; **i:** 375.

40 Potter BJ, Chapman RWG, Nunes RM *et al.* Transferrin metabolism in alcoholic liver disease. *Hepatology* 1985; **5:** 714.

41 Powell LW, Halliday JW, Cowlishaw JL. Relationship between serum ferritin and total body iron stores in idiopathic haemochromatosis. *Gut* 1978; **19:** 538.

42 Powell LW, Kerr JFR. Reversal of 'cirrhosis' in idiopathic haemochromatosis following long-term intensive venesection therapy. *Aust. ann. med.* 1970; **19:** 54.

43 Prieto J, Barry M, Sherlock S. Serum-ferritin in patients with iron overload and with acute and chronic liver diseases. *Gastroenterology* 1975; **68:** 525.

44 Raphael B, Cooperberg AA, Niloff P. The triad of hemochromatosis, hepatoma and erythrocytosis. *Cancer* 1979; **43:** 690.

45 Rivers J, Garrahy P, Robinson W *et al.* Reversible cardiac dysfunction in hemochromatosis. *Am. Heart J.* 1987; **113:** 216.

46 Roudot-Thoraval F, Halphen M, Lardé D *et al.* Evaluation of liver iron content by computed tomography: its value in the follow-up of treatment in patients with idiopathic hemochromatosis. *Hepatology* 1983; **6:** 974.

47 Schafer AI, Cheron RG, Dluhy R *et al.* Clinical consequences of acquired transfusional iron overload in adults. *N. Engl. J. Med.* 1981; **304:** 319.

48 Selden C, Owen M, Hopkins JMP *et al.* Studies on the concentration and intracellular localization of iron proteins in liver biopsy specimens from patients with iron overload with special reference to their role in lysosomal disruption. *Br. J. Haematol.* 1980; **44:** 593.

49 Seymour CA, Peters TJ. Organelle pathology in primary and secondary haemochromatosis with special reference to lysosomal changes. *Br. J. Haematol.* 1978; **40:** 239.

50 Sheldon JH. *Haemochromatosis.* Oxford University Press 1935.

51 Simon M, Fauchet R, Hespel JP *et al.* Idiopathic haemochromatosis: a study of biochemical expression in 247 heterozygous members of 63 families; evidence for a single major HLA-linked gene. *Gastroenterology* 1980; **78:** 703.

52 Stark DD, Moseley ME, Bacon BR *et al.* Magnetic resonance imaging and spectroscopy of hepatic iron overload. *Radiology* 1985; **154:** 137.

53 Stremmel W, Lotz G, Niederau C *et al.* Iron uptake by rat duodenal microvillous membrane vesicles: evidence for carrier-mediated transport system. *Eur. J. clin. Invest.* 1987; **17:** 136

54 Tavill AS, Bacon BR. Hemochromatosis: how much iron is too much? *Hepatology* 1986; **6:** 142.

55 Tonz O, Weiss S, Strahm HW *et al.* Iron absorption in cystic fibrosis. *Lancet* 1965; **ii:** 1096.

56 Walton C, Kelly WF, Laing I *et al.* Endocrine abnormalities in idiopathic haemochromatosis. *Q. J. Med.* 1983; **52:** 99.

57 Williams R, Scheuer PJ, Sherlock S. The inheritance of idiopathic haemochromatosis: a clinical and liver biopsy study of 16 families. *Q. J. Med.* 1962; **31:** 249.

58 Williams R, Smith PM, Spicer EJF *et al.* Venesection therapy in idiopathic haemochromatosis. *Q. J. Med.* 1969; **38:** 1.

59 Williams R, Williams HS, Scheuer PJ *et al.* Iron absorption and siderosis in chronic liver disease. *Q. J. Med.* 1967; **36:** 151.

60 Zuyderhoudt FMJ, Sindram JW, Marx JM *et al.* The amount of ferritin and hemosiderin in the livers of patients with iron-loading diseases. *Hepatology* 1983; **3:** 232.

22 · Wilson's Disease

This rare disease, predominantly of young people, is characterized by cirrhosis of the liver, bilateral softening and degeneration of the basal ganglia of the brain, and greenish-brown pigmented rings in the periphery of the cornea (Kayser−Fleischer rings). Kinnier Wilson (1912) [46] was the first to define it in an article entitled 'Progressive lenticular degeneration: a familial nervous disease associated with cirrhosis of the liver'.

Aetiology

Increased amounts of copper, deposited in the tissues, are responsible for the liver and neurological changes, the Kayser−Fleischer rings in the cornea and lesions in kidneys and other organs (fig. 22.1) [2, 4].

Biliary copper excretion is low [11]. Urinary copper excretion is increased. The serum copper level, however, is almost invariably reduced. Ceruloplasmin, an α_2-globulin responsible for

transfer of copper in the plasma, is reduced [2].

The normal daily dietary intake of copper is 4 mg of which 2 mg is absorbed and excreted in bile so that the patient is in balance. In Wilson's disease, only 0.2 to 0.4 mg can be excreted in bile with 1 mg in the urine so that a positive copper balance develops.

Inheritance is autosomal recessive and both parents must carry the abnormal gene (22.2). This mode of inheritance suggests that a single gene defect is responsible for the impaired biliary copper excretion and reduced caeruloplasmin level. The Wilson's disease gene has been assigned to chromosome 13 in linkage disequilibrium with a polymorphic locus encoding esterase D, a red cell enzyme [13]. This discovery should eventually lead to the isolation and characterization of the Wilson's disease gene.

The disease is worldwide but particularly in Jews of eastern European origin, Arabs, Italians, Japanese, Chinese, Indians and any

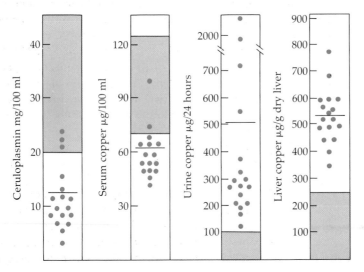

Fig. 22.1. Copper studies in 17 patients with Wilson's disease presenting as chronic active hepatitis. Horizontal lines indicate mean values. Hatched areas represent the normal ranges for serum ceruloplasmin (20−45 mg/dl) and serum copper (69−125 μg/dl) and delineate the levels above which urine copper concentrations (> 250 μg/g dry weight) are compatible with the diagnosis of Wilson's disease (Scott et al. 1978).

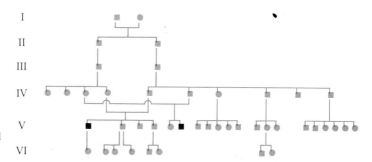

Fig. 22.2. Pedigree showing two instances of second cousin marriages, each having an affected offspring (Bearn 1953).

community having a high inter-marriage rate [3]. The prevalance is about 1 in 30 000 with a carrier frequency of about 1 in 90 [27].

Mutation of a structural gene responsible for the synthesis of copper-carrying protein could result in reduction in both biliary copper excretion and ceruloplasmin synthesis [8]. This is unlikely as biliary copper excretion and ceruloplasmin synthesis are independent pathways deriving their copper from separate copper pools.

The normal neonate also shows reduced serum caeruloplasmin and greatly elevated hepatic copper concentrations. In the neonatal guinea pig, the neonatal copper binding protein soon reverts to the adult form [34] but this persists in Wilson's disease. There might be a controller gene mutation, resulting in perpetuation of the fetal mode of copper homeostasis into childhood [9].

Clinical failure of caeruloplasmin synthesis is unlikely to be important as Wilson's disease can exist with normal caeruloplasmin values and levels do not correlate with duration or severity.

An abnormal or absent carrier protein necessary to present copper for incorporation into caeruloplasmin and for its excretion into bile has been suggested but never identified. Similarly an abnormal high affinity copper-binding protein preventing traffic of copper out of the liver has been suggested but, again, never isolated.

The reduced biliary excretion of copper [11] could reflect a defect in hepato-cellular mobilization by lysosomes [36]. The lysosomal change is, however, non-specific and similar lysosomal appearances are seen in other copper storage states such as cholestasis.

Bedlington terriers have an abnormality in biliary copper excretion and provide an animal model for Wilson's disease [17].

Pathology

LIVER

The liver shows all grades of change from peri-portal fibrosis through submassive necrosis to a coarse, macronodular cirrhosis [38].

Liver cells are ballooned, show multiple nuclei, clumped glycogen and glycogen vacuolation of the nuclei (fig. 22.3). Fatty change is usual. Kupffer cells are large. In some patients a particularly florid picture is seen with Mallory's bodies, simulating acute alcoholic hepatitis. Inflammatory reaction is inconspicuous. Hepatic histology is not diagnostic, but in a young person with cirrhosis such a picture should always suggest Wilson's disease.

Rubeanic acid or rhodanine stains for copper may be unreliable as the metal is patchily distributed, being absent from regenerating nodules. The copper is usually peri-portal in distribution and associated with atypical lipofuscin deposits.

Electron microscopy [26]

Autophagic vacuoles are seen and mitochondria are large and abnormal even in asymptomatic patients. Fatty change can be related to the mitochondrial alterations. Collagen fibrils infiltrate between cells and light

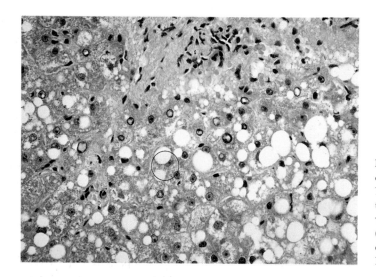

Fig. 22.3. Hepato-lenticular degeneration (Wilson's disease). Liver cells adjoining a fibrous tissue band show gross vacuolation of their nuclei (glycogenic degeneration) and occasionally fatty change. (Stained H & E, ×65) (Sherlock 1962).

and dark liver cells are seen. Copper is deposited in lysosomes which also show lipofuscin deposition.

OTHER ORGANS

The *kidney* shows fatty and hydropic change with copper deposition in the proximal convoluted tubules.

The *Kayser–Fleischer* ring is due to a copper-containing pigment deposited in Descemet's membrane at the periphery of the posterior surface of the cornea.

Clinical picture

The picture is a composite one due to general poisoning of the tissues with copper. The emphasis falls on different parts at different ages (fig. 22.4). In children the liver is chiefly involved (*hepatic form*). Later neuropsychiatric changes become increasingly important (*neurological form*). Patients presenting after age 20 usually have neurological symptoms [37]. The two types may overlap. Most patients have developed symptoms or been diagnosed between the ages of 5 and 30 [37].

The *Kayser–Fleischer* ring (fig. 22.5) is a greenish-brown ring at the periphery of the cornea. The upper pole is first affected. Slit-lamp examination by an expert may be necessary to show it. It is usually present with neurological abnormalities. It may be absent in young people with an acute presentation [29]. A rather similar ring may rarely be found with prolonged cholestasis and cryptogenic cirrhosis [10, 12].

Rarely the posterior layer of the capsule of the lens may show greyish-brown 'sunflower' cataracts, similar to those due to copper-containing foreign bodies [6].

HEPATIC FORMS

Fuminant hepatitis. This is characterized by progressive jaundice, ascites and hepatic and renal failure, usually in a child or young person [20, 24]. The liver cell necrosis is presumably related to accumulation of copper. Acute intravascular haemolysis may be due to destruction of erythrocytes by a sudden flux of copper from the necrotic hepatocytes (fig. 22.6) [21]. Haemolysis of similar type is reported in sheep with copper intoxication, and in humans in accidental copper poisoning.

Kayser–Fleischer rings may be absent. Urinary and serum copper levels are very high. Serum ceruloplasmin is usually low. However,

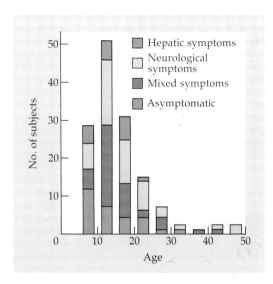

Fig. 22.4. Type of symptom complex at onset by age in 142 British and Chinese patients with Wilson's disease (Strickland *et al.* 1973).

it may be normal or raised as ceruloplasmin is an acute phase reactant, increased by underlying active liver disease. Serum transaminases and alkaline phosphatase levels are inappropriately low for fulminant viral hepatitis [20, 30].

Chronic active hepatitis. The condition presents at 10–30 years of age as a chronic active hepatitis with jaundice, high transaminase values and hypergammaglobulinaemia (fig. 22.7) [29]. Neurological changes appear some 2–5 years later. The picture may resemble other forms of chronic active hepatitis very closely. This emphasizes the need to screen all such patients for Wilson's disease.

Cirrhosis. The patient may present with insidiously developing cirrhosis. Clinical features include vascular spiders, splenomegaly, ascites and portal hypertension. The disease can exist without any neurological signs. In some patients the cirrhosis is well compensated. Hepatic biopsy may be necessary for diagnosis. If possible the copper content of the biopsy should be estimated quantitatively.

All young patients with chronic liver disease showing any mental peculiarity, any slurring of the speech, early ascites or haemolysis and especially with a family history of cirrhosis should be screened for Wilson's disease.

Hepato-cellular carcinoma is very rare and copper may be protective [45].

NEUROPSYCHIATRIC FORMS

The neurological condition may be acute and rapidly progressive. Early changes include a flexion–extension tremor of the wrists, grimacing, difficulty in writing and a slurred speech. The limbs show a fluctuating rigidity. The intellect is fairly well preserved although 61% of patients have some psychiatric disturbance

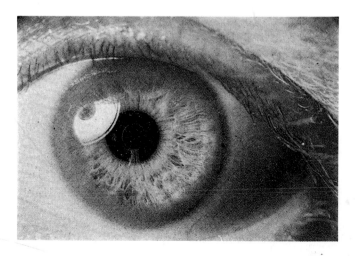

Fig. 22.5. Kayser–Fleischer ring. A brownish deposit is seen at the periphery of the cornea.

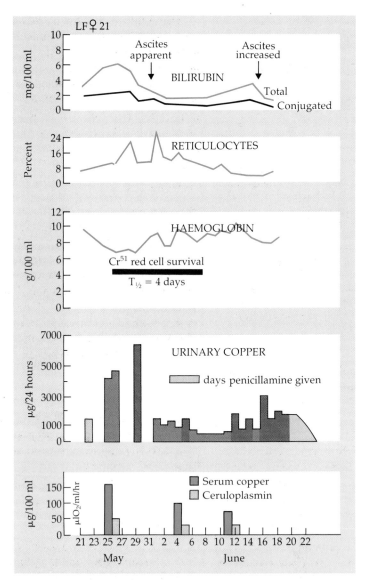

Fig. 22.6. Haemolytic crisis in Wilson's disease, marked by a rise in serum (mainly unconjugated) bilirubin and followed by reticulocytosis. The haemoglobin fell and red cell survival was reduced. Urinary copper was very high even without the administration of penicillamine. Serum copper was higher than that usually found in Wilson's disease. Ascites developed. The second episode of haemolysis, which was noted in June, was marked by a slight rise in serum bilirubin and a fall in haemoglobin (McIntyre *et al.* 1967).

usually presenting as a slow deterioration of the personality.

More usually the neurological changes are chronic: onset is in early adult life with tremor, gross and of a wing-beating type, exaggerated by voluntary movement. Sensory loss and pyramidal tract signs are absent. The expression is fatuous. Dystonia carries a very poor prognosis.

The EEG shows generalized non-specific changes. The asymptomatic siblings of patients with an abnormal EEG showed similar changes.

RENAL CHANGES

Aminoaciduria, glycosuria, phosphaturia, uricosuria and failure to excrete *p*-amino-hippurate (PAH) reflect renal tubular changes. These are presumably due to copper deposition in the proximal renal tubules.

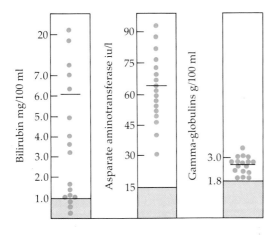

Fig. 22.7. Biochemical tests in 17 patients with Wilson's disease presenting as chronic active hepatitis. Horizontal lines indicate mean values. Normal ranges are denoted by hatching (serum bilirubin 0.2−0.8 mg/dl; aspartate aminotransferase 4−15 i.u./l; gamma-globulins 0.7−1.8 g/dl) (Scott et al. 1978).

Renal tubular acidosis is frequent and may be related to stone formation [44].

OTHER CHANGES

Rarely, the lunulae of the nails are blue [5] due to increased copper. Skeletal changes include demineralization, premature osteo-arthritis, subarticular cysts and fragmentation of bone about the joints. Changes in the spine are common and due to calcium pyrophosphate dihydrate deposition [19]. Gallstones are related to haemolysis [25]. Hypoparathyroidism is an association, possibly due to copper deposition [5].

Laboratory tests

Serum ceruloplasmin and copper levels are usually reduced [4, 14]. Distinction must be made from acute or chronic hepatitis with reduced serum ceruloplasmin due to failure of synthesis [33]. Malnutrition also reduces serum ceruloplasmin. The level may be raised by oestrogen administration, oral contraceptive drugs, biliary obstruction or pregnancy.

Twenty-four-hour urinary copper excretion is increased. Results may be difficult to evaluate unless strict precautions are taken to collect into copper-free containers.

In those in whom liver biopsy is contraindicated and where the serum ceruloplasmin level is normal, incorporation of orally administered radio-copper into ceruloplasmin may be diagnostic [28].

LIVER BIOPSY

The copper content must be measured by neutron activation [31]. Before use, the needle must be washed with EDTA and rinsed in 5% dextrose to remove copper. The normal is less than 55 μg/g dry liver weight, and concentrations greater than 250 μg are usual in homozygous Wilson's disease (fig. 22.8). High values may even be found in those with normal hepatic histology [17]. High values are also found in all forms of long-standing cholestasis (fig. 22.8).

SCANNING

Cranial CT scanning may show ventricular enlargement before neurological changes appear [16]. MR is more sensitive and allows better anatomical localization [1].

DETECTION OF SYMPTOM-FREE HOMOZYGOTES

All siblings of sufferers must be screened [17, 28]. A homozygote is suggested by such features as hepatomegaly, splenomegaly, vascular spiders and a slight rise in serum transaminase values. The Kayser−Fleischer rings may or may not be seen. Serum ceruloplasmin will usually be reduced to below 20 mg/100 ml. Liver biopsy with copper analysis is confirmatory.

Some difficulty may arise in distinguishing the homozygote from the heterozygote but the distinction is usually clear cut. The homozygote must be treated with penicillamine, even if symptom-free. The heterozygote does not require treatment. Thirty-six symptom-free

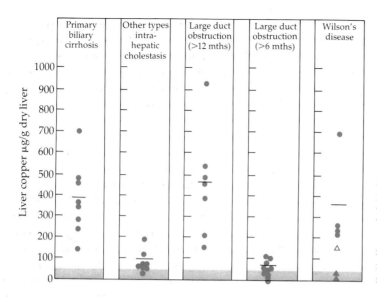

Fig. 22.8. Liver copper levels in patients with Wilson's disease and various types of cholestasis. Wilson's disease: △ heterozygote, ▲ siblings, probably homozygous normal (these three patients not included in the calculation of the mean) (Smallwood *et al.* 1968).

homozygotes have been treated and remain well, whereas seven left untreated have all developed the disease and five are dead of Wilson's disease [35].

Treatment

Penicillamine is the treatment of choice [40]. This chelates copper and increases urinary excretion to as much as 1000–3000 μg daily. Treatment is started with 1.2 g d-penicillamine hydrochloride by mouth in four doses taken before meals. Improvement is slow and at least six months' continuous therapy should be given. If there is no improvement, the dose may be increased to 1.5 and even to 2 g daily. Improvement is marked by fading and disappearance of the Kayser–Fleischer rings. Speech is clearer, tremor and rigidity lessen. Mentality is more normal. Handwriting is a good test of progress. Liver function improves. Hepatic biopsy shows lessening of activity and reversion to an inactive cirrhosis. Serum ceruloplasmin values fall. Failure to improve implies that irreparable tissue damage was present before treatment started. Failure should not be admitted until two years' massive therapy has been

Maintenance is usually 1.5–2g daily in the adult. This should not be reduced until the

Table 22.1. Treatment of Wilson's disease

Penicillamine 1.5–2 g daily
Yearly liver copper until decoppered
Then liver biopsy every 3–5 years

patient is decoppered. This may be indicated by a 24-hour urinary copper excretion below 100 mg by atomic absorption spectrophotometry. The liver copper level should also be within normal limits. This may take many years (fig. 22.9). A maintenance of 1 g daily is then continued with further liver biopsies performed at three- to five-year intervals to confirm decoppering. A fulminant course may follow non-compliance of penicillamine treatment by a previously well-controlled patient [43].

In contrast to other conditions, reactions to penicillamine are unusual in patients with Wilson's disease. They include rashes, leucopenia, aplastic anaemia, proteinuria and an SLE-like syndrome. They are usually solved by stopping the drug and recommencing in increasing doses under prednisolone cover. Clinical pyridoxine deficiency is a theoretical possibility but exceedingly rare. When large doses are being given, pyridoxine supplements can be added.

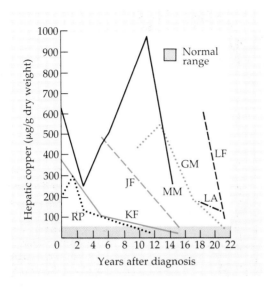

Fig. 22.9. Liver copper levels in seven penicillin-treated patients with Wilson's disease (some reduced their dose). Many years passed before the liver copper reached the normal range (shaded area).

Triene (tetraethylene tetramine dihydro-chloride) may be tried in those unable to take penicillamine [27, 42] but has side effects.

Elemental zinc (50 mg) as acetate three times a day between meals inhibits gastrointestinal absorption of copper [39]. It may be tried only in patients who have not responded to a long course of penicillamine or have had an irreversible reaction to both penicillamine and triene [18].

Physiotherapy is of value in the re-education of the patient's gait, writing and movement generally.

A low copper diet is of little value but high copper-containing foods, including chocolate, peanuts, mushrooms, liver and shell fish, should be avoided.

Hepatic transplantation may be indicated for the fulminant form (which is usually fatal), the young cirrhotic in severe hepato-cellular failure who fails to improve after 2 to 3 months' penicillamine, or the patient who develops severe liver failure with haemolysis after unwisely stopping therapy [23, 32]. The metabolic defect is corrected and the results are very satisfactory

(see Chapter 33). Before transplant, renal failure may be treated by post-dilution and continuous arterio-venous haemofiltration which removes large quantities of copper as large molecules of copper/penicillamine complex [23].

Prognosis

add in pathophysiology.

Untreated Wilson's disease is progressive and fatal. The great danger is that the patient remains undiagnosed and dies untreated.

In the acute neurological form the prognosis is poor, for cystic changes in the basal ganglia are irreversible. In the more chronic form the outlook depends on early diagnosis, preferably before symptoms have appeared. The final prognosis also depends on the response to six months' continuous penicillamine treatment. In one series, 16 asymptomatic patients were treated and have remained alive and asymptomatic, and three-quarters of 22 symptomatic patients treated for longer than two years are now asymptomatic. Dystonia carries a poor prognosis, being little affected by chelation therapy. Successful pregnancies have been reported in well-treated cases and penicillamine causes little problem to the fetus [41].

In chronic active hepatitis, response to treatment can be poor, nine of 17 patients dying in one series [29]. The fulminant cases are frequently fatal despite chelation therapy [24]. Jaundice, ascites, and a high serum bilirubin, aspartate transaminase and prothrombin time are ominous signs [22].

Death is from liver failure, bleeding oesophageal varices or intercurrent infections in those bedridden from neurological disability.

References

1 Aisen AM, Martel W, Gabrielsen TO *et al.* Wilson disease of the brain: MR imaging. *Radiology* 1985; **157**: 137.

2 Bearn AG. Wilson's disease. An inborn error of metabolism with multiple manifestations. *Am. J. Med.* 1957; **22**: 747.

3 Bearn AG. A genetic analysis of thirty families with Wilson's disease (hepato-lenticular degeneration). *Ann. hum. Genet.* 1960; **24**: 33.

4 Bearn AG, Kunkel HG. Biochemical abnormalities in Wilson's disease. *J. clin. Invest.* 1952; **51**: 616.

5 Bearn AG, McKusick VA. Azure lunulae. An unusual change in the finger nails in two patients with hepatolenticular degeneration (Wilson's disease). *J. Am. med. Assoc.* 1958; **166**: 904.

6 Cairns JE, Williams HP, Walshe JM. 'Sunflower cataract' in Wilson's disease. *Br. med. J.* 1969; **iii**: 95.

7 Carpenter TO, Carnes DL. Jr, Anast CS. Hypoparathyroidism in Wilson's disease. *N. Engl. J. Med.* 1983; **309**: 873.

8 Cox DW, Fraser FC, Sass-Kortsak A. A genetic study of Wilson's disease: evidence for heterogeneity. *Am. J. hum. Genet.* 1972; **24**: 646.

9 Epstein O, Sherlock S. Is Wilson's disease caused by a controller gene mutation resulting in perpetuation of the fetal mode of copper metabolism into childhood? *Lancet* 1981; **i**: 303.

10 Flemming CR, Dickson ER, Wahner HW *et al.* Pigmented corneal rings in non-Wilsonian liver disease. *Ann. intern. Med.* 1977; **86**: 285.

11 Frommer D. The binding of copper by bile and serum. *Clin. Sci.* 1971; **41**: 485.

12 Frommer D, Morris J, Sherlock S *et al.* Kayser–Fleischer-like rings in patients without Wilson's disease. *Gastroenterology* 1977; **72**: 1331.

13 Frydman M, Bonné-Tamir B, Farrer LA *et al.* Assignment of the gene for Wilson's disease to chromosome 13: linkage to the esterase D locus. *Proc. Natl. Acad. Sci. USA* 1985; **82**: 1819.

14 Gibbs K, Walshe JM. A study of the caeruloplasmin concentrations found in 75 patients with Wilson's disease, their kinships and various control groups. *Q. J. Med.* 1979; **48**: 447.

15 Johnson GF, Morell AG, Stockert RJ *et al.* Hepatic lysosomal copper protein in dogs with inherited copper toxicosis. *Hepatology* 1981; **1**: 243.

16 Kendall BE, Pollock SS, Barr NM *et al.* Wilson's disease: clinical correlation with cranial computed tomography. *Neuroradiology* 1981; **22**: 1.

17 Levi AJ, Sherlock S, Scheuer PJ *et al.* Presymptomatic Wilson's disease. *Lancet* 1967; **ii**: 575.

18 Lipsky MA, Gollan JL. Treatment of Wilson's disease: In D-penicillamine we trust—what about zinc? *Hepatology* 1987; **7**: 593.

19 McClure J, Smith PS. Calcium pryophosphate dihydrate deposition in the intervertebral discs in a case of Wilson's disease. *J. clin. Pathol.* 1983; **36**: 764.

20 McCollough AJ, Fleming CR, Thistle JL *et al.* Diagnosis of Wilson's disease presenting as fulminant hepatic failure. *Gastroenterology* 1983; **84**: 161.

21 McIntyre N, Clink HM, Levi AJ, *et al.* Hemolytic anemia in Wilson's disease. *N. Engl. J. Med.* 1967; **276**: 439.

22 Nazer H, Ede RJ, Mowat AP *et al.* Wilson's disease: clinical presentation and use of prognostic index. *Gut* 1986; **27**: 1377.

23 Rakela J, Kurtz SB, McCarthy JT *et al.* Fulminant Wilson's disease treated with post dilution hemofiltration and orthotopic liver transplantation. *Gastroenterology* 1986; **90**: 2004.

24 Roche-Sicot J, Benhamou J-P. Acute intravascular hemolysis and acute liver failure associated as a first manifestation of Wilson's disease. *Ann. intern. Med.* 1977; **86**: 301.

25 Rosenfield N, Grand RJ, Watkins JB *et al.* Cholelithiasis and Wilson's disease. *J. Pediatr.* 1978; **92**: 210.

26 Schaffner F, Sternlieb I, Barka T *et al.* Hepatocellular changes in Wilson's disease: histochemical and electron microscopic studies. *Am. J. Pathol.* 1962; **41**: 315.

27 Scheinberg IH, Jaffe ME, Sternlieb I. The use of trientine in preventing the effects of interrupting penicillamine therapy in Wilson's disease. *N. Engl. J. Med.* 1987; **317**: 209.

28 Scheinberg H, Sternlieb I. *Wilson's disease.* WB Saunders, Philadephia. 1983.

29 Scott J, Gollan JL, Samourian *et al.* Wilson's disease, presenting as chronic active hepatitis. *Gastroenterology* 1978; **74**: 645.

30 Shaver WA, Bhartt H, Combes B. Low serum alkaline phosphatase activity in Wilson's disease. *Hepatology* 1986; **6**: 859.

31 Smallwood RA, Williams HA, Rosenoer VM. *et al.* Liver-copper levels in liver disease. Studies using neutron activation analysis. *Lancet*; **ii**: 1310.

32 Sokol RJ, Francis PD, Gold SH *et al.* Orthotopic liver transplantation for acute fulminant Wilson's disease. *J. Pediatr.* 1985; **107**: 549.

33 Spechler SJ, Koff RS. Wilson's disease: diagnostic difficulties in the patient with chronic hepatitis and hypoceruloplasminemia. *Gastroenterology* 1980; **78**: 103.

34 Srai SKS, Burroughs AK, Wood B *et al.* The ontogeny of liver copper metabolism in the guinea pig: clues to the etiology of Wilson's disease. *Hepatology* 1986; **6**: 427.

35 Sternlieb I. Wilson's disease indications for liver transplants. *Hepatology* 1984; **4**: 15S.

36 Sternlieb I, van den Hamer CJA, Morell AG *et al.* Lysosomal defect of hepatic copper excretion in Wilson's disease (hepatolenticular degeneration). *Gastroenterology* 1973; **64**: 99.

37 Strickland GT, Frommer D, Leu M-L *et al.* Wilson's disease in the United Kingdom and Taiwan. 1. General characteristics of 142 cases and prognosis. II. A Genetic analysis of 88 cases. *Q. J. Med.* 1973; **42**: 619.

38 Stromeyer FW, Ishak KG. Histology of the liver in Wilson's disease. *Am. J. clin. Pathol.* 1980; **73**: 12.

39 Van Caillie-Bertrand M, Degenhart HJ, Visser HKA *et al*. Oral zinc sulphate for Wilson's disease. *Arch. Dis. Child.* 1985; **60:** 656.

40 Walshe JM. Treatment of Wilson's disease with penicillamine. *Lancet* 1960; **i:** 188.

41 Walshe JM. Pregnancy in Wilson's disease. *Q. J. Med.* 1977; **46:** 73.

42 Walshe JM. Treatment of Wilson's disease with trientine (triethylene tetramine) dihydrochloride. *Lancet* 1982; **ii:** 643.

43 Walshe JM, Dixon AK. Dangers of non-compliance in Wilson's disease. *Lancet* 1986; **i:** 845.

44 Wieber DO, Wilson DM, McLeod RA *et al*. Renal stones in Wilson's disease. *Am. J. Med.* 1979; **67:** 249.

45 Wilkinson ML, Portmann B, Williams R. Wilson's disease and hepatocellular carcinoma: possible protective role of copper. *Gut* 1983; **24:** 767.

46 Wilson AK. Progressive lenticular degeneration: a familial nervous disease associated with cirrhosis of the liver. *Brain* 1912; **34:** 295.

23 · Nutritional and Metabolic Liver Diseases

Clinical nutritional liver injury

Hepatic necrosis and fibrosis can be produced in experimental animals by appropriate diets, particularly those low in protein and essential amino acids [15]. Worldwide, protein malnutrition is extremely common [30]. The liver suffers in common with other organs.

The most clearly defined syndrome is *kwashiorkor*, but this represents only one end of the malnutrition spectrum. The liver is involved in *wasting diseases*, especially with chronic diarrhoea such as ulcerative colitis, and the hepatic changes in the *alcoholic* may be, at least in part, nutritional [26].

In *starvation* and hunger oedema, the liver shrinks, increased lipochrome pigment is seen in the liver cells, but there is no fatty change [27]. Liver biopsies from malnourished children show reduction in liver protein [30]. Liver biopsies from patients with *anorexia nervosa* are essentially normal. Previous malnutrition may 'condition' the liver to toxic and infective agents, but this has not been proved. Increased mortality from virus hepatitis, particularly in pregnancy, may occur in protein-deficient communities.

Fatty liver

This is defined as fat, largely triglyceride, exceeding 5% of the liver weight. Liver biopsy and imaging procedures, such as ultrasound and CT, are resulting in increasing numbers of patients being identified with excess fat in the liver. Theoretically, fatty liver could come from dietary fat transported to the liver as medium-chain triglycerides or via chylomicrons and lipolysis from adipose tissue (fig. 23.1). Fatty acids could accumulate in the liver due to increased mitochondrial synthesis or to reduced oxidation. Finally, export of triglycerides from the hepatocyte demands packaging with an apoprotein, phospholipid and cholesterol to form very low density lipoprotein (VLDL). The liver is also responsible for the degradation of lipoproteins [12].

Fatty liver could thus be due to increased delivery of fatty acids to the liver, increased or decreased oxidation of fatty acids or a defect in removal of triglyceride as very low density lipoproteins.

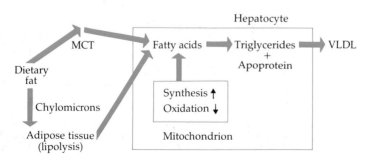

Fig. 23.1. Factors in fatty liver.

DIAGNOSIS

Fatty liver may present as diffuse, smooth hepatomegaly in appropriate circumstances such as obesity, diabetes or alcoholism.

Ultrasound may show a bright echo pattern but can be normal. Reflective echoes from fibrosis or cirrhosis are difficult to distinguish. CT shows a low density with reduced attenuation. Portal vein radicals appear prominent in a scan unenhanced with contrast. The attenuation is less than that of the spleen or kidneys (fig. 23.2). CT scan is useful to follow the effects of therapy [23].

Liver biopsy is the best method of diagnosing fatty liver. Appropriate stains such as oil red O on frozen sections are essential to diagnose lesser degrees of fatty change. Liver biopsy appearances are not diagnostic of the cause of the fatty change.

In most instances, the fat is maximal in hepatocytes in zone 3 (central). A zone 1 (peri-portal) distribution is found in protein calorie malnutrition, kwashiorkor, total parenteral nutrition, phosphorous poisoning, methotrexate injury and various other toxic states.

CLASSIFICATION

Increased fat in the liver is divided into two morphological categories; macroscopic and microscopic (figs 23.3, 23.4, 23.5). The two may be combined.

Macroscopic (large droplet)

In haematoxylin-eosin-stained liver sections, the hepatocytes contain punched out, empty vacuoles. The nucleus is displaced to the periphery of the cell (fig. 23.4).

Fat in the hepatocyte *per se* is not damaging. The serious association is with steatonecrosis (alcoholic hepatitis) (table 23.1). This is marked by zone 3 (Dissë space) pericellular fibrosis (creeping collagenosis) often with hepatocyte swelling and deposits of Mallory's hyaline in hepatocytes which are surrounded by neutrophils. This lesion is due to some factor in addition to that which causes fatty liver. It is pre-cirrhotic and can be diagnosed only by liver biopsy.

Clinical features. The patient is usually symptom free. He may complain of right upper quadrant heaviness and discomfort, worse on

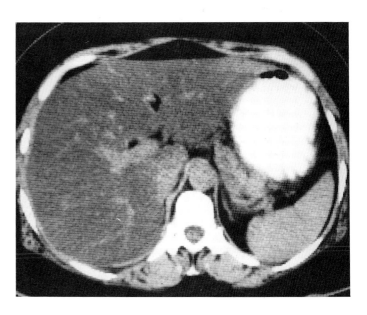

Fig. 23.2. CT fatty liver (without contrast: unenhanced). Liver is enlarged smooth and less dense than spleen. The intrahepatic portal vein radicles are more prominent than normal.

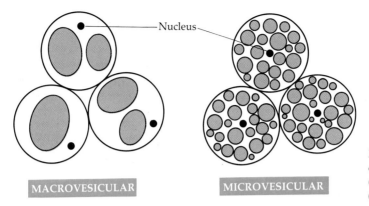

Nucleus

MACROVESICULAR

MICROVESICULAR

Fig. 23.3. Fatty liver may be classified into microvesicular (large droplet) and microvesicular (small droplet types).

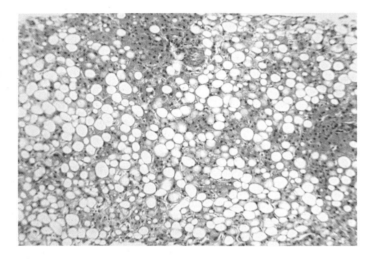

Fig. 23.4. Microvesicular fat. The liver cells appear empty. The change is maximal in zone 1 ('central'). Stained haemotoxylin-eosin ×135.

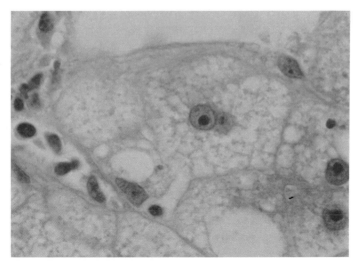

Fig. 23.5. Microvesicular fat. The hepatocyte has a foamy appearance. The nucleus is central with a dense nucleolus.

Table 23.1. The aetiology of large droplet macrovesicular fatty liver

Nutritional
   Kwashiorkor
   Gastrointestinal disease
   Pancreatic disease
   Obesity*
   Intestinal bypass*
   Prolonged parenteral nutrition*

Metabolic diseases
   Type II diabetes mellitus*
   Galactosaemia
   Glycogenoses
   Fructose intolerance
   Wilson's disease
   Tyrosinaemia
   Hyperlipidaemias
   Abetalipoproteinaemia
   Wolman's disease
   Weber–Christian disease
   Acylcoenzyme A dehydrogenase deficiency

Drug-related
   Alcohol*
   Corticosteroids
   Direct hepatotoxicity (Chapter 18)
   High dose oestrogens*
   Amiodarone*

General
   Fever
   Systemic disease
   Viral infections
   Cryptogenic

* Steatonecrosis ('alcoholic hepatitis') can develop.

movement. Pain over the liver is usually related to rapid accumulation of fat associated with alcoholism or with diabetes.

The liver is usually, but not always, smoothly enlarged.

Biochemical tests. These correlate poorly with hepatic histology. Serum transaminases and alkaline phosphatase show mild increases. Bilirubin and serum albumin are usually normal. Fatty liver is one of the commonest causes of a raised serum transaminase value detected in 'healthy' blood donors.

Cryptogenic fatty liver

When common causes, such as obesity, alcoholism and diabetes have been excluded a hard core remains with no obvious aetiology. Some may be pre-diabetic [4] or give a family history of diabetes. Patients usually have no symptoms other than anxiety. Serum transaminases may be slightly increased. Treatment is by reassurance and avoiding over-investigation.

Microvesicular fat

Hepatic histology shows zone 3 microvesicular fat. Cell necrosis is variable and minor, although, occasionally, there may be massive zone 3 necrosis. Hepatocytes show central nuclei with prominent nucleoli. Inflammation is minimal, and centrizonal cholestasis is occasionally found. Frozen sections stained for fat are necessary for diagnosis in mild cases. Electron microscopy shows the mitochondria swollen, pleomorphic and varying in shape.

The microvesicular fat diseases can be related to a widespread hepatic metabolic disturbance, particularly involving mitochondria and ribosomes. Increases in blood ammonia and low citrulline values can be related to reduction of mitochondrial Krebs' cycle enzymes. The amino acid profile shows high glutamine, alanine and lysine levels. Hypoglycaemia is frequent.

Triglyceride accumulation reflects disordered lipoprotein secretion and assembly. Synthesis of the apoprotein of VLDL is depressed with interference with the exit of lipid from the liver. Mitochondrial injury also depresses fatty acid oxidation.

This group has many members (table 23.2) [25]. They all show the same general pattern. The onset is marked by fatigue, nausea, vomiting with variable jaundice, impairment of consciousness, coma and fits (table 23.3). Renal failure and disseminated intravascular coagulation may be complications. The liver is not the only organ involved, and triglyceride accumulations may be found in the renal tubules and occasionally in myocardium and pancreas. Liver failure is not the usual cause of

Table 23.2. The microvesicular fat diseases

Acute fatty liver of pregnancy
Reye's syndrome
Vomiting disease of Jamaica
Sodium valproate toxicity
Tetracycline toxicity
Congenital defects of urea cycle enzymes
Genetic defects of mitochondrial fatty acid oxidation
Alcoholic foamy fat syndrome
Delta virus hepatitis in northern South America

Table 23.3. Features of the microvesicular fat diseases (Sherlock, 1983)

Vomiting
Variable jaundice
Coma
Disseminated intravascular coagulation
Renal failure
Raised blood ammonia values
Hypoglycaemia
Rise in serum fatty acids
Liver biopsy:
   microvesicular fat
   necrosis and cellular infiltration not prominent
Electron microscopy:
   mitochondrial abnormalities

death. Coma may be related to increases in blood ammonia levels or to cerebral oedema.

The mode of initiation of these diseases is diverse and in most instances not fully understood. Viral, toxic and nutritional factors have been implicated.

Focal fatty liver [9]

This condition is recognized by ultrasound, when areas of increased echogenicity are seen. The CT scan shows peripheral areas of low attenuation (figs 23.6, 23.7). Needle biopsy under CT guidance confirms the diagnosis. The lesions are usually multiple and resolve with time. They may recur. Patients at risk include diabetics, alcoholics, the obese, those on hyperalimentation and sufferers from Cushing's syndrome.

Kwashiorkor syndrome

Children may develop a syndrome of protein malnutrition called kwashiorkor, which, in the Ga language of the Gold Coast, means 'red boy'. It has a world wide distribution in under-privileged, overpopulated communities, especially tropical and subtropical [7, 30]. It is rare in Europe and indeed in the temperate areas of any continent.

PATHOLOGY

Deficiency of dietary protein affects particularly organs concerned with the elaboration of proteins and protein-containing enzymes.

The acinar cells of the pancreas, salivary and lacrymal glands, and glands of the small intestinal wall are atrophied. There is muscle wasting. The parotid glands may enlarge during recovery.

The liver shows extensive zone 1 fatty change. This might be secondary to the pancreatic damage and analogous to the fatty liver of depancreatized dogs. Alternatively, it may be due to dietary protein deficiency. The liver loses protein and gains water, sharing in the general oedema [30]. The very fatty liver may be related to mobilization of fat from adipose tissue. The hepatic glucose-6-phosphatase level is reduced. Although hepatic glycogen is increased this suggests failure to handle dietary

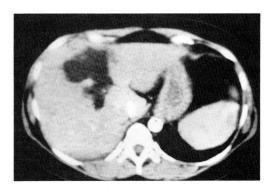

Fig. 23.6. Focal fatty liver. CT scan shows a low attenuation filling defect in the right lobe of liver. This lesion disappeared spontaneously.

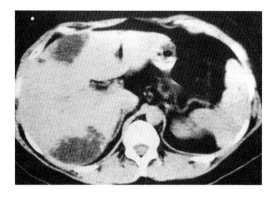

Fig. 23.7. The same patient. A further CT scan performed six months later showed two further areas of focal filling defects anteriorly and posteriorly in the right lobe of the liver.

carbohydrate which may then be converted into fat. Electron microscopy shows surprisingly mild changes [31].

The hepatic change is not specific. It might be an epiphenomenon: the fatty infiltration bears very little relation to clinical severity and causes little disturbance of liver function [30]. There is no progressive fibrosis or cirrhosis [11].

CLINICAL FEATURES

Children are most commonly affected 6–18 months after weaning when they are fed on an almost pure carbohydrate diet. Even before weaning, the milk of the undernourished mother may have been poor in protein, and this lack is emphasized by the demands of growth. Malaria and hookworm disease or an additional insult such as aflatoxin may contribute.

The acute breakdown is often initiated by a diminished food intake due to deprivation of mother love or to an infection [29]. The child is incredibly miserable with arrested growth, generalized oedema and cold extremities. The hair shows characteristic depigmentation, becoming pale and, losing its crisp black curliness, thin, straight and soft. The characteristic der-

matosis starts in the inguinal region and napkin area and spreads to sites of pressure and irritation. The dusky red patches have been likened to crazy paving. The skin desquamates and becomes pallid.

Appetite is decreased and diarrhoea is prominent, especially in the severe case, the stools showing undigested food. The liver may be enlarged or of normal size.

Severe protein malnutrition in *adults*, resembling kwashiorkor, can be related to ineffective utilization of dietary protein due to pancreatic exocrine deficiency or enteric bacterial colonization [17, 22].

Laboratory findings include reduced haemoglobin and plasma protein concentrations. Pancreatic enzymes are diminished.

Analysis of liver biopsy material shows reduction of pseudo-cholinesterase, D-amino acid oxidase and xanthine oxidase [25]. Enzymes subserving respiration and oxidative phosphorylation are well preserved.

Serum enzymes are depressed in keeping with all protein production [25]. Serum transaminase and plasma-free fatty-acid levels are increased [18].

The liver in obesity

Fatty liver is usual when body weight exceeds 70% of ideal. The quantity approximates to the increase in body weight.

Lipolysis from expanded fat depots is markedly increased and more fatty acids are supplied to the liver. This leads to an imbalance of triglyceride synthesis and secretion. There is also an imbalance between protein and calorie intake. Free fatty acids might damage biological membranes in the hepatocyte.

The fatty change is macrovesicular and in zone 3. It is generally benign. However, occasionally the liver shows the changes of acute alcoholic hepatitis (steatonecrosis) [1, 6, 10, 21]. The fibrotic change is often related to another condition such as diabetes or alcoholism [6]. However, as fatty liver and steatonecrosis are found in obese, non-diabetic children [20] they are likely to be caused by obesity alone. Liver function tests reflect the underlying histological change [14].

Overall, the liver changes of obesity are benign and non-progressive. Weight loss by low-calorie dieting or starvation is accompanied by improvement in fatty change and return of liver function tests to normal [13].

EFFECTS OF JEJUNO-ILEAL BYPASS

The hepatic changes of obesity are enhanced. Hepatic lipid concentration increases, and the morphological changes of alcoholic liver disease can develop [16]. Progressive inflammation, fibrosis, zone 3 sclerosis and cirrhosis can develop within two years of the operation in 1–17%. The patient may die in hepatic failure. Reversal of the bypass may not be effective treatment although liver fat decreases [28].

The liver changes are probably related to rapid weight loss, protein-calorie malnutrition, bacterial overgrowth in the blind loop of intestine, malabsorption and other complex nutritional deficiencies. They can also follow gastric partitioning operations.

Obese subjects are prone to super-saturated bile and hence to cholesterol gallstone formation. During weight reduction, bile acid pool size falls and biliary cholesterol saturation may increase.

Parenteral nutrition [3]

Cholestasis has developed in infants given long-term parenteral nutrition for neonatal intestinal obstruction [8]. In adults, increases in serum transaminases, alkaline phosphatase and bilirubin values follow fat-free total parenteral nutrition for two weeks or longer. Liver biopsies show fatty change and mild peri-portal cholestasis. Abnormal biochemical tests also complicate enteral elemental diets in adults [5].

Hepatic fatty change occurs particularly with high glucose feeding and when the rate of infusion exceeds the hepatic oxidative capacity so that fat is synthesized. In addition, apo-

protein production is reduced. Similar effects follow intravenous fat emulsions. These changes do not develop if the infusion is balanced in terms of carbohydrate and fat.

Gallbladder biliary sludging and pigment gallstones may follow prolonged total parenteral nutrition, especially in infants [8, 19]. It is detected by ultrasound.

Vitamins

The fat-soluble vitamins A, D and K are not absorbed if biliary bile acid excretion is inadequate. Deficiencies therefore complicate cholestasis (Chapter 13).

Hypervitaminosis A leads to perisinusoidal fibrosis, central vein sclerosis and focal congestion with perisinusoidal lipid storage cells. Vitamin A fluorescence may be shown in frozen sections [24]. Portal hypertension and ascites are consequences. Similar changes can complicate *retinoid* treatment for psoriasis or acne.

Vitamin E deficiency causes a neuromuscular syndrome in patients with cholestasis.

Alcoholics may show thiamine deficiency. Clinical evidence of this in non-alcoholic patients with liver disease is very rare. Similarly folic acid may be reduced in alcoholics.

Low circulating levels of PLP, the active form of vitamin B6 compounds, in cirrhosis is probably due to increased degradation.

References

1 Adler M, Schaffner F. Fatty liver hepatitis and cirrhosis in obese patients. *Am. J. Med.* 1979; **67**: 811.
2 Allison F, Bennett MJ, Variend S *et al.* Acylo-enzyme A dehydrogenase deficiency in heart tissue from infants who died unexpectedly with fatty change in the liver. *Brit. med. J.* 1988; **296**: 11.
3 Baker AL, Rosenberg IH. Hepatic complications of total parenteral nutrition. *Am. J. Med.* 1987; **82**: 489.
4 Batman PA, Scheuer PJ. Diabetic hepatitis pre-

ceding the onset of glucose intolerance. *Histopathology* 1985; **9:** 237.

5 Bower RH. Hepatic complications of parenteral nutrition. *Semin. Liver Dis.* 1983; **3:** 216.

6 Braillon A, Herse MA, Degott C *et al.* Liver in obesity. *Gut* 1985; **26:** 133.

7 Brock JF. Survey of the world situation on kwashiorkor. *Ann. NY Acad. Sci.* 1954; **57:** 696.

8 Case records of the Massachusetts General Hospital. *N. Engl. J. Med.* 1984; **310:** 774.

9 Clain JE, Stephens DH, Charboneau JW. Ultrasonography and computed tomography in focal fatty liver. *Gastroenterology* 1984; **87:** 948.

10 Clain DJ, Lefkowitch JH. Fatty liver disease in morbid obesity. *Gastroenterol. Clin. N. Am.* 1987; **16:** 239.

11 Cook GC, Hutt MSR. The liver after kwashiorkor. *Br. med. J.* 1967; **iii:** 454.

12 Cooper AD. Role of the liver in the degradation of lipoproteins. *Gastroenterology* 1985; **88:** 192.

13 Drenick EJ, Simmons F, Murphy JF. Effect of hepatic morphology of treatment of obesity by fasting, reducing diets and small bowel bypass, *N. Engl. J. Med.* 1970; **282:** 829.

14 Galambos JT, Wills CE. Relationship between 505 paired liver tests and biopsies in 242 obese patients. *Gastroenterology* 1978; **74:** 1191.

15 Himsworth HP, Glynn LE. Massive hepatic necrosis and diffuse hepatic fibrosis (acute yellow atrophy and portal cirrhosis): their production by means of diet. *Clin. Sci.* 1944; **5:** 93.

16 Hocking MP, Duerson MC, O'Leary JP *et al.* Jejunoileal bypass for morbid obesity. *N. Engl. J. Med.* 1983; **308:** 995.

17 Jones EA, Craigie A, Tavill AS *et al.* Protein metabolism in the intestinal stagnant loop syndrome. *Gut* 1968; **9:** 466.

18 Lewis B, Hansen JDL, Wittman W *et al.* Plasma free fatty acids in kwashiorkor and the pathogenesis of the fatty liver. *Am. J. clin. Nutr.* 1964; **15:** 161.

19 Messing B, Bories C, Kunstlinger F *et al.* Does parenteral nutrition induce gallbladder sludge formation and lithiasis? *Gastroenterology* 1983; **84:** 1012.

20 Moran JR, Ghishan FK, Halter SA *et al.* Steatohepatitis in obese children. A cause of chronic liver dysfunction. *Am. J. Gastroenterol.* 1983; **78:** 374.

21 Nasrallah SM, Wills CE Jr, Galambos JT. Hepatic morphology in obesity. *Dig. Dis. Sci.* 1981; **26:** 325.

22 Neale G, Antcliff AC, Welbourn RB *et al.* Protein malnutrition after partial gastrectomy. *Q. J. Med.* 1967; **36:** 469.

23 Nomura F, Ohnishi K, Ochiai T *et al.* Obesity related non-alcoholic fatty liver: CT features and follow-up studies after low calorie diet. *Radiology* 1987; **162:** 845.

24 Russell RM, Boyer JL, Bhageri SA *et al.* Hepatic injury from chronic hypervitaminosis A resulting in portal hypertension and ascites. *N. Engl. J. Med.* 1974; **291:** 435.

25 Sherlock S. Acute fatty liver of pregnancy and the microvesicular fat diseases. *Gut* 1983; **24:** 265.

26 Sherlock S. Nutrition and the alcoholic. *Lancet* 1984; **i:** 436.

27 Sherlock S, Walshe VM. Hepatic structure and function. In *Studies of Undernutrition, Wuppertal, 1946 9.* Medical Research Council Special Report, 1951 Series No 275, p. 111.

28 Styblo T, Martin S, Kaminski DL. The effects of reversal of jejunoileal bypass operations on hepatic triglyceride content and hepatic morphology. *Surgery* 1984; **96:** 632.

29 Waterlow JC. Kwashiorkor revisited: the pathogenesis of oedema in Kwashiorkor and its significance. *Trans. R. Soc. trop. Med. Hyg.* 1984; **78:** 436.

30 Waterlow JC, Cravioto J, Stephen JML. Protein malnutrition in man. *Adv. Protein Chem.* 1960; **15:** 131.

31 Webber BL, Freiman I. The liver in kwashiorkor. *Arch. Pathol.* 1974; **98:** 400.

Carbohydrate metabolism in liver disease

HYPOGLYCAEMIA

This is usually due to reduction in hepatic glucose release. The hepatectomized dog rapidly develops hypoglycaemia [1] and this is seen in acute liver failure (Chapter 8). In fulminant hepatitis it may be intractable [2]. Hypoglycaemia is rare in chronic liver disease, even terminally. Very rarely it is found in cirrhotic patients after a porta-caval anastomosis. Reactive hypoglycaemia, 1½–2 hours after glucose, has been seen in two patients with active chronic hepatitis; blood insulin levels were high. Alcohol can also induce hypoglycaemia, especially in cirrhotic patients.

Hypoglycaemia may complicate Reye's syndrome in children, primary hepatic carcinoma, glycogen storage disease and hereditary fructose intolerance.

References

1 Mann FC, Magath TB. Studies on the physiology of the liver. II. The effect of the removal of the liver on the blood sugar level. *Arch. intern. Med.* 1922; **30:** 73.

2 Samson RI, Trey G, Timme AH *et al.* Fulminating hepatitis with recurrent hypoglycaemia and hemorrhage. *Gastroenterology* 1967; **53:** 291.

The liver in diabetes mellitus

Insulin and the liver

The liver is the principal organ for the degradation of insulin. Peripheral tissues take up insulin to a lesser extent and also remove glucagon. Hyperinsulinaemia is a characteristic association of cirrhosis and is due to failure of degradation and not to hypersecretion or extrahepatic portal–systemic bypassing [8, 9, 15].

In diabetes, glucose-6-phosphatase increases in the liver, facilitating glucose release into the blood. The opposing enzymes which phosphorylate glucose are hexokinase, which is unaffected by insulin, and glucokinase, which decreases in diabetes. As a result the liver continues to produce glucose even with severe hyperglycaemia. Under these circumstances the normal liver would shut off and deposit glycogen. Fructose-1–6-phosphate activity is also increased in diabetes. Gluconeogenesis is thus favoured.

Substances released from the pancreas into the portal blood are known to increase hepatic regeneration (*hepato-trophic substances*). Insulin is the main hepato-trophic substance although glucagon may also be important. Blood glucagon is increased in liver disease, probably due to pancreatic over-secretion.

Liver changes

A low liver glycogen is unusual even in autopsy material. Needle biopsy shows normal or increased amounts of glycogen in the livers of severe untreated diabetes [7]. Even higher values follow the administration of insulin, provided hypoglycaemia is prevented.

Histologically the zonal structure is normal. In sections stained H & E, the glycogen-filled cells appear pale and fluffy. Zone 1 cells always contain less than zone 3 and this is accentuated by glycogenolysis. In type 1, the liver cells appear bloated and oedematous: glycogen is maintained or even increased [7].

Glycogenic infiltration of the liver cell nuclei (fig. 23.8) is shown as a vacuolization, the nature of which is confirmed by glycogen stains. It is not specific but is found in about two-thirds of diabetics.

Fatty change of large droplet type is common in the obese type 2 diabetic, but is minimal in type 1 (fig. 23.9). It is mainly in zone 1.

Mechanisms. Diabetes is marked by insulin deficiency and glucagon excess (fig. 23.10). This enhances lipolysis and inhibits glucose uptake so increasing triglyceride formation by adipose tissue. Hepatic uptake of free fatty acids increases. In the liver, glycogen degradation and gluconeogenesis are increased while glucose utilization is inhibited. Ketoacidosis enhances the lipolysis. These factors are responsible for the fatty liver of diabetics.

Steatonecrosis resembling alcoholic hepatitis, but without polymorph infiltration, can be seen particularly in type 2 diabetes [5], even preceding glucose intolerance [2]. This collagenosis of Dissë's space can develop in both types of diabetes and may be aetiologically similar to that seen in systemic capillaries in diabetes [10]. Cirrhosis can develop and is twice as common in diabetics as in the general population.

Liver changes in the various types of diabetes mellitus

JUVENILE TYPE 1 OR
INSULIN-DEPENDENT

There are usually no clinical features referable to the liver. Occasionally, however, the liver is greatly enlarged, firm and with a smooth, tender edge. Some of the nausea, abdominal pain and vomiting of diabetic ketosis may be due to hepatomegaly [6]. Hepatic enlargement is

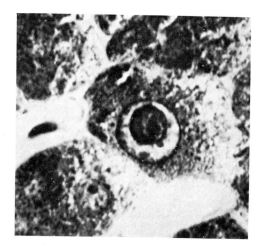

Fig. 23.8. Glycogen infiltration of an hepatic nucleus. Cells contain much glycogen. Best's carmine for glycogen, ×1150.

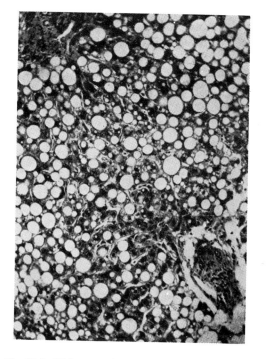

Fig. 23.9. Diabetes mellitus. Liver biopsy sections show great increase in fat in the liver cells. H & E, ×145 (Sherlock *et al.* 1951).

found particularly in young people and children with severe, uncontrolled diabetes. In adults, **479** hepatomegaly occurs with prolonged acidosis.

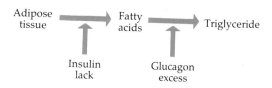

Fig. 23.10. The mechanism of microvesicular fatty change in type 2 diabetes.

In one large series, hepatomegaly was noted in only 9% of well-controlled diabetics, in 60% of uncontrolled diabetics and in 100% of patients in ketosis [6]. The liver returns to a normal size when the diabetes is brought under complete control. The enlargement is due to increased glycogen. Insulin therapy in the presence of a very high blood sugar level augments still further the glycogen content of the liver and in the initial stages of treatment, hepatomegaly may increase. The liver cells in severe acidosis may contain more water than usual: it is probably retained to keep the glycogen in solution.

The blood glucose levels and hepatic glucose output fall promptly with insulin [3]. In ketosis, hepatic insulin sensitivity is lost.

TYPE 2 OR
INSULIN-INDEPENDENT

The liver may be enlarged with a firm smooth non-tender edge. Enlargement is due to increased deposition of liver fat largely related to the obesity.

The blood glucose level and the hepatic glucose output respond poorly to a small dose of insulin [2, 3].

Diabetes in childhood

The liver may be enlarged and this enlargement has been attributed both to fatty infiltration and to increased amounts of glycogen. Aspiration biopsy studies show that the fatty change is slight but that the liver does contain an excess of glycogen. The hepatic changes are similar to those already described in the type 1, insulin-sensitive diabetic.

Sometimes a huge liver is associated with retarded growth, obesity, florid facies and hypercholesterolaemia (*Mauriac syndrome*) [12]. Splenomegaly, portal hypertension and hepato-cellular failure do not occur.

Liver function tests

In well-controlled diabetics, routine tests are usually normal and any change is due to a cause other than diabetes. Acidosis may produce mild changes including hyperglobulinaemia and a slightly raised serum bilirubin level. These return to normal with diabetic control.

80% of diabetics with a fatty liver have abnormal results for one or more serum biochemical test such as transaminases, alkaline phosphatase and gammaglutamyl transpeptidase.

Hepatomegaly, whether due to increased amounts of glycogen in type 1 or to fatty change in type 2, does not correlate with the results of the liver function tests.

Hepato-biliary disease and diabetes

Any real increase of cirrhosis in diabetics seems unlikely. In most instances, the cirrhosis is diagnosed first, before impaired glucose tolerance is recognized.

Diabetes mellitus is associated with hereditary haemochromatosis. It is also associated with auto-immune chronic active hepatitis and with the histocompatibility antigens HLA-B8 DW3, which are common to both.

Gallstones are frequent in type 2 diabetics [1]. Bile acid synthesis rate decreases but cholesterol synthesis does not change. The saturation index of hepatic bile therefore increases and this is further raised if insulin therapy is given. Reduced gallbladder contractability, a consequence of diabetic visceral neuropathy, contributes. Elective surgery is not dangerous but emergency biliary surgery in diabetics is associated with an increased mortality and a high risk of wound infections.

Sulfonylurea therapy can be complicated by cholestatic or granulomatous liver disease.

Peripheral monocytes from cirrhotic patients have reduced numbers of insulin receptors [4]. Adipocytes show defects in insulin sensitivity [16]. Insulin degradation is reduced due to hepatocyte disease and to intra-hepatic portal–systemic shunting [14]. Cirrhotic patients therefore often have an impaired oral and intravenous glucose tolerance test and increased resistance to exogenous insulin (fig. 23.11) [13]. This is in spite of raised blood insulin levels and indicates peripheral insulin resistance (13). Reduced liver mass is contributory [11].

The glucose intolerance of cirrhotic patients can be distinguished from genuine diabetes mellitus as the fasting blood glucose is usually normal and blood insulin levels are increased. Clinical features of diabetes are not seen. Insulin therapy is not required.

High carbohydrate feeding may be necessary in the management of cirrhosis, especially if there is encephalopathy. This always takes precedence over any impairment of glucose tolerance whether genuine diabetes or secondary to the liver disease.

Cirrhotics are twice as likely as the general population to have diabetes. The cirrhosis may have unmasked a genetically determined diabetic trait.

Diagnosis of cirrhosis in the presence of diabetes is usually easy, for diabetes alone does not cause vascular spiders, jaundice, hepatosplenomegaly and ascites. If necessary liver biopsy is diagnostic.

References

1 Abrams JJ, Ginsberg H, Grundy SM. Metabolism of cholesterol and plasma triglycerides in non-ketotic diabetes mellitus. *Diabetes* 1982; **29**: 788.

2 Batman PA, Scheuer PJ. Diabetic hepatitis preceeding the onset of glucose intolerance. *Histopathology* 1985; **9**: 237.

3 Bearn AG, Billing BH, Sherlock S. Hepatic glucose output and hepatic insulin sensitivity in diabetes mellitus. *Lancet* 1951; **ii**: 698.

4 Blei AT, Robbins DC, Drobny E *et al.* Insulin resistance and insulin receptors in hepatic cirrhosis. *Gastroenterology* 1982; **83**: 1191.

5 Falchuk KR, Fiske SC, Haggitt RC *et al.* Pericentral

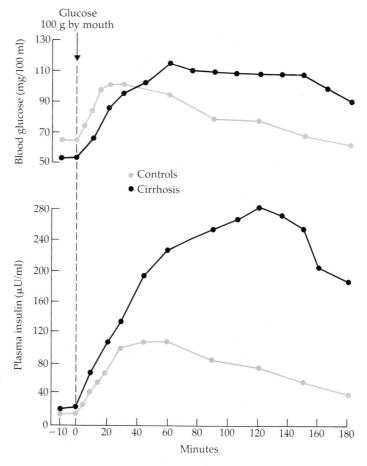

Fig. 23.11. The oral glucose tolerance test in cirrhosis. The cirrhotic patients showed a normal fasting blood glucose but some impaired tolerance. Plasma insulin levels rose slowly in controls and there was insulin resistance (Megyesi *et al.* 1967).

hepatic fibrosis and intracellular hyalin in diabetes mellitus. *Gastroenterology* 1980; **78**: 535.

6 Goodman JI. Hepatomegaly and diabetes mellitus. *Ann. intern. Med.* 1953; **39**: 1077.

7 Hildes JA, Sherlock S, Walsh V. Liver and muscle glycogen in normal subjects, in diabetes mellitus and in acute hepatitis. *Clin. Sci.* 1949; **7**: 287.

8 Johnston DG, Alberti KGM, Faber OK *et al.* Hyperinsulinism of hepatic cirrhosis: diminished degradation or hypersecretion? *Lancet* 1977; **i**: 10.

9 Johnston DG, Alberti GMK, George K *et al.* C-peptide and insulin in live disease. *Diabetes* 1978; **27**: 201.

10 Latry P, Bioulac-Sage P, Echinard E *et al.* Perisinusoidal fibrosis and basement membrane-like material in the livers of diabetic patients. *Hum. Path.* 1987; **18**: 775.

11 Marchesini G, Bianchi GP, Forlani G *et al.* Insulin resistance is the main determinant of impaired glucose tolerance in patients with liver cirrhosis. *Dig. Dis. Sci.* 1987; **32**: 1118.

12 Mauriac P. Hepatomégalie, nanismé, obesité dans le diabète infantile: pathogenie du syndrome. *Presse med.* 1946; **54**: 826.

13 Megyesi C, Samols E, Marks V. Glucose tolerance and diabetes in chronic liver disease. *Lancet* 1967; **ii**: 1051.

14 Ohnishi K, Mishira A, Takashi M *et al.* Effects of intra- and extrahepatic portal systemic shunts on insulin metabolism. *Dig. Dis. Sci.* 1983; **28**: 201.

15 Smith-Laing G, Sherlock S, Faber OK. Effects of spontaneous portal–systemic shunting on insulin metabolism. *Gastroenterology* 1979; **76**: 685.

16 Taylor R, Heine RJ, Collins J *et al.* Insulin action in cirrhosis. *Hepatology* 1985; **5**: 64.

The glycogenoses

These are diseases with excessive and/or abnormal glycogen in the tissues [13]. Various forms have different enzymatic or structural defects.

Needle biopsy specimens should be examined histologically, quantitative glycogen analysis is helpful and a portion should be sent, appropriately preserved, to a centre where *in vitro* study of the enzymes present and of glycogen structure can be made (table 23.4). The diagnosis cannot be made on hepatic histology alone. All forms seem to be inherited, usually as an autosomal recessive except type VI which is sex-linked. The types vary greatly in their severity and in their clinical picture. The critical abnormality is usually insufficient glucose production by the liver, which results in hypoglycaemia when the blood glucose level is not supported by an inflow of glucose from the intestinal tract. The other abnormalities follow this defect and from the metabolic reactions to hypoglycaemia (fig. 23.12).

Type I (Von Gierke's disease)

This type involves liver and kidney but not muscle and heart. The inheritance is autosomal recessive. Siblings may be involved, but transmission through successive generations has not been shown.

Type 1a is due to deficiency in the liver of glucose-6-phosphatase. In *type 1b*, the defect is in glucose-6-phosphatase at the membrane of the endoplasmic reticulum [16]. The clinical features of 1a and 1b are generally similar. Type 1b may affect adults.

Pericellular zone 3 fibrosis and Mallory bodies have been described in type 1a glycogenosis [14].

Type 1c is due to a defect in hepatic microsomal phosphate/pyrophosphate translocase T-2 [3].

HEPATIC CHANGES

The liver is enlarged, smooth and brown. The liver cells and their nuclei are laden with glycogen, but this is not diagnostic. In formol-fixed material, glycogen is washed out leaving an appearance of clear, plant-like cells. Excess fat is usually present. The glycogen is usually stable, persisting many days *post mortem* and despite severe ketosis or prolonged anaesthesia. Cirrhosis does not develop. Hepatocellular adenomas and, rarely, carcinomas are late developments [11].

CLINICAL FEATURES

In early infancy the symptoms include irritability, pallor, cyanosis, feeding difficulties and seizures usually associated with hypoglycaemia. Episodes of diarrhoea and vomiting are frequent.

Presentation is as massive hepatomegaly at about two years old. The spleen is not enlarged—a point of distinction from the lipoidoses, the cirrhoses and congenital hepatic fibrosis.

Table 23.4. The hepatic glycogen storage diseases

Type	Enzyme defect	Tissues involved
I	Glucose-6-phosphatase	Liver, kidney intestines
II	Lysosomal alpha-1,4 glucosidase (acid maltase)	Generalized
III	Amylo-1,6 glucosidase (debranching enzyme)	Liver, muscle WBC
IV	Amylo-1,4,1,6 transglucosidase (branching enzyme)	Generalized
VI	Liver phosphorylase	Liver, WBC
VIII	Phosphorylase activation	Liver
IXa, IXb	Phosphorylase kinase	Liver, WBC, RBC

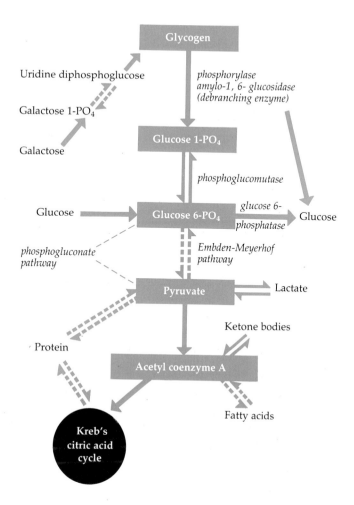

Fig. 23.12. Metabolic pathways in glycogen breakdown (Sokal 1962).

Untreated patients have a doll-like facies and hypotonia with delayed motor milestones.

Type 1 glycogenosis can present in adults as hypoglycaemic symptoms and/or hepatomegaly [3].

Hypoglycaemic episodes and fasting ketosis are usual.

The child is short and fat with particularly fat cheeks. Mental development is usually normal.

Excessive bleeding is due to abnormal platelet function. In type 1b infectious complications are due to neutropenia and neutrophil dysfunction related to abnormal glucose-6-phosphatase transport [1].

INVESTIGATIONS

Routine liver function tests are usually normal. Occasionally transaminases are raised.

The fasting blood glucose level is low. Ketosis is related to defective glucose metabolism. Hyperlipaemia, hypercholesterolaemia and a fatty liver are common. Plasma uric acid levels are raised and gout develops after puberty. There is chronic lactic acidosis.

Diagnosis depends on showing that the blood glucose fails to rise adequately when hepatic glycogenolysis is stimulated. *Glucagon* (20 µg/kg body weight) is given intramuscularly after a fast of 10–12 hours, or 3–4 hours if hypoglycaemia is severe. Results are classified according to the blood glucose response. Normals show a rise of 35 mg/100 ml, subnormals 15–35 mg/100 ml, and absent or minimal less than 15 mg/100 ml. Lactic acid changes are classified as normal with increases of less than 10 mg/100 ml or abnormal with increases of more than 10 mg/100 ml.

These patients cannot utilize galactose or fructose as a source of blood glucose and intravenous lactose and fructose tests may also be performed.

The erythrocyte glycogen level is increased.

If a test is positive, liver biopsy should be taken for histology, including histochemistry, quantitative glycogen analysis and enzyme analysis.

Classification into the actual type can then be attempted.

TREATMENT

Repeated glucose feeds, often given as a continual nocturnal infusion, are needed to prevent hypoglycaemia [9]. The optimal rate of enteral carbohydrate infusion to maintain normoglycaemia and suppress organic acidaemia is 8.5 mg carbohydrate per kilogram per minute [19]. Uncooked corn starch, a slow release source of glucose, is an alternative regime [5]. Parenteral hyperalimentation may be useful [4]. Allopurinol may be given for the high serum uric acid. Hepatic transplantation has been successfully performed for hepatic adomas in type 1a [6].

PROGNOSIS

Many patients die in early childhood, often with infections. There are great variations in severity and some patients seem to recover completely. The disease tends to become milder after puberty. Later deaths are due to gouty nephropathy or to hepato-cellular tumours. Haemorrhage into an adenoma may necessitate resection [8].

Type II (Pompe's disease)

This primary lysosomal disease is due to deficiency of lysosomal acid α-1,4 glucosidase which prevents degradation of glycogen within lysosomes.

There is weakness of skeletal muscle, cardiomegaly, hepatomegaly and macroglossia. Mental development is normal. Infantile, childhood and adult onset forms exist. The infantile is the most severe. Glucagon and adrenaline tests are normal and hypoglycaemia does not occur. Hyperlipidaemia is conspicuous.

All organs show vacuolated cells due to the enlarged lysosomes which contain the glycogen. Vacuolated lymphocytes are found in peripheral blood and marrow. The liver cells at autopsy show particularly prominent vacuoles.

Type III (Cori's disease) (fig. 23.13)

Clinically this resembles type 1 glycogenosis. Acidosis, hypoglycaemia and hyperlipidaemia may be present. Blood glucose does not rise after glucagon, but galactose and fructose tolerance are normal. Serum transaminases are usually increased. Symptoms may be mild and by adult life only the hepatomegaly may remain. The prognosis is fair to good.

Peri-portal fibrosis occurs but cirrhosis is rare. Liver biopsy is rarely necessary for diagnosis which is made by measuring debrancher activity in a mixed white blood cell pellet.

Glycogen is increased in muscle and liver and the debranching enzyme, amylo-1,6 glucosidase, is absent.

Corn starch therapy may improve growth and liver function [2].

Type IV (Andersen's disease)

This very rare form of generalized glycogenosis is associated with low normal tissue levels of glycogen. The glycogen structure is abnormal due to deficiency of the branching enzyme amylo-1,4,1,6 transglucosidase.

A cirrhosis develops which may be associated with many giant cells. It can resemble that of

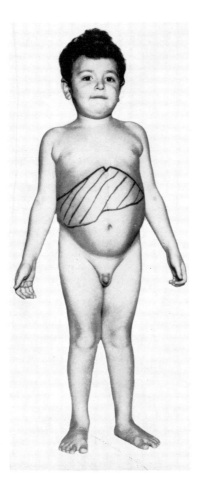

Fig. 23.13. Type III glycogen storage disease (Cori's disease). A boy of four years with enormous hepatomegaly but without splenomegaly. At the age of 20, this young man is well and has just finished his military service.

the alcoholic. The chief distinction is the presence of intracellular deposits of abnormal glycogen partially removed by diastase digestion. This may show abnormal staining properties turning purplish with iodine instead of the usual reddish-brown. It stains strongly with PAS. The cirrhosis is presumably due to a reaction to this abnormal glycogen. This abnormal material is found in every organ examined [18].

^{21}P magnetic resistance spectroscopy can be used for diagnosis, to monitor compliance with diet and to detect heterozygotes [17].

The child develops hepatosplenomegaly, ascites and finally liver failure. Enzyme deficiencies in skin fibroblasts have been shown and may allow diagnosis and detection of heterozygotes [10]. The features of cirrhosis are present. Death is in early childhood.

Hepatic transplantation should be considered.

Type VI (Hers' disease)

This involves only the liver and is marked by deficiency of phosphorylase. Growth retardation and hepatomegaly are marked. Hypoglycaemia and acidosis are usually found. Mental function is normal. Survival into adult life is usual.

Variants have been described as type VIII and type XI glycogenosis [12]. Here, although phosphorylase is reduced it can be increased to normal by glucagon or adrenaline, or *in vitro* by substitution of an activation system. In these patients the low hepatic phosphorylase activity is not the result of deficiency of the enzymes.

Type IXa and IXb

This benign condition is due to phosphorylase kinase deficiency. It presents with short stature and hepatomegaly. The outlook is excellent and the patient catches up growth and hepatomegaly becomes less marked. It is diagnosed by measuring phosphorylase kinase in red blood cells. Autosomal and X-linked forms exist.

Low molecular weight glycogen

This very rare condition is associated with cirrhosis, early death and a widespread deposition in tissues, including the liver, of a polysaccharide material of low molecular weight.

Hepatic glycogen synthetase deficiency [7]

This very rare condition is associated with glucose intolerance, hypoglycaemia and mental retardation. Analysis of liver biopsy material shows complete absence of the enzyme glycogen synthetase.

References

1 Ambruso DR, McCabe ERB, Anderson D *et al.* Infectious and bleeding complications in patients with glycogenosis lb. *Am. J. Dis. Child.* 1985; **139:** 691.

2 Borowitz SM, Greene HL. Cornstarch therapy in a patient with type III glycogen storage disease. *J. Paediatr. Gastroenterol. Nutr.* 1987; **6:** 631.

3 Burchell A, Jung RT, Lang CC *et al.* Diagnosis of type 1a and type 1c glycogen storage diseases in adults. *Lancet* 1987; **i:** 1059.

4 Burr IM, O'Neill JA, Karson DT *et al.* Comparison of the effects of total parenteral nutrition, continuous intragastric feeding and portacaval shunt on a patient with type 1 glycogen storage disease. *J. Paediatr.* 1974; **85:** 792.

5 Chen Y-T, Cornblath M, Sidbury JB. Corn starch therapy in type 1 glycogen-storage disease. *N. Engl. J. Med.* 1984; **310:** 171.

6 Coire CI, Qizilbash AH, Castelli MF. Hepatic adenomata in type 1a glycogen storage disease. *Arch. Pathol. lab. Med.* 1987; **111:** 166.

7 Dykes JRW, Spencer-Peet J. Hepatic glycogen synthetase deficiency. Further studies on a family. *Arch. Dis. Child.* 1972; **47:** 558.

8 Fink AS, Appleman HD. Hemorrhage into a hepatic adenoma and type 1a glycogen storage disease: a case report and review of the literature. *Surgery* 1985; **97:** 117.

9 Greene HL, Slonim AE, O'Neill JA *et al.* Continuous nocturnal intragastric feeding for management of type 1 glycogen-storage disease. *N. Engl. J. Med.* 1976; **294:** 423.

10 Howell RR, Kaback MM, Brown BI. Type IV glycogen storage disease: branching enzyme deficiency in skin fibroblasts and possible heterozygote detection. *J. Paediatr..* 1971; **78:** 638.

11 Howell RR, Stevenson RE, Ben-Menachem Y *et al.* Hepatic adenomata with type 1 glycogen storage disease. *J. Am. Med. Assoc.* 1976; **236:** 1481.

12 Hug G, Schubert WK, Chuck G *et al.* Liver phosphorylase. Deactivation in a child with progressive brain disease, elevated hepatic glycogen and increased urinary catecholamines. *J. Am. med. Assoc.* 1967; **42:** 139.

13 Huijing F. Glycogen metabolism and glycogen-storage diseases. *Physiol Rev.* 1975; **55:** 609.

14 Itoh S, Ishida Y, Matsuo S. Mallory bodies in a patient with type 1a glycogen storage disease. *Gastroenterology* 1987; **92:** 520.

15 Krivit W, Sharp HL, Lee JC. Low molecular weight glycogen as a cause of generalised glycogen storage disease. *N. Engl. J. Med.* 1973; **54:** 88.

16 Kuzuya T, Matsuda A, Yoshida S *et al.* An adult case of type 1b glycogen-storage disease. *N. Engl. J. Med.* 1983; **308:** 566.

17 Oberhaensli RD, Rajagopalan B, Taylor DJ *et al.* Study of hereditary fructose intolerance by use of ^{31}P magnetic resonance spectroscopy. *Lancet* 1987; **ii:** 931.

18 Schochet SS Jr, McCormick WF, Zellweger H. Type IV glycogenosis (amylopectinosis) light and electron microscopic observations. *Arch. Pathol.* 1970; **90:** 354.

19 Schwenk WF, Haymond MW. Optimal rate of enteral glucose administration in children with glycogen storage disease type 1. *N. Engl. J. Med.* 1986; **314:** 680.

Hereditary fructose intolerance

An autosomal recessive defect of aldolase B severely impairs the enzymatic cleavage of fructose 1-phosphate in liver, renal cortex and intestinal epithelium. Exposure to fructose induces cytoplasmic accumulation of fructose 1-phosphate and hence fructose intoxication [1].

The acute syndrome is marked by abdominal pain, vomiting and hypoglycaemia. The chronic syndrome is one of severe metabolic derangement with failure to thrive, vomiting, hepatomegaly and liver and renal tubular dysfunction. Fructosaemia, fructosuria and hypophosphataemia are features. Hepatic histology shows similar findings to galactosaemia with the ultimate development of cirrhosis.

Older children learn to avoid fructose and sucrose and isolated hepatomegaly may be the only abnormality.

Treament is by a diet without sucrose and fructose. Sometimes the symptoms persist in older children and are marked by growth retardation when even more strict fructose restriction may be necessary [2].

References

1 Froesch ER, Wolf HP, Baitsch H *et al.* Hereditary fructose intolerance: inborn defect of hepatic fructose-1-phosphate splitting aldolase. *Am. J. Med.* 1963; **34:** 151.

2 Mock DM, Perman JA, Thaler MM *et al.* Chronic fructose intoxication after infancy in children with hereditary fructose intolerance: a cause of growth retardation. *N. Engl. J. Med.* 1983; **309**: 764.
3 Oberhaensli RD, Rajagopalan B, Taylor DJ *et al.* Study of hereditary fructose intolerance by use of ^{31}P magnetic resonance spectroscopy. *Lancet* 1987; **ii**: 931.

Glutaric aciduria type II

This disturbance of organic acid metabolism presents in infants or adults as recurrent hypoglycaemia with elevated serum free fatty acid [1]. The liver shows fatty change, glycogen depletion and patchy necrosis.

Reference

1 Dusheiko G, Kew MC, Joffe BI *et al.* Recurrent hypoglycaemia associated with glutaric aciduria type II in an adult. *N. Engl. J. Med.* 1979; **301**: 1405.

Galactosaemia

The liver and red blood cells lack the specific enzyme, galactose-1-phosphate-uridyl transferase, essential for galactose metabolism [1]. Toxic effects are related to the accumulation in the tissues of galactose-1-phosphate. The mechanism of toxicity is uncertain.

Transferase deficiency is inherited as an autosomal recessive. A significant reduction of the transferase is found in heterozygotes.

CLINICAL PICTURE

The disease starts *in utero*. The infant presents with feeding difficulties, with vomiting, diarrhoea and malnutrition, often with jaundice. Ascites and hepatosplenomegaly are noted. Cataracts develop. Death may result in the first few weeks, but survivors become mentally retarded and finally show the features of cirrhosis, portal hypertension and, later, ascites.

HEPATIC CHANGES [5]

Those dying in the first few weeks show diffuse hepato-cellular fatty change. In the next few months the liver shows pseudoglandular or ductular structures around the canaliculi which may contain bile. Regeneration is conspicuous, necrosis scanty and a macronodular cirrhosis results. Giant cells may be numerous.

DIAGNOSIS [4]

The biochemical changes [1] include galactosaemia, galactosuria, hyperchloraemic acidosis, albuminuria and aminoaciduria. Diagnosis is made by finding a urinary reducing substance which is glucose oxidase negative. Definite diagnosis comes from determining galactose-1-phosphate uridyl transferase levels in the erythrocytes.

The condition should be considered in all young patients with cirrhosis and even in the adult if there are suggestive features such as cataract. Galactosaemia has been diagnosed as late as 63 years [3]. A survey of a group of juvenile cirrhotics with this disease, however, failed to reveal a single case and this must be a rare cause of adult cirrhosis [2].

PROGNOSIS AND TREATMENT

Great improvement results from withdrawal of dietary milk and milk products from the diet. If the child survives to five years of age, recovery may be complete apart from persistent cataracts or cirrhosis. Those living into childhood and adult life without treatment may be only partially enzyme-deficient. Alternatively they may have developed another pathway for handling galactose [1]. The consumption of galactose-containing foods also decreases with age.

References

1 Cohn RM, Segal S. Galactose metabolism and its regulation. *Metabolism* 1973; **22**: 627.
2 Fisher MM, Spear S, Samols E *et al.* Erythrocytic galactose-1-phosphate uridyl transferase levels in hepatic cirrhosis. *Gut* 1964; **5**: 170.
3 Hsia DY-Y, Walker FA. Variability in the clinical manifestations of galactosaemia. *J. Pediatr.* 1961; **59**: 872.

4 Monk AM, Mitchell AJH, Milligan DWA *et al.* The diagnosis of classical galactosaemia. *Arch. Dis. Child.* 1977; **52**: 943.
5 Smetana HF, Olen E. Hereditary galactose disease. *Am. J. clin. Pathol.* 1962; **93**: 3.

Mucopolysaccharidoses

These are a group of lysosomal storage diseases each of which is due to a deficiency of a specific lysosomal enzyme involved in the degradation of dermatin sulphate, heparin sulphate or keratin sulphate.

Hepatocyte and Kupffer cell swelling and vacuolization are due to storage of poorly degraded mucopolysaccharide.

In addition, hepatic fibrosis outlining the hepatic lobule (zone 1) may be seen. The mechanism is unknown, but is possibly due to abnormal accumulation of a hepatotoxic metabolite of mucopolysaccharide.

Hurler's syndrome (gargoylism) (MPU) is inherited as an autosomal recessive and is characterized by deficiency of the lysosomal degrading enzyme, alpha-L-iduronidase, in liver, cultured skin fibroblasts and leucocytes. It is characterized by coarse facial features, dwarfism, limitation of joint movement, deafness, abdominal hernias, hepatosplenomegaly, cardiac abnormalities and mental retardation.

The liver in the mucopolysaccharidoses is large and firm. Fibrosis and cirrhosis may be present. Microscopically, liver cells and Kupffer cells are swollen, empty or vacuolated [1]. The vacuoles consist of lysosomes containing mucopolysaccharide. The material is demonstrated by a colloidal iron stain.

Diagnosis may be made by finding increased urinary or leucocyte mucopolysaccharides. Culture of skin biopsies shows fibroblasts containing mucopolysaccharides.

Reference

1 Van Hoof F. Mucopolysaccharidoses and mucolipidoses *J. clin. Pathol.* 1974; **27** (suppl. 8); 64.

Familial hypercholesterolaemia

This is an autosomal dominant disease due to absence of a gene which codes for the LDL receptor on cell membranes [2]. The liver contains 60% of such receptors. Sufferers have increased plasma total cholesterol and LDL from birth, cutaneous xanthomas develop and most homozygotes die from coronary artery disease before the age of 30.

Hypercholesterolaemia is controlled by reduction in dietary saturated fats and administration of bile acid sequestrants such as cholestyramine. One child has been successfully treated by simultaneous heart transplant for the coronary disease and liver transplant to provide low-density lipoprotein receptors [1, 3]. Follow-up showed decreases in LDL and plasma cholesterol [4].

References

1 Bilheimer DW, Goldstein JL, Grundy SM *et al.* Liver transplantation to provide low-density-lipoprotein receptors and lower plasma cholesterol in a child with homozygous familial hypocholesterolemia. *N. Engl. J. Med.* 1984; **311**: 1638.
2 Brown MS, Goldstein JL. Lipoprotein receptors in the liver: control signals for plasma cholesterol traffic. *J. clin. Invest.* 1983; **72**: 743.
3 Starzl TE, Bilheimer DW, Bahnson HT *et al.* Heart—liver transplantation in a patient with familial hypercholesterolaemia. *Lancet* 1984; **i**: 1382.
4 Valdivielso P, Escolar JL, Cuervas-Mons V *et al.* Lipids and lipoprotein changes after heart and liver transplantation in a patient with homozygous familial hypercholesterolemia. *Ann. intern. Med.* 1988; **108**: 204.

Hepatic amyloidosis

This waxy infiltration of the organs was termed amyloidosis because it resembled starch in its staining [13].

The diseases have in common extracellular deposition of a number of relatively insoluble proteins as fibrils with typical staining properties. All forms are related to overproduction of a protein which can assume a fibrillar form;

Table 23.5. Classification of the amyloid diseases

Type	Pathology	Protein
Primary	Pericollagen	AL
With multiple myeloma	Pericollagen	AL
Secondary	Perireticulin	AA
With familial Mediterranean fever	Perireticulin	AA

they can be termed β-fibrilloses [5]. The amyloid is deposited in association with glycoprotein composed of globular sub-units. At least six different proteins can be concerned.

The amyloidoses may be classified according to the protein deposited (table 23.5).

In the case of primary amyloidosis and the amyloidosis accompanying multiple myeloma the protein consists of immunoglobulin light chains of kappa or lambda types and is termed AL [5].

In the case of secondary amyloidosis and the amyloidosis complicating familial Mediterranean fever (FMF) the protein shares antigenicity and structure with the acute phase protein of human serum and is termed AA. During the acute phase response, interleukin 1 is produced through activated macrophages. This causes reduced hepatic albumin synthesis, with production of acute phase proteins including serum amyloid A protein (SAA) [3]. A persistently high SAA level is a prerequisite for AA amyloidosis, but not every patient with such levels will develop the disease. Predisposing factors include failure of AA degradation, a low serum albumin level, activity of proteolytic enzymes from macrophages and genetics [2].

Amyloid fibrils may resolve. This emphasizes the importance of searching for precipitating chronic diseases in patients with amyloidosis.

The amyloid fibrils are deposited along pre-existing fibres which may be reticulin, giving perireticulin amyloidosis, or collagen, giving pericollagen amyloidosis [6].

Perireticulin amyloidosis (AA) is primarily a disease of small blood vessels, capillaries (including sinusoids) and small veins. Parenchymal tissue is replaced only secondarily to the spillover of amyloid beyond capillary structures.

Pericollagen amyloidosis (AC) affects vessels, connective tissue round vessels, the stroma of various organs, sarcolemma and neurilemma. Hepatic involvement is constant, but the concept that parenchymal amyloid is AA and vascular is AL is not always true, and the two may overlap [1].

Primary amyloidosis ('atypical') (AL). This is rare and occurs without pre-existing disease. The liver is rarely involved by deposits in the walls of the small hepatic arterioles in the portal tracts. The deposits may stain poorly with Congo red. Parenchymal deposits are also seen.

Amyloidosis complicating myeloma (AL). This occurs in about 15% of patients. The deposits are usually in the atypical ('primary') distribution.

Familial Mediterranean fever (FMF) (AA) [5]. Although of perireticulin type, the hepatic sinusoids, surprisingly, are spared. Hepatic involvement is seen only in the arterioles. The glomeruli, spleen and pulmonary alveoli bear the brunt of the disease. Renal failure is fatal.

Secondary (acquired, perireticular) (AA). This is the commonest form, involving spleen, kidneys, liver and adrenal glands, in that order of frequency. It follows chronic diseases such as tuberculosis, pleuro-pulmonary suppuration, long-standing rheumatoid arthritis, ulcerative colitis, Crohn's disease, leprosy, some neoplasms and Hodgkin's disease. Affected organs have a firm waxy consistency and develop a deep red-brown colour on the addition of dilute iodine.

Globular amyloid. Eosinophilic globules 5–40 μm in diameter are found in the space of Dissë and aggregated within the portal tracts. There are no distinctive clinical or laboratory features distinguishing this type from classical hepatic amyloidosis. It is, however, not associated with multiple myeloma [7]. Globular amyloid usually co-exists with classical (AA) systemic amyloidosis.

CLINICAL FEATURES OF HEPATIC INVOLVEMENT

Hepato-cellular failure and portal hypertension are rare. Jaundice is present in about 5%. Biochemical tests are usually normal apart from a slight rise in alkaline phosphatase. Amyloidosis is suspected when an enlarged, smooth, non-tender liver is detected in a patient with a predisposing cause; however, occasionally the liver may not be enlarged. An enlarged spleen, infiltrated with amyloid, may be found.

Severe intra-hepatic cholestasis may rarely complicate kappa and lambda AL amyloidosis [8, 12]. It is presumably due to the intense amyloid deposition interfering with bile passage into canaliculi and small bile ducts. The prognosis is very poor for the cholestatic type.

There may be a nephrotic syndrome, albuminuria or progressive renal failure.

DIAGNOSTIC METHODS

Aspiration liver biopsy is the most satisfactory technique for diagnosis. Hepatic amyloidosis is diffuse and the sampling error is negligible. The procedure is said to be dangerous, but this has been over-emphasized.

Histologically, the amyloid is shown as homogeneous, amorphous, eosinophilic material (fig. 23.14). It stains with Congo red or methyl violet (fig. 23.15) and reddish-brown with iodine. All these reactions are transient and remain for only a few weeks. Polarization microscopy of Congo red stained sections shows the amyloid as green birefringent fibrils [6]. Amyloid may also be shown by fluorescent microscopy.

The amyloid is deposited between the columns of liver cells and the sinusoidal wall in the space of Dissë. The liver cells themselves are not involved but are compressed to a variable extent. The mid-zonal and portal areas are most heavily infiltrated.

Occasionally, in primary amyloidosis or complicating multiple myeloma, the amyloid is found only in the portal tracts in the walls of hepatic arterioles, around the interlobular arteries and lying free in clumps.

Electron microscopy confirms fibrils 10 nm long that do not branch.

Percutaneous renal biopsy is used for the diagnosis of renal involvement.

Rectal biopsy is safe and useful. The amyloid is deposited in the walls of arterioles.

Hepatic scan. Multiple filling defects simulate metastases.

In patients with AA, *immuno-electrophoresis* can detect a monoclonal protein in serum or urine in about 90% of patients [6].

PROGNOSIS

This depends on the causative condition and on the extent of the kidney involvement. Ninety per cent of patients with secondary amyloid disease are dead within two years of diagnosis, usually from the toxaemia of their chronic infection. In the few patients who live long enough, death occurs from secondarily contracted amyloid kidneys. These patients never die of liver failure.

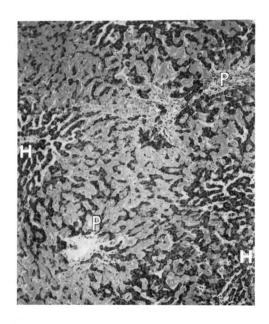

Fig. 23.14. Amyloid material is deposited in the sinusoidal wall, especially in the periportal zones. The liver cell trabeculae are narrowed. H = central hepatic veins; P = portal tracts. Best's carmine, ×70.

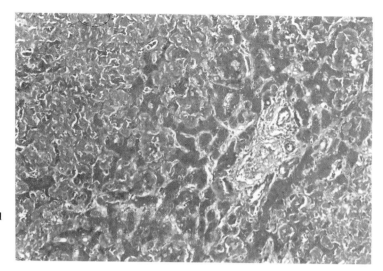

Fig. 23.15. Amyloid is shown as amorphous dark staining material between liver cells and sinusoids (stained methyl violet × 40 alpha antitrypsin).

TREATMENT

AA amyloid is treated by controlling the underlying disease. If tuberculosis is cured then amyloid may disappear [14]. Similarly, clinical improvement in rheumatoid arthritis may be paralleled by disappearance of clinical signs of amyloidosis. There is no specific treatment.

AL amyloid may be treated by melphalan-β prednisone which reduces the synthesis of precursor proteins [4, 10].

Colchicine, which blocks amyloid induction and prevents fibril deposition, is of value in the amyloidosis complicating SMF [11].

References

1 Chopra S, Rubinow A, Koff RS *et al.* Hepatic amyloidosis: a histopathologic analysis of primary (AL) and secondary (AA) forms. *Am. J. Pathol.* 1984; **115**: 186.

2 Cohen AS, Connors LH. The pathogenesis and biochemistry of amyloidosis. *J. Pathol.* 1987; **151**: 1.

3 Dinarello CA. Interleukin-I and the pathogenesis of the acute phase response. *N. Engl. J. Med.* 1984; **311**: 1413.

4 Gertz MA, Kyle RA. Response of primary hepatic amyloidosis to melphalan and prednisone: a case report and review of the literature. *Mayo Clin. Proc.* 1986; **61**: 218.

5 Glenner GG. Medical progress: amyloid deposits and amyloidosis. The β-fibrilloses. *N. Engl. J. Med.* 1980; **302**: 1283.

6 Heller H, Missmahl H-P, Sohar E *et al.* Amyloidosis: its differentiation into perireticulin and pericollagen types. *J. Path. Bact.* 1964; **88**: 15.

7 Kanel GC, Uchida T, Peters RL. Globular hepatic amyloid—an unusual morphologic presentation. *Hepatology* 1981; **1**: 647.

8 Konikoff F, Mor C, Stern S *et al.* Cholestasis and liver failure with lambda-AL amyloidosis. *Gut* 1987; **28**: 903.

9 Kyle RA, Greipp PR. Amyloidosis (AL): clinical and laboratory features in 229 cases. *Mayo Clin. Proc.* 1983; **58**: 665.

10 Kyle RA, Greipp PR, Garton JP *et al.* Primary systemic amyloidosis. Comparison of melphalan/prednisone versus colchicine. *Am. J. Med.* 1985; **79**: 708.

11 Ravid M, Robson M, Kedar I. Prolonged colchicine treatment in four patients with amyloidosis. *Ann. intern. Med.* 1977; **87**: 568.

12 Skander MP, Harry DS, Lee FI. Severe intrahepatic cholestasis and rapidly progressive renal failure in a patient with immunocyte-related amyloidosis. *J. clin. Gastroenterol.* 1987; **9**: 219.

13 Virchhow R. Über den Gang der Amyloiden Degeneration. *Virchows Archiv.* 1855; **8**: 364.

14 Waldenström H. On the formation and disappearance of amyloid in man. *Acta chir. Scand.* 1928; **63**: 479.

α₁-Antitrypsin deficiency [10]

α₁-antitrypsin is synthesized in the rough

endoplasmic reticulum of the liver. It comprises 80–90% of the serum α_1-globulin and is an inhibitor of trypsin and other proteases *in vitro*.

Its genetic control is by a single autosomal dominant gene responsible for 24 different alleles distinguished by starch gel electrophoresis, isoelectric focusing in polyacrylamide gel or by monoclonal antibodies against variants of a α_1-antitrypsin. The single gene locus coding for α_1-antitrypsin is on the long arm of chromosome 14 [4]. This is the same chromosome that codes for immunoglobulin light chains.

The alleles are labelled alphabetically. Pi (protease inhibitor) M is the predominant normal type and the serum α_1-antitrypsin value is 200–400 mg/dl. Genetic deficiency with liver disease is seen in the PiZZ and Pi-nul phenotypes and their serum α_1-antitrypsin value is 20–160 mg/dl or even 0 in the Pi-nul phenotype. Intermediate phenotypes PiSZ, PiMZ, and PiMS exist with serum α_1-antitrypsin levels of 50–60% of normal.

Liver disease is associated with the Pi gene and with rare variants such as PiM$_1$ or PiM duarte.

PATHOGENESIS OF LIVER DISEASE

This is uncertain. The glycoprotein may have a protective function in tissues, inhibiting many proteolytic enzymes. When α_1-trypsin is deficient, these enzymes may produce more tissue damage. The liver damage, however, is unrelated to the deposition of α_1-trypsin globules in the liver. An additional factor has been postulated in those suffering liver damage. This might control protease/anti-protease balance in tissues.

CLINICAL PICTURE

Patients with only 10% of serum α_1-antitrypsin may remain well throughout life, or can develop pulmonary emphysema. Ten to 20% of α_1-antitrypsin deficient homozygotes will develop liver dysfunction.

Many present with hepatitic-cholestatic jaundice of variable severity in the first four months of life. This may be fatal, but usually subsides by about the age of six or seven months, leaving hepatomegaly. A period of relative well-being is followed in childhood and early adult life by cirrhosis and its complications [8]. The patient may present as a problem of portal hypertension or ascites.

The prognosis for neonatal cholestasis related to α_1-antitrypsin deficiency may not be so poor as previously believed. In one eight-year follow-up, only two of 14 patients with neonatal cholestasis had developed cirrhosis and the rest were apparently healthy [14]. The chances of complete recovery remain uncertain.

Cirrhosis may remain compensated for many years but can pursue a relentless course with 25% dying during childhood [1].

The condition is rare in adults. In an adult liver clinic, only five homozygotes (ZZ phenotype), α_1-antitrypsin deficient patients, were found in 469 patients with chronic liver disease and all five gave a history of neonatal jaundice [7].

An increased prevalence of heterozygotes (MZ) has been found in patients with cryptogenic cirrhosis or chronic active hepatitis [10]. The significance is unknown. Intermediate PiMZ and PiSZ persons are predisposed to liver disease and hepato-cellular cancer, but the risk is relatively small, perhaps 10 to 15% [2].

Rarely, both pulmonary and hepatic disease affect the same patient [3, 8].

Hepato-cellular cancer may be a complication particularly in males [6].

LIVER HISTOLOGY

The acute picture is of neonatal hepatitis except that giant cells are not prominent. After twelve weeks, intracellular globules which are diastase resistant and stain brilliantly with PAS are seen in *peri-portal* liver cells (fig. 23.16) [12]. The globules stain positively with the specific α_1-antitrypsin immunoperoxidase method. The liver contains increased amounts of copper.

Electron microscopy discloses clumps of protein in dilated rough endoplasmic reticulum. These fluoresce when exposed to an anti-body against α_1-antitrypsin [3].

DIAGNOSIS

The condition should be suspected with neo-natal jaundice. It should also be considered in any patient with cirrhosis, whatever the age, particularly with a past history of infantile liver disease or with associated chest infections. α_1-antitrypsin deficiency can present as cryp-togenic cirrhosis in persons over the age of 50 [15].

Confirmation comes by measuring serum α_1-antitrypsin. The exact phenotype should be determined.

There is a 75% chance that a subsequent affected child will run the same clinical course.

The deficiency may be diagnosed prenatally by amniotic fluid or cultured amniotic cells using synthetic oligomer probes for DNA analysis [13].

First trimester prenatal diagnosis is possible by analysis of fetal DNA [9]. This is justified in families where there is a history of severe disease.

TREATMENT

Replacement therapy with plasma-derived or synthetic α_1-antitrypsin has been used to treat the pulmonary disease [17].

Hepatic transplantation has been successfully performed [11]. The recipient's phenotype rapidly changes to that of the donor [16].

References

1 Alagille D. Alpha-1-antitrypsin deficiency. *Hepatology* 1984; **4**: 115.
2 Carlson J, Eriksson S. Chronic 'cryptogenic' liver disease and malignant hepatoma in intermediate alpha i-antitrypsin deficiency identified by a Pi Z-specific monoclonal antibody. *Scand. J. Gastroenterol.* 1985; **20**: 835.
3 Cohen KL, Rubin PE, Echevarria RE *et al.* Alpha$_1$-antitrypsin deficiency, emphysema and cirrhosis in an adult. *Ann. intern. Med.* 1973; **78**: 227.
4 Cox DW, Markovic VD, Teshima IE. Genes for immunoglobulin heavy chains and for 1-antitrypsin are localised to specific regions of chromosome 14q. *Nature* 1982; **279**: 428.
5 Crowley JJ, Sharp HL, Freier E *et al.* Fatal liver disease associated with alpha 1-antitrypsin deficiency PiM$_1$ PiM$_{duarte}$. *Gastroenterology* 1987; **93**: 242.
6 Eriksson S, Carlson J, Velez R. Risk of cirrhosis and primary liver cancer in alpha 1-antitrypsin deficiency. *N. Engl. J. Med.* 1986; **314**: 736.
7 Fisher RL, Taylor L, Sherlock S. α-1-antitrypsin deficiency in liver disease: the extent of the problem. *Gastroenterology* 1976; **71**: 646.
8 Glasgow JFT, Lynch MJ, Hercz A *et al.* Alpha$_1$ antitrypsin deficiency in association with both cirrhosis and chronic obstructive lung disease in two sibs. *Am. J. Med.* 1973; **54**: 181.
9 Hejtmancik JF, Ward PA, Sifers RN *et al.* Prenatal diagnosis of alpha 1-antitrypsin deficiency by restriction fragment length polymorphisms, and

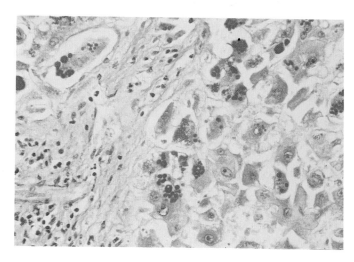

Fig. 23.16. α_1-anti-trypsin deficiency. Liver biosy shows bright red deposits in periportal liver cells when stained by periodic acid Schiff after diastrase digestion. PAS, ×100.

comparison with oligonucleotide probe analysis. *Lancet* 1984; **ii:** 767.

10 Hodges JR, Millward-Sadler GH, Barbatis C *et al.* Heterozygous MZ alpha-1-antitrypsin deficiency in adults with chronic active hepatitis and cryptogenic cirrhosis. *N. Engl. J. Med.* 1981; **304:** 557.

11 Hood JM, Koep LJ, Peters RL *et al.* Liver transplantation for advanced liver disease with alpha-1-antitrypsin deficiency. *N. Engl. J. Med.* 1980; **302:** 272.

12 Jeppsson J-O, Larsson C, Eriksson S. Characterisation of α_1-antitrypsin in the inclusion bodies from the liver in α_1-antitrypsin deficiency. *N. Engl. J. Med.* 1975; **293:** 576.

13 Kidd VJ, Golbus MS, Wallace RB *et al.* Prenatal diagnosis of alpha-1-antitrypsin deficiency by direct analysis of the mutation site in the gene. *N. Engl. J. Med.* 1984; **310:** 639.

14 Sveger T. Prospective study of children with α_1-antitrypsin deficiency: eight-year-old follow up. *J Pediat.* 1984; **104:** 91.

15 Thatcher BS, Winkelman EI, Tuthill RJ. Alpha-1-antitrypsin deficiency presenting as cryptogenic cirrhosis in adults over 50. *J. clin. Gastroenterol.* 1985; **7:** 405.

16 Van Furth R, Kramps JA, Van Der Putten ABMM *et al.* Change in alpha-1-antitrypsin phenotype after orthotopic liver transplant. *Clin. exp. Immunol.* 1986; **66:** 669.

17 Wewers MD, Casolaro MA, Sellers SE *et al.* Replacement therapy for alpha-1-antitrypsin deficiency associated with emphysema. *N. Engl. J. Med.* 1987; **316:** 1055.

Hereditary tyrosinaemia

This autosomal recessive disorder is due to lack of the enzyme *p*-hydroxyphenyl pyruvate hydroxylase, but this is probably not the only defect [1].

It is characterized by cirrhosis, severe hypophosphataemic rickets, renal tubular defects and a derangement of tyrosine metabolism with hyper-amino-acidaemia. Hepato-cellular carcinoma is a complication.

Regenerating nodules may be seen as high attenuating foci on CT [2].

Patients with the acute type usually die in spite of restricting dietary tyrosine; the chronic will respond to this treatment.

Liver transplantation cures the metabolic disease and dietary restrictions become unnecessary [3].

References

1 Carson NAJ, Biggart JD, Bittles AH *et al.* Hereditary tyrosinaemia: clinical, enzymatic and pathological study of an infant with the acute form of the disease. *Arch Dis. Child.* 1976; **51:** 106.

2 Day DL, Letourneau JG, Allan BT *et al.* Hepatic regenerating nodules in hereditary tyrosinemia. *Am. J. Roentgenol.* 1987; **149:** 391.

3 Van Thiel DH, Gartner LM, Thorp FK *et al.* Resolution of the clinical features of tyrosinemia following orthotopic liver transplantation for hepatoma. *J. Hepatol.* 1986; **3:** 42.

Cystic fibrosis of the pancreas

This common condition has a carrier rate of 1:40. A genomic sequence, close to the cystic fibrosis locus, has been cloned and characterized [3]. The primary defect may be in the cleavage of cholecystokinin to the active octapeptide (CCK-8) so resulting in failure of stimulation of exocrine secretion [5].

Fatty change is the commonest abnormality. A focal biliary fibrosis due to eosinophilic material obstructing intra-hepatic bile ducts has been described [1]. However, in most instances, hepatic abnormalities are due to intra-hepatic biliary strictures secondary to the pancreatic disease [4]. These result in zone 1 (portal) fibrosis and biliary cirrhosis. They are usual in those with hepatomegaly and serum biochemical abnormalities. They result in abdominal pain [6]. Biliary strictures may be amenable to endoscopic or surgical relief. Gallbladder disease, including gallstones, is seen in 3.6% [7]. Cholecystectomy is safe.

Postnatal jaundice is associated with meconium ileus.

Clinical features of cirrhosis rarely become apparent until the pulmonary and pancreatic diseases have been overt for many years.

The cirrhosis is usually clinically silent but may cause portal hypertension.

The prognosis seems to be determined by the respiratory state rather than the liver.

Liver transplantation has been performed but the problem of sepsis, both pulmonary and elsewhere, persists [2].

References

1 Bodian M. *Fibrocytic Disease of the Pancreas.* p. 104. Heinemann, London, 1952.

2 Cox KL, Ward RE, Furgiuele TL *et al.* Orthotopic liver transplantation in patients with cystic fibrosis. *Pediatrics* 1987; **4:** 571.

3 Estivill X, Farrall M, Scambler PJ *et al.* A candidate for the cystic fibrosis locus isolated by selection for methylation-free islands. *Nature* 1987; **326:** 840.

4 Gaskin KJ, Waters DLM, Howman-Giles R *et al.* Liver disease and common-bile duct stenosis in cystic fibrosis. *N. Engl. J. Med.* 1988; **318:** 340.

5 Gosden CM, Gosden JR. Fetal abnormalities in cystic fibrosis suggest a deficiency in proteolysis of cholecystokinin. *Lancet* 1984; **ii:** 541.

6 Patrick MK, Howman-Giles R, De Silva M *et al.* Common bile duct obstruction causing right upper abdominal pain in cystic fibrosis. *J. Pediatr.* 1986; **108:** 101.

7 Stern RC, Rothstein FC, Doershuk CF. Treatment and prognosis of symptomatic gallbladder disease in patients with cystic fibrosis. *J. Pediatr. Gastroenterol. Nutr.* 1986; **5:** 35.

Liver and thyroid

The liver metabolizes thyroxine by oxidative deamination, deiodination, conjugation and finally biliary excretion. There is an entero-hepatic circulation, but only about 3% thyroxine is reabsorbed.

The liver contains 35% of the body's exchangeable thyroxine (T4), and 5% of the tri-iodothyronine (T3)—there is a ready exchange with the bound hormone in plasma. The liver converts T4 to T3 [8]. Reversed T3 (rT3) is probably produced in extra-hepatic tissues [11]. The liver also produces thyroxine-binding globulin.

Thyrotoxicosis

Jaundice in thyrotoxic patients may be due to heart failure. Thyrotoxicosis may also aggravate an underlying defect in serum bilirubin metabolism, such as Gilbert's syndrome. This may account for some instances of jaundice in thyrotoxics who are not in heart failure and who have a normal liver biopsy [6].

Hepatic blood flow in hyperthyroidism is little if at all increased in spite of an increased cardiac output. The increased hepatic metabolism, however, is reflected in an increased hepatic oxygen consumption which is elevated even more than the general metabolic rate.

Liver biopsy is normal in those not in congestive failure. Electron microscopy [9] shows enlarged mitochondria, hypertrophied smooth endoplasmic reticulum and decreased glycogen.

Minor abnormalities of liver function are seen in hyperthyroidism [3]. There is little evidence of significant hepatic functional and structural changes in an otherwise normal liver.

Myxoedema

Ascites without congestive heart failure in patients with myxoedema has been attributed to centrizonal congestion and fibrosis [2]. The pathogenesis is unknown. It disappears on giving thyroid.

Jaundice may be related to neonatal thyroid deficiency.

Changes in hepato-cellular disease

Most patients with liver disease are clinically euthyroid although standard function tests may give misleading results [4]. The radio-iodine uptake may be abnormally low. Serum total T4 may be raised or decreased in association with varying levels of thyroid hormone binding proteins. Estimation of the free thyroxine index is usually normal.

In *acute hepatitis B*, there is a decreased T4 to T3 conversion in peripheral tissues [5].

In fulminant hepatitis, the T3/T4 ratio is particularly low and this may have prognostic value [7].

In *alcoholic liver disease* raised serum levels of thyrotrophin (TSH) and free T4 are associated with normal or low T3 values [10]. The conversion of T4 to T3 is reduced. This suggests a compensatory increase in TSH in response to relative T3 deficiency. The total and free T3 levels are reduced in proportion to the degree of liver damage [2]. Plasma rT3 levels are high.

In *primary biliary cirrhosis and chronic active hepatitis* thyroxine-binding globulins are increased and these may be markers of inflammatory activity [11]. Although average total T4 and T3 would be increased, the corresponding free hormone concentrations are reduced, probably because of decreased thyroid function associated with the high incidence of thyroiditis in these patients [1].

References

1 Babb RR. Associations between diseases of the thyroid and the liver. *Am. J. Gastroenterol.* 1984; **79:** 421.
2 Baker A, Kaplan M, Wolfe H. Central congestive fibrosis of the liver in myxedema ascites. *Ann. intern. Med.* 1972; **77:** 927.
3 Beckett GJ, Kellett HA, Gow SM *et al.* Subclinical liver damage in hyperthyroidism and in thyroxine replacement therapy. *Br. Med. J.* 1985; **291:** 427.
4 Chopra IJ, Solomon DH, Chopra U *et al.* Alterations in circulating thyroid hormones and thyrotropin in hepatic cirrhosis: evidence for euthyroidism despite subnormal serum triiodothyronine. *J. clin. Endocrinol. Metabol.* 1974; **39:** 501.
5 Gardner DF, Carithers RLJ, Utiger RD. Thyroid function tests in patients with acute and resolved hepatitis B virus infection. *Ann. intern. Med.* 1982; **96:** 450.
6 Greenberger NJ, Milligan FD, De Groot LJ *et al.* Jaundice and thyrotoxicosis in the absence of congestive heart failure. *Am. J. Med.* 1964; **36:** 840.
7 Itoh S, Yamaba Y, Oda T *et al.* Serum thyroid hormone, triiodothyronine, thyroxine, and triiodothyronine/thyroxine ratio in patients with fulminant, acute, and chronic hepatitis. *Am. J. Gastroenterol.* 1986; **6:** 444.
8 Klachko DM, Johnson ER. The liver and circulating thyroid hormones. *J. clin. Gastroenterol.* 1983; **5:** 465.
9 Klion FM, Segal R, Schaffner F. The effect of altered thyroid function on the ultrastructure of the human liver. *Am. J. Med.* 1971; **50:** 317.
10 Nomura S, Pittman CS, Chambers JB Jr *et al.* Reduced peripheral conversion of thyroxine to triiodothyronine in patients with hepatic cirrhosis. *J. clin. Invest.* 1975; **56:** 643.
11 Schussler GC, Schaffner F, Korn F. Increased serum thyroid hormone binding and decreased free hormone in chronic active liver disease. *N. Engl. J. Med.* 1978; **299:** 510.

Liver and growth hormone

The liver and kidneys degrade growth hormone. Patients with cirrhosis have raised peripheral growth hormone levels [4].

Paradoxical growth hormone may contribute to insulin resistance and glucose intolerance in cirrhosis [2].

Serum somatomedins are produced by the liver and values are low in cirrhosis [3]. In spite of the chronic elevation of peripheral growth hormones acromegaly does not develop.

In *acromegaly* the liver enlarges in line with other viscera. The splanchnic blood flow is normal so that tissue perfusion must be reduced relative to the increment in hepatic mass [1].

References

1 Preisig R, Morris TQ, Shaver JC *et al.* Volumetric, hemodynamic and excretory characteristics of the liver in acromegaly. *J. clin. Invest.* 1966; **65:** 1379.
2 Shankar TP, Fredi JL, Himmelstein S *et al.* Elevated growth hormone levels and insulin resistance in patients with cirrhosis of the liver. *Am. J. Med. Sci.* 1986; **291:** 248.
3 Takano K, Hizuka N, Shizume K *et al.* Serum somatomedin peptides measured by somatomedin A radioreceptor assay in chronic liver disease. *J. clin. Endocrinol. Metabol.* 1977; **45:** 828.
4 Zanoboni A Zanoboni-Muciaccia W. Elevated basal growth hormone levels and growth hormone response to TRH in alcoholic patients with cirrhosis. *J. clin. Endocrinol. Metabol.* 1977; **45:** 576.

Hepatic porphyrias

Hepatic porphyrias are associated with abnormalities in the biosynthesis of haem (fig. 23.17) [3].

Three are inherited as dominants: *acute intermittent* porphyria, *hereditary coproporphyria* and *variegate* porphyria. All are marked by neuropsychiatric attacks with vomiting, abdominal colic, constipation and peripheral neuropathy. All are exacerbated by countless enzyme-inducing drugs including barbiturates, sulphonamides, oestrogens, oral contraceptives, griseofulvin, chloroquine and possibly alcohol.

Hormones are important inducers and

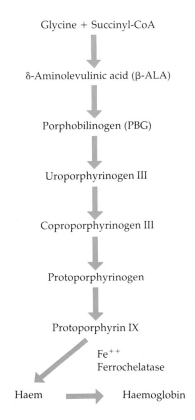

Glycine + Succinyl-CoA

δ-Aminolevulinic acid (β-ALA)

Porphobilinogen (PBG)

Uroporphyrinogen III

Coproporphyrinogen III

Protoporphyrinogen

Protoporphyrin IX

Fe^{++}
Ferrochelatase

Haem ⟶ Haemoglobin

Fig. 23.17. The biosynthesis of porphyrins.

women develop attacks in pregnancy and pre-menstrually.

During the attacks, large amounts of the colourless porphyrin precursors, porphobilinogen and delta aminolaevulinic acid (ALA), are excreted in the urine. In all three, an acute attack is treated by glucose loading. Infusions of haematin which regress or inhibit hepatic ALA synthetase may be valuable in the acute attack [2].

Haem arginate which suppresses overproduction of haem precursors and improves hepatic oxidative metabolism may be useful [9].

The fourth type, *porphyria cutanea tarda*, is probably hereditary and may be associated with actual hepato-cellular disease. It is not exacerbated by barbiturates and acute attacks are not seen.

ACUTE INTERMITTENT PORPHYRIA

The basic deficiency is in hepatic uroporphyrinogen I synthetase. A diagnostic deficiency may be shown in red cells. The enzyme delta aminolaevulinic acid-synthetase (ALA-S) is secondarily induced in the liver by heam through a negative feedback mechanism.

Photosensitivity is absent. The urine darkens on standing and gives a positive urobilinogen test. It contains slight increases in ALA-S and porphobilinogen. Latent cases develop acute attacks on various drugs and in the later stages of pregnancy.

HEREDITARY COPROPORPHYRIA

The deficiency is in coproporphyrinogen oxidase. Attacks are similar to those of other hepatic porphyrias. ALA-S activity is increased in the liver. Faecal and urinary coproporphyrin are increased with a corresponding increase in protoporphyrin.

PORPHYRIA VARIEGATA

The defect is in protoporphyrinogen oxidase. ALA-S is increased in the liver. This variant is frequently encountered in South Africa and New England [14]. The features are intermediate between acute intermittent porphyria and hereditary coproporphyria. Protoporphyrin is increased in the stools at all times.

PORPHYRIA CUTANEA TARDA

The deficiency is in uroporphyrinogen decarboxylase. Alcoholism is a common association and a precipitating factor and so is sex hormone treatment. It may be a toxic effect of chlorinated hydrocarbons. Sensitivity to drugs such as barbiturates is absent.

This is the most common porphyria and is usually latent and the patient symptom-free.

It is characterized clinically by photosensitive skin, blistering and scarring, pigmentation and hypertrichosis. Acute attacks are absent. There is usually evidence of liver dysfunction.

Uroporphyrin is increased in the urine.

Liver biopsy [12] shows subacute hepatitis or cirrhosis. Iron overload has never been adequately explained and may or may not be related to co-existent HLA-linked haemochromatosis [1, 11]. Uroporphyrin can be shown by red fluorescence in ultraviolet light.

The incidence of hepato-cellular carcinoma is increased [15].

Exacerbation of symptoms accompanies deterioration of liver function. At this time, porphyrins which would normally be excreted into the bile may be directed via the kidneys to the urine. Where the liver is healthy, the porphyrin is excreted harmlessly into the bile; when it is diseased, it is retained in the blood. The porphyria itself may be hepato-toxic.

Chloroquine causes an exacerbation which may be followed by a remission of a few months [7].

Venesection has a good effect probably related to removal of excess iron. About six months is taken to clinical remission and 13 months to biochemical remission.

ERYTHROPOIETIC PROTOPORPHYRIA

The defect is in haem synthetase. The inheritance is dominant. Protoporphyrin is increased in tissues and urine.

This type is characterized by skin photosensitivity. Protoporphyrin is increased in tissues and urine, perhaps secondary to abnormalities in haem synthesis.

Liver biopsies examined by fluorescent microscopy or phase microscopy [10] show focal deposits of pigment containing protoporphyrin. Complications include gallstones containing protoporphyrin.

Deaths have been reported in liver failure [16] particularly after alcohol excess [6]. These are related to accumulation of the protoporphyrin within the hepatocyte [4].

Haematin infusions, by reducing porphyrin production, may be useful therapeutically [5].

Cholestyramine increases protoporphyrin excretion and may reduce hepatotoxicity [13]. Iron therapy decreases erythrocyte and stool protoporphyrin levels and improves liver function [8].

HEPATOERYTHROPOIETIC PORPHYRIA

This very rare type is due to a deficiency of uroporphyrinogen decarboxylase [18]. It is marked by hepatosplenomegaly and cirrhosis. Liver biopsies fluoresce but there is no iron excess.

SECONDARY COPROPORPHYRIAS

Heavy metal intoxication, especially with lead, causes porphyria with ALA-S and coproporphyrin in the urine. Erythrocyte protoporphyrins are increased. Coproporphyrinuria may also be seen with sideroblastic anaemia, various liver diseases, the Dubin—Johnson syndrome and as a complication of drug therapy.

A patient has been described with a *hepatic adenoma* who developed photosensitivity with skin blisters and showed uroporphyrin and coproporphyrin in the urine [17]. Family history was negative. The tumour was removed and contained considerable quantities of proto-, copro- and uroporphyrin. Post-operatively the skin lesions disappeared and the urinary excretion of porphyrins returned to normal.

References

1 Beaumont C, Fauchet R, Phung LN *et al.* Porphyria cutanea tarda and HLA-linked hemochromatosis: evidence against a systematic association. *Gastroenterology* 1987; **92**: 1833.
2 Bissell DM. Treatment of acute hepatic porphyria with hematin. *J. Hepatol.* 1988; **6**: 1.
3 Bloomer JR. The hepatic porphyrias: pathogenesis, manifestations and management. *Gastroenterology* 1976; **71**: 689.
4 Bloomer JR, Enriquez R. Evidence that hepatic crystalline deposits in a patient with protoporphyria are composed of protoporphyrin. *Gastroenterology* 1982; **82**: 569.
5 Bloomer JR, Pierach CA. Effect of hematin administration to patients with protoporphyria and liver disease. *Hepatology* 1982; **2**: 817.
6 Bonkovsky HL, Schned AR. Fatal liver failure in

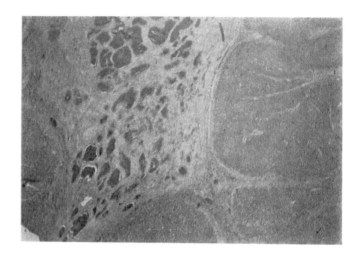

Fig. 23.18. The cirrhosis accompanying hereditary haemorrhagic telangiectasia. Note spaces filled with blood at the periphery of the lobules.

protoporphyria: synergism between ethanol excess and the genetic defect. *Gastroenterology* 1986; **90:** 191.

7 Felsher BF, Redeker AG. Effect of chloroquine on hepatic uroporphyrin metabolism in patients with porphyria cutanea tarda. *Medicine (Baltimore)* 1966; **45:** 575.

8 Gordeuk VR, Brittenham GM, Hawkins CW *et al.* Iron therapy for hepatic dysfunction in erythropoietic protoporphyria. *Ann. intern. Med.* 1986; **105:** 27.

9 Herrick A, McColl KEL, McLellan A *et al.* Effect of haem arginate therapy on porphyrin metabolism and mixed function oxygenase activity in acute hepatic porphyria. *Lancet* 1987; **ii:** 1178.

10 Klatskin G, Bloomer JR. Birefringence of hepatic pigment deposits in erythropoietic protoporphyria. Specificity of polarization microscopy in the identification of hepatic protoporphyrin deposits. *Gastroenterology* 1974; **67:** 294.

11 Kushner JP, Edwards CQ, Dadone MM *et al.* Heterozygosity for HLA-linked hemochromatosis as a likely cause of the hepatic siderosis associated with sporadic porphyria cutanea tarda. *Gastroenterology* 1985; **88:** 1232.

12 Lefkowitch JH, Grossman ME. Hepatic pathology in porphyrea cutanea tarda. *Liver* 1983; **3:** 19.

13 McCullough AJ, Barron D, Mullen KD *et al.* Fecal protoporphyrin excretion in erythropoietic protoporphyria: effect of cholestyramine and bile acid feeding. *Gastroenterology* 1988; **94:** 177.

14 Muhlbauer JE, Pathak MA, Tishler PV *et al.* Variegate porphyria in New England. *J. Am. med. Assoc.* 1982; **247:** 3095.

15 Salata H, Cortes JM, Enriquez de Salamanca R *et al.* Porphyria cutanea tarda and hepatocellular carcinoma-frequency of occurrence and related factors. *J. Hepatol.* 1985; **1:** 477.

16 Singer JA, Plaut AG, Kaplan MM. Hepatic failure and death from erythropoietic protoporphyria. *Gastroenterology* 1978; **74:** 588.

17 Tio Tiong Hoo, Leijnse B, Jarrett A *et al.* Acquired porphyria from a liver tumour. *Clin. Sci.* 1957; **16:** 517.

18 Toback AC, Sassa S, Poh-Fitzpatrick MB *et al.* Hepatoerythropoietic porphyria: clinical, biochemical, and enzymatic studies in a three-generation family lineage. *N. Engl. J. Med.* 1987; **316:** 645.

Hereditary haemorrhagic telangiectasia

Hepatomegaly is a common feature of this disease. The liver may show telangiectasia and cirrhosis. Bands of fibrous tissue surrounding the regenerative nodules contain numerous thin-walled telangiectases (fig. 23.18) [2]. Benign fibro-vascular lesions are always suggestive [1]. It has been suggested that the telangiectases interfere with the nutrition of liver cells [2].

Occasionally large intra-hepatic arteriovenous aneurysms lead to portal hypertension, haemorrhage from varices and high output heart failure.

References

1 Daly JJ, Schiller AL. The liver in hereditary haemorrhagic telangiectasia (Osler−Weber−Rendu disease). *Am. J. Med.* 1976; **60:** 723.

2 Martin GA. Lebercirrhöse bei Morbus Osler, Cirrhosis hepatis telangiectatica. *Gastroenterologia, Basel* 1955; **73:** 157.

24 · The Liver in Infancy and Childhood

Biochemical tests in infancy

Fractionation into unconjugated and conjugated *serum bilirubin* is important in neonates [96]. Because of overlap, the proportion of serum bilirubin conjugates does not distinguish between extra-hepatic biliary obstruction and hepato-cellular disease [83].

Serum bilirubin levels are a guide to the development of kernicterus. Serial levels are useful in the assessment of prolonged jaundice.

Serum cholesterol. Extremely high levels may be recorded in prolonged cholestasis, particularly intra-hepatic.

Serum alkaline phosphatase levels are influenced by bone metabolism as well as by cholestasis. Levels are increased in the first month of life as well as around puberty.

Serum 5 nucleotidase or gamma glutamyl transpeptidase levels may be estimated if there is doubt concerning the origin of a raised serum alkaline phosphatase level.

Serum transaminase values are about twice the normal adult level during the first month of life.

Bile acid metabolism [62, 92]. Bile acid secretion evolves during the final trimester of pregnancy and in the early neonatal period. In the infant, conjugation and pool size are reduced as are secretion, intraluminal concentration and ileal active transport. Serum bile acids are increased.

The main bile acid in neonates is glycocholic. After one to three months, glycochenodeoxycholic predominates [77]. The neonate shows immaturity of hepatic 12 α-hydroxylation.

Secretion of bile acids by the hepatocyte may be reduced and atypical bile acids produced which may not be functionally adequate. This picture of *'Physiological cholestasis'* is enhanced in the low birth-weight neonate. It may contribute to cholestasis produced by other factors such as *E. coli*, endotoxaemia and prolonged parenteral nutrition.

LIVER SIZE

Liver span in normal infants and children is measured by percussion of the upper border and percussion/palpation of the lower border (table 24.1) [75].

CIRCULATORY FACTORS AND HEPATIC NECROSIS

In the fetus the right lobe of the liver is supplied largely by the portal vein whereas the left receives highly oxygenated placental blood, rich in endogenous and exogenous materials. It is not surprising therefore that studies in the fetal mouse have shown higher levels of cytochrome P_{450} gene expression in the left than right lobe [16]. This lobar heterogeneity disappears as the pattern of adult liver circulation develops.

At the time of birth, loss of placental blood can be followed by atrophy of the left lobe of the liver.

Table 24.1. Approximate mean liver span of infants and children based on four studies on 470 subjects (Naveh & Berant 1984)

Age	Span (cm)
Birth	5.6–5.9
2 months	5
1 year	6
2 years	6.5
3 years	7
4 years	7.5
5 years	8
12 years	9

Right-sided hepatic necrosis may be seen in post-mature infants dying about the time of birth [22]. This is related to poor placental blood supply and anoxia at the time of delivery.

Disseminated mid-zonal necrosis is found with congenital cardiac defects [85]. This may be due to decrease in total hepatic blood flow. In others the zone 3 changes of congestive heart failure may be seen. Cholestasis in the first week can be related to congenital cardiac defects and 'shock'.

Localized necrosis of the liver may be due to trapping in defects of the anterior abdominal wall.

Copper is increased in the fetal liver, more so in the left lobe than the right [33].

Neonatal jaundice

A simple classification is made into those cases where the increase in serum bilirubin is predominantly unconjugated (total serum bilirubin >3.0 mg with less than 30% direct reacting), and those where the increase is in the conjugated fraction (tables 24.2, 24.3) [96].

Unconjugated hyperbilirubinaemia (table 24.2)

This is common in the newborn. The development of hepatic conjugating and transport systems for bilirubin is delayed in the neonate. Factors which further depress hepatic function or add to the load of bilirubin on the liver lead to marked hyperbilirubinaemia. In the neonatal period this is complicated by the development of bilirubin encephalopathy (*kernicterus*).

'Physiological' and prematurity jaundice

Jaundice, reaching its peak within 2–5 days of delivery and disappearing in two weeks, is common in normal infants. It is more serious in low birth-weight infants where it may persist for as long as two weeks. The urine contains both urobilin and bilirubin and the stools are paler than normal. Serum unconjugated bilirubin is moderately or markedly raised.

Table 24.2. Unconjugated hyperbilirubinaemia in neonates related to onset

Birth to 2 days
  Haemolytic disease

3–7 days
  Physiological±prematurity
                hypoxia
                acidosis

1–8 weeks
  Congenital haemolytic disorders
  Breast milk jaundice
  Lucey–Driscoll
  Crigler–Najjar
  Hypothyroidism
  Perinatal complications: haemorrhage, sepsis
  Upper gastrointestinal obstruction

The cause is multi-factorial. Haemolysis of surplus erythrocytes, relative deficiency of hepatic bilirubin-conjugating enzymes and increased absorption of bilirubin from the intestines are important. Bilirubin binding to albumin is reduced particularly in premature infants [83]. The hyperbilirubinaemia is enhanced by hypoxia and hypoglycaemia. Drugs such as water-soluble vitamin K analogues add to the jaundice.

MANAGEMENT

Phototherapy. Hyperbilirubinaemia may be prevented or controlled by exposure of the infant to light of wavelength near 450 nm. This is probably due to the light converting bilirubin IX alpha photochemically to a relatively stable geometric isomer [87]. Structural isomerization also takes place with a production of a non-reversible product called *lumirubin* [29]. Side effects include increased insensible water loss, haemolysis and bronzing of the skin. The eyes must be protected.

Phototherapy should not be routine but is of value in selected cases. It is also useful in the Crigler–Najjar syndrome.

Exchange transfusion is given if the serum bilirubin level is 340 mmol/1 (20 mg/dl). It is rarely necessary with the advent of photo-therapy.

Enzyme induction, using phenobarbitone, is effective when given to the mother. Antipyrine similarly reduces infantile serum bilirubin levels but without causing drowsiness.

Haemolytic disease of the newborn

Antigens in fetal red cells may provoke the development of maternal antibodies which, passing into the fetal circulation, lead to haemolysis of fetal red blood corpuscles. The incompatibility usually concerns the rhesus blood factors and rarely the ABO or other blood groups.

Characteristically, the firstborn escapes the disease unless the mother's blood has been sensitized by a previous transfusion of Rh-positive blood. A normal first pregnancy sensitizes the mother's blood sufficiently to provoke haemolytic disease in subsequent infants. The clinical forms of the disease vary in severity, but the underlying pathological lesions are essentially similar.

The infant is jaundiced during the first two days of life. Serum unconjugated bilirubin is increased. The critical period occurs in the first few days when the more deeply jaundiced infants may develop *kernicterus*.

Diagnosis may be suspected by antenatal examination of the mother's blood for specific antibodies and confirmed by a positive Coombs' test in the infant and by blood-typing on mother and child.

KERNICTERUS (BILIRUBIN ENCEPHALOPATHY)

This grave condition is a complication of prematurity jaundice and of haemolytic disease. It can complicate neonatal hepatitis.

Within the first five days of life, the jaundiced infant becomes restless or lethargic and febrile, developing a stiff neck and head retraction which proceeds to opisthotonus. There is stiffness of the limbs with pronated arms, eye squinting, lid retraction, twitching or convulsions and a high-pitched cry.

Death may supervene rapidly in 12 hours and 70% of affected infants die within seven days of the onset. The remaining 30% may survive, but are maimed by mental defect, cerebral palsy or athetosis, unless they eventually die from intercurrent infections.

Autopsy reveals yellow staining of the basal ganglia predominantly and also of other areas of the brain and spinal cord with unconjugated bilirubin which, being lipid-soluble, has an affinity for nervous tissue. Unconjugated bilirubin is able to disturb cerebral metabolism.

Kernicterus is related to circulating free bilirubin crossing the blood–brain barrier. Reduction of serum bilirubin–albumin binding may play a part and indeed albumin infusions have been used therapeutically. The blood–brain barrier may be damaged by hyperosmolarity or hypercarbia. Any organic anion which competes for bilirubin binding sites on albumin will increase kernicterus although the serum bilirubin level falls. Such anions include salicylates, sulphonamides, free fatty acids and haematin.

Kernicterus is seen in the neonate but not in the adult.

CONGENITAL HAEMOLYTIC DISORDERS

These can all lead to unconjugated hyperbilirubinaemia in the first two days of life. They include the red cell enzyme deficiencies—glucose 6PD and pyruvate kinase—congenital spherocytosis and pyknocytosis.

Glucose-6-phosphate dehydrogenase deficiency. Infants develop jaundice, usually on the second or third day of life. The precipitating haemolytic agent may be a drug such as salicylate, phenacetin, or sulphonamides transmitted in the maternal breast milk. This condition is frequent in the Mediterranean area, in the Far East and in Nigeria [13].

BREAST MILK JAUNDICE

Hyperbilirubinaemia (serum bilirubin more

than 12 mg-dl) affects 34% of new-born breast-fed babies compared with only 15% of those who are formula-fed [80]. It may be due to increased β–glucuronidase in breast milk which leads to increased unconjugated bilirubin in the intestine and to its subsequent absorption [37]. Increased free fatty acids in breast milk might inhibit conjugation [41].

The condition lasts from two weeks to more than two months after delivery. Discontinuation of breast feeding results in a fall of the serum bilirubin level.

TRANSIENT FAMILIAL HYPERBILIRUBINAEMIA (Lucey–Driscoll type) [66]

This appears in the first few days of life and persists to the second or third week. It affects every sibling. It is believed to be due to an inhibitor of bilirubin conjugation present in maternal and infantile serum.

CRIGLER–NAJJAR HYPERBILIRUBINAEMIA (Chapter 12)

This may present in the first few days of life.

HYPOTHYROIDISM [68]

This is three times more common in girls than boys. Mild anaemia is common and the infant is sluggish. The diagnosis is confirmed by finding low serum thyroxine and tri-iodothyronine levels with high thyroid stimulating hormone and by observing the effects of therapy. The mechanism of the jaundice is unknown.

PERINATAL COMPLICATIONS

Haemorrhage with release of blood into the tissues provides a bilirubin load which may exacerbate jaundice, particularly in the premature. Anaemia depresses hepato-cellular function. Cephalohaematoma is a common association. The prothrombin time should be measured and vitamin K given.

Sepsis, whether umbilical or elsewhere, leads to unconjugated hyperbilirubinaemia in the first few days of life. Blood, urine and, if necessary, cerebrospinal fluid are cultured and appropriate antibodies given.

UPPER GASTROINTESTINAL OBSTRUCTION [34]

About 10% of infants with congenital pyloric stenosis are jaundiced due to unconjugated bilirubin. The mechanism may be similar to that postulated for the increase in jaundice when patients with Gilbert's syndrome are fasted.

Hepatitis and cholestatic syndromes (conjugated hyperbilirubinaemia)

The reaction of the neonatal liver to different insults is similar. Proliferation of giant cells is always a part and this reflects an increased regenerative ability. In some instances the condition may be the so-called 'idiopathic' hepatitis formerly called giant cell hepatitis. In others a specific virus such as type B hepatitis or another infection can be identified. Metabolic disturbances, such as galactosaemia, can cause a giant cell reaction. Cholestatic syndromes are also seen which may be associated with hepatitis and, in these, hepatic histology may include a giant cell reaction. In all these conditions the conjugated 'direct reacting' bilirubin is more than 30% of the total (table 24.3).

It is extremely important to recognize those that are immediately treatable, such as congenital syphilis or bacterial infections—which will respond to antibiotics, and galactosaemia or tyrosinosis—which will require exclusion diets. The main bile duct atresias, which might benefit from surgical treatment, must be diagnosed.

Diagnosis of the hepatitic–cholestatic syndromes (tables 24.3, 24.4)

Family history is important in diagnosing galactosaemia, α$_1$-antitrypsin deficiency, tyro-

Table 24.3. Conjugated hyperbilirubinaemia in neonates

Infection
   Viruses (CMV rubella, Coxsackie, herpes,
     hepatitis A, B) (Chapter 16)
   Syphilis
   Bacteria (*E. coli*)

Metabolic (Chapter 23)
   Galactosaemia
   α_1-antitrypsin deficiency
   Tyrosinosis
   Cystic fibrosis
   Hereditary fructose intolerance
   Total parenteral nutrition
   Niemann–Pick disease

Idiopathic
   'Neonatal' hepatitis
   Congenital hepatic fibrosis
   Byler's disease

Biliary atresia
   Intra-hepatic
   Extra-hepatic
Erythroblastosis with cholestasis

Table 24.4. Aetiology of cholestasis in neonates

Week 1
Inspissated bile syndrome (erythroblastosis with
   cholestasis)
Bacterial infections
Vascular causes
   'Shock', congenital heart disease

After Week 1
Bile duct anomalies
Genetic
   galactosaemia, α_1-antitrypsin deficiency, etc.
Infections (same as immune deficiency in adults)
   TORCH screen (toxoplasmosis, rubella,
     cytomegala, herpes)
Total parenteral hyperalimentation

---

sinosis, cystic fibrosis and hereditary fructose intolerance.

Virus infections in the mother during pregnancy, such as rubella, hepatitis, or genital herpes, must be recorded.

At the onset it is valuable to test the blood of mother, father and other siblings by appropriate methods and to store the sera for later use. The *routine biochemical tests* of the adult are of little value in the diagnosis of jaundice in infancy and childhood. A serum alkaline phosphatase level three times normal and a serum cholesterol value exceeding 250 mg/100 ml suggest intra-hepatic biliary atresia. A serum $\alpha-$glutamyl transpeptidase value exceeding 300 units/L, particularly if rising, is also suggestive, but not diagnostic, of atresia [36]. A direct reacting bilirubin value exceeding 4 mg (68 mmol) suggests extra-hepatic biliary obstruction.

Serum tyrosine is measured if tyrosinosis is suspected and serum α_1-antitrypsin values noted for the diagnosis of α_1-antitrypsin deficiency.

Biliary isotopic scanning is useful in establishing patency of the biliary passages but is not reliable in diagnosing atresia [20].

Serological methods. The serum is tested for HBsAg, IgMantiHBc, IgM anti-HAV and for syphilis. Antibodies to herpes simplex, rubella, toxoplasma, cytomegala and adenovirus and Coxsackie viruses are estimated in both baby and mother. Blood cultures are performed if *E. coli* infection is suspected.

Urine tests. Cultures are taken for Gram-negative organisms and for cytomegala infection. Aminoaciduria is noted. Reducing substances are sought if galactosaemia is suspected.

Liver biopsy. Needle biopsy of the liver is easy and well tolerated in neonates, infants and children. Interpretation of the histological appearances is always difficult due to the overlap between hepatitis and cholestatic syndromes, both of intra-hepatic and extra-hepatic origin. Neonatal changes in the liver include giant cells and extra-medullary erythropoiesis. These subside by about three months.

Portal zone duct proliferation and a biliary type of fibrosis are helpful in diagnosing extra-hepatic atresia. A relative paucity of portal zone bile ducts supports the diagnosis of intra-hepatic cholestasis but is not constant.

The PAS positive bodies of α_1-antitrypsin deficiency may be seen after two months.

Electron microscopy is essential if metabolic disease is suspected.

Ultrasonography shows absence of the gall-bladder in biliary atresia [20]. It can also diagnose choledochal cyst.

CT scan is also of value.

Percutaneous and endoscopic cholangiography. The percutaneous technique is of great value when liver biopsy findings are equivocal and the HIDA test suggests biliary atresia. Endoscopic cholangiography is rarely employed, largely due to the lack of suitably sized instruments.

Virus hepatitis

Immunity is reduced in the neonate and virus infections similar to those seen in the immuno-deficient adult are frequent. The infection is very liable to persist and chronic hepatitis and cirrhosis ensue. Similarly, older children with immunological deficits such as agammaglo-bulinaemia or who are receiving treatment with immunosuppressive drugs for such conditions as leukaemia or nephritis are also at risk.

HEPATITIS B

This disease develops in babies of mothers who suffer the acute disease during the later part of pregnancy, within two months of delivery, or, rarely, who are chronic carriers. The mother is usually, but not always, hepatitis B 'e' antigen positive. Antigenaemia is usually found between six weeks and six months of birth, suggesting transmission from the mother's blood during delivery or later during her care of the infant. The condition is probably not spread by breast milk.

Umbilical cord sera may rarely be positive for HBsAg and HBV particles, and placental transmission is possible. Positivity does not necessarily imply infectivity by this route, for the umbilical cord sera may have been contaminated by maternal blood.

Hepatitis B also is acquired in early childhood from intra-familial spread.

The natural history of hepatitis B contracted at birth is very variable. Follow-up of children at four to nine years showed the majority to be asymptomatic with mild histological changes in the liver. With histological regression the child converts from HBeAg positive to anti-HBe [14, 15, 88]. Others, particularly males, rarely develop chronic active hepatitis, cirrhosis and hepato-cellular cancer [46]. Core antigen is detected in the cytoplasm of the hepatocyte in those with aggressive disease compared with presence in the nuclei or absence in the inactive. In Italy, superinfection with hepatitis delta virus may influence the progression towards cirrhosis [11, 12].

On liver biopsy in the acute stage a giant cell hepatitis is seen (fig. 24.1). Later the usual picture is chronic persistent hepatitis and only occasionally chronic active hepatitis and cirrhosis.

Prophylaxis

See Chapter 16.

Treatment

See Chapters 16, 17.

HEPATITIS A

Asymptomatic hepatitis A can spread in nurseries for neonates. The source may be infected blood [78] or a nurse carrier [54]. The babies spread the hepatitis A to adults in the nursery and to the community.

HEPATITIS NON-A, NON-B

Non-A, non-B hepatitis, both transfusion-related and sporadic, can affect children [12], and can lead to cirrhosis in multiple transfused thalassaemic children [18].

CYTOMEGALOVIRUS

This is a very common virus infection (Chapter 27). The incidence in small children is 5—10%

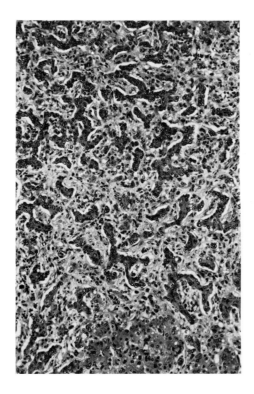

Fig. 24.1. Virus hepatitis in an infant of three months. Necrosis of liver cells and multinucleated giant liver cells are seen. Bile thrombi stained very darkly. (Stained H & E, ×115.)

in those living in good hygienic conditions rising to 80% in the under-privileged.

It is usually acquired placentally from an asymptomatic mother. It can also be transmitted in breast milk and from blood products. Many congenital infections are asymptomatic.

The disease may, however, be fulminant with intense jaundice, purpura, hepatosplenomegaly and neurological and pulmonary defects. Survivors may run a prolonged course with persistent jaundice and hepatomegaly.

In one series, three of 22 children died and one has cirrhosis [15].

HERPES SIMPLEX

The liver may be involved in the course of a fulminating viraemia, contracted at birth from maternal genital herpes. Jaundice is due to viral involvement of the liver, which shows white nodules. Histologically, these represent necrosis with little or no inflammatory reaction. Giant cells are absent, but inclusion bodies may be found.

Antivirals are often given too late when massive hepatic necrosis and fulminant failure have developed and the mortality is 70%.

CONGENITAL RUBELLA SYNDROME

This disease, if contracted in the first trimester of pregnancy, may cause fetal malformations. The infection may also persist through the neonatal period and on into later life. The liver with the brain, lung, heart and other organs can be involved in the generalized virus infection.

The hepatitis is marked by jaundice commencing within the first one to two days and by hepatosplenomegaly. A cholestatic picture may sometimes be seen. Serum transaminase levels are slightly elevated..

Hepatic histology shows bile in swollen Kupffer cells and ductules with a focal hepatocellular necrosis and portal fibrosis. Erythroid haemopoietic tissue is relatively increased and may persist. A typical giant cell hepatitis can be seen [91]. The virus can be identified from the liver at necropsy or by biopsy.

Usually the hepatitis resolves completely with restitution of a normal liver structure. Alternatively it may pursue a chronic undulant course culminating in death at 3–8 weeks. At autopsy a cirrhosis has been seen and rubella may be one cause of childhood cirrhosis and of extra- and intra-hepatic biliary atresia.

ADENOVIRUSES

These may disseminate in babies with decreased resistance due to thymic alymphoplasia and agammaglobulinaemia [105]. A marked coagulative necrosis with inclusion-bearing cells may be seen in the liver. Under similar circumstances this lesion can also complicate *varicella*.

507

Non-viral causes of hepatitis

CONGENITAL SYPHILIS

This condition is very rare. Visceral involvement is late in acquired syphilis but common in fetal infection [65]. Tremendous numbers of treponemata can be found in the liver. Such involvement leads to a fine pericellular cirrhosis with a marked connective tissue reaction. Jaundice is usual.

CONGENITAL TOXOPLASMOSIS

This protozoon is transmitted to the fetus from an inapparent maternal infection. Jaundice develops within a few hours of birth with hepatomegaly, encephalomyelitis, hydrocephalus, microcephaly, choroidoretinitis and intracerebral calcification. It is diagnosed by finding toxoplasmosis IgM antibodies.

The liver shows infiltration of portal zones with mononuclear cells. Extramedullary haemopoiesis with increased stainable iron is conspicuous. Histiocytes containing toxoplasma may be present. The jaundice is difficult to relate to the extent of liver damage and haemolysis may be contributory.

BACTERIAL INFECTION

In the neonate, an immature reticulo-endothelial system with decreased complement and opsonins impairs the ability of the liver and spleen to phagocytose bacteria.

The upsurgence of Gram-negative infections, particularly *E. coli* in nurseries, has led to an increase in cholestatic jaundice due to this cause.

The origins include umbilical sepsis, exchange blood transfusion, pneumonia, otitis media or even gastroenteritis. Diagnosis may be difficult as focal signs are minimal or absent. Jaundice appears suddenly in a child who does not look ill. Hepatomegaly need not be present and splenomegaly is never great. The leucocyte count exceeds 12 000. A blood culture is usually positive. The umbilical stump should be cultured. Liver function tests are of little value.

Hepatic histology is non-contributory. It shows non-specific changes with Kupffer cell hypertrophy and portal zone infiltrates. Culture of liver biopsies is usually negative. The jaundice seems to be due to a combination of haemolysis, hepato-cellular dysfunction and even cholestasis, presumably due to endotoxaemia.

Prognosis depends on early treatment and age of onset, the mortality being 80% below the age of one week and 25% later. Antibiotics are given, depending on the nature of the infection.

Portal vein occlusion may be diagnosed years later.

Liver abscesses in older children are associated with blood-spread organisms. A third have acute blastic leukaemia [25].

URINARY TRACT INFECTIONS

Jaundice may be associated with urinary tract infections both in infants and children. Infants are usually affected in the first week of life. They are often male, but have no underlying abnormality of the renal tract. Endotoxin is believed to contribute to the hepatic dysfunction.

The infants fail to thrive, show fever, jaundice and moderate hepatomegaly. Bilinuria is found. Liver biopsy shows a non-specific hepatitis. Urine culture is an essential investigation in any jaundiced child or infant.

'Idiopathic' neonatal hepatitis

AETIOLOGY

When identifiable causes of neonatal and infantile hepatitis, have been excluded, there remain about 75% of patients in whom the aetiology remains unknown. These are sometimes called 'idiopathic' giant cell hepatitis, or neonatal hepato-cellular cholestasis. The condition is often familial, the inheritance being autosomal recessive. It is possible that the familial incidence reflects common exposure to a toxic agent.

This may be a cause of stillbirth or the infant may die soon after or before jaundice has had time to develop. More usually a fluctuant jaundice appears during the first two weeks or even up to four months. The liver and sometimes the spleen are enlarged and the stools pale. The child may appear well and continue to gain weight or may fail to thrive. Serum transaminase is usually above 800 units/100 ml. Hypoprothrombinaemia may be profound. Stools are pale and urine contains bilirubin.

HEPATIC HISTOLOGY [84]

The normal zonal architecture is lost. The most prominent feature is the large multinucleated cell containing 20–40 nuclei in a cytoplasmic mass. Liver cells may be aggregated into acini, simulating bile ducts. Necrosis is not conspicuous and, if present, focal. Haemosiderosis is constant and foci of erythropoiesis are obvious. Fibrosis is peri-portal and also extends between groups of liver cells. Cholestasis is seen both in small proliferated ductules in the portal zone and between necrotic liver cells.

PROGNOSIS AND TREATMENT

Prognosis is variable. In a 10-year follow-up of 29 patients only two died and only two had signs of persisting liver disease [28].

Treatment is symptomatic. Medium-chain triglycerides may be useful to promote nutrition. The haemorrhagic diathesis must be controlled. Corticosteroid therapy is useless.

Infantile cholangiopathies (biliary atresias)

These diseases commence in intra-uterine life (fig. 24.2). They are often classified as congenital, although, in most instances, the abnormality is due to an extraneous, often infectious,

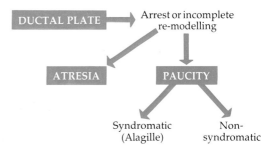

Fig. 24.2. Infantile cholangiopathy. Intra-uterine mechanisms of biliary atresia.

cause acting during the normal process of intra-uterine development or shortly after birth. The importance of infection is supported by the histology of ductular tissue taken from the hepatic hilum early when the Kasai operation is being performed. This shows acute and subacute inflammation suggesting bile duct obliteration secondary to sclerosing cholangitis [71]. Reo-virus III induces similar changes in the neonatal monkey [19]. Other infective causes include cytomegalovirus [35] and rubella [91]. Alpha-I-antitrypsin deficiency and an increase in a bile acid, such as trihydroxycoprostanic may be related in some cases.

Vascular malformations of the hepatic artery have been suggested as causing ischaemic fibrosis of the extra-hepatic biliary tree.

The biliary atresias are rarely familial [56].

A chromosomal abnormality, namely trisomy 17–18, and Down's syndrome have been associated with neonatal hepatitis and atresia [5], but these are rare.

The diseases result not from the failure of bile ducts to form, but from their destruction at some moment during embryonic development [27]. Hepatic histology may indicate the stage at which the damage started [27]. At the early stage of the ductal plate, abnormal cylindrical ducts show atrophy or necrosis of lining cells; later the changes are of regression and involution in normally shaped ducts.

These diseases are often grouped together as 'infantile obstructive cholangiopathy' [58]. There are all grades of destruction from complete absence of bile ducts, termed atresia, to drastic reduction of numbers, termed *paucity of bile ducts*. The extent of the process and its continuation into extra-uterine life is reflected in the prognosis. The baby with complete atresia is usually dead by five years old. The baby with paucity of bile ducts may survive into adult life.

Finally, there is the Alagille syndromatic form of paucity of bile ducts [3]. Here the characteristic facies, skeletal defects, cardiovascular and eye changes make the diagnosis.

Extra-hepatic biliary atresia

The abnormality may be in any part of the biliary system. Multiple defects are common and other congenital lesions may be present. In some bile ducts are absent at birth, but in others the ducts may have been formed but sclerosis starts in the perinatal period and there is a dynamic evolution to bile duct destruction.

DEVELOPMENTAL ASPECTS

The biliary passages may fail to develop from the primitive foregut bud. The gallbladder may also be absent or the biliary tract represented only by a gallbladder connecting directly with the duodenum. The more usual defect is failure of vacuolation of the solid biliary bud. This is usually partial and rarely extends throughout the biliary tree.

PATHOLOGY

The ducts may be absent or replaced by fibrous strands. The site and extent of the atresia are variable. Bile is absent from the extra-hepatic biliary system, including the gallbladder.

The cystic duct only may be involved, the gallbladder becoming a mucous cyst; this has no clinical significance. Involvement of the common bile duct or hepatic duct gives rise to the characteristic syndrome of biliary atresia with deep cholestatic jaundice.

Liver biopsy shows cholestasis with a variable number of giant cells; proliferated bile ductules are conspicuous with biliary type fibrosis. The picture is virtually diagnostic.

CLINICAL FEATURES

Extra-hepatic biliary atresia complicates one in 10 000 live births. There are more females than males, and all races are affected. The condition is not inherited.

The baby becomes icteric by the first week and the icterus continues unremittingly. When deeply jaundiced the infant even cries yellow tears. Pruritus is severe and the child suffers increasingly from it. The urine is dark. The stools are pale, although some pigment may reach the intestine, presumably through the intestinal secretions. Serum transaminase values rarely exceed 300 units. Nutrition is well maintained for the first two months and then falls off, the child usually dying before three years. The serum cholesterol level may rise very high and skin xanthomas appear (fig. 24.3). The prolonged steatorrhoea can result in osteomalacia (*biliary rickets*). Death is usually due to intercurrent infection, to liver cell failure, or to bleeding related to vitamin K deficiency or to oesophageal varices. Ascites is a late and terminal event.

PROGNOSIS

Prognosis is poor unless the cystic duct only is involved or the bile ducts are hypoplastic and not entirely obliterated. Where surgical relief is possible recovery may be complete, but very few patients are amenable to surgical treatment.

SURGERY

If the proximal bile ducts are patent but end blindly before the duodenum the condition is *correctable* by Roux en Y jejunal anastomosis to the common hepatic duct. This is an exceedingly rare circumstance (<5%).

In the vast majority of infants the atresia is *non-correctable* because extra-hepatic ducts are not patent. In these circumstances the Kasai operation (hepatic porto-enterostomy) must be considered [49]. The entire ductal system is resected in the porta hepatis and proximal transected common hepatic duct anastomosed to the intestine. The basis for subsequent biliary drainage is the presence of minuscule biliary ductules in the scarred 'non-patent' extra-hepatic bile ducts. These communicate with the intra-hepatic biliary system and when surgically transected may drain bile from the liver into the interposed intestine.

The operation must be done early (preferably less than four weeks and certainly less than four months) as the small intra-hepatic ducts disappear with time. Bile flow is re-established in 40−80% with a five-year survival with a normal serum bilirubin value of 33% [67]. It should be performed in a centre experienced in the procedure [50]. Post-operative cholangitis, progressive portal hypertension and liver failure are serious post-operative complications. The physician has to be quite sure that the baby is not suffering from the biliary hypoplasia syndrome, when the prognosis is relatively good and jaundice will lessen without porto-enterostomy.

Hepatic transplantation must be considered. Any preceding abdominal operation, such as the Kasai procedure, enhances blood transfusion requirements and increases abdominal infections, but mortality is unaffected [21]. Indications include abnormal blood coagulation, varices, ascites and recurrent cholangitis. The child's quality of life and family support must be considered. A portal vein less than 5 mm in diameter contraindicates the operation. The child must weigh more than 10 kg. The one-year survival is 80%. The long-term outlook is unknown. About 50% of babies suitable for transplantation die for lack of a donor (see Chapter 35).

The intra-hepatic atresia (paucity of bile ducts) syndrome

Intra-hepatic cholestasis in early life may be related to a known cause such as α_1-antitrypsin deficiency. The characteristic PAS positive cells can be seen in a liver biopsy from the age of two months. Congenital abnormalities of bile salt metabolism, such as Byler's disease, can present in the first six months of life.

Primary sclerosing cholangitis can affect infants (see Chapter 15) [87].

In the majority however, no clear aetiology is evident. The early histological appearances may resemble 'idiopathic neonatal hepatitis'. This progresses histologically to bile duct disappearance and biliary cirrhosis. This suggests that hepatitis, often viral, in the neonatal period or even *in utero* may be the first change, ultimately leading to biliary hypoplasia [42]. In most instances the causative virus cannot be identified, although occasionally an association with congenital cardiac defects, nerve deafness or rising titres of rubella antibody suggests that this virus is at fault. Reo-virus 3 [70], Epstein−Barr and cytomegalovirus [35] have also been incriminated.

CLINICAL PRESENTATION

Jaundice usually appears within three days of birth, but may be delayed to 3−4 weeks, or even up to six years.

BIOCHEMICAL CHANGES

The findings are those of chronic cholestasis with very high serum δ-glutamyl transpeptidase levels. Serum cholesterol levels are very high and xanthomas appear after about the first year of life (fig. 24.3). Serum bile acids are increased. Hepatic copper concentrations increase markedly and urinary copper is also elevated [31].

HEPATIC HISTOLOGY [48]

The early changes, at less than 90 days, are those of cholestasis, bile duct paucity, inflammation and fibrosis. Giant cells may be conspicuous. Electron microscopy shows abnormal canaliculi suggesting a primary ductal defect.

Later the picture is of hypoplasia of intra-hepatic bile ducts, increasing portal fibrosis

511

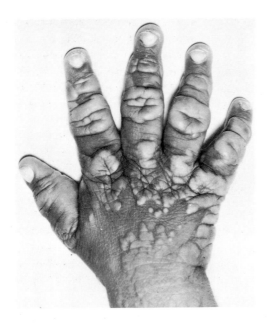

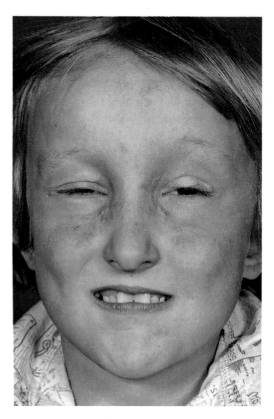

Fig. 24.3. Intra-hepatic biliary atresia (Alagille's syndrome) in a child of four years. Cholesterol deposits are noted on the hands, particularly on the extensor surfaces. Note also skin pigmentation and white nailbeds. This child spontaneously lost the xanthomas and is alive and reasonably well at 13 years.

and eventually cirrhosis. Hepatic copper is increased [31].

ARTERIO-HEPATIC DYSPLASIA (ALAGILLE SYNDROME) [3, 72, 101]

This is sometimes called syndromatic paucity of intra-hepatic bile ducts. It is seen world-wide.

Chronic intra-hepatic cholestasis presents in infancy or early childhood [86]. Inheritance is autosomal dominant with variable expression and penetrance.

The face is triangular with a prominant broad forehead, deep set eyes, a flattened nose and a pointed mandible (fig. 24.4). Hepato-spleno-megaly is usual. Skeletal changes include short distal phalanges and butterfly vertical bodies. The eyes show various abnormalities including retinal pigmentation and posterior embry-

Fig. 24.4. Alagille syndrome of biliary atresia. A five year old boy showing triangular facies, deep set eyes and a flattened nose. This patient had poor vision. At 16 years he is well with normal intelligence but dwarfed.

otoxon. Renal abnormalities have been noted [97].

Liver biopsy shows few, if any, interlobular bile ducts with a reduced number of portal zones [38]. The ratio of interlobular ducts to portal spaces is less than 0.09. There is little fibrosis so that neither cirrhosis nor secondary portal hypertension develop. However, both the liver biopsy and the electron microscopical appearances are not diagnostic of Alagille's syndrome.

Patients survive into adult life with varying degrees of growth and mental retardation, xanthomatosis and pruritus (fig. 24.5) [42]. Hepatocellular carcinoma may be a complication [1, 52]. On the whole, the condition improves

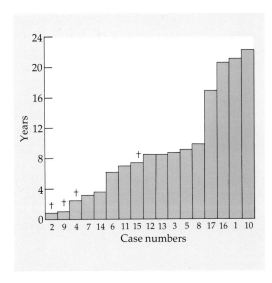

Fig. 24.5. Histogram showing the ages to date of 17 children with chronic intra-hepatic cholestasis (Heathcote *et al.* 1976).

with time. In one series followed long-term, only 21 of 80 patients died, liver failure being responsible in only four [6]. The patient can have normal children.

SYMPTOMATIC TREATMENT OF CHOLESTATIC SYNDROMES [2]

Steatorrhoea can be attributed to reduction in duodenal bile salt concentration. Calcium and vitamin D are not absorbed and biliary rickets results [55]. Vitamin A deficiency is frequent. Hepatic storage is normal and faulty absorption is the cause [79]. Vitamin A (50 000 units), vitamin D (50 000 units) and vitamin K1 (5 mg) must be given by intramuscular injection every four weeks. The child is encouraged to drink skimmed milk.

Vitamin E deficiency is particularly important in cholestatic infants (Chapter 13) [74]. It results in a degenerative neuro-muscular syndrome with areflexia. Vitamin E 10 mg/kg should be given intramuscularly every two weeks. Oral D-α tocopheryl polyethylene glycol-1000 succinate 15−25 i.u./kg/day may also be useful [90]. Once a neurological condition has developed, it is arrested, but not reversed, by intra-muscular vitamin E [89].

Medium chain triglyceride (coconut oil) is added to puréed fruit and vegetables and used in cooking. Portagen (Mead−Johnson) is a valuable food but is costly and not always available.

The tendency to bone thinning absolutely contraindicates the use of corticosteroids, which also stunt growth. In any case they are not of permanent value. In partial cholestasis cholestyramine (Questran) is given to the limit of tolerance levels. It may be flavoured with apple purée, tomato juice or chocolate syrup. It is valuable in controlling pruritus and in reducing skin xanthomas. Serum lipids, bile salts and bilirubin are reduced.

PROLONGED PARENTERAL NUTRITION

The cholestasis affects premature low birth-weight or severely compromised babies. Diagnosis is made by exclusion as the infants usually have other causes of cholestasis [104].

After one to two weeks, serum conjugated bilirubin rises steadily, increasing with duration of therapy.

Liver biopsy shows non-specific changes with features of extra-hepatic biliary obstruction. Biliary sludge and gallstones develop. Cholestasis continues as long as the parenteral nutrition but usually resolves within weeks or months or stopping. If therapy cannot be stopped, biliary cirrhosis develops and this may be fatal.

The cholestasis is related to loss of the entero-hepatic circulation of bile acids and consequent reduced bile formation, biliary stasis and sludging.

ABNORMAL BILE ACIDS

Atypical bile acids, not normally found in the adult, and similar to those of cholestatic states, have been identified in meconium [8]. Such acids synthesized by the developing liver and combined with defective sulphation might damage the biliary tract.

Abnormal synthesis of labile *sulphated chol-enoic acids* has been associated with cholestasis and giant-cell hepatitis in a three-month-old boy [17]. Inheritance was autosomal recessive.

Coprostanicacidemia results from a defect in the conversion of coprostanic to varinic acid. It is associated with progressive cholestasis and death by two years.

Zellweger's cerebro-hepato-renal syndrome is a fatal autosomal recessive condition with severe cholestasis. It is probably related to a block in mitochondrial side-chain oxidation—the first step in bile acid synthesis.

BYLER'S DISEASE

See Chapter 13.

IDIOPATHIC HYPOPITUITARISM

This is associated with severe hypoglycaemia, hepatomegaly and persistent direct hyperbilirubinaemia during the neonatal period [51].

SPONTANEOUS PERFORATION OF THE BILE DUCTS

This occurs between birth and three months, usually in the anterior wall of the common bile duct close to the junction with the cystic duct. This is a junctional site, particularly prone to faulty development. The child seems relatively well, but then develops non-bile-stained vomiting and acholic stools. Jaundice is mild, intermittent and variable. Abdominal hernias develop and the scrotum becomes green. Percutaneous cholangiography shows the blocked cystic duct with the hepatic duct leak. The results of surgery are good.

GALLBLADDER DISEASE AND GALLSTONES [93]

In babies, total parenteral nutrition is a frequent accompaniment of biliary sludge in the gallbladder and cholestasis. In babies bile duct perforation is associated with gallstones secondary to bile stasis.

Pigment gallstones may be found in the lower common bile duct without obvious cause. Acute gastroenteritis with bacterial overgrowth, dehydration or a minor atypical termination of the common bile duct may contribute.

A similar picture may complicate neonatal jaundice due to such conditions as hepatic prematurity or haemolytic disease. This has been termed the *inspissated bile syndrome*.

Surgical or endoscopic washing of the bile ducts is curative without the need for cholecystectomy [26].

In older children, cholecystitis and gallstones may be associated with blood dyscrasias or congenital anomalies of the biliary tract, such as choledochal cysts or biliary atresia. Immunoglobulin A deficiency has been linked with biliary sludge and gallstones in children [24].

Older children with gallstones often have a strong family history.

Reye's syndrome

In 1963 Reye and associates described this syndrome of acute encephalopathy and fatty change in the viscera [81].

AETIOLOGY AND EPIDEMIOLOGY

The syndrome has followed almost any known viral disease and can be encountered in epidemic form, often in winter or spring. There are two phases, an infective followed by an encephalopathic. Influenza B or A or varicella are the commonest antecedent infections.

Preceding salicylate administration has been incriminated [47] and numbers have fallen since they have been avoided for respiratory infections in children. Other possible modifying exogenous factors include aflatoxin, multiple hornet stings [102] and insecticides. The viral–host reaction is said to be modified by such factors.

There are geographic differences in Reye's syndrome [59]. In the United States, for instance, the median age is 11 years compared with 4 months in Britain where there is no clear association with influenza.

There is an acute mitochondrial insult with decreased activity of mitochondrial enzymes in liver [45]. A rise in blood ammonia with low citrulline values can be related to reduction of Krebs' cycle enzymes. The serum amino acid profile shows high glutamine, alanine and leucine levels. Hypoglycaemia may be related to inhibition of the citric acid cycle. Accumulation of triglycerides within hepatocytes reflects interference with the exit of lipid through depression of synthesis of the apoprotein of very low density lipoproteins. Mitochondrial injury also depresses fatty acid oxidation. Plasma free fatty acids are increased.

CLINICAL FEATURES

Sexes are equally affected, usually below 14 years old; young adults have been described [69]. Three to 7 days after a viral-type illness the child develops intractable vomiting and progressive, neurological deterioration. The encephalopathy is marked by erratic behaviour, irritability and listlessness progressing through lethargy to stupor and coma. Jaundice is rare.

Milder (grade 1) Reye's syndrome presents simply as vomiting with abnormal liver function tests after an upper respiratory infection or varicella [64].

In severe cases, medullary coning and brain death results 4–60 hours after the onset.

LIVER BIOPSY

This shows microvesicular fat. Electron microscopy shows swelling and distortion of the mitochondria to be followed by showers of peroxisomes.

Succinate dehydrogenase activity is low or absent.

OTHER ORGANS

The kidneys show proximal tubular fat. The myocardium is fatty and there is marked cerebral oedema. Electron microscopy of the neurones shows similar mitochondrial changes to those seen in the liver.

LABORATORY FINDINGS

Characteristic features are an increase in blood ammonia and serum transaminase levels. Hypoglycaemia is found in about 50%, usually in those seriously ill and less than 2 years old. Serum prothrombin time, more than 3 seconds prolonged, together with a serum ammonium value greater than 100 µg/dl predict a serious course [44].

TREATMENT

The patient presents as a problem in liver disease, but it is the cerebral oedema that is lethal. Treatment is directed towards this, combined with intense supportive care. There is no specific treatment.

Reye's-like syndromes [59]

A number of metabolic defects produce a picture clinically, biochemically and light-microscopically resembling Reye's syndrome. In general, however, there is a family history and episodes are recurrent. Five urea-cycle defects have been incriminated [45], disturbances in the mitochondrial β-oxidation pathway of fatty acids have also been described, particularly deficiencies of medium and long-chain acyl-co-A dehydrogenase [9, 99].

A child less than three years old should not be accepted as having Reye's syndrome unless genetic defects have been excluded. This demands special diagnostic facilities. Specimens of urine and serum should be obtained and frozen so that they may be subsequently analysed in specialist centres. Electron microscopy of a liver biopsy may also be useful as, in contrast to Reye's syndrome, mitochondrial morphology in the metabolic errors is normal.

Cirrhosis in infancy and childhood

The cirrhosis of infants and children has many aetiologies. As in the older age group, many are cryptogenic.

A number, presenting in later childhood and

at puberty, show the picture of *chronic active autoimmune hepatitis*. These patients usually respond to prednisolone treatment (Chapter 17).

Neonatal 'giant cell' hepatitis may be followed by cirrhosis and this may also apply to some of the neonatal virus infections such as chronic rubella, hepatitis B, or non-A, non-B.

Iron overload is usually related to transfusions in anaemic children. However, hereditary haemochromatosis can affect children as early as 2 years [30, 39]. Diagnosis is made by transferrin saturation and liver biopsy. Females and males are equally affected. Cardiac involvement is often fatal. Hypergonadism is frequent.

Wilson's disease, galactosaemia, Fanconi's disease, type IV glycogen disease and *fibro-cystic disease* may be followed by cirrhosis.

In the tropics the kwashiorkor syndrome is not followed by cirrhosis whereas *veno-occlusive disease* is followed by zone 3 fibrosis and finally a cirrhosis.

Congenital hepatic fibrosis may cause portal hypertension but the hepatic lesion is not a cirrhosis.

Cholestatic syndromes are followed by biliary cirrhosis and this is also so of α_1-*antitrypsin deficiency*.

Cardiac cirrhosis is unusual in childhood except complicating constrictive pericarditis.

CLINICAL FEATURES

Portal hypertension is usually prominent. The spleen tends to be larger than in the adult. Presentation with splenomegaly and hepatomegaly at a school medical examination or while in hospital for another condition is not unusual. Vascular spiders are conspicuous. Growth is uninterrupted; indeed the adolescent growth spurt may be particularly great so that the child is above normal height (fig. 24.6).

At puberty, both sexes may show acne and facial mooning with cutaneous striae, girls have amenorrhoea and boys gynaecomastia.

This relatively inactive stage can continue for years. Decompensation is followed by deepening jaundice and very high serum globulin and

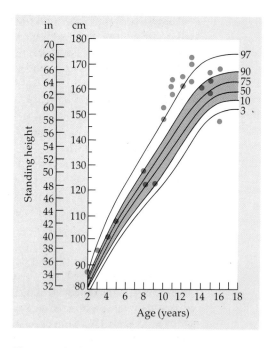

Fig. 24.6. Cirrhosis in female children. The age and height are in agreement. Note that children between 10 and 13 years are taller than 90% of the population (Sherlock 1958).

transaminase values. When pre-coma appears it is accompanied by mania, screaming, fits and psychic outbursts. Ascites is usual at this late stage. Sclerotherapy of oesophageal varices is well tolerated [7].

The prognosis is very variable depending on the aetiology. The outlook is better than for an adult with an equivalent degree of clinical decompensation.

Indian childhood cirrhosis

This condition is seen in rural, middle-class, Hindu families throughout India. It has also been reported in an American sibship [60]. Both sexes are affected between the ages of 1 and 3 years. The familial incidence suggests genetic factors although it may indicate a common environmental origin. Death is usually due to liver failure and occurs within a year of diagnosis.

Hepatic histology shows profound injury to individual liver cells which may contain Mallory's hyaline bodies and which are surrounded by polymorph accumulations. A fine, micronodular cirrhosis results. The picture resembles acute alcoholic hepatitis, but without the fatty change.

Hepatic copper is markedly increased, and this is largely located in the cytoplasm. The livers of unaffected siblings do not show excess copper [76].

Ingestion of animal milk contaminated by brass and copper household utensils provides the excess copper [10]. Prevention is by changing the feeding of the child.

Wilson's disease is excluded by absence of Kayser—Fleischer rings and normal serum caeruloplasmin values.

Penicillamine proves of no value in the advanced disease [94]. However, those without jaundice and ascites show a significantly improved survival.

Fetal alcohol syndrome

Hepatomegaly and raised transaminase values may be found. The liver may show fatty changes with portal and perisinusoidal fibrosis resembling those seen in the adult with alcoholic liver disease [61].

Peliosis hepatis (see Chapter 18)

Hamartomas

These benign, congenital lesions present as an abdominal mass in the first two years of life. They may be an incidental finding at autopsy. They must be distinguished from malignant tumours. They are not true neoplasms. They consist of abnormal arrangements of all the cells of the normal liver, particularly bile ducts and fibroblasts. They contain central veins. They are nearly always cystic. They require no treatment.

Tumours of the liver (see also Chapter 28)

Primary tumours in infants and children are rare, two-thirds are diagnosed before the second year of life. They may arise from liver cells and/or from supporting structures. Secondary tumours are extremely rare and are usually associated with a neuroblastoma of the adrenals.

Adenomas

These rare tumours do not become malignant, and over the years may even regress [103]. They consist of sheets of liver cells and have a fibrous capsule. They should be treated conservatively.

Hepato-cellular carcinoma

These usually present after five years old. Males are more frequently affected than females. The tumours are often single, large and metastasize late. Cirrhosis may be absent.

Hepatitis B carriage is a very important accompaniment [106]. Hepato-cellular carcinoma has developed in a boy aged 5 following perinatal transmission of hepatitis B [98].

Hepato-cellular carcinoma may also complicate giant cell hepatitis, biliary atresia and the polycystic diseases, including congenital hepatic fibrosis.

The patients present with weight loss, abdominal swelling usually in the right upper quadrant, pain, ascites and jaundice. Calcification in the tumour may be noted.

Treatment

The only hope is surgical resection and this is rarely possible. However, following lobectomy, growth and development are normal. Chemotherapy may be useful in reducing tumour size before resection.

The fibrolamellar form has a much better prognosis and resection is more often possible.

Hepatoblastoma [57]

This rare embryonal tumour with epithelial and mesenchymal elements usually presents before 3 years of age and is usually fatal within 5 years.

It has been reported in association with hemi-hypertrophy, Wilms' tumour, fetal alcohol syndrome and with polyposis coli in the mother [53]. It may produce human chorionic gonadotrophins resulting in precocious puberty [9, 73].

Hypercholesterolaemia can be associated [73].

Chemotherapy may prolong life so that resection may be possible. Hepatic transplantation has led to falls of human chorionic gonadotrophins [43].

Infantile haemangio-endothelioma

This is a usually benign, vascular tumour of infancy. It consists of endothelium-lined channels of capillary size. It may be associated with skin haemangiomas. Anaemia is usual.

It presents usually before 6 months of age as abdominal mass or hepatomegaly [23]. Cardiac failure may be related to arterio–venous shunts within the tumour. A systolic bruit may be heard in the epigastrium. Rupture can cause haemoperitoneum. Associated congenital defects are frequent.

Severe anaemia has been attributed to micro-angiopathic haemolysis related to the abnormal, tortuous narrow anastomotic vessels within the tumour. Thrombocytopenia may also be seen.

Treatment

Congestive cardiac failure must be treated vigorously to allow time for the tumour to involute spontaneously [100]. Ligation of the hepatic artery or preferably embolization after arteriography should be performed.

Diagnosis of hepatic tumours

Biochemical tests may be normal. The most usual abnormality is an increase in serum 5'-nucleotidase and α_2-globulin levels. Serum α_1-fetoprotein may be present.

The site and extent of the tumour must be defined by splenic venography, coeliac angiography and scanning. Haemangio-endotheliomas show a blush in the liver on selective coeliac angiography.

Needle hepatic biopsy is usually a safe method of confirming the diagnosis.

Treatment

The only procedure offering hope of cure in the primary carcinoma group is resection. This will cure the benign lesions. Cure may even follow in the malignant group for the tumour is usually single, often large and metastasizes late. In any case palliation is usual. Subsequent growth and development are normal after hepatic lobectomy.

The prognosis is very poor if resection is impossible.

Hepatic transplantation

This is particularly important in children with liver disease and is considered Chapter 35.

References

1 Adams PC. Hepatocellular carcinoma associated with arteriohepatic dysplasia. *Dig. Dis. Sci.* 1986; **31**: 438.
2 Alagille D. Management of paucity of inter-lobular bile ducts. *J. Hepatol.* 1985; **1**: 561.
3 Alagille D, Odièvre M, Gautier M *et al.* Hepatic ductular hypoplasia associated with characteristic facies, vertebral malformations, retarded physical, mental and sexual development and cardiac murmur. *J. Pediatr.* 1975; **86**: 63.
4 Alagille D, Estrada A, Hadchouel M *et al.* Syndromic paucity of interlobular bile ducts (Alagille syndrome or arteriohepatic dysplasia): review of 80 cases. *J. Pediatr.* 1987; **110**: 195.
5 Alpert LI, Strauss L, Hirschhorn K. Neonatal hepatitis and biliary atresia associated with

trisomy 17—18 syndrome. *N. Engl. J. Med.* 1969; **270**: 16.

6 Alvarez F, Landrieu P, Laget P *et al.* Nervous and ocular disorders in children with cholestasis and vitamin A and E deficiencies. *Hepatology* 1983; **3**: 410.

7 Atkinson JB, Woolley MM. Treatment of esophageal varices by sclerotherapy in children. *Am. J. Surg.* 1983; **146**: 103.

8 Back P, Walter K. Developmental pattern of bile acid metabolism as revealed by bile acid analysis of meconium. *Gastroenterology* 1980; **78**: 671.

9 Beach R, Bett P, Radford M *et al.* Production of human chorionic gonadotrophin by a hepatoblastoma resulting in precocious puberty. *J. clin. Pathol.* 1984; **37**: 734.

10 Bhave SA, Pandit AN, Tanner MS. Comparison of feeding history of children with Indian childhood cirrhosis and paired controls. *J. pediatr. Gastroenterol. Nutr.* 1987; **6**: 562.

11 Botolotti F, Calzia R, Cadrobbi P *et al.* Liver cirrhosis associated with chronic hepatitis B virus infection in childhood. *J. Pediatr.* 1986; **108**: 224.

12 Botolotti F, Cadrobbi P, Armigliato M *et al.* Acute non-A, non-B hepatitis in childhood. *J. pediatr. Gastroenterol. Nutr.* 1988; **7**: 22.

13 Capps FPA, Gilles HM, Jolly H *et al.* Glucose-6-phosphate dehydrogenase deficiency and neonatal jaundice in Nigeria. Their relation to the use of prophylactic vitamin K. *Lancet* 1963; **ii**: 379.

14 Chang M-H, Hsu H-C, Lee C-Y *et al.* Neonatal hepatitis: a follow-up study. *J. pediatr. Gastroenterol Nutr.* 1987; **6**: 203.

15 Chang M-H, Hwang L-Y, Hsu H-C *et al.* Prospective study of asymptomatic HBsAg carrier children infected in the perinatal period: clinical and liver histologic studies. *Hepatology* 1988; **8**: 374.

16 Chianale J, Dvorak C, Farmer DL *et al.* Cytochrome P-450 gene expression in the functional units of the fetal liver. *Hepatology* 1988; **8**: 318.

17 Clayton PT, Leonard JV, Lawson AM *et al.* Familial giant-cell hepatitis associated with synthesis of 3 beta, 7 alpha-dihydroxy-and 3 beta, 7 alpha, 12 alpha-trihydroxy-5-cholenoic acids. *J. clin. Invest.* 1987; **79**: 1031.

18 Colombo C. Cirrhosis associated with multiple transfusions in thalassaemia. *J. pediatr. Gastroenterol. Nutr.* 1985; **4**: 849.

19 Cornelius CE, Rosenberg DP. Animal model of human disease. Neonatal biliary atresia. *Am. J. Pathol.* 1985; **118**: 168.

20 Cox KL, Stadalnik RC, McGahan JP *et al.* Hepatobiliary scintigraphy with technetium-99 m disoferin in the evaluation of neonatal cholestasis. *J. pediatr. Gastroenterol. Nutr.* 1987; **6**: 885.

21 Cuervas-Mons V, Rimola A, Van Thiel DH *et al.* Does previous abdominal surgery alter the outcome of pediatric patients subjected to orthotopic liver transplantation? *Gastroenterology* 1986; **90**: 853.

22 Daamen CGF, Schaberg A. Hemilateral liver degeneration in perinatal death. *J. Pathol.* 1969; **97**: 29.

23 Dachman AH, Lichtenstein JE, Friedman AC *et al.* Infantile hemangioendothelioma of the liver: a radiologic-pathologic-clinical correlation. *Am. J. Roentgenol.* 1983; **140**: 1091.

24 Danon YL, Dinari G. Garty B-Z *et al.* Cholelithiasis in children with immunoglobulin A deficiency: a new gastroenterologic syndrome. *J. Pediatr. Gastroenterol Nutr.* 1983; **2**: 663.

25 Dehner LP, Kissane LM. Pyogenic hepatic abscesses in infancy and childhood. *J. Pediatr.* 1969; **74**: 763.

26 Descos B, Bernard O, Brunelle F *et al.* Pigment gallstones of the common bile duct in infancy. *Hepatology* 1984; **4**: 678.

27 Desmet VJ. Intrahepatic bile ducts under the lens. *J. Hepatol.* 1985; **1**: 545.

28 Dick MC, Mowat AP. Hepatitis syndrome in infancy—an epidemiological survey with 10 year follow up. *Arch. Dis. Child.* 1985; **60**: 512.

29 Ennever J, Costarino AT, Polin RA *et al.* Rapid clearance of a structural isomer of bilirubin during phototherapy. *J. clin. Invest.* 1987; **79**: 1674.

30 Escobar GJ, Heyman MB, Smith WB *et al.* Primary hemochromatosis in childhood. *Pediatrics* 1987; **80**: 549.

31 Evans, J, Newman S, Sherlock S. Liver copper levels in intrahepatic cholestasis of childhood. *Gastroenterology* 1978; **75**: 875.

32 Evans J, Zerpa H, Nuttall L *et al.* Copper chelation therapy in intrahepatic cholestasis of childhood. *Gut* 1983; **24**: 4.

33 Faa G, Liguori C, Columbano A *et al.* Uneven copper distribution in the human newborn liver. *Hepatology* 1987; **7**: 838.

34 Felsher BF, Carpio NM, Woolley MM *et al.* Hepatic bilirubin glucuronidation in neonates with unconjugated hyperbilirubinaemia and congenital gastrointestinal obstruction. *J. lab. clin. Med.* 1974; **83**: 90.

35 Finegold MJ, Carpenter RJ. Obliterative cholangitis due to cytomegalovirus: a possible precursor of paucity of intrahepatic bile ducts. *Hum. Pathol.* 1982; **13**: 662.

36 Fung KP, Lau SP. Gamma-glutamyl transpeptidase activity and its serial measurement in differentiation between extra-hepatic biliary atresia and neonatal hepatitis. *J. pediatr. Gastroenterol. Nutr.* 1985; **4**: 208.

37 Gourley GR, Arend RA. β glucuronidase and hyperbilirubinaemia in breast-fed and formula-fed babies. *Lancet* 1986; **i:** 644.

38 Hadchouel M, Hugon RN, Gautier M. Reduced ratio of portal tracts to paucity of intrahepatic bile ducts. *Arch. Pathol. lab. Med.* 1978; **102:** 402.

39 Haddy TB, Castro OL, Rana SR. Hereditary hemochromatosis in children, adolescents, and young adults. *Am. J. pediatr. Hematol/Oncol.* 1988; **10:** 23.

40 Hansen TWR, Bratlid D. Bilirubin and brain toxicity. *Acta Pediatr. Scand.* 1986; **75:** 513.

41 Hargreaves T. Effect of fatty acids on bilirubin conjugation. *Arch. dis. Child.* 1973; **48:** 446.

42 Heathcote J, Deodhar KP, Scheuer PJ *et al.* Intrahepatic cholestasis in childhood. *N. Engl. J. Med.* 1976; **295:** 801.

43 Heimann A, White PF, Riely CA *et al.* Hepatoblastoma presenting as isosexual precocity. *J. clin. Gastroenterol.* 1987; **9:** 105.

44 Heubi JE, Daughterty CC, Partin JS *et al.* Grade 1 Reye's syndrome—outcome and predictors of progression to deeper coma grades. *N. Engl. J. Med.* 1984; **311:** 1539.

45 Heubi JE, Partin JC, Partin JS *et al.* Reye's syndrome: current concepts. *Hepatology* 1987; **7:** 155.

46 Hsu H-C, Lin Y-H, Chang M-H *et al.* Pathology of chronic hepatitis B virus infection in children: with special reference to the intrahepatic expression of hepatitis B virus antigens. *Hepatology* 1988; **8:** 378.

47 Hurwitz ES, Barrett MJ, Bregman D *et al.* Public health service study of Reye's syndrome and medications. Report of the main study. *J. Am. med. Assoc.* 1987; **257:** 1905.

48 Kahn E, Daum F, Markowitz J *et al.* Nonsyndromatic paucity of interlobular bile ducts: light and electron microscopic evaluation of sequential liver biopsies in early childhood. *Hepatology* 1986; **6:** 890.

49 Kasai M, Watanabe I, Ohi R. Follow-up studies of long-term survivors after hepatic portoenterostomy for 'non-correctable' biliary atresia. *J. pediatr. Surg.* 1975; **10:** 173.

50 Kobayashi A, Itabashi F, Ohbe Y. Long-term prognosis in biliary atresia after hepatic portoenterostomy: analysis of 35 patients who survived beyond 5 years of age. *J. Pediatr.* 1984; **105:** 243.

51 Kaufman FR, Costin G, Thomas DW *et al.* Neonatal cholestasis and hypopituitarism. *Arch. Dis. Child.* 1984; **59:** 787.

52 Kaufman SS, Wood RP, Shaw B Jr, *et al.* Hepatocarcinoma in a child with the Alagille syndrome. *Am. J. Dis. Child.* 1987; **141:** 698.

53 Kingston JE, Herbert A, Draper GJ *et al.* Association between hepatoblastoma and polyposis

coli. *Arch. Dis. Child.* 1983; **38:** 959.

54 Klein BS, Michaels JA, Rytel MW *et al.* Nosocomial hepatitis A: a multinursery outbreak in Winsconsin. *J. Am. med. Assoc.* 1984; **252:** 2716.

55 Kooh SW, Jones G, Reilly BJ *et al.* Pathogenesis of rickets in chronic hepatobiliary disease in children. *J. Pediatr.* 1979; **94:** 870.

56 Lachaux A, Descos B, Plchau H *et al.* Familial extrahepatic biliary atresia. *J. pediatr. Gastroenterol. Nutr.* 1988; **7:** 280.

57 Lack EE, Neave C, Vawter GF. Hepatoblastoma: a clinical and pathologic study of 54 cases. *Am. J. surg. Pathol.* 1982; **6:** 693.

58 Landing BH. Considerations of the pathogenesis of neonatal hepatitis, biliary atresia and choledochal cyst—the concept of infantile obstructive cholangiopathy. *Prog. paediatr. Surg.* 1974; **6:** 113.

59 Leading Article. Reye's syndrome and aspirin: epidemiological associations and inborn errors of metabolism. *Lancet* 1987; **ii:** 429.

60 Lefkowitch JH, Honig CL, King ME *et al.* Hepatic copper overload and features of Indian childhood cirrhosis in an American sibship. *N. Engl. J. Med.* 1982; **307:** 271.

61 Lefkowitch JH, Rushton AR, Feng-Chen K-C. Hepatic fibrosis in fetal alcohol syndrome. Pathologic similarities to adult alcoholic liver disease. *Gastroenterology* 1983; **85:** 951.

62 Lester R. Bile acid metabolism in the newborn. *J. Pediatr. Gastroenterol. Nutr.* 1983; **2:** 335.

63 Lewis HM, Campbell RHA, Hambelton G. Use or abuse of phototherapy for physiological jaundice of newborn infants. *Lancet* 1982; **ii:** 408.

64 Lichtenstein PK, Heubi JE, Daughterty CC *et al.* Grade I Reye's syndrome: a frequent cause of vomiting and liver dysfunction after varicella and upper-respiratory-tract infection. *N. Engl. J. Med.* 1983; **309:** 133.

65 Long WA, Ulshen MH, Lawson EE. Clinical manifestations of congenital syphilitic hepatitis: implications for pathogenesis. *J. Pediatr. Gastroenterol. Nutr.* 1984; **3:** 551.

66 Lucey JF, Arias IM, McKay RJ Jr. Transient familial neonatal hyperbilirubinemia. *Am. J. Dis. Child.* 1960; **100:** 787.

67 McClement JW, Howard ER, Mowat AP. Results of surgical treatment for extrahepatic biliary atresia in United Kingdom 1980—2. *Br. med. J.* 1985; **290:** 345.

68 MacGillivray MH, Crawford JD, Robey JS. Congenital hypothyroidism and prolonged neonatal hyperbilirubineamia. *Pediatrics* 1967; **40:** 283.

69 Meythaler JM, Varma RR. Reye's syndrome in adults. Diagnostic considerations. *Arch. intern. Med.* 1987; **147:** 61.

70 Morecki R, Glaser JH, Cho S *et al.* Biliary atresia and reovirus type 3 infection. *N. Engl. J. Med.* 1982; **307**: 481.

71 Morecki R, Glaser JH, Johnson AB *et al.* Detection of reovirus type 3 in the porta hepatis of an infant with extra-hepatic biliary atresia: ultrastructural and immunocytochemical study. *Hepatology* 1984; **4**: 1137.

72 Mueller RF. The Alagille syndrome (arteriohepatic dysplasia). *J. Med. Genet.* 1987; **24**: 621.

73 Muraji T, Woolley MM, Sinatra F *et al.* The prognostic implication of hypercholesterolemia in infants and children with hepatoblastoma. *J. pediatr. Surg.* 1985; **20**: 228.

74 Perlmutter DH, Gross P, Jones HR *et al.* Intramuscular vitamin E repletion in children with chronic cholestasis. *Am. J. Dis. Child.* 1987; **141**: 170.

75 Naveh Y, Berant M. Assessment of liver size in normal infants and children. *J. pediatr. Gastroenterol. Nutr.* 1984; **3**: 346.

76 Nayak NC, Marwaha N, Kalva V *et al.* The liver in siblings of patients with Indian childhood cirrhosis: a light and electron microscopic study. *Gut* 1981; **22**: 295.

77 Niijima S-I. Studies on the conjugating activity of bile acids in children. *Pediatr. Res.* 1985; **19**: 302.

78 Noble RC, Kane MA, Reeves SA *et al.* Post transfusion hepatitis A in a neonatal intensive care unit. *J. Am. med. Assoc.* 1984; **252**: 2711.

79 Ong DE, Amédée-Manesme O. Liver levels of vitamin A and cellular retinol-binding protein for patients with biliary atresia. *Hepatology* 1987; **7**: 253.

80 Osborn LM, Reiff MI, Bolus R. Jaundice in the full-term neonate. *Pediatrics* 1984; **73**: 520.

81 Reye RDK, Morgan G, Baral J. Encephalopathy and fatty degeneration of the viscera. A disease entity in childhood. *Lancet* 1963; **ii**: 749.

82 Ritter DA, Kenny JD. Bilirubin binding in premature infants from birth to three months. *Arch. Dis. Child.* 1986; **61**: 352.

83 Rosenthal P, Henton D, Felber S *et al.* Distribution of serum bilirubin conjugates in pediatric hepatobiliary diseases. *J. Pediatr.* 1987; **110**: 201.

84 Scheuer PJ, Liver disease in childhood and heredofamilial disorders. In *Liver Biopsy Interpretation* 4th edn. 1988, Ballière Tindall, London.

85 Shiraki K. Hepatic cell necrosis in the newborn: a pathogenic study of 147 cases with particular reference to congenital heart disease. *Am. J. Dis. Child.* 1970; **119**: 395.

86 Shulman SA, Hyams JS, Gunta R *et al.* Arteriohepatic dysplasia (Alagille syndrome): extreme variability among affected family members. *Am. J. med. Genet.* 1984; **19**: 325.

87 Sisto A, Feldman P, Garel L *et al.* Primary sclerosing cholangitis in children: study of five cases and review of the literature. *Pediatrics* 1987; **80**: 918.

88 Sodeyama T, Kiyosawa K, Akahane Y *et al.* Evolution of HBeAg/anti-HBe status and its relationship to clinical and histological outcome in chronic HBV carriers in childhood. *Am. J. Gastroenterol.* 1986; **81**:239.

89 Sokol RJ, Guggenheim MA, Iannaccone ST *et al.* Improved neurologic function after long-term correction of vitamin E deficiency in children with chronic cholestasis. *N. Engl. J. Med.* 1985; **313**: 1580.

90 Sokol RJ, Heubi JE, Butler-Simon N *et al.* Treatment of vitamin E deficiency during chronic childhood cholestasis with oral alpha-tocopheryl polyethylene glycol-1000 succinate. *Gastroenterology* 1987; **93**: 975.

91 Stern H, Williams BM. Isolation of rubella virus in a case of neonatal giant-cell hepatitis. *Lancet* 1966; **i**: 293.

92 Suchy FJ, Bucuvalas JC, Novak DA. Determinants of bile formation during development: ontogeny of hepatic bile acid metabolism and transport. *Sem. Liv. Dis.* 1987; **7**: 77.

93 Takiff HJ, Fonkalsrud EW. Gallbladder disease in childhood. *Am. J. Dis. Child.* 1984; **138**: 565.

94 Tanner MS, Bhave SA, Pradhan AM *et al.* Clinical trials of penicillamine in Indian childhood cirrhosis. *Arch. Dis. Child.* 1987; **62**: 1118.

95 Taubman B, Hale DE, Kelley RI. Familial Reye-like syndrome: a presentation of medium chain acyl-coenzyme A dehydrogenase deficiency. *Pediatrics* 1987; **79**: 382.

96 Thaler MM. Jaundice in the newborn: algorithmic diagnosis of conjugated and unconjugated hyperbilirubinemia. *J. Am. med. Assoc.* 1977; **237**: 58.

97 Tolia V, Dubois RS, Watts FB Jr *et al.* Renal abnormalities in paucity of interlobular bile ducts. *J. pediatr. Gastroenterol.* 1987; **6**: 971.

98 Tong MJ, Govindarajan S. Primary hepatocellular carcinoma following perinatal transmission of hepatitis B. *West. J. Med.* 1988; **148**: 205.

99 Treem WR, Witzleben CA, Piccoli DA *et al.* Medium-chain and long-chain acyl CoA dehydrogenase deficiency: clinical, pathologic and ultrastructural differentiation from Reye's syndrome. *Hepatology* 1986; **6**: 1270.

100 Vorse HB, Smith I, Luckstead EF *et al.* Hepatic hemangiomatosis of infancy. *Am. J. Dis. Child.* 1983; **137**: 672.

101 Watson GH, Miller V. Arteriohepatic dysplasia: familial pulmonary arterial stenosis with neonatal liver disease. *Arch. Dis. Child.* 1973; **48**: 459.

102 Weizman Z, Mussafi H, Ishay JS *et al.* Multiple

hornet stings with features of Reye's syndrome. *Gastroenterology* 1985; **89:** 1407.

103 Wheeler DA, Edmondson HA, Reynolds TB. Spontaneous liver cell adenoma in children. *Am. J. Clin. Path.* 1986; **85:** 6.

104 Whitington PF. Cholestasis associated with total parenteral nutrition in infants. *Hepatology* 1985; **5:** 693.

105 Wigger HJ, Blanc WA. Fatal hepatic and bronchial necrosis in adenovirus infection with thymic alymphoplasia. *N. Engl. J. Med.* 1966; **275:** 870.

106 Wu TC, Tong MJ, Hwang B *et al.* Primary hepatocellular carcinoma and hepatitis B infection during childhood. *Hepatology* 1987; **7:** 46.

25 · The Liver in Pregnancy

Normal pregnancy

Physical examination in pregnant women may show palmar erythema and vascular spiders. The liver is impalpable. Serum biochemical tests in the last trimester show modest increases in alkaline phosphatase, cholesterol and α_1- and α_2-globulins. Most of the alkaline phosphatase is of placental origin and the serum γ-GT value is normal. Serum bile acids are slightly increased [18]. The transport maximum for bromsulphalein (BSP) is reduced [6]. These results, taken together, suggest that a normal pregnancy is mildly cholestatic. Bilirubin and transaminase levels are within normal limits. Serum albumin, urea and uric acid concentrations are reduced.

Needle liver biopsy in normal pregnancy gives virtually normal histological appearances [11]. Electron microscopy shows some increase in endoplasmic reticulum.

Liver blood flow is within the normal range [22]. In pregnancy, blood volume and cardiac output increase. The liver blood flow comprises 35% of the cardiac output in non-pregnant females and only 28% of the cardiac output in pregnancy. The excess blood volume is shunted through the placenta.

Hepatic haemorrhage

This usually complicates pre-eclampsia or eclampsia with accompanying disseminated intravascular coagulation and intra-hepatic vascular lesions. It may also be spontaneous, usually, but not always, in the last trimester.

Hepatic adenomas, often with peliosis hepatis, developing after long-term use of oral contraceptives may rupture during pregnancy.

Clinical features include sudden, constant, right upper quadrant or epigastric pain, usually radiating to the back and right shoulder with vomiting and circulatory collapse. Haemoglobin, haematocrit and platelet values fall. Ultrasound or, preferably, CT scanning of the liver are invaluable in diagnosing intra-hepatic haemorrhage, subcapsular haematoma and free peritoneal fluid (Chapter 5) [19]. Hepatic angiography is useful in identifying the site of a tear and its blood supply. The laceration usually involves the right lobe of the liver and varies from an ooze to a large tear.

If recognized early, and particularly at the stage of unruptured subcapsular haematoma, conservative management may be adequate with careful monitoring and blood product replacement [8, 10]. Surgery is reserved for those who cannot be haemodynamically stabilized. Hepatic angiography followed by selective transcatheter embolization is the most effective treatment [17]. The mortality rate for the mother is about 50% and for the fetus about 60%. Early recognition and conservative management will undoubtedly improve these results.

Hyperemesis gravidarum

This is rare and occurs in the first trimester. Serum conjugated bilirubin increases. It can recur in successive pregnancies (16).

Jaundice in pregnancy

The jaundice may be peculiar to pregnancy such as acute fatty liver of pregnancy, cholestatic jaundice in pregnancy, or jaundice complicating the toxaemias. The jaundice may be an intercurrent one affecting the pregnant woman such as virus hepatitis or gallstones. Finally, the effect of pregnancy on underlying chronic liver disease must be considered (table 25.1).

Jaundice occurs in about one out of every 1500 gestations, an incidence of 0.067% [9]. At least 41% of all cases with jaundice are due to viral hepatitis and about 21% to intra-hepatic cholestasis of pregnancy. Common bile duct obstruction accounts for less than 6% of all cases. These results are from Switzerland and different statistics can be expected from other parts of the world.

Acute fatty liver of pregnancy

The first full description is usually attributed to Sheehan [34] who, in 1940, described obstetric acute liver atrophy as a specific cause of jaundice in pregnancy. The condition is rare [4].

AETIOLOGY

Acute fatty liver is a member of the microvesicular fat disease group [35]. This is marked by swollen hepatocytes with central nuclei, containing microvesicular fat droplets, with absence of liver cell necrosis and with periportal sparing (figs 25.1, 25.2). The disease can be related to a widespread hepatic metabolic disturbance particularly involving mitochondria and ribosomes. The mode of initiation is ill understood. Viral, toxic and nutritional factors have been implicated. As in Reye's syndrome, a preceding acute respiratory infection has been described. Large doses of intravenous tetracycline, a known inhibitor of protein synthesis, were associated with acute fatty liver of pregnancy, but this is very rare nowadays. Nutritional factors are even less clearly defined.

CLINICAL FEATURES

The onset is between the 30th and 38th week of pregnancy and is marked by nausea, repeated vomiting and abdominal pain followed about a week later by jaundice (tables 25.2, 25.3). In some patients, preceding hypertension, peripheral oedema and proteinuria suggest pregnancy toxaemia. The condition is more common with twins and male births and in primiparae [4]. In those severely affected, the course is marked by coma, renal failure and haemorrhages.

Ascites is found in 50%, perhaps related to portal hypertension.

SERUM BIOCHEMICAL CHANGES

High serum uric acid levels are usual, and these may be related to tissue destruction and

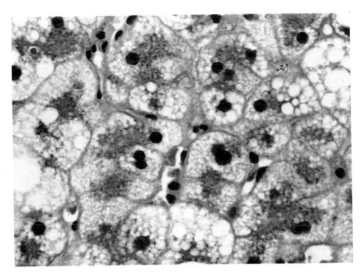

Fig. 25.1. Acute fatty liver of pregnancy. Hepatocytes have a foamy appearance with a central dense nucleus. (Stained H & E, ×120.)

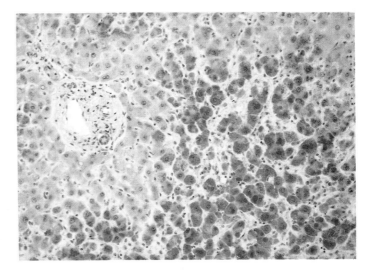

Fig. 25.2. Acute fatty liver of pregnancy: zone 3 hepatocytes are full of microvesicular fat droplets. Portal zones are normal and inflammation is minimal. (Stained oil red, ×40.)

lactic acidosis. This is not a usual feature of viral hepatitis or other types of acute liver failure.

Hyperbilirubinaemia is found in the absence of demonstrable haemolysis, in contradistinction to pregnancy toxaemia where jaundice is rare except with haemolysis. The serum aspartate transaminase values are raised, but gammaglobulin levels are normal.

Serum ammonia levels are increased and there is a generalized hyperaminoacidaemia.

Hypoglycaemia can be profound.

HAEMATOLOGICAL FINDINGS

Leucocytosis, more than 12 000 per mm^3, is found in 90%. Blood films reveal a characteristic picture of neutrophilia, thrombocytopenia and

Table 25.1. Jaundice in pregnancy

	Notes
Peculiar to pregnancy	
Acute fatty liver	Presents vomiting, variable prognosis, no recurrence
Recurrent cholestasis	Good prognosis, familial, recurs, fetal wastage
Toxaemias	Rare cause of jaundice
	Hepatic haemorrhage may be a complication
Hyperemesis	Rare cause of jaundice
Intercurrent	
Viral hepatitis	Prognosis as in non-pregnant, fetal wastage
	A—no effect on fetus
	B—transmitted to fetus
	Non-A, non-B often fatal in Africa and Asia
Gallstones	Rare cause of jaundice, ultrasound diagnosis
Underlying chronic liver disease	Rare to become pregnant, prognosis variable, still-births increased

Table 25.2. Acute fatty liver of pregnancy. Symptoms and signs recorded before hospital admission in twelve patients (Burroughs *et al.* 1982)

Patient	1	2	3	4	5	6	7	8	9	10	11	12
Malaise	+	+	+	+	+	+	+	+	+	+	+	+
Anorexia		+		+		+		+	+			
Nausea/vomiting	+	+	+	+	+	+	+	+	+	+	+	+
Coffee-ground vomiting	+					+	+			+		
Heartburn						+	+	+	+			
Abdominal pain/tenderness			+	+	+	+	+	+	+			
Hypertension	+		+	+	+		+	+	+		+	
Peripheral oedema	+		+	+	+			+		+	+	+
Proteinuria	+		+		+	+			+	+		+
Jaundice (days from onset of symptoms)	10	7	16	8	2	14	7	15	8	18	11	post delivery

normoblasts. Films also show giant platelets and basophilic stippling. This combination of features is not seen in pre-eclampsia or viral hepatitis and provides a strong pointer towards the diagnosis of acute fatty liver of pregnancy.

Severe bleeding is frequent but a firm diagnosis of disseminated intravascular coagulation is found in only 10%. Platelet half-life is reduced. Depression of antithrombin 3 may be particularly marked.

LIVER BIOPSY APPEARANCES

Needle biopsy may be required to make the distinction from acute viral hepatitis, although, if blood coagulation is impaired, this procedure may be postponed until the recovery stage. There is natural reluctance to perform liver biopsy in a pregnant woman with impaired clotting. If necessary, this can be done using the transjugular approach. The microscopical picture is of microvesicular fat droplets with swollen hepatocytes with dense central nuclei and peri-portal sparing. Cytoplasmic fat-filled microvacuoles may be clearly recognized only on frozen sections stained for fat with such methods as oil-red O [2, 31, 32]. Occasionally, liver cell necrosis is marked especially in fatal cases.

Electron microscopy confirms vacuoles and may show a honeycomb appearance in the smooth endoplasmic reticulum and variations in mitochondrial size and shape.

Ultrasound shows hyperechogenicity in 50% and the CT is hypodense in 30%. These non-invasive techniques may be useful diagnostically [5, 21].

COURSE AND PROGNOSIS (table 25.3)

Formerly the prognosis for mother and baby was very grave. Improved results have followed early diagnosis of the less severely affected [2, 30].

Death is usually due to extra-hepatic causes such as disseminated intravascular coagulation with massive haemorrhage and renal failure, which are seen in the less severely affected.

Subsequent pregnancies in survivors have been normal without any recurrence of symptoms or abnormalities in liver or renal function tests [4]. Future pregnancies are safe.

MANAGEMENT

The routine for acute renal and hepatic failure is adopted (Chapter 8). Oesophagitis with bleeding is a frequent complication and H_2 antagonists should be given.

Early delivery, using oxytocin or, if necessary, Caesarean section, probably improves maternal and fetal survival [13].

Table 25.3. Subsequent pregnancies in patients with acute fatty liver of pregnancy (AFLP) (Burroughs *et al.* 1982)

	Interval from pregnancy with AFLP	
Patient reported by:	First pregnancy	Second pregnancy
Burroughs (*Patient 3*)	4 years (induced 38 weeks)	7 years (spontaneous at term)
Burroughs (*Patient 4*)	1¼ years (spontaneous at term)	6¼ years (spontaneous at term)
Burroughs (*Patient 5*)	2 years (spontaneous at term)	6 years (Caesarian at 38 weeks)
Burroughs (*Patient 7*)	10 months (spontaneous at term)	
MacKenna (*Patient 1*)	no date available (spontaneous at term)	
MacKenna (*Patient 2*)	1½ years (spontaneous at term)	
Davies (*Patient 2*)	3 years	
Davies (*Patient 3*)	2 years	
Breen (*Patient 1*)	*c.* 2 years	
Breen (*Patient 2*)	3¾ years (Caesarian at 38 weeks)	5½ years (spontaneous at term)
Breen (*Patient 3*)	1½ years (spontaneous at term)	
Jenkins	2 years	

Fresh frozen plasma and intravenous albumin are given. Haemodialysis is used if necessary.

Pregnancy toxaemias

MILD

Increases in serum alkaline phosphatase and transaminase values are frequently found. Minor signs of disseminated intravascular coagulation, such as a reduction in platelets, are also common. Liver biopsies usually show fibrin deposits in peri-portal sinusoids if immunofluorescent staining is used [29]. These may be present without clinical or light microscopical evidence of hepatic involvement.

SEVERE

Jaundice is infrequent and often terminal. It is usually haemolytic with disseminated intravascular coagulation. Failure of renal bilirubin excretion may contribute.

Severe toxaemia may present with epigastric pain, nausea, vomiting, right upper quadrant tenderness and hypertension. The whole picture can develop in the absence of hypertension and proteinuria [1].

Hepatic histology. The peri-portal fibrin deposits and haemorrhage progress to small necrotic foci, infarcts and haematomas. Centrizonal necrosis and haemorrhage represent shock. An inflammatory reaction is characteristically absent (fig. 25.3).

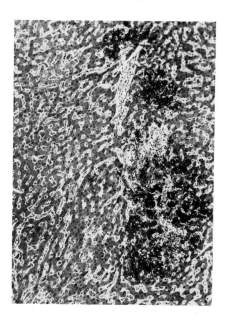

Fig. 25.3. The liver in eclampsia. Focal periportal necrosis of liver cells; the lesion contains fibrin. (Stained Mallory's phosphotungstic acid, ×80.)

Rupture of the liver is associated with shock. *Ultrasound* and *CT* show focal filling defects.

The *HELLP syndrome* of haemolysis, elevated liver enzymes and low platelets is a variant occurring in patients with severe hypertension [39].

Pregnancy toxaemia and acute fatty liver. There is considerable overlap between the two conditions (table 25.4). Patients with acute fatty liver have a 40% chance of showing some features of pregnancy toxaemia, such as hypertension and proteinuria and even some perisinusoidal fibrin deposition. Less often, the patient with clear pregnancy toxaemia lacks proteinuria and hypertension, yet the liver biopsy in addition to fibrin deposition shows some microvesicular fat. The aetiology of both these rare conditions is unclear and clarification of the overlap awaits their identification.

Cholestasis of pregnancy

This type of intra-hepatic cholestasis appears in the last trimester of pregnancy [7, 24].

In its mildest form, jaundice is absent and pruritus is the only abnormality. In many patients it accounts for generalized itching in the last weeks of pregnancy. Pruritus usually commences in the last trimester, but can start as early as the second or third month. Jaundice is rarely deep. The urine is dark and the stools pale. General health is preserved and there is no pain. The liver and spleen are impalpable. After delivery, jaundice disappears and within 1−2 weeks the pruritus has ceased. The condition recurs with subsequent pregnancies. Consecutive pregnancies in multiparous patients are associated with variability in the severity and in the time of onset [22].

LABORATORY CHANGES

Serum shows an increase in conjugated bilirubin and alkaline phosphatase values. Serum transaminases are normal or slightly increased, although occasionally very high values are found. These changes return to normal after delivery. Increased serum bile acid levels are common in pregnant women, particularly in those of Mediterranean or Asian origin [18]. They predict pruritus in pregnancy.

Steatorrhoea is usual. It correlates with the severity of the cholestasis [28].

The prothrombin time is prolonged due to vitamin K deficiency. Cholestyramine enhances the hypoprothrombinaemia.

Hepatic histology, obtained by needle biopsy, shows mild focal and irregular cholestasis. Electron microscopy shows the changes in the microvilli of the bile canaliculi common to all forms of cholestasis.

AETIOLOGY

The biliary excretion of oestriol and oestrogenic compounds is reduced. It is, however, uncertain whether these changes are causal or secondary to cholestasis. The finding of abnormal steroids in plasma may reflect the increased concentration of total neutral steroids. None of these compounds selectively alters bile canalicular membranes or other hepatocyte subcellular structures in man.

Over-production of oestrogens may reduce

Table 25.4. Acute fatty liver of pregnancy and toxaemias contrasted: overlaps exist

	Acute fatty liver	Toxaemia
Abdominal pain	50%	100%
Jaundice	100%	40%
Serum transaminases (× normal)	<10	>10
Scans	Diffuse change	Focal abnormalities
Liver biopsy	Microvesicular fat	Fibrin (perisinusoidal)
Liver failure	Present	Absent

bile flow in normal pregnancy. However, there is no evidence that any specific oestrogenic steroid or oestrogen metabolite is responsible for the cholestasis. Any changes in progesterone conjugation and metabolism are probably secondary to cholestasis.

Occasionally, rises in serum bile acids seem to precede those in bilirubin and alkaline phosphatase. Again the changes seem to be secondary to cholestasis and not causative.

EPIDEMIOLOGY

Cholestasis of pregnancy is often familial, and has been reported in mothers, sisters and daughters, some of whom develop pruritus when given oral contraceptives [10, 25]. Male family members may show the cholestatic tendency when given oestrogens [26]. Findings support a Mendelian dominant inheritance.

The condition is particularly common in Scandinavia, Northern Europe generally and in Chile. It does not seem to affect Asiatic or black women [24]. Prevalence varies widely and figures from 1 in 750 to 1 in 7000 pregnancies have been quoted.

In Chile, cholestasis seems to be associated with Araucanial Indian descent, rather than with Chilean Caucasoids. The histocompatibility antigen HLA-BW 16 seems to be more frequent than in control women [27]. This histocompatibility antigen may be a genetic characteristic common to some Aboriginal populations in North and South America.

The aetiology of cholestasis of pregnancy remains unknown.

DIAGNOSIS

In the first pregnancy, the diagnosis from viral hepatitis and other conditions causing jaundice may be difficult. Absence of constitutional symptoms, prominent pruritus and biochemical tests suggesting cholestasis are helpful. Tests for acute hepatitis A and B are negative. Ultrasound helps to exclude such conditions as obstruction to main bile ducts by tumour or gallstones. Liver biopsy is rarely necessary, but

the appearances are diagnostic. Failure of the pruritus to stop after delivery with continuing high serum alkaline phosphatase values suggest underlying primary biliary cirrhosis and liver biopsy and serum mitochondrial antibody tests should be performed. After delivery, the woman may show a cholestatic response to small doses of oestrogens [10].

PROGNOSIS AND MANAGEMENT

The condition is benign and prognosis for mother and baby is excellent. However, there is an increased incidence of prematurity, fetal distress and stillbirths [23, 36]; perhaps related to bile salts crossing the placenta [36]. Postpartum haemorrhage is also increased, probably related to vitamin K deficiency. There seems to be no long-term sequelae for the mother apart, perhaps, from an increased incidence of gallbladder disease. The condition will almost certainly return in subsequent pregnancies.

Management includes cholestyramine for relief of pruritus and intramuscular vitamin K_1 to control hypoprothrombinaemia. The mother requires careful nutritional support. Termination is indicated only for fetal distress. The mother is warned that the condition will almost certainly return in a subsequent pregnancy and that she may develop pruritus if she takes oral contraceptive drugs.

Viral hepatitis

This is the commonest cause of jaundice in pregnant women. They are not more susceptible to hepatitis and the incidence in epidemics is usually the same in the pregnant and non-pregnant. It is equal in all trimesters. Clinical course, biochemical tests and hepatic histology tend to be the same as the disease in the general population.

In general, disease is managed in a similar fashion in the pregnant and non-pregnant. The course of severe hepatitis is not influenced by termination of pregnancy and this should be avoided because it adds the strain of operation to an already failing liver.

Pregnant women who are exposed to hepatitis A must be given immunoglobulin prophylaxis.

All pregnant women, not only those in high risk groups, should be screened for hepatitis B (Chapter 16) [12, 15].

In certain countries, particularly India, Pakistan and the Middle East, acute epidemic non-A, non-B hepatitis often becomes fulminant and fatal in pregnant women (14).

Maternal neonatal transmission is recorded in infants born to women with acute non-A, non-B hepatitis during the third trimester of pregnancy. Virus hepatitis in the mother is said to induce abortion or premature delivery—fetal survival depending on the stage of maturity at birth and not on the mother's disease [7, 36]. Others have observed no increase in fetal wastage.

Fulminant *herpes simplex* can affect the pregnant woman, the picture resembling acute fatty liver of pregnancy.

Gallstones

At all ages, gallstones are more frequent in women than men, and especially so below the age of 50. Gallstones are also associated with obesity and parity, but not with number of pregnancies. Oestrogens have a mildly cholestatic effect with reduction of hepatic bile acid secretion and the production of more lithogenic bile. The gallbladder empties incompletely in late pregnancy leaving a large, residual volume which may cause retention of cholesterol crystals. Sludge develops in the gallbladder, but usually disappears within a week of delivery [20]. All these factors explain the association of gallstones with pregnancy. Stones in the common bile duct may coincide with pregnancy and cause jaundice, although the association is surprisingly rare.

The clinical picture of gallstones in pregnancy does not differ from that in the non-pregnant and the management should be the same. Ultrasound is useful for diagnosis [9].

Hepato-toxic drugs and the pregnant woman

The pregnant woman can react to drugs causing jaundice in a similar fashion to the non-pregnant. Sensitivity to chlorpromazine with consequent cholestatic jaundice is infrequent. When it does affect the pregnant, however, it may be particularly prolonged.

The effect of drugs in potentiation of jaundice or kernicterus in the newborn must be considered. In particular, drugs such as sulphonamides which displace bilirubin from its binding site to serum albumin should be avoided. Drugs such as phenacetin given to the mother may precipitate jaundice in an infant with glucose-6-phosphate dehydrogenase deficiency.

Effect of pregnancy on pre-existing chronic liver disease

The full-time parturition of a woman suffering from hepatic cirrhosis is unusual. It is rare for such a patient to conceive. The liver disease *per se* is not an indication for termination. Patients with chronic active hepatitis (autoimmune 'lupoid' hepatitis) are younger, often physically attractive women. Amenorrhoea is usual at the onset but, as the disease becomes less active with corticosteroid therapy, menses return and they may become pregnant. Liver function may deteriorate during pregnancy, but after delivery soon returns to its previous level. The fetal loss rate is about 33% and babies may be born prematurely, but will be normal [36]. The coincidence of liver disease with pregnancy should not *per se* indicate termination. Special care should be taken during the pregnancy. Corticosteroids must be continued. Management in a specialist obstetric unit with hepatological back-up is essential.

Bleeding from oesophageal varices is a risk in those with portal hypertension, whether due to cirrhosis or a portal vein obstruction. Patients who have previously bled are particularly at risk. It is treated along similar lines to those adopted in the non-pregnant.

Pregnancy is not contraindicated in those with well-treated Wilson's disease, and penicillamine does not pose an undue risk to the fetus [38].

Primary biliary cirrhosis may present as cholestatic jaundice in, or shortly after, pregnancy.

Successful pregnancy has been reported in a patient with Alagille's syndrome [33].

References

1 Aarnoudse JG, Houthoff HJ, Weits J et al. A syndrome of liver damage and intravascular coagulation in the last trimester of normotensive pregnancy. A clinical and histopathological study. Br. J. Obstet. Gynaecol. 1986; **93;** 145.

2 Bernuau J, Degott C, Nouel O et al. Non-fatal acute fatty liver of pregnancy. Gut 1983; **24;** 340.

3 Britton RC. Pregnancy and esophageal varices. Am. J. Surg. 1982; **143:** 421.

4 Burroughs AK, Seong NH, Dojcinov DM et al. Idiopathic acute fatty liver of pregnancy in 12 patients. Q. J. Med. 1982; **51:** 481.

5 Campillo B, Bernuau J, Witz M-O et al. Ultrasonography in acute fatty liver of pregnancy. Ann. intern. Med. 1986; **105:** 383.

6 Combes B, Shibata H, Adams R et al. Alterations in sulfobromophthalein sodium-removal mechanisms from blood during normal pregnancy. J. clin. Invest. 1963; **42;** 1431.

7 Haemmerli UP. Jaundice during pregnancy with special emphasis on recurrent jaundice during pregnancy and its differential diagnosis. Acta med. Scand. 1966; **179** (suppl): 444.

8 Henny CP, Lim AE, Brummelkamp WH et al. A review of the importance of acute multidisciplinary treatment following spontaneous rupture of the liver capsule during pregnancy. Surg. Gynecol. Obstet. 1983; **156;** 593.

9 Hiatt JR, Hiatt JCG, Williams RA et al. Biliary disease in pregnancy: strategy for surgical management. Am. J. Surg. 1986; **151:** 263.

10 Holzbach RT, Sivak DA, Braun WE. Familial recurrent intrahepatic cholestasis of pregnancy: a genetic study providing evidence for transmission of a sex-limited, dominant trait. Gastroenterology 1983; **85:** 175.

11 Ingerslev M, Teilum G. Jaundice during pregnancy. Acta Obstet. Gynecol. Scand. 1951; **31:** 74.

12 Jonas MM, Schiff ER, O'Sullivan MJ et al. Failure of centers for disease control criteria to identify hepatitis B infection in a large municipal obstetrical population. Ann. intern. Med. 1987; **107:** 335.

13 Kaplan MM. Current concepts. Acute fatty liver of pregnancy. N. Engl. J. Med. 1985; **313:** 367.

14 Khuroo MS, Teli MR, Skidmore S et al. Incidence and severity of viral hepatitis in pregnancy. Am J. Med. 1981; **70:** 252.

15 Kumar ML, Dawson NV, McCullough AJ et al. Should all pregnant women be screened for hepatitis B? Ann. intern. Med. 1987; **107:** 273.

16 Larrey D, Rueff B, Feldmann G et al. Recurrent jaundice caused by recurrent hyperemesis gravidarum. Case report. Gut 1984; **25:** 1414.

17 Loevinger EH, Vujic I, Lee WM et al. Hepatic rupture associated with pregnancy: treatment with transcatheter embolotherapy. Obstet. Gynecol. 1985; 65: 281.

18 Lunzer M, Barnes P, Byth K et al. Serum bile acid concentrations during pregnancy and their relationship to obstetric cholestasis. Gastroenterology 1986; **91:** 825.

19 Manas KJ, Welsh JD, Rankin RA et al. Hepatic hemorrhage without rupture in preeclampsia. N. Engl. J. Med. 1985; **312:** 424.

20 Maringhini A, Marceno MP, Lanzarone F et al. Sludge and stones in gall bladder after pregnancy. Prevalence and risk factors. J. Hepatol. 1987; **5:** 218.

21 McKee CM, Weir PE, Foster JH et al. Acute fatty liver of pregnancy and diagnosis by computed tomography. Br. med. J. 1986; **292:** 291.

22 Munnell EW, Taylor HC Jr. Liver blood flow in pregnancy—hepatic vein catheterization. J. clin. Invest. 1947; **26:** 952.

23 Reid R, Ivey KJ, Recoret RH. Fetal complications of obstetric cholestasis. Br. med. J. 1976; **i:** 870.

24 Reyes H. The enigma of intrahepatic cholestasis of pregnancy: lessons from Chile. Hepatology 1982; **2:** 87.

25 Reyes H, Ribalta J, Gonzáles-Cerón M. Idiopathic cholestasis of pregnancy in a large kindred. Gut 1976; **17:** 709.

26 Reyes H, Ribalta J, Gonzáles MC et al. Sulfobromophthalein clearance tests before and after ethinyl estradiol administration, in women and men with familial history of intrahepatic cholestasis of pregnancy. Gastroenterology 1981; **81:** 226.

27 Reyes H, Wegmann ME, Segovia N et al. HLA in Chileans with intrahepatic cholestasis of pregnancy. Hepatology 1982; **2:** 463.

28 Reyes H, Radrigan ME, Gonzalez MC et al. Steatorrhea in patients with intrahepatic cholestasis of pregnancy. Gastroenterology 1987; **93:** 584.

29 Riely CA, Romero R, Duffy TP. Hepatic dysfunction with disseminated intravascular coagulation in toxaemia of pregnancy: a distinct clinical syndrome. Gastroenterology 1981: **80;** 1346.

30 Riely CA, Latham PS, Romero R et al. Acute fatty liver of pregnancy. A reassessment based on ob-

servations in nine patients. *Ann. intern. Med.* 1987; **106:** 703.

31 Rolfes DB, Ishak KG. Liver disease in toxemia of pregnancy. *Am. J. Gastroenterol.* 1986; **81:** 1138.

32 Rolfes DB, Ishak KG. Acute fatty liver of pregnancy: a clinicopathologic study of 35 cases. *Hepatology* 1985; **5:** 1149.

33 Romero R, Reece EA, Riely C *et al.* Arteriohepatic dysplasia in pregnancy. *Am. J. Obstet. Gynecol.* 1983; **147:** 108.

34 Sheehan HL. The pathology of acute yellow atrophy and delayed chloroform poisoning. *J. Obstet. Gynaecol. Br. Emp.* 1940; **47:** 49.:

35 Sherlock S. Acute fatty liver of pregnancy and the microvesicular fat diseases. *Gut* 1983; **24:** 265.

36 Steven MM. Pregnancy and liver disease. *Gut* 1981; **22:** 592.

37 Steven MM, Buckley JD, Mackay IR. Pregnancy in chronic active hepatitis. *Q. J. Med.* 1979; **48:** 519.

38 Walshe JM. Pregnancy in Wilson's disease. *Q. J. Med.* 1977; **46:** 73.

39 Weinstein L. Syndrome of hemolysis, elevated liver enzymes, and low platelet count: a severe consequence of hypertension in pregnancy. *Am. J. Obstet. Gynecol.* 1982; **142:** 159.

40 Whelton MJ, Sherlock S. Pregnancy in patients with hepatic cirrhosis. Management and outcome. *Lancet* 1968; **ii:** 995.

26 · The Liver in Systemic Disease; Hepatic Trauma

The liver in the collagen diseases

The liver has no significant role in aetiology. If hepatomegaly is present, it is probably due to amyloidosis in chronic rheumatoid arthritis, or to cardiac failure with rheumatic fever or systemic lupus erythematosus. Splenomegaly reflects reticulo-endothelial hyperplasia rather than portal hypertension.

Primary biliary cirrhosis is associated with collagen diseases.

BIOCHEMISTRY

Serum α- and β-globulins may be elevated and serum albumin values slightly depressed. Serum, bilirubin, transaminase and alkaline phosphatase levels are normal or mildly disturbed.

DISEASES

Polyarteritis nodosa. The hepatic arterioles may show characteristic lesions with, occasionally, small hepatic infarcts [15]. Hepatic arteriography may be useful in diagnosis. Hepatic arterial aneurysms are sometimes found. Nodular regenerative hyperplasia may be a complication [9].

Hepatitis B carriage may be associated with polyarteritis nodosa [2], with migrating arthralgias or with polymyositis [7]. Immune complexes containing HBsAg can be shown in the tissues.

Giant cell arteritis can be found with granulomatous liver disease [5] and with hepatic arteritis [10].

Polymyalgia rheumatica. Changes include granulomatous hepatitis and lymphocytic infiltration [6]. These usually remit with corticosteroid treatment.

Rheumatoid arthritis. The liver shows nonspecific changes, such as mild fatty infiltration, focal necroses or complicating amyloidosis. Kupffer cells are hyperplastic. The serum alkaline phosphatase increase is of hepatic origin.

Still's disease. Patients may show mild chronic hepatitis with portal bridging [13].

Felty's syndrome. Lymphocytic infiltration of the sinusoids with nodular regenerative hyperplasia of normal-appearing liver cells may lead to portal hypertension and variceal bleeding [14].

Cryoglobulinaemia and vasculitis. Hepatomegaly and increased hepatic enzymes are found in patients with essential mixed cryoglobulinaemia. Histology varies from mild non-specific changes to chronic active hepatitis and cirrhosis. Some, but not all, patients have serological evidence of hepatitis B infection [1]. Mixed cryoglobulinaemia is also a feature of primary liver disease such as acute and chronic hepatitis and primary biliary cirrhosis. It is difficult to know which is the cart and which is the horse.

Weber—Christian disease (relapsing febrile nodular non-suppurative panniculitis). Severe fatty change may be seen with Mallory's hyaline. These changes are related to reduced lipoprotein synthesis in the deformed rough endoplasmic reticulum [3].

SYSTEMIC LUPUS ERYTHEMATOSUS (SLE)

Subclinical liver disease, as measured by liver enzyme increases, is seen in about a quarter, but in only 8% are these unexplained, and possibly related to SLE itself [8]. Liver biopsy shows no serious lesions, and only rarely has chronic hepatitis been described [12].

Autoimmune 'lupoid' hepatitis is not a subset of SLE but belongs in the spectrum of chronic active hepatitis [15].

The lupus anticoagulant may lead to hepatic vein thrombosis [11].

Rarely a severe hepatic arteritis is present. Rupture of the liver has been reported [4].

Jaundice with SLE is usually haemolytic.

References

1 Case Records of the Massachusetts General Hospital (case 40—1984) *N. Engl. J. Med.* 1984; **311:** 904.

2 Druëke T, Barbanel C, Jungers P *et al.* Hepatitis B antigen-associated periarteritis nodosa in patients undergoing long-term hemodialysis. *Am. J. Med.* 1980; **68:** 86.

3 Kimura H, Kako M, Yo K *et al.* Alcoholic hyalins (Mallory bodies) in a case of Weber—Christian disease: electron microscopic observations of liver involvement. *Gastroenterology* 1980, **78:** 807.

4 Levitin PM, Sweet D, Brunner CM *et al.* Spontaneous rupture of the liver; an unusual complication of SLE. *Arthritis Rheum.* 1977; **20:** 748.

5 Litwack KD, Bohan A, Silverman L. Granulomatous liver disease and giant cell arteritis: case report and literature review. *J. Rheumatol.* 1977; **4:** 307.

6 Long R, James O. Polymyalgia rheumatica and liver disease. *Lancet* 1974; **i:** 77.

7 Mihas AA, Kirby D, Kents P. Hepatitis B antigen and polymyositis. *J. Am. med. Assoc.* 1978; **239:** 221.

8 Miller MH, Urowitz MB, Gladman DD *et al.* The liver in systemic lupus erythematous. *Q. J. Med.* 1984; **53:** 401.

9 Nakanuma Y, Ohta G, Sasaki K. Nodular regenerative hyperplasia of the liver associated with polyarteritis nodosa. *Arch. path. lab. Med.* 1984; **108:** 133.

10 Ogilvie AL, James PD, Toghill PJ. Hepatic artery involvement in polymyalgia arteritica. *J. clin. Pathol.* 1981; **34:** 769.

11 Pomeroy C, Knodell RG, Swaim WR *et al.* Budd—Chiari syndrome in a patient with the lupus anticoagulant. *Gastroenterology* 1984; **86:** 158.

12 Runyon BA, La Brecque DR, Anuras S. The spectrum of liver disease in systemic lupus erythematosus. *Am. J. Med.* 1980; **69:** 187.

13 Tesser JRP, Pisko EJ, Hartz JW *et al.* Chronic liver disease and Still's disease. *Arth. Rheumat.* 1982; **25:** 579.

14 Thorne C, Urowitz MB. Wanless I *et al.* Liver disease in Felty's syndrome. *Am. J. Med.* 1982; **73:** 35.

15 Weinblatt ME. Teser JRP, Gilliam JH, III. The liver in rheumatic diseases. *Semin. Arth. Rheum.* 1982; **11:** 399.

Liver changes in organ transplant recipients

Virus hepatitis. There is an increased prevalence of persistent carriage of hepatitis B in patients on long-term haemodialysis for end-stage kidney disease, and in those having renal transplants. Immunosuppression facilitates the viraemia [5].

Other types of virus hepatitis, such as non-A, non-B, herpes and cytomegala are also frequent in these patients (see Chapter 16).

Vascular changes. These are probably related to prolonged administration of such drugs as 6-mercaptopurine or azathioprine. They include idiopathic portal hypertension due to perisinusoidal fibrosis [3] and veno-occlusive disease. Peliosis hepatis is associated with subendothelial thickening at the junction of the sinusoid and centrizonal vein [2].

Cholestasis is also related to azathioprine therapy.

Nodular transformation of normal hepatocytes may be shown by reticulin stains of a liver biopsy; it is of unknown aetiology.

Hepatic changes after bone-marrow transplantation. A graft-versus-host reaction may involve skin, gut and liver [4]. Veno-occlusion can also be seen (see also Chapters 4 and 35) [1, 6].

References

1 Berk PD, Popper H, Krueger GRF *et al.* Veno-occlusive disease of the liver after allogeneic bone marrow transplantation. *Ann. intern. Med.* 1979; **90:** 158.

2 Degott C, Rueff B, Kreis H *et al.* Peliosis hepatis in recipients of renal transplants. *Gut* 1978; **19:** 748.

3 Nataf C, Feldmann G, Lebrec D *et al.* Idiopathic portal hypertension (perisinusoidal fibrosis) after renal transplantation. *Gut* 1979; **20:** 531.

4 Shulman HM, Sullivan KM, Weiden PL *et al.* Chronic graft-versus-host syndrome in man. A long-term clinicopathologic study of 20 Seattle patients. *Am. J. Med.* 1980; **69:** 204.

5 Ware AJ, Luby JP, Hollinger B *et al.* Etiology of

liver disease in renal-transplant patients. *Ann. intern. Med.* 1979; **91**: 364.

6 Woods WG, Dehner LP, Nesbit ME *et al.* Fatal veno-occlusive disease of the liver following high dose chemotherapy, irradiation and bone marrow transplantation. *Am. J. Med.* 1980; **68**: 285.

Hepatic granulomas

Hepatic granulomatous lesions, having a common histological pattern but sometimes differing in detail are found in a number of diseases (table 26.1). The lesions are reticulo-endothelial in origin. Although seen anywhere in the liver they are most frequent near the portal tracts. They are sharply defined and do not disturb the normal pattern of the liver. They consist basically of pale-staining, epithelioid cells with surrounding lymphocytes (fig. 26.1). Giant cells, central caseation and necrosis may be present. Older lesions may be surrounded by a fibrous capsule, and healing is accompanied by hyaline change (figs 26.2, 26.3). In general they reflect a disturbance of cellular immunity. They cause little hepatic functional disturbance.

The importance of granulomas is not in the hepatic functional disturbance they may cause, but as a means of diagnosing the causative condition. Hepatic biopsy can be used to obtain confirmation of the diagnosis. The percentage of granulomas obtained is surprisingly high considering the random scattering of lesions and the small size of the biopsy sample.

Aetiology

Hepatic granulomas are found in 4–10% of needle liver biopsy specimens. In 10% of these no cause is found even after noting specific histological characteristics, staining for possible causative organisms, and culture of the specimen [16]. The granulomas vary in size, between 50 and 300 µm. This must be related to that of an aspiration liver biopsy specimen having a width of 100 µm. Serial sections must therefore be cut and stained if granulomas are to be identified. Hepatic granulomas are always part of a generalized disease process.

They are associated with a multitude of diseases [7]. Sarcoidosis and tuberculosis account for 50–65% and others include brucellosis and other bacterial infections, histoplasmosis and other fungal infections, syphilis, leprosy, cytomegalovirus infection, infectious mononucleosis, schistosomiasis and other parasitic infestations. Other causes include berylliosis, lymphomas, intra-abdominal neoplasms, Crohn's disease and primary biliary cirrhosis.

Drug reactions may be granulomatous and causes include sulphonamides, allopurinol [21],

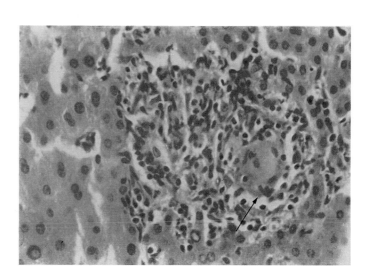

Fig. 26.1. A well-demarcated hepatic granuloma in a portal tract shows a giant cell, pale staining epithelioid cells and a rim of lymphocytes. (Stained H & E, ×160.)

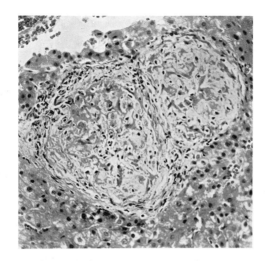

Fig. 26.2. Healing hepatic sarcoid. Two adjacent lesions are acquiring a structureless hyaline appearance and are surrounded by a connective tissue capsule. (Stained H & E, ×90.)

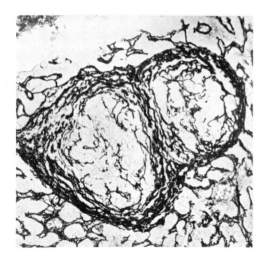

Fig. 26.3. Same section stained to show reticulin formation around the granulomas. (Stained modified silver, ×90.)

carbamazepine [9], quinine [6] and phenylbutazone [3]. They are frequent in sufferers from AIDS (table 26.2).

In some patients the granulomas may have been found by chance in a needle biopsy specimen. The interpretation is difficult. Many of these patients may, in fact, be suffering from sarcoidosis or tuberculosis with minimal clinical evidence. In these symptomless patients the granuloma must be ignored but the patient should be observed over the next year or so.

GRANULOMATOUS 'HEPATITIS'

Hepatic granulomas may be associated with a severe, prolonged, febrile syndrome [11, 18]. Some patients are eventually diagnosed as lymphoma, others defy diagnosis. The sufferer is often a middle-aged or elderly male. The granulomas are not widespread and pulmonary involvement is unusual. Biochemical tests of liver function are moderately impaired with increases in serum alkaline phosphatase, and slight increases in serum transaminases and globulins. Serum bilirubin is normal. A trial of antituberculous chemotherapy may be justified in these patients. Prednisone treatment may be beneficial but clearly this should not be given without the fullest possible investigation.

SARCOIDOSIS

Sarcoidosis is a disease of unknown aetiology, characterized by widespread granulomatous lesions involving most organs [4]. Involvement of lungs, lymph nodes, eyes, skin and of the neurological system may be associated with well recognized clinical features, although this is not always so.

The liver is frequently affected although granulomas are often asymptomatic [10]. Overt evidences of hepatic insufficiency are rare. The liver is palpable in only 20% of patients. Occasionally the picture is of active liver disease with marked hepatic functional abnormalities and liver cell destruction, and fibrosis on liver biopsy [10]. In general, however, the evidence of hepatic involvement arises not by the clinical picture but from the result of liver biopsy. This technique confirms sarcoidosis in about 60%. This agrees with autopsy figures showing hepatic involvement in about two-thirds.

Liver biopsy is indicated when another more accessible tissue, such as lymph gland or skin, is not available for biopsy [17].

Table 26.1. Differential diagnosis of some diseases with granulomas

Disease	Clinical accompaniments	Diagnostic aids
Sarcoidosis	Lung changes, uveitis, skin lesions, splenomegaly, lymphadenopathy	Chest X-ray. Kveim and tuberculin tests. Serum angiotensin converting enzyme
Tuberculosis	Pulmonary disease. Choroidal tubercles. Meningitis	Broncho-alveolar lavage Chest X-ray. Tuberculin test. Isolation of organism
Erythema nodosum	Sarcoidosis, primary tuberculosis, streptococcal infection, drug sensitivity	Chest X-ray. Kveim and tuberculin tests. Antistreptolysin titre
Brucellosis	Fever. Lassitude. Hepatosplenomegaly	Blood culture. Complement fixation test
Berylliosis	Industrial exposure. Loss of weight. Skin lesions	Chest X-ray. Urinary beryllium. Beryllium skin patch test
Syphilis	Skin lesions. Cerebral involvement	Treponema test
Leprosy	Skin and nerve lesions	Lepromin skin test
Histoplasmosis	Non-specific	Complement fixation test. Histoplasmin skin test. Chest X-ray
Ascariasis	Gastrointestinal and pulmonary symptoms	Faeces examination. Eosinophilia
Infectious mononucleosis	See Chapter 27	Blood film. Monospot, IgM EB antibodies
Tularaemia	Septicaemic and pulmonary features	Complement fixation test. Isolation of causal organism
Lymphoma	Pyrexia, weight loss, splenomegaly, lymphadenopathy	Chest X-rays. Lymph node biopsy. CT scan
Primary biliary cirrhosis	See Chapter 18	Mitochondrial antibodies
Hypogamma-globulinaemia	Recurrent bacterial infections	Serum immunoglobulins
Granulomatous disease of childhood	Skin granulomas. Recurrent bacterial infections	Chest X-ray, nitroblue tetrazolium test

Hepatic histology

Rounded, well demarcated lesions can occur anywhere, but most often in the portal zones. The distinction is particularly striking in sections stained for glycogen, although the pallor makes them distinctive even in H & E-stained sections.

The granuloma (fig. 26.1) contains a central area of eosinophilic necrosis, often containing nuclear debris. There is no caseation. The delicate reticulin framework is maintained, whereas this is destroyed in tuberculous lesions. Surrounding are the clusters of basophilic epithelioid cells. Also conspicuous are giant cells in which the nuclei may be peripheral or scattered through the cell. The cytoplasm may be vacuolated, or may contain non-specific inclusions of various types. A thin,

Table 26.2. Hepatic granulomas in patients with AIDS

Infections
  Mycobacterium avium-intracellulare
  Mycobacterium tuberculosis
  Cytomegalovirus
  Histoplasmosis
  Toxoplasmosis
  Cryptococcosis

Neoplasms
  Hodgkin's and non-Hodgkin's lymphoma

Drugs
  Sulphonamides
  Antibiotics
  Anti-fungal
  Isoniazid
  Tranquillizers

peripheral ring of lymphocytes surrounds the lesion. Acid-fast bacilli are not seen.

Proliferation of Kupffer cells, even in areas remote from granulomas, demonstrates the wide-spread reticulo-endothelial activity.

Healing is by sclerosis. The granuloma is converted into an acellular mass of hyaline material with a fibrous capsule (figs 26.2, 26.3); many disappear.

Since the hepatic lesions are focal, and fibrosis is restricted to healing lesions, sarcoidosis does not produce the diffuse fibrosis and nodular regeneration of cirrhosis. It is, therefore, difficult to accept the occasional reports of cirrhosis following sarcoidosis, and a fortuitous combination seems more likely. The association with jaundice and hepatic failure is very rare and unexpected.

Corticosteroid therapy seems to have little effect on the liver biopsy appearances.

Biochemical changes

The reticulo-endothelial involvement causes a rise in serum IgG. The alkaline phosphatase may be slightly raised. Serum bilirubin level is normal. Serum angiotensin-converting enzyme is increased.

Portal hypertension

The patients are usually young, blacks of both sexes or females greater than 40. The portal hypertension is presinusoidal due to portal (zone 1) granulomas. Sinusoidal block may be superimposed due to fibrosis [19, 20]. Corticosteroids do not prevent the portal hypertension.

In some, thrombotic occlusion of a portal or splenic vein may be found. Rarely, oesophageal bleeding is a real problem. These patients tolerate surgical shunts well.

Budd−Chiari syndrome

Sarcoidosis has been reported in association with hepatic vein occlusion. The hepatic veins are narrowed by sarcoid granulomas leading to venous stasis and extensive thrombotic occlusions [15]. Similar Budd−Chiari syndrome has been caused by idiopathic granulomatous venulitis involving hepatic vein radicles [24].

Cholestasis

Rarely patients with sarcoidosis, usually male and black, show features of chronic cholestasis. This is presumably due to involvement of the bile ducts in the granulomatous tissue (fig. 26.4). The distinction from primary biliary cirrhosis can be difficult and sometimes impossible (see Chapter 14).

TUBERCULOSIS

Miliary dissemination accompanies the primary complex, and is also common with chronic adult tuberculosis. Aspiration liver biopsies in patients with tuberculosis have shown positive results in about 25%. In another series 24 of 30 patients with extrapulmonary tuberculosis showed granulomas by liver biopsy [8].

Aspiration biopsy has been used in the diagnosis of tuberculous meningitis when other methods have failed, and also in miliary tuberculosis at the stage of an indeterminate pyrexia. In such cases, Ziehl−Neelsen stains should be performed, and an unfixed portion

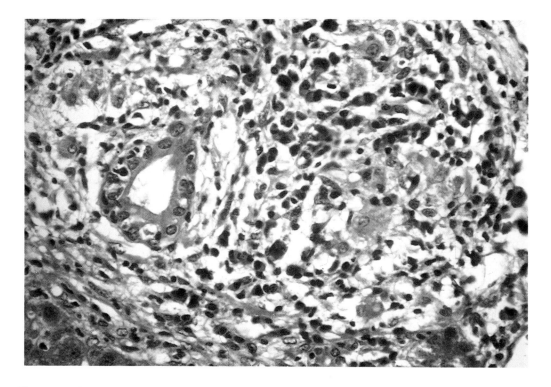

Fig. 26.4. Chronic cholestasis in sarcoidosis. A damaged bile duct is surrounded by an inflammatory infiltrate including lymphocytes. (Stained H & E, ×160).

of the biopsy cultured for tubercle bacilli.

The distinction between these granulomas and those of sarcoidosis may be impossible. Distinctive features of tuberculosis are the presence of acid-fast bacilli and caseation with destruction of the reticulin framework. There is irregularity of the contour with a particularly dense cuff of lymphocytes. Less numerous lesions with a tendency to coalesce also suggest tuberculosis.

Miliary granulomas are found after BCG vaccination, especially in the immuno-suppressed [2].

Granulomas containing *atypical mycobacteria*, usually *M. avian intracellulare*, may complicate AIDS (Chapter 27). Granulomas have also been related to the atypical mycobacterium, *Scrofulaceum patel.*

BRUCELLOSIS

Hepatic granulomas complicate *Br. abortus* infection. *Br. suis* is more invasive with hepatic suppuration sometimes followed by calcification in the liver and spleen.

Hepatic tenderness and mild elevations of transaminases and alkaline phosphatase may be found in the acute stage [1].

Hepatic histology usually shows a non-specific reactive hepatitis. Granulomas may be associated. These cannot be distinguished from those of sarcoidosis, although they tend to be smaller and less clearly demarcated (fig. 26.5). Healing results in scarring. Brucellosis leads to miliary granulomas and the subsequent healing is never diffuse enough to justify the term cirrhosis.

In *Br. melitensis* the picture may be of scattered inflammatory cells and necrotic hepato-

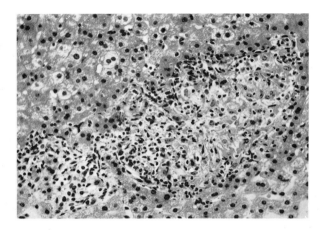

Fig. 26.5. Brucellosis. Granulomas in the liver. The smaller is little more than a collection of round cells. (Stained H & E, ×170.)

cytes without granulomas. *Br. suis* can lead to hepatic abscesses after years of dormancy [23].

A small portion of the unfixed biopsy specimen should be cultured and is occasionally positive for *Br. abortus* or *Br. melitensis*.

INDUSTRIAL CAUSES

Beryllium poisoning leads to pulmonary granulomas. Hepatic involvement consists of miliary granulomas, as in sarcoidosis. Aspiration liver biopsy material is, therefore, valueless in differential diagnosis.

Pulmonary and hepatic granulomas may be due to inhalation of *cement* and *mica dust* [14] and in vineyard sprayers to *copper* [13].

Lipogranulomas [22] may be found in a non-fatty liver. Perivenular clusters of lipid droplets are surrounded by a light infiltrate of lymphocytes and macrophages. These are due to deposition of mineral oils, widely used in the food industry.

OTHER CONDITIONS WITH HEPATIC GRANULOMAS

Similar granulomas are found in the liver of patients suffering from acquired secondary syphilis.

In lepromatous *leprosy*, hepatic granulomas indistinguishable from sarcoidosis may be found in 62% compared with the tuberculoid form when only 21% are positive [5]. Lepra bacilli are sometimes present [5].

Histoplasmosis. The liver is second only to the spleen in frequency of involvement. In the granulomatous form, the lesions are histologically identical with those of sarcoidosis, except for the presence of the intracellular fungus in the Kupffer cells. Liver biopsy can be used in the diagnosis of histoplasmosis. Sections should be stained for *Histoplasma capsulatum* and an unfixed portion of the biopsy should be cultured. Histoplasmosis leads to discrete hepatic calcification [12].

Coccidioidomycosis and *blastomycosis* also produce sarcoid-like hepatic granulomas and the organism may be demonstrated.

Q fever. Characteristic 'doughnut' granulomas are seen (see Chapter 27).

Hepatic granulomas can be due to migrating larvae of *Ascaris lumbricoides*. Hepatic granulomas may also be found in children suffering from *Toxocara canis*.

Acute *cytomegalovirus* infection produces a mononucleosis syndrome. Transient well-formed hepatic granulomas may be associated.

Hepatic granulomas may also be seen in *schistosomiasis*, but the presence of ova usually makes the diagnosis easy.

In the early stages of *primary biliary cirrhosis* the liver may show widespread hepatic granulomas. This histological picture may be indistinguishable from sarcoidosis.

Whipple's disease may be accompanied by hepatic granulomas, with bacillary inclusions negative for periodic acid Schiff stain after protein digestion.

NON-SPECIFIC RETICULO-ENDOTHELIAL PROLIFERATIONS 'REACTIVE HEPATITIS'

Focal accumulations of mononuclear and epithelioid cells are found in a great variety of diseases. They are perhaps most frequent in virus infections, including infectious mononucleosis, during the recovery phase of hepatitis, especially non-A, non-B, when they contain iron, and in influenza. Occasionally, they are noted in pyogenic infections and septicaemias where polymorphonuclear leucocytes are also present.

Their distinction from small sarcoid granulomas may be difficult, especially since they may also be seen in sarcoidosis. If such an accumulation of cells is found in a liver biopsy section, the whole block should be sectioned serially to identify typical granulomas.

Generalized proliferation of Kupffer cells is another frequent histological finding of doubtful diagnostic value. As well as occurring in primary reticulo-endothelial conditions, it occurs in infections and in malignant disease arising in any part of the body. Generalized Kupffer cell proliferation is also seen in a liver containing local lesions—such as malignant deposits or an amoebic abscess.

References

1 Cervantes F, Bruguera A, Carbonell J *et al.* Liver disease in brucellosis. A clinical and pathological study of 40 cases. *Postgrad. med. J.* 1982; **58:** 346.

2 Flipping T, Mukherji B, Dayal Y. Granulomatous hepatitis as a late complication of BCG immunotherapy. *Cancer* 1980; **46:** 1759.

3 Ishak KG, Kirchner JP, Dhar JK. Granulomas and cholestatic-hepatocellular injury associated with phenylbutazone: report of two cases. *Am. J. dig. Dis.* 1977; **22:** 611.

4 James DG, Jones Williams W. *Sarcoidosis and other granulomatous disorders.* WB Saunders, Philadelphia, 1985.

5 Karat ABA, Job CK, Rao PSS. Liver in leprosy: histological and biochemical findings. *Br. med. J.* 1971; **i:** 307.

6 Katz B, Weetch M, Chopra S. Quinine-induced granulomatous hepatitis. *Br. med. J.* 1983; **286:** 264.

7 Klatskin G. Hepatic granulomata: problems in interpretation. *Mount Sinai J. Med. (NY)* 1977; **44:** 798.

8 Korn RJ, Kellow WF, Heller P *et al.* Hepatic involvement in extrapulmonary tuberculosis. *Am. J. Med.* 1965; **27:** 60.

9 Levy M, Goodman MW, van Dyne BJ *et al.* Granulomatous hepatitis secondary to carbamazepine. *Ann. intern. Med.* 1981; **95:** 64.

10 Maddrey WC, Johns CJ, Boitnott JK *et al.* Sarcoidosis and chronic hepatic disease: a clinical and pathological study of 20 patients. *Medicine (Baltimore)* 1970; **49:** 375.

11 Neville E, Piyasena KHG, James DG. Granulomas of the liver. *Postgrad. med. J.* 1975; **51:** 361.

12 Okudaira M, Straub M, Schwarz J. The etiology of discrete splenic and hepatic calcifications in an endemic area of histoplasmosis. *Am. J. Pathol.* 1961; **39:** 599.

13 Pimentel JC, Menezes AP. Liver granulomas containing copper in vineyard sprayer's lung. *Ann. Rev. respir. Dis.* 1975; **111:** 189.

14 Pimentel JC, Menezes AP. Pulmonary and hepatic granulomatous disorders due to the inhalation of cement and mica dusts. *Thorax* 1978; **33:** 219.

15 Russe EW, Bansky G, Pfaltz M *et al.* Budd–Chiari syndrome in sarcoidosis. *Am. J. Gastroenterol.* 1986; **81:** 71.

16 Scheuer PJ. In *Liver Biopsy Interpretation.* 4th edn. 1988; Ballière Tindall, London, p. 223.

17 Scadding JG, Sherlock S. Liver biopsy in sarcoidosis. *Thorax* 1948; **3:** 79.

18 Simon HB, Wolff SM. Granulomatous hepatitis and prolonged fever of unknown origin: a study of 13 patients. *Medicine (Baltimore)* 1973; **52:** 1.

19 Tekeste H, Latour F, Levitt RE. Portal hypertension complicating sarcoid liver disease: case report and review of the literature. *Am. J. Gastroenterol.* 1984; **79:** 389.

20 Valla D, Pessegueiro-Miranda H, Degott C *et al.* Hepatic sarcoidosis with portal hypertension. A report of seven cases with a review of the literature. *Q. J. Med.* 1987; **63:** 531.

21 Vanderstigel M, Zafrani ES, Lejonc JL *et al.* Allopurinol hypersensitivity syndrome as a couse of hepatic fibrin-ring granulomas. *Gastroenterology* 1986; **9:** 188.

22 Wanless IR, Geddie WR. Mineral oil lipogranu-lomata in liver and spleen. *Path. lab. Med.* 1985; **109**: 283.

23 Williams RK, Crossley K. Acute and chronic hep-atic involvement of brucellosis. *Gastroenterology* 1982; **83**: 455.

24 Young ID, Clark RN, Manley PN *et al.* Response to steroids in Budd—Chiari syndrome caused by idiopathic granulomatous venulitis. *Gastroenter-ology* 1988; **94**: 503.

Hepato-biliary associations of inflammatory bowel disease

The liver is involved in many ways in the patient with ulcerative colitis and other forms of chronic intestinal disease such as Crohn's disease. In one large clinic over half the patients with ulcerative colitis showed liver function abnormalities. The surgeon sees acute fatty liver when operating on patients with fulmi-nant colitis, biliary strictures in those with sclerosing cholangitis, or gallstones in patients with ileal resection. In treating ulcerative colitis the physician sees chronic active (autoimmune) hepatitis or chronic cholestasis in those with pericholangitis and sclerosing cholangitis. The pathologist may encounter hepatic granulomas or amyloidosis in a liver biopsy from a patient with inflammatory bowel disease. Involvement of the liver in patients with malabsorption has been discussed in Chapter 23.

Sclerosing cholangitis (Chapter 15) [2, 6] pre-sents in many forms and is being increasingly diagnosed as more endoscopic and trans-hepatic cholangiograms are being done. *Gall-stones* are present in up to a third of patients with Crohn's disease of the terminal ileum [1].

Ulcerative colitis, rarely, has been compli-cated by the *Budd—Chiari syndrome* [3].

Fatty change

This is very frequent. As with other types of fatty infiltration, the incidence is higher when autopsy rather than biopsy material is used for diagnosis. It may be focal but usually starts in zone 1 and spreads to zone 3. Cirrhosis is not a sequel.

This change is related to the anorexia, anaemia, faecal protein loss and malnutrition of severe colitis.

Massive hepatic steatosis can complicate adult coeliac disease [8].

Carcinoma of the bile ducts (Chapter 34)

This has been reported in ulcerative colitis with or without accompanying biliary disease. The ulcerative colitis is usually of long stand-ing. The bile duct carcinoma develops inde-pendently of the extent and severity of the colitis. It may develop many years after procto-colectomy. It must be considered in any patient with ulcerative colitis developing deep, persist-ent cholestatic jaundice. Differentiation from sclerosing colitis is often impossible without surgical exploration.

PROGNOSIS

This is considerably better than originally thought. If the large duct obstruction can be relieved, liver cell function can be preserved and the patients may remain asymptomatic for periods of more than five years.

Chronic active hepatitis and cirrhosis

Five per cent of cirrhotic patients have ulcera-tive colitis, a greater incidence than in the general population. In some the cirrhosis is of chronic active autoimmune type. The colitis is then part of the general spectrum of this *multi-system disease*. In these patients, and in contrast to sclerosing cholangitis, the colitis tends to present with the cirrhosis and to be severe but often not subsequently relapsing. The recog-nition of the cirrhosis may precede the diar-rhoea.

In others the cirrhosis is inactive and is diagnosed after many years of chronic relapsing colitis. Initially the colitis is predominant and the cirrhosis mild but as the years pass the positions reverse.

The cirrhosis might be related to the long

course of the illness, many hospital attendances, injections, infusions, blood transfusions, all carrying the hazard of viral hepatitis. This cannot be the whole answer for the cirrhosis may precede the colitis.

The latter stages of pericholangitis and sclerosing cholangitis may be associated with piecemeal necrosis of liver cells and scar formation. This can proceed to a biliary cirrhosis. Severe bile duct lesions can exist without biochemical evidence of cholestasis [4]. Every patient with chronic liver disease and also ulcerative colitis should have percutaneous or endoscopic cholangiography performed to exclude primary sclerosing cholangitis. This is a much more common association than with autoimmune chronic active hepatitis.

Liver abscess

Patients with Crohn's disease may develop liver abscesses, usually multiple and with a predisposing abdominal focus of infection rather than a biliary one [5, 7]. Streptococci, especially *S. milleri*, are often responsible.

References

1 Baker AL, Kaplan MM, Norton RA et al. Gallstones in inflammatory bowel disease. Am. J. dig. Dis. 1974; 19: 109.
2 Chapman RW. Primary sclerosing cholangitis. J. Hepatol 1985; 1: 179.
3 Chesner IM, Muller S, Newman J. Ulcerative colitis complicated by Budd-Chiari syndrome. Gut 1986; 27: 1096.
4 Clements D, Rhodes JM, Elias E. Severe bile duct lesions without biochemical evidence of cholestasis in a case of sclerosing cholangitis. J. Hepatol 1986; 3: 72.
5 Greenstein AJ, Sachar DB, Lowenthal D et al. Pyogenic liver abscess in Crohn's disease. Q. J. Med. 1985; 56: 505.
6 La Russo NF, Wiesner RH, Ludwig J et al. Current concepts. Primary sclerosing cholangitis. N. Engl. J. Med. 1984; 310: 899.
7 Mir-Madjlessi SH, McHenry MC, Farmer RG. Liver abscess in Crohn's disease. Report of four cases and review of the literature. Gastroenterology 1986; 91: 987.
8 Naschitz JE, Yeshurun D, Zuckerman E et al. Massive hepatic steatosis complicating adult celiac disease: report of a case and review of the literature. Am. J, Gastroenterol. 1987; 82: 1186.

Hepatic trauma

CAUSES

Hepatic trauma is usually due to road traffic accidents, to penetrating wounds from stabbing or to gunshots. It may be a sequel of birth injury. Spontaneous rupture may occur in the last trimester of pregnancy, usually complicated by toxaemia.

Non-penetrating injury may be due to deceleration (leading to splits and tears from shearing) or to direct violence causing contusion or disruption of the liver substance. It may complicate cardio-pulmonary resuscitation [1].

Injury to the hepatic parenchyma is usually the main problem, and injuries to portal vein, hepatic artery, hepatic vein or retro-hepatic vena cava are rare [3].

DIAGNOSIS

This may be difficult as physical signs may be minimal. Pattern bruising of the abdominal wall indicates severe abdominal compression.

Diagnostic peritoneal aspiration can be misleading, ultrasonography and CT scanning are invaluable. CT may show laceration, subcapsular fluid (blood or bile) and fragmentation (fig. 26.6). Hepatic parenchymal gas may indicate infection but may also be seen simply after blunt trauma [7].

If CT shows minimal or absent haemoperitoneum and an intact or nearly intact hepatic capsule, surgical intervention will not be necessary [2]. There should, however, be no hesitation in performing laparotomy if serious liver trauma is suspected.

The possibility of other organs being damaged, such as spleen, intestines, lungs, kidneys, or the coincidence of head injuries and fractures, must be remembered.

Blunt abdominal trauma may lead to haemobilia, usually secondary to hepatic arterial aneurysm (see Chapter 11) [8]. Angiography is a necessary investigation.

In children, blunt abdominal trauma results in injury to the liver, usually the right lobe and frequently posteriorly [14]. Associated thoracic injuries are common.

MANAGEMENT

This is usually surgical. Transfusion facilities must be adequate.

At the time of emergency laparotomy definitive surgical treatment is often impossible. In such circumstances, haemorrhage in the damaged area may be controlled, and the patient transferred immediately to a specialized unit where definitive operative treatment can be carried out [11]. In general, packing is to be avoided as the mortality, particularly from abscess, increases [4].

Mild splits, lacerations and penetrating wounds can usually be managed by simple haemostasis and drainage.

Deeper lacerations with tearing of intrahepatic vessels and bile ducts are treated by ligating the bleeding vessels and repairing the liver with deep sutures.

Porta-hepatis injuries are rare and control of bleeding is of prime importance [10]. Bleeding is controlled by digital compression of the hepatic artery and portal vein in the lesser omentum. Selective hepatic arteriography is useful in defining treatment. Hepatic arterial embolectomy with gel foam must be considered (fig. 26.6) [6].

Repair of major venous injuries requires adequate exposure. The mid-line abdominal incision is extended, cephaled, and a median sternal split made. This allows control of the hepatic vein and any tear of the sub-diaphragmatic inferior vena cava. Repairs of the inferior vena cava or hepatic vein are sutured or side-clamped. Portal vein injuries are rare and have the worse prognosis. They are treated by suture, end-to-side anastomosis or, if necessary, acute portal vein ligation [4, 5].

In the majority of cases hepatic trauma can be managed by local pressure and aggressive debridement with hepatic segmentectomy, not necessarily following the anatomists' neat lines. With damaged liver exposed, ragged areas of questionable viability can be excised, local haemostasis obtained and efficient drainage established. Excellent results have been noted after resection of as much as 400 g of liver tissue. Hepatic resection and lobectomy

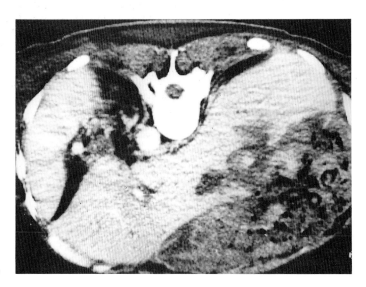

Fig. 26.6. CT (intravenous contrast enhanced) of a patient with a gun shot injury to the anterior part of the liver. A low attenution haematoma with disorganized liver tissue and gas indicates infection. Successful treatment was by drainage of pus debridement, with gel foam angiographic embolization of a feeding hepatic artery branch.

are required in only a small number of cases.

Repeated ultrasound examinations are important in following the patient [5].

Coagulopathy is a frequent and serious complication of severe liver trauma. Other post-operative problems include jaundice, infection of a haematoma and hypoproteinaemia. Abscess is a late and often fatal complication [9].

PROGNOSIS

The overall mortality is 10.5% with 78.1% of all deaths occurring in the peri-operative period from shock or transfusion-related coagulopathies [3].

The prognosis depends on the extent of the hepatic injury and the number of organs involved. Injuries to the hepatic veins, portal vein or retrohepatic inferior vena cava are highly lethal. Shotgun injuries are most serious, followed by blunt trauma, gunshot wounds and lastly stab wounds.

RUPTURE OF THE GALLBLADDER

Rupture or contusion of the gallbladder can follow blunt abdominal trauma [12]. It is rare because the gallbladder is cushioned by surrounding bony and visceral structures. The gallbladder is usually distended at the time of rupture. Early diagnosis is difficult. The condition is recognized by fever, jaundice, increasing distension and ascites. Paracentesis shows bile-stained fluid. Later, encysted bile accumulations are recognized by ultrasound and CT scanning [13]. The perforation is confirmed by percutaneous or endoscopic cholangiography. HIDA scanning may be useful.

Treatment is by cholecystectomy.

References

1 Adler SN, Klein RA, Pellechia C et al. Massive hepatic hemorrhage associated with cardiopulmonary resuscitation. Arch. intern. Med. 1983; 143: 813.

2 Federle MP. CT of upper abdominal trauma. Semin. Roentgenol. 1984; 19: 269.

3 Feliciano DV, Jordan GL Jr, Bitondo CG et al. Management of 1000 consecutive cases of hepatic trauma (1979–1984). Ann. Surg. 1986; 204: 438.

4 Ivatury RR, Nallathambi M, Gunduz Y et al. Liver packing for uncontrolled haemorrhage: a reappraisal. J. Trauma 1986; 26: 744.

5 Ivatury RR, Nallathambi M, Lankin DH et al. Portal vein injuries. Noninvasive follow-up of venorrhaphy. Ann. Surg. 1987; 206: 733.

6 Jander JP, Laws JL, Kogutt MS et al. Emergency embolization in blunt hepatic trauma. Am. J. Roentgenol. 1977; 129: 249.

7 Panicek DM, Paquet DJ, Clark KG et al. Hepatic parenchymal gas after blunt trauma. Radiology 1986; 159: 343.

8 Sax SL, Athey PA, Lamki N et al. Sonographic findings in traumatic hemobilia: report of two cases and review of the literature. J. clin. Ultrasound 1988; 16: 29.

9 Scott CM, Grasberger RC, Heeran TF. Intraabdominal sepsis after hepatic trauma. Am. J. Surg. 1988; 155: 284.

10 Sheldon GF, Lim RC, Yee ES et al. Management of injuries to the porta hepatis. Ann. Surg. 1985; 202: 539.

11 Smadja C, Traynor O, Lumgart LH. Delayed hepatic resection for major liver injury. Brit. J. Surg. 1982; 69: 361.

12 Soderstrom CA, Maekawa K, Du Priest RW Jr et al. Gall bladder injuries resulting from blunt abdominal trauma. Ann. Surg. 1981; 193: 60.

13 Spigos DG, Tan WS, Larson G et al. Diagnosis of traumatic rupture of the gall bladder. Am. J. Surg. 1981; 141: 731.

14 Stalker HP, Kaufman RA, Towbin R. Patterns of liver injury in childhood: CT analysis. Am. J. Roentgenol. 1986; 147: 1199.

27 · The Liver in Infections

Pyogenic liver abscess

Pyogenic liver abscess used to be due to portal infection, often in young people secondary to acute appendicitis. This is less frequent, because of earlier diagnosis and treatment. Abscesses secondary to obstruction and infection of the biliary tree, and affecting an older age group, have, however, continued to increase. Immunosuppression as in AIDS, intensive chemotherapy or transplant recipients [3, 11] is increasing the number of liver abscesses due to opportunist organisms.

Earlier diagnosis has followed increased use of scanning and cholangiographic techniques. Failures are usually due to the clinician not considering the diagnosis.

Classification

Portal pyaemia

Pelvic or gastrointestinal infection may result in portal pylephlebitis or in septic emboli. This may follow appendicitis, empyema of the gall-bladder, diverticulitis, regional enteritis [12], *Yersinia* ileitis [4], perforated gastric or colonic ulcers, leaking anastomoses, pancreatitis or infected haemorrhoids.

Neonatal umbilical vein sepsis may spread to the portal vein with subsequent hepatic abscesses.

Biliary

The biliary tree is the commonest source of infection. Septic cholangitis can complicate any form of biliary obstruction, especially if partial. The abscesses are commonly multiple. Causes include gallstones, cancer, sclerosing cholangitis, congenital biliary anomalies (especially Caroli's disease), biliary strictures [6, 14] and the sump syndrome following side-to-side choledochoduodenostomy [15].

Direct infection

Solitary liver abscess may follow a penetrating wound or direct spread from an adjacent septic focus such as a perinephric abscess. It may follow a secondary infection of an amoebic abscess, metastasis, cyst or intra-hepatic haematoma. Automobile accidents or other blunt trauma may lead to hepatic abscess formation [8].

Miscellaneous

Iatrogenic causes include liver biopsy, percutaneous biliary drainage or hepatic artery injury or perfusion.

Cryptogenic

In about one-half, there is no obvious predisposing cause. This is especially so in the elderly.

BACTERIOLOGY

The commonest infecting organisms are Gram-negative. *E. coli* is found in two-thirds. *Str. faecalis* and *Pr. vulgaris* are also frequent. Recurrent pyogenic cholangitis may be due to *Salmonella typhi*.

Anaerobic organisms have become increasingly important, and include bacteroides, aerobacteria, actinomyces and anaerobic and micro-aerophilic streptococci. This emphasizes the need to culture all possibly infective material, including blood, pus, bile and swabs, under strictly anaerobic as well as aerobic conditions.

Streptococcus milleri Lancefield group F, which is neither a true anaerobe nor a micro-aerobe, is a very common causative organism [7, 13].

Staphylococci are found in nearly a half, especially in those who have received chemotherapy, when they are usually resistant. Friedländer's bacillus, pseudomonas and *Cl. welchii* may also be found.

Rare causes include *yersiniosis* [4], *septicaemic melioidosis* and *Pasteurella multocida* [5].

Infection is often multiple.

The abscess may be sterile, but this is usually due to lack of adequate, particularly anaerobic, culture techniques or to previous antibiotics.

PATHOLOGY

The enlarged liver may contain multiple yellow abscesses, 1 cm in diameter, or a single abscess encased in fibrous tissue.

When there is an associated pylephlebitis, the portal vein and its branches may contain pus and blood clots. The abscesses are particularly in the right lobe. There may be peri-hepatitis or even adhesion formation.

In bacteroides infections, the pus has a foul odour and the abscess wall is ill defined.

When infection is spread by the bile ducts, multiple foci correspond to the bile duct system.

A chronic solitary liver abscess may persist for as long as two years before death or diagnosis.

There may be small pyaemic abscesses elsewhere, such as lungs, kidneys, brain and

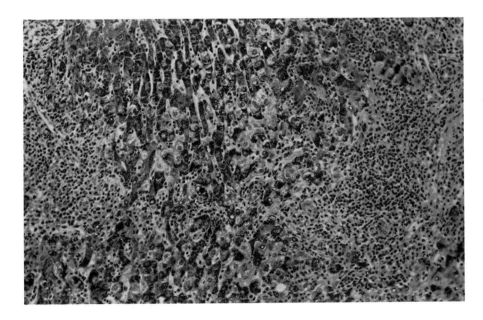

Fig. 27.1. Pylephlebitis complicating acute appendicitis. The portal tracts show an acute inflammatory exudate in which polymorphonuclear leucocytes are conspicuous. The walls of the portal vein radicles are thickened and the lining epithelium is desquamating. The inflammatory cells are invading the adjoining liver parenchyma and the periportal liver cells are necrosing. Culture of this biopsy grew *E. coli*. (Stained Best's carmine, ×145.)

spleen. Direction extension from the liver may lead to subphrenic or pleuro-pulmonary suppuration. Extension to the peritoneum or rupture of a sinus pointing under the skin are rare. A small amount of ascites is present in about a third of patients.

Histologically, areas remote from the abscess show signs of infection in the portal tracts surrounding disintegrating liver cells being infiltrated by polymorphs (fig. 27.1).

CLINICAL FEATURES

In the pre-antibiotic era, the picture was of spiking fever and right upper quadrant pain, often with prostration and shock. Nowadays, the presentation is less acute, with malaise, low-grade fever and dull abdominal pain increased by movement. It is particularly likely to be occult in the elderly.

The onset may be insidious and the duration at least one month before diagnosis. Multiple abscesses are associated with more acute sys temic features and the cause is more ofte identified. The single abscess is more insidious and often 'cryptogenic'. If there is sub-diaphragmatic irritation or pleuro-pulmonary spread of infection, the patient may complain of right shoulder pain and an irritating cough. The liver is enlarged and tender, and pain may be accentuated by percussion over the lower rib cage.

The spleen is palpable in chronic cases. Ascites is rare. Jaundice is late unless there is suppurative cholangitis.

Recovery may be followed by portal hypertension due to thrombosis of the portal vein.

INVESTIGATIONS

Jaundice is usually mild, but may be marked in the cholangitic types. It is more common than with amoebic abscess.

Serum alkaline phosphatase is usually raised. The ESR is very high. Polymorph leucocytosis is usual.

Blood cultures may show the causative infection or infections in 50% [2].

Fluoroscopic examination

This may show a high, immobile, right diaphragm, with alterations in contour and a plural effusion. A penetrating film may show a fluid level, indicating gas-producing organisms.

Localization of the abscess

Ultrasound is a useful routine test and this distinguishes a solid tumour from a fluid-filled lesion. CT scanning is particularly valuable in localization (figs 27.2, 27.3, 27.4).

Cholangitic abscesses may be diagnosed by percutaneous trans-hepatic cholangiography [9]. Endoscopic cholangiography may also be useful in localizing an abscess (fig. 27.5) [1].

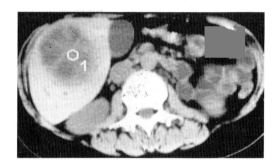

Fig. 27.2. Thallassaemic Greek patient post-splenectomy. CT scan shows a filling defect in the right lobe of the liver with marker over it (1).

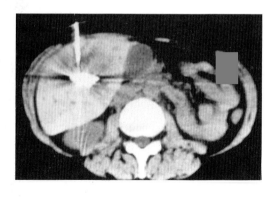

Fig. 27.3. Same patient with directed puncture of the abscess which resolved without surgery.

Aspirated material may be obtained for culture and is positive in 90% [2]. It should be cultured aerobically, anaerobically and in carbon dioxide enriched media for *S. milleri*. Aspiration is usually done percutaneously under ultrasound or CT direction.

TREATMENT

Prevention is by early treatment of acute abdominal infections and the adequate drainage, usually percutaneous or endoscopic, of intra-abdominal purulent collections under adequate antibiotic cover.

Antibiotics are rarely effective alone, and should not be continued where drainage is mandatory. The course should be intensive and the choice of antibiotic depends on the causative organism.

Once a single abscess is localized, it must be drained. If amoebiasis is suspected, metronidazole should be given before aspiration. Otherwise, the treatment of choice is aspiration, which can be repeated [10, 16].

Sometimes a percutaneously inserted pigtail catheter drain is necessary.

With multiple abscesses, the largest is aspirated and the smaller lesions usually resolve with chemotherapy. Occasionally, percutaneous drainage of each is necessary [8].

High dose antibiotics alone, given for at least six months, may be successful particularly if the infection is streptococcal [9].

Open surgical drainage is rarely indicated.

Biliary obstruction must be relieved. This is usually done by the endoscope with papillotomy and, if necessary, the insertion of a biliary endoprosthesis. Even with eventual cure, fever may continue for one to two weeks [2].

PROGNOSIS

The high mortality is largely due to failure to diagnose and to drain the abscess. The advent of percutaneous needle aspiration and antibiotic therapy has now lowered the mortality to 1.5% [16]. The prognosis is better for a unilocular abscess in the right lobe. If adequately treated the survival is 90%. The outcome for multiple abscesses throughout the liver especially if of biliary origin is very poor; only one-fifth survive. When there is delay in diagnosis of jaundice, continued fever, multiple infections shown by blood culture and old age, the prognosis is worse.

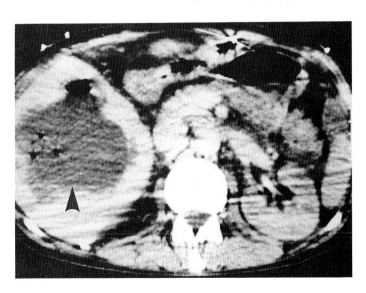

Fig. 27.4. CT shows a large pyogenic abscess with thick shaggy walls in the inferior part of the right lobe of the liver (arrow). The abscess contains gas.

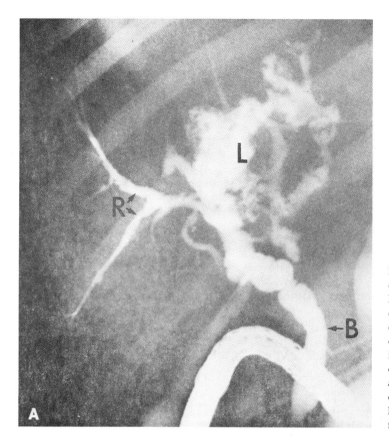

Fig. 27.5. Retrograde cholangiogram in pyogenic liver abscess. The common bile duct (B) is dilated. The main divisions of the right hepatic duct (R) are seen to be irregular in calibre. The left main hepatic duct (L) is grossly disorganized and surrounded by areas of extravasation of dye into the liver substance. [Fig. 27.5B on facing page.]

References

1 Ascione A, Elias E, Scott J et al. Endoscopic retrograde cholangiography (ERC) in non-amebic liver abscesses. *Am. J. dig. Dis.* 1978; **23**: 39.

2 Barnes PF, DeCock KM, Reynolds TN et al. A comparison of amebic and pyogenic abscesses of the liver. *Medicine (Baltimore)* 1987; **66**: 472.

3 Brown RKJ, Memsic LDF, Pusey EJ et al. Hepatic abscess in liver transplantation. *Clin. nucl. Med.* 1986; **11**: 233.

4 Capron J-P, Delmarre J, Delcenserie R et al. Liver abscess complicating yersinia pseudotuberculosis ileitis. *Gastroenterology* 1981; **81**: 150.

5 Cortez JC, Shapiro M, Awe RJ. *Pasteurella multocida* liver abscess. *Am. J. med. Sci.* 1986; **292**: 107.

6 Fischer MG, Beaton HL. Unsuspected hepatic abscess associated with biliary tract disease. *Am. J. Surg.* 1983; **146**: 658.

7 Gleeson DC, Fielding J, Heath DA. *Streptococcus milleri* liver abscesses associated with leiomyosarcoma of the ileum. *Postgrad. med. J.* 1983; **59**: 323.

8 Greenwood LH, Collins TL, Yrizarry JM. Percutaneous management of multiple liver abscesses. *Am. J. Roentgenol.* 1982; **139**: 390.

9 Matlow A, Vellend H. Medical treatment of multiple streptococcal liver abscesses. *J. clin. Gastroenterol.* 1983; **5**: 143.

10 McDonald MI, Corey GR, Gallis HA et al. Single and multiple pyogenic liver abscesses. Natural history, diagnosis, and treatment, with emphasis on percutaneous drainage. *Medicine (Baltimore)* 1984; **63**: 291.

11 McDonald GB, Shulman HM, Wolford JL et al. Liver diseases after human marrow transplantation. *Semin. Liver Dis.* 1987; **7**: 210.

12 Mir-Madjlessi SH, McHenry MC, Farmer RG. Liver abscesses in Crohn's disease. Report of four cases and review of the literature. *Gastroenterology* 1986; **91**: 987.

13 Moore-Gillon JC, Eykyn SJ, Phillips I. Microbiology of pyogenic liver abscess. *Br. med. J.* 1981; **283**: 819.

14 Reddy KR, Jeffers L, Livingstone AS et al. Pyogenic liver abscess complicating common bile duct stenosis secondary to chronic calcific pancreatitis. *Gastroenterology* 1984; **86**: 953.

15 Rumans MC, Katon RM, Lowe DK. Hepatic abscesses as a complication of the sump syndrome: combined surgical and endoscopic therapy. Case

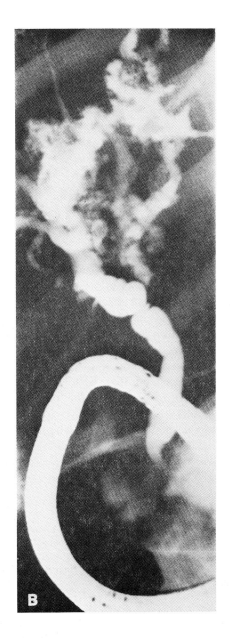

report and review of the literature. *Gastroenterology* 1987; **92**: 791.
16 Sheinfeld AM, Steiner AE, Rivkin LB *et al.* Transcutaneous drainage of abscesses of the liver guided by computed tomography. *Surg. Gynecol. Obstet.* 1982; **155**: 662.

Other infections

Giardiasis is rarely associated with hepatic
551 granulomas and cholangitis [4].

Campylobacter colitis can be related to a nonspecific acute hepatitis [3].

Cat scratch disease is believed due to a pleomorphic bacillus. It causes hepatic nodules, biopsy of which reveals necrotising granulomata containing the organism [2]. CT shows focal hepatic defects and mediastinal and peri-portal lymphenopathy [5].

Listeria monocytogenes can cause liver abscesses [1].

References

1 Jenkins D, Richards JE, Rees Y *et al.* Multiple listerial liver abscesses. *Gut* 1987; **28**: 1661.
2 Lenoir AA, Storch GA, De Schryver-Kecskemeti K *et al.* Granulomatous hepatitis associated with cat scratch disease. *Lancet* 1988; **i**: 1132.
3 Reddy KR, Farnum JB, & Thomas E. Acute hepatitis associated with campylobacter colitis. *J. clin. Gastroenterol.* 1983; **5**: 259.
4 Roberts-Thomas IC, Anders RF, Bhathal PS, Granulomatous hepatitis and cholangitis associated with giardiasis. *Gastroenterology* 1982; **83**: 480.
5 Rocco VK, Roman RJ, Eigenbrodt EH. Cat scratch disease. Report of a case with hepatic lesions and a brief review of the literature. *Gastroenterology* 1985; **89**: 1400.

Hepatic amoebiasis

Entamoeba histolytica exists in a free-living vegetative form and as cysts which survive outside the body and are highly infectious. The cystic form passes unharmed through the stomach and small intestine and changes into the vegetative, trophozoite form in the colon. Here, it invades the mucosa, forming typical flask-shaped ulcers. Amoebae are carried to the liver in the portal venous system. Occasionally, they pass through the hepatic sinusoids into the systemic circulation with the production of abscesses in lungs and brain.

Amoebae multiply and block small intrahepatic portal radicles with consequent focal infarction of liver cells. They contain a proteolytic enzyme which destroys the liver parenchyma. The lesions produced are single or multiple and of variable size.

The amoebic abscess is usually about the

size of an orange. The most frequent site is in the right lobe, often supero-anteriorly, just below the diaphragm. The centre consists of a large necrotic area which has liquefied into thick, reddish-brown pus. This has been likened to anchovy or chocolate sauce. Although it is referred to as amoebic pus, it is not strictly so because it is produced by lysis of liver cells. Fragments of liver tissue may be recognized in it. Initially, the abscess has no well-defined wall, but merely shreds of shaggy, necrotic liver tissue. Histologically, the necrotic areas consist of degenerate liver cells, leucocytes, red blood cells, connective tissue strands and debris. Amoebae may be identified in scrapings from the wall.

Small lesions heal with scars, but larger abscesses show a chronic wall of connective tissue of varying age.

There is no justification for retaining the term 'acute amoebic hepatitis' [6]. Histologically, the liver remote from the isolated abscesses or micro-abscesses is normal. The amoebic lesion from the outset is not diffuse but focal. These hepatolytic areas remain silent and are symptomatic only when they have progressed to a larger abscess [6].

Many factors determine the balance between healing or progression. The virulence and resistance of the host must play a part. There may be a specific pathogenic organism responsible for amoebic liver abscess. Starch-gel electrophoresis of pus from amoebic liver abscess showed specific zymodemes, differing from those found in the faeces of symptom-free cyst passers [8]. Another factor is secondary bacterial infection, which occurs in about 20%. The pus then becomes green or yellow and foul smelling.

EPIDEMIOLOGY

Colonic amoebae have a world-wide distribution, but the actual disease is one of the tropics and subtropics. Endemic areas are Africa, South East Asia, Mexico, Venezuela and Colombia.

In temperate climates, symptomless carriers of toxic strains are found but colonic ulcers are not seen. It is a frequent commensal in homosexual men [2]. Various factors might explain the change in virulence in the tropics.

In the tropics a new arrival is heavily exposed. Spread of infection by faeces is easier when sanitation is poor. Locals are less prone to hepatic amoebiasis than Europeans, presumably because of partial immunity induced by repeated contact.

The latent period between the intestinal infection and hepatic involvement has not been explained.

Liver abscesses may be induced in hamsters by intra-peritoneal inoculation of amoebae and by direct inoculation of human, sterile pus containing amoebae.

CLINICAL FEATURES

Note must be made of any residence or illness suffered in tropical or subtropical areas. Amoebic dysentery is present in only 10% and cysts in the stool of only 15% of patients with hepatic amoebiasis. A past history of dysentery is rare. Hepatic amoebiasis has been recorded as long as 30 years after the primary bowel infection. It is most frequent in young males aged 30−50. Multiple abscesses are frequent in such areas as Mexico and Taiwan.

The onset is usually gradual but, rarely, may be sudden with rigors and sweating. Fever is variously intermittent, remittent or even absent unless an abscess becomes secondarily infected; it rarely exceeds 40°C. Deep abscesses may present simply as fever without signs referable to the liver.

Jaundice is unusual and if present is mild. Occasionally, however, if bile ducts are compressed it is the presenting feature usually in those with large and multiple abscesses [7].

The patient looks ill, with a peculiar sallowness of the skin, like faded suntan.

Pain in the liver area may commence as a dull ache, later becoming sharp and stabbing. If the abscess is near the diaphragm, there may be referred shoulder pain accentuated by deep breathing or coughing. Alcohol makes the pain worse, as do postural changes. The patient tends to lean to the left side; this opens up the right intercostal space and diminishes the tension on the liver capsule. The pain increases at night. Pain and tenderness are greatest when the lesion is expanding rapidly.

A swelling may be visible in the epigastrium or bulging the intercostal spaces. Hepatic tenderness is virtually constant. It may be elicited over a palpable liver edge or by percussion over the lower right chest wall [6]. The spleen is not enlarged.

Examination of the lungs may show consolidation of the right lower zone, signs of pleurisy or an effusion. Pleural fluid may be blood stained.

Examination of faeces. Cysts and vegetative forms are rare and found usually in the early stages.

CLASSIFICATION [6]

Acute. The patients are younger with negative, or low *E. histolytica* antibodies. Liver scan shows multiple focal lesions.

Chronic. This usually follows many years' residence in an endemic area. The abscess is large and single in the right lobe. Antibody titres are very high.

SEROLOGICAL TESTS [5]

Numerous tests are available. They remain positive for a long time after clinical cure. However, an amoebic abscess is unlikely to be present if serological tests are negative. The haemagglutination test is sensitive and valuable in community surveys. Counter-immunoelectrophoresis is useful for rapid screening for amoebic liver abscess. An enzyme-linked, immuno-sorbent assay (ELISA) is sensitive for serum diagnosis and useful for stool and aspirates from liver abscesses [7].

BIOCHEMICAL TESTS

In the chronic case, serum alkaline phosphatase values are usually about twice normal. In-creases in transaminases are found only in those who are acutely ill or with severe complications. A rise in serum bilirubin is unusual except in those with superinfection or rupture into the peritoneum.

RADIOLOGICAL FEATURES

Chest radiographs may show a high right diaphragm, obliteration of the costo-phrenic and cardio-phrenic angles by adhesions, pleural effusions or right basal pneumonia. Perpendicular string-like adhesions may pass from the diaphragm to the lung base. A right lateral abscess may cause widening of the intercostal spaces. A central or inferior abscess may show few signs.

The upper abdomen may demonstrate an enlarged liver shadow, with a raised right diaphragm, which may be immobile on screening (fig. 27.6). The abscess is commonly situated in a supero-anterior position causing a bulge in the antero-medial part of the right diaphragm.

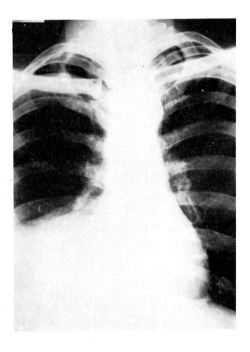

Fig. 27.6. Amoebic abscess of liver. Note the elevated right diaphragm with overlying reaction in the chest.

An abscess in the left lobe of the liver may show a crescentic deformity of the lesser curve of the stomach.

Modern *scanning methods* have shown multiple abscesses more frequently than formerly described.

Ultrasound (fig. 27.7) is most useful in diagnosis and in following progress. Changes are not specific for amoebic liver abscess [9].

CT shows the abscess with a somewhat irregular edge and less echogenic than the surrounding liver. It is more sensitive than ultrasound for small abscesses.

MR imaging can be used to diagnose amoebic abscess and to follow treatment [1].

Arteriography shows an avascular mass, with distortion of the normal vascular architecture.

DIAGNOSTIC CRITERIA [6]

Certain criteria are of value in reaching a diagnosis of hepatic amoebiasis [6]:

1 an enlarged tender liver in a young male;
2 response to metronidazole;
3 leucocytosis without anaemia in those with a short history, and less marked leucocytosis and

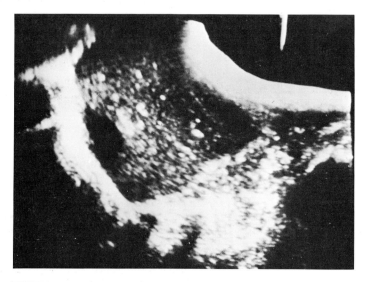

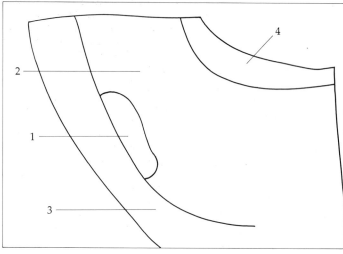

Fig. 27.7. Amoebic liver abscess. Ultrasound demonstrates an amoebic abscess (1) in the liver (2) lying posteriorly against the diaphragm (3). The anterior abdominal wall (4) is also shown.

anaemia in those with a long history;

4 suggestive radiological findings particularly in the postero-anterior and lateral chest X-ray;

5 demonstration of amoebic pus possibly containing trophozoites by aspiration or because of rupture into an adjacent viscous or serous cavity;

6 scanning showing a filling defect;

7 a positive amoebic haemagglutination test.

COMPLICATIONS

Two-thirds of ruptures are intra-peritoneal and one-third intra-thoracic [3].

Rupture into the lungs or pleura causes empyema, hepato-bronchial fistula or pulmonary abscess. The patient coughs up pus, develops pneumonitis or lung abscess or a pleural effusion.

Rupture into the pericardium is a complication of amoebic abscess in the left lobe.

Intra-peritoneal rupture results in acute peritonitis. If the patient survives the initial effect, long-term results are good. Abscesses of the left lobe may perforate into the lesser sac.

Rupture into the portal vein, bile ducts or gastrointestinal tract is rare.

Secondary infection is suspected if prostration is particularly great, and fever and leucocytosis high. Aspiration reveals yellowish, often foetid, pus and culture reveals the causative organism.

TREATMENT

Metronidazole 750 mg three times a day for 5—10 days is the treatment of choice for amoebic dysentery or liver abscess. An intravenous (costly) preparation is available for those unable to take the drug orally. Complications of metronidazole include nausea, diarrhoea, metallic taste, dizziness and discoloration of urine. Alcohol should not be permitted during treatment. Failures are very few, and may be related to persistence of intestinal amoebiasis, drug resistance or inadequate absorption.

The time taken for the abscess to disappear depends on its size and varies from 10 to 300 days [9].

Aspiration is rarely required. It may be necessary with very large abscesses or where there is lack of response to five days' metronidazole treatment. The site is chosen by the presence of bulging intercostal spaces or abdominal wall, by tenderness or radiology. If possible, aspiration should be done under ultrasound or CT control. The needle should be at least 10 cm long, of 1—2 mm diameter, and with a fitted stilette. A tense abscess in the left lobe which is likely to rupture into the peritoneum demands aspiration.

Surgery is reserved for those with secondary infection of the abscess cavity.

To prevent relapse, a course of a luminal amoebocide such as diloxanide furoate (500 mg three times a day for 10 days) or iodoquin (650 mg three times a day for 20 days) should be given to cover amoebae persisting in the gut.

References

1 Elizondo G, Weissleder R, Stark DD *et al.* Amebic liver abscess: diagnosis and treatment evaluation with MR imaging. *Radiology* 1987; **165**: 795.

2 Goldmeier D, Sargeaunt PG, Price AB et al. Is *Entamoeba histolytica* in homosexual men a pathogen? *Lancet* 1986; **i**: 641.

3 Greaney GC, Reynolds TB, Donovan AJ. Ruptured amebic liver abscess. *Arch. Surg.* 1985; **120**: 555.

4 Katzenstein D, Rickerson V, Braude A. New concepts of amebic liver abscess derived from hepatic imaging, serodiagnosis, and hepatic enzymes in 67 consecutive cases in San Diego. *Medicine (Baltimore)* 1982; **61**: 237.

5 Krogstad DJ, Spencer HC Jr, Healy GR. Current concepts in parasitology: amebiasis. *N. Engl. J. Med.* 1978; **298**: 262.

6 Lamont NMcE, Pooler NR. Hepatic amoebiasis. A study of 250 cases. *Q. J. Med.* 1958; **27**: 389.

7 Nigam P, Gupta AK, Kapoor KK *et al.* Cholestasis in amoebic liver abscess. *Gut* 1985; **26**: 140.

8 Sargeaunt PG; Jackson TFHG, Simjee A. Biochemical homogeneity of entamoeba histolytica isolates, especially those from liver abscess. *Lancet* 1982; **i**: 1386.

9 Simjee AE, Patel A, Gathiram V *et al.* Serial ultrasound in amoebic liver abscess. *Clin. Radiol.* 1985; **36**: 61.

Tuberculosis of the liver

Although the liver is frequently involved by haematogenous spread, the lesions tend to heal spontaneously. Hepatic tuberculosis is therefore seldom of clinical importance and rarely diagnosed.

The basic lesion is the *granuloma* which is very frequent in the liver of a patient with both pulmonary and extra-pulmonary tuberculosis (Chapter 26). The lesions usually heal without scarring but sometimes with focal fibrosis and calcification.

Tuberculomata are very rare. They may be multiple, consisting of white, irregular, caseous abscesses surrounded by a fibrous capsule. Their naked eye distinction from Hodgkin's disease, secondary carcinoma or actinomycosis may be difficult. Occasionally, the necrotic area calcifies.

Tuberculous cholangitis is extremely rare, resulting from spread of caseous material from the portal tracts into the bile ducts. The caseous central areas become bile stained.

Tuberculous pylephlebitis results from rupture of caseous material, often in portal lymph nodes, into the portal vein. It is rapidly fatal.

Tuberculous glands at the hilum may lead to biliary stricture [1].

CLINICAL FEATURES

These may be few or absent. An associated pyrexia is usually due to concomitant, active tuberculosis elsewhere rather than to hepatic disease. The condition may present as a pyrexia of unknown origin. Jaundice may appear in overwhelming miliary tuberculosis, particularly in the racially susceptible. Rarely multiple caseating granulomas lead to massive hepatosplenomegaly and death in liver failure [6].

BIOCHEMICAL TESTS

Serum alkaline phosphatase levels may be raised. Hyperglobulinaemia reflects chronic infection and hepatic granulomas.

DIAGNOSIS

This is difficult. Liver biopsy is essential. The main indications are unexplained fever, hepatomegaly or hepatosplenomegaly [4]. A small portion of the tissue obtained should be stained for acid-fast bacilli and also cultured. Positives are obtained in about 50%.

A *plain X−ray* of the abdomen may reveal hepatic calcification. Local hepatic tuberculosis can cause a lobulated hypoechoic mass on CT. Biopsy reveals the acid-fast bacilli [2, 3].

Extra-hepatic features of tuberculosis may not be obvious.

Treatment is that of haematogenous tuberculosis. No specific treatment of the liver is indicated.

THE EFFECT ON THE LIVER OF TUBERCULOSIS ELSEWHERE

Amyloidosis may complicate chronic tuberculosis. Fatty change is due to wasting and toxaemia. Drug jaundice may follow therapy, especially with isoniazid.

OTHER MYCOBACTERIA

Atypical mycobacteria can produce a granulomatous hepatitis, particularly as part of the AIDS syndrome (see p. 579). *Mycobacterium scrofulaceum* can cause a granulomatous hepatitis, characterized by a rise in alkaline phosphatase, tiredness and low grade fever. Liver biopsy culture produces the organism [5].

References

1 Alvarez SZ, Carpio R. Hepatobiliary tuberculosis. *Dig. Dis. Sci.* 1982; **28:** 193.
2 Blangy S, Cornud F, Sibert A *et al.* Hepatitic tuberculosis presenting as tumoral disease on ultrasonography. *Gastrointest. Radiol.* 1988; **13:** 52.
3 Gallinger S, Strasberg SM, Marcus HI *et al.* Local hepatic tuberculosis, the cause of a painful hepatic mass: case report and review of the literature. *Canad. J. Surg.* 1986; **29:** 451.
4 Maharaj B, Leary WP, Pudifin DJ. A prospective study of hepatic tuberculosis in 41 black patients. *Q. J. Med.* 1987; **63:** 517.

5 Patel KM. Granulomatous hepatitis due to mycobacterium scrofulaceum: report of a case. *Gastroenterology* 1981; **81**: 156.

6 Sharma SK, Shamin SQ, Bannerjee CK *et al.* Disseminated tuberculosis presenting as massive hepato-splenomegaly and hepatic failure. *Am. J. Gastroenterol.* 1981; **76**: 153.

Hepatic actinomycosis

This disease is due to the fungus *Actinomyces israelii*.

Hepatic involvement is a sequel to intestinal actinomycosis, especially of the caecum and appendix. It spreads by direct extension or, more often, by the portal vein, but can be primary. Large greyish-white masses, superficially resembling malignant metastases, soften and form collections of pus, separated by fibrous tissue bands, simulating a honeycomb. The liver becomes adherent to adjacent viscera and to the abdominal wall, with the formation of sinuses. These lesions contain the characteristic 'sulphur granules', which consist of branching filaments with eosinophilic, clubbed ends.

Clinically, the patient is toxic, febrile, sweating, wasted and anaemic. There is local, sometimes irregular, enlargement with tenderness of one or both lobes of the liver. The overlying skin may have the livid, dusky hue seen over a taut abscess which is about to rupture. Multiple irregular sinus tracks develop, from which bile may exude. Similar sinuses may develop from the ileo-caecal site or from the chest wall if there is pleuro-pulmonary extension.

The *diagnosis* is obvious at the stage of sinus tracks, because the organism can be isolated from the pus. If actinomycosis is suspected before this stage, aspiration liver biopsy should be avoided, because of the danger of developing a persistent sinus. In the early stages, the condition presents as pyrexia with hepatosplenomegaly, anaemia and non-specific hepatic cellular infiltrates [1].

It may be months before multiple abscesses are detected, often by ultrasound, CT or isotope scans [2]. Anaerobic blood cultures may be positive.

Treatment. Penicillin should be given in masssive doses for six weeks. Because of the thick fibrous capsule surrounding the abscess, parenterally administered penicillin may reach the area with difficulty. It should be supplemented by local instillation of penicillin wherever possible.

References

1 Meade RH III Primary hepatic actinomycosis. *Gastroenterology* 1980; **78**: 355.

2 Mongiardo N, De Rienzo B, Zanchetta G *et al.* Primary hepatic actinomycosis. *J. Infection* 1986; **12**: 65.

Other fungal infections

These usually affect the immuno-compromised host including sufferers from AIDS, acute leukaemia [8] and cancer [13].

The liver is involved, together with other organs, particularly kidney, spleen, heart, lungs and brain. Fever, a raised serum transaminase or alkaline phosphatase indicate needle liver biopsy.

Ultrasound shows multiple hypoechoic areas throughout the liver and spleen, often with a target (bulls-eye) configuration [11]. CT shows multiple non-enhancing low attenuation lesions [8]. The scanning appearances are not diagnostic.

The histological picture is usually granulomatous and the causative organism can be identified by appropriate stains and cultures, so allowing selection of appropriate anti-fungal treatment [7].

Candidiasis. The liver is affected in up to three-quarters of compromised hosts with disseminated *Candida albicans* infection who come to autopsy [7]. Hepatic granulomas and micro-abscesses are the commonest histological lesions. Candida can be demonstrated in the liver.

Disseminated aspergillosis may attack the immuno-compromised patients with respiratory, renal or hepatic failure [10].

Hepatic cryptococcosis usually affects the immuno-compromised but sometimes it may be seen in the otherwise normal. Liver biopsy shows granulomas with yeast-like organisms, stained by Grocott's technique.

The picture may resemble sclerosing cholangitis when bile is positive for the fungus [1].

Disseminated coccidioidomycosis may involve the liver and be diagnosed by liver biopsy [5].

Torulopsis glabrata hepatic abscesses and fungaemia have developed in a severely diabetic patient with biliary stricture due to chronic pancreatitis [4].

Syphilis of the liver

CONGENITAL

The liver is heavily affected by any transplacental infection. It is firm, enlarged and swarming with spirochaetes. Initially, there is a diffuse hepatitis, but gradually fibrous tissue is laid down between the liver cells and in the portal tracts, and this leads to a true pericellular cirrhosis.

Since hepatic involvement is but an incident in a widespread spirochaetal septicaemia, the clinical features are seldom those of the liver disease. The fetus may be stillborn or die soon after birth. If the infant survives, other manifestations of congenital syphilis are obvious, apart from the hepatosplenomegaly and mild jaundice. Syphilis nowadays is a very rare cause of neonatal jaundice.

In older children who have survived without this florid neonatal picture, the hepatic lesion may be a gumma.

Diagnosis can be confirmed by blood serology which is always positive. Needle liver biopsy has been used for diagnosis and to assess the effects of treatment. Electron microscopy confirms the presence of spirochaetes.

SECONDARY

In the secondary septicaemic stage, spirochaetes invade the liver with the production of miliary granulomas [3].

Rarely, jaundice and hepatitis are seen [12].

Serology is positive. Serum alkaline phosphatase levels are very high. Liver biopsy shows non-specific changes with moderate infiltration with polymorphs and lymphocytes, some hepatocellular disarray, but no cholestasis (fig. 27.8). Portal-to-central zonal necrosis can be seen. Spirochaetes are not usually detected.

The response to treatment is rapid [2].

TERTIARY

Gummas may be single or multiple. They are usually situated in the right lobe. They consist of a caseous mass, circumscribed by a fibrous capsule, from which fibrous tissue spreads out interstitially. Healing occurs with the production of deep scars and coarse lobulation (*hepar lobatum*). Despite this distortion, the liver architecture is not disturbed and the lesion is not a true cirrhosis.

Hepatic gummas are usually discovered incidentally at laparotomy or autopsy. Occasionally, the enlarged nodular liver may be confused with cirrhosis or hepatic metastases. Liver function tests are unhelpful and the presence of positive serology is insufficient evidence of hepatic syphilis. Aspiration liver biopsy of an accessible nodule provides histological confirmation. The response to adequate penicillin may be diminution in size of a gumma over prolonged periods of time.

Jaundice complicating penicillin treatment

Rarely, the patient shows an idiosyncrasy to treatment with penicillin. Jaundice, chills and fever, often with a rash (*erythema of Milan*), occur about nine days after starting therapy. This forms part of the Herxheimer reaction. The mechanism of the jaundice is unclear.

References

1 Bucuvalas JC, Bove KE, Kaufman RA et al. Cholangitis associated with *Cryptococcus neoformans*. *Gastroenterology* 1985; **88**: 1055.
2 Campisi D, Whitcomb C. Liver disease in early syphilis. *Arch. intern. Med.* 1979; **139**: 365.

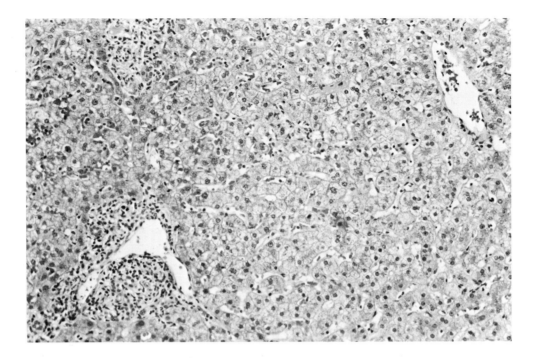

Fig. 27.8. Liver in secondary syphilis. Mononuclear cell infiltration can be seen in portal zones and in the sinusoids. (Stained H & E, ×160.)

3 Case Records of the Massachusetts General Hospital Case 27—1983. *N. Engl. J. Med.* 1983; **309:** 35.

4 Friedman E, Blahut RJ, Bender MD. Hepatic abscesses and fungemia from *Torulopsis glabrata.* Successful treatment with percutaneous drainage and amphotericin B. *J. clin. Gastroenterol.* 1987; **9:** 711.

5 Howard PF, Smith JW. Diagnosis of disseminated coccidioidomycosis. *Arch. intern. Med.* 1983; **143:** 1335.

6 Korinek JK, Guarda LA, Bolivar R *et al.* Trichosporon hepatitis. *Gastroenterology* 1983; **85:** 732.

7 Lewis JH, Patel HR, Zimmerman HJ. The spectrum of hepatic candidiasis. *Hepatology* 1982; **2:** 479.

8 Maxwell AJ, Mamtora H. Fungal liver abscesses in acute leukaemia—a report of two cases. *Clin. Radiol.* 1988; **39:**197.

9 Pareek SS. Liver involvement in secondary syphilis. *Am. J. dig. Dis.* 1979; **24:** 41.

10 Park GR, Drummond GB, Lamb D *et al.* Disseminated aspergillosis occurring in patients with respiratory, renal and hepatic failure. *Lancet* 1982; **1:** 179.

11 Pastakia B, Shawker TH, Thaler M *et al.* Hepatosplenic candidiasis: wheels within wheels. *Radiology* 1988; **166:** 417.

12 Schlossberg D. Syphilitic hepatitis: a case report and review of the literature. *Am. J. Gastroenterol.* 1987; **82:** 552.

13 Thaler M, Pastakia FB, Shawker TH *et al.* Hepatic candidiasis in cancer patients: the evolving picture of the syndrome. *Ann. intern. Med.* 1988; **108:** 88.

Weil's disease (leptospirosis)

In 1886, Weil [6] described a disease characterized by intense prostration, fever, jaundice, renal injury and a haemorrhagic tendency. This was later shown to be due to a leptospira, *L. icterohaemorrhagiae*, and to be transmitted by rats. Later various other leptospira were related to human disease. These do not cause a distinct clinical pattern and the whole group should be designated leptospirosis and Weil's disease applied only to infections with *L. icterohaemorrhagiae*. There are at least 22 serological types, most of them causing disease in man.

MODE OF INFECTION

The renal tubules of rats form the principal reservoir of infection for man. Living leptospira are continually excreted and are capable of surviving for months in pools, canals or damp soil. The portal of entry in man is thought to be the respiratory or gastrointestinal canal, or through abrasions in the skin. The highest incidence is therefore in adult males, particularly agricultural workers, sewer workers, coalminers, ditch diggers, soldiers and fish cutters.

PATHOLOGY

Liver [1, 2] necrosis is minimal and focal. Dissociation of the cells one from another is probably a post-mortem phenomenon. The centrizonal necrosis of acute virus hepatitis is absent. Active hepato-cellular regeneration, shown by mitoses and nuclear polyploidy, is out of proportion to cell damage. Kupffer cells proliferate.

Peri-portal infiltration with leucocytes is constant and centrizonal bile thrombi are prominent if the patient is deeply jaundiced. The histological changes do not parallel the severity of icterus. Cirrhosis is not a sequel.

Kidney shows tubular necrosis.

Skeletal muscles show punctate haemorrhages and focal necrosis of muscle fibres.

Heart may show haemorrhages in all layers. Pericarditis may complicate the uraemia.

Haemorrhage into tissues, especially skin and lungs, is apparently due to capillary injury and thrombocytopenia.

The jaundice is complex. Hepato-cellular dysfunction is probably important, although serious, even fatal, deeply jaundiced patients may show minimal changes in the liver. Jaundice is magnified by the concomitant renal failure, preventing urinary bilirubin excretion. Tissue haemorrhage and intravascular haemolysis increase the bilirubin load on the liver. Hypotension with diminished hepatic blood flow is contributory.

The uraemia is related to pigment in the tubules, a direct effect of the spirochaetes on the kidney and lowered renal blood flow.

CLINICAL FEATURES (fig. 27.9) [2]

The disease is most prevalent in late summer and autumn. The incubation period is 6−15 days. The course may be divided into three stages: the first or septicaemic phase lasts for about seven days, the second or toxic stage for a similar period, and the third or convalescent period begins in the third week.

The first or septicaemic stage is marked by the presence of the spirochaete in the circulating blood.

The onset is abrupt, with prostration, high fever, even rigors. The temperature rises rapidly to 39.5−40.5°C and falls by lysis within 3−10 days.

Abdominal pain, nausea and vomiting may simulate an acute abdominal emergency, and severe muscular pains, especially in the back or calves, are common.

Central nervous system involvement is shown by severe headache, mental confusion and sometimes meningism. The cerebrospinal fluid confirms the meningeal infection, there being an increase in protein, with a leucocytosis. If jaundice is present, there is xanthochromia, the infection increasing the permeability of the meninges to bile pigments.

The eyes show a characteristic suffusion.

There is a haemorrhagic tendency usually in those with a severe attack. Bleeding may occur from nose, gut or lung, with skin petechiae or ecchymoses.

Pneumonitis with cough, sore throat and rhonchi occurs in 40% of sufferers.

Jaundice appears between the fourth and seventh day in 80% of patients [2, 3]. It is a grave sign, for the disease is never fatal in the absence of icterus. The liver is enlarged, but not the spleen.

The urine shows albumin, urobilin and bile pigment. The stools are well coloured.

There is a leucocytosis of 10 000−30 000/mm^3 with a relative increase in polymorphs. Thrombocytopenia may be profound.

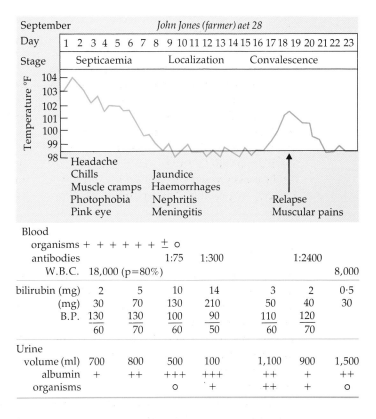

Fig. 27.9. The clinical course of a patient with Weil's disease.

Blood							
organisms	+ + + + + + ± o						
antibodies		1:75	1:300			1:2400	
W.B.C.	18,000 (p=80%)						8,000
bilirubin (mg)	2	5	10	14	3	2	0·5
(mg)	30	70	130	210	50	40	30
B.P.	130/60	130/70	100/60	90/50	110/60	120/70	
Urine							
volume (ml)	700	800	500	100	1,100	900	1,500
albumin	+	++	+++	+++	++	+	++
organisms			o	+	++	+	o

The second or immune stage in the second week is characterized by a normal temperature but without clinical improvement. This is the stage of deepening jaundice, with increasing renal and myocardial damage. Albuminuria persists, there is a rising blood urea, and oliguria may proceed to anuria. Death may be due to renal failure. A markedly elevated creatinine phosphokinase level reflects myositis.

Severe prostration is accompanied by a low blood pressure and a dilated heart. There may be transient cardiac arrhythmias and electro-cardiographic evidence of a prolonged P–R or Q–T interval, with T-wave changes. Death may be due to circulatory failure.

During this stage, the leptospira can be found in the urine, and rising antibody titres demonstrated in the serum.

The third or convalescent stage starts at the beginning of the third week. Clinical improvement is shown by a brightening of the mental state, fading of the jaundice, a rise in blood pressure and an increased urinary volume, with a drop in the blood urea concentration. Albuminuria is slow to disappear. Permanent renal and hepatic damage have not been reported.

Temperature may rise during the third week (fig. 27.9), associated with muscle pains. Such relapses occur in 20% of cases.

There is great variation in the clinical course ranging from a mild illness, clinically indistinguishable from influenza, to a prostrating, fatal disease with anuria.

INVESTIGATIONS

In the first week, the spirochaetes are found in the blood, becoming less evident with the development of antibodies at the end of the first week. Thereafter, they may be isolated from the urine.

Diagnosis in the first week

1 Thick, dry, blood films are used for staining for spirochaetes and for dark field examination.
2 Blood culture is performed but results take several days.
3 Acute-phase serological antibodies are measured as a base line for subsequent rising titres.
4 The leucocyte count is raised—a point of distinction from viral hepatitis.
5 Blood is injected intra-peritoneally into guinea pigs, who develop jaundice and fever within a few days. Spirochaetes are demonstrated in liver and other tissues.

Diagnosis after the first week

From the 10th to the 20th day, leptospira may be shown in the urine. Injection into a guinea pig may be positive, but the organisms are not often viable from urine.

Serological antibodies appear after the first week and usually reach a peak in the fourth week. They may persist for years.

The IgM specific dot-ELISA technique is useful for rapid serodiagnosis [4].

The leptospiral agglutination test is usually positive in a titre of at least 1 in 300 and a rising titre can be demonstrated. Cross-agglutination occurs between the various serotypes and the infecting type may not be ascertained without actual isolation of the leptospira.

Aspiration liver biopsy. In spite of the bleeding tendency, biopsies have been performed. The histological picture is not specific for leptospirosis, because the dissociation of liver cells, histiocytic proliferation and peri-portal changes are seen in other severe infections. The histological picture, however, is quite distinct from acute virus hepatitis. A portion of the liver biopsy may be used for culture of the leptospira.

Spinal fluid shows increased protein and leucocytes. It is often xanthochromic.

Liver function tests are non-contributory. The serum bilirubin level is raised and the alkaline phosphatase and transaminases slightly increased.

DIFFERENTIAL DIAGNOSIS

In the early stages, Weil's disease is confused with septicaemic bacterial infections or typhus fever. When jaundice is evident, there may be difficulty in excluding acute virus hepatitis (table 27.1). Important distinguishing points are the sudden onset and albuminuria of Weil's disease.

Spirochaetal jaundice would be diagnosed

Table 27.1. The diagnosis of Weil's disease from virus hepatitis during the first week of illness

	Weil's disease	Virus hepatitis
Onset	Sudden	Gradual
Headache	Constant	Occasional
Muscle pains	Severe	Mild
Conjunctival infection	Present	Absent
Prostration	Great	Mild
Disorientation	Common	Rare
Haemorrhagic diathesis	Common	Rare
Nausea and vomiting	Present	Present
Abdominal discomfort	Common	Common
Bronchitis	Common	Rare
Albuminuria	Present	Absent
Leucocyte count	Polymorph leucocytosis	Leucopenia with lymphocytosis
Inoculation of blood into guinea-pig	Spirochaetes present	Spirochaetes absent

more often if blood samples for agglutinins were taken from patients with obscure icterus and fever.

PROGNOSIS

Mortality is about 16%. This depends on the depth of jaundice, renal and myocardial involvement, and the extent of haemorrhages. Death is usually due to renal failure. The mortality is negligible in non-icteric patients, and is lower under 30 years old. Since many mild infections are probably unrecognized, the overall mortality may well be considerably less.

Although transient relapses in the third and fourth weeks are common, final recovery is complete.

PREVENTION

Specific immune serum has proved preventative in exposed laboratory workers.

Protective clothing, such as rubber boots and gloves, should be provided for workers in industries with a high incidence of Weil's disease, and adequate measures taken to control rodents. Bathing in stagnant water should be avoided.

TREATMENT

Penicillin, 6 million units intravenously for seven days, in severe and even late leptospirosis shortens hospital stay, and reduces duration of fever and rises in creatinine [5].

There is, however, no conclusive evidence of its value [2, 3]. It will be less effective after the first four days of illness, i.e., at the time when the diagnosis is usually made and treatment instituted.

Other types of leptospirosis

There are many species of leptospira pathogenic to man, varying in antigenic constitution and geographic distribution [2]. In general these infections are less severe than those due to *L. icterohaemorrhagiae*. *L. canicola* infection, for instance, is characterized by headache, meningitis and conjunctival infection. Albuminuria is only found in 40%, and jaundice in only 18% of patients. The frequent presentation is that of 'benign aseptic meningitis'. The disease affects young adults who have usually been in close contact with an infected dog. Fatalities in man are virtually unknown.

Diagnosis is confirmed in a similar way to Weil's disease. A convenient method is the demonstration of rising antibody titres. The spinal fluid shows a lymphocytic fluid in most cases, even in the absence of meningitis.

References

1 Arean VM. The pathologic anatomy and pathogenesis of fatal human leptospirosis (Weil's disease). *Am. J. Pathol.* 1962; **40**: 393.
2 Edwards GA, Domm BM. Human leptospirosis. *Medicine (Baltimore)* 1960; **39**: 117.
3 Heath CW Jr, Alexander AD, Galton MM. Leptospirosis in the United States. Analysis of 483 cases in man. 1949–1961. *N. Engl. J. Med.* 1965; **273**: 857.
4 Pappas MG, Ballou WR, Gray MR *et al.* Rapid serodiagnosis of leptospirosis using the IgM-specific Dot-ELISA. Comparison with the microscopic agglutination test. *Am. J. trop. Med. Hyg.* 1985; **34**: 346.
5 Watt G, Padre LP, Tuazon ML *et al.* Placebo-controlled trial of intravenous penicillin for severe and late leptospirosis. *Lancet* 1988; **1**: 433.
6 Weil A. Über eine eigenthumliche mit Milztumor, Icterus und Nephritis einhergehene, acute Infektionskrankheit. *Dtsch. Arch. klin. Med.* 1886; **39**: 209.

Relapsing fever

This arthropod-borne infection is caused by spirochaetes of the genus *Borrelia recurrentis*. It is encountered throughout the world except in New Zealand, Australia and some parts of the west Pacific.

The borrelia multiply in the liver, invading liver cells and causing focal necrosis. Just before the crisis the borrelia roll up and are ingested by reticulo-endothelial cells. This effect is related to immunologically competent lymphocytes. Surviving borrelia remain in the liver, spleen, brain and bone-marrow until the next relapse [2].

The incubation period is 3–15 days. The onset is acute with chills, a continuous high temperature, headache, muscle pains and profound prostration. The patient is flushed, sometimes with injected conjunctivae, and epistaxes. In severe attacks, tender hepatosplenomegaly and jaundice develop. The jaundice is similar to that seen in Weil's disease. Sometimes a rash develops on the trunk. There may be bronchitis.

These symptoms continue for 4–9 days and then the temperature falls, often with collapse of the patient. This peripheral collapse may be fatal, but more usually the symptoms and signs then rapidly abate. The patient remains afebrile for about a week, when there is a relapse. There may be a second or even a third milder relapse before the disease ends.

DIAGNOSIS

Spirochaetes can rarely be found in thick blood films. Agglutination and complement fixation tests are available [2]. Organisms may be identified by lymph node aspiration, or from the bite site.

TREATMENT

Tetracyclines and streptomycin are more effective than penicillin. Mortality is 5%.

References

1 Bryceson ADM, Parry EHO, Perine PL et al. Louseborn relapsing fever: a clinical and laboratory study of 62 cases in Ethiopia and a reconsideration of the literature. Q. J. Med. 1970; 39: 129.
2 Felsenfeld O, Wolf RH. Immunoglobulins and antibodies in borrelia turicetae infections. Acta Trop. 1969; 26: 156.

Lyme disease

This is due to a tick-borne spirochaete, *Borrelia burgdorfii*. It has caused hepatitis with numerous liver cell mitoses [1]. It responds to oral doxycycline therapy.

References

1 Goellner MH, Agger WA, Burgess JH et al. Hepatitis due to recurrent Lyme disease. Ann. intern. Med. 1988; 108: 707.

Q fever

This rickettsial disease has predominantly pulmonary manifestations. Occasionally hepatitis may be prominent and clinical features may mimic anicteric virus hepatitis.

The liver shows a granulomatous hepatitis. Portal areas contain abundant lymphocytes and the limiting plate is destroyed. Kupffer cells are hypertrophied. The granulomas have a characteristic ring of fibrinoid necrosis surrounded by lymphocytes and histiocytes. In the centre of the granuloma is a clear space giving a 'doughnut' appearance (fig. 27.10). The diagnosis is made by showing a rising titre of complement-fixing antibodies to *C. burnetti* 2–3 weeks after the infection.

Rocky mountain spotted fever

Jaundice and rises in serum enzymes sometimes occur. Liver histology shows portal zone inflammation with large mononuclear cells. Hepato-cellular necrosis is inconspicuous but erythrophagocytosis is marked. Rickettsiae may be demonstrated in the portal zones by immunofluorescence microscopy [1].

References

1 Adams JS, Walker DH. The liver in rocky mountain spotted fever. Am. J. clin. Pathol. 1981; 75: 156.
2 Dupont HL, Hornick RB, Levin HS et al. Q fever hepatitis. Ann. intern. Med. 1971; 74: 198.
3 Westlake P, Price LM, Russell M et al. The pathology of Q fever hepatitis. A case diagnosed by liver biopsy. J. clin. Gastroenterol. 1987; 9: 357.

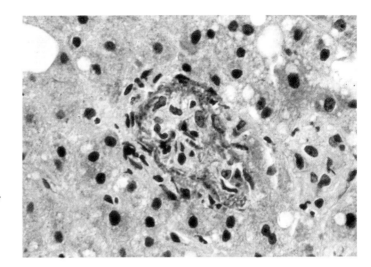

Fig. 27.10. Liver biopsy in Q fever showing a granuloma with fibrin rings having a clear centre. (Stained martius scarlet blue (MSB) ×350.)

Schistosomiasis (Bilharziasis)

Hepatic schistosomiasis is usually a complication of the intestinal disease, since emboli of schistosoma ova reach the liver from the intestines via the mesenteric veins. *S. mansoni* and *S. japonicum* affect the liver. *S. haematobium* can sometimes involve the liver.

Schistosomiasis affects more than two hundred million people in 73 countries. *S. japonicum* is prevalent in Japan, China, Indonesia and the Philippines. *S. mansoni* is found in Africa, the Middle East, the Caribbean, and northern parts of South America.

PATHOGENESIS

Eggs, excreted in the faeces, hatch out in water to free-swimming embryos which enter appropriate snails and develop into fork-tailed cercariae. These re-enter human skin in contact with infected water. They burrow down to the capillary bed, whence there is widespread haematogenous dissemination. Those reaching the mesenteric capillaries enter the intrahepatic portal system, where they grow rapidly.

The extent and severity of chronic liver disease correlates with the intensity and duration of egg production by fertile worm pairs and hence with the number of eggs excreted per gram of stool. However, when liver disease is advanced, many patients have low faecal egg counts because of senescence of adult worms or previous therapy.

S. japonicum is more pathogenic than *S. mansoni* and produces hepatosplenic schistosomiasis more often and faster.

In the liver, the ova penetrate and obstruct the portal branches and are deposited either in the large radicles, producing the coarser type of bilharzial hepatic fibrosis, or in the small portal tracts, producing the fine diffuse form.

The granulomatous reaction to the schistosoma ovum is an immunological one of delayed hypersensitivity type [10]. The granulomas seem to be related to antigen released by the egg.

Portal fibrosis is related to the adult worm load. The classic, clay-pipe stem cirrhosis is due to fibrotic bands originating from the granulomas. The collagen deposited in the enlarged portal triads and fibrotic septa is type 1, 3 and B [4].

Collagen may be deposited in the space of Disse independently of any granuloma.

Wide, irregular, thin-walled vascular spaces are found in 85% of cases and form a characteristic feature in the thickened portal tracts. These angiomatoids are useful in distinguishing the bilharzial liver from other forms of hepatic fibrosis. Remnants of ova are also diagnostic. There is little or no bile duct proliferation. The extent of nodular regeneration and disturbance of the hepatic architecture is not sufficient to justify the term 'cirrhosis'. If cirrhosis is present it can usually be attributed to other aetiological factors such as hepatitis B or hepatitis non-A, non-B.

Splenic enlargement is mainly due to the resulting portal venous hypertension, although there is also reticulo-endothelial hyperplasia. Very few ova are found in the spleen. Portal−systemic collateral channels are numerous.

There are associated bilharzial lesions in the intestines and elsewhere. Fifty per cent of patients with rectal schistosomiasis have granulomas in the liver.

CLINICAL FEATURES

Schistosomiasis shows three stages of infection. Itching follows the entry of the cercariae through the skin. This is followed by a stage of fever, urticaria and eosinophilia. Finally the third stage of deposition of ova results in intestinal, urinary and hepatic involvement.

Initially liver and spleen are firm, smooth and easily palpable. This is followed by hepatic fibrosis and eventually portal hypertension which may appear years after the original infection.

Oesophageal varices develop. Bleeding episodes are recurrent but rarely fatal.

The liver shrinks in size and the spleen becomes much larger. Dilated abdominal wall veins and a venous hum over the liver are indications of the portal venous obstruction. Ascites and oedema may develop. The blood shows a leucopenia and anaemia. The faeces at this stage contain few, if any, parasites.

Patients tolerate blood loss well and hepatic encephalopathy is unusual. This is because hepato-cellular function remains good although there is a large portal−systemic collateral circulation.

Aspiration liver biopsy (fig. 27.11). A 'squash' preparation in glycerol shows eggs or their

remnants in 94% of livers from those with faecal eggs.

Remnants of ova may sometimes be seen but appearances are not usually diagnostic and the liver biopsy serves mainly to exclude other types of liver disease.

Rectal biopsy is useful but bleeding may be a complication in those with marked portal hypertension.

DIAGNOSTIC TESTS

The best method of detecting active infection is stool examination. However, in long-standing or treated infections, very few eggs may be found. Examination of a rectal mucosal biopsy crushed in saline 'rectal snip' is helpful in detecting very light or recently treated infections.

Serological tests are not used routinely. When positive, they indicate past exposure without specifying the time. A negative ELISA excludes schistosomal infection.

CT shows dense bands following the portal vein from the porta hepatis to the liver edge; these enhance with contrast [8].

Portal hypertension

The portal hypertension is presinusoidal and presumably related to the portal zone reaction. In advanced schistosomiasis, hepatic arterial hypertension contributes to increased sinusoidal pressure [1]. Retrograde flow develops in the portal vein. Hepatic blood flow is not significantly reduced.

At the stage when haemorrhage occurs from varices the granulomatous reaction may have subsided and the picture is predominantly that of fibrosis.

Biochemical changes

Serum alkaline phosphatase may be raised. Hypoalbuminaemia can be related to poor nutrition and to the effects of repeated gastrointestinal haemorrhages. Serum transaminases are virtually normal.

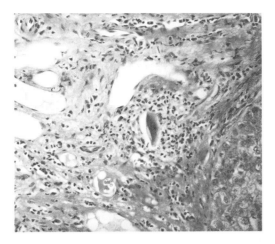

Fig. 27.11. Bilharzial liver. An ovum of *S. Mansoni* has lodged in a portal tract which shows a granulomatous reaction. (Stained H & E, ×64.)

TREATMENT

Chemotherapy [5]

Praziquantel, 40−75 mg per kg once only, is the drug of choice for all forms of schistosomiasis. Side effects are few; they include spasmodic abdominal pain for 1−2 hours and responding to antispasmodic drugs, headache and occasional vomiting. Fever and eosinophilia are also occasional complications.

Oxamniquine 20 mg/kg per day for three days is effective only against *S. mansoni*. Drowsiness, giddiness and headaches are side effects.

Control is by mass education on hygiene and on the avoidance of infected water. Killing the snails is very difficult and the introduction of more effective therapy such as praziquantel, particularly for those excreting the largest number of eggs, will eventually reduce the number of persons responsible for transmitting the disease [5, 6].

Surgery

Oesophageal transection, using the stapler technique (see Chapter 10), controls emergency bleeding in 90% [3].

In the later stages, haemorrhage from oesophageal varices may be treated by porta−caval shunt, usually the selective type [7]. In spite of good pre-operative liver function, the patients often develop encephalopathy after the shunt and, on the whole, these patients are not such good candidates for surgery as might be anticipated. There is a place for repeated endoscopic sclerosis of oesophageal varices [2].

References

1 Alves CAP, Alves AR, Abreu ION *et al.* Hepatic artery hypertrophy and sinusoidal hypertension in advanced schistosomiasis. *Gastroenterology* 1977; **72:** 126.
2 Bessa SM, Helmy I. Injection sclerotherapy for esophageal varices caused by schistosomal fibrosis. *Surgery* 1985; **97:** 164.
3 Bessa SM, Helmy I, Haman SM *et al.* Esophageal transection by the EEA stapler for bleeding esophageal varices in schistosomal hepatic fibrosis. *Surg. Gyn. Obstet.* 1988; **166:** 17.
4 Biempica L, Dunn MA, Kamel IA *et al.* Liver collagen-type characterization in human schistosomiasis. *Am. J. trop. Med. Hyg.* 1983; **32:** 316.
5 Davis A. Recent advances in schistosomiasis. *Q. J. Med.* 1986; **58:** 95.
6 De Cock KM. Hepatosplenic schistosomiasis: a clinical review. *Gut* 1986; **27:** 734.
7 Ezzat FA, Aly MA, Bahgat OO *et al.* Distal splenorenal shunt for management of variceal bleeding in patients with schistosomal hepatic fibrosis. *Ann. Surg.* 1986; **204:** 566.
8 Fataar S, Bassiony H, Satyanath S. CT of hepatic schistosomiasis mansoni. *Am. J. Roentgenol.* 1985; **145:** 63.
9 Sleigh AC, Mott KE, Hoff R *et al.* Three year prospective study of the evolution of Manson's schistosomiasis in North-East Brazil. *Lancet* 1985; *ii:* 63.
10 Warren KS. Regulation of the prevalence and intensity of schistosomiasis in man: immunology or ecology? *J. infect. Dis.* 1973; *127:* 595.

Malaria

In the *erythrocytic stage*, the parasite is engulfed by reticulo-endothelial cells. The liver suffers from the general effects of the toxaemia and pyrexia [1].

The *pre-erythrocytic stage* (exo-erythrocytic) schizogony takes place in the liver without obvious effect on its function. The hepatocyte is invaded by the sporozoite. The nucleus of the parasite divides many times and, at last (in 6–12 days according to the species), a spherical or irregular body containing thousands of ripe merozoites is formed. This pre-erythrocytic schizont bursts and the merozoites are discharged into the sinusoids and invade red blood corpuscles. In quartan or benign tertian malaria, a few merozoites return to the liver cells to initiate the exo-erythrocytic or relapse cycle. In malignant tertian this does not happen and there are no true relapses. So far only *P. falciparum* and *P. vivax* have been found in the liver of man. The tissue stage of human malaria is confined to the liver cells.

PATHOLOGICAL CHANGES

Liver biopsy studies show reticulo-endothelial proliferation, both of Kupffer cells and in the portal tracts (zone 1). Focal accumulations of histiocytes, forming non-specific granulomatous lesions, may be seen in the sinusoids. Brown 'malarial' pigmentation, representing iron and haemofuscin, is seen in the Kupffer cells. Malarial parasites are not demonstrable. Hepato-cellular change is slight. The cells may be swollen, with nuclei of variable size and shape and increased mitoses.

The zone 3 necrosis described in malignant (*P. falciparum*) malaria is probably a post-mortem phenomenon. Sinusoids may contain parasitized clumped erythrocytes.

The reaction of the liver to the malarial parasite is reticulo-endothelial, with minor effects on the liver cells. Fibrosis does not follow and malaria is not pre-cirrhotic. The high incidence of cirrhosis in malarial areas may be attributed to other factors operating in the region concerned.

CLINICAL FEATURES

There are usually no clinical features specific for the liver. Occasionally, in acute malignant malaria, there may be mild jaundice, hepatomegaly and tenderness over the liver [2].

HEPATIC FUNCTION CHANGES

The haemolysis and mild liver cell damage are associated with increases of the serum bilirubin concentration, but rarely above 3 mg/dl. Serum transaminases increase slightly.

Reticulo-endothelial proliferation is associated with a rise in the serum globulin concentration.

References

1 Hollingdale MR. Malaria and the liver. *Hepatology* 1985; **5**: 327.
2 Ramachandran S, Perera MVF. Jaundice and hepatomegaly in primary malaria. *J. trop. Med. Hyg.* 1976; **79**: 207.

Kala azar

Leishmaniasis is a reticulo-endothelial disease. Peri-portal cellular infiltrations and macrophage accumulations are scattered throughout the liver and within them the Leishman–Donovan bodies may be identified (fig. 27.12). There is some portal zone fibrosis [1]. The picture is similar in the American, Mediterranean or Oriental types [1].

Kala azar presents with fever, splenomegaly, a firm tender liver, pancytopenia, anaemia and polyclonal gammopathy. Aspiration of the bone marrow is usually positive.

Reference

1 Da Silva JR, De Paola D. Hepatic lesions in American kala-azar: a needle-biopsy study. *Ann. trop. Med. Parasitol.* 1961; **55**: 249.

Hydatid disease

Hydatid disease is due to the larval or cyst stage of infection by the tapeworm. *Echinococcus granulosus*, which lives in dogs. Man, sheep and cattle are intermediate hosts and the dog is the common definitive host.

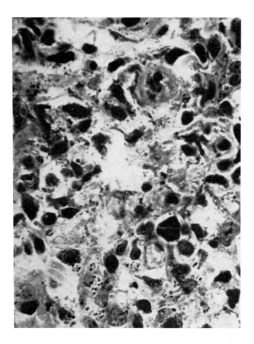

Fig. 27.12. Kala Azar. Leishman–Donovan bodies lying within histiocytic accumulations. (Stained Leishman, ×775.)

BIOLOGY (fig. 27.13)

Man is infected by contact with the excreta of dogs, often during childhood. The dog is infected by eating the viscera of sheep, which contain hydatid cysts. Scolices, contained in the cysts, adhere to the small intestine of the dog and become adult taenia which attach to the intestinal wall. The terminal segment of the worm, the proglottis, contains about 500 ova when shed into the lumen of the bowel. The infected faeces of the dog contaminate grass and farmland, and the contained ova are ingested by sheep, pigs, camels or man. The ova adhere readily to the coats of dogs, so man is infected by handling dogs, as well as by eating contaminated vegetables.

The ova have chitinous envelopes which are dissolved by gastric juice. The liberated ovum burrows through the intestinal mucosa and is carried by the portal vein to the liver, where it develops into an adult cyst. Most cysts are caught in the hepatic sinusoids and, in fact, 70% of eventual hydatid cysts are in the liver. A few ova pass through the liver and right side of the heart and are held up in the pulmonary capillary bed and so give rise to pulmonary hydatid cysts. A few ova reach the general systemic circulation, giving rise to cysts in such organs as spleen, brain and bone.

THE DEVELOPMENT OF THE HEPATIC CYST (fig. 27.14)

In the course of its slow development from the ovum, the adult cyst provokes a *cellular response* in which three zones can be distinguished—a peripheral zone of fibroblasts, an intermediate layer of endothelial cells, and an inner zone of round cells and eosinophils.

The peripheral zone, derived from the host tissues, becomes the *adventitia* or ectocyst, a thick layer which may calcify. The intermediate and inner zones become hyalinized (the *laminated layer*). Finally, the cyst becomes lined with the *germinal layer*, which gives rise to pedunculated nodes of multiplying cells which project into the lumen of the cyst as *brood capsules*. Scolices develop from the brood capsules and eventually indent it. The attachment of the brood capsules to the germinal layer becomes progressively thinner until the capsule bursts, releasing the scolices into the cyst fluid. These fall to the bottom by gravity and are termed *hydatid sand*. When ingested by the dog, the cycle begins again.

The cyst fluid is a transudate of serum. It contains protein and is antigenic. If released into the circulation eosinophilia or anaphylaxis may result.

Daughter and even granddaughter cysts develop by fragmentation of the germinal layer. The majority of cysts in adult patients are thus multilocular.

ENDEMIC REGIONS

The disease is common in sheep-raising countries, where dogs have access to infected offal. These include South Australia, New Zealand, Africa, South America, southern

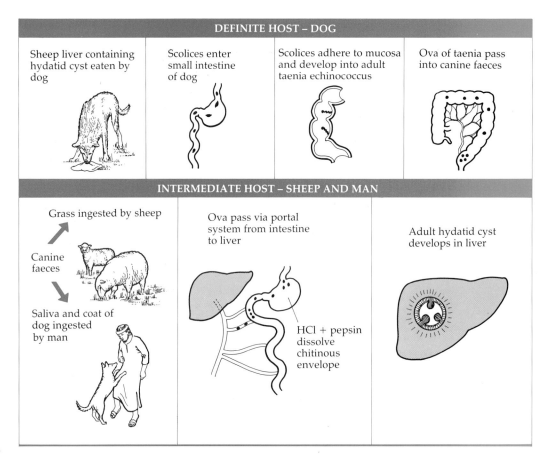

Fig. 27.13. The life cycle of the hydatid parasite (Douglas 1948).

Europe, especially Cyprus, Greece and Spain and the Middle and Far East. The disease is rare in in Britain, apart from some areas in Wales. The disease in Alaska and northern Canada may be more benign.

THE DISTRIBUTION OF CYSTS IN THE LIVER

Hydatid cysts usually involve the right lobe on its antero-inferior or postero-inferior surface. If the right lobe is involved anteriorly, the costal margin is pushed forward; if posteriorly, the diaphragm is pushed upwards. When the left lobe is involved, it is usually anterior and the swelling presents in the epigastrium.

CLINICAL FEATURES

These depend on the site, the stage of development and whether the cyst is alive or dead.

The rest of the liver hypertrophies and hepatomegaly results.

The *uncomplicated hydatid cyst* may be silent and found incidentally at autopsy. It should be suspected if a rounded, smooth swelling, continuous with the liver, is found in a patient who is not obviously ill. The only complaints may be a dull ache in the right upper quadrant and sometimes a feeling of abdominal distension. The tension in the cyst is always high and fluctuation is never marked.

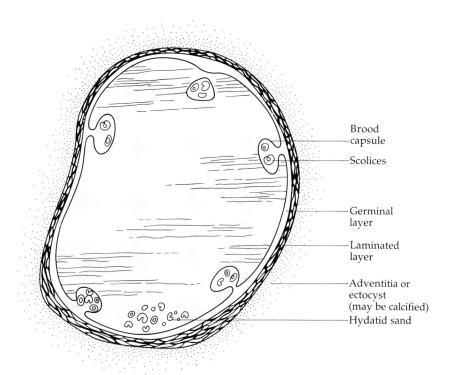

Brood capsule
Scolices
Germinal layer
Laminated layer
Adventitia or ectocyst (may be calcified)
Hydatid sand

Fig. 27.14. The basic constitution of a hydatid cyst.

COMPLICATIONS

Rupture. Intra-peritoneal rupture is frequent and leads to multiple cysts throughout the peritoneal cavity with intestinal obstruction and gross abdominal distension.

The pressure in the cyst greatly exceeds that in bile and rupture into bile ducts is frequent. This may lead to cure or to cholestatic jaundice with recurrent cholangitis.

Colonic rupture leads to elimination *per rectum* and to secondary infection.

The cysts may adhere to the diaphragm, rupture into the lungs and result in expectoration of daughter cysts. Pressure on and rupture into the hepatic veins leads to the Budd–Chiari syndrome. Secondary involvement of the lungs may follow.

Infection. Secondary invasion by pyogenic organisms follows rupture into biliary passages, giving the picture of a pyogenic abscess; the parasite dies. Occasionally, the entire cyst content undergoes aseptic necrosis and again the parasite dies. This amorphous yellow debris must be distinguished from the pus of secondary infection.

Other organs. Cysts can occur in lung, kidney, spleen, brain or bone, but mass infestation is rare in man; the liver is usually the only organ involved. If a hydatid cyst is found elsewhere, there is always concomitant infestation of the liver.

Hydatid allergy. Cyst fluid contains a fine protein which sensitizes the host. This may lead to severe anaphylactic shock but more commonly leads to recurrent urticaria or 'hives'.

Membranous glomerulitis may be related to glomerular deposits of hydatid antigen [5].

DIAGNOSIS

Serological tests

Hydatid fluid contains specific antigens, leak-age of which sensitizes the patient with the production of antibodies.

The Casoni skin test has been abandoned because of non-specificity and difficulty in obtaining satisfactory test fluid.

The indirect haemagglutination test and complement fixation tests are positive in about 85% of patients.

All serological tests can give false negative and false positive results.

Results may be negative for all tests if the cyst has never leaked, if it contains no scolices or if the parasite is dead.

Eosinophilia of greater than 7% is found in about 30% of patients.

Radiological changes

These include a raised, poorly moving right diaphragm, hepatomegaly and calcification. Calcium is laid down in the ectocyst as a dis-tinct round or oval opacity (fig. 27.15) or merely as shreds. Other rare causes of hepatic calcifi-cation include haemangioma, primary liver cancer, tuberculoma, intra-hepatic gallstones, amoebic abscess and gumma. Calcification in adjacent structures such as suprarenal, kidney, gallbladder, peritoneum, diaphragm, costal cartilages and in an old subphrenic abscess must be excluded.

Floating bodies are occasionally seen within hydatid cysts, indicating the presence of free-moving daughter cysts. Infected gas-containing cysts may show a fluid level.

Hepatic cysts may cause displacement of ad-joining structures such as the stomach or hepatic flexure of the colon.

Characteristic radiological changes may be seen in the lungs, spleen, kidney or bone.

Selective coeliac angiography shows stretch-ing and elongation of the hepatic arteries and avascular areas in the hepatogram.

Ultrasound or CT scanning demonstrates

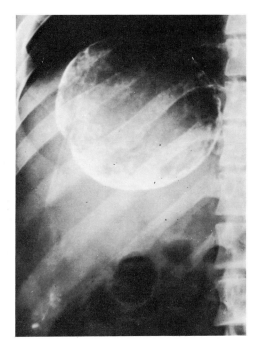

Fig. 27.15. X-ray of the abdomen shows a calcified hydatid cyst in the liver.

cysts which may be single or multiple, uni- or multi-located, thin or thick walled (figs 27.16, 27.17, 27.18). Infected cysts are poorly defined. Hydatid cysts may also be shown by MR imaging [4]. Portable US scanners may be used for mass screening in endemic areas [8].

ERCP may show cysts in the bile ducts (fig. 27.19).

Exploratory aspiration is dangerous because of a risk of anaphylaxis and peritoneal dis-semination. Fine needle aspiration can be used to obtain diagnostic fluid.

Needle liver biopsy is absolutely contra-indicated.

PROGNOSIS

The uncomplicated hepatic hydatid cyst carries a reasonably good prognosis. The risk of complications is, however, always present. Intra-peritoneal or intrapleural rupture is grave, but rupture into the biliary tree is not so serious

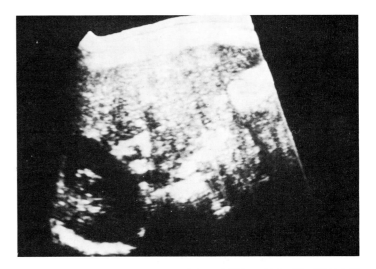

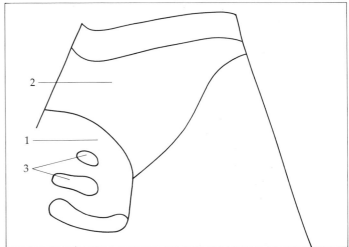

Fig. 27.16. Ultrasound shows a hydatid cyst (1) in the right lobe of the liver (2). Daughter cysts (3) can be seen inside the larger cyst.

because spontaneous cure may follow the biliary colic. Infection used to be fatal, but the outlook is now improved by chemotherapy. Calcification is unwelcome if surgery is attempted, because of the difficulty in collapsing the cyst cavity.

TREATMENT

Dogs are denied access to infected offal and hands are washed after handling dogs. Dogs in affected areas must be regularly de-wormed.

The risks of rupture and secondary infection are so great that unless they are small and

multiple, hepatic hydatids should be treated surgically if the patient's condition permits. There is no completely satisfactory surgical approach but the operation is best performed by an expert in management. The object is to remove the cyst completely, without soiling and infecting the peritoneum, and with complete obliteration of the resulting dead space. Complete removal of the cyst, with its adventitia, is ideal to avoid spilling the contents.

The cyst is first aspirated through its most superficial part (detected by scanning) and alcohol, 20% saline or silver nitrate injected into it as a scolicidal agent. Sclerosing cholangitis

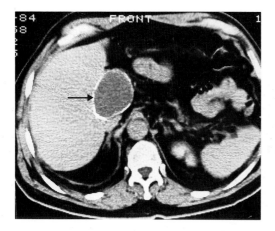

Fig. 27.17. CT scan shows calcified hydatid cyst (arrow) in quadrate lobe of the liver (contrast-enhanced scan).

can complicate injection of these agents particularly if formalin is used and this has now been abandoned [12].

The usual operation is cystectomy with removal of the germinal and laminated layers and preservation of the host-derived ectocyst [6]. The ectocyst cavity, left after removal of the parasitic endocyst, is difficult to obliterate. The choice lies between leaving it open (with or without a drain), tightly closing it after filling it with saline, or doing omentoplasty.

Radical pericystectomy is more complex and haemorrhagic.

Occasionally, the cyst is removed by hemi-hepatectomy or segmentectomy. Recurrence is the major complication and is usually due to spillage at operation. Serial scans are used in follow-up.

Cholangitis is treated by biliary drainage, usually by endoscopy with papillotomy and cyst removal. Otherwise, a surgical biliary drain may be necessary. The technical problem is great.

Rupture into the peritoneal cavity

The cyst contents are removed from the peritoneal cavity as far as possible by sucking and swabbing. The scolices, however, usually settle down in the peritoneal cavity and form daughter cysts so that recurrence is almost inevitable.

MEDICAL TREATMENT

Mebendazole diffuses through the cyst membrane and interferes with glucose metabolism and microtubular function in the parasite. Clinical improvement and reduction in cyst size have followed 400–600 mg daily for 21–30 days. However, viable cysts can persist even

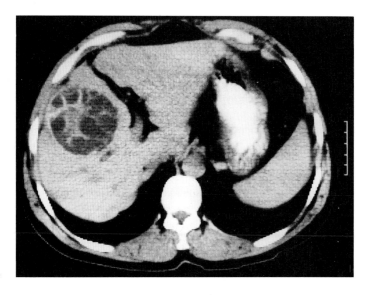

Fig. 27.18. CT scan shows hydatid cyst in right lobe of liver showing patchy calcification of the wall and containing multiple septae produced by daughter cysts (contrast enhanced scan).

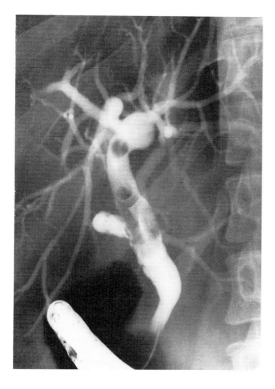

Fig. 27.19. Endoscopic cholangiography shows hydatid cysts in the common bile duct.

in hydatid disease of the liver. *Gastrointest. Radiol.* 1987; **12**: 39.

5 Ibarrola AS, Sobrini B, Guisantes J *et al.* Membranous glomerulonephritis secondary to hydatid disease. *Am. J. Med.* 1981; **70**: 311.

6 Langer B. Surgical treatment of hydatid disease of the liver. *Br. J. Surg.* 1987; **74**: 237.

7 Luder PJ, Witassek F, Weigand K *et al.* Treatment of cystic echinococcosis (echinococcus granulosus) with mebendazole: assessment of bound and free drug levels in cyst fluid and of parasite vitality in operative specimens. *Eur. J. Clin. Pharmacol.* 1985; **28**: 279.

8 Macpherson CNL, Romig T, Zeyhle E *et al.* Portable ultrasound scanner versus serology in screening for hydatid cysts in a nomadic population. *Lancet* 1987; **ii**: 259.

9 Manivel JC, Bloomer JR, Snover DC. Progressive bile duct injury after thiabendazole administration. *Gastroenterology* 1987; **93**: 245.

10 Morris DL, Chinnery JB, Georgiou G *et al.* Penetration of albendazole sulphoxide into hydatid cysts. *Gut* 1987; **28**: 75.

11 Saimot AG, Meulemans A, Cremieux AC *et al.* Albendazole as a potential treatment for human hydatidosis. *Lancet* 1983; **ii**: 652.

12 Teres J, Gomez-Moli J, Bruguera M *et al.* Sclerosing cholangitis after surgical treatment of hepatic echinococcal cysts: report of three cases. *Am. J. Surg.* 1984; **148**: 694.

after twelve months' therapy [7]. Recurrence is not unusual and the concentration of drug achieved in large cysts is very uncertain. Albendazole is also said to be effective, and with less toxicity [11]. It freely diffuses across parasitic membranes [10].

Thiabendazole is also used but can cause progressive bile duct injury [9].

Medical treatment has not replaced surgery.

References

1 Beggs I. The radiology of hydatid disease. *Am. J. Roentgenol.* 1985; **145**: 639.

2 Douglas DM. Hydatid disease. *Edinb. med. J.* 1948; **55**: 78.

3 Gemmell MA, Lawson JR, Roberts MG. Control of echinococcosis/hydatidosis: present status of worldwide progress. *Bull. World Health Org.* 1986; **64** (3): 333.

4 Hoff FL, Aisen AM, Walden ME *et al.* MR imaging

Ascariasis

The roundworm *Ascaris humbricoides* is large (10–20 cm long) and usually too big to enter the biliary passages. Occasionally, however, it lodges in the common bile duct and produces partial bile duct obstruction and secondary cholangitic abscesses [2, 3].

Ova segment in the liver having arrived via the portal vein or possibly by retrograde flow in the bile ducts. They exert an immunological granulomatous reaction and eggs, giant cells and granulomas are surrounded by a dense eosinophil infiltrate (fig. 27.20).

Ascaris infestation is particularly common in the Far East, India and South Africa. The ascaris may be a nucleus for intra-hepatic gallstone formation [6]. Biliary colic is a complication.

The worm usually dies in the common bile duct and may even calcify, when it can be demonstrated in a plain X-ray of the abdomen.

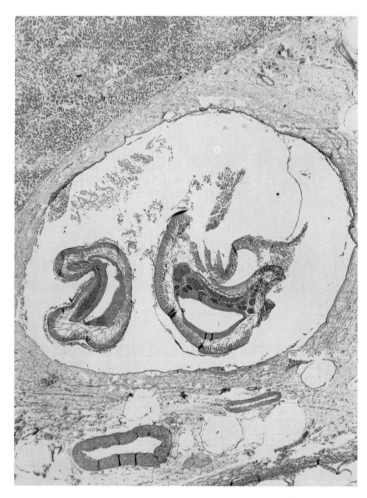

Fig. 27.20. Section shows a dead ascaris in an intrahepatic blood vessel in a portal zone. There is surrounding fibrous tissue reaction. (Stained H & E, ×40.)

Haemobilia may complicate biliary ascariasis and also secondary hepatic abscess formation [5].

Ultrasound shows long linear echogenic structures or strips which characteristically move [3]. *Endoscopic* cholangiography shows the ascaris as a linear filling defect (fig. 27.21). Worms can be seen moving into and out of the biliary tree from the duodenum [1].

Treatment with piperazine citrate (75 mg/kg daily for two days maximum 3.5 g) will usually kill the ascaris but the worm remains in the bile ducts. Endoscopic removal after papillotomy is usually possible. If necessary, piperazine may be given into the biliary tree by a nasobiliary tube [1].

References

1 Kamath PS, Joseph DC, Chandran R *et al.* Biliary ascariasis: ultrasonography, endoscopic retrograde cholangiopancreatography, and biliary drainage. *Gastroenterology* 1986; **91:** 730.

2 Khuroo MS, Ali Zargar S. Biliary ascariasis. A common cause of biliary and pancreatic disease in an endemic area. *Gastroenterology* 1985; **88:** 418.

3 Khuroo MS, Ali Zargar S, Mahajan R *et al.* Sonographic appearances in biliary ascariasis. *Gastroenterology* 1987; **93:** 267.

4 Manialawi MS, Khattar NY, Helmy MM *et al.* Endoscopic diagnosis and extraction of biliary ascaris. *Endoscopy* 1986; **18:** 204.

5 Rosenbaum JM, Johnston C. Hemobilia with multiple liver abscesses and ascariasis. *Am. J. Dis. Child.* 1966; **112:** 82.

6 Shulman A. Non-Western patterns of biliary stones and the role of ascariasis. *Radiology* 1987; **162:** 425.

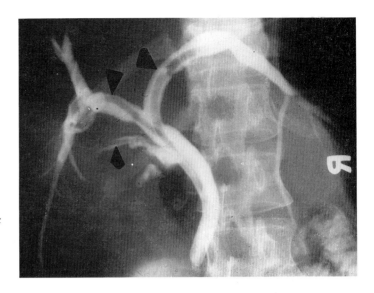

Fig. 27.21. *Asciariasis*: Endoscopic cholangiography shows linear filling defects in the bile ducts due to ascaris worms (Khuroo *et al.* 1985).

Trichiniasis

This disease is caused by eating raw, infected pork with subsequent dissemination of trichinella larvae throughout the body.

Hepatic histology may show invasion of hepatic sinusoids by trichinella larvae and fatty change [1].

Diagnosis is difficult unless it occurs in an epidemic. The presence of eosinophilia is suggestive. Muscle pain and tenderness may warrant muscle biopsy.

Treatment. Laparotomy is indicated if the biliary tract is obstructed. Treatment on the whole is unsatisfactory. Mebendazole may be effective in the migratory stage but is of doubtful value later.

Reference

1 Guattery JM, Milne J, House RK. Observations on hepatic and renal dysfunction in trichinosis. Anatomic changes in these organs occurring in cases of trichinosis. *Am. J. Med.* 1956; **21**: 567.

Toxocara canis (visceral larva migrans)

This parasite is spread by cats and dogs. The second stage can infect the liver of man, forming granulomas [1]. Hepatomegaly, recurrent pneumonia, eosinophilia and hypergamma-globulinaemia are associated findings. The serum fluorescent antibody test is positive.

Treatment may be tried with diethyl carbamazine or thiabendazole.

Reference

1 Zinkham WH. Visceral larva migrans. *Am J. Dis. Child.* 1978; **132**: 627.

Liver flukes

Cysts are consumed and larvae develop in the duodenum and eventually reach the bile ducts. Their route is uncertain. They might invade the biliary passages from the duodenum against the direction of biliary flow. The flukes probably invade the liver through its peritoneal coat and are carried via the parenchyma to the bile ducts. During the migratory phase they cause fever and eosinophilia. When they reach the biliary passages they may cause obstruction, the clinical picture simulating choledocholithiasis with complicating suppurative cholangitis.

CLONORCHIS SINENSIS

The Chinese liver fluke is found mainly in eastern Asia. It can present years after the patient has left his country of origin as the biliary flukes persist for decades. It gains access to the body by the ingestion of cysts contained in improperly cooked or raw fish. In uncomplicated cases the changes are confined to the walls of the bile duct with abundant adenomatous formation; fibrosis increases with time. Cholangiocarcinoma is a serious complication [6].

Complications arise from obstruction to the main bile ducts with secondary infection, usually by *E. coli*, followed by intra-hepatic stone formation, cholangitis and multiple abscess formation. Percutaneous cholangiography has been used to show the flukes. Faeces contain the ova.

FASCIOLA HEPATICA

The common sheep fluke is found mostly in mid- and western Europe and in the Caribbean. The animal infestation rate in Britain is high: 30–90% of all sheep and cattle excrete the ova. This increases in wet summers when the intermediate host, the snail *Lymnaea trunculata*, is also more numerous. The encysted cercariae from these snails survive on herbage and patients are affected usually by eating contaminated watercress.

The clinical picture in the acute stage is of cholangitis with fever, right upper quadrant pain and hepatomegaly. Eosinophilia and a raised serum alkaline phosphatase are noted. The picture may simulate choledocholithiasis.

Percutaneous or endoscopic *cholangiography* shows several irregular linear or rounded filling defects in the bile ducts or segmental stenosis, with an inflammatory pattern [2]. Worms can be aspirated in bile.

Liver biopsy shows infiltration of the portal zones with histiocytes, eosinophils and polymorphs. Hepatic granulomas and ova in the liver may occasionally be seen [4].

Diagnosis is suspected by finding the clinical picture of biliary tract disease with eosinophilia [4]. It is confirmed by finding ova in the faeces. These, however, may not be detected until twelve weeks after the infection when parasites have attained sexual maturity. They disappear later. The serum fasciola complement fixation test is positive [4].

CT shows peripheral filling defects, sometimes crescentic, in the liver due to the migrating fluke (fig. 27.22) [5].

Treatment of all liver flukes is by praziquantel 25 mg/kg three times a day for one day, or bithionol 30–50 mg/kg on alternate days for 10–15 doses.

Treatment of intra-hepatic stones is difficult. They are usually unaffected by biliary solvents. Endoscopic papillotomy may be useful in high risk patients [1]. Endoprostheses inserted trans-hepatically or endoscopically may be useful to treat biliary obstruction [7]. Surgery may be necessary.

References

1 Choi TK, Wong J. Endoscopic retrograde cholangiopancreatography and endoscopic papillotomy in recurrent pyogenic cholangitis. *Clin. Gastroenterol.* 1986; **15**: 393.

2 Condomines J, Reñe-Espinet JM, Espinos-Perez JC et al. Percutaneous cholangiography in the diagnosis of hepatic fascioliasis. *Am. J. Gastroenterol.* 1985; **80**: 384.

3 Hou PC, Pang LSC. *Clonorchis sinensis* infestation in man in Hong Kong. *J. Pathol. Bact.* 1964; **87**: 245.

4 Jones AE, Kay JM, Milligan HP et al. Massive infection with fasciola hepatica in man. *Am. J. Med.* 1977; **63**: 836.

5 Pagola Serrano MA, Vega A, Ortega E et al. Computed tomography of hepatic fascioliasis. *J. Comp. Assist. Tomogr.* 1987; **11**: 269.

6 Schwartz DA. Cholangiocarcinoma associated with liver fluke infection: a preventable source of morbidity in Asian immigrants. *Am. J. Gastroenterol.* 1986; **81**: 76.

7 Van Sonnenberg E, Casola G, Cubberley DA et al. Oriental cholangio-hepatitis: diagnostic imaging and interventional management. *Am. J. Roentgenol.* 1986; **146**: 327.

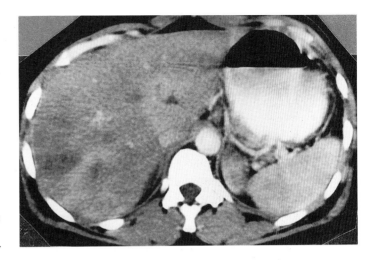

Fig. 27.22. Fascioliasis hepatica: CT in the migratory stage shows multiple, sometimes linear, filling defects at the periphery of the liver (courtesy A.T. McCormack).

Peri-hepatitis

This upper abdominal peritonitis is associated with genital infections, particularly *C. trachomatis* and *N. gonorrhoeae* [1]. It affects young, sexually active women and simulates biliary tract disease. Diagnosis is by laparoscopy. The liver surface shows white plaques, tiny haemorrhagic spots and 'violin string' adhesions.

Reference

1 Simson JNL. Chlamydial perihepatitis (Curtis–Fitz–Hugh syndrome) after hydrotubation. *Br. med. J.* 1984; **289:** 1146.

Hepato-biliary changes in the acquired immunodeficiency syndrome (AIDS)

There are probably no direct effects of HIV (human immunodeficiency virus) on the liver. Many diseases, however, affect the immunodeficient and provide a confusing picture. All parts of the hepato-biliary system can show changes and may be involved by more than one process (table 27.2). In general, there is little difference in the hepato-biliary disease seen in the homosexual, drug abuser, or blood product-related AIDS except for the prevalence of B markers. The hepato-biliary system is usually involved as part of the general disease.

Liver biopsy is often done in AIDS patients. However, this rarely influences therapy or leads to improved survival [11] and is rarely diagnostic. Liver involvement does not contribute significantly to morbidity or mortality [4]. However, once AIDS-specific changes, such as *Mycobacterium avium intra-cellulare* (MAI), are seen in liver biopsies, the mean survival is only 69 days.

NON-SPECIFIC HEPATIC CHANGES

These are related to chronic debilitating disease. Hepatomegaly and fever are frequent. Serum shows an increase in transaminases (up to four times) and in alkaline phosphatase.

Hepatic histology shows macrovesicular fat and mild portal and peri-portal lymphocytes [5]. Occasionally Kupffer cells contain iron and focal necrosis may be seen. On the whole lymphocytes are deficient. Granulomas are frequent.

INFECTIONS

These are largely opportunistic and part of generalized infection. Liver biopsy in patients with hepatomegaly, fever and abnormal biochemical tests gives the cause in about 25% [6].

Table 27.2. Hepato-biliary changes in AIDS

Non-specific
  Hepatomegaly
  Abnormal biochemistry
  Histology:
    fatty change
    portal inflammation
    Kupffer cell iron
    diminished lymphocytes

Infections
  Mycobacterium avium-intracellulare
  Mycobacterium tuberculosis
  Cytomegalovirus
  Herpes simplex
  Epstein–Barr
  *Cryptococcus neoformans**
  Histoplasmosis
  *Candida albicans**
  Coccidiomycosis
  Microsporidia*
  Toxoplasmosis

Hepatitis B
  Impaired response to vaccine and antiviral therapy
  Fulminant rare

Tumours
  Hodgkin's and non-Hodgkin's lymphoma
  Kaposi sarcoma (rare)

Hepatotoxic drugs
  Sulphonamides
  Antibiotics
  Isoniazid
  Antifungals
  Tranquillizers

* Associated biliary tract disease

Mycobacterium avium intracellulare is the most commonly diagnosed hepatic infection. It is shown by poorly formed granulomas without lymphocyte cuffing, giant cells or central caseation. Staining for acid-fast baccili shows the presence of large numbers in clusters of foamy histiocytes or within Kupffer cells (figs 27.23, 27.24). The bacilli can be seen without the presence of granulomas. *Cytomegalovirus* and *herpes simplex* infections are usually part of disseminated disease. Granulomas can be seen.

Diagnosis is made by demonstrating the large intranuclear and small cytoplasmic inclusions in Kupffer cells, bile duct epithelium and, occasionally, hepatocytes. *Epstein–Barr virus* can also cause hepatic changes, particularly in children [3]. The picture is usually that of an acute hepatitis but occasionally may be markedly cholestatic.

Fungal infections are usually part of disseminated disease. They include *Cryptococcosis neoformans*, histoplasmosis and coccidiomycosis and *Candida albicans*. The protozoan, *Microsporidia*, can cause hepatitis and may be diagnosed only by electron microscopy [14]. *Abnormalities of the biliary tract* including intra- and extra-hepatic sclerosing cholangitis [8], papillary stenosis [11] and acalculous cholecystitis [2] have been associated with cryptosporidial (fig. 27.25), cytomegalovirus and microsporidial infections [14].

RELATION TO HEPATITIS B

In homosexuals or drug abuser patients with AIDS, markers of past or present HBV infection are found in approximately 90%. Those positive for HBsAg tend to be HBe antigen positive despite having minimal biochemical and histological evidence of inflammation [10]. Delta is present depending on the location [13]. They respond poorly to hepatitis B vaccination [1] and to antiviral treatment [9].

Fulminant hepatitis has not been reported in AIDS patients.

DRUG-RELATED LIVER INJURY

AIDS patients are exposed to many potential hepatotoxins including sulphonamides, antibiotics, anti-fungals and tranquillizers [6]. This adds complexity to the diagnosis of an AIDS patient presenting with fever and abnormal biochemical tests of liver function.

TUMOURS

Kaposi's sarcoma frequently involves the liver, but is usually detected at autopsy rather than

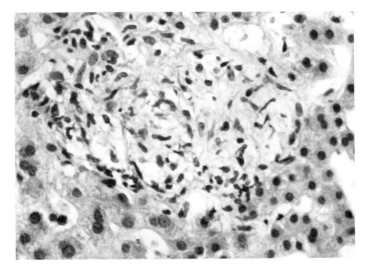

Fig. 27.23. An ill-defined poorly cellular granuloma in the liver of a patient with AIDS. (Stained H & E, ×220.)

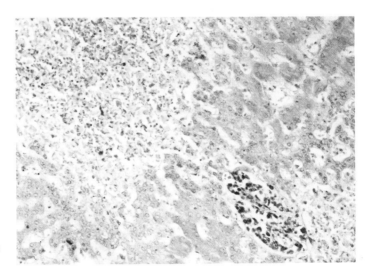

Fig. 27.24. Same patient. Liver stained for acid-fat bacilli shows two granulomas containing many red-staining bacilli (*Mycobacterium avian intracellulare*).

by biopsy. It is shown macroscopically as purple-brown, soft nodules. Histology shows multifocal areas of vascular endothelial proliferation with pleomorphic spindle cells and extravasated erythrocytes.

Non-Hodgkins's lymphoma is of the monoclonal B-cell type [7]. Hepatic granulomas are associated with Hodgkin's and non-Hodgkin's lymphomas.

581

References

1 Carne CA, Weller IVD, Waite J *et al.* Impaired responsiveness of homosexual men with HIV antibodies to plasma derived hepatitis B vaccine. *Br. med. J.* 1987; **294**: 866.
2 Cockerill FR, Hurley DV, Malagelada J−R *et al.* Polymicrobial cholangitis and Kaposi's sarcoma in blood product transfusion-related acquired immune deficiency syndrome. *Am. J. Med.* 1986; **80**: 1237.

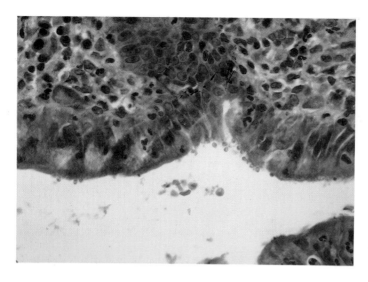

Fig. 27.25. Cryptosporidiosis of the gallbladder in a patient with AIDS. (Stained H & E, ×160.)

3 Duffy LF, Daum F, Kahn E *et al.* Hepatitis in children with acquired immune deficiency syndrome. *Gastroenterology* 1986; **90**: 173.

4 Glasgow BJ, Anders K, Layfield LJ *et al.* Clinical and pathologic findings of the liver in the acquired immune deficiency syndrome (AIDS). *Am. J. clin. Pathol.* 1985; **83**: 582.

5 Gordon SC, Reddy KR, Gould EE *et al.* The spectrum of liver disease in the acquired immunodeficiency syndrome. *J. Hepatol.* 1986; **2**: 475.

6 Lebovics E, Dworkin BM, Heier SK *et al.* The hepatobiliary manifestations of human immunodeficiency virus infection. *Am. J. Gastroenterol.* 1988; **83**: 1.

7 Levine AM, Meyer PR, Begandy MK *et al.* Development of B-cell lymphoma in homosexual men. *Ann. intern. Med.* 1984; **100**: 7.

8 Margulis SJ, Honig CL, Soave R *et al.* Biliary tract obstruction in the acquired immunodeficiency syndrome. *Ann. intern. Med.* 1986; **105**: 207.

9 McDonald JA, Caruso L, Karayiannis P *et al.* Diminished responsiveness of male homosexual chronic hepatitis B carriers with HTLV-111 antibodies to recombinant alpha interferon. *Hepatology* 1987; **7**: 719.

10 Rustgi VK, Hoofnagle JH, Gerin JG *et al.* Hepatitis B virus infection in the acquired immunodeficiency syndrome. *Ann. intern. Med.* 1984; **101**: 795.

11 Schneiderman DJ, Arenson DM, Cello JP *et al.* Hepatic disease in patients with the acquired immune deficiency syndrome (AIDS). *Hepatology* 1987; **7**: 925.

12 Schneiderman DJ, Cello JP, Laing FC. Papillary stenosis and sclerosing cholangitis in the acquired immunodeficiency syndrome. *Ann. intern. Med.* 1987; **106**: 546.

13 Soloman RE, Kaslow RA, Phair JP *et al.* Human immunodeficiency virus and hepatitis delta virus in homosexual men. A study of four cohorts. *Ann. intern. Med.* 1988; **108**: 51.

14 Terada S, Reddy KR, Jeffers LJ *et al.* Microsporidan hepatitis in the acquired immunodeficiency syndrome. *Ann. intern. Med.* 1987; **107**: 61.

Jaundice of infections

BACTERIAL PNEUMONIA

Jaundice is an unusual complication of pneumonia. It is, however, still frequent in Africans, where it may be related partly to haemolysis in those deficient in glucose 6-phosphate dehydrogenase [6]. The jaundice is also both hepato-cellular and cholestatic.

Liver biopsy shows non-specific changes; electron microscopy [5] shows bile canalicular dilatation with loss of microvilli, suggesting cholestasis. There is also evidence of toxic liver injury. Increased numbers of fat-storing lipocytes are seen during the acute stage.

SEPTICAEMIA AND SEPTIC SHOCK

Liver function abnormalities including modest increases in serum alkaline phosphatase, transaminases and bile salts, are not uncommon in patients with severe infections, septicaemia, toxic shock and endotoxaemia [1, 2, 3]. In two-thirds, jaundice is a feature and, if it persists, carries a bad prognosis [1].

Hepatic histology shows non-specific hepatitis including mid-zonal and peripheral necrosis [2]. Cholestasis may be marked and in severe cases is shown as inspissated bile within dilated and proliferated portal and peri-portal bile ductules [4]. Cultures of the liver are sterile.

The causes are multifactorial. Hepatic hypoperfusion plays a part. The cholangiolar lesions might be related to interference with canalicular exchange of water and electrolytes, to endotoxaemia, to staphylococcal exotoxin or to interference with the peribiliary vascular plexus as a result of shock [1, 3].

References

1 Bank JG, Foulis AK, Ledingham I McA *et al.* Liver function in septic shock. *J. clin. Pathol.* 1982; **35:** 1249.
2 Caruana JA Jr, Montes M, Camara DS *et al.* Functional and histopathologic changes in the liver during sepsis. *Surg. Gynecol. Obstet.* 1982; **154:** 653.
3 Gourley GR, Chesney PJ, Davis JP *et al.* Acute cholestasis in patients with toxic-shock syndrome. *Gastroenterology* 1981; **81:** 928.
4 Lefkowitch JH. Bile ductular cholestasis: an ominous histopathologic sign related to sepsis and 'cholangitis tenta'. *Hum. Pathol.* 1982; **13:** 19.
5 Theron JJ, Pepler WJ, Mekel RCPM. Ultrastructure of the liver in Bantu patients with pneumonia and jaundice. *J. Pathol.* 1972; **106:** 113.
6 Tugwell P, Williams AO. Jaundice associated with lobar pneumonia. *Q. J. Med.* 1977; **46:** 97.

28 · Hepatic Tumours

The liver is affected by both simple and malignant growths (table 28.1). The simple ones are usually anatomical curiosities of no clinical importance. Malignant disease of the liver, however, is common, secondary deposits in the liver being much more common than primary cancers.

Hepato-cellular carcinoma

The frequency depends on the geographic area from which statistics are taken (table 28.2). In temperate climates it is a rare condition, being found in under 1% of autopsies. In the East African Bantu, however, four out of every five autopsies show hepato-cellular cancer. The highest frequency is in the African and Oriental races in whom there is nearly always an associated cirrhosis. It is the second commonest cancer encountered in South East Asia. The condition is increasing in the West, and in California the frequency has multiplied three times in 20 years [105].

The importance of the various aetiological factors depends on whether the area is a high or low incidence one.

EXPERIMENTAL LIVER CANCER

A bewildering number of carcinogens can initiate tumours in animals, but their relevance to man is uncertain. They include P-dimethyl-amino-azobenzene (butter yellow), nitrosamines, aflatoxin and senecio alkaloids [35].

There are multiple steps from initiation to progression and finally to expression of the cancer. The carcinogen binds covalently to DNA. The development of cancer depends on the ability of the host to repair the DNA or on its tolerance to the carcinogen.

MYCOTOXINS

The most important mycotoxin is aflatoxin produced by a contaminating mould, *Aspergillus flavus* [31]. It is highly carcinogenic to the rainbow trout, the mouse, the guinea-pig and the monkey. There is variation in the susceptibility of different species. Aflatoxin and similar toxic moulds can readily contaminate food such as ground nuts or grain especially when stored in tropical conditions.

Estimated minimum aflatoxin intake from foods in various areas of Africa correlates with the frequency of primary liver cancer (table 28.3).

It is possible that aflatoxin acts as a co-carcinogen with hepatitis B. It is also possible that aflatoxin suppresses the cellular immune response and may increase the hepatitis B carriage rate, and hence the risk of development of primary liver cancer [79].

RELATION TO CIRRHOSIS

Cirrhosis may be a premalignant condition irrespective of the aetiology [59, 64]; this is understandable. The nodular hyperplasia progresses to carcinoma. Liver cell *dysplasia*, marked by cellular enlargement, nuclear pleomorphism and multinucleate cells affecting groups or whole nodules, may be an intermediate step [2]. Dysplasia is found in 60% of cirrhotic livers harbouring hepato-cellular carcinoma and in only 10% of non-cirrhotic livers. Repetitive mitosis favours carcinogenesis. The liver regeneration might promote carcinogenesis by increased expression of oncogenes. Genetic aberrations of specific oncogenes might lead to malignant transformation of the hepatocyte.

Table 28.1. Primary tumours of the liver

Benign	Malignant
Hepato-cellular	
Adenoma	Hepato-cellular carcinoma
	Fibro-lamellar
	Hepatoblastoma
Biliary	
Adenoma	Cholangiocarcinoma
Cystadenoma	Combined hepato-cellular cholangiocarcinoma
Papillomatosis	Cystadenocarcinoma
Mesodermal	
Haemangioma	Angiosarcoma (haemangio-endothelial sarcoma)
	Epithelioid haemangio-endothelioma
	Sarcoma
Other	
Mesenchymal hamartoma	
Lipoma	
Fibroma	

Table 28.2. Worldwide incidence of primary liver cancer reported by cancer registries (Doll *et al.* 1966)

Area	Rate per 100 000 males per year
Group 1	
Mozambique	98.2
China	17.0
South Africa	14.2
Hawaii	7.2
Nigeria	5.9
Singapore	5.5
Uganda	5.5
Group 2	
Japan	4.6
Denmark	3.4
Group 3	
England and Wales	3.0
USA	2.7
Chile	2.6
Sweden	2.6
Iceland	2.5
Jamaica	2.3
Puerto Rico	2.1
Columbia	2.0
Yugoslavia	1.9

The cirrhosis is usually of large nodule type. In one series of 1073 hepato-cellular carcinomas, 658 (61.3%) also showed cirrhosis. However, in 30% of African patients with hepatitis B-related hepato-cellular cancer, cirrhosis was not present. In the United Kingdom, about 30% of patients with hepato-cellular carcinoma have no cirrhosis and survival is significantly better.

There are pronounced geographical differences in the frequency of cancer in cirrhotic livers [25]. There is a particularly high association in South Africa and Indonesia, where cancer is reported in more than 30% of cirrhotic livers, whereas frequencies of 10–20% are reported from India, Britain and North America.

RELATION TO HEPATITIS B

In 1970 a positive association was reported between liver cell cancer and a positive hepatitis B test [117]. World wide, the problem of hepatitis B carriage correlates with frequency of primary liver cancer [8]. In Britain, for instance, the mortality for primary liver cancer is 1–2 per 100 000 and the carriage rate for hepatitis B surface antigen is 0.1 per 100 000, whereas in

Table 28.3. Aflatoxin ingestion and hepatoma incidence (Linsell & Peers 1977)

Country	Locale	Aflatoxin intake (ng/kg/day)	Hepatoma rate (per 10/year)
Kenya	High altitude	3.5	1.2
Thailand	Songkhla	5.0	2.0
Swaziland	High veld	5.1	2.2
Kenya	Mid-altitude	5.9	2.5
Swaziland	Mid-veld	8.9	3.8
Kenya	Low altitude	10.0	4.0
Swaziland	Lebombo	15.4	4.3
Thailand	Ratburi	45.6	6.0
Swaziland	Low veld	43.1	9.2
Mozambique	Inhambane	222.4	13.0

Table 28.4. Association of HBV with hepato-cellular carcinoma (Lutwick 1979)

Country	Test(s)	Hepatoma associated with HBV (%)	Control associated with HBV (%)*
Uganda	HBsAg	40	1
Taiwan	HBsAG	80	15
USA	HBsAg	21	0.4
Senegal	Anti-HBc	93	42
Hong Kong	Anti-HBc	70	36
USA	Anti-HBc	24	4
Uganda and Zambia	HBsAg, anti-HBs, anti-HBc	96	63
USA	HBsAg, anti-HBs, anti-HBc	74	20
Senegal	HBsAg, anti-HBs, anti-HBc	61	11*

* Control group age and sex matched with either cancer or no cancer.
HBsAg; hepatitis B surface antigen; anti-HBs=antibody to hepatitis B surface antigen; anti-HBc=antibody to hepatitis B core antigen.

China the primary liver cancer mortality is approximately 17 per 100 000 and the hepatitis B antigen carrier rate 7.5–14 per 100 000 (table 28.4).

The incidence of HBsAg positivity is higher in hepato-cellular carcinoma patients compared with a control population or those with other tumours. A prospective study from Taiwan showed that HBsAg positive persons were 390 times more likely to develop hepato-cellular carcinoma than HBsAg negative ones [8].

Populations with a high incidence of HBsAg carriage and primary liver cancer migrating to low incidence areas continue to show evidence of hepatitis infection and a high liver cancer mortality. This has been shown particularly in Chinese-Americans [128].

HBsAg may be negative or in low titre, but anti-HBc is usually present. This is particularly so in African and Asian patients, 95% of whom have a positive anti-HBc. The risk of hepato-cellular cancer is greater when the carrier state is acquired in early life.

Pre-cancerous changes, particularly dysplasia of small cell type, have a strong association with HBsAg [2, 45].

In the hepatitis B positive patient, integration of viral with host DNA may be the initiating event [9]. This induces changes in cellular and HBV gene expression due to either chromo-somal rearrangements or insertional mutagen-esis [12]. The 'initiation' of infected hepatocytes would then be linked to cell regeneration as shown for experimental carcinogenesis (fig. 28.1). Cells with integrated sequences escape the cytotoxic immune effect. Interaction with chemical carcinogens and hormones would favour the clonal proliferation of these hepato-cytes.

The Alexander cell tumour line, derived from a human hepato-cellular cancer, secretes HBsAg [6]. Animals such as the woodchuck [107] or the Peking Duck are infected with viruses simi-lar to hepatitis B (HEPADNA viruses) and also develop hepato-cellular cancer.

STAGES IN HEPATOCELLULAR CANCER

Integration

Division

Co carcinogen

Transformation

Focal clonal growth

CANCER   Autonomy

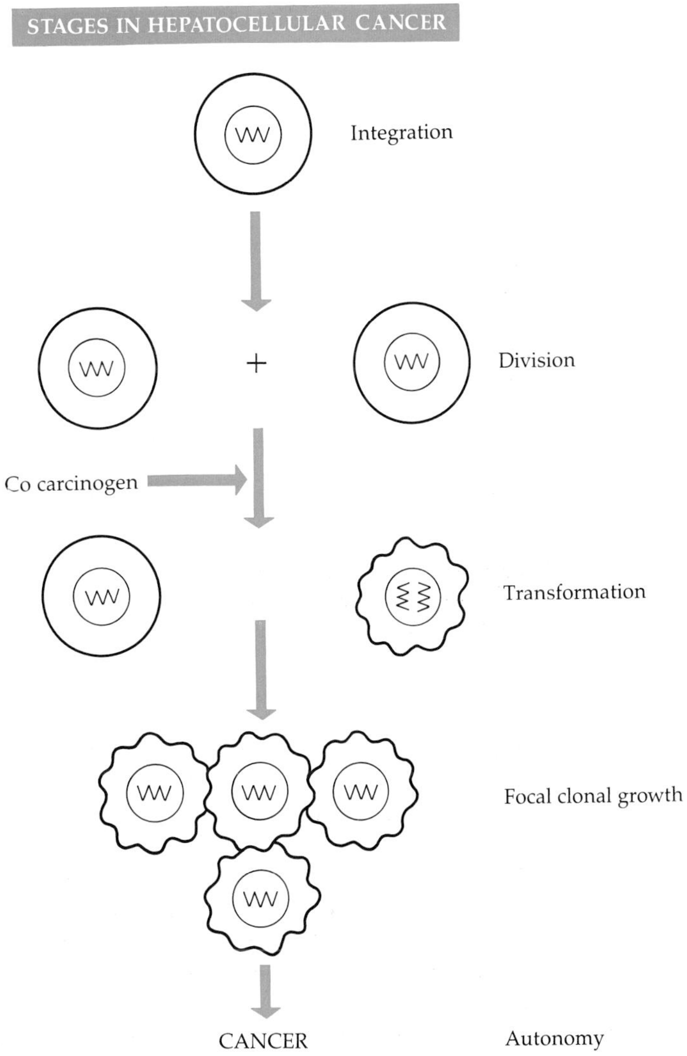

Fig. 28.1. Stages in hepato-cellular cancer in a hepatitis B carrier (Shafitz *et al.*).

587

RELATION TO ALCOHOL

In temperate climates, alcohol has been associated with hepato-cellular cancer, particularly in older patients. There is a fourfold risk of primary hepato-cellular cancer in alcoholics in northern Europe and North America [42]. Cirrhosis is always present and alcohol is probably not a hepatic carcinogen *per se.*

Alcohol may be a co-carcinogen with the hepatitis B virus (fig. 28.2). Hepatitis B markers are highly prevalent in alcoholic cirrhotic patients complicated by hepato-cellular cancer. Alcohol-mediated enzyme induction may increase the conversion of co-carcinogens to carcinogens, so contributing to hepato-carcinogenesis. Alcohol may also promote carcinogenesis through depression of immune responses. Carcinogen-mediated DNA alkylation is impaired by alcohol.

The development of hepato-cellular cancer in alcoholic cirrhotics is sometimes accompanied by the finding of integrated hepatitis B viral DNA in malignantly transformed hepatocytes [12]. However, hepato-cellular cancer can develop in alcoholics with no evidence of past or present hepatitis B infection.

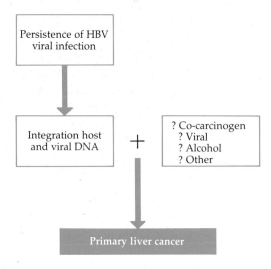

Fig. 28.2. Factors leading to the development of primary liver cancer in the hepatitis B-positive patient.

RACE AND SEX

There is no clear evidence of genetic predisposition. In particular, HLA antigens fail to show a relationship either to hepato-cellular carcinoma or to hepatitis B infection [63].

World wide, hepato-cellular cancer is three times more frequent in males than females. This may partly be due to the higher carriage rate of hepatitis B in males. Expression of androgen receptors on cancerous hepatocytes may be augmented and oestrogen receptors suppressed [96]. The significance of this in terms of hormone dependence remains uncertain.

SEX HORMONE THERAPY

See Chapter 18.

MISCELLANEOUS FACTORS

Hepato-cellular cancer is a rare complication of autoimmune chronic active hepatitis and cirrhosis [14].

It is also rare in patients with Wilson's disease or primary biliary cirrhosis [136].

Hepato-cellular cancer is a frequent cause of death in haemochromatosis. It is increased in α_1-antitrypsin deficiency [32] and type 1 glycogen storage disease.

Hepato-cellular cancer can complicate massive immuno-suppressive therapy in patients having renal transplants.

HBsAg positive patients infected with the delta agent have a reduced incidence of hepato-cellular cancer, perhaps because the course is more severe and death supervenes before the cancer has had time to develop [108].

The association of hepato-cellular cancer with non-A, non-B virus infection is uncertain. Cases have been reported after post-transfusion non-A, non-B hepatitis [67, 75, 110].

Clonorchiasis may be followed by hepato-cellular and cholangio-cellular carcinoma.

The relationship between schistosomiasis and liver cancer has not been established.

In Africa and Japan, hepato-cellular cancer is

associated with membranous obstruction to the inferior vena cava [121].

In HBsAg negative patients, tobacco smoking is a dose-dependent risk factor for hepato-cellular cancer [132].

Conclusions

World wide, hepatitis B is the most important factor for the development of hepato-cellular cancer. Co-factors contribute. However, in low prevalence areas, other factors are concerned [60, 140]. In the United Kingdom, for instance, 40% are found in the absence of detectable markers of present or past hepatitis B infection [28]. The mechanisms in such cases and in particular the role of cirrhosis *per se* remain obscure.

Pathology

The tumour is usually white, sometimes necrotic, bile stained or haemorrhagic. Large hepatic or portal veins within the liver are often thrombosed and contain tumour. The morphological division is into three types: expanding with discrete margins, spreading (infiltrative) and multifocal [96]. The expanding type tends to affect the non-cirrhotic liver and in Japan may be encapsulated. In the West and Africa, most tumours are either spreading or multifocal.

Hepato-cellular carcinoma (figs 28.3, 28.4)

The cells resemble normal liver, with compact finger-like processes or solid trabeculae. The tumour simulates normal liver with varying degrees of success. The cells sometimes secrete bile and contain glycogen. There is no inter-cellular stroma and the tumour cells line the blood spaces.

The tumour cell is usually smaller than the normal liver cell; it is polygonal, with granular cytoplasm. Occasionally, atypical giant cells are found. The cytoplasm is eosinophilic, becoming basophilic with increasing malignancy. The nuclei are hyperchromatic and vary in size. Predominantly eosinophilic tumours may

sometimes be seen. The centres of the tumours are often necrotic. Peri-portal lymphatic involvement with malignant cells is an early feature. PAS positive, diastase resistant globular inclusions are found in about 15%, usually in those with high α-fetoprotein levels [19]. They may represent hepatocyte-produced glyco-proteins. α1-antitrypsin and α-fetoprotein have also been shown.

It may be extremely difficult to differentiate simple from malignant hepatic tumours. All gradations exist from benign to malignant hepato-cellular tumours. Dysplasia is an intermediate appearance [2]. The small dysplastic cell may be particularly precancerous [45].

Electron microscopy. 'Cytoplasmic' hyaline is described in human hepato-cellular carcinoma cells [62]. The cytoplasmic inclusions are filamentous bodies and also autophagic vacuoles.

Clear cell hepato-cellular carcinoma

Histology shows tumour cells with clear non-staining cytoplasm, often foamy or vacuolated. Lipids, and sometimes glycogen are present in

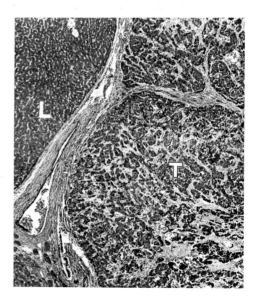

Fig. 28.3. Hepato-cellular carcinoma. The tumour cells (T) are arranged in trabeculae simulating normal liver which is seen on the left of the section (L). (Stained H & E, ×22.)

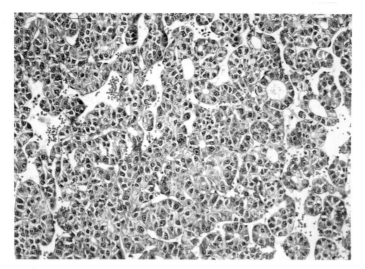

Fig. 28.4. Hepato-cellular carcinoma. The tumour cells are smaller than normal with granular cytoplasm and large hyper-chromatic nuclei. Mitoses are conspicuous. Atypical giant cell may be seen. Stroma is scanty and the tumour cells have blood spaces between them. (Stained H & E, ×90.)

excess abundant cytoplasm. The condition is often associated with hypoglycaemia and hypercholesterolaemia and has a variable prognosis [112].

SPREAD

Intra-hepatic. Metastases in the liver may be multiple or in one lobe. Spread is by the blood vessels, for the tumour cells abut on vascular spaces, which they readily penetrate. Lymphatic permeation and direct infiltration also occur.

Extra-hepatic. Involvement of small or large hepatic or portal veins or the vena cava may be seen. Metastases have also been found in oesophageal varices even if sclerosed [47]. Lung metastases may develop by this route [3]. Tumour emboli result in pulmonary thrombosis. Systemic spread results in deposits anywhere, but especially in bone. Regional lymph nodes at the porta hepatis are frequently involved and the mediastinal and cervical chains can also be infiltrated.

Large pulmonary metastases are rare. The tumour may involve the peritoneum with resulting haemorrhagic ascites; this may be terminal.

The histology of metastases. The secondary tumour may faithfully reproduce the structure of the primary, even forming bile. Sometimes, however, the cell type diverges widely. Bile or glycogen in cells of a metastasis suggests a hepatic primary.

Clinical features

Age. All ages are affected. In races such as the Chinese and the Bantu the sufferers are often below 40 years old. In temperate climates the patients are usually over 40 years.

Sex. Males exceed females in a ratio of 4–6:1.

Associated cirrhosis must be established. Primary carcinoma of the liver should be suspected if a patient with cirrhosis deteriorates or, for no obvious reason, develops right upper quadrant pain, or if a local lump can be palpated in the liver. It should be considered if there is no improvement when ascites or pre-coma is adequately treated.

Rapid decline in a patient with haemochromatosis or with chronic liver disease and a positive HBsAg also suggests a complicating carcinoma.

The patient complains of malaise and abdominal fullness. He loses weight. The temperature is rarely higher than 38°C.

Pain is frequent but rarely severe and is felt as a non-specific, continuous dull ache in the epigastrium, right upper quadrant or back.

Severe pain is due to peri-hepatitis or involvement of the diaphragm.

Gastrointestinal symptoms such as anorexia, flatulence and constipation are common.

Dyspnoea is a late symptom and may be due to the large size of the tumour compressing or directly involving the diaphragm, or to pulmonary metastases.

Jaundice is by no means constant and rarely deep. The depth has little relation to the extent of hepatic involvement. Very rarely the tumour may invade main bile ducts resulting in progressive cholestatic jaundice [66]. Intra-bile duct tumour casts may be seen and haemobilia may be the immediate cause of death.

The liver is enlarged, not only downwards into the abdomen but also upwards into the thorax. A hard irregular lump may be felt in the right upper quadrant, continuous with the liver. If the left lobe is involved, the mass is epigastric. Sometimes multiple masses are palpable, but they are not usually tender. However, tenderness may be so severe that the patient cannot tolerate palpation.

A friction rub, due to peri-hepatitis, is occasionally heard over the tumour. An arterial murmur (fig. 28.5) [12] is due to increased arterial vascularity. In the absence of acute alcoholic hepatitis such a murmur is diagnostic of hepato-cellular carcinoma.

Ascites is found in about half the patients. The protein content is high. Malignant cells may be found but interpretation of these in peritoneal fluid is difficult. LDH and carcino-embryonic antigen may be increased. The fluid may be blood stained. Rupture causes *haemo-peritoneum.* This may present insidiously or as an acute abdomen with severe pain. Prognosis is very poor.

Portal vein thrombosis adds to ascites. *Hepatic vein* block may occur. Tumour may grow into the right atrium [62].

Haemorrhage from oesophageal varices is frequent and usually terminal. Failure to control variceal bleeding in a cirrhotic patient is often due to a complicating hepato-cellular carcinoma with portal vein invasion.

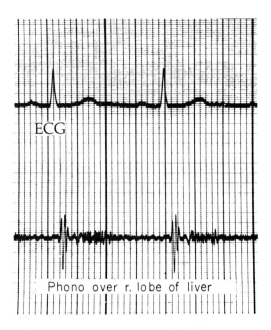

Fig. 28.5. Hepato-cellular carcinoma in the right lobe. Phonogram of the right lobe of the liver showing a systolic murmur (Clain *et al.* 1966).

CLINICAL FEATURES OF METASTASES

Lymph glands may be felt, especially in the right supra-clavicular region. *Pulmonary metastases* may result in a pleural effusion. Massive pulmonary emboli may lead to dyspnoea and to pulmonary hypertension [137]. Massive arterio−portal fistulae can develop [46]. *Osseous metastases* may appear in ribs and vertebrae. *Brain secondaries* give the features of a brain tumour.

SYSTEMIC EFFECTS [84]

Florid endocrine changes are associated more often with the hepatoblastoma of childhood than with adult primary liver cell carcinoma.

Painful *gynaecomastia* [127] with increased secretion of oestrogen may be seen.

Hypercalcaemia [86], sometimes due to pseudo-hyperparathyroidism, has been reported. The tumour may contain a parathormone-like material and serum parathormone levels are raised. Hepatic arterial embolization may be useful therapeutically [4].

Hypoglycaemia can be found in up to 30% of patients [83]. This may be due to demand for glucose by an enormous tumour mass and so is often associated with an undifferentiated rapidly progressing tumour. Rarely the hypo-glycaemia is seen with a well-differentiated, slowly progressive cancer. In this type glucose-6-phosphatase and phosphorylase are reduced or absent in the tumour while the glycogen content in tumour and adjacent tissues is in-creased. This suggests an acquired glycogen storage disease as the mechanism of the hypo-glycaemia. In this group control is difficult even with an enormous carbohydrate intake.

Insulin-like production by the tumour has been reported. This is an unlikely explanation of the hypoglycaemia for plasma insulin or insulin-like activity are not increased when the blood glucose level is low.

Hyperlipidaemia is rare, but about a third have increased serum cholesterol levels when maintained on a low cholesterol diet. In one patient, the hyperlipidaemia and the hyper-cholesterolaemia were caused by production of an abnormal lipoprotein with β mobility.

Hyperthyroidism may be due to inappropri-ate thyroid-stimulating hormone production [44].

Pseudo-porphyria with markedly elevated levels of porphobilinogen in urine and serum may be related to porphyrin production by the carcinoma [106].

BIOCHEMICAL CHANGES

These may be only those of cirrhosis. The serum alkaline phosphatase is markedly elevated and serum transaminase levels increase.

Electrophoresis of serum proteins may show a γ and an α_2 component. A serum macro-globulin of myeloma type is a rare finding.

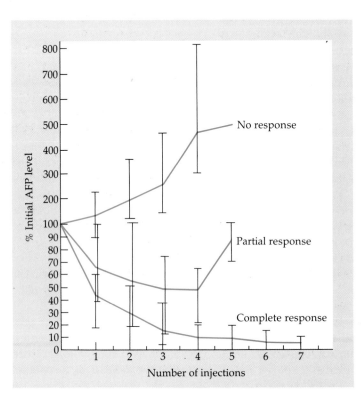

Fig. 28.6. Primary hepato-cellular carcinoma. Mean and range of AFP levels expressed as a percentage of the level at presentation in patients showing complete, partial and no response to adriamycin therapy (Johnson *et al.* 1978).

SEROLOGICAL MARKERS

Serum alpha-1-fetoprotein

Alpha-l-fetoprotein (AFP) is a normal component of plasma in human fetuses older than six weeks and is maximum between twelve and sixteen weeks of fetal life. The normal adult value of up to 20 ng/ml is reached 10 weeks after birth. Progressive increases are found in the blood of some patients with hepato-cellular carcinoma and AFP can be shown in the tumour [90]. Rising levels are of particular diagnostic value. Increases up to 500 ng/ml may be found in acute and chronic hepatitis and alcoholic hepatitis. Levels exceeding this are virtually confined to hepato-cellular carcinoma and germ cell tumours.

The level has no relation to the size of the liver tumour. However, AFP doubling time is closely related to tumour doubling time [120]. Resection of the primary tumour, or liver transplant, results in a fall in serum AFP. Persisting low levels indicate residual tumour and increases indicate rapid tumour growth. Serial values are useful in assessing therapy (fig. 28.6).

Serum AFP is a valuable screening procedure for hepato-cellular cancer in a patient with cirrhosis. However, values may be normal in the early stages. Positive results are found more frequently in patients from high incidence areas such as Hong Kong, Greece or South Africa than in the UK or USA.

Carcino-embryonic antigen values are particularly high with hepatic metastases. Because of lack of specificity it is of little value in the diagnosis of hepato-cellular cancer. Lack of specificity also applies to increases of *serum alpha-l-antitrypsin* and *alpha-acid glycoprotein*.

Serum ferritin increase is due to production of ferritin by the tumour rather than to liver necrosis. Ferritin is an acute phase reactant and is increased in active hepato-cellular disease; increases do not necessarily mean hepato-cellular cancer.

Des-gamma-carboxyprothrombin is a vitamin K dependent prothrombin precursor synthesized in the normal hepatocyte. It requires carboxylation of its glutamic acid residues, a process the hepato-cellular carcinoma cell cannot perform. Values in hepato-cellular cancer therefore exceed 50 ng/ml. They are normal in chronic hepatitis, cirrhosis and metastatic carcinoma [123].

Serum vitamin B_{12} binding protein may be very high [60] and this probably arises from the tumour. The serum B_{12} level is increased as is the unsaturated vitamin B_{12} binding capacity.

HEPATITIS B MARKERS

Tests for HBsAg should always be performed. Titres may be low and can even be negative by the ELISA method. Other markers such as anti-HBc may be positive and, if so, this increases the likely relationship to hepatitis B.

HAEMATOLOGICAL CHANGES

The leucocyte count is usually raised to about 10 000 per mm^3 with 80% polymorphonuclears. Eosinophilia is an occasional finding. The platelet count may be high—an unusual feature of uncomplicated cirrhosis.

The erythrocyte count is usually normal and anaemia is mild. Erythrocytosis is seen in 1%. It is probably due to increased erythropoietin production by the tumour [91]. Increased serum erythropoietin levels may even be found with a normal haemoglobin and packed cell volume [63].

Blood coagulation may be disturbed. Fibrinolytic activity tends to be decreased. This may be due to liberation by the tumour of an inhibitory substance. Increase in plasma fibrinogen levels may be secondary to this effect.

Dysfibrinogenaemia may represent reversion to a fetal form of fibrinogen [40]. Ground-glass cells in hepato-cellular carcinoma may contain fibrinogen and be producing it [125].

Tumour localization

Plain X-ray may show calcification (sunburst lesion) (fig. 28.14).

HEPATIC SCANNING

Isotope scan shows tumours larger than 3 cm in diameter as filling defects.

The ultrasound pattern may show increased or decreased reflectivity or a mixed echo picture. Real time ultrasound shows the tumour as a hypo-echoic shadow with ill-defined margins and non-uniform echoes. The diagnosis may be confirmed by ultrasound/guided biopsy. Sensitivity and specificity are high. False positives in cirrhosis are due to increased echogenicity in large nodules [22]. The method is particularly suitable for diagnostic screening [130]. Lesions less than 2 cm in diameter can be detected (fig. 28.7).

CT scan shows a hypo-dense lesion which does not enhance with contrast (fig. 28.8). CT may show rupture of the tumour, but no invasion of adjacent structures. It is particularly valuable for demonstrating the extent of hepatic involvement. It is highly diagnostic but less sensitive than angiography.

Dynamic bolus enhancement improves sensitivity. The margins after contrast may be sharp or ill-defined. Portal vein involvement can be shown [85].

Lipiodol introduced into the hepatic artery is cleared from non-cancerous tissue but remains in the tumour almost permanently so that lesions as small as 3 mm may be detected by CT (fig. 28.9) [95].

MRI may detect smaller lesions than CT [29]. It is particularly useful if fatty liver co-exists. Calcification may be seen [30].

Single photoemission CT (SPECT) may have little advantage over ultrasound as a screening method but may be complementary [69].

VASCULAR RADIOLOGY

Hepatic angiography

This is very valuable for localization, for diagnosis, to determine operability and to follow the effects of therapy. The tumour is supplied by the hepatic artery, and selective coeliac and superior mesenteric arteriography results in filling of the lesion (fig. 28.10).

Superselective contrast infusion angiography is of particular value in identifying small tumours (fig. 28.11). Difficulty may arise in distinction from regeneration nodules in the cirrhotic liver [126]. The appearances can be related to the gross anatomy of the tumour. The arterial pattern is bizarre with pooling, stretching and displacement of vessels. The vessels may be sclerosed, have an irregular lumen and be fragmented. Arterio—venous shunts can be shown often with retrograde filling of the portal

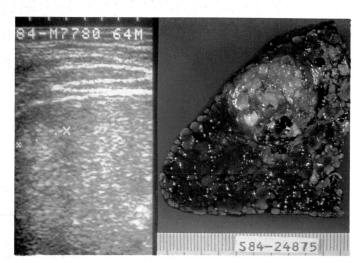

Fig. 28.7. Ultrasound shows a small hepato-cellular carcinoma (marked xx). This was surgically resected and the specimen is shown (Courtesy J F Liaw).

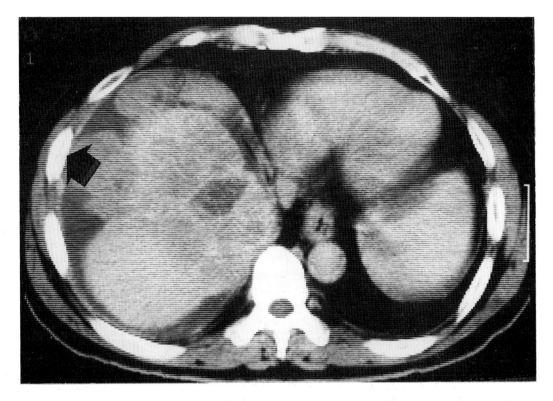

Fig. 28.8. CT scan in hepato-cellular cancer shows tumour bursting through capsule (arrow). Ascites is also present.

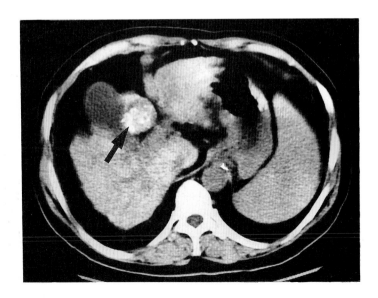

Fig. 28.9. CT scan after injection of lipiodol into the hepatic artery shows contrast remaining in a small hepato-cellular carcinoma (arrow). The liver is cirrhotic and the spleen is enlarged.

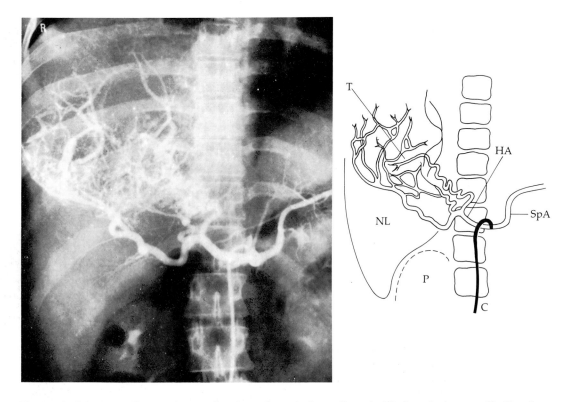

Fig. 28.10. Selective coeliac arteriogram showing catheter in the coeliac axis (C), the splenic artery (SpA) and the hepatic artery (HA). An abnormal arterial pattern (T) is shown in the tumour. The normal liver (NL) is not outlined by contrast media. P is pyelogram.

trunk (fig. 28.12). There may be delayed emptying of the lesion. The portal vein may be distorted if there is tumour invasion.

Splenic venography

This shows displacement of the main portal veins by the tumour. It demonstrates whether the portal vein is patent or obstructed by tumour. In the hepatogram phase the tumour shows as a non-filled zone.

Needle liver biopsy

Histological confirmation is particularly important if small space-occupying lesions have been detected by ultrasound or CT. If possible, the biopsy needle should be directed into the lesion under imaging control (Chapter 3) [118].

The possibility that biopsy will facilitate spread along the needle tract exists but is exceedingly rare.

Fine needle aspiration, using a heparinized 22-gauge needle, yields cytological specimens which will diagnose moderately and poorly differentiated hepato-cellular cancers (fig. 28.13), but the cytological diagnosis of well differentiated tumours is difficult [93].

Diagnosis

Increased awareness of the condition has improved the accuracy of diagnosis. Although the likelihood is greater in such areas as Africa or South East Asia, primary liver cancer is being increasingly recognized world wide.

Clinically, abdominal pain or weight loss with hepatomegaly or ascites are the common

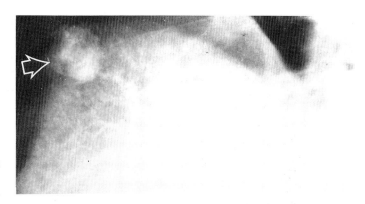

Fig. 28.11. Super selective hepatic angiography shows a very small hepato-cellular carcinoma (arrow).

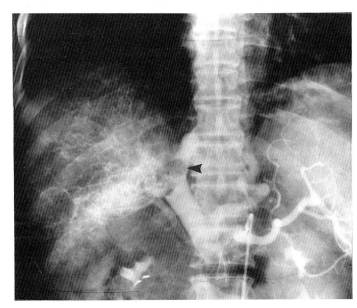

Fig. 28.12. Coeliac angiogram in patient with known cirrhosis, sudden deterioration in function and rising serum alpha-fetoprotein level. Abnormal vessels are seen in right lobe above the hilum with massive and immediate arterio-portal shunting. Appearances are diagnostic of primary liver cancer. Defect in portal vein (arrow head) represents tumour invasion rather than clot (Sherlock & Dick, 1987).

presentations. Deterioration in a patient with known chronic liver disease especially with hepatitis B markers positive, and with a rising serum AFP is suspicious. A space-occupying lesion may be demonstrated by scanning and final confirmation comes from hepatic histology obtained by needle biopsy.

Early detection

This results in diagnosis of tumours at the stage where surgical resection is possible. In Shanghai, serum AFP testing of over 2 million people yielded 351 subclinical cases of hepato-cellular cancer, a discovery rate of 16/100 000 [131].

Combination of AFP with high resolution, linear array real-time ultrasonography increases the diagnostic yield [76]. CT and angiography are useful for confirmation [126].

HBsAg positive patients with chronic hepatitis or cirrhosis, particularly if Oriental males more than 45 years old, should be screened by alpha-fetoprotein or des-gamma-carboxyprothrombin and real-time ultrasound at six-monthly intervals. This routine is clearly

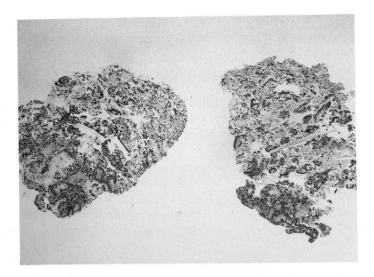

Fig. 28.13. Fine needle aspiration under untrasound guidance yielded a clump of hepato-cellular carcinoma cells.

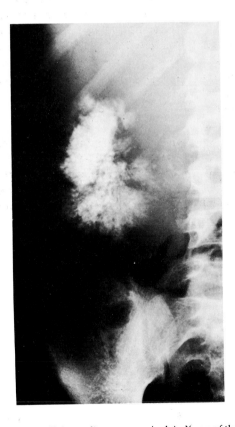

Fig. 28.14. Primary liver cancer. A plain X-ray of the abdomen shows calcification (sunburst lesion).

not practical or so successful for all cirrhotic patients. In my experience, in the UK the tumour seems to start as an explosion and within six months of a normal ultrasound examination and serum alpha-fetoprotein level has progressed to an inoperable state.

Prognosis

The outlook is usually hopeless. The prognosis depends on the stage of disease and the speed of tumour growth. Small tumours (less than 3 cm diameter) are associated with a one-year survival of 90.7%, a two-year of 55% and a three-year of 12.8% [29]. The speed of growth varies from time to time. Patients with massive tumours are unlikely to survive three months. Occasionally, with a slow growing tumour, and particularly the small encapsulated type, survival is 2–3 years or even longer [70]. The massive type runs a shorter course than the nodular. Pulmonary metastases and increased serum bilirubin levels adversely affect survival [15]. Patients less than 45 years old survive longer than older ones. A tumour size exceeding 50% of the liver and a serum albumin less than 3 g/dl are ominous features [97].

Prognosis seems to be related to geographic location. The downhill course is particularly rapid in southern Europe, South Africa and Hong Kong. In Japan, small encapsulated tumours are recognized and patients survive for eight months even if untreated [98].

Treatment

PREVENTION

If hepatitis B infection could be controlled by a vaccine (Chapter 16), the incidence of primary liver cancer would fall world wide but especially in areas with high prevalence of hepatitis B carriage.

Better agricultural methods and improved storage and transport of cereals will reduce contamination by mycotoxins.

RESECTION

The liver has a remarkable capacity for regeneration. After partial resection, DNA synthesis increases and the remaining liver cells become larger (hypertrophy) and undergo increased mitosis (hyperplasia). Up to 90% of the non-cirrhotic liver may be removed with eventual survival. The opportunities for resection have followed on advances in tumour localization.

The resectability rate for all hepatic tumours is very low. Multicentric involvement of both lobes, invasion of the inferior vena cava, portal vein or adjacent structures, jaundice and ascites are contraindications to surgery. Cirrhosis is not a definite contraindication, but the chances of resection are reduced and survival is less. The resectability rate depends upon the size of the tumour and its geographic origin. In South Africa, for instance, very few hepato-cellular carcinomas are operable, whereas in Japan the small, often encapsulated, hepato-cellular cancer can be removed (table 28.5).

Before surgery, the tumour must be localized by scanning and arteriography. Intra-operative hepatic ultrasound is of indispensable valuie in detecting small tumours [119]. The left lobe is resected with relative ease. The right lobe is more difficult. The overall operative mortality is 5–10%, and a three-year overall actuarial survival rate 56% [56]. Results are best in the paediatric age group.

In Japan and China, small tumours are being increasingly diagnosed due to more intensive screening and more are found to be operable (table 28.5) [131]. Results are improving so that in 1986, 56 of 63 tumours were resectable with a one-year survival of 48.6 months [66].

CHEMOTHERAPY

Adriamycin (doxorubicin). This drug induces remissions in about one-third of patients with primary liver cancer [58]. Grade A patients, that is those without jaundice, ascites or high transaminase values, have a survival of 43%

Table 28.5. Surgical resection for hepatocellular carcinoma

Country	Author	No. treated	Op. or hosp. mortality %	% 1-year survival	% resectable
Africa	Kew	—	—	—	5
UK	Dunk	46	—	—	6.5
France	Bismuth	270	15	66	12.9
USA*	Lim	86	36	22.7	22
Hong Kong	Lee	935	20	45	17.6
Japan	Okuda	2411	27.5	33.5	11.9
China	Li	?	11.4	58.6	?
Taiwan	Lees	?	6	84	?

* Chinese-Americans.

compared with grade B patients of 18%. Hepatitis B antigen negative patients may respond better than those who are positive. Therapy is monitored by α-fetoprotein levels (fig. 28.6).

The dose is 60 mg/m² body surface (diluted with 5% dextrose) given intravenously every three weeks. The maximum dose is 550 mg. This is reduced by half if the serum bilirubin level is raised, if the white cell count is less than 2000 or if the platelets are less than 100 000. An electrocardiogram is taken before each dose. Side effects include mild nausea, vomiting, haematuria and alopecia (the hair regrows later). Marrow depression and cardiotoxicity are very rare.

Mitozantrone gives rather similar results, about 45.4% have clinical benefit with a response rate of 27.3%. The dose is 12 mg/m² intravenously diluted in 5% dextrose over 10−30 minutes every 21 days [27]. Side effects, particularly vomiting and hair loss, are reduced, but nausea and cardiotoxicity can occur. Myelosuppression is rarely a clinical problem.

HEPATIC ARTERIAL THERAPY

The tumour is largely supplied by the hepatic artery which may be catheterized percutaneously via the femoral artery and coeliac axis. This allows procedures which reduce the blood supply to the cancer and which permit chemotherapeutic agents to be delivered in high concentration to the tumour.

Embolization

Hepatic arterial branches supplying the tumour can be embolized using gel foam (figs 28.15, 28.16). The portal vein must be patent. The tumour undergoes complete or incomplete necrosis [1]. The procedure usually requires general anaesthesia and antibiotic cover is given. It is often painful and abscess formation, fever and misplaced injections are other complications. The tumour rapidly acquires a fresh arterial circulation. The one-year survival is about 42% [97]. Embolization gives the best

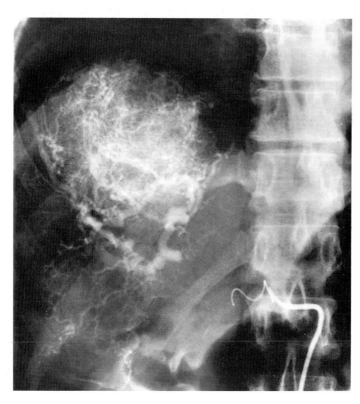

Fig. 28.15. Selective hepatic angiography shows a large hepato-cellular carcinoma in the right lobe of the liver.

results in the treatment of hepatic carcinoid tumours [1]. Where there is a marked reduction in symptoms and tumour size (figs 28.17, 28.18) therapy can be repeated as required. Embolization can be followed by chemotherapy or resection. Hepatic arterial embolization may be used to cut off the blood supply to a ruptured tumour (where the portal vein is patent) [114].

Variceal haemorrhage secondary to hepatic arterial–portal venous shunting and a hyperkinetic portal hypertension may be treated by transcatheter embolization of the fistula [88].

Arterial chemotherapy

A therapeutic agent, such as mitomycin C, may be prepared in microcapsular form and delivered to the tumour by selective hepatic intra-arterial infusion [94].

Long duration of therapy may be achieved by combining the therapeutic agent with iodized oil (lipiodol) [129]. This is slowly re-leased from the lipiodol which remains in the tumour [84]. The lipiodol in the tumour is localized by a CT scan (fig. 28.9) and assessment of size and effects of therapy is possible.

Direct intratumour injection

Small (less than 2 to 3 cm) tumours may be treated by direct, percutaneous injection of absolute alcohol [101]. This may be a preliminary to resection.

Monoclonal directed chemotherapy

Radio-isotopes bound to antibodies against components of the cancer may be given intravenously or via the hepatic artery. I^{131}-ferritin and α-fetoprotein antibodies have been used in this way [79, 102]. At present results are inconclusive.

A liver tumour membrane marker has been identified in a rat bearing a primary liver cancer

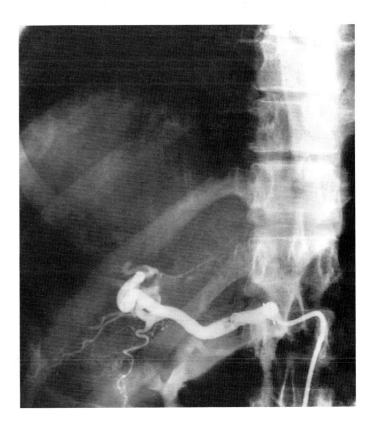

Fig. 28.16. Same patient as Fig. 28.15. Hepatic arterial embolization with gel foam occlusion of blood supply to the tumour.

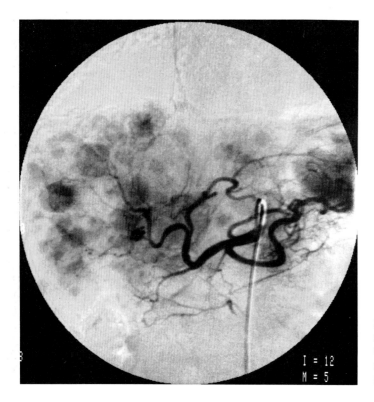

Fig. 28.17. Coeliac angiography in a patient with primary carcinoid tumour of ileum and multiple, symptomatic liver metastases (Sherlock & Dick, 1987).

and a monoclonal antibody produced against it. This antibody is used to direct anti-tumour drugs to the cancer [5]. This interesting approach offers prospects for the future.

Immunotherapy

The growth of the cancer may be related to inability of the tumour-bearing host to mount an immune response adequate for lysis of sufficient numbers of tumour cells. The immunological response may be stimulated by lymphokine activated killer (LAK) cells produced by treating the patient's mononuclear cells with gamma interleukin 2 [50]. The tumour is then lysed. This approach is in its early stages in man.

Alpha interferon is very toxic if given in the amounts necessary to treat human hepatocellular cancer [35]. Combination with other chemotherapeutic agents may be possible in the future.

Hepatic transplantation

This is being used but with generally unsatisfactory results (Chapter 23). If the patient survives the surgery, recurrence and mestastases are usual and this may be enhanced by the immunosuppression necessary to prevent rejection [122].

Conclusions

Hepato-cellular cancer remains a fatal disease (fig. 28.19). The few long-term survivors are those lucky enough to have had complete surgical removal of a small tumour.

Fibro-lamellar carcinoma of the liver

This tumour is found in young people (aged 5–35) of both sexes [23, 48]. It presents as an abdominal mass, sometimes with pain. It is unrelated to sex hormones. The liver is non-cirrhotic.

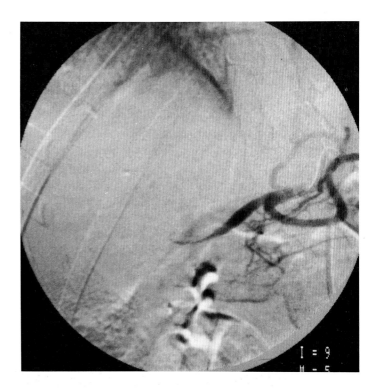

Fig. 28.18. Same patient as Fig. 28.17 after selective hepatic arterial embolization to ablate tumour functions (Sherlock & Dick, 1987).

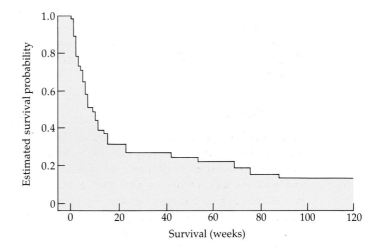

Fig. 28.19. Estimated survival probability of UK patients with hepato-cellular carcinoma (Dunk *et al*, 1987).

Histologically, clumps of deeply eosinophilic tumour cells containing hyaline and pale bodies are interspersed with bands of mature fibrous tissue (fig. 28.20). Electron microscopy shows **603** the cytoplasm packed with mitochondria and thick compact bands of collagen in parallel arrays. The tumour cells are believed to be oncocytes. The hepatocytes contain excess of copper-associated protein, presumably produced by the cancer cell [73].

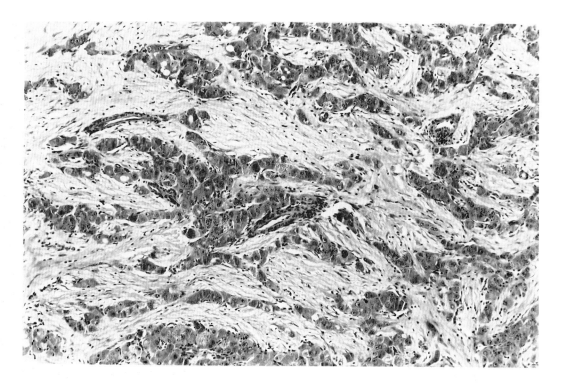

Fig. 28.20. Fibrolamellar carcinoma: clumps of eosinophilic cells are interspersed with bands of mature connective tissue. (Stained H & E, ×275.)

Serum α-fetoprotein is normal. Serum calcium levels may be raised with pseudo-hyperparathyroidism. Serum vitamin B_{12} binding protein [103] and neurotensin [21] may also be increased.

CT and ultrasound appearances resemble those of hepato-cellular carcinoma although the margin tends to be well defined. On angiography, arterio–venous shunting and retrograde opacification of the portal vein are unusual.

Prognosis is better than for other forms of liver cancer (survival 32 to 62 months), although the tumour may metastasize.

Treatment is by surgical resection or transplantation [90].

Hepatoblastoma

This rare tumour develops in both sexes and presents before the age of two years as progressive enlargement of the abdomen with anorexia, failure to gain weight, fever and, rarely, jaundice [68]. Associated features include sexual precocity due to secretion of an ectopic gonadotrophin by the tumour, cystathioninuria, hemihypertrophy and renal adenomas. Serum α-fetoprotein levels are markedly increased. Imaging shows a space-occupying lesion in the liver with displacement of adjacent organs. There may be focal calcification. Angiography shows the features of primary liver cancer with a diffuse parenchymal blush persisting into the venous phase, encasement of vessels, pooling of contrast and an ill-defined margin.

Hepatoblastoma is one of a group of malignant tumours of childhood whose histological features recapitulate the developmental stages of the liver. Teratoid features may therefore be seen [85]. The usual picture is of fetal type and embryonal cells in acini-pseudo-rosettes or papillary formations. Sinusoids contain haematopoietic cells. The mixed epithelial–mesenchymal type shows primitive mesenchyma, osteoid tissue and, rarely, cartilage, rhadomyoblasts or squamous foci [135].

If a resection is possible, the prognosis is better than for primary hepato-cellular carcinoma, 36% of patients surviving five years.

Intra-hepatic cholangiocarcinoma

Aetiological factors include clonorchiasis, the fibrocystic diseases (Chapter 30), anabolic steroids and thorotrast [39].

The tumour is firm to hard and of whitish colour.

Histologically, this is a glandular tumour arising from intra-hepatic bile ducts. The tumour cells resemble bile ducts; sometimes they have a papillary arrangement. There is no bile secretion. The stroma differs from that of hepato-cellular carcinoma as it consists of fibrous tissue with little or no capillary formation (fig. 28.21). The cell type is cuboidal and peri-portal lymphatic permeation may be seen. Focal calcification is rare.

Keratin is a good marker of biliary epithelium and is found in 90% of cholangiocarcinomas. α-fetoprotein is not detected in the tumour [39].

The tumour affects older persons. The clinical features are those of hepatic malignancy with jaundice prominent. Serum α-fetoprotein is not increased.

CT scan shows the tumour as a space-occupying lesion of low attenuation. It is usually hypovascular. Treatment is unsatisfactory, and there is no response to chemotherapy.

Combined hepato-cellular-cholangiocarcinoma

This primary liver cancer shows the features of both hepato-cellular and biliary epithelial differentiation [39]. Some represent coincidental occurrence of both hepato-cellular and cholangiocarcinoma in the same patient. Some contain transition elements between hepato-cellular and cholangiocarcinoma, and some are examples of fibro-lamellar tumours.

Within the tumour, intracellular α-fetoprotein

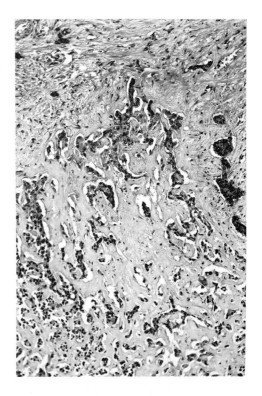

Fig. 28.21. Bile duct carcinoma. The tumour cells are arranged in tubular fashion simulating bile ducts. The cell type is columnar. Stroma is dense, fibrous avascular. (Stained H & E, ×90.)

is found in 29% and keratin markers of bile duct epithelium in 52%.

The *clinical features* and course are those of hepato-cellular carcinoma. Cirrhosis may or may not be present.

Cystadenocarcinoma

This rare tumour occurs in adults, more often female. It presents as abdominal fullness with pain and weight loss.

Grossly the appearance is of multilocular cysts containing muddy bile-stained, mucinous material. Histologically the cysts are lined by malignant epithelial cells with papillary enfoldings and dense fibrous stroma. The origin may be from a benign cystadenoma or even a congenital cyst.

Imaging shows a space-occupying lesion, usually large, with cystic features [52].

The prognosis is better than for cholangiocarcinoma with survival of up to 5 years after resection [54]. Hepatic transplantation may also be possible.

Angiosarcoma (haemangio-endothelioma)

This very rare and highly malignant tumour is difficult to distinguish from primary hepatocellular cancer. The liver is enlarged and full of knobbly cavernous growths.

Histologically, blood-filled cavernous sinuses are lined with layers of highly malignant, anaplastic, endothelial cells which in parts may resemble the earliest stages of embryonic vascular development. Many well-differentiated tumours resemble peliosis hepatis. They may have a Kupffer cell origin.

Giant cell formations, solid sarcomatous foci, and intrasinusoidal spread with invasion of portal venous and hepatic venous radicles are prominent. Adjacent liver shows cholangioproliferation and hypertrophy of sinusoidal lining cells. Factor VIII-related antigen may be identified in tumour cells.

The disease affects older age groups. It presents with the signs of hepato-cellular liver disease, weight loss and fever.

The clinical course is rapidly downhill with cachexia and blood-stained ascites. A bruit may be heard over the liver. Platelets may be consumed in the tumour and disseminated intravascular coagulation has been reported. Occasionally the course is chronic with ascites and hepatomegaly over many years [17].

Scanning shows multiple defects in the liver. The right diaphragm is high.

The *prognosis* is very poor, and the tumour is only rarely radiosensitive.

Thorotrast. This consists of a colloidal solution of thorium dioxide with the isotope radiothorium which is mainly an α-ray emitter and has a half-life of 1.39×10 years. It was formerly used as a contrast medium in radiology. Primary hepatic tumours have developed years after intravascular administration [13, 111]. Hepato-cellular or bile duct carcinoma has a latent period of about 20 years and haemangio-endothelioma about 15 years. Plain X-ray of the abdomen shows continued presence of the isotope in liver and spleen and this is confirmed by autoradiographs of liver tissue. Total body counting may be used to quantitate radioactivity in the patient's body. Microradiology has been used to demonstrate deposition of thorium in the liver at autopsy. Cirrhosis can develop even without liver tumours.

Other *aetiological factors* in angiosarcoma [80] include vinyl chloride (page 386), arsenic (page 386) and androgenic-anabolic steroids [34] (page 402) (see fig. 18.31). Angiosarcoma and malignant schwannoma can complicate hepatic neurofibromatosis [73].

Epithelioid haemangio-endothelioma [52]

This rare tumour of adults may present incidentally, with jaundice or with haemoperitoneum.

Microscopically, tumour cells are dendritic and epithelioid and infiltrate sinusoids and intra-hepatic veins of all sizes. The matrix may show inflammation, sclerosis and calcification. Tumour cells synthesize factor VIII. Prognosis is more favourable than for angiosarcoma, but the tumour can metastasize. No specific therapeutic recommendations can be made.

Undifferentiated sarcoma of the liver

This is an extremely rare tumour diagnosed from anaplastic hepato-cellular carcinoma, angiosarcoma or epithelioid haemangio-endothelioma only on hepatic histology. Spread of a sarcoma from a nearby structure such as the thoracic cage, diaphragm or retroperitoneum must be excluded.

The tumour may present in an infantile form (Chapter 24), but can affect the adult [37].

The histology is typical of sarcoma. Reticulin stains show the characteristic uniform distribution of fibres.

The prominent clinical features are pyrexia and an abdominal mass. Hypoglycaemia may develop. The course is rapidly downhill with a survival of about two months.

Imaging shows a solid and cystic lesion with multiple loculi. Calcification and invasion of the right atrium and inferior vena cava may be noted. Angiography shows variable vascularity depending on the degree of cystic transformation.

Chemotherapy is useless and hepatic transplantation is rarely possible.

Benign tumours of the liver

ADENOMA

These are very rare. They present as right upper quadrant masses or as acute intra-peritoneal haemorrhage. They have an association with sex hormone therapy (Chapter 18) and with pregnancy.

CHOLANGIOMA

This is a very rare, simple tumour of bile duct origin. It has the structure of a cystadenoma and it must be distinguished from a simple cyst or polycystic disease of the liver. A mixed type of tumour is also recorded with both proliferating bile ducts and hepatic cells.

BILIARY CYSTADENOMA [54]

Tumour is usually large and affects the right lobe. It may be pedunculated. The cysts contain clear yellow or mucinous brown material.

This tumour affects largely middle-aged women. Symptoms include abdominal mass and pain. Rarely, the biliary tree is obstructed. Resection may be possible.

BILIARY PAPILLOMATOSIS

See Chapter 34.

HAEMANGIOMA

This is the commonest benign tumour of the liver, being found in about 5% of autopsies. It is being increasingly diagnosed with the greater use of scanning procedures. It is usually single and small, but occasionally may be multiple or very large.

The tumour is commonly subcapsular, on the convexity of the right lobe of the liver, and is occasionally pedunculated. On section it appears round or wedge-shaped, dark red in colour and has a honeycomb pattern, with a fibrous capsule which may be calcified. Histologically, a communicating network of spaces contains red corpuscles.

The tumour is lined by flat endothelial cells and contains scanty fibrous tissue. Occasionally, there is a marked fibrous component.

Clinical. The majority are asymptomatic and discovered incidentally. Symptoms from giant tumours (>4 cm diameter) include abdominal mass and pain due to thrombosis. Symptoms may be due to pressure on adjacent organs. Rarely, a vascular hum is heard over the lesion.

RADIOLOGY [11]

A *plain X-ray* may show a calcified capsule.

Ultrasound shows a solitary echogenic spot with smooth well-defined borders. Posterior acoustic enhancement due to increased sound transmission through the blood of the cavernous sinuses is characteristic [11].

CT scan, enhanced by contrast, shows distinctive puddling of contrast in venous channels (figs 5.9, 28.22). The contrast diffuses from the periphery to the centre, until opacification is homogeneous after 30 to 60 minutes. Calcification may be seen due to previous bleeding or thrombus formation.

MRI shows the tumour as a markedly high intensity area. T-2 is prolonged over 8 msec. MRI is of special value in diagnosing small haemangiomas [55].

Angiography is only necessary in cases not showing typical CT appearance. Lesions displace large hepatic arterial branches to one side. The hepatic arteries are not enlarged, taper normally and divide to normal small vessels before filling the vascular spaces. The spaces tend to adopt a circular or 'C' shape due to the

607

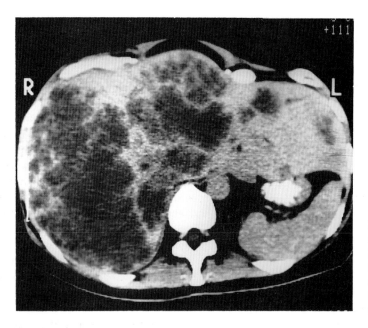

Fig. 28.22. Haemangioma: CT shows a giant benign haemangioma in the right lobe of the liver. A few small lesions are seen in the left lobe. The lesions filled in completely one hour after intravenous contrast.

central fibrosis. Haemangiomas may show prolonged opacification even up to 18 seconds. They may be recognized incidentally during angiography for another condition.

Needle liver biopsy (directed). Using a fine-cut biopsy technique this is usually safe [120] but unnecessary in view of the diagnostic imaging appearances.

Treatment is usually unnecessary as the lesions do not increase in size or in clinical manifestations. The possibility of rupture is not an indication for surgery. If there is severe pain or rapid expansion resection (usually lobectomy or segmentectomy) is safe [10, 114].

MESENCHYMAL HAMARTOMA [26]

This usually presents in the first two years of life as a massive cystic lesion of the right lobe of liver. It can affect adults. It arises from tissues in the portal zones and histology shows an admixture of hepatocytes, biliary epithelium, mesenchymal elements and cysts [70]. Extra medullary haematopoiesis may be seen.

Treatment is by surgical resection, but aspiration and careful follow-up may be considered in some cases.

NON-METASTATIC HYPERNEPHROMA [133]

Hepatosplenomegaly with reduction in serum albumin, increased serum globulins and alkaline phosphatase can complicate hypernephroma without hepatic metastases. Liver biopsy shows non-specific cellular infiltration. The changes may regress if the renal tumour is resected. The mechanism of the hepatic changes is unknown.

Hepatic metastases

The liver is the most frequent site of blood-borne metastases, irrespective of whether the primary is drained by systemic or portal veins. It is involved in about a third of all cancers, including half of those of stomach, breast, lung and those arising from the portal territory. Other frequent primary sites include oesophagus, pancreas and those of malignant melanoma.

PATHOGENESIS [138]

Invasion from tumours in adjacent organs, retrograde lymphatic permeation and extension along the lumen of blood vessels are all unusual.

Portal emboli come from malignant neoplasms arising in the organs of the portal vascular territory. Primary tumours in the uterus and ovaries, prostate or bladder, may involve contiguous tissue drained by the portal vein and hence give embolic metastases to the liver; these are extremely rare.

Microscopically, *hepatic arterial embolization* is difficult to identify, because the picture is confused by the succeeding intra-hepatic metastases. It must be frequent.

PATHOLOGY

There may be only one or two microscopic nodules or the whole liver may be enormous and full of metastases. Liver weights of 5000 g are not unusual and one liver is said to have weighed 21 500 g. The deposits are usually white and well demarcated. The consistency depends on the ratio of cancer cells to fibrous stroma. Occasionally the centre may be soft, necrotic and haemorrhagic. On the surface of the liver they show characteristic umbilication; this results from necrosis of the centre, which has outgrown its blood supply. Perihepatitis may be seen over peripheral lesions. A zone of venous hyperaemia may surround the deposits. Portal vein invasion is usual, and arteries are rarely involved by tumour thrombus although they may be encased.

The tumour cells metastasize rapidly and widely through the liver, both by perivascular lymphatics and by direct invasion of the portal venous radicles.

Injection studies show that, in contrast to hepato-cellular carcinoma, metastases may have a decreased rather than increased blood supply from the hepatic artery. This is particularly so in those of gastrointestinal origin.

HISTOLOGY

The secondary deposits in the liver may reproduce the histology of the primary lesions. However, this is not necessarily so, and in many instances the primary tumour may be well differentiated, while the secondary deposits in the liver may be extremely anaplastic and give no hint of their origin (fig. 28.23).

CLINICAL FEATURES

These may be due to the hepatic metastases, to the distant primary growth or more usually to a combination of both.

The patients complain of malaise, lassitude and loss of weight. Abdominal distension and a dragging sensation are due to the enlarged liver. Occasionally the pain is sharp and intermittent, simulating biliary colic. Fever and sweats may occur.

Depending upon the weight loss, the patient may be emaciated, with an enlarged abdomen.

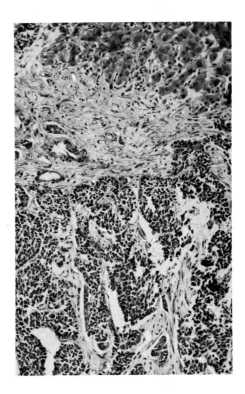

Fig. 28.23. Anaplastic secondary carcinoma of the liver. The tumour is composed of sheets of undifferentiated malignant cells. Normal liver cells are seen to the left. There was a small bronchial primary growth which was not revealed by chest X-ray. (Stained H & E, ×110.)

The liver may be normal sized or so large that it protrudes visibly in the right upper abdomen. The tumour deposits are hard and may be umbilicated. Friction may be heard over them. The deposits are not vascular, so an arterial bruit is not heard. Splenomegaly is frequent, even in those with a patent portal vein. Jaundice is mild and may be absent. Deep jaundice implies invasion of major bile ducts.

Oedema of the legs with dilated veins coursing upwards over the abdominal wall suggests that the inferior vena cava is obstructed on the posterior aspect of the liver.

Glands in the right supra-clavicular region may be involved.

A pleural effusion may indicate pulmonary metastases and similar localizing signs may provide clinical evidence of the primary growth.

Ascites reflects peritoneal involvement and occasionally a thrombosed portal vein. Bleeding may be secondary to portal hypertension. Rarely obstructive jaundice may be seen due to metastases from breast, colon [134], or small cell lung cancer [57].

Secondary malignant deposits are by far the commonest causes of a really large liver.

Hypoglycaemia is a rare complication. The primary is usually a sarcoma [139]. Rarely, extensive tumour infiltration and parenchymal infarction may lead to the picture of fulminant hepatic failure [43].

When *malignant carcinoid* of the small intestine or bronchus is associated with vaso-motor abnormalities and pulmonary stenosis, there are always many hepatic metastases.

Unless the bile ducts are completely obstructed, the faeces are well coloured, and if the primary lesion is in the alimentary tract they may give a positive reaction for blood.

LABORATORY INVESTIGATIONS

Biochemical tests

Even with an enormous liver, sufficient functioning tissue remains. The smaller intrahepatic bile ducts may be compressed yet no jaundice develops. The area with uninvolved ducts may excrete the bilirubin from the occluded areas. Serum total bilirubin values greater than 2 mg/100 ml suggest involvement of major bile ducts at the hilum.

Biochemical tests suggesting hepatic metastases include a raised serum alkaline phosphatase or lactic dehydrogenase level. Transaminase levels may be increased. If serum bilirubin, alkaline phosphatase, lactic dehydrogenase and transaminase levels are all normal, there is a 98% probability that metastases are absent [60].

Serum albumin concentration is normal or slightly decreased. The *serum globulin* level may be normal, slightly raised or even, occasionally, very high. Electrophoresis may show a raised α_2- or γ-globulin.

Serum carcino-embryonic antigen may be present [82].

The *ascitic fluid* shows increased protein, occasionally the presence of carcino-embryonic antigen and increases in lactic dehydrogenase three times over the serum value.

Haematology

A polymorph leucocytosis is fairly common: even values up to 40 000−50 000 per mm^3 are sometimes recorded. There may be a mild anaemia.

NEEDLE LIVER BIOPSY

The chances of a positive result are increased if the biopsy needle is directed into the lesion under ultrasound, CT or peritoneoscopic guidance. Tumour tissue is characteristically white and friable. If a cylinder of tissue is not obtained it is worth examining any blood clot or debris for malignant cells. Even if tumour cells are not aspirated, the presence of proliferated and abnormal bile ducts and polymorphs in oedematous portal tracts and focal sinusoidal dilatation suggest an adjacent metastasis [38].

Histology will not always enable the site of the primary to be detected especially if the tumour is undifferentiated (fig. 28.23). Cytological examination of aspiration fluid and touch preparations of the biopsy may slightly increase the yield of cancer cells.

The chance of obtaining a positive result increases with the extent of tumour, size of liver, and the presence of a palpable nodule. If liver metastases are suspected, a pre-operative needle biopsy is well worth while. A positive may make surgery unnecessary.

PERITONEOSCOPY

The liver surface is seen, metastases identified and any suspicious nodule biopsied.

RADIOLOGY

A *plain film* of the abdomen demonstrates the large liver. The diaphragm may be elevated and its contour irregular. *Calcification* in hepatic tumours is rare but is noted with primary cancer or haemangiomas and in secondaries, for instance from the colon, breast, thyroid or bronchus.

Chest radiograph may show associated pulmonary metastases.

Barium swallow may show oesophageal varices and the *meal* displacement to the left and rigidity of the lesser curve of the stomach. *Barium enema* may reveal depression of the hepatic flexure and transverse colon. The barium meal, colonoscopy, enema and fibre-optic endoscopy are helpful in demonstrating any primary tumour.

SCANNING

Scanning usually detects lesions greater than 2 cm in diameter.

Ultrasound usually shows echogenic lesions. It is useful, simple and inexpensive [115], but less powerful for examination of the posterior segment of the liver [41]. Intra-operative ultrasound is of great value in detecting metastases.

CT shows metastases as hypovascular lesions (fig. 28.24). Those from the colon generally have a large avascular centre with a dense peripheral ring-like accumulation of contrast. About 29% of patients undergoing apparently curative

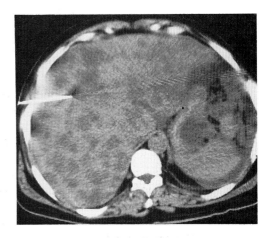

Fig. 28.24. CT scan of widespread hepatic metastases from a primary in the colon. A biopsy needle is directed into one of them.

resection for colorectal cancer will have occult hepatic metastases demonstrated by CT scanning. Contrast enhancement adds to the positivity rate.

Magnetic resonance using the spin-echo technique may show metastases where CT studies are negative [24].

SPECIAL DIAGNOSTIC PROBLEMS

The patient with a known primary growth may be suspected of having liver secondaries but they cannot be confirmed clinically. Suggestive evidence includes slightly increased serum bilirubin, transaminase and alkaline phosphatase levels. If the serum alkaline phosphatase and transaminases are normal there is a 90% chance of there being no hepatic metastases. Aspiration needle biopsy, scanning and peritoneoscopy are useful.

The other problem, of more academic interest, is obvious involvement of the liver when the primary is unknown. Breasts, thyroid and lungs must be considered as possible primaries. Positive stool blood suggests gastrointestinal cancer, and fibro-endoscopy, sigmoidoscopy, barium meal and enema are useful. Removal of skin tumours and the presence of melanomas suggest malignant melanoma. Suspected carcinoma of the body of the pancreas merits ERCP. Needle liver biopsy is usually positive and may indicate the site of the primary. However, even this may show only the presence of a squamous, scirrhous, columnar or anaplastic growth, the site of the primary remaining unknown.

PROGNOSIS

This depends on the site of the primary and the malignancy. In general, patients are dead within one year of diagnosis of hepatic metastases. Secondaries from tumours of colon and rectum have the best outlook. Patients with hepatic metastases at the time of colonic resection have a mean survival of 12 months with an eight month median.

TREATMENT

This remains very unsatisfactory. Those that have the best prognosis without therapy, for instance, secondaries from the rectum, do best with therapy. Most of the published results of therapy have no controls. Nevertheless, therapy has to be offered if only to give the patient and relatives some hope. Chosen treatment should be the one having the greatest prospect of slowing tumour growth and with the least undesirable side effects.

Intravenous bolus 5-fluorouracil (5-FU) has very few side effects but no significant effect on survival time.

Other treatment includes combined therapy using 5-FU or mitozantrone plus methotrexate and methyl CCNU. Side effects are greater and the results again uncontrolled. Best results are associated with breast metastases.

Metastases are resistant to radiation and immunotherapy. In the carcinoid syndrome, heroic surgery should be considered. The tumours shell out rather easily. Embolization via the hepatic artery is probably preferable [1]. Embolization with gel foam into a peripheral

artery has also been used for other types of hepatic metastases [19].

Hepatic arterial infusion chemotherapy

Primary and secondary hepatic tumours are supplied mainly by the hepatic artery, although the portal vein may play a small part [77]. Cytotoxic drugs may be delivered directly to the tumour by hepatic artery catheterization. The catheter is usually introduced surgically into the hepatic artery via the gastro-duodenal artery. The gallbladder is removed. The agent is usually 5-fluorodeoxy uridine (FUDR), which has an 80 to 95% extraction rate during the first pass through the liver. It is delivered continuously via an implantable pump for periods of two weeks in each month [104]. ^{29m}-technetium (TC) macroaggregated albumin, introduced into the hepatic artery, is taken up by the tumour and this may be used to predict the response to FUDR and show appropriate hepatic arterial perfusion [111].

This treatment leads to regression of the cancer in 20% and symptomatic improvement in 50%. For colorectal cancer, the survival is 26 months against 8 months in historical controls. A randomized trial showed a higher response rate compared with systemic treatment [65]. Side effects include sepsis and catheter failure, peptic ulcer, chemical cholecystitis and hepatitis, and sclerosing cholangitis.

Hepatic arterial perfusion may be used as an adjuvant to surgical resection [48, 104].

Surgical resection of colorectal cancer metastases

The secondaries grow slowly, can be single, and are mostly found in the subcapsular regions. Resection may be feasible in about 5 to 10% of patients. Pre-operative imaging is essential, but despite this, a surgeon must be prepared at the time of operation to increase the resection by at least a quarter and to abandon cure in an eighth [41]. A lobectomy or segmentectomy is usually performed. The operative mortality is about 5% [31]. This may be too high and tumours should probably only be resected by surgeons whose operative mortality approaches zero.

In a Multi-Institutional Study of 607 patients having metastases resected, 43% showed a recurrence in the liver and 31% in the lungs [51]. 36% recurred in the first year and 25% were alive and disease free at 5 years. In another series, 21% of patients survived 10 years—a most impressive figure. There is an increased risk of recurrence if a resection margin free of tumour is not obtained and if the metastases are bilobar.

The whole picture is confused and controlled trials are required to establish the contribution of surgery to survival of patients with hepatic metastases.

References

1 Allison DJ, Jordon H, Hennessy O. Therapeutic embolisation of the hepatic artery: a review of 75 procedures. *Lancet* 1985; i: 595.

2 Anthony PB. Liver cell dysplasia: what is its significance. *Hepatology* 1987; 7: 394.

3 Arakawa M, Kage M, Matsumoto S *et al*. Frequency and significance of tumour thrombi in oesophagal varices in hepatocellular carcinoma associated with cirrhosis. *Hepatology* 1986; 6: 419.

4 Attali P, Houssin D, Roche A *et al*. Hepatic arterial embolization for malignant hypercalcemia in hepatocellular carcinoma. *Dig. Dis. Sci.* 1984; 29: 466.

5 Baldwin RW, Byres VS. Monoclonal antibodies in cancer treatment. *Lancet* 1986; i: 603.

6 Bassendine MF, Arborgh BAM, Shipton U *et al*. Hepatitis B surface antigen and alpha fetoprotein secreting human primary liver cell cancer in athymic mice. *Gastroenterology* 1980; 79: 528.

7 Bassendine MF, Seta L, Salmeron J *et al*. Incidence of hepatitis B virus infection in alcoholic liver disease. HBsAg negative chronic active liver disease and primary liver cell cancer in Britain. *Liver* 1983; 3: 65.

8 Beasley RP. Hepatitis B virus as the etiologic agent in hepatocellular carcinoma—epidemiologic considerations. *Hepatology* 1982; 2: 215.

9 Bengmark S, Hafström L. The natural history of primary and secondary malignant tumours of the liver. II. The prognosis for patients with hepatic metastases from gastric carcinoma verified by laparotomy and postmortem examination. *Digestion* 1969; 2: 179.

10 Bornman PC, Terblanche J, Blumgart RL. Giant hepatic hemangiomas: diagnostic and therapeutic dilemmas. *Surgery* 1987; 101: 445.

11 Brant WE, Floyd JL, Jackson DE *et al*. The radiological evaluation of hepatic cavernous hemangioma *J. Am. Med. Assoc.* 1987; 257: 2471.

12 Brechot C, Pourcel C, Louise A *et al*. Presence of integrated hepatitis B virus DNA sequence in cellular DNA of human hepatocellular carcinoma. *Nature* 1980; 286: 533.

13 Brechot C. Hepatitis B virus (HBV) and hepatocellular carcinoma. *J. Hepatol.* 1987; 4: 269.

14 Burroughs AK, Bassendine MF, Thomas HC *et al*. Primary liver cell cancer in autoimmune chronic liver disease. *Br. med. J.* 1981; 282: 273.

15 Butler J, Attiyeh FF, Daly JM. Hepatic resection for metastases of the colon and rectum. *Surg. Gyn. Obstet.* 1986; 162: 109.

16 Chlebowski RT, Tong M, Weissman J *et al*. Hepato-cellular carcinoma: diagnostic and prognostic features in North American patients. *Cancer* 1984; 53: 2701.

17 Chowdhury AR, Black M, Lorber SH *et al*. Hemangio-endotheliomatosis of the liver: a twelve year follow-up. *Gastroenterology* 1977; 72: 157.

18 Clain D, Wartnaby K, Sherlock S. Abdominal arterial murmurs in liver disease. *Lancet* 1966; ii: 516.

19 Clouse ME, Lee RGL, Duszlak EJ *et al*. Peripheral hepatic artery embolization for primary and secondary hepatic neoplasms. *Radiology* 1983; 147: 407.

20 Cohen C. Intracytoplasmic hyaline globules in hepatocellular carcinomas. *Cancer* 1976; 37: 1754.

21 Collier NA, Weinbren K, Bloom SR. Neurotensin secretion by fibrolamellar carcinoma of the liver. *Lancet* 1984; i: 538.

22 Cottone M, Marceno MP, Maringhini A *et al*. Ultrasound in the diagnosis of hepatocellular carcinoma associated with cirrhosis. *Radiology* 1983; 147: 517.

23 Craig JR, Peters RL, Edmondson HA *et al*. Fibrolamellar carcinoma of the liver: a tumor of adolescents and young adults with distinctive clinico-pathologic features. *Cancer* 1980; 46: 372.

24 Demas BE, Hricak H, Goldberg HI *et al*. Magnetic resonance imaging diagnosis of hepatic matastases in the presence of negative CT studies. *J. clin. Gastro.* 1985; 7: 553.

25 Doll R, Payne P, Waterhouse J. *Cancer Incidence in Five Continents*. International Union against Cancer and Springer-Verlag, Heidelberg. 1966.

26 Dooley JS, Li AKC, Scheuer PJ *et al*. A giant cystic mesenchymal hamartoma of the liver: diagnosis, management, and study of cyst fluid. *Gastroenterology* 1983; 85: 958.

27 Dunk AA, Scott SC, Johnson PJ *et al.* Mitoxantrone as a single agent therapy in hepatocellular carcinoma. A phase II study. *J. Hepatol.* 1985; **1:** 395.

28 Dunk AA, Spiliadis, Sherlock S *et al.* Hepatocellular carcinoma and the hepatitis B virus: a study of British patients. *Q. J. Med.* 1987; **62:** 109.

29 Ebara M, Ohto M, Watanabe Y *et al.* Diagnosis of small hepatocellular carcinoma. Correlation of MR imaging and tumour histologic studies. *Radiology* 1986; **159:** 371.

30 Ebara M, Ohto M, Shinagawa T *et al.* Natural history of minute hepatocellular carcinoma smaller than three centimeters complicating cirrhosis. *Gastroenterology* 1986; **90:** 289.

31 Ekberg H, Tranberg K-G, Andersson R *et al.* Determinants of survival in liver resection for colorectal secondaries. *Br. J. Surg.* 1986; **73:** 727.

32 Enwonwu CO. The role of dietary aflatoxin in the genesis of hepatocellular cancer in developing countries. *Lancet* 1984; **ii:** 956.

33 Eriksson S, Carlson J, Velez R. Risk of cirrhosis and primary liver cancer in ATT deficiency. *N. Engl. J. Med.* 1986; **314:** 736.

34 Falk H, Thomas LB, Popper H *et al.* Hepatic angiosarcoma associated with androgenic-anabolic steroids. *Lancet* 1979; **ii:** 1120.

35 Farber E. Pre-cancerous steps in carcinogenesis: their physiological adaptive nature. *Biochem. Biophys. Acta.* 1984 **738:** 171.

36 Forbes A, Johnson PJ, Williams R. Recombinant human gamma interferon in primary hepatocellular carcinoma. *J. R. Soc. Med.* 1985; **78:** 826.

37 Forbes A, Portmann B, Johnson P *et al.* Hepatic sarcomas in adults: a review of 25 cases. *Gut* 1987; **28:** 668.

38 Gerber MA, Thung SN, Bodenheimer HC Jr *et al.* Characteristic histologic triad in liver adjacent to metastatic neoplasm. *Liver* 1986; **6:** 85.

39 Goodman ZD, Ishak KG, Langloss JM *et al.* Combined hepatocellular-cholangiocarcinoma: a histologic and immunohistochemical study. *Cancer* 1985; **55:** 124.

40 Gralnik HR, Givelber H, Abrams E. Dysfibrinogenemia associated with hepatoma. *N. Engl. J. Med.* 1978; **299:** 221.

41 Gunven P, Makuuchi M, Takayasu K *et al.* Preoperative imaging of liver metastases. Comparison of angiography, CT scan and ultrasonography. *Ann. Surg.* 1985; **202:** 573.

42 Hardell L, Bengtsson NO, Jonsson U *et al.* Aetiological aspects of primary liver cancer with special regard to alcohol, organic solvents and acute intermittent porphyria—an epidemiological investigation. *Br. J. Cancer* 1984; **50:** 389.

43 Harrison HB, Middleton HM III, Crosby JH *et al.* Fulminant hepatic failure: an unusual presentation of metastatic liver disease. *Gastroenterology* 1981; **80:** 820.

44 Helzberg JH, McPhee MS, Zarling EJ *et al.* Hepatocellular carcinoma: an unusual course with hyperthyroidism and inappropriate thyroid-stimulating hormone production. *Gastroenterology* 1985; **88:** 181.

45 Henmi A, Uchida T, Shikata T. Karyometric analysis of liver cell dysplasia and hepato-cellular carcinoma. Evidence against precancerous nature of liver cell dysplasia. *Cancer* 1985; **55:** 2594.

46 Hertzanu Y, Mendelsohn DB, Epstein BM. Massive arterioportal fistula in hepatocellular carcinoma. *Am. J. Gastroenterol.* 1984; **79:** 403.

47 Hiraoka T, Iwai K, Yamashita R *et al.* Metastases from hepatocellular carcinoma in sclerosed oesophagal varices in cirrhotic patients. *Br. J. Surg.* 1986; **73:** 932.

48 Hodgson WJB, Mittelman A, Katz S *et al.* Treatment of colorectal hepatic metastases by intrahepatic chemotherapy alone or as an adjuvant to complete or partial removal of metastatic disease. *Ann. Surg.* 1986; **203:** 420.

49 Hodgson HJF. Fibrolamellar cancer of the liver. *J. Hepatol.* 1987; **5:** 24.

50 Hsieh KH, Shu S, Lee CS *et al.* Lysis of primary hepatic tumours by lymphokine activated killer cells. *Gut* 1987; **28:** 117.

51 Hughes KS, Simon R, Songhorabodi S *et al.* Resection of the liver for colorectal carcinoma metastases: a multi-institutional study of patterns of recurrence. *Surgery* 1986; **100:** 278.

52 Iemoto Y, Kondo Y, Nakano T *et al.* Biliary cystadenocarcinoma diagnosed by liver biopsy performed under ultrasonographic guidance. *Gastroenterology* 1983; **84:** 399.

53 Ishak KG, Sesterhenn IA, Goodman MZD *et al.* Epithelioid hemangioendothelioma of the liver: a clinicopathologic and follow-up study of 32 cases. *Hum. Pathol.* 1984; **15:** 839.

54 Ishak KG, Willis GW, Cummins SD *et al.* Biliary cystadenoma and cystadenocarcinoma: report of 14 cases and review of the literature. *Cancer* 1977; **39:** 322.

55 Itai Y, Ohtomo K, Furui S *et al.* Non-invasive diagnosis of small cavernous hemangioma of the liver. Advantage of MRI. *Am. J. Roentgenol.* 1985; **145:** 1195.

56 Iwatsuki S, Shaw B W Jr, Starzi TE. Experience with 150 liver resections. *Ann. Surg.* 1983; **197:** 247.

57 Johnson DH, Hainsworth JD, Greco FA. Extrahepatic biliary obstruction caused by small-cell lung cancer. *Ann. intern. Med.* 1985; **102:** 487.

58 Johnson PJ, Williams R, Thomas H *et al.* Induction of remission in hepatocellular carcinoma with doxorubicin. *Lancet* 1978; **i:** 1006.

59 Johnson PJ, Williams R. Cirrhosis and the aetiology of hepatocellular carcinoma. *J. Hepatol.* 1987; **5**: 140.

60 Kamby C, Dirksen H, Vejborg I *et al.* Incidence and methodologic aspects of the occurrence of liver metastases in recurrent breast cancer. *Cancer* 1987; **59**: 1524.

61 Kane SP, Murray-Lyon IM, Paradina FJ *et al.* Vitamin B_{12} binding protein as a marker for hepatocellular carcinoma. *Gut* 1978; **19**: 1105.

62 Keeley AF, Iseri OA, Gottlieb LS. Ultrastructure of hyaline cytoplasmic inclusions in a human hepatoma: relationship to Mallory's alcoholic hyalin. *Gastroenterology* 1972; **62**: 280.

63 Kew MC, Gear AJ, Baumgarten I *et al.* Histocompatibility antigens in patients with hepatocellular carcinoma and their relationship to chronic hepatitis B virus infection in these patients. *Gastroenterology* 1979; **77**: 537.

64 Kew MC, Popper H. Relationship between hepatocellular carcinoma and cirrhosis. *Semin. Liver Dis.* 1984; **4**: 136.

65 Kew MC, Fisher JW. Serum erythropoietin concentrations in patients with hepatocellular carcinoma. *Cancer* 1986; **58**: 2485.

66 Kinami Y, Takashima S, Miyazaki I. Hepatic resection for hepatocellular carcinoma associated with liver cirrhosis. *World J. Surg.* 1986; **10**: 294.

67 Kiyosawa K, Akahane Y, Nagata A *et al.* Hepatocellular carcinoma after non-A, non-B posttransfusion hepatitis. *Am. J. Gastroenterol.* 1984; **79**: 777.

68 Kojiro M, Kawabata K, Kawano Y *et al.* Hepatocellular carcinoma presenting as intrabile duct tumour growth: a clinicopathologic study of 24 cases. *Cancer* 1982; **49**: 2144.

69 Kudo M, Hirasa M, Takakuwa H *et al.* Small hepatocellular carcinomas in chronic liver disease: detection with SPECT. *Radiology* 1986; **159**: 697.

70 Lack EE, Neave C, Vawter GF. Hepatoblastoma: a clinical and pathological study of 54 cases. *Am. J. surg. Pathol.* 1982; **6**: 693.

71 Lack EE. Mesenchymal hamartoma of the liver. A clinical and pathological study of nine cases. *Am. J. Pediatr. Hematol/Onocology* 1986; **8**: 91.

72 Lam KC, Ho JCI, Yeung RTT. Spontaneous regression of hepatocellular carcinoma. A case study. *Cancer* 1982; **50**: 332.

73 Lederman SM, Martin EC, Laffey KT *et al.* Hepatic neurofibromatosis, malignant shwannoma and angiosarcoma in von Recklinghauses's disease. *Gastroenterology* 1987; **92**: 234.

74 Lefkowitch JH, Muschel R, Price JB *et al.* Copper and copper-binding protein in fibrolamellar liver cell carcinoma. *Cancer* 1983; **51**: 97.

75 Lefkowitch JH, Apfelbaum TF. Liver cell dys-

plasia and hepatocellular carcinoma in non-A, non-B hepatitis. *Arch. Path. Lab. Med.* 1987; **III**: 170.

76 Liaw Y-F, Tai D-I, Chu C-M *et al.* Early detection of hepatocellular carcinoma in patients with chronic type B hepatitis. *Gastroenterology* 1986; **90**: 263.

77 Lin G, Hagerstrand I, Lunderquist A. Portal blood supply of liver metastases. *Am. J. Roentgenol.* 1984; **143**: 53.

78 Linsell CA, Peers FG. Aflatoxin and liver cell cancer. *Trans. R. Soc. trop. Med. Hyg.* 1977; **71**: 471.

79 Liu YK, Zang KZ, Wu YD *et al.* Treatment of advanced primary hepatocellular carcinoma by I^{131}-anti-AFP. *Lancet* 1983; **i**: 531.

80 Locker GY, Doroshow JH, Zwelling LA *et al.* The clinical features of hepatic angiosarcoma: a report of four cases and a review of the English literature. *Medicine (Baltimore)* 1979; **58**: 48.

81 Lutwick LI. Relation between aflatoxins and hepatitis-B virus and hepatocellular carcinoma. *Lancet* 1979; **i**: 755.

82 McCartney WH, Hoffer PB. Carcinoembryonic antigen assay in hepatic metastasis detection: an adjunct to liver scanning. *J. Am. med. Assoc.* 1976; **236**: 1023.

83 McFazdean AJS, Yeung RTT. Further observations on hypoglycemia in hepatocellular carcinoma. *Am. J. Med.* 1969; **47**: 220.

84 Maki S, Konno T, Maeda H. Image enhancement in a computerized tomography for sensitive diagnosis of liver cancer and semiquantitation of tumour. Selective drug targeting with oily contrast medium. *Cancer* 1985; **56**: 751.

85 Manivel C, Wick MR, Abenoza P *et al.* Teratoid hepatoblastoma. The nosologic dilemma of solid embryonic neoplasms of childhood. *Cancer* 1986; **37**: 2168.

86 Margolis S, Homcy C. Systemic manifestations of hepatoma. *Medicine (Baltimore)* 1972; **51**: 381.

87 Mathieu D, Grenier P, Larde D *et al.* Portal vein involvement in hepatocellular carcinoma: dynamic CT features. *Radiology* 1984; **152**: 127.

88 Morse SS, Sniderman KW, Galloway S *et al.* Hepatoma, arterioportal shunting and hyperkinetic portal hypertension: therapeutic embolization. *Radiology* 1985; **155**: 77.

89 Nagasue N, Yukaya H, Ogawa Y *et al.* Hepatic resection in the treatment of hepatocellular carcinoma: a report of 60 cases. *Br. J. Surg.* 1985; **72**: 292.

90 Nagorney DM, Adson MA, Weiland LH *et al.* Fibrolamellar hepatoma. *Am. J. Surg.* 1985; **149**: 113.

91 Nakao K, Kimura K, Miura Y *et al.* Erythrocytosis associated with carcinoma of the liver (with

erythropoietin assay of tumor extract). *Am. J. med. Sc.* 1966; **251**: 161.

92 Nishioka M, Ibata T, Okita K *et al.* Localisation of α-fetoprotein in hepatoma tissues by immunofluorescence. *Cancer Res.* 1972; **32**: 162.

93 Noguchi S, Yamamoto R, Tatsuta M *et al.* Cell features and patterns in fine-needle aspirates of hepatocellular carcinoma. *Cancer* 1986; **58**: 321.

94 Ohnishi K, Tsuchiya S, Nakayama T *et al.* Arterial chemoembolization of hepatocellular carcinoma with mitomycin C microcapsules. *Radiology* 1984; **152**: 51.

95 Ohnishi S, Murakami T, Moriyama T *et al.* Androgen and estrogen receptors in hepatocellular carcinoma and in the surrounding noncancerous liver tissue. *Hepatology* 1986; **6**: 440.

96 Ohnishi H, Uchida H, Yoshimura H *et al.* Hepatocellular carcinoma detected by iodized oil. Use of anticancer agents. *Radiology* 1985; **154**: 25.

97 Okuda K, and Liver Cancer Study Group of Japan. Primary liver cancers in Japan. *Cancer* 1980; **45**: 2663.

98 Okuda K, Obata H, Nakajima Y *et al.* Prognosis of primary hepatocellular carcinoma. *Hepatology* 1984; **4**: 3S.

99 Okuda K, Peters RL, Simson IW. Gross anatomic features of hepatocellular carcinoma from three disparate geographic areas. *Cancer* 1984; **54**: 2165.

100 Okuda K. Primary liver cancer. Quadrennial review lecture. *Dig. Dis. Sci.* 1986; **31**: (suppl) 133S.

101 Okuda K. Early recognition of hepatocellular carcinoma. *Hepatology* 1986; **6**: 729.

102 Order SE, Stillwagon GB, Klein JL *et al.* Iodine[131] antiferritin, a new treatment modality in hepatoma. *J. clin. Oncol.* 1985; **3**: 1573.

103 Paradinas RJ, Melia WM, Wilkinson ML *et al.* High serum vitamin B12 binding capacity as a marker of the fibrolamellar variant of hepatocellular carcinoma. *Br. med. J.* 1982; **285**: 840.

104 Patt YZ, McBride CM, Ames FC *et al.* Adjuvant perioperative hepatic arterial mitomycin C and floxuridine combined with surgical resection of metastatic colorectal cancer of the liver. *Cancer* 1987; **59**: 867.

105 Peters RL, Afroudakis AP, Tatter D. The changing incidence of association of hepatitis B with hepatocellular carcinoma in California. *Am. J. clin. Pathol.* 1977; **68**: 1.

106 Pierach CA, Bossenmaier IC, Cardinal RA *et al.* Pseudoporphyria in a patient with hepatocellular carcinoma. *Am. J. Med.* 1984; **76**: 545.

107 Popper H, Gerber MA, Thung SN. The relation of hepatocellular carcinoma to infection with hepatitis B and related viruses in man and animals. *Hepatology* 1982; **2**: 1S.

108 Raimondo G, Craxi A, Longo G *et al.* Delta infection in hepatocellular carcinoma positive for hepatitis B surface antigen. *Ann. intern. Med.* 1984; **101**: 342.

109 Ramming KP, O'Toole K. The use of implantable cheminfusion pump in the treatment of hepatic metastases of colorectal cancer. *Arch. Surg.* 1986; **121**: 1440.

110 Resnick RH, Stone K, Antonioli D. Primary hepatocellular carcinoma following non-A, non-B post-transfusion hepatitis. *Dig. Dis. Sci.* 1983; **28**: 908.

111 Ridge JA, Sigurdson ER. Distribution of fluorodeoxyuridine uptake in the liver and colorectal metastases of human beings after arterial infusion. *Surg. Gyn. Obstet.* 1987; **164**: 319.

112 Ross JS, Kurian S. Clear cell hepatocarcinoma: sudden death from hypoglycemia. *Am. J. Gastroenterol.* 1985; **80**: 188.

113 Rubel LR, Ishak KG. Thorotrast-associated cholangiocarcinoma: an epidemiologic and clinicopathologic study. *Cancer* 1982; **50**: 1408.

114 Sato Y, Fujiwara K, Furui S *et al.* Benefit of transcatheter arterial embolization for ruptured hepatocellular carcinoma complicating liver cirrhosis. *Gastroenterology* 1985; **89**: 157.

115 Schreve RH, Terpstra OT, Ausema L *et al.* Detection of liver metastases: a prospective study comparing liver enzymes, scintigraphy, ultrasonography and computed tomography. *Br. J. Surg.* 1984; **71**: 947.

116 Schwartz SI, Husser WC. Cavernous hemangioma of the liver. A single institution report of 16 resections. *Ann. Surg.* 1987; **205**: 456.

117 Sherlock S, Fox FA, Niazi SP *et al.* Chronic liver disease and primary liver-cell cancer with hepatitis-associated (Australia) antigen in serum. *Lancet* 1970; **i**: 1243.

118 Sherlock S, Dick R. The impact of radiology on hepatology. *Am. J. Roentgenol.* 1986; **147**: 1116.

119 Sheu J-C, Lee C-S, Sung J-L *et al.* Intra-operative hepatic ultrasonography—an indispensable procedure in resection of small hepatocellular carcinomas. *Surgery* 1985; **97**: 97.

120 Sheu J-C, Sung J-L, Chen D-S *et al.* Growth rate of asymptomatic hepatocellular carcinoma and its clinical implications. *Gastroenterology.* 1985; **89**: 259.

121 Simpson IW. Membranous obstruction of the inferior vena cava and hepatocellular carcinoma of South Africa. *Gastroenterology.* 1982; **82**: 171.

122 Solbiati L, Livraghi T, De Pra L *et al.* Fine-needle biopsy of hepatic hemangioma with sonographic guidance. *Am. J. Roentgenol.* 1985; **144**: 471.

123 Soulier J-P, Gozin D, Lefrere J-J. A new method to assay des-gamma-carboxyprothrombin. Results obtained in 75 cases of hepatocellular carcinoma. *Gastroenterology* 1986; **91**: 1258.

124 Starzl TE, Iwatsuki S, Shaw BW Jr *et al.* Treatment

of fibrolamellar hepatoma with partial or total hepatectomy and transplantation of the liver. *Surg. Gyn. Obstet.* 1986; **162:** 145.

125 Strohmeyer FW, Ishak KG, Gerber MA *et al.* Ground-glass cells in hepatocellular carcinoma may contain fibrinogen. *Am. J. clin. Path.* 1980; **74:** 254.

126 Sumida M, Ohto M, Ebara M *et al.* Accuracy of arteriography in the diagnosis of small hepatocellular carcinoma. *Am. J. Roentgenol.* 1986; **147:** 531.

127 Summerskill WHJ, Adson MA. Gynecomastia as a sign of hepatoma. *Am. J. dig. Dis.* 1962; **74:** 250.

128 Szmuness W, Stevens CE, Ikram H *et al.* Prevalence of hepatitis-B virus infection and hepatocellular carcinoma in Chinese-Americans. *J. infect. Dis.* 1978; **137:** 822.

129 Takayasu K, Shima Y, Muramatsu Y *et al.* Hepatocellular carcinoma: treatment with intraarterial iodized oil with and without chemotherapeutic agents. *Radiology* 1987; **162:** 345.

130 Tanaka S, Kitamura T, Ohshima A *et al.* Diagnostic accuracy of ultrasonography for hepatocellular carcinoma. *Cancer* 1986; **58:** 344.

131 Tang ZY, Yang BH. Early detection of subclinical hepatocellular carcinoma *In* Tang, *Subclinical Hepatocellular Carcinoma*, 27th edn. Beijing: China Academic Publishers 1985; 12.

132 Trichopoulos D, Day NE, Kaklamani E *et al.* Hepatitis B virus, tobacco smoking and ethanol consumption in the etiology of hepatocellular carcinoma. *Int. J. Cancer* 1987; **39:** 45.

133 Walsh PN, Kissane JM. Nonmetastatic hypernephroma with reversible hepatic dysfunction. *Arch. intern. Med.* 1968; **122:** 214.

134 Warshaw AL, Welch JP. Extrahepatic biliary obstruction by metastatic colon cancer. *Ann. Surg.* 1978; **188:** 593.

135 Weinberg AG, Finegold MJ. Primary hepatic tumours of childhood. *Hum. Pathol.* 1983; **14:** 512.

136 Wilkinson ML, Portmann B, Williams R. Wilson's disease and hepatocellular carcinoma: possible protective role of copper. *Gut* 1983; **24:** 767.

137 Willett IR, Sutherland RC, O'Rourke MF *et al.* Pulmonary hypertension complicating hepatocellular carcinoma. *Gastroenterology* 1984; **87:** 1180.

138 Willis RA. Secondary tumours of the liver. In *The spread of tumours in the human body* 3rd edn. London: Butterworths 1973: 178.

139 Younus S, Soterakis J, Sossi AJ *et al.* Hypoglycemia secondary to metastases to the liver. *Gastroenterology* 1977; **72:** 334.

140 Zaman SN, Melia WM, Johnson RD *et al.* Risk factors in development of hepatocellular carcinoma in cirrhosis: prospective study of 613 patients. *Lancet* 1985; **i:** 1357.

29 · Investigation of the Biliary Tract: Therapeutic Imaging

Bile secretion

The liver secretes approximately 600 dl bile per day. There is a diurnal variation, more being excreted in the day than at night. Bile is secreted at a pressure of 15–25 cm H_2O and ceases when the pressure in the common bile duct rises to 35 cm H_2O. The sphincter of Oddi offers a resistance to bile flow of 10–25 cm H_2.

Protein is present in small amounts and there are variable amounts of mucin. The reaction of bile is neutral or slightly alkaline.

The cholesterol, phospholipid, bile salts and probably bilirubin form soluble macromolecular complexes or micelles. These allow the non-polar, insoluble cholesterol to be carried in solution (Chapter 31). Bile is usually sterile but occasionally *E. coli*, staphylococci or enterococci may be isolated.

The mechanisms and control of biliary secretion are discussed in Chapters 13 and 31. Secretion is largely by a bile salt-dependent mechanism and ductular flow is controlled by secretin. The place of nervous and vascular reflexes is unknown.

The entero-hepatic circulation of bile salts is discussed in Chapters 2 and 31.

FUNCTIONS OF BILE

Bile salts form micelles or vesides, solubilize triglycerides and assist in its absorption, together with calcium, cholesterol and fat-soluble vitamins, from the intestine.

Bile is the main route for excretion of bilirubin and cholesterol. The products of steroid hormones, particularly sex, thyroid and adrenal, are also excreted in bile.

Bile is the main route of excretion of some drugs and poisons such as the salts of heavy metals, atropine, strychnine and salicylates. This may be related to molecular size (fig. 18.1). Larger molecules, after being made soluble by such processes as conjugation, are excreted into the bile. Smaller molecules are excreted in the urine.

Bile salts absorbed from the intestine stimulate the liver to make more bile. Bile salts activate intestinal and pancreatic lipolytic and proteolytic enzymes.

Gallbladder function [56]

Hepatic bile is stored in the gallbladder where its volume is reduced by the absorption of an essentially isotonic NaCl, HCO_3 solution. The concentration of bile salts, bilirubin and cholesterol, for which the gallbladder wall is essentially impermeable, may increase 10-fold or more. This reduction is achieved by active transport of NaCl and HCO_3 along with a nearly isotonic amount of water from bile into the blood.

The rate of trans-cellular sodium transport across the gallbladder epithelium depends on the rate of entry by passive diffusion across the luminal cell membrane and on active sodium extrusion across the basal–lateral cell membrane by a sodium pump. Water absorption is passive and secondary to active solute movement. Ions also move across the epithelium by the paracellular pathway. The gallbladder mucosa also secretes water and electrolytes, possibly to lubricate its wall.

The transport is influenced by gastro-intestinal peptides, prostaglandins, bile acids and the autonomic nervous system [57].

Changes in epithelial transport are particularly important in acute cholecystitis where the gallbladder neck is obstructed by a stone with a reversal of the direction of fluid transport across the gallbladder mucosa. This leads to distention of the gallbladder which stimulates prostaglandin synthesis by the gallbladder wall. Necrosis and gallbladder perforation follow [54].

The gallbladder is appreciably permeable to lipid-soluble molecules and this may lead to gradual but significant alteration of bile composition, by absorption of biliary lipids and of unconjugated bilirubin which have been formed by bacterial enzymatic breakdown of conjugated bilirubin [56]. Even some of the bile acids, particularly those conjugated with glycine or those which have undergone bacterial deconjugation, may be absorbed. This might promote gallstone formation (Chapter 31).

Because of micelle (vesicle) formation, the bile salts do not exert their expected osmotic activity. The concentrated bile therefore remains isoosmotic with serum despite the fact that it has nearly twice the number of ionic particles per litre.

Motor functions of the biliary tract

The choledochal sphincter (*sphincter of Oddi*) [28] is short, about 5 mm long, and lies within the intraduodenal portion of the common bile duct. Manometry at the time of endoscopic cholangiography shows that the bile duct pressure exceeds that in the duodenum by 10 mmHg and, at rest, the sphincter of Oddi pressure zone is 5–10 mmHg greater than the common bile duct pressure. The sphincter contracts 4–6 times a minute with peristalsis towards the duodenum. It can act independently of the rest of the duodenal musculature. It can withstand a pressure of 10–15 mmHg in the common bile duct.

When the sphincter contracts, bile is diverted into the cystic duct for storage in the gallbladder. When the gallbladder is full, and if there is no specific stimulus for its evacuation, the sphincter relaxes and bile trickles into the duodenum. The sphincter creates a gradient between the bile or pancreatic ducts and the duodenum and prevents reflux of duodenal content into them [11].

Gallbladder motility may be studied by timed aspiration of bile from the duodenum, but this lacks precision. Cineradiography of the biliary tract has been used to show peristalsis of the common bile duct. Cholescintigraphy using ^{99m}Tc-HIDA has also been used to study gallbladder emptying [27]. Gallbladder contraction may also be investigated by real-time ultrasonography so obviating the need for radiation exposure or intestinal intubation.

Cholecystokinin (CCK) is a peptide hormone contained in neuroendocrine cells of the duodenum and jejunum (called I cells) from where it is released into the blood stream, presumably by stimulation by intraluminal hydrogen ions, fats and some amino acids. It binds to receptors on gallbladder smooth muscle and on acinar cells and induces gallbladder contraction and stimulates pancreatic enzyme secretion. The gallbladder empties within one to two minutes with complete emptying within fifteen minutes. The sphincter of Oddi is relaxed. In man, the gallbladder contracts in response to physiological concentrations of CCK [23]. It responds to sham feeding if the vagus nerves are intact [17]. At least in the dog, post-contractile gallbladder filling may be controlled in part by pancreatic polypeptide [8]. Other gallbladder stimulants include pituitrin while atropin is a relaxant.

Using a modified duodenal perfusion technique, it seems likely that gallbladder storage and emptying alternate frequently, a phenomenon more analogous to a bellows than the conventional concept of a simple pump [29].

CCK and glucagon suppress sphincter of Oddi motor activity, whereas pentagastrin increases it. Secretin causes the largest response, excitation followed by inhibition. The sphincter of Oddi is contracted by morphia (which also lessens bile duct contractions), secretin and analgesics generally. Opioid peptides participate in the neuromuscular control of the sphincter of Oddi, at least in the cat [3]. Enkephalins stimulate the sphincter. Naloxone infusion decreases sphincter pressure and antagonizes morphine contraction. Increased tone is little affected by the usual antispasmodics such as atropin. Amyl nitrate may relax the sphincter. Of the analgesics, pentazocine (fortral) causes least rise in biliary pressure.

Biliary dyskinesia
See Chapter 31.

Gallbladder stasis

Interference with the neural and hormonal stimulation of the biliary tract may result in gallbladder stasis. Gallbladder dilatation is seen in diabetes [26] and after vagotomy. It develops during the last trimester of pregnancy and after oral contraceptive steroids. Prolonged periods of fasting promote gallbladder stasis by failure of neural and hormonal stimulation and a similar sequence follows long-term parenteral nutrition [41]. Gallbladder stasis facilitates gallstone production (see Chapter 31).

Somatostatin is a potent inhibitor of gallbladder emptying in humans but this may be important in the development of gallstone in patients with somatostatinomas [18].

Duodenal intubation and drainage

These procedures are rarely performed to assess biliary function. Cholesterol crystals, calcium bilirubinate granules and microspheroliths are found in abnormal amounts in patients with gallbladder disease, particularly after CCK stimulation [4].

Cholesterol monohydrate crystals in the bile may distinguish patients with or without gallstones even when the stones are not visualized by conventional means [12].

An increased bacterial flora in the upper gastrointestinal tract may be found in patients with cholangitis and this may even produce a 'blind loop' syndrome [41].

Ultrasound

Ultrasonography is an important screening investigation in patients with cholestasis (figs 29.1, 29.2). The presence of dilated hepatic ducts characterizes large bile duct obstruction. The intra-hepatic bile ducts exceed 6 mm in diameter. They are seen as two fluid-filled structures in a parasagittal plane. The dilated common duct assumes a comma shape as it passes dorsally through the head of the pancreas. The technique is 94% accurate if a serum bilirubin level exceeds 10 mg/dl. False negatives are seen if the cholestasis is of short duration and the ducts are less dilated. Ultrasound rarely diagnoses the cause of the obstruction, largely due to failure to visualize the complete biliary tract. The lower end particularly is not seen because of overlying gas in the duodenum and bowel. The gallbladder is ideal for sonography. The examination should be performed fasting which results in a distended gallbladder full of bile. Gallstones cast intense echoes with obvious posterior acoustic shadows. They change in position with that of the patient. Stones 3 mm in size and upwards may be

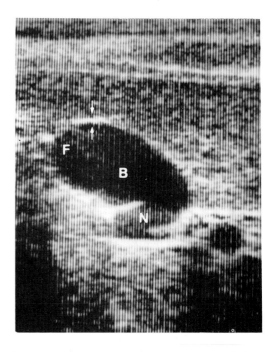

Fig. 29.1. Ultrasound appearances of the gallbladder. F = fundus, B = body, N = neck. (Courtesy of K. Okuda.)

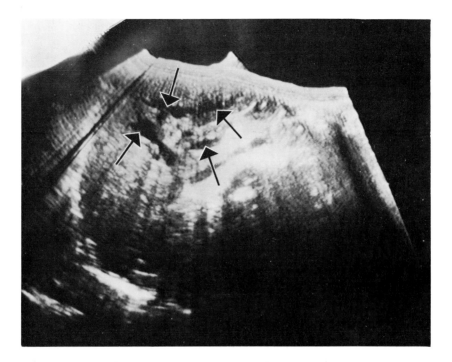

Fig. 29.2. Ultrasound shows dilated intra-hepatic bile ducts in a patient with carcinoma of the head of the pancreas.

visualized (fig. 29.3). Diagnostic accuracy is said to be 96% but less experienced operators will not achieve this success and there are many diagnostic pitfalls [19].

Acute cholecystitis is suggested by gallstones, thickening of the gallbladder wall and bile sludging, but the appearances are not diagnostic. Bile sludge may also be seen with biliary obstruction, prolonged fasting and parenteral nutrition. Sometimes it forms sludge balls which do not cast acoustic shadows [2].

Dilatation of the gallbladder may be shown. Cancer of the gallbladder may be suspected. Congenital biliary anomalies such as Caroli's disease or choledochal cysts may be demonstrated.

Intra-operative ultrasound is of particular value in the localization of focal lesions, such as metastases so allowing accurate planning of surgical resections.

Polyps in the gallbladder are visualized. If less than 1 cm in size they are not significant, if greater than 2 cm there is a risk of cancer.

Ultrasound allows guided percutaneous access to the gallbladder for sampling bile, drainage or antegrade cholangiography, and even gallstone dissolution or removal.

Computerized axial tomography (CT scan)

In cholestatic jaundice, CT scanning will show dilated bile ducts. It distinguishes obstructive from non-obstructive jaundice with an accuracy rate of 90%, but as a screening procedure has no advantages over ultrasound. It is, however, more likely to give the cause of the obstruction (figs 29.4, 29.5). The lower end of the common bile duct is well seen. Any pancreatic or hilar lesion will be identified. It shows air in the bile ducts (fig. 29.6) and can be used following previous biliary bypass surgery.

CT scanning is of limited use in gallbladder disease as it will not consistently demonstrate gallstones and may fail to visualize the thickness of the gallbladder wall.

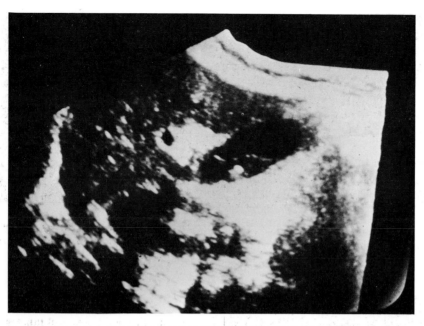

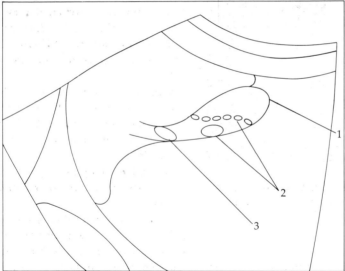

Fig. 29.3. Ultrasound in acute cholecystitis. A distended gallbladder (1) contains stones (2). A stone is impacted in the cystic duct (3).

CT may be used to distinguish cholesterol gallstone with a low density (less than 50 HU) from brown-black gallstones with a high density (greater than 150 HU).

Radiology

The shape and position of the gallbladder depend on the individual's somatotype; it may be found as high as the eleventh rib or below the iliac crest. It usually lies parallel to the spine, at the eleventh and twelfth ribs, and its body is cut by the shadow of the oblique lower margin of the liver. In one-quarter of normal subjects, part may overlap the shadow of the second and third lumbar vertebrae. The gallbladder always lies above the transverse colon and the fundus is usually in apposition to the

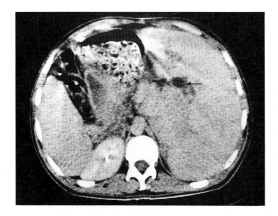

Fig. 29.4. CT scan (enhanced by contrast) showing dilated intra-hepatic bile ducts (arrowed).

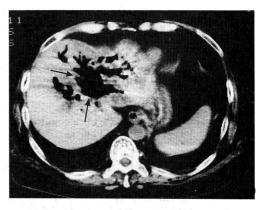

Fig. 29.6. CT scan (enhanced by contrast) showing air in a dilated biliary tree (arrowed) in a patient with a biliary–enteric surgical anastomosis.

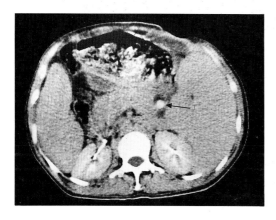

Fig. 29.5. Same patient as fig. 29.4 a (lower 'cut') showing the cause of the biliary obstruction to be a gallstone in the common bile duct (arrowed).

PLAIN FILM OF THE ABDOMEN

Diagnostic yield is low and this test is tending to be omitted. However, it may reveal gallstones, a calcified gallbladder or, rarely, the outline of a distended gallbladder. A soft tissue shadow may be seen with carcinoma of the gallbladder.

With obstruction to the cystic duct, calcium carbonate may be excreted with the bile (milk of calcium bile or 'limey bile'). The wall of the gallbladder may also calcify (porcelain gallbladder).

Gas in the biliary tree (fig. 29.7) may be due to a spontaneous or post-operative biliary fistula.

Gas may regurgitate through an incompetent sphincter of Oddi with cholecystitis, stricture or gallstones or after sphincterotomy. Gas-gangrene infection is a very rare cause (emphysematous cholecystitis) [24].

Cholecystography and cholangiography

The contrast materials are iodine-containing, conjugated and detoxicated by the liver, and excreted in the bile. With renal disease hepato-biliary excretion increases. Conversely, with hepato-cellular disease, renal excretion predominates and a pyelogram results. In such

duodenal cap. It overlies and is well anterior to the right renal shadow. Similarly, the more medially placed common bile duct overlies the pelvis of the kidney, but is anterior to it.

The dimensions of the common bile duct depend on techniques employed. Using endoscopic cholangiography, the common bile duct is usually less than 11 mm and values greater than 18 mm are pathological [35]. By ultrasound, values are less, the common bile duct being 2–5 mm and values greater than this are abnormal.

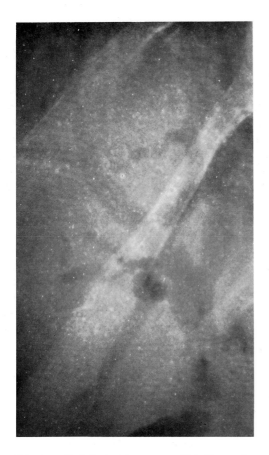

Fig. 29.7. Choledochojejunostomy. Plain X-ray of the abdomen shows gas outlining the biliary tract.

patients high blood levels of contrast are reached. However, with the newer contrast materials of low osmolarity, hypersensitivity and renal changes are extremely rare.

ORAL

Three films are necessary: control, fasting after oral contrast, and after gallbladder contraction by a fatty meal or CCK. The gallbladder and common bile duct will be shown in 85% of patients. Films are taken in erect and prone positions. The erect is useful in demonstrating translucent stones.

Normal visualization, without stones, gives a 95% probability that the gallbladder is normal.

Cholecystography should not be done if the serum conjugated bilirubin level is above 2 mg/100 ml. Failure of gallbladder filling within 14 hours may be due to defective intestinal absorption of contrast, previous cholecystectomy, a diseased or intra-hepatic gallbladder, an obstructed cystic duct or poor liver function.

Uses of cholecystography

Gallstones will be detected with a false-negative rate of 1% [11].

Oral cholecystography is of particular value in lesions of the gallbladder wall which are best shown after CCK injection [11] as small fixed radiolucent zones unaffected by posture. The most usual are cholesterol deposits. Adenomyomatosis is shown as small fundal outpouchings. *Rokitansky—Aschoff sinuses* are shown as a dotted second contour around the gallbladder. Abnormalities in shape, size and contractility of the gallbladder may be seen. The common bile duct is usually visualized.

Intravenous with tomography

The contrast (meglumine iotroxate; biliscopin) is concentrated by the liver so that cystic, hepatic and common bile ducts are regularly demonstrated before the gallbladder.

Intravenous cholangiography has become obsolete because of its poor diagnostic accuracy, morbidity and the advent of ultrasound.

Biliary scintigraphy

The technetium-labelled compound is cleared from the plasma by hepato-cellular organic anion transport and excreted in the bile. The biliary radiopharmaceuticals have so improved that one of the newest, diethyliodo HIDA (Iod HIDA) is easily prepared and only 5% of the injected dose is excreted in the urine. Effective concentration in the bile duct is achieved in patients with total serum bilirubin levels exceeding 20 mg/dl. Resolution is much less than with other forms of bile duct visualization and the role of cholescintigraphy is therefore limited.

The method may be used to determine patency of the cystic duct in suspected *acute cholecystitis* (fig. 29.8). The contrast is followed until it reaches the duodenum. If the gallbladder fails to visualize in three to four hours, despite common bile duct patency and intestinal visualization, the probability of acute cholecystitis is 99% [13]. Acalculous cholecystitis may be diagnosed. Combination with ultrasound may improve the discrimination between intra-hepatic and extra-hepatic *cholestasis* [32].

The patency of *biliary—enteric shunts*, whether surgical or prostethic, may be established.

Biliary leaks, whether operative, post-operative or traumatic can be identified. The method is of particular value after hepatic transplantation [25].

Choledochal cysts can be diagnosed although ultrasound or CT scanning are just as satisfactory.

In the *neonate*, biliary scanning is used to differentiate between atresia and neonatal hepatitis (fig. 29.9). It may be combined with ultrasound.

Functional obstruction of the sphincter of Oddi after cholecystectomy may be suggested by delayed and reduced excretion of contrast with a slower emptying rate.

Endoscopic retrograde cholangio-pancreatography (ERCP) [9, 15]

The ampulla of Vater is visualized endoscopically, the common bile duct or pancreatic duct is cannulated and contrast material injected (fig. 29.10). Diseases of oesophagus, stomach, duodenum, pancreas and biliary tract including duodenal diverticulae and fistulae may be diagnosed. Manometry of the sphincter area is possible. Immediate treatment may be instituted for instance, sphincterotomy for common duct stones. However, endoscopes are costly and the technique demands an experienced team. Usually the patient must be under observation for 24 hours after the procedure which is done under light sedation (atropine and diazepam) and local (never general) anaesthesia. Duodenal ileus is maintained by intermittent intravenous hyoscine N-butylbromide (Buscopan) or glucagon. The fibrescope, usually sideviewing JFB3 or JF1T duodenoscope, is passed. The papillary region is reached. The stomach and duodenum having been surveyed, biopsy and cytology specimens and photographs are taken as necessary. The papilla is identified and any lesion in the area biopsied. The cannula is then introduced under direct vision into the papilla and bile duct and contrast (diatrizoate sodium or angiografin 65%) injected under fluoroscopic control.

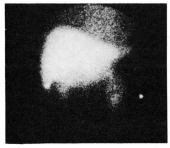
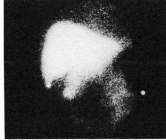
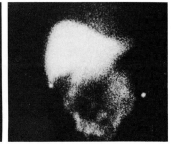

Fig. 29.8. ^{99m}Tc-HIDA Gamma camera scan. Serial scans show the uptake of HIDA by the liver (5 min, *left*) and into the common bile duct (25 min, *centre*) and finally into the duodenum (35 min, *right*). This patient had acute cholecystitis. The gallbladder did not fill.

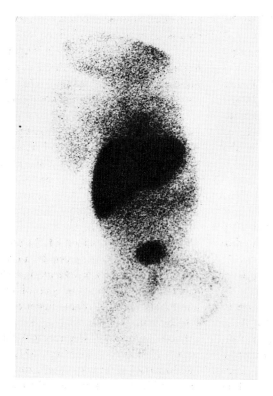

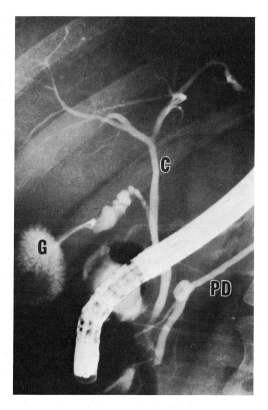

Fig. 29.9. Two-week-old infant with severe jaundice. Cholescintogram, using diethyl iodo HIDA, shows radionuclide concentrated in liver, with some in urinary bladder. Biliary atresia was confirmed. (Sherlock & Dick, 1986.)

Fig. 29.10. ERCP, normal appearances. PD = pancreatic duct; G = gallbladder; C = common bile duct.

Posturing is needed to fill the intra-hepatic biliary tree, cystic and common bile ducts and gallbladder (fig. 29.10). Changes in the position of the patient and tilting of the radiological table at the end of the injection distribute contrast material through the duct system. In difficult cases a balloon catheter in the duct may be used to block contrast leakage and so obtain better filling [58]. The pancreatic duct is similarly cannulated and photographed. Patients with suspected biliary obstruction or cholangitis are given antibiotics before the examination and afterwards if the biliary obstruction has not been relieved or a diseased gallbladder remains *in situ*.

An aseptic technique is maintained throughout. Cannulas are sterilized with ethylene oxide gas and the endoscopes thoroughly cleansed with soap and water and disinfected with activated glutaraldehyde. The danger of spreading disease is shown by a single endoscope which, although cleaned in an automatic machine, remained contaminated with *P. aeruginosa* so resulting in biliary infection in ten patients with one fatality [1]. This could have been prevented by manually suctioning alcohol through the endoscope before drying.

The history of minor reactions to intravenous contrast is not important but those who have had a major allergic reaction to iodinated contrast should be premedicated with corticosteroids and antihistamines [34].

The success rate is 75 to 85% but depends on experience. Other causes of failure include papillary stenosis or tumour, peri-ampullary diverticulum or previous ulceration. A Billroth

II gastrectomy poses difficulties which may be avoided with appropriate manipulation and the use of a forward viewing endoscope [38].

Interpretation is not always very easy. Contrast may obscure small stones. Air bubbles may be confusing. The sphincter zone is difficult to interpret. Poor mixing of contrast with bile and failure to fill the biliary tree, particularly in non-dependent parts, may add to the difficulty.

COMPLICATIONS

The complication rate is 3% and mortality 0.1−0.2%. Complications are directly related to the skill and experience of the operator and to the presence of underlying pancreatic or biliary disease.

Cholangitis is the commonest cause of death and the second most common complication. Bacteraemia is reported in 0−14% [46]. Pre-existing biliary infection and stasis are more important aetiologically. Prophylactic antibiotics are important in prevention together with early decompression of any biliary obstruction.

Serum amylase levels rise considerably after ERCP and acute pancreatitis is the commonest

complication. It always follows successful pancreatic cannulation and injection, usually in those with pancreatic disease. There is no correlation between acinar filling and pancreatitis. Infection plays a minor role. Pancreatic pseudo-cyst is an absolute contraindication to ERCP.

Biliary leakage and haemorrhage have been seen in those with tumours. It is also possible to damage the papilla and to perforate the duodenum.

CLINICAL INDICATIONS

ERCP adds to the speed of diagnosis of the jaundiced patient as it can be performed irrespective of depth of icterus or state of liver function. It outlines the site of any biliary obstruction and in many instances indicates the cause (fig. 29.11).

It can be used to diagnose gallbladder and common bile duct stones (fig. 29.12). ERCP is of particular value in those with biliary disease and undilated intra-hepatic ducts. Diagnoses include primary sclerosing cholangitis, Caroli's disease and other congenital anomalies, biliary strictures, both simple and malignant and haemobilia.

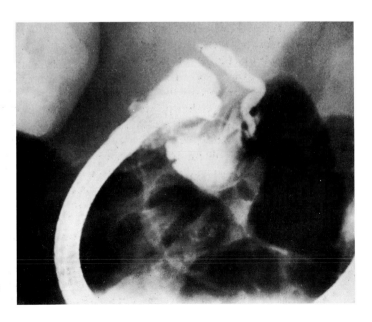

Fig. 29.11. ERCP showing nipple-like obstruction at the hilum of the liver due to bile duct carcinoma.

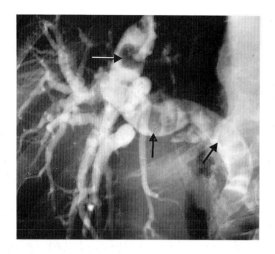

Fig. 29.12. Endoscopic retrograde cholangiography shows multiple gallstones in the common bile duct.

ERCP may be performed after biliary surgery in the investigation of benign post-cholecystectomy symptoms or to define more serious sequelae such as residual calculi, biliary strictures and choledochoduodenal fistulae.

ERCP may be used to diagnose pancreatic disease, particularly in those with coincident hepato-biliary problems such as alcoholic pancreatitis with biliary obstruction (fig. 19.10).

ERCP is used in the investigation of the patient with obscure epigastric pain. It allows visualization of stomach and duodenum as well as pancreatic and biliary ducts, all at one sitting.

Pure pancreatic juice or bile may be obtained for culture, aspiration cytology or chemical analysis.

Endoscopic sphincterotomy [6]

Haemoglobin and blood coagulation must be checked. Following ERCP, a sphincterotomy of the ampulla of Vater may be performed. A skilled team is required with adequate equipment and in a hospital with facilities to treat any complication. The sphincterotomy is done with a diathermy knife inserted deep into the bile duct. The bow is tightened and under fluoroscopic control a cut 15 to 20 mm long is produced sufficiently deep to oblate the biliary sphincters (figs 29.13, 29.14). The valve-like function of the ampulla is destroyed, allowing

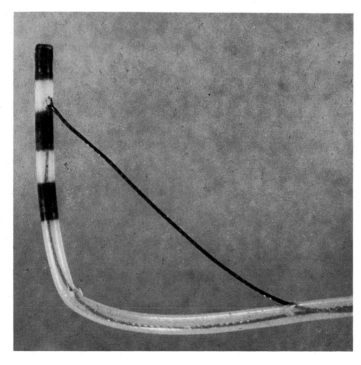

Fig. 29.13. Catheter and electrocautery used for endoscopic sphincterotomy.

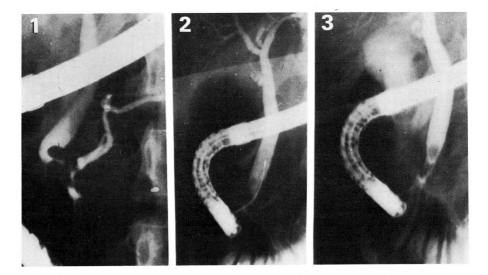

Fig. 29.14. Endoscopic sphincterotomy. Endoscopic retrograde cholangiography shows (1) residual gallstones at the lower end of the common bile duct, (2) the electrocautery is in position at the lower end of the common bile duct, (3) post-sphincterotomy the stone has passed and air bubbles are seen in the common bile duct.

reflux of air into the biliary system. The pressure in the common bile duct falls.

The success rate is about 93% [30]. Causes for failure include a large peri-ampullary diverticulum, a Billroth II partial gastrectomy and an unusual anatomy of the bile ducts.

COMPLICATIONS

These occur in 10% and in 2–3% are life threatening, usually requiring surgical treatment. Mortality is 0.5 to 2%.

Bleeding, usually from the retro-duodenal artery, is the commonest problem. It usually settles, but if not, surgery can be difficult. Cholangitis has been reduced by the insertion of a post-operative peri-nasal biliary drain. Retro-peritoneal duodenal or biliary perforation is another possibility.

Late results show that two-thirds of patients develop air in the biliary tract and free reflux of bile from the duodenum. Bacterial overgrowth in the bile is present whether or not there are symptoms; the significance of this is unknown. In one three-year follow-up, mild symptoms with an increase in serum gamma GT level and with slight hepatic histological changes were

noted [20]. The long-term results of loss of sphincter function are unresolved.

INDICATIONS

Choledocholithiasis is the commonest therapeutic indication. Endoscopy is the treatment of choice for frail, elderly patients with *post-cholecystectomy retained stones*. In one series, there was only one death out of 59 patients having endoscopic treatment and who were judged to be unsuitable for surgery; 90% were jaundiced, 32% had cholangitis and the mean age was 78 years. Sphincterotomy is of particular value as an emergency in patients with *acute biliary disease* (jaundice, cholangitis, gallstone pancreatitis). Those patients who are young and fit can then come to cholecystectomy electively. The question of eventual cholecystectomy remains controversial. 45 patients having clearance of duct stones but with the gallbladder left *in situ* were followed for 2 to 7 years and only six required cholecystectomy [10].

The role of endoscopic sphincterotomy in young, fit patients who have not had a cholecystectomy remains to be determined. It is, however, preferred by the patient, necessitates only 2 to 6 days in hospital and is therefore considerably less costly.

Stone extraction is done with wire baskets (fig. 29.15), or balloon-tipped catheters. In 90% the common bile duct is successfully cleared of stones [9]. If all the stones cannot be extracted, a peri-nasal biliary catheter must be left to drain the duct and antibiotics must be given (fig. 29.16). Stones larger than 15 mm may be difficult to extract and crushing baskets may be used. Peri-nasal intra-biliary infusion of solutions such as mono-octanoin may reduce the size of the stone and allow extraction, but is only 50–60% successful [31].

Extra corporeal shock wave lithotripsy of common bile duct stones fragments them and allows them to pass through the sphincterotomy [51].

Papillary stenosis (see Chapter 31).

Choledochoduodenostomy stenosis. Sphincterotomy at the main papilla may be used to treat the rare sump syndrome. Enlargement of the stenotic stoma may also be attempted by diathermy incision and balloon dilatation.

Foreign bodies in the bile ducts. Ascaris or *Fasciola hepatica* worms may be removed through a sphincterotomy.

Acute biliary pancreatitis (see Chapter 31).

Endoscopic therapy in the bile duct may be preceded by sphincterotomy to allow the passage of a perinasal biliary drain or to allow the introduction of a stent into the common bile duct. It would, of course, be preferable if such procedures could be performed without the need for sphincterotomy as complications would be less. This might be achieved by dilating the papilla with an angioplasty-type balloon perhaps combined with better crushing devices for stones [30].

Nasobiliary drainage

A previous sphincterotomy may or may not be necessary. Using the endoscope, the common bile duct is cannulated and the guide wire passed through it into the distal intra-hepatic ducts. The cannula is removed and a 300 cm 5F thin wall, pigtail catheter with multiple side

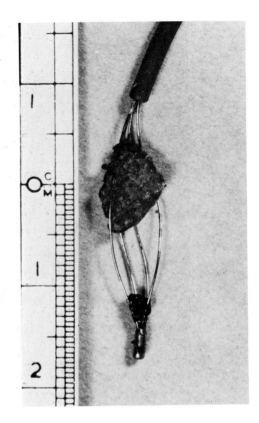

Fig. 29.15. Dormia basket containing a gallstone which has been extracted from the common bile duct via a T tube.

holes is threaded over the wire which is then removed. The cannula is brought out through the nose. This allows decompression of the biliary tree through the catheter. Hilar lesions are difficult to cannulate. Duodenal obstruction adds to technical difficulties. There are less complications than with percutaneous biliary drainage in terms of infection, bile leak and bleeding.

This is used as a preliminary to sphincterotomy in poor risk patients with choledocholithiasis and acute suppurative cholangitis or with gallstone pancreatitis (fig. 29.16).

A nasal biliary drain may be left in position when, after sphincterotomy, it has been impossible to clear all the stones from the common bile duct.

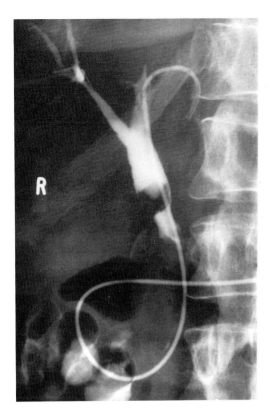

Fig. 29.16. Perinasal biliary tube with stones in the common bile duct.

A nasal biliary drain allows cholangiography of the bile ducts to check complete clearance of stones.

A nasal biliary drain may be used to perfuse the common bile duct with gallstone solvents such as mono-octanoic acid.

Nasal biliary drainage may be used to aspirate bile for chemical and bacteriological studies.

Endoscopic biliary prostheses

After successful endoscopic sphincterotomy, a guide wire is inserted through a cannula and through the obstruction, the stent is passed over it and advanced through the lesion and pushed above the obstruction. A large calibre stent (3.3 mm diameter 10 French) provides effective decompression, but requires a special endoscope (JF-IT; duo-XL; F32A) [47, 55]. The endotheses are kept in position by barbs or by pigtails at one or both ends. Two may be used if necessary (fig. 29.17). In skilled hands the success rate is 80%. Complications include blockage of the stent, in the early stages by haemorrhage and later by sludge. Obstruction is indicated by a recurrence of jaundice and cholangitis. Patency may be maintained by irrigation or wire probes. Regular antibiotics are probably required.

The stent can be easily removed and exchanged via the endoscope and this is necessary at about three-monthly intervals.

Indications

Malignant biliary obstruction. Inoperable carcinomas of pancreas, ampulla and even hilum can be relieved. In one series of 277 patients with carcinoma of the pancreas, the procedure was successful in 89%, but 18% were dead within 30 days. There were major complications in 4%, but no procedure-related death or surgery. Occlusion of the stent occurred in 30% in three months. The hospital stay was only 3.5 days and the average survival 129 days [48].

Benign strictures whether post-cholecystectomy or part of primary sclerosing cholangitis may be relieved by the introduction of a biliary prosthesis.

Failed endoscopic sphincterotomy for common duct stones. A stent may be introduced into the common bile duct where it has been impossible to remove all stones and when the patient is unfit for surgery.

External biliary fistulas. Post-operative leaks from the cystic duct or injuries to the common bile duct may be treated by introduction of a biliary stent which may render further operations unnecessary [43].

BALLOON DILATATION

Following endoscopic cholangiography, a catheter bearing a balloon may be introduced into the common bile duct and dilated. This may be used for sphincterotomy or for a benign stricture, whether traumatic or secondary to

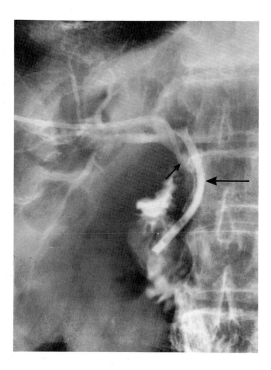

Fig. 29.18. Radiograph of a patient with carcinoma of the pancreas, showing drainage of radio-opaque contrast medium from the intra-hepatic bile ducts into duodenum, through an endoprosthesis (large arrow). The tip of an external drainage catheter lies in the bile duct above the endoprosthesis (Dooley *et al.* 1984).

Percutaneous trans-hepatic cholangiography [15]

Contrast is injected percutaneously into bile ducts within the liver. The procedure is done in the radiology department with intravenous diazepam premedication and under local anaesthesia. Preliminary antibiotics are given 24 hours before the procedure. The 'skinny' Chiba needle is 0.7 mm (22 gauge) outside diameter. It does not have an outer sheath and is very flexible so that the patient is able to breathe normally with it *in situ*.

The needle is introduced in the seventh, eighth or ninth right intercostal space at a point of maximal dullness to percussion. Ultrasound [28] or CT scan guidance adds to the success. It is advanced parallel to the table top as far as the spine, bisecting a sagittal line between the dome of the diaphragm and the duodenal cap identified by an air bubble. Contrast is injected continuously as the needle is withdrawn. Bile ducts are identified by centripetal flow, the contrast remaining for some time. Portal and hepatic veins are recognized by the direction of flow and rapid disappearance of contrast medium. Lymphatics can be filled when contrast enters the hepatic parenchyma. Such deposits take 5–10 minutes to be cleared by the lymphatic channels. Up to six needle 'passes' are allowed before the procedure is abandoned. After injection into obstructed and dilated ducts the patient is tilted upright so that the common bile duct has an opportunity to fill. If hilar obstruction is found, a percutaneous cholangiogram of both right and left hepatic duct systems should be done. The technique is relatively safe so that surgery need not inevitably follow. If dilated ducts are encountered, external biliary drainage using a slightly wider needle should continue until the obstruction is relieved. Trans-hepatically-aspirated bile should be cultured [52]. The patient must be observed carefully in hospital.

The technique is easy and the success rate is 100% if intra-hepatic bile ducts are dilated. With undilated ducts, such as in primary biliary cirrhosis, sclerosing cholangitis or with some

primary sclerosing cholangitis [42]. It may be a useful preliminary to insertion of a prosthesis.

CHOLEDOCHOSCOPY [16]

This procedure allows the surgeon to see directly into the lumen of the intra-hepatic and extra-hepatic biliary system. The scope is introduced at surgery into the common bile duct. Although its use undoubtedly decreases the retained stone rate, it has never achieved popularity. It may, however, be of value when used post-operatively through a hepatico-cutaneous-jejunostomy to remove residual Oriental intra-hepatic stones [5].

632

cases of choledocholithiasis the success rate drops to 90% but can rise to 96% in specially skilled hands.

CLINICAL INDICATIONS

Percutaneous cholangiography is an extremely valuable method of demonstrating the main biliary system, particularly in cholestatic patients with intra-hepatic biliary dilatation shown by ultrasound. The site and nature of any biliary obstruction can usually be determined. Exfoliative cytology and biliary biopsy may be performed [37].

COMPLICATIONS

These include biliary leaks with peritonitis, haemorrhage, septicaemias (usually Gram-negative) in those with cholangitis, and puncture of adjacent organs.

THERAPEUTIC USES

External biliary drainage

Theoretically this would be expected to bring the patient with biliary obstruction, particularly malignant, to surgery in better condition and so lessen the incidence of post-operative renal failure. There are, however, many complications including fluid and electrolyte loss with metabolic acidosis, infections along the cannula tract, haemobilia and dislodgement of the drainage tube [7, 33].

Short-term drainage (about nine days) is said to lessen morbidity and mortality [21], but this is not a universal finding [33]. It may have a place for two or three days in a patient with severe cholangitis and biliary obstruction but naso-biliary drainage via the endoscope is probably preferable.

Long-term external biliary drainage may be used to treat jaundice and pruritus in those in whom it is impossible to relieve the biliary obstruction by any other means. In a multi-centre controlled trial of 731 patients with malignant biliary obstruction, palliative ex-

ternal biliary drainage was successful in 96% with a complication rate of 10% and a 30-day mortality of 29%. Survival was 2.9 months in those treated by percutaneous trans-hepatic biliary drainage and 2.4 months in those that were given palliative bypass surgery.

Percutaneous biliary endoprosthesis [14, 40]

The biliary obstruction is relieved by the passage of an endoprosthesis through it. The procedure is done under local anaesthesia with sedation. Pre-operative broad-spectrum antibiotics are given.

A percutaneous cholangiogram is performed. Under lateral fluoroscopy, an intra-hepatic bile duct is chosen and a sheathed needle inserted into it. A guide wire is then manipulated through the stricture. The polythene endoprosthesis with side holes (2–2.6 mm) is then inserted over the guide wire and through the stricture allowing free drainage of bile into the lower common bile duct (figs 29.18, 29.19). A

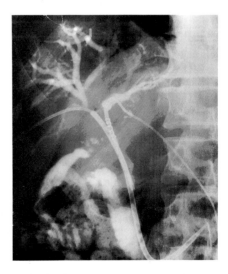

Fig. 29.19. Cholangiocarcinoma at confluence of hepatic ducts. An endoprosthesis has been passed percutaneously from right to left (Carey-Coon's on right, Burcharth prosthesis on left). Note external drainage catheters above stent for 24 hour follow-up cholangiogram (Sherlock & Dick, 1986).

further external drainage tube above the endo-prosthesis allows biliary decompression for 12–48 hours. A cholangiogram is then taken to check patency of the endoprosthesis and the external drainage tube withdrawn (fig. 29.20). The patient remains in bed for 24 hours.

Results and complications. Success rate is 85% (fig. 29.21). Failures are due to inability to find the lumen of the stricture with the guide wire. Complications include peritonitis, bile leaks, cholangitis, intra-peritoneal haemorrhage and infections.

Indications. The advantages of percutaneous biliary endoprostheses are ease of insertion, avoidance of surgery, the short period in hospital and low cost. The disadvantage is that they allow no possibility of radical resection of a tumour. Any other relevant problem, such as pyloric obstruction, is not treated. Biopsies of the bile ducts obtained trans-hepatically are often inconclusive and histological confirmation is not made. In general, therefore, it is the older, poorer risk patient who receives the non-surgical prosthesis and the younger, fitter patient who has surgery.

Hilar carcinomas are particularly suitable as they are rarely resectable. This also applies to large carcinomas of the head of the pancreas shown by imaging and radiology. With ampullary carcinomas, if the patient is in reasonable condition, the treatment is surgical.

Benign biliary stricture, where reconstructive surgery is thought unlikely to succeed, can often be relieved dramatically. Similar good results can be seen in some patients with primary sclerosing cholangitis.

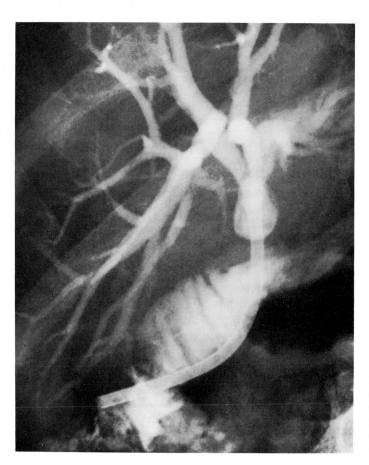

Fig. 29.20. Patient with hilar stricture due to bile duct carcinoma. An endoprosthesis is in position allowing biliary drainage into the duodenum (Dooley *et al.* 1979).

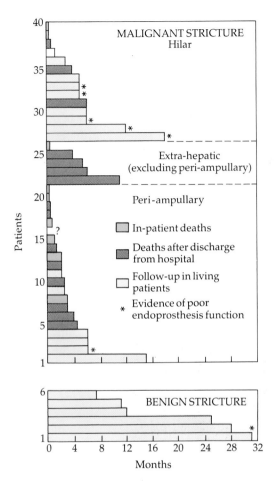

Fig. 29.21. Follow-up in 46 patients after the successful insertion of a biliary endoprosthesis. (Dooley *et al.* 1984).

Balloon dilatation

Benign strictures of the distal bile ducts have been successfully treated by percutaneous trans-hepatic balloon dilatation (fig. 32.7) [42].

CHOICE BETWEEN PERCUTANEOUS TRANS-HEPATIC CHOLANGIOGRAPHY OR ERCP (table 29.1)

Using one or both of these procedures, the biliary tree can be visualized in virtually every patient in whom mechanical cholestasis has to be excluded. ERCP is more satisfactory with undilated ducts. Post-cholecystectomy problems, the diagnosis of gallstones and the suspicion of pancreatic lesions should indicate ERCP as the first choice. It may be performed where there are coagulation problems or if ascites is present.

With its increasing availability, ERCP is becoming the first choice. Any large hospital should have both techniques available and a surgeon should always have a cholangiogram in front of him when exploring the biliary tract. The techniques are complementary rather than competitive.

ERCP has the advantage that, where necessary, sphincterotomy and stone extraction may be conducted at the time of the examination. Both techniques can be used to introduce endoprostheses into the biliary tract. In general, percutaneous cholangiography is better for high obstructions and ERCP for those at the distal end of the common bile duct.

In a randomized trial in patients with malignant obstructive jaundice, the insertion of a stent by the endoscopic route proved preferable

Table 29.1. Comparison of percutaneous trans-hepatic (PTC) and endoscopic retrograde cholangio-pancreatography (ERCP)

	PTC	ERCP
Technique	Easy	Difficult
Time taken (min.)	15	15–60
Anatomical difficulties	Few	Many
Cost	Low	High
Complications (%)	5	5
	Biliary leak	Pancreatitis
	Cholangitis	Cholangitis
Success (%)		
Overall	95	75–85
Dilated ducts	100	80
Undilated ducts	90	80
Pancreatic duct	0	80
Endoprosthesis insertion (%)		
Overall	>75	50
High	70	<40
Low	85	60

to the percutaneous one because of the absence of the complications of haemorrhage and bile leaks [50].

PERCUTANEOUS CHOLECYSTOTOMY

The gallbladder is punctured percutaneously under real-time and fluoroscopic control and a Teflon catheter introduced [39]. This technique has been used as an emergency for patients with acute cholecystitis and common duct obstruction, sometimes combined with biliary decompression through the cystic duct into the common bile duct [45]. Biliary leak is a risk but probably less with a diseased, adherent gall-bladder than with the thin-walled normal one.

Solvents have also been introduced directly into the gallbladder for stone dissolution (see Chapter 31).

OPERATIVE AND POST-OPERATIVE CHOLANGIOGRAPHY

Routine operative cholangiography is not necessary at cholecystectomy unless there are indications suggesting that stones are present in the common bile duct [13, 22, 49]. These include a history of jaundice, dilated bile ducts, palpable gallstones or a raised serum bilirubin, alkaline phosphatase or gamma GT level. After exploration of the common bile duct, cholan-giography should always be performed using high kVp technique and full strength contrast [53].

Debris may cause filling defects less sharply defined than those caused by gallstones. Air bubbles may simulate stones. Small stones may be obliterated by the contrast medium.

Operative ultrasound may obviate the use of operative cholangiography and choledochos-copy in excluding retained stones.

Post-operative cholangiography, using con-trast injected gently, should be undertaken routinely before final removal of a T-tube draining the biliary tree. During the injection, biliary duct contents, including bacteria, prob-ably regurgitate into the blood. This is parti-

cularly marked in the presence of biliary obstruction.

A surprising number of operative and post-operative cholangiograms are technically un-satisfactory, through failure to visualize intra-hepatic bile ducts or the trans-duodenal or sphincteric segment of the ducts. It is essen-tial not to use too dense contrast to fill the biliary tree and to ensure correct positioning and exposure. Practice is necessary.

T-tube extraction of gallstones
See Chapter 31.

Barium meal

A barium meal or enema may be useful in diagnosing obstructive jaundice by disclosing a primary neoplasm or revealing pressure de-formities or internal fistulae. Gallstones keep a constant relationship to the first or second part of the duodenum.

A pancreatic carcinoma may cause pressure effects on adjacent organs.

Internal biliary fistulae or a lax sphincter may allow the passage of intestinal barium into the biliary tree, confirming a suspicion aroused in the plain film by the presence of gas in the biliary tract.

References

1 Allen JI, Allen MO, Olson MM *et al.* Pseudomonas infection of the biliary system resulting from the use of a contaminated endoscope. *Gastroenterology* 1987; **92:** 759

2 Barkin JS, Fayne SD, Stolzenberg J *et al.* Endo-scopic retrograde cholangio-pancreatography findings of a gallbladder filling defect caused by sludge. *Am. J. Gastroenterol.* 1987; **82:** 254.

3 Behar J, Biancani P. Neural control of the sphincter of Oddi: physiologic role of enkephalins on the regulation of basal sphincter of Oddi motor activity in the cat. *Gastroenterology* 1984; **86:** 134.

4 Burnstein MJ, Vassal KP, Strasberg SM. Results of combined biliary drainage and cholecystokinin cholecystography in 81 patients with normal oral cholecystograms. *Ann. Surg.* 1982; **196:** 627.

5 Choi TK, Lee MJR, Lui R *et al.* Post-operative flexible choledochoscopy for residual primary

intrahepatic stones. *Ann. Surg.* 1986; **203**: 260.

6 Classen M. Endoscopic papillotomy: new indications, short- and long-term results. *Clin. Gastroenterol.* 1986; **15**: 457.

7 Clouse ME, Evans D, Costello P *et al.* Percutaneous transhepatic biliary drainage complications due to multiple duct obstructions. *Ann. Surg.* 1983; **198**: 25.

8 Conter RL, Roslyn JJ, Den Besten L *et al.* Pancreatic polypeptide enhances postcontractile gallbladder filling in the prairie dog. *Gastroenterology* 1987; **92**: 771.

9 Cotton PB, Williams CB. *Practical Gastrointestinal Endoscopy*, 2nd edn. Blackwell Scientific Publications, Oxford 1982.

10 Cotton PB, Vallon AG. Duodenoscopic sphincterotomy for removal of bile duct stones in patients with gallbladders. *Surgery* 1982; **91**: 628.

11 De Lacey G, Gajjar B, Twomey B *et al.* Should cholecystography or ultrasound be the primary investigation for gallbladder disease. *Lancet* 1984; **i**: 205.

12 Delchier J-C, Benfredj P, Preaux A-M *et al.* The usefulness of microscopic bile examination in patients with suspected microlithiasis: a prospective evaluation. *Hepatology* 1986; **6**: 118.

13 Dick R. State of the art: operative and postoperative (T-tube) cholangiography. In *Imaging in Hepatobiliary Disease*, eds JS Dooley, R Dick, M. Viamonte Jr, S Sherlock. Blackwell Scientific Publications, Oxford 1987.

14 Dooley JS, Dick R, George P *et al.* Percutaneous trans-hepatic endoprosthesis for bile duct obstruction: complications and results. *Gastroenterology* 1984; **86**: 905.

15 Dooley JS, Dick R, Viamonte M Jr, Sherlock S. *Imaging in Hepatobiliary Disease*. Blackwell Scientific Publications, Oxford 1987.

16 Escat J, Glucksman DL, Maigne C *et al.* Choledochoscopy in surgery for choledocholithiasis. *Am. J. Surg.* 1984; **147**: 670.

17 Fisher RS, Rock E, Malmud LS. Gallbladder emptying response to sham feeding in humans. *Gastroenterology* 1986; **90**: 1854.

18 Fisher RS, Rock E, Levin G *et al.* Effects of somatostatin on gallbladder emptying. *Gastroenterology* 1987; **92**: 885.

19 Fitzgerald EJ, Toi A. Pitfalls in the ultrasonographic diagnosis of gallbladder diseases. *Postgrad. med. J.* 1987; **63**: 525.

20 Greenfield C, Cleland P, Dick R *et al.* Biliary sequelae of endoscopic sphincterotomy. *Postgrad. med. J.* 1985; **61**: 213.

21 Gundry SR, Strodel WE, Knol JA *et al.* Efficacy of pre-operative biliary tract decompression in patients with obstructive jaundice. *Arch. Surg.* 1984; **119**: 703.

22 Hauer-Jensen M, Karesen R, Nygaard K *et al.* Predictive ability of choledocholithiasis indicators: a prospective evaluation. *Ann. Surg.* 1985; **202**: 64.

23 Hopman WPM, Kerstens PJSM, Jansen JBMJ *et al.* Effect of graded physiologic doses of cholecystokinin on gallbladder contraction measured by ultrasonography. *Gastroenterology* 1985; **89**: 1242.

24 Jacob H, Appelman R, Stein HD. Emphysematous cholecystitis. *Am. J. Gastroenterol.* 1979; **71**: 325.

25 Jamieson NV, Friend PJ, Wraight EP. A two year experience with 99m TC HIDA cholescintigraphy in teaching hospital practice. *Surg. Gynecol. Obstet.* 1986; **163**: 29.

26 Keshavarzian A, Dunne M, Iber FL. Gallbladder volume and emptying in insulin-requiring male diabetics. *Dig. Dis. Sci.* 1987; **32**: 824.

27 Krishnamurthy GT, Bobba VR, Kingston E. Radionuclide ejection fraction: a technique for quantitative analysis of motor function of the human gallbladder. *Gastroenterology* 1981; **80**: 482.

28 Lameris JS, Obertop H, Jeekel J. Biliary drainage by ultrasound-guided puncture of the left hepatic duct. *Clin. Radiol.* 1985; **36**: 269.

29 Lanzini A, Jazrawi RP, Northfield TC. Simultaneous quantitative measurements of absolute gallbladder storage and emptying during fasting and eating in humans. *Gastroenterology* 1987; **92**: 852.

30 Leese T, Neoptolemos JP, Carr-Locke DL. Successes, failures, early complications and their management following endoscopic sphincterotomy: results in 394 consecutive patients from a single centre. *Br. J. Surg.* 1985; **72**: 215.

31 Leuschner U. Endoscopic therapy of biliary calculi. *Clin. Gastroenterol.* 1986; **15**: 333.

32 Lieberman DA, Krishnamurthy GT. Intrahepatic versus extrahepatic cholestasis. Discrimination with biliary scintigraphy combined with ultrasound. *Gastroenterology* 1986; **90**: 734.

33 McPherson GAD, Benjamin IS, Hodgson HJF *et al.* Pre-operative percutaneous transhepatic biliary drainage: the results of a controlled trial. *Br. J. Surg.* 1984; **71**: 371.

34 Moreira VF, Meroño E, Larraona JL *et al.* ERCP and allergic reactions to iodized contrast media. *Gastrointest. Endosc.* 1985; **31**: 293.

35 Niederau C, Sonnenberg A, Mueller J. Comparison of the extrahepatic bile duct size measured by ultrasound and by different radiographic methods. *Gastroenterology* 1984; **87**: 615.

36 Oddi R. D'une disposition a sphincter spéciale de l'ouverture du canal cholédoque. *Arch. ital. Biol.* 1887; **8**: 317.

37 Okamura J, Monden M, Horikawa S *et al.* Exfoliative cytology and biliary biopsy using a percutaneous transhepatic biliary tube. *J. surg. Oncol.* 1983; **22**: 121.

38 Osnes M, Rosseland AR, Aabakken L. Endoscopic retrograde cholangiography and endoscopic papillotomy in patients with a previous Billroth-II resection. *Gut* 1986; **27:** 1193.

39 Pearse DM, Hawkins IF Jr, Shaver R *et al.* Percutaneous cholecystostomy in acute cholecystitis and common duct obstruction. *Radiology* 1984; **152:** 365.

40 Pereiras RV Jr, Rheingold OJ, Hutson D *et al.* Relief of malignant obstructive jaundice by percutaneous insertion of a permanent prosthesis in the biliary tree. *Ann. intern. Med.* 1978; **89:** 589.

41 Roslyn JJ, Pitt HA. Mann LL *et al.* Gallbladder disease in patients on long-term parenteral nutrition. *Gastroenterology* 1983; **84:** 148.

42 Salamonowitz E, Castaneda-Zuniga WR, Lund G *et al.* Balloon dilatation of benign biliary strictures. *Radiology* 1984; **151:** 613.

43 Sauerbruch T, Weinzierl M, Holl J *et al.* Treatment of post-operative bile fistulas by internal endoscopic biliary drainage. *Gastroenterology* 1986; **90:** 1998.

44 Scott AJ, Khan GA. Partial biliary obstruction with cholangitis producing a blind loop syndrome. *Gut* 1968; **9:** 187.

45 Shaver RW, Soong J. Percutaneous placement of a transcystic duct internal biliary drainage catheter. *Gastrointest. Radiol.* 1983; **8:** 149.

46 Shorvon PJ, Eykyn SJ, Cotton PB. Progress report: gastrointestinal instrumentation, bacteraemia, and endocarditis. *Gut* 1983; **24:** 1078.

47 Siegel JH. Improved biliary decompression with large caliber endoscopic prostheses. *Gastrointest. Endosc.* 1984; **30:** 21.

48 Siegel JH, Snady H. The significance of endoscopically placed prosthesis in the management of biliary obstruction due to carcinoma of the pancreas: results of non-operative decompression in 277 patients. *Am. J. Gastroenterol.* 1986; **81:** 634.

49 Simpson CJ, Gray GR, Gillespie G. Early endoscopic sphincterotomy for retained common bile duct stones. *J. R. Coll. Surg. Edinb.* 1985; **30:** 288.

50 Speer AG, Cotton PB, Russell RCG *et al.* Randomised trial of endoscopic versus percutaneous stent insertion in malignant obstructive jandice. *Lancet* 1987; **ii:** 57.

51 Staritz M, Rambow A, Floth A *et al.* Fragmentation of giant common bile duct stones by extracorporeal shockwave lithotripsy (device of the second generation). *J. Hepatol.* 1987; **5:** S63.

52 Suzuki Y, Kobayashi A, Ohto M *et al.* Bacteriological study of transhepatically aspirated bile: relation to cholangiographic findings in 295 patients. *Dig. Dis. Sci.* 1984; **29:** 109.

53 Thompson WM, Halvorsen RA, Foster WL *et al.* Optimal cholangiographic technique for detecting bile duct stones. *Am. J. Roentgenol.* 1986; **146:** 537.

54 Thornell E. Mechanisms in the development of acute cholecystitis and biliary pain: a study on the role of prostaglandins and effects of indomethacin. *Scand. J. Gastroenterol.* 1982; **suppl. 76:** 1.

55 Tytgat GNJ, Bartelsman JFWM, Den Hartog Jager FCA. Upper intestinal and biliary tract endoprosthesis. *Dig. Dis. Sci.* 1986; **31 (suppl):** 57S–76S.

56 Wheeler HO. Concentrating function of the gallbladder. *Am. J. Med.* 1971; **51:** 588.

57 Wood JR, Svanik J. Gall-bladder water and electrolyte transport and its regulation. *Gut* 1983; **24:** 579.

58 Yoshimoto H, Ikeda S, Tanaka M *et al.* Endoscopic retrograde cholangiography with a balloon catheter: analysis of 100 consecutive cases. *Radiology* 1986; **159:** 53.

30 · Cysts and Congenital Biliary Abnormalities

Fibropolycystic disease

Cystic lesions of the liver and bile ducts are being increasingly diagnosed. This can be related to the improved methods of imaging the liver and bile ducts and of liver biopsy. Application of such methods makes it clear that the fibropolycystic diseases do not exist as single entities, but as members of a family [35]. The members are found in various combinations (fig. 30.1). They consist of polycystic liver disease, microhamartoma, congenital hepatic fibrosis, congenital intra-hepatic biliary dilatation (Caroli's disease), and choledochal cysts (fig. 30.2). Clinically, fibropolycystic diseases have three effects, again present in different proportions: those of a space-occupying lesion, of portal hypertension and of cholangitis. All may be complicated by cancer, usually biliary [1, 33]. They are usually inherited. Fibrocystic disease of the kidneys is associated to a variable extent. Embryologically the cysts develop at the 23 mm stage from the original segments of the blind bile ducts probably due to malformation of the ductal plate [10, 14, 15].

Malignant change may complicate hepatic fibrosis, hepatic duct cysts and Caroli's syndrome [1].

Childhood fibropolycystic diseases

These are recessively inherited and may be perinatal, neonatal or infantile (table 30.1). Prognosis depends on the extent of renal involvement. Morphometry shows that the neonatal and infantile forms represent one disorder [18]. Choledochal cysts may be associated with any of them.

The importance of the renal problem relative to the hepatic one varies from patient to patient.

Adult fibropolycystic disease

The liver cysts are probably developmental and similar to and frequently associated with polycystic kidneys.

The cysts may arise from defective development of the intra-hepatic bile ducts in the portal tracts. This may occur at about the 23 mm stage of fetal life, when the original segment of blind bile ducts is being replaced by a second generation of highly active, proliferating bile ducts. The original group may become distorted and degenerate into cysts. These, frequently localized, cystic areas are accompanied by normal second generation bile ducts elsewhere, so there is no biliary dysfunction.

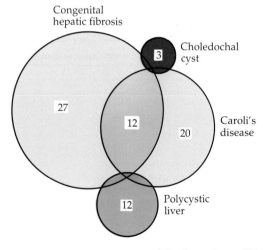

Fig. 30.1. Venn diagram showing one series in which 51 patients had more than one fibropolycystic disease. The combination of CHF and Caroli's disease was most striking (Summerfield *et al.* 1986).

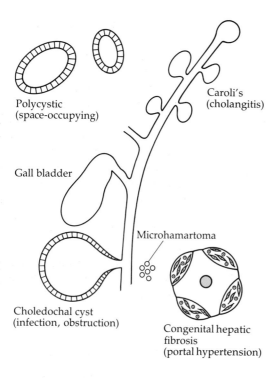

Polycystic
(space-occupying)

Caroli's
(cholangitis)

Gall bladder

Microhamartoma

Choledochal cyst
(infection, obstruction)

Congenital hepatic
fibrosis
(portal hypertension)

outer surface may be considerably deformed. A cyst may vary in size from a pin's head to a child's head, the largest having a capacity of over a litre. They are rarely greater than 10 cm in diameter. The larger ones are probably derived by rupture of septa between adjacent cysts, and the cut liver may display a honeycomb appearance. The cavities are thin walled and contain clear or brown fluid due to altered blood. They never contain bile because they are not in continuity with the biliary tract. They may be complicated by haemorrhage or infection.

Histologically (fig. 30.3) the lobular architecture is unchanged and the liver cells are normal. The cystic areas are related to the bile ducts in the portal areas. They are surrounded by a fibrous tissue capsule and lined by columnar or cuboidal epithelium. Microhamartomas may be present.

Frequently, there is cystic disease of other organs, including kidneys, spleen, pancreas, ovary and lungs. About half the patients with polycystic disease of the liver have polycystic kidneys. Only about 29% of the patients with polycystic kidney have polycystic liver.

PATHOLOGY

Depending on the number and size of the cysts, the liver may be normal or greatly enlarged. Cysts may be scattered diffusely or restricted to one lobe, usually the left. The

CYST FLUID

Fluid has been obtained using needle aspiration under ultrasound guidance [28]. The con-

Table 30.1. Hepatic fibropolycystic disease

Subtype	Inheritance	Presentation	Hepatic	Portal hypertension	Renal
Adult fibropolycystic	Dominant	Adult	Cysts	Rare	Cysts
Childhood fibropolycystic					
Perinatal	Recessive	Birth	Fibrosis± Ducts dilated+	—	90% tubules
Neonatal	Recessive	1 month	Fibrosis++ Ducts dilated+	—	60% tubules
Infantile	Recessive	3–6 months	Fibrosis++ Ducts dilated+	Common	25% tubules
Hepatic fibrosis	Recessive	Child or adult	Fibrosis+++ Ducts dilated+	Usual	0–10% tubules
Intra-hepatic biliary dilatation		Cholangitis any age	Dilated ducts only	—	—

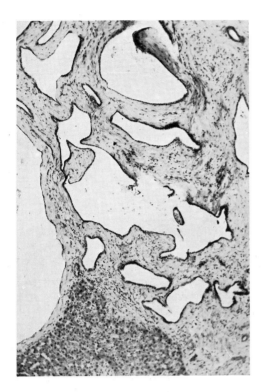

Fig. 30.3. Polycystic disease of the liver. The cysts vary in size and are lined by flattened epithelium. H & E, ×63.

stituents resemble the bile salt-independent fraction of human bile. This supports the concept that the cyst fluid is formed by the functioning secretory bile duct epithelium lining the cysts.

CLINICAL FEATURES

In many patients the liver lesion is diagnosed at autopsy. Sometimes the patient presents with some other disease or with polycystic kidneys.

Patients with symptoms and signs are usually in the fourth or fifth decade. The patient complains of abdominal distension and dull abdominal pain. Pressure on the stomach and duodenum causes epigastric discomfort, nausea, flatulence and occasional vomiting. Rarely, severe pain simulates biliary colic. Severe pain may also be due to rupture of or haemorrhage into a cyst.

Ascites and obstructive jaundice are very rare [42].

The symptoms are more often due to associated polycystic kidney disease.

On examination the liver may be impalpable or so large that it seems to fill the whole abdomen. The edge is firm and nodules can be palpated. There may be difficulty in diagnosing cysts from other types of liver nodule.

Bilaterally enlarged irregular *kidneys* may suggest the associated renal cysts.

Hepatic function is excellent for the liver cells are uninvolved. Serum alkaline phosphatase and γ-GT may be increased but bilirubin is normal.

Portal venous obstruction is usually absent, but occasionally can result in oesophageal varices with bleeding [29]. The spleen is not enlarged.

IMAGING

Ultrasound is the most satisfactory method of diagnosis. The space-occupying lesion does not enhance with intravenous contrast (fig. 30.4). CT scanning is equally useful (fig. 30.5).

DIFFERENTIAL DIAGNOSIS

Polycystic liver may be suspected in an apparently well person, often over 30 years of age, with nodular hepatomegaly, but no evidence of hepatic dysfunction, associated with polycystic kidney or a family history of this condition.

The condition may be confused with *hydatid disease* (Chapter 27).

Metastases are accompanied by failure in health, rapid increase in size of the liver, and, possibly, evidence of a primary neoplasm.

Cirrhosis may be accompanied by signs of hepato-cellular disease and the spleen is usually enlarged.

PROGNOSIS AND TREATMENT

Polycystic disease of the liver is compatible with long life.

The prognosis is determined by the extent of

641

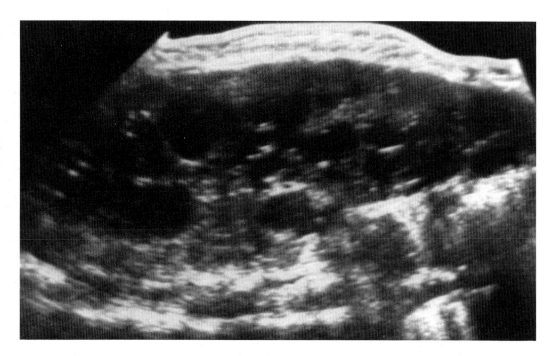

Fig. 30.4. Adult polycystic liver: ultrasound shows numerous space-occupying lesions.

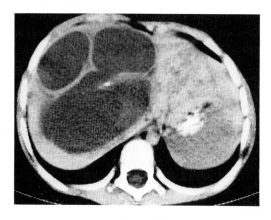

Fig. 30.5. CT scan (enhanced contrast) showing polycystic liver.

associated renal cystic disease. Carcinoma is very rare. Surgery is rarely necessary and aspiration under ultrasound control is easy and effective in controlling symptoms [30]. However, the fluid usually returns. The introduction of 2–3 ml of absolute alcohol into the cyst may delay recurrence [40]. Large cysts, greater than 10 cm, may be excised if symptomatic and accessible. Surgical treatment is by wide unroofing [19].

Congenital hepatic fibrosis [16]

This condition consists, histologically, of broad, densely collagenous fibrous bands surrounding otherwise normal hepatic lobules (figs 30.6, 30.7) [16]. The bands contain large numbers of microscopic, well-formed bile ducts, some containing bile. Arterial branches are normal or hypoplastic, while the veins appear reduced in size. Inflammatory infiltration is not seen. Rarely the intra-hepatic ducts are dilated and contain concretions [5]. Caroli's syndrome may be associated, also choledochal cyst.

The disease appears both sporadically and in a familial form. It is inherited as an autosomal recessive.

Portal hypertension is common. Occasionally this may be due to defects in the main portal veins. More often it is caused by hypoplasia or

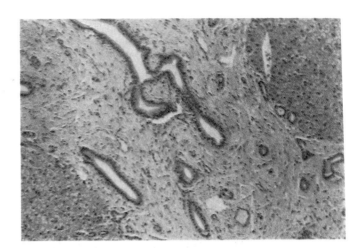

Fig. 30.6. Congenital hepatic fibrosis. Portal area shows dense mature fibrous tissue with a number of abnormal bile ducts. (Stained H & E, ×40).

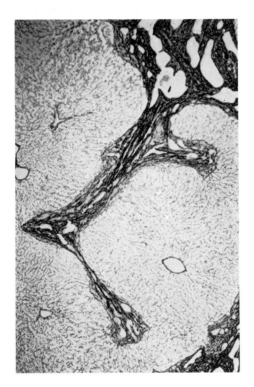

Fig. 30.7. Congenital hepatic fibrosis. Broad bands of fibrous tissue containing bile ducts separate and surround liver lobules. Silver impregnation, ×36. (Kerr *et al*. 1961.)

fibrous compression of portal vein radicles in the fibrous bands surrounding the nodules.

Associated renal conditions include renal dysplasia, adult type polycystic kidneys [36] and nephrophthisis (medullary cystic disease) [2].

CLINICAL FEATURES

The condition is usually misdiagnosed as cirrhosis. The patient is usually diagnosed between the ages of three and 10 years but recognition may be delayed until adult life. Sexes are equal. The patient presents with haemorrhage from oesophageal varices, a symptomless, large, very hard liver or splenomegaly (fig. 30.8) (table 30.2).

Occasionally a large cyst may obstruct a bile duct causing cholestatic jaundice. Other congenital anomalies, especially of the biliary system, may be present.

Carcinoma, both hepato-cellular and cholangiolar, may be a complication [33].

INVESTIGATIONS

Serum protein, bilirubin and transaminase levels are usually normal, but serum alkaline phosphatase values are sometimes increased.

Liver biopsy is essential for diagnosis. Because of the tough consistency of the liver this may fail, and a wedge, operative sample may be necessary.

Portal venography reveals the collateral circulation and a normal or distorted intra-hepatic portal tree [16].

643

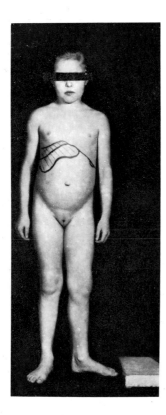

Fig. 30.8. Girl of eight years. Hepatosplenomegaly discovered at routine examination. Liver biopsy showed congenital fibrosis. Note normal development.

Ultrasound shows very bright areas of sound reflectivity due to the dense bands of fibrous tissue. Percutaneous or endoscopic *cholangiography* shows tapered intra-hepatic radicles, suggesting fibrosis.

Intravenous pyelography may show cystic changes or medullary sponge kidney.

PROGNOSIS AND TREATMENT

Congenital hepatic fibrosis must be distinguished from cirrhosis since hepato-cellular function is preserved and the prognosis is considerably better.

Following haemorrhage these patients are excellent candidates for porta-caval anastomosis.

Death can be due to renal failure, but renal transplantation has been successful [20].

Table 30.2. The presentation of sixteen patients with congenital hepatic fibrosis

Presentation	No.	Age (yr)
Large abdomen	9	2½–9
Haematemesis or melaena	5	3–6
Jaundice	1	10
Anaemia	1	16

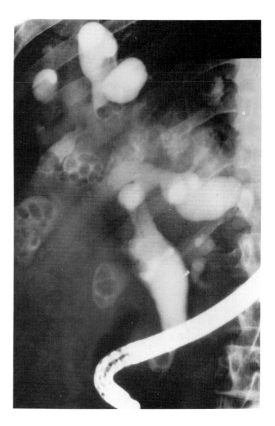

Fig. 30.9. Caroli's disease. Endoscopic cholangiography shows bulbous dilatations of the intra-hepatic bile ducts some of which contain multiple gallstones.

Congenital intra-hepatic biliary dilatation (Caroli's disease) [5]

This rare syndrome is characterized by congenital, segmental, saccular dilatations of the intra-hepatic bile ducts. The dilated ducts connect with the main duct system and are liable to become infected and contain stones (fig. 30.9).

Caroli's disease is not familial. Kidney lesions are usually absent, but renal tubular ectasia and larger cysts have been associated.

Mode of inheritance is unknown.

CLINICAL FEATURES

The condition presents at any age, but usually in childhood or early adult life, as abdominal pain, hepatomegaly, and fever with Gram-negative septicaemia [22]. About 75% are male.

Jaundice is mild or absent but may increase during the episodes of cholangitis.

Bile in the duodenum is reduced and Caroli's disease can cause steatorrhoea in childhood [17]. Portal hypertension is absent.

Biliary drainage may be excessive, and flow increased by an infusion of secretin which increases ductular flow. It is likely that the high resting flow arises from the cysts [41].

IMAGING

Ultrasound and CT scanning may be helpful but endoscopic or percutaneous cholangiography is diagnostic (figs 30.9, 30.10) [21]. The common bile duct is normal, but the intra-hepatic ducts are marked by bulbous dilatations with normal ducts between. The abnormality may be unilateral [23]. The appearances contrast with those of primary sclerosing cholangitis where the common bile duct is irregular with strictures and the intra-hepatic ducts show irregularities with dilatations. The changes in cirrhosis are smooth distortion of main bile ducts around regeneration nodules.

Cholangiocarcinoma may be a complication [5, 9].

TREATMENT

Antibiotics are given to treat the cholangitis as it appears, and drainage of the common bile duct, whether endoscopic or surgical, may be required to remove calculi.

Unilateral involvement may be treated by hepatic resection [23]. Hepatic transplantation must be considered, but the infection is usually a contraindication.

The prognosis is poor but episodes of cholangitis can extend over many years.

Death from renal failure is very unusual.

Congenital hepatic fibrosis and Caroli's disease

These conditions may co-exist [35]. Both result from similar malformations of the embryonic ductal plate at different levels of the biliary tree. Presentation may be as abdominal pain and cholangitis or as oesophageal varices (fig. 30.11). Patients with congenital hepatic fibrosis often show biliary abnormalities on cholangiography, and patients with Caroli's disease may show the histological lesions of congenital hepatic fibrosis.

A neonate, at autopsy, showed the features of congenital hepatic fibrosis, Caroli's disease

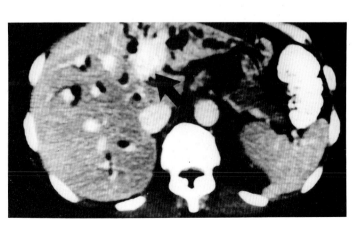

Fig. 30.10. Caroli's disease. CT scan after intravenous contrast shows dilated intra-hepatic bile ducts with adjacent enhanced radicles of the portal vein.

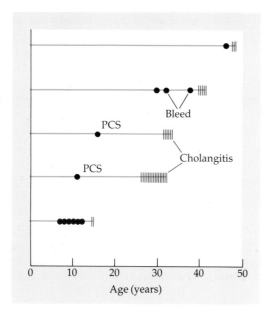

Fig. 30.11. The evolution of symptoms in five patients with co-existent CHF and Caroli's disease who had both variceal haemorrhages and cholangitis. Haemorrhage always occurred first, followed, a mean of ten years later, by cholangitis. PCS = porta-caval shunt. (Summerfield *et al.* 1986).

and infantile type of polycystic disease of the kidneys [8].

Congenital biliary dilatation (choledochal cyst)

This is a dilatation of the common bile duct. The gallbladder, cystic duct and hepatic ducts above the dilatation are not enlarged. Multiple cysts may be present. Histologically the cyst wall consists of fibrous tissue lacking epithelium or smooth muscle.

Choledochal cysts are *classified* (fig. 30.12) [7] into:

Type 1: which is by far the commonest (93%) and is a segmental or diffuse fusiform dilatation of the extra-hepatic biliary ducts.

Type 2: the cyst forms a diverticulum of an extra-hepatic bile duct.

Type 3: this is a choledochocele of the distal

common bile duct mostly within the duodenal wall.

Type 4: this comprises type 1 anatomy with an intra-hepatic bile duct cyst.

Rarely a solitary cystic dilatation of an intra-hepatic bile duct is seen [37].

The lesion presents as a partially retro-peritoneal, cystic tumour varying from 2–3 cm in size, to a capacity of 8 litres. The cyst contains thin, dark brown fluid. It is sterile but may become secondarily infected. The cyst can burst.

In the adult, recurrent pancreatitis can be associated [11]. Biliary cirrhosis is a late complication. Choledochal cysts may obstruct the portal vein leading to portal hypertension. Malignant tumours in the cyst or bile ducts are complications [7]. Gallstones may form in the gallbladder.

CLINICAL FEATURES

The *infantile form* presents as prolonged cholestasis. In infancy the cyst may perforate. The aetiological factors are similar to those of biliary atresia (see Chapter 23). The *adult form* is marked by the classical clinical triad of symptoms namely intermittent jaundice, pain and abdominal tumour. Repeated episodes of pancreatic juice, refluxing into the bile ducts, may be causative.

The adult type presents most frequently in females less than 10 years old, but can affect adults [2], and survival up to 79 years has been recorded. There is a preponderance in the Japanese and other Oriental races.

The jaundice is intermittent, of cholestatic type, and associated with fever. The pain is colicky and mainly experienced in the right upper abdomen. The tumour is cystic and in the right upper quadrant of the abdomen. It characteristically varies in size and in tenseness.

Choledochal cysts may be associated with congenital hepatic fibrosis or Caroli's disease.

In infancy the cyst may perforate, causing bile peritonitis. Anomalous pancreatico-biliary drainage is important particularly if the duct

646

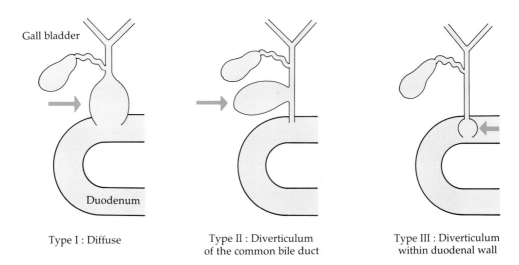

Type I : Diffuse   Type II : Diverticulum of the common bile duct   Type III : Diverticulum within duodenal wall

Fig. 30.12. Classification of congenital biliary dilatation (choledochal cyst).

junction is right angular or acute [26, 38]. It may be associated with biliary and gallbladder carcinoma [32].

IMAGING

Plain X-ray of the abdomen may show a soft tissue mass. In infants, the cyst may sometimes be revealed by HIDA scanning or ultrasound which allows diagnosis *in utero* and after delivery. In older children, CT is preferable. False negatives are found with all techniques [34]. The diagnosis is confirmed by percutaneous or endoscopic cholangiography (fig. 30.13).

TREATMENT

Because of the risk of subsequent adenocarcinoma or squamous cell carcinoma, excision is the method of choice [24]. Biliary tract continuity is maintained by choledochojejunostomy with Roux-en-Y anastomosis.

Anastomosis of the cyst to the intestinal tract is simpler but post-operative cholangitis and subsequent biliary stricturing and stone formation are frequent. The risk of carcinoma remains, perhaps related to dysplasia and metaplasia of the epithelium [31, 39, 45].

Microhamartoma (von-Meyenberg complexes)

These are usually asymptomatic, diagnosed incidentally or found at autopsy. Rarely, they may be associated with portal hypertension. Kidneys may show medullary sponge change. Microhamartomas can be associated with polycystic disease.

Histologically, microhamartomas consist of groups of rounded biliary channels, lined by cuboidal epithelium and often containing inspissated bile (fig. 30.14). Biliary structures are embedded in mature collagenous stroma. They are usually located in, or near, portal tracts. The appearances suggest congenital hepatic fibrosis, but in a localized form.

IMAGING

In a hepatic arteriogram, multiple microhamartomas lead to stretching of the arteries and blushing in the venous phase.

Carcinoma secondary to fibropolycystic disease

Tumours may arise in association with all

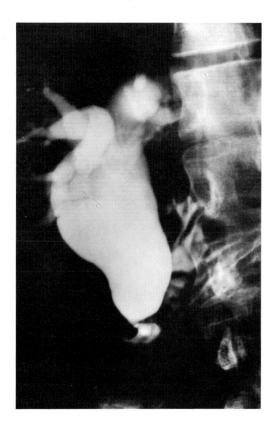

Fig. 30.13. Endoscopic cholangiogram in a 21-year-old woman with type 1 choledochal cyst showing a grossly dilated common bile duct from which contrast medium drained freely. This patient presented with acute pancreatitis.

members of the fibropolycystic family. These include microhamartomas, congenital hepatic fibrosis, Caroli's disease [9], and choledochal cyst. Carcinoma is rare in association with non-parasitic cysts or polycystic liver disease. Malignant change is more likely where epithelium is exposed to the bile.

Solitary non-parasitic liver cyst

This is being increasingly diagnosed due to the increase in various scanning techniques. It is probably a variant of polycystic disease.

The lining wall has partitions, which suggest an origin from conglomerate polycystic disease. The fibrous capsule contains aberrant bile ducts and blood vessels. The contents vary from colourless to brown altered blood. It appears as a smooth, glistening, greyish-blue cyst usually on the antero-inferior aspect of the right lobe. The tension is low in contrast to the high pressure of hydatid cysts.

Symptoms are rare and related to abdominal distension, or pressure effects on adjacent organs including the bile ducts causing intermittent jaundice. The patient should be reassured.

Symptoms follow rupture or haemorrhage into the cyst. They are extremely rare. Surgical excision is indicated only for complications.

Other cysts

These are all very rare, small and superficial. Their contents vary with the cause. Bile cysts may follow prolonged extra-hepatic biliary obstruction of all types.

Hepatic cysts can arise from glands adjacent to bile ducts especially in patients with portal hypertension [44]. These can cause obstructive jaundice.

Blood cysts follow haemorrhage into a simple cyst. They can also follow trauma to the liver. Small cystic spaces containing blood may follow needle biopsy.

Lymphatic cysts are due to obstruction or congenital dilatation of liver lymphatics. They are usually on the surface of the liver.

Malignant pseudocysts result from degeneration and softening of secondary malignant growths. Biliary cystadenocarcinoma is a cause.

Congenital anomalies of the biliary tract

The liver and biliary tract develop from a bud-like outpouching of the ventral wall of the primitive foregut just cranial to the yolk sac. Two solid buds of cells form the right and left lobes of the liver while the original elongated diverticulum forms the hepatic and common bile ducts. The gallbladder arises as a smaller bud of cells from this same diverticulum. The biliary tract is patent in early intra-uterine

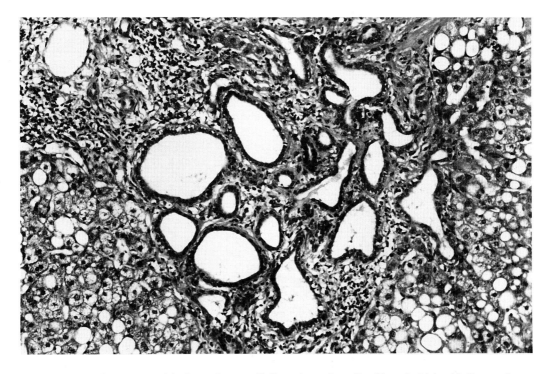

Fig. 30.14. Microhamartoma of the liver. Groups of biliary channels are lined by cuboidal epithelium and are embedded in mature fibrous tissue (Summerfield *et al.* 1986). H & E, ×180.

life but becomes solid later by epithelial proliferation within the lumen. Eventually re-vacuolization takes place, starting simultaneously in different parts of the solid gallbladder bud and spreading until the whole system is re-canalized. At five weeks the ductal communications of gallbladder, cystic duct and hepatic ducts are completed and at three months the fetal liver begins to secrete bile [17].

The majority of the congenital anomalies can be related to alterations in the original budding from the foregut or to failure of vacuolization of the solid gallbladder and bile diverticulum (table 30.3).

These congenital defects are usually of no importance and cannot be related to symptoms [4]. Occasionally they may predispose to bile stasis, inflammation and gallstones. They are of importance to the radiologist and to the biliary and hepatic transplant surgeon.

Anomalies of the biliary tree and liver may be associated with congenital lesions elsewhere, including cardiac defects, polydactyly and polycystic kidneys. They can also be related to maternal virus infections, such as rubella.

Absence of the gallbladder

This is a rare congenital anomaly. Multiple congenital defects are usually present. Two types can be recognized.

Type I is the failure of the gallbladder and cystic duct to develop as an outgrowth from the hepatic diverticulum of the foregut. This type is often found with other anomalies of the biliary passages.

Type II is the failure of the gallbladder to vacuolize from its solid state. This is usually associated with atresia of the extra-hepatic ducts. The gallbladder is not absent but *rudimentary*. This type is therefore found in infants

Table 30.3. Classification of congenital anomalies of the biliary tract

Anomalies of the primitive foregut bud
Failure of bud
  Absent bile ducts
  Absent gallbladder
Accessory buds or splitting of bud
  Accessory gallbladder
  Bilobed gallbladder
  Accessory bile ducts
Bud migrates to left instead of right
  Left-sided gallbladder

Anomalies of vacuolization of the solid biliary bud
Defective bile duct vacuolization
Congenital obliteration of bile ducts
Congenital obliteration of cystic duct
Choledochal cyst
Defective gallbladder vacuolization
  Rudimentary gallbladder
Fundal diverticulum
Serosal type of Phrygian cap
Hour-glass gallbladder

Persistent cysto-hepatic duct
Diverticulum of body or neck of gallbladder

Persistence of intra-hepatic gallbladder

Aberrant folding of gallbladder anlage
Retroserosal type of Phrygian cap

Accessory peritoneal folds
Congenital adhesions
Floating gallbladder

Anomalies of hepatic and cystic arteries
Accessory arteries
Abnormal relation of hepatic artery to cystic duct

who present the picture of congenital biliary atresia.

Failure to identify the gallbladder at operation is not proof of its absence. The gallbladder may be intra-hepatic, buried in extensive adhesions, or atrophied following previous cholecystitis.

Cholangiography and scanning are diagnostic [27]. There are no specific symptoms.

Double gallbladder

Double gallbladder is very rare [6]. In embryonic life, little pockets often arise from the hepatic or common bile ducts. Occasionally these persist and form a second gallbladder having its own cystic duct (fig. 30.15). This may enter the hepatic substance directly. If the pouch forms from the cystic duct the two gallbladders share a cystic duct (Y-shaped cystic duct) (fig. 30.15).

Double gallbladder can be recognized by imaging. The accessory organ is frequently diseased.

Bilobed gallbladder [12] is an extremely rare congenital anomaly. Embryologically, the single bud forming the gallbladder becomes paired but primary connection is maintained, thus forming two separate and distinct fundi with a single cystic duct.

The anomaly is of no clinical significance.

Accessory bile ducts

These are rare. The extra duct is usually the right hepatic and joins the common hepatic duct somewhere between the junction of the right and left hepatic ducts and the entry of the cystic duct. It may, however, join the cystic duct, the gallbladder or the common bile duct.

Cholecysto-hepatic ducts are due to persistence of fetal connections between the gallbladder and the liver parenchyma with failure of recanalization of the right and left hepatic ducts [13]. Continuity is maintained by the cystic duct entering a remaining hepatic duct or common hepatic duct or the duodenum directly.

Accessory ducts are of importance to the biliary and transplant surgeon as they may be inadvertently ligated or cut with resultant biliary stricture or fistula.

Left-sided gallbladder

In this rare anomaly the gallbladder lies under the left lobe of the liver to the left óf the falciform ligament [25]. The embryonic bud from the hepatic diverticulum migrates to the

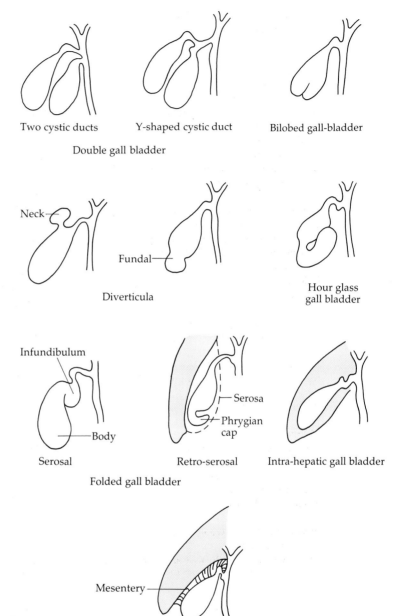

Two cystic ducts   Y-shaped cystic duct   Bilobed gall-bladder

Double gall bladder

Neck

Fundal

Diverticula

Hour glass
gall bladder

Infundibulum

Body

Serosal

Serosa

Phrygian
cap

Retro-serosal

Intra-hepatic gall bladder

Folded gall bladder

Mesentery

Fig. 30.15. Congenital anomalies
of the gallbladder.

Floating gall bladder

left instead of to the right. Alternatively, it may be due to independent development of a second gallbladder from the left hepatic duct with failure of development or regression of the normal structure on the right side.

In transposition of the viscera, the gallbladder bears its normal relationship to the liver but lies on the left side of the abdomen.

A left-sided gallbladder is of little clinical significance.

Rokitansky–Aschoff sinuses of the gallbladder

These consist of hernia-like protrusions of the gallbladder mucosa through the muscular layer (intramural diverticulosis). Although potentially congenital they are particularly prominent with chronic cholecystitis when intraluminar pressure rises. They may be seen in an oral cholecystogram as a halo-like stippling surrounding the gallbladder.

Folded gallbladder

The gallbladder is deformed so that the fundus appears folded 'bent down to the breaking point after the manner of a *Phrygian cap*' [8]. A Phrygian cap is a conical cap or bonnet, with the peak bent or turned over in front, worn by the ancient Phrygians, and identified with the Cap of Liberty (*Oxford English Dictionary*).

Two varieties are recognized:

Kinking between body and fundus (retroserosal; Phrygian cap) (fig. 30.15). This is due to aberrant folding of the gallbladder within the embryonic fossa.

Kinking between body and infundibulum (serosal) (fig. 30.15). This is due to aberrant folding of the fossa itself in the early stages of development. The bend in the gallbladder is fixed by development of fetal ligaments, vestigial septa or constrictions of the lumen following delayed vacuolization of the solid epithelial anlage.

These kinked gallbladders empty at a normal rate and are of no clinical significance [4]. The importance lies in the correct interpretation of cholecystograms.

Hour-glass gallbladder. This probably represents an exaggerated form of Phrygian cap, presumably of the serosal type. The constancy of position of the fundus during contraction and the small size of the opening between the two parts indicate that this is probably a fixed, congenital malformation.

Diverticula of the gallbladder and ducts

Diverticula of body and neck may arise from persistent cysto-hepatic ducts which run in embryonic life between the gallbladder and the liver.

The *fundal variety* arises from incomplete vacuolization of the solid gallbladder of embryonic life. An incomplete septum pinches off a small cavity at the tip of the gallbladder (fig. 30.15).

These diverticula are rare and of no clinical significance. The congenital variety should be distinguished from *pseudo-diverticula* developing in the diseased gallbladder as a result of partial perforation. The pseudo-diverticulum in these cases usually contains a large gallstone.

Intra-hepatic gallbladder

The gallbladder is included and buried in hepatic tissue up to the second month of intra-uterine life, thereafter assuming an extrahepatic position. In some instances the intrahepatic condition may persist. The gallbladder is higher than normal and more or less buried but never entirely covered by liver tissue. It is frequently diseased, for the embedded organ has difficulty in contracting and so becomes infected, with subsequent gallstone formation.

Congenital adhesions to the gallbladder

These are very frequent. Developmentally these peritoneal sheets are due to an extension of the anterior mesentery, which forms the lesser omentum. The sheet may run from the common bile duct laterally over the gallbladder down to the duodenum, to the hepatic flexure of the colon and even to the right lobe of the liver, perhaps closing the foramen of Winslow. In a milder form, a band of tissue runs from the lesser omentum across to the cystic duct and anterior to the gallbladder; or a loose veil forms a mesentery to the gallbladder ('floating gallbladder').

These adhesions are of no clinical importance. Surgically, their presence should be remembered, so that they are not mistaken for inflammatory adhesions.

Floating gallbladder and torsion of the gallbladder

The gallbladder possesses a supporting membrane in 4–5% of specimens. The peritoneal coat surrounding the gallbladder continues as two approximated leaves to form a fold or mesentery to support the gallbladder from under the surface of the liver. This fold may allow the gallbladder to hang for as much as 2–3 cm below the inferior hepatic surface.

The mobile gallbladder is apt to twist, and *torsion* results. The blood supply is impaired in the small pedicle and infarction follows.

The condition usually occurs in thin, elderly women. With ageing, omental fat lessens and visceroptosis increases. The gallbladder with mesentery becomes more pendulous and can twist. It can affect all ages, including children.

Torsion is followed by sudden, severe, constant epigastric and right costal margin pain passing through to the back with vomiting and collapse. Characteristically a palpable tumour appears, having the features of an enlarged gallbladder. Within a few hours it may disappear. The treatment is cholecystectomy.

Recurrent partial torsion leads to acute episodes. Ultrasound or CT shows a gallbladder situated low in the abdomen and even in the pelvis. It is suspended by a very long, down-curved cystic duct. Early cholecystectonmy is indicated.

Anomalies of the cystic duct and cystic artery

In 20% of subjects the cystic duct does not join the common hepatic duct directly but first runs parallel to it, lying in the same sheath of connective tissue. Occasionally it makes a spiral turn around the duct.

These variations are extremely important to the surgeon. Unless the cystic duct is carefully dissected and its union with the common hepatic duct identified, the common hepatic duct

may be ligated, with disastrous consequences.

The *cystic artery* can arise not, as normally, from the right hepatic artery but from the left hepatic artery or even from the gastroduodenal artery. Accessory cystic arteries usually arise from the right hepatic artery. Again, the surgeon must be careful to identify the cystic artery precisely.

References

1 Bloustein PA. Association of carcinoma with congenital cystic conditions of the liver and bile ducts. *Am. J. Gastroenterol.* 1977; **67**: 40.
2 Boichis H, Passwell J, David R *et al.* Congenital hepatic fibrosis and nephronophthisis. A family study. *Q. J. Med.* 1973; **42**: 221.
3 Bova JG, Dempsher CJ, Sepulveda G. Cholangiocarcinoma associated with a type 2 choledochal cyst. *Gastrointest. Radiol.* 1983; **8**: 41.
4 Boyden EA. 'Phrygian cap' in cholecystography. A congenital anomaly of the gall bladder. *Am. J. Roentgenol.* 1935; **33**: 589.
5 Caroli J, Corcos V. La dilatation congénitale des voies biliaries intrahépatiques. *Rev. Medicochir. Mal. Foie* 1964; **39**: 1.
6 Clot M, Thierrée RA, Tod R. Vésicule biliare double. Une observation. *Presse Med.* 1972; **1**: 2313.
7 Crittenden SL, McKinley MJ. Choledochal cyst—clinical features and classification. *Am. J. Gastroenterol.* 1985; **80**: 643.
8 Davies CH, Stringer DA, Whyte H *et al.* Congenital hepatic fibrosis with saccular dilatation of intrahepatic bile ducts and infantile polycystic kidneys. *Pediatr. Radiol.* 1986; **16**: 302.
9 Dayton MT, Longmire WP Jr, Tompkins RK. Caroli's disease: a premalignant condition? *Am. J. Surg.* 1983; **145**: 41.
10 Desmet VJ. Intrahepatic bile ducts under the lens. *J. Hepatol.* 1985; **1**: 545.
11 Goldberg PB, Long WB, Oleaga JA *et al.* Choledochocele as a cause of recurrent pancreatitis. *Gastroenterology* 1980; **78**: 1041.
12 Hobby JAE. Bilobed gall-bladder. *Br. J. Surg.* 1970; **57**: 870.
13 Jackson JB, Kelly TR. Cholecystohepatic ducts: case report. *Ann. Surg.* 1964; **159**: 581.
14 Jorgensen M. Three-dimensional reconstruction of intra-hepatic bile ducts in a case of polycystic disease of the liver in an infant. *Acta pathol. microbiol. Scand.* 1972; (A)**80**: 201.
15 Jorgensen M. A stereological study of intrahepatic bile ducts. 4. Congenital hepatic fibrosis. *Acta pathol. microbiol. Scand.* 1972; (A)**82**: 21.

16 Kerr DNS, Harrison CV, Sherlock S *et al.* Congenital hepatic fibrosis. *Q. J. Med.* 1961; **30:** 91.

17 Kocoshis SA, Riely CA, Burrell M *et al.* Cholangitis in a child due to biliary tract anomalies. *Dig. Dis. Sci.* 1980; **25:** 59.

18 Landing BH, Wells TR, Claireaux AE. Morphometric analysis of liver lesions in cystic diseases of childhood. *Hum. Pathol.* 1980; **11:** 549.

19 Litwin DEM, Taylor BR, Greig P *et al.* Nonparasitic cysts of the liver. The case for conservative surgical management. *Ann. Surg.* 1987; **205:** 45.

20 McGonigle RJS, Mowat AP, Bewick M *et al.* Congenital hepatic fibrosis and polycystic kidney disease: role of porta-caval shunting and transplantation in three patients. *Q. J. Med.* 1981; **50:** 269.

21 Missavage AE, Sugawa C. Caroli's disease: role of endoscopic retrograde cholangio-pancreatography. *Am. J. Gastroenterol.* 1983; **78:** 815.

22 Murray-Lyon IM, Shilkin KB, Laws JW *et al.* Non-obstructive dilatation of the intrahepatic biliary tree with cholangitis. *Q. J. Med.* 1972; **41:** 477.

23 Nagasue N. Successful treatment of Caroli's disease by hepatic resection: report of six patients. *Ann. Surg.* 1984; **200:** 718.

24 Nagorney DM, McIlrath DC, Adson MA. Choledochal cysts in adults: clinical management. *Surgery* 1984; **96:** 656.

25 Newcombe JF, Henley FA. Left-sided gallbladder. *Arch. Surg.* 1964; **88:** 494.

26 Oguchi Y, Okada A, Nakamura T *et al.* Histopathologic studies of congenital dilatation of the bile duct as related to an anomalous junction of the pancreatico-biliary ductal system: clinical and experimental studies. *Surgery* 1988; **103:** 168.

27 O'Sullivan J, O'Brien PA, MacFeely L *et al.* Congenital absence of the gall bladder and cystic duct: non-operative diagnosis. *Am. J. Gastroenterol.* 1987; **82:** 1190.

28 Patterson M, Gonzalez-Vitale JC, Fagan CJ. Polycystic liver disease: a study of cyst fluid consituents. *Hepatology* 1982; **2:** 475.

29 Ratcliffe PJ, Reeders S, Theaker JM. Bleeding oesophageal varices and hepatic dysfunction in adult polycystic kidney disease. *Br. med. J.* 1984; **288:** 1330.

30 Roemer CE, Ferrucci JT, Mueller PR *et al.* Hepatic cysts: diagnosis and therapy by sonographic needle aspiration. *Am. J. Roentgenol.* 1981; **136:** 1065.

31 Rossi RL, Silverman ML, Braasch JW *et al.* Carcinomas arising in cystic conditions of the bile ducts. A clinical and pathologic study. *Ann. Surg.* 1987; **205:** 377.

32 Sameshima Y, Uchimura M, Muto Y *et al.* Co-existent carcinoma in congenital dilatation of the bile duct and anomalous arrangement of the pancreatico-bile duct. Carcinogenesis of coexistent gall bladder carcinoma. *Cancer* 1987; **60:** 1883.

33 Scott J, Shousha S, Thomas HC *et al.* Bile duct carcinoma: a late complication of congenital hepatic fibrosis. Case report and review of literature. *Am. J. Gastroenterol.* 1980; **73:** 113.

34 Sherman P, Kolster E, Davies C *et al.* Choledochal cysts: heterogeneity of clinical presentation. *J. pediatr. Gastroenterol. Nutr.* 1986; **5:** 867.

35 Summerfield JA, Nagafuchi Y, Sherlock S *et al.* Hepatobiliary fibropolycystic disease: a clinical and histological review of 51 patients. *J. Hepatol.* 1986; **2:** 141.

36 Tazelaar HD, Payne JA, Patel NS. Congenital hepatic fibrosis and asymptomatic familial adult-type polycystic kidney disease in a 19-year-old woman. *Gastroenterology* 1984; **86:** 757.

37 Terada T, Nakanuma Y. Solitary cystic dilation of the intrahepatic bile duct: morphology of two autopsy cases and a review of the literature. *Am. J. Gastroenterol.* 1987; **82:** 1301.

38 Todani T, Watanabe Y, Fujii T *et al.* Anomalous arrangement of the pancreatobiliary ductal system in patients with a choledochal cyst. *Am. J. Surg.* 1984; **147:** 672.

39 Todani T, Watanabe Y, Toki A *et al.* Carcinoma related to choledochal cysts with internal drainage operations. *Surg. Gynec. Obstet.* 1987; **164:** 61.

40 Trinkl W, Sassaris M, Hunter FM. Nonsurgical treatment for symptomatic nonparasitic liver cyst. *Am. J. Gastroenterol.* 1985; **80:** 907.

41 Turnberg LA, Jones EA, Sherlock S. Biliary secretion in a patient with cystic dilation of the intrahepatic biliary tree. *Gastroenterology* 1968: **54:** 1155.

42 Van Erpecum KJ, Janssens AR, Terpstra JL. *et al.* Highly symptomatic adult polycystic disease of the liver. A report of fifteen cases. *J. Hepatol.* 1987; **5:** 109.

43 Venu RP, Geenen JE, Hogan WJ *et al.* Role of endoscopic retrograde cholangio-pancreatography in the diagnosis and treatment of choledochocele. *Gastroenterology* 1984; **87:** 1144.

44 Wanless IR, Zahradnik J, Heathcote EJ. Hepatic cysts of periductal gland origin presenting as obstructive jaundice. *Gastroenterology* 1987; **93:** 894.

45 Yoshikawa K, Yoshida K, Shirai Y *et al.* A case of carcinoma arising in the intrapancreatic terminal choledochus 12 years after primary excision of a giant choledochal cyst. *Am. J. Gastroenterol.* 1986: **81:** 378.

31 · Gallstones and Inflammatory Gallbladder Diseases

Composition of gallstones

Gallstones can be analysed by infra-red spectroscopy [87]. There are three major types, cholesterol, black and brown (fig. 31.1) (table 31.1). In the western world gallstones are composed mainly of cholesterol (11—98%). Other constituents include calcium salts of bilirubin and trace amounts of fatty acids, phospholipids, bile acids and glycoproteins. Crystallography confirms that the cholesterol is in monohydrate and anhydrous forms and is the major constituent, with calcium carbonate and phosphate, palmitate and amorphous material also identified [125]. The nature of the nucleus of the stone is uncertain—pigment, glycoprotein and amorphous material have all been suggested.

The problem is to explain how, in normal persons, insoluble cholesterol is kept in solution in bile and what leads, in some people, to its precipitation to form gallstones.

Composition of bile

Biliary cholesterol is in the free unesterified form. Concentration is unrelated to serum cholesterol level and depends only to a limited extent on the bile acid pool size and bile acid secretory rate.

Biliary phospholipids. These are insoluble in water and include lecithin (90%) with small quantities of lysolecithin (3%) and phosphatidyl ethanolamine (1%). Phospholipids are hydrolysed in the gut and there is no enterohepatic circulation. Bile acids determine excretion and enhance synthesis.

Bile acids (fig. 31.2). The primary bile acids are the trihydroxy, cholic acid, and the dihydroxy, chenodeoxycholic acid. These are converted by bacterial action, usually in the colon, to the secondary bile acids, deoxycholic acid and lithocholic acid. Cholic, cheno- and deoxycholic acids are absorbed and undergo an entero-hepatic circulation which takes place

Table 31.1. Classification of gallstones

Type	Cholesterol	Black	Brown
Location	Gallbladder, ducts	Gallbladder, ducts	Ducts
Major constituents	Cholesterol	Bilirubin, calcium salts	Calcium
Consistency	Crystalline with nucleus	Hard	Soft, friable
% Radio-opaque	15%	60%	0%
Associations			
Infections	Rare	Rare	Usual
Other diseases	See fig. 31.3	Haemolysis, cirrhosis	Chronic partial biliary obstruction

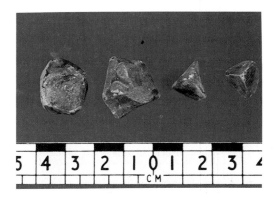

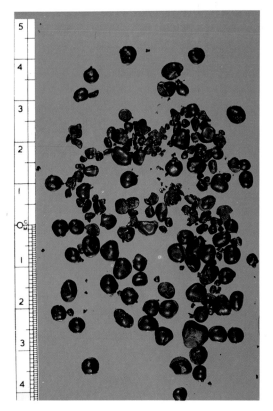

Fig. 31.1. Gallstones: (a) cholesterol gallstones and (b) pigment gallstones.

6—10 times daily [33]. Lithocholic acid is poorly absorbed and there is little to be found in the bile.

The total bile acid pool is 3—5 g and the average daily production of cholic acid about 330 mg and chenodeoxycholic acid 162 mg.

The control of bile acid synthesis is complex; it is probably a negative feedback mechanism through the amount of bile salts and cholesterol reaching the liver from the gut. Bile acid synthesis is decreased by addition of bile salts and increased by interruption of the entero-hepatic circulation.

Factors in gallstone formation

Three major factors determine the formation of cholesterol gallstones (fig. 31.3). These are altered hepatic bile which becomes supersaturated with cholesterol, nucleation of cholesterol monohydrate crystals and the function of the gallbladder.

ALTERED HEPATIC BILE COMPOSITION

Bile is 85—95% water. Cholesterol is insoluble in water and must be maintained in solution. This may be by the formation of micelles that have a hydrophilic external surface and a hydrophobic internal surface. Cholesterol is incorporated into the hydrophobic interior. Phospholipids are inserted into the walls of the micelles so that they are enlarged; these 'mixed micelles' are thus able to hold more cholesterol [3, 21]. This micellar theory is not as simple as originally thought and the distinction between lithogenic bile, which is outside the micellar liquid zone and is supersaturated with cholesterol, and non-lithogenic bile which is unsaturated, is not clear cut. In particular, supersaturated bile is frequently found in healthy individuals during fasting [56].

It seems that biliary cholesterol may also be solubilized by *vesicles*. These have been shown by ultracentrifugation and electron microscopy in fresh supersaturated and unsaturated bile [138]. The cholesterol is carried in the bile in a stable vesicular form in association with phospholipids but not bile acids. This biliary non-micelle complex has a major cholesterol transport function especially at low bile acid concentrations [93], and when the bile is highly saturated with cholesterol [52]. The unilamellar vesicles are presumably secreted from the

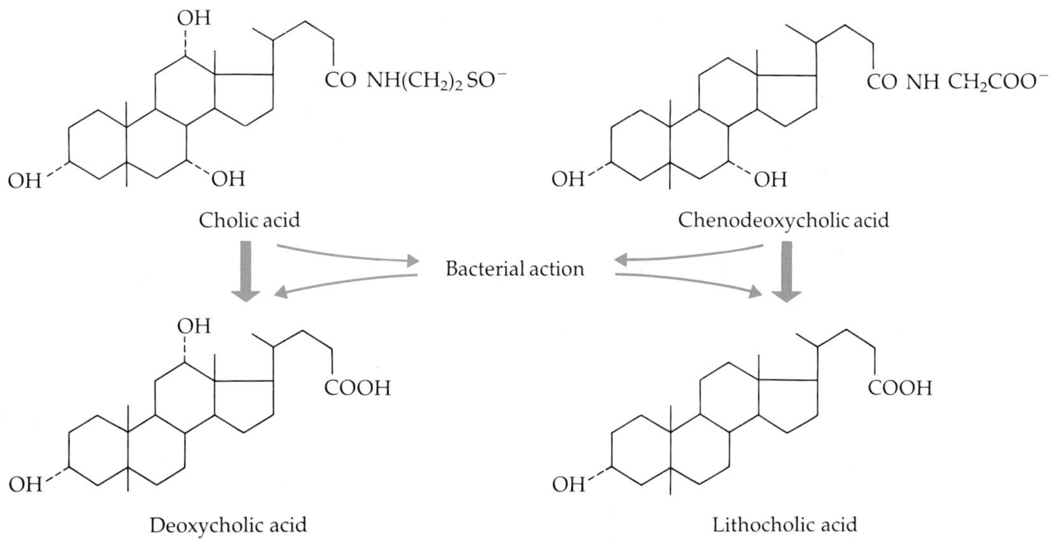

OH
CO NH(CH2)2 SO−
OH
OH
Cholic acid
CO NH CH2COO−
OH
OH
Chenodeoxycholic acid
Bacterial action
OH
COOH
OH
Deoxycholic acid
COOH
OH
Lithocholic acid

Fig. 31.2. The chemical structures of the primary (cholic and chenodeoxycholic) and secondary (deoxycholic and lithocholic) bile acids.

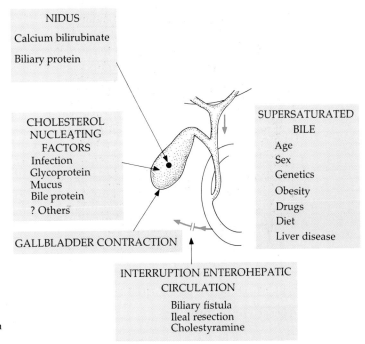

NIDUS
Calcium bilirubinate
Biliary protein
CHOLESTEROL NUCLEATING FACTORS
Infection
Glycoprotein
Mucus
Bile protein
? Others
SUPERSATURATED BILE
Age
Sex
Genetics
Obesity
Drugs
Diet
Liver disease
GALLBLADDER CONTRACTION
INTERRUPTION ENTEROHEPATIC CIRCULATION
Biliary fistula
Ileal resection
Cholestyramine

Fig. 31.3. Factors in cholesterol gallstone formation are supersaturation of the bile, cholesterol crystal nucleation, gallbladder function, the nidus and the entero-hepatic circulation of bile salts.

hepatocyte into the canaliculi where bile salts initiate the process of micellar solubilization of the biliary cholesterol.

Nevertheless, in most gallstone sufferers in the Western world, gallstone formation can be related to supersaturation of bile with cholesterol due to an increased proportion of cholesterol with a decreased proportion of bile

acids [100]. In the majority of patients a diminished hepatic secretion rate of bile acids is the primary defect, and this is related to a reduced total body pool of bile acids [142]. The bile acids circulate more frequently within the entero-hepatic circulation, thereby suppressing synthesis.

CHOLESTEROL NUCLEATION

Nucleation of cholesterol monohydrate crystals is the crucial first step in the process leading to gallstone formation. The distinguishing feature between those who form gallstones and those who do not is the ability of the bile to nucleate cholesterol to form crystals. The time taken for this process is significantly shorter in those with gallstones than in those without [55]. Nucleation time can also be related to the transport of cholesterol in the form of cholesterol/phospholipid vesicles [122].

Compared to control bile, gallbladder bile from patients with cholesterol gallstones contains a potent nucleating factor(s). This might be closely linked to increased pro-nucleating protein which has also been demonstrated in such bile [43].

Gallbladder mucin, secreted by epithelial cells, may play a role in cholesterol nucleation [120].

Antinucleating factors have also been invoked. These have been found in the protein fraction of gallbladder bile and include apolipoproteins A 1 and A 2 [62].

Cholesterol gallstones have bilirubin at their centres, and the protein pigment complex might provide a surface for nucleation of cholesterol crystals from gallbladder bile [74].

GALLBLADDER FUNCTION

The gallbladder has to be capable of emptying and clearing itself of any sludge or debris that might initiate stone formation [15]. Ultrasound shows that prior to stone formation the gallbladder contains a highly viscous mixture of cholesterol, calcium, bilirubin and mucous glycoprotein-forming sludge [68].

Cholecystokinin (CCK) contracts and empties the gallbladder and induces fluid secretion with dilution of gallbladder contents. A decrease in CCK receptors may be an early event in the pathogenesis of gallstone formation by causing a decrease in gallbladder motility [118, 139].

Cholesterol absorption by the gallbladder reduces the cholesterol saturation of bile [105].

ROLE OF INFECTION

Infection is of little importance in uncomplicated gallstone formation. The bile is often sterile and culture of the gallstone yields no growth. Conceivably bacteria might deconjugate bile salts, making the bile more acid and less able to maintain cholesterol in solution. Infection in the gallbladder provides epithelial nuclei on which gallstones may form.

AGE

There is a steady increase in gallstone prevalence with advancing years, probably due to the increased cholesterol content in bile. The presentation is usually in the 50s and 60s.

Gallstones of pigment and cholesterol type are reported in childhood [64].

GENETICS

Families of patients with gallstones have an increased frequency of gallstones, irrespective of their age and weight [44].

SEX AND OESTROGENS

Gallstones are twice as common in women as in men, and this is particularly so before the age of 50 [39].

The incidence is higher in multiparous than in nulliparous women. Incomplete emptying of the gallbladder in late pregnancy leaves a large residual volume and thus retention of cholesterol crystals, and this favours gallstone formation [19].

In women younger than 30 years, gallstones

are usually associated with pregnancy and obesity [67].

Oestrogens also have a mildly cholestatic effect, with reduction of hepatic bile acid secretion and the production of more lithogenic bile.

The bile becomes more lithogenic when women are placed on birth control pills [13]. Women on long-term oral contraceptives have a twofold increased incidence of gallbladder disease over controls [16]. Post-menopausal women taking oestrogen-containing drugs have a highly significant (2.5 times) increase in gallbladder disease [17]. Oestrogen and progesterone receptors have been found in the human gallbladder.

OBESITY

This seems to be more common among gallstone sufferers than in the general population and is a particular risk factor in women less than 50 years old [114]. Obesity is associated with increased cholesterol synthesis and excretion [115]. 50% of markedly obese patients were found to have gallstones at surgery [5].

DIETARY FACTORS

In Western countries, gallstones have been linked to dietary fibre deficiency. This would increase the secondary bile acids, such as desoxycholic acid, in bile and render it more lithogenic. Carbohydrate in refined form increases bile cholesterol saturation [133]. A moderate amount of alcohol seems to protect against gallstones. Vegetarians get fewer gallstones irrespective of their tendency to be slim anyway [97].

Increasing dietary cholesterol increases biliary cholesterol but there is no epidemiological or dietary data to link cholesterol intake with gallstones [114]. Indeed, newly synthesized cholesterol is probably a more important source of biliary cholesterol.

EPIDEMIOLOGY (table 31.2)

Black Africans and the Eastern world are largely free of cholelithiasis. The prevalence, however, is rising as life styles change. In Japan, the change from traditional to Western diets has been associated with a change from bilirubin to cholesterol gallstones.

American Indians have the highest known prevalence. This is related to supersaturation of the bile with cholesterol [141]. Gallstones are also very frequent in the United States generally, in the United Kingdom, France, Germany, Sweden and almost all the Western world.

CIRRHOSIS OF THE LIVER

About 30% of patients with cirrhosis have gallstones and the increased prevalence is also seen in primary biliary cirrhosis [18, 88]. Stones are usually of black pigment type. Such stones were found at cholecystectomy in 79% of patients with cirrhosis compared with 26% of non-cirrhotics [113]. The mechanisms are uncertain. All patients with hepatocellular disease show a variable degree of haemolysis. Although the bile acid secretion is reduced the stones are pigment ones. Phospholipid secretion and

Table 31.2. Comparison of gallstone prevalence between countries and races [11]

Very high	High	Moderate	Low
North American Indians	USA Whites	USA Blacks	Greece
Chile	Great Britain	Japan	Egypt
Sweden	Norway		Zambia
Czechoslovakia	Australia		
	Italy		

cholesterol excretion are also lowered so that the bile is not supersaturated. It has greater cholesterol binding powers than in controls.

Cholecystectomy and bile duct exploration are poorly tolerated, liver failure being frequently precipitated. Such operations should be done only for life-threatening complications of biliary tract disease, such as empyema, perforation and ascending cholangitis. Endoscopic procedures are preferable.

OTHER FACTORS [12]

Ileal resection breaks the entero-hepatic circulation of bile salts, reduces the total bile salt pool and is followed by gallstone formation.

Long-term cholestyramine therapy increases bile salt loss with a reduced bile acid pool and gallstone formation.

Cholesterol-lowering diets high in unsaturated fat and plant sterols but low in saturated fats and cholesterol result in increased gallstone formation.

Clofibrate enhances biliary cholesterol excretion and makes the bile more lithogenic.

Cancer of the gallbladder (see Chapter 34).

Parenteral nutrition leads to a dilated, sluggish gallbladder containing stones [104].

Summary

The formation of gallstones depends on the production of bile in which cholesterol cannot be maintained in solution. This might be related to increased secretion of cholesterol or perhaps to reduction in total bile acid pool. The gallbladder is important in providing nuclei for stone formation and acting as a reservoir allowing growth of the stone. Infection in the gallbladder provides nuclei for stones and alters the chemical composition of the bile, favouring precipitation. Changes in motor and other functions of the gallbladder may be important.

Pigment gallstones

This term is used for stones containing less than 25% cholesterol. They are 2–5 mm in diameter, irregular or smooth, amorphous or crystalline on cross-section. They represent about a quarter of gallstones removed at cholecystectomy. About half are radio-opaque. There are two types, black and brown [74, 137].

Black pigment stones are largely composed of calcium bilirubinate but also have calcium phosphate and carbonate as major constituents. They are usually limited to the gallbladder. They accompany chronic haemolysis, usually hereditary spherocytosis or sickle cell disease, and mechanical prostheses in the circulation. They show an increased prevalence with all forms of cirrhosis including biliary [18]. They are also encountered in the elderly, often male, without an underlying clinical disorder.

Brown pigment stones also have calcium bilirubinate as their major constituent but calcium palmitate and cholesterol are other major constituents. They are usually radiolucent. They are found in the intra-hepatic and extra-hepatic bile ducts and in the gallbladder. They are virtually 100% associated with stricture, sclerosing cholangitis and Caroli's syndrome. Recurrent bile duct stones are usually of this type.

In oriental countries, they are associated with parasitic infestations of the biliary tract such as *Clonorchis sinensis* or *Ascaris lumbricoides*. The stones are frequently intra-hepatic [84].

Radiology of gallstones (see Chapter 29)

Only about 10% of gallstones are radio-opaque, compared with 90% of renal calculi. Visualization is due to the calcium content of the stone. Mixed stones may or may not have sufficient calcium to be rendered visible.

Gallstones are usually multiple and faceted, although occasionally a single, rounded, ring stone fills the whole gallbladder (fig. 31.4).

They usually have a peripheral rim of calcium and a clear centre. Occasionally the structure is laminated due to alternate deposition of cholesterol and calcium bilirubin. Rarely, gallstones contain gas which shows stellate, translucent areas (*Mercedes–Benz sign*).

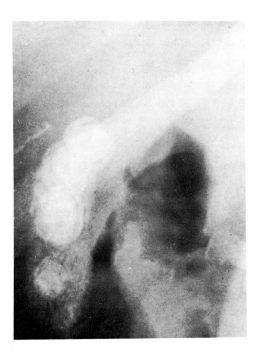

Fig. 31.4. Plain X-ray of the abdomen shows calcified gallstones with alternate deposition of cholesterol and calcium salts. These stones would not be suitable for medical dissolution.

Oral cholecystography is highly accurate in detecting calculi with a false-negative rate of 1% [28]. Failure may be associated with a non-functioning gallbladder and less often with contrast material concealing the stones or with a hepato-cellular dysfunction.

The stones appear as negative shadows which move with changes of posture. In the erect position they may float on the contrast column medium as a translucent layer (floating gall-stones).

Biliary isotopic scanning (see Chapter 29) is useful in showing patency of the bile ducts which, with failure to fill the gallbladder, is used as evidence of acute cholecystitis. Hepato-cellular disease must be taken into account.

CT shows cholesterol gallstones having a density of less than 20 Hounsfield units.

Ultrasound or CT scanning may show a thickened gallbladder wall and the presence of stones (see fig. 29.3). They are particularly valuable in

the acute situation. Ultrasound and oral cholecystography are about equally effective but 1% of stones will be missed by either technique [28].

ERCP and percutaneous cholangiography are the most satisfactory methods for the diagnosis of both gallbladder and bile duct stones (fig. 31.5).

The natural history of gallstones (fig. 31.6)

Disease of the gallbladder is rare unless it complicates gallstones.

Gallstones can be dated from the atmospheric radiocarbon produced by nuclear bomb explosions. This suggests a time lag of about 12 years between initial stone formation and symptoms culminating in cholecystectomy [83].

Stones in the gallbladder are symptomless (*silent gallstones*) unless they migrate into the neck of the gallbladder or into the common bile duct.

Migration of the stones to the neck of the gallbladder causes *obstruction of the cystic duct* resulting in chemical irritation of the gallbladder mucosa by the retained bile, and this is succeeded by bacterial invasion. According to

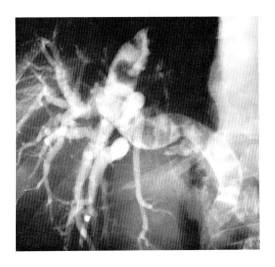

Fig. 31.5. Endoscopic retrograde cholangiography shows multiple gallstones in the common bile duct.

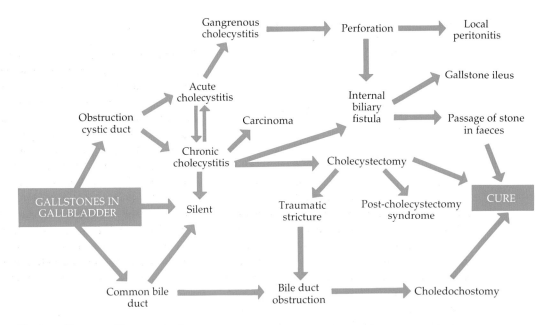

Fig. 31.6. The natural history of gallstones.

the severity of the changes, *acute* or *chronic cholecystitis* results. Acute cholecystitis may gradually subside or progress to acute gangrene and perforation of the gallbladder or to empyema.

If it subsides spontaneously, chronic inflammatory changes persist with subsequent acute exacerbations.

Chronic cholecystitis can be silent. Usually, however, there are dyspeptic symptoms, and the patient may eventually come to cholecystectomy. This is usually curative, but may rarely lead to the *post-cholecystectomy syndrome* or the unfortunate sequel of *traumatic stricture of the bile duct*.

Internal biliary fistula follows the migration of a gallstone from the acutely, or more usually chronically, inflamed gallbladder into an adjacent viscus. The stone may be passed in the faeces, or impact in the alimentary tract, causing *gallstone ileus*.

Gallstones traversing the common bile duct may pass uneventfully into the duodenum, or remain clinically silent in the duct, but usually result in partial *obstruction to the common bile duct* with intermittent obstructive jaundice.

Infection behind the obstruction is common, with consequent *cholangitis*, and this may ascend to the liver, giving rise to abscesses.

Silent gallstones

Gallstones may be symptomless and diagnosed by chance by imaging or during investigation for some other condition. The future course of action is controversial. Physicians usually believe in leaving well alone. The surgeon is more likely to take a positive attitude. Follow-up studies however, show that only a small proportion develops symptoms. In one study only about 10% of patients with asymptomatic gallstones develop symptoms within five years and only 5% require surgery [80]. Only about half the patients with symptomatic gallstones come to cholecystectomy within six years of diagnosis. Patients with gallstones seem to tolerate their symptoms for long periods of time, preferring this to cholecystectomy. If symptoms develop, they are unlikely to present as an emergency.

Prophylactic cholecystectomy should not be performed [98]. It should not be done to prevent gallbladder cancer, a tumour associated with gallstones, as the risk is small and less than that of cholecystectomy [30].

Treatment of gallstones in the gallbladder

Cholecystectomy

This removes the gallstones and the factory making them. About 500 000 cholecystectomies are performed yearly in the United States and this operation is a billion dollar industry. The mortality rate of elective cholecystectomy is 0.1% in patients under 50 years and 0.5% in those over 50 [143]. It is a safe and effective treatment for gallstones. Elderly patients (greater than 75 years old) having emergency surgery, often with gallbladder perforation and biliary peritonitis, provide a high risk group [27]. To prevent this, early elective surgery is recommended in patients with *symptomatic* gallstones, especially if elderly.

The operation demands adequate assistance, exposure, illumination and the facilities for operative cholangiography if necessary. This is performed only if clinical, radiological and operative findings predict that stones will be found in the common bile duct [53]. When the common duct is explored, choledochoscopy is useful and reduces the chance of overlooking common duct calculi.

Medical dissolution

ORAL BILE SALTS

The total bile salt pool is reduced in gallstone patients. Attempts at expansion and at increasing bile salts in bile might therefore be of use in dissolving gallstones and this can be achieved by giving chenodeoxycholic acid or ursodeoxycholic acid which decrease hepatic secretion of cholesterol into bile, so inducing desaturation [73, 134]. Ursodeoxycholic acid also dissolves biliary cholesterol by liquid crystal formation [92].

INDICATIONS

The patient must be compliant and prepared for at least two years' treatment. Symptoms must be mild to moderate and silent stones should not be treated. On cholecystography, the stones must be radiolucent and preferably floating. Unfortunately no imaging technique determines the composition of gallstones. CT is more sensitive and the stones should not be more dense than bile (less than 20 Hounsfield units). Ultrasound is of little value in assessing stone solubility or patency of the cystic duct. 15% of radiolucent stones are composed of pigment where bile acid therapy would be useless. This can only be determined by CT. Stones should be less than 15 mm in diameter.

CHENODEOXYCHOLIC ACID

The dose is 12−15 mg/kg/day in the non-obese. The markedly obese have increased biliary cholesterol and so require 18−20 mg kg/day. Diarrhoea is a side effect and the dose should be increased gradually starting with 500 mg daily. A bedtime dose gives the maximum effect. Other side effects include a dose-dependent rise in serum aspartate transaminase levels which usually subside. Values must be monitored monthly for three months, then at six, twelve, eighteen and twenty-four months.

URSODEOXYCHOLIC ACID

This is derived from the Japanese white-collared bear. It is the 7-beta epimer of chenodeoxycholic acid. The dose is 8−10 mg/kg per day with more being needed if the patient is markedly obese. It dissolves about 30% of radiolucent gallstones completely and faster than using chenodeoxycholic acid [35, 135]. Side effects are absent.

During treatment, the stones may undergo surface calcification [10] but this is probably of little significance.

Results

Gallstone dissolution can be shown by oral cholecystography plus ultrasound or by two negative ultrasound examinations. Ultrasound is more sensitive as residual small fragments may be present after the oral cholecystogram shows no stones. These fragments may provide the nidus for new stone formation. Recurrences develop in 25 to 50% of patients at a rate of 10% per year. They are most likely in the first two years and unlikely after the first three years.

The effect on symptoms is variable and inconsistent [111].

Conclusions

The disadvantages of oral bile acid therapy to dissolve gallbladder stones includes restriction to non-calcified and, if possible, pure cholesterol stones. Dissolution rate is slow. Side effects are possible and there is a probable lifetime commitment to therapy. These must be weighed against the established advantages of cholecystectomy, with a very low mortality and an immediate cure in most instances. At present, ursodeoxycholic acid therapy should be reserved for those who are symptomatic and will co-operate. They should have small, lucent gallstones in a functioning gallbladder and poor general health, including obesity, age or associated conditions should prevent surgery.

Ursodeoxycholic acid may have a role in softening fragments before shock-wave therapy or to dissolve them after the shock.

Possible combinations of ursodeoxycholic acid, 6.5 mg per/kg per day, with chenodoxycholic acid, 7.5 mg/kg per day are less costly and probably as effective [41].

Future developments [41] should include better methods of predicting the composition of gallstones, particularly the calcium and pigment content, and detection of early gallstones in high risk groups. Better dissolving agents are required which have no side effects. These should achieve high concentration in bile, be efficiently reabsorbed from the intestine without intestinal bacterial biotransformation, should act on calcium, pigment and mucous constituents of the stone and should also improve gallbladder emptying.

Solvent dissolution

A percutaneous trans-hepatic number 7 French catheter is inserted under real-time ultrasound guidance into the gallbladder and the solvent pumped in and out (fig. 31.7) [4]. The solvent used is methyltentbutyl ether, a gasoline additive of low viscosity and with power to dissolve cholesterol stones rapidly [4]. The solvent (5–10 ml) envelops the stone but does not overflow into the cystic duct. Computer-assisted pumps have been devised. These eliminate the tedium of manually filling and emptying the gallbladder [144].

The gallstones are dissolved in 4–16 hours and the patient is observed in hospital overnight. Side effects include pain and nausea. Duodenitis and haemolysis are serious consequences of spill of solvent into the duodenum. An ether smell develops on the breath and the patient may become drowsy. Common bile-duct stones should probably not be treated because of leak of solvent into duodenum with consequent systemic absorption [31]. This method may be useful to remove fragments remaining after such procedures as shock-wave therapy. Access to the gallbladder will allow injection of other solutions such as EDTA which would remove non-cholesterol stone fragments [86] and this must be evaluated.

Shock-wave therapy

Gallstones in the gallbladder may be disintegrated into sludge or fragments by high energy shock-waves generated extracorporeally [108]. The original technique demanded a costly Dornier lithotripter, the patient being immersed in water and under general anaesthesia. Second generation lithotripters, similar to those used for disintegrating kidney stones, use acoustically generated shock-waves focused by an acoustic lens onto the stone [123]. A water

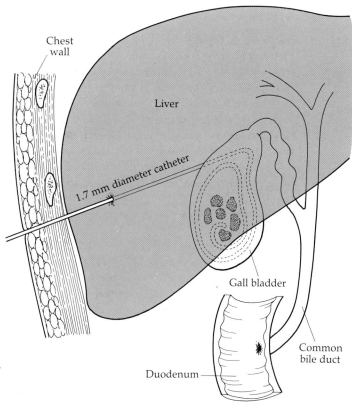

Fig. 31.7. Technique of percutaneous transhepatic gallbladder catheter placement for MBTE dissolution of gallstones (Allen *et al.* [4]).

bath is unnecessary as is general anaesthesia. Afterwards, a mixture of chenodeoxycholic acid and ursodeoxycholic acid (7–8 mg/kg/day of each) is given for three months to dissolve the fragments [106].

Patients selected must be symptomatic having had one attack of biliary colic. The stones must be radiolucent or with only a slim rim of calcium and in a functioning gallbladder as assessed by cholecystography. Only patients having one, two or three stones, each maximum diameter 25 mm, can be treated. Heavily calcified stones are unsuitable. There are many exclusions and only 5–10% of those referred for therapy prove suitable.

One hundred and thirty-one solitary stones were treated and three, six and twelve months later ultrasound showed disappearance in 70, 75 and 100%, respectively. Twenty-four patients with multiple stones were treated and the

values were 27, 50 and 75%, respectively at three, six and twelve months [106]. Only one patient had insufficient fragmentation so that cholecystectomy became necessary. About a third of those treated have episodes of biliary colic; mild pancreatitis is rare. Skin patechiae and haematuria are other complications.

Shock-wave therapy has also been applied to giant common bile duct stones [124]. The procedure is done after ERCP and papillotomy have been performed and with a naso-biliary tube *in situ*. The stone is focused by two-dimensional ultrasound. The procedure is particularly applicable to patients with stones too large for Dormia basket removal, too hard for mechanical lithotripsy or too inaccessible because of their intra-hepatic position. After therapy, fragments are removed endoscopically. The procedure was successful in 16 of 20 patients.

Conclusions

Shock-wave therapy offers a new dimension for the treatment of gallstones. Problems are cost and the small percentage of patients who prove suitable. The procedure must be confined to those with symptomatic gallstones and not to those whose stones are silent. The diseased gallstone factory is left *in situ* and one year after stopping bile acids gallstones will have recurred in 11%. So far serious complications have not been reported, but there is a possibility of tissue injury to lungs, gas-filled bowel, normal liver or pancreas. There is also a possibility that relatively safe gallbladder stones will be converted to more serious ones in the common bile duct. The procedure must be measured against other treatments such as cholecystectomy and, for choledocholithiasis, endoscopic papillotomy and stone removal.

Mechanical lithotripsy of common bile duct stones

The lithotripter is introduced into the common bile duct [101]. Preliminary endoscopic papillotomy is usually necessary but in young persons this may not be necessary, particularly if the papilla can be dilated via the endoscope. The stones are grasped and if they cannot be extracted they are crushed with a lithotripter and the fragments removed with the conventional Dormia basket. The success rate is 82.1% [101].

Acute cholecystitis

AETIOLOGY

In 96% of patients the cystic duct is obstructed by a gallstone (fig. 31.8). The imprisoned bile salts have a toxic action on the gallbladder wall. Lipids may penetrate the Rokitansky–Aschoff sinuses and exert an irritant reaction. The rise in pressure compresses blood vessels in the gallbladder wall; infarction and gangrene follow.

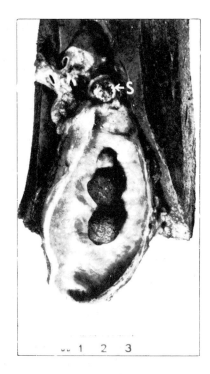

Fig. 31.8. Three gallstones lie in a greatly thickened, chronically inflamed gallbladder. A further calculus (S) is lodged in the cystic duct. Scale is in cm.

Pancreatic enzymes may also cause acute cholecystitis, presumably by regurgitation in the presence of obstruction of a common biliary and pancreatic channel. Such pancreatic regurgitation may account for some instances of acute cholecystitis developing in the absence of gallbladder stones.

Bacterial inflammation is an integral part of acute cholecystitis. Bacterial deconjugation of bile salts may produce toxic bile acids which can injure the mucosa.

PATHOLOGY

The gallbladder is greyish-red in colour with a lustreless surface. There are vascular adhesions to adjacent structures. The gallbladder is usually distended, but after previous inflammation the wall becomes thickened and contracted. It contains turbid fluid which may be frankly purulent (*empyema of the gallbladder*). A gallstone may be lodged in the neck (fig. 31.8).

Histology shows haemorrhage and moderate oedema reaching a peak about the fourth day and diminishing by the seventh day. As the acute reaction subsides it is replaced by fibrosis.

Related lymph glands at the neck of the gallbladder and along the common bile duct are enlarged.

Bacteriology. Cultures of both gallbladder wall and bile usually show organisms of intestinal type, including anaerobes, in about three-quarters of cases.

CLINICAL FEATURES

These vary from those of mild inflammation to fulminating gangrene of the gallbladder wall. The acute attack is often an exacerbation of underlying chronic cholecystitis.

The sufferers are often obese, female and over 40, but no type, age or sex is immune.

Pain often occurs late at night or in the early morning, usually in the right upper abdomen or epigastrium and is referred below the angle of the right scapula, the right shoulder, or rarely to the left side. It may simulate angina pectoris.

The pain usually rises to a plateau and can last 30–60 minutes without relief, unlike the short spasm of biliary colic [38]. Attacks may be precipitated by late-night, heavy meals or fatty foods, or even by such simple acts as abdominal palpation or yawning. The wretched, perspiring sufferer lies motionless in a curled-up posture, often with local heat applied to the abdomen.

Distension pain is due to the gallbladder contracting to overcome the blocked cystic duct. This visceral pain is deep seated, central and unaccompanied by muscular rigidity and superficial or deep tenderness.

Peritoneal pain is superficial with skin tenderness, hyperaesthesia and muscular rigidity. The fundus of the gallbladder is in apposition to the diaphragmatic peritoneum, which is supplied by the phrenic and last six intercostal nerves. Stimulation of the anterior branches produces right-upper quadrant pain and of the posterior cutaneous branch leads to the characteristic right infrascapular pain.

The spinal nerves extend a short distance into the mesentery and gastro-hepatic ligament around the major bile ducts, and stimulation of these nerves is interpreted as pain and referred to the back and right upper quadrant. This explains the pain of stones in the common bile duct and of cholangitis.

Digestive system. Flatulence and nausea are common, but vomiting is unusual, unless there is a stone in the common bile duct.

EXAMINATION

The patient appears ill, with shallow, jerky respirations. The temperature rises with bacterial invasion. Jaundice usually indicates associated stones in the common bile duct.

The abdomen moves poorly. Spread of infection to peritoneal surfaces leads to gastric and duodenal distension. Hyperaesthesia is maximal in the 8th and 9th right thoracic segments, and the right upper abdominal muscles are rigid. The gallbladder is usually impalpable; occasionally a tender mass of gallbladder and adherent omentum may be felt. Murphy's sign is positive. The liver edge is tender.

The *leucocyte count* is raised to about $10\,000/mm^3$, with moderate increase in polymorphs.

A *plain film* of the abdomen should be taken.

Isotopic biliary scanning is of value (Chapter 29). A completely normal gallbladder rules out acute cholecystitis, whereas a well opacified common bile duct without filling of the gallbladder is reasonable evidence of an obstructed cystic duct.

Ultrasound or CT scanning may show a thickened gallbladder wall and the presence of stones. Either technique is of particular value in this acute situation.

In the very severely ill, peri-nasal endoscopic biliary drainage or percutaneous aspiration [79] may be life saving (fig. 31.10). Drainage is combined with intensive antibiotic therapy both systemic and directly into the bile ducts. The patient is thus brought to surgery or endoscopic sphincterotomy in much better condition.

DIFFERENTIAL DIAGNOSIS

Acute cholecystitis is liable to be confused with other causes of sudden pain and tenderness in the right hypochondrium. These include referred pain from muscular and spinal root lesions.

Below the diaphragm, acute retrocaecal appendicitis, intestinal obstruction, a perforated peptic ulcer or acute pancreatitis may be confusing.

Diaphragmatic pleurisy may be associated with tenderness in the gallbladder area and this is also characteristic of Bornholm disease. Myocardial infarction should always be considered.

PROGNOSIS

Spontaneous recovery follows disimpaction of the stone in 85% of patients. However, the gallbladder remains shrunken, fibrotic, full of stones and non-functioning. Recurrent acute cholecystitis may follow, but there may be surprisingly long, clinically silent periods.

Rarely, acute cholecystitis proceeds rapidly to gangrene or empyema of the gallbladder, fistula formation, hepatic abscesses or even generalized peritonitis. The acute fulminating disease is becoming less common because of earlier antibiotic therapy and more frequent cholecystectomies for recurrent gallbladder symptoms.

Acute emergency surgery in the aged (over 74 years old) carries a bad prognosis with many complications [27].

TREATMENT

General measures include bed rest, intravenous fluids, a light diet and relief of pain with pethidine (demerol) and buscopan.

Antibiotics (table 31.3) [32, 126]

Antibiotics prevent such complications as peritonitis, cholangitis and septicaemia. During the first 24 hours, 30% of gallbladder cultures are positive. This rises to 80% after 72 hours.

In the presence of acute inflammation and biliary obstruction, antibiotics may not achieve satisfactory levels in the bile and diseased tissues. Concurrent hepatic disease affects biliary excretion and dangerous blood levels can develop.

Common infecting organisms in bile are *E. coli*, *Strep. faecalis* and *Klebsiella*, often in combination. *Pseudomonas* and *proteus* are found in patients who are receiving antibiotics. Anaerobes are present, if sought, and are usually found with aerobes. They include bacteroides and clostridia.

Antibiotics achieve different biliary levels (table 31.3). In general, the penicillins achieve satisfactory biliary levels. Erythromycin is excreted mainly in bile but has the wrong bacteriological spectrum. Intravenous mezlocillin results in biliary concentrations sufficient to

Table 31.3. Antibiotic concentration in bile [32]. Note that biliary obstruction and hepato-cellular disease may reduce the concentration. The sensitivity of the causative organisms must also be considered

Poor	Moderate	Good
Gentamicin	Ampicillin	Mezlocillin
		Mecillinam
	Amoxycillin	Piperacillin
Cefotaxime	Metronidazole	Cefamandole
		Cefoperazone
Sulphonamides	Co-trimoxazole	Erythromycin
Amikacin	Carbenicillin	Tetracycline
Cefuroxime	Clindamycin	Rifampicin
Ticarcillin		
Cefazidime		
Cephazolin		

inhibit most biliary pathogens, even in jaundiced patients [32] in combination with an aminoglycoside such as gentamycin.

Surgery

There is much to be said for early cholecystectomy (p. 663), morbidity, mortality and cost being less than with medical management [57]. If performed during the first three days, cholecystectomy has a mortality of about 0.5%.

In about 50% of patients, the acute attack resolves without surgery. However, 20% have to be admitted later and require urgent surgery and about 30% are treated expectantly but deteriorate, so that urgent surgery is necessary. If the operation is performed later, the patient's condition has deteriorated and there are difficulties in anatomical definition. In high risk, critically ill patients percutaneous, trans-hepatic cholecystostomy may be life saving [65].

About 10% of patients with acute cholecystitis will have associated common duct stones. These are diagnosed by jaundice, dark urine and pale stools, fever, a serum bilirubin raised three times and an alkaline phosphatase two times above normal with operative findings of large cystic and common bile duct with possible palpable stones [53]. These indicate exploration of the common duct unless inflammation around the porta hepatis renders dissection and identification of structures difficult.

Perforation of the gallbladder

Acute calculous cholecystitis may proceed to complete necrosis of the gallbladder wall and perforation. The gallstone may erode the necrotic wall; alternatively, dilated infected Rokitansky−Aschoff sinuses may provide a weak point for rupture.

Rupture usually takes place at the fundus which is the least well vascularized part of the gallbladder. Rupture into the free peritoneal cavity is rare and, more usually, adhesions form between adjacent organs with local abscess formation. Rupture into adjacent viscera leads to internal biliary fistula.

The patient presents with nausea, right upper quadrant pain and vomiting. A right upper quadrant mass is palpable in 50%, and a similar number are febrile. The diagnosis is often overlooked.

CT and ultrasound are of value in showing peritoneal fluid, abscess and gallstones. There are three clinical types [103].

Acute with bile peritonitis. These patients rarely give a history of gallbladder disease. They frequently have systemic conditions associated with vascular insufficiency or immunodeficiency such as atherosclerosis, diabetes mellitus, collagen diseases, corticosteroid use, decompensated cirrhosis or are postoperative. The diagnosis should be suspected in any immunocompromised young male presenting as an acute abdomen.

Prognosis is poor with a mortality of about 30%.

Treatment is by massive antibiotics and restoration of the fluid balance. The gangrenous gallbladder wall is removed or drained percutaneously or surgically. Any abscess must also be drained.

Subacute with pericholecystic abscess. These patients have chronic gallstone disease and the picture is intermediate between the acute and chronic types.

Chronic with cholecystenteric fistula formation (see p. 678).

Emphysematous cholecystitis

The term is used to denote infection of the gallbladder with gas-producing organisms, *E. coli, Clostridium welchii*, or aerobic or anaerobic streptococci. The primary lesion is occlusion of the cystic duct or cystic artery and infection is secondary. [77].

The condition classically affects male diabetics who develop features of severe toxic acute cholecystitis. An abdominal mass may be palpable.

Radiology. In the plain film the gallbladder is seen as a sharply outlined pear-shaped gas shadow. Occasionally air may be seen infiltrating the wall and surrounding tissue. Gas is not apparent in the cystic duct which is blocked by a gallstone. In the erect position, a fluid level is seen in the gallbladder; this is never seen with an internal biliary fistula.

Treatment. Antibiotics are given in large doses. Cholecystostomy and drainage are done either surgically or by the percutaneous ultrasound-guided method.

Chronic calculous cholecystitis

This is the commonest type of clinical gallbladder disease. The association of chronic cholecystitis with stones is almost constant.

Aetiological factors, therefore, include all those related to gallstones (fig. 31.3). The chronic inflammation may follow acute cholecystitis, but usually develops insidiously.

PATHOLOGY

The gallbladder is usually contracted with a thickened, sometimes calcified, wall but may be cystic. The contained bile is turbid with a sediment of debris, called biliary sludge. The contained stones are seen lying loosely embedded in the wall or in meshes of an organizing fibrotic network. One stone is usually lodged in the neck (fig. 31.8). The mucosa is ulcerated and scarred. Histologically the mucosa is thickened and congested with lymphocytic infiltration and occasionally complete destruction of the mucosa.

CLINICAL FEATURES

Chronic cholecystitis is difficult to diagnose because of the ill-defined symptoms. A familial incidence of gallstones, previous attacks of jaundice, multiparity and obesity form a suggestive background. Rarely, episodes of acute cholecystitis punctuate the course. The patient may experience episodes of biliary colic.

Abdominal distension or epigastric discomfort, especially after a fatty meal, may be temporarily relieved by belching. Nausea is common, but vomiting is unusual unless there are stones in the common bile duct. Apart from

a constant dull ache in the right hypochondrium and epigastrium, pain may be experienced in the right scapular region, substernally or at the right shoulder. Post-prandial pain may be relieved by alkalis.

Local tenderness over the gallbladder and a positive Murphy sign are very suggestive.

INVESTIGATIONS

The temperature, leucocyte count, haemoglobin and erythrocyte sedimentation rate are within normal limits. A plain X-ray of the abdomen, ultrasonography or CT scan may reveal gallstones. On cholecystography the gallbladder is usually non-functioning. ERCP is helpful in demonstrating stones in the gallbladder or common bile duct and the size of the common bile duct.

DIFFERENTIAL DIAGNOSIS

Fat intolerance, flatulence and post-prandial discomfort are common symptoms. Even if associated with imaging evidence of gallstones, the calculi are not necessarily responsible, for stones are frequently present in the symptom-free.

Other disorders producing a similar clinical picture must be excluded before cholecystectomy is advised, otherwise symptoms persist post-operatively. These include peptic ulceration, hiatus hernia, irritable bowel syndrome, chronic urinary tract infections and functional dyspepsias. A careful appraisal of the patient's psychological make-up is necessary.

The oral cholecystogram or ultrasound is only 95% accurate. There is a possibility that symptomatic gallbladder disease may not only be over-diagnosed but may sometimes be unrecognized.

PROGNOSIS

This chronic disease is compatible with good life expectancy. However, once symptoms, particularly biliary colic, are experienced, the patients tend to remain symptomatic and prolonged remission is unusual [131]. Gallbladder cancer is a very rare, later development.

TREATMENT

Medical measures may be tried if the diagnosis is uncertain and a period of observation is desirable. This is especially so when indefinite symptoms are associated with a well-functioning gallbladder. The general condition of the patient may contraindicate surgery. The place of medical dissolution and shocking of radiolucent stones has already been discussed.

Obesity should be corrected. Fat intake will depend upon the functional state of the gallbladder: if it is non-functioning, a low-fat diet is advisable. Cooked fats are badly tolerated and should be avoided.

Cholecystectomy (see p. 663)

This is indicated if the patient is symptomatic, particularly with repeated episodes of pain. The common bile duct should be explored if stones are likely to be present.

The T-tube is in position in the common bile duct for not longer than two days as a longer time increases morbidity. Culture of the bile is done, for post-operative deaths are often due to septicaemia. Cholangiography precedes its removal.

Intravenous fluids are not usually necessary as fluids may be taken by mouth almost immediately and a light diet eaten on the second day.

Slight and transient increases in serum bilirubin and alkaline phosphatase levels can be expected in the normal post-operative cholecystectomy course [109]. Greater increases indicate such complications as mild peritonitis or injury to the bile ducts. Pancreatitis is another post-operative complication.

Acalculous cholecystitis

ACUTE

671 Between 6 and 17% of gallbladders removed

for acute cholecystitis contain no stones and the percentage may be increasing [47]. In about half a predisposing cause will be found. The most frequent is an associated critical condition [90], such as non-biliary surgical operations [29], multiple injuries [36], burns, recent childbirth or severe sepsis [54]. A severe form was seen in American soldiers, severely wounded in Vietnam, and suffering from bacteriaemia [71].

Multiple factors must contribute. Dehydration may increase bile viscosity. Parenteral nutrition and assisted ventilation cause cholestasis [93]. Opiates increase sphincter of Oddi pressure and hence luminal pressure in the gallbladder. Bacteriaemia results in biliary infection [90]. Shock impairs cystic arterial blood flow.

In elderly patients, gallbladder ischaemia with superadded infection is probably important [37].

Clinical features are those of acute calculous cholecystitis but males are more affected than females and the mortality is twice as high [47]. In the critically ill, gangrene and perforation of the gallbladder are common [29]. Unless considered, the diagnosis may not be suspected. Treatment is by prompt cholecystectomy. In critically ill patients, cholecystostomy under ultrasound guidance may be life saving [34].

CHRONIC

This is a difficult diagnosis as the clinical condition resembles others, particularly the irritable bowel syndrome and the functional dyspepsias. Ultrasound scans and oral cholecystograms are normal. Nevertheless, chronic inflammation can be present in the gallbladder without gallstones and relief will follow cholecystectomy.

Oral cholecystography after intravenous cholecystokinin (CCK) is associated with reproduction of the pain within five to ten minutes. The gallbladder shows poor contraction and incomplete emptying [50, 70].

TYPHOID CHOLECYSTITIS

Circulating typhoid bacilli are filtered by the liver and excreted in the bile. The biliary tract, however, is infected in only about 0.2% of patients with typhoid fever.

Acute typhoid cholecystitis is becoming very rare. Signs of acute cholecystitis appear at the end of the second week or even during convalescence, and are sometimes followed by perforation of the gallbladder.

Chronic typhoid fever cholecystitis and the typhoid carrier state. The typhoid carrier passes organisms in the faeces derived from a focus of infection in the gallbladder or biliary tract. Chronic typhoid cholecystitis is symptomless.

The carrier state is not cured by antibiotic therapy. Cholecystectomy is successful if there is not an associated infection of the biliary ducts. Chronic typhoid cholecystitis is not an important cause of gallstones.

Biliary carriers of other salmonellae have been reported and treated with ampicillin and cholecystectomy.

OTHER INFECTIONS

Opportunist. Patients with AIDS develop sclerosing cholangitis with gallbladder involvement due to infections with opportunist organisms such as cytomegalovirus and cryptosporidia [110].

Actinomycosis can very rarely involve the gallbladder.

Giardiasis can result in biliary dysfunction [48].

Staphylococcal infection can be associated with acalculous cholecystitis [132].

OTHER ASSOCIATIONS

A *chemical cholecystitis* may follow long-term infusion of cytotoxic drugs, such as FUDR, into the hepatic artery [116].

Diseases involving the *cystic artery*, such as polyarteritis nodosa, may lead to cholecystitis [72].

The gallbladder may be involved in *Crohn's*

disease [78]. *Sjögren's disease* has been reported with acute gallbladder dilatation [128].

CHOLESTEROSIS OF THE GALLBLADDER

Cholesterol esters and other lipids are deposited in the submucosal and epithelial cells as small, yellow, lipid specks and, together with the intervening red bile-stained mucosa, give the appearance of a ripe strawberry. The deposits are at first found only on the mucosal ridges but later they extend into the troughs. As more lipid is deposited, it projects into the lumen as polyps which may become pedunculated. The change is confined to the gallbladder and never extends to the ducts.

The lipid is seen in reticulo-endothelial xanthoma cells of the mucosa, which is not inflamed. The cholesterosis is related to the biliary, not blood cholesterol concentration.

The aetiology is uncertain [60]. The bile is supersaturated with cholesterol and indeed half the patients do develop gallstones. The gallbladder mucosa may simply be taking up excess cholesterol from bile. Other possibilities are a defect in sub-mucosal macrophages or synthesis of surplus lipid by the mucous membrane.

Cholesterolosis is common, being found in about 10% of autopsies, most frequently in middle-aged women.

There is controversy concerning the relation of cholesterolosis to symptoms.

However, cholesterolosis may sometimes cause right upper quadrant pain and features causing confusion with the irritable bowel syndrome. Diagnosis is difficult. Cholecystography, preferably with CCK, shows filling defects in the gallbladder in only a third [23], and ultrasonography is usually negative.

The pain is reproduced by intravenous CCK in those patients who are relieved by cholecystectomy [70].

XANTHOGRANULOMATOUS CHOLECYSTITIS

This is an uncommon inflammatory disease of the gallbladder characterized by a focal or diffuse destructive inflammatory process with lipid-laden macrophages. Macroscopically, areas of xanthogranulomatous cholecystitis appear as yellow masses within the wall of the gallbladder [102]. The gallbladder wall is invariably thickened and cholesterol or mixed gallstones are usually present.

The pathogenesis is uncertain, but an inflammatory response to extravasated bile, possibly from ruptured Rokitansky–Aschoff sinuses, is likely [49].

Symptoms often begin as an episode of acute cholecystitis and persist for up to five years. There is extension of yellow tissue into adjacent organs. Fistulae from gallbladder to skin or duodenum may develop [102]. At operation, carcinoma seems likely and frozen sections are usually required to make the differentiation.

Post-cholecystectomy problems

Poor results after cholecystectomy can be expected in about one-third of patients. These may be due to wrong diagnosis. About 95% of those *with gallstones* are freed of symptoms or improved post-operatively. Results are good if stones are found. Their absence questions the original diagnosis. The patients may have been suffering from a psychosomatic or some other disorder. A biliary cause is likely if stones are found at cholecystectomy and if a period of relief follows the operation. The colon and pancreas are common alternative culprits.

Symptoms may be related to technical difficulties at the time of surgery. These include traumatic *biliary stricture* (Chapter 32), and *residual calculi*. A *cystic duct remnant*, greater than 1 cm, is very frequent after cholecystectomy. It is an infrequent cause of symptoms in the absence of common duct stones [58]. These patients benefit from removal of the cystic duct or gallbladder remnant.

Amputation neuromas can be demonstrated in some patients but removal offers no relief and this seems unlikely to be the cause of the symptoms.

Chronic pancreatitis, a common association of choledocholithiasis may persist post-operatively.

Cholangiography—endoscopic or percutaneous—is of particular value in the investigation of post-cholecystectomy symptoms. Residual calculi, stricture, ampullary stenosis, a cystic duct stump or normal appearances are significant findings.

Papillary stenosis or dysfunction

This diagnosis remains controversial. *Papillary stenosis* is often associated with present or past duct gallstones. Cholestatic biochemical tests may be present. Functional abnormalities may be shown by biliary manometry, the basal sphincter pressure being raised [8] and this is increased by morphia. Endoscopic cholangiography shows dilatation of the common bile duct and delayed drainage of contrast material into the duodenum [130]. In such patients endoscopic sphincterotomy is indicated but only 70% get good long-term results [25], and prediction of success is impossible.

Others have little evidence of organic stenosis but still may have functional disturbance of the sphincter (*biliary dyskinesia*). In these patients manometry may show abnormal motility disturbances and an abnormal response to cholecystokinin [136]. In such patients increases in bile duct pressure induced by morphine coincide with pain [127]. In these patients, endoscopic balloon dilatation of the sphincter may be tried. It is certainly less irrevocable than sphincterotomy.

Gallstones in the common bile duct (choledocholithiasis)

The majority of stones in the common bile duct have migrated from the gallbladder and are associated with calculous cholecystitis. Migration is related to the size of the stone relative to the cystic and common bile duct [129]. The stones grow in the common bile duct so causing biliary obstruction and facilitating the migration of further stones from the gallbladder.

Secondary stones that are not of gallbladder origin usually follow partial biliary obstruction due to such causes as residual calculus, traumatic stricture, sclerosing cholangitis or congenital biliary abnormalities. Infection may be the initial event [22]. Stones are brown, single or multiple, oval and conforming to the long axis of the duct. They tend to impact in the ampulla of Vater and may project into the duodenum.

EFFECTS OF COMMON BILE DUCT STONES

Bile duct obstruction is usually partial for the calculus exerts a ball-valve action at the lower end of the common bile duct. In the anicteric, hepatic histology is virtually normal. In the icteric, it shows cholestasis. In chronic cases, the bile ducts show concentric scarring (fig. 31.9) and eventually secondary sclerosing cholangitis and biliary cirrhosis.

Cholangitis. The stagnant bile is readily infected, probably from the intestines. The bile becomes opaque and dark brown (*biliary sludge*). Rarely the infection is more acute and the bile is purulent. The common bile duct is thickened and dilated, with desquamated or ulcerated mucosa, especially in the ampulla of Vater. The cholangitis may spread to the intrahepatic bile ducts and, in severe and prolonged infections, cholangitic abscesses are seen. The cut section of liver shows cavities containing bile-stained pus, communicating with the bile ducts. *E. coli* is the commonest infecting organism. Others include bacteroides, streptococci, lactobacilli and clostridia.

Acute or chronic pancreatitis may result from stones in the ampulla of Vater, with bile regurgitation along the pancreatic duct.

CLINICAL SYNDROMES

Choledocholithiasis presents as three clinical situations. The stones may be *silent* and symptomless, discovered only by imaging or at the time of a routine cholecystectomy for chronic calculous cholecystitis. In the elderly, they may present simply as mental and physical debility [24]. Secondly, the stones may cause an *acute cholangitis* with jaundice. Finally, the stones may be *residual*, detected early or late post-

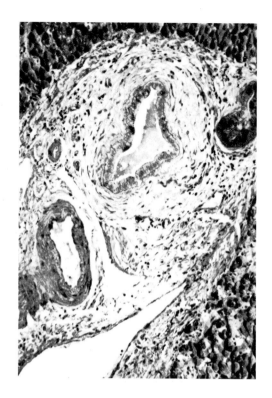

Fig. 31.9. Portal zone from operative liver biopsy of a patient with sclerosing cholangitis secondary to choledocholithiasis. The duct wall shows concentric fibrosis and the whole portal area is fibrosed. (Stained PAS, ×126.)

cholecystectomy, where again they can be silent or causing symptoms.

Acute jaundice and cholangitis

The classical picture is of an elderly, obese woman, with a previous history of flatulent indigestion, fat intolerance and mid-epigastric pain, presenting with jaundice, abdominal pain, chills and fever.

The cholestatic *jaundice* is usually mild, but is occasionally deep or absent. The bile duct obstruction is rarely complete and the amount of pigment fluctuates in the stools.

Pain occurs in about three-quarters of the patients. It is always severe, colicky, intermittent and needing analgesics for its relief. Sometimes it is a constant, sharp, severe, mounting pain. The site may be right upper quadrant or epigastric. It radiates to the back and to the right scapula. It is associated with vomiting. Palpation of the epigastrium is painful. *Fever* occurs in about a third of the patients, ranging from a continuous pyrexia to occasional spikes of 38–38.5°C.

Urine is dark and infected when the patient is febrile.

The *bile* shows a mixed growth of intestinal organisms, predominantly *E. coli*. The bacterial overgrowth in the small intestine is confirmed by a positive bile salt 'breath' test which confirms that deconjugating bacteria are present.

The *serum* shows the findings of cholestatic jaundice. The serum conjugated bilirubin is raised to about 3–10 mg/100 ml.

If the stones obstruct the main pancreatic duct, the serum amylase concentration may rise sharply.

Haematological changes. The polymorph leucocyte count may be raised; the level depends on the acuteness and severity of the cholangitis.

Blood culture should be performed repeatedly during the febrile period and the antibiotic sensitivity of any organism determined. Although the usual organisms encountered are the intestinal ones, such as *E. coli* and anaerobic streptococci, other unusual ones such as the *Aeromonas* species must be sought.

X-rays of the abdomen may show calculi in the gallbladder, and more medially and posteriorly in the common bile duct. Endoscopic or percutaneous *cholangiography* confirms the presence of stones.

Ultrasound may show dilated intra-hepatic ducts although more often these are undilated. Stones in the lower end of the common bile duct are often missed by ultrasound but are shown by *CT scanning*.

DIAGNOSIS

This is not difficult if jaundice follows biliary colic and febrile episodes. Too often, however, there is only vague indigestion, no fever, no gallbladder tenderness and an unhelpful white blood count. Alternatively, the patient may present with painless jaundice. The condition must then be differentiated from other forms of cholestasis, including neoplastic, and acute virus hepatitis (table 12.2). The bile in total biliary obstruction due to carcinoma is rarely infected.

Residual common duct stones

Between 5 and 10% of patients having a cholecystectomy with exploration of the common bile duct will have retained stones. Calculi in the hepatic ducts are specially liable to be overlooked. Residual bile duct calculi may be suspected if the patient experiences pain when a T-tube draining the bile duct is temporarily clamped. Cholangiography reveals filling defects. Sepsis and cholangitis occur post-

Table 31.4. Management of choledocholithiasis

		Patient type	
Category	Gallbladder	Young, fit	Old, frail
Silent	Present	Nil	Nil
Cholangitis and jaundice	Present	Endoscopy later cholecystectomy (surgery—T-tube)*	Endoscopy only (surgery—T-tube)*
Residual (No T-tube)	Absent	Endoscopy (surgery—T-tube)*	Endoscopy (surgery—T-tube)*
Residual (T-tube)	Absent	Remove via T-tube	Remove via T-tube

* ERCP not available.

operatively. In many instances, however, the residual bile duct calculi remain silent.

Management of common duct stones

This depends on the clinical situation—emergency or elective—on the age and general condition of the patient and on the facilities and available clinical expertise (table 31.4). Antibiotics are only temporarily effective in controlling the cholangitis if the bile duct remains obstructed. Other measures include control of fluid and electrolyte balance, correction of anaemia and intramuscular vitamin K_1, if the patient is jaundiced.

In the severely ill, pre-operative biliary drainage for a few days either by the percutaneous trans-hepatic route (Chapter 29) or by endoscopic cannulation of the common bile duct with drainage of bile trans-nasally (fig. 31.10) is useful. Drainage is combined with intensive antibiotic therapy both systemic and directly into the bile ducts. The patient is thus brought to surgery or endoscopic sphincterotomy in a much better condition.

Surgical management

The common bile duct must be explored and all calculi removed. The chronically infected gallbladder should also be removed to prevent further migration of stones into the bile ducts. The bile duct is drained with a T-tube of adequate size (no. 16 French).

The operative recognition of stones in the bile duct is difficult. Percutaneous and endoscopic cholangiography are valuable preoperative procedures. Stones can be missed by simple palpation, but probing with bougies is uncertain and carries the risk of causing a false passage to the duodenum. Stenosis of the sphincter of Oddi may result. If stones are present at the lower end of the common bile duct, the duodenum should be opened and the papilla examined from below.

Direct cholangiography should be performed routinely at the time of operation and again post-operatively before removal of the tube draining the common duct. Choledochoscopy is useful but adds to the operative time.

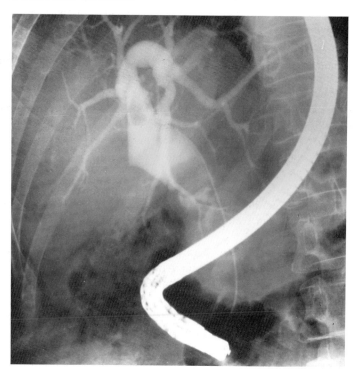

Fig. 31.10. Choledocholithiasis with acute cholangitis. Biliary drainage has been achieved by a tube in the common bile duct introduced via the endoscope.

If there are operative difficulties in the poor-risk patient, no attempt is made to remove all the stones which will later be recovered through the T-tube. In patients with large and many stones, a drainage choledochoduodenostomy may be helpful.

Non-surgical management

This is discussed fully in Chapter 29. Endoscopic removal with sphincterotomy is frequently used particularly in the elderly and frail (table 31.4).

The presence of a T-tube allows extraction with a basket or sometimes the stone can be pushed into the duodenum.

Medical solvent dissolution [91] and shock treatment are being increasingly used.

Cholangitis

This is usually associated with partial biliary obstruction due to choledocholithiasis, biliary stricture, sclerosing cholangitis, congenital biliary dilatations and, rarely, neoplastic biliary obstruction [14].

Malaise and fever are followed by shivering and sweating (*Charcot's intermittent biliary fever*). Malaise, fever, pain, vomiting and pruritus increase with the jaundice. In those previously anicteric, the urine darkens and the stools may become pale. The syndrome is due to oedema of the bile duct mucous membrane, so that partial biliary obstruction becomes complete. There is septicaemia with a positive blood culture for *E. coli* and other intestinal organisms. As the oedema subsides so the partial biliary obstruction is relieved and the temperature falls. Associated renal failure may be related to endotoxins.

Multiple abscesses may develop in the liver (Chapter 27).

ACUTE OBSTRUCTIVE CHOLANGITIS

This is the most severe form of cholangitis. In addition to the classical symptoms of cholangitis the patient is lethargic, prostrated and shocked. Purulent material accumulates under increasing pressure in the biliary tract. A Gram-negative septicaemia is associated with endotoxic shock.

Treatment: this is by fluid and electrolyte replacement, and broad spectrum antibiotics. Biliary decompression is achieved by percutaneous trans-hepatic or nasal endoscopic biliary drainage [96] (fig. 31.10). The mortality is then only 5%. This routine is followed by definitive cholangiography and treatment, whether endoscopic or surgical removal of calculi, balloon dilatation or intra-duct infusions of solvents.

Intra-hepatic gallstones

Stones in the intra-hepatic ducts are particularly common in certain parts of the world such as the Far East and Brazil [84] where they are associated with parasitic infestation. Gallstones form in chronically obstructed bile ducts due to such conditions as traumatic biliary stricture, primary sclerosing cholangitis, or Caroli's disease. They are usually of brown pigment type and are associated with stones in the common bile duct. Secondary hepatic infection results in multiple abscesses.

Intra-hepatic calculi are difficult to treat and recurrences are frequent. Lavage of the duct is often performed trans-hepatically or endoscopically after T-tube drainage. In some instances, choledocho-intestinal anastomosis or even hepatic lobectomy may be necessary [119].

Mirizzi syndrome

Impaction of a gallstone in the cystic duct or neck of the gallbladder can cause partial common hepatic duct obstruction [82]. Recurrent cholangitis follows and the stone may erode into the common hepatic duct creating a single cavity.

Diagnosis is by percutaneous or endoscopic cholangiography (fig. 31.11). Ultrasound shows gallstones lying outside the hepatic duct [99]. Surgery consists of removing the cystic duct,

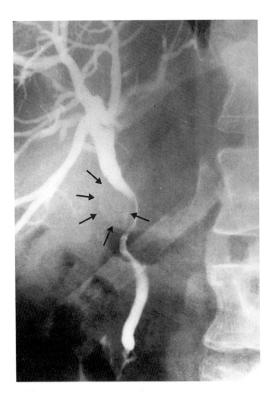

Fig. 31.11. Percutaneous cholangiography in Mirizzi syndrome shows a large gallstone impacted in the cystic duct (arrowed) which has caused partial obstruction to the common hepatic duct.

the diseased gallbladder and the impacted stone with drainage of the common bile duct via the cystic duct stump [99].

Biliary fistulae

EXTERNAL

These follow procedures such as cholecystotomy, trans-hepatic biliary drainage or T-tube choledochotomy. Very rarely they follow gallstones, carcinoma of the gallbladder or trauma.

Bile has a higher sodium and bicarbonate content than plasma. Patients with external biliary fistulae run a risk of severe hyponatraemic acidosis and rise in blood urea levels.

Distal biliary obstruction contributes to the failure of the fistula to heal and the placement of an endoscopic or percutaneous biliary stent is followed by healing and without the need for further difficult re-operations [121].

INTERNAL

These may follow cholecystoenterostomy. In 80% they are due to long-standing calculous cholecystitis. The inflamed gallbladder, containing stones, adheres and ruptures into a segment of the intestine, usually into the duodenum and less often the colon. The ejected gallstones may be passed or cause intestinal obstruction (*gallstone ileus*), usually in the terminal ileum.

Post-operative biliary strictures, especially after multiple efforts at repair, may be complicated by fistula formation, usually hepaticoduodenal or hepatico-gastric. The fistulae are short, narrow and liable to block.

Biliary fistulae may also follow rupture of a chronic duodenal ulcer into the gallbladder or common bile duct. Fistulae may also develop between the colon and biliary tract in ulcerative colitis or regional ileitis, especially if the patient is receiving corticosteroid therapy [26].

Rarely, in a patient with duct stones, a fistula can develop between the hepatic duct and portal vein with massive bilaemia, shock and death [6].

Clinical features

There is a long history of biliary disease. The fistula may be symptomless and, when the gallstones have discharged into the intestine successfully, the fistula closes. Such instances are often diagnosed only at the time of a later cholecystectomy.

About one-third give a history of jaundice or are jaundiced on admission [107]. Pain may be absent or as severe as biliary colic. The features of cholangitis may be present. In cholecystocolic fistula the common bile duct may be filled with calculi, putrefying matter and faeces, which cause the severe cholangitis. Bacteria deconjugate bile salts in the colon producing severe diarrhoea. Weight loss is profound.

Radiological features

These include gas in the biliary tract (fig. 29.7) and the presence of a gallstone in an unusual position. A barium meal, in the case of a cholecysto-duodenal, or a barium enema, in the case of a cholecysto-colic fistula, may fill the biliary tree. Small bowel distension may be noted.

ERCP may be diagnostic [59].

Treatment

Fistulae due to gallbladder disease must be treated surgically. Adherent viscera are separated and closed and cholecystectomy and drainage of the common bile duct performed. The operative mortality is high, being about 13% [107].

Gallstone ileus

A gallstone over 2.5 cm in diameter entering the intestine causes obstruction, usually of the ileum, less often of the duodeno-jejunal junction, duodenal bulb, pylorus or even colon. The impacted gallstone may excite an inflammatory reaction in the intestinal wall, or cause intussusception.

Gallstone ileus is very rare but is the cause of a quarter of all cases of non-strangulated intestinal obstruction in patients over 65 [66].

The patient is usually an elderly, afebrile female possibly with a preceding history suggestive of chronic cholecystitis. The onset is insidious, with nausea, occasional vomiting, colicky abdominal pain and a somewhat distended but flaccid abdomen. Finally, a complete intestinal obstruction leads to rapid physical deterioration.

A plain film of the abdomen (fig. 31.12) may reveal loops of distended bowel with fluid levels and possibly the obstructing stone. Gas may be seen in the biliary tract and gallbladder, indicating a biliary fistula.

CT scan may show a gallstone in the ileum or duodenum.

Leucocytosis is not usual unless there is associated cholangitis with pyrexia.

The prognosis is poor and proportional to age.

Treatment

After the patient's general condition has been restored by i.v. fluids and electrolytes, the intestinal obstruction should be relieved surgically. This may be done by manual propulsion of the stone or by enterotomy. Additional surgical procedures such as cholecystectomy and fistula repair should be avoided and later biliary surgery performed only in those with recurrent biliary disease [140]. Mortality is about 19%.

Gallstone pancreatitis

Small gallstones in the ampulla allow bile to regurgitate into the pancreas and produce acute haemorrhagic pancreatitis. The stones are usually small and pass into the faeces [1]. The inflammation then subsides.

Management is usually expectant and followed by cholecystectomy and duct clearance as an elective procedure. In those who continue to deteriorate, endoscopic sphincterotomy to remove the obstructing stone or ablate the stenotic sphincter is indicated [117].

Haemobilia [144]

Haemorrhage into the biliary tract may follow trauma, including surgical and needle liver biopsy, aneurysms of the hepatic artery or one of its branches, extra- or intra-hepatic tumours of the biliary tract, gallstone disease, inflammation of the liver, especially helminthic or pyogenic, rarely varicose veins related to portal hypertension and sometimes in association with primary liver cancer. Iatrogenic disease such as liver biopsy and percutaneous transhepatic cholangiography now accounts for 40.8% [144].

Clinical features are pain related to the passage of clots, jaundice and haematemesis and melaena. Minor degrees may be shown only by positive occult blood tests in faeces. Fever or a

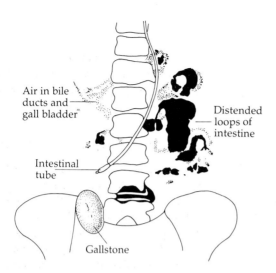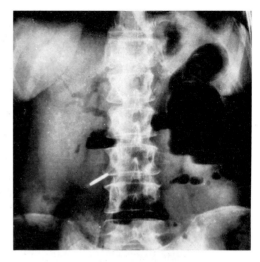

Fig. 31.12. Plain X-ray of the abdomen shows air in the biliary tree indicating a cholecyst-enteric fistula, a radio-opaque gallstone just medial and to the right of the 5th lumbar vertebra and distended loops of small intestine indicating ileus.

palpable mass each occur in about 40% of patients.

Diagnosis is suspected whenever upper gastrointestinal bleeding is associated with biliary colic, jaundice or a right upper quadrant mass or tenderness. Angiography is useful for confirmation and anatomic definition of haemobilia. ERCP or percutaneous cholangiography may show the clot in the ducts (fig. 31.13).

Treatment. Many clear spontaneously. Otherwise the treatment consists of angiographic embolization. Surgical exploration and drainage of the common bile duct may be indicated if bleeding and colic do not subside.

Biliary peritonitis

AETIOLOGY

Post-cholecystectomy. Bile may leak from small bile channels between the gallbladder and liver or through an imperfectly ligated cystic duct. If the biliary pressure is raised, perhaps by a residual common duct stone, leakage is facilitated and the subsequent paraductal bile accumulation favours the development of biliary stricture.

Rupture of the gallbladder. Empyema or gangrene of the gallbladder may lead to rupture and the formation of an abscess; this is localized by previous inflammatory adhesions.

Trauma. Crushing or gunshot wounds may involve the biliary tree. Needle biopsy of the liver or percutaneous cholangiography may rarely be complicated by puncture of the gallbladder or of a dilated intra-hepatic bile duct in a patient with deep cholestasis. Oozing of bile rarely follows operative liver biopsy.

Spontaneous. Biliary peritonitis may develop in patients with prolonged, deep obstructive jaundice without demonstrable breach of the biliary tree. This is presumably due to bursting of minute bile ducts. It may also develop in infancy [68].

CLINICAL PICTURE

This depends on whether the bile is localized or free in the peritoneal cavity, sterile or infected. Free rupture of bile into the peritoneal cavity causes severe shock. Due to the irritant effect of bile salts, large quantities of plasma are poured into the ascitic fluid. The onset is with excruciating, generalized, abdominal

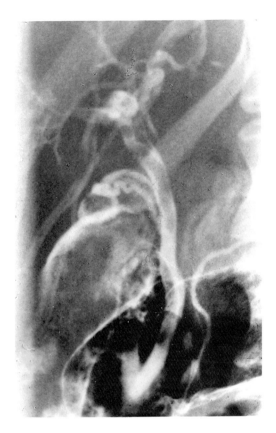

Fig. 31.13. ERCP in haemobilia shows filling defects, representing blood clot in the bile ducts.

pain. Examination shows a shocked, pale, motionless patient, with low blood pressure and persistent tachycardia. There is board-like rigidity of the diffusely tender abdomen. Paralytic ileus is a frequent complication. Biliary peritonitis should always be considered in any patient with unexplained intestinal obstruction. In a matter of hours secondary infection follows and the temperature rises while abdominal pain and tenderness persist. Anaerobic infection is common and increases the shock.

Laboratory findings are non-contributory. There may be haemoconcentration. Abdominal paracentesis reveals bile, usually infected. Serum bilirubin rises and this is followed by increase in alkaline phosphatase levels.

Prognosis is poor with a mortality of 60%.

TREATMENT

Fluid replacement is imperative. Paralytic ileus may demand intestinal intubation. Antibiotics are given to prevent secondary infection and the peritoneal cavity is drained.

Spontaneous rupture of the bile ducts

Common bile duct: perforation is exceedingly rare and leads to biliary peritonitis. The factors concerned are similar to those for perforated gallbladder. They include increases of intra-ductal pressure, calculous erosion and necrosis of the duct wall secondary to thrombosis [61]. Therapy includes surgical repair with cholecystectomy and decompression of the biliary system.

Intra-hepatic duct: perforations are usually secondary to common duct obstruction. Sometimes, a minute cholangitic liver abscess may perforate. The lesion is usually minute and in the left lobe or anterior surface of the right lobe over the gallbladder fossa. Diagnosis is difficult but may be made by percutaneous or operative cholangiography.

Association of gallstones with other diseases

COLORECTAL AND OTHER CANCERS

Population surveys show that gallstone sufferers do not seem at increased risk for other malignancies except perhaps that of the gallbladder and this risk is very small [76]. Faecal bile acids and cholesterol metabolites may promote colorectal oncogenesis [112]. Cholecystectomy may allow greater exposure of conjugated primary bile acids to anaerobic intestinal bacteria and so the increased production of carcinogens. Cholecystectomy and gallstones and colorectal cancer have been linked, although the association was not confirmed in recent studies [2, 40]. The association may be related to increased diagnostic efforts in symptomatic post-cholecystectomy patients, so detecting incidentally early colo-rectal cancers.

DIABETES MELLITUS

About 30% of all diabetics over 20 years old have gallstones, compared with 11.6% of the general population of the same age. The older diabetic tends to be obese, an important factor in gallstone formation. Chronic pancreatitis and gallstones are associated and chronic pancreatitis can produce mild diabetes.

Patients with diabetes may have large, poorly contracting and poorly filling gallbladders [63]. A 'diabetic neurogenic gallbladder' syndrome has been postulated [45].

Patients with diabetes mellitus undergoing cholecystectomy, whether emergency or elective have increased complications. These are probably related to associated diseases such as cardiovascular or renal and to more advanced age [94].

References

1 Acosta JM, Ledesma CL. Gallstone migration as a cause of acute pancreatitis. *N. Engl. J. Med.* 1974; **290**: 484.
2 Adami HO, Meirik O, Gustavsson S *et al.* Colorectal cancer after cholecystectomy: absence of risk increase within 11–14 years. *Gastroenterology* 1983; **85**: 859.
3 Admirand WH, Small DM. The physiochemical basis of cholesterol gallstone formation in man. *J. clin. Invest.* 1968; **47**: 1043.
4 Allen MJ, Borody TJ, Bugliosi TF *et al.* Rapid dissolution of gallstones by methyl tert-butyl ether. *N. Engl. J. Med.* 1985; **312**: 217.
5 Amaral JF, Thompson WR. Gallbladder disease in the morbidly obese. *Am. J. Surg.* 1985; **149**: 551.
6 Antebi E, Adar R, Zweig A *et al.* Bilemia: an unusual complication of bile duct stones. *Ann. Surg.* 1973; **177**: 274.
7 Barbara L, Sama C, Labate AMM *et al.* A population study on the prevalence of gallstone disease: the Sirmione study. *Hepatology* 1987; **7**: 913.
8 Bar-Meir S, Halpern Z, Bardan E *et al.* Frequency of papillary dysfunction among cholecystectomized patients. *Hepatology* 1984; **4**: 328.
9 Bateson MC, Bouchier IAD. Prevalence of gallstones in Dundee: an necropsy study. *Br. med. J.* 1975; **4**: 427.
10 Bateson MC, Bouchier IAD, Maudgal DP *et al.* Calcification of radiolucent gallstones during treatment with ursodeoxycholic acid. *Br. med. J.* 1981; **283**: 645.
11 Bateson MC. Gallstone epidemiology. *Curr. Gastroenterol.* 1986; **5**: 120.
12 Bennion LJ, Grundy SM. Risk factors for the development of cholelithiasis in man. *N. Engl. J. Med.* 1978; **299**: 1161.
13 Bennion LJ, Ginsberg RL, Garnick MB *et al.* Effects of oral contraceptives on the gall bladder bile of normal women. *N. Engl. J. Med.* 1976; **294**: 189.
14 Boey JH, Way LW. Acute cholangitis. *Ann. Surg.* 1980; **191**: 264.
15 Bolondi L, Gaian S, Testa S *et al.* Gall bladder sludge formation during prolonged fasting after gastrointestinal tract surgery. *Gut* 1985; **26**: 734.
16 Boston Collaborative Drug Surveillance Program. Oral contraceptives and venous thromboembolic disease: surgically confirmed gall-bladder disease and breast tumours. *Lancet* 1973; **i**: 1399.
17 Boston Collaborative Drug Surveillance Program. Gallbladder disease, venous disorders, breast tumours: relation to estrogens. *N. Engl. J. Med.* 1974; **290**: 15.
18 Bouchier IAD. Postmortem study of the frequency of gallstones in patients with cirrhosis of the liver. *Gut* 1969; **10**: 705.
19 Braverman DZ, Johnson ML, Kern F Jr. Effects of pregnancy and contraceptive steroids on gall bladder function. *N. Engl. J. Med.* 1980; **302**: 362.
20 Burnstein MJ, Ilson RG, Petrunka CN *et al.* Evidence for a potent nucleating factor in the bile of patients with cholesterol gallstones. *Gastroenterology* 1983; **85**: 801.
21 Carey MC, Small DM. The physical chemistry of cholesterol solubility in bile: relationship to gallstone formation and dissolution in man. *J. clin. Invest.* 1978; **61**: 998.
22 Cetta FM. Bile infection documented as initial event in the pathogenesis of brown pigment biliary stones. *Hepatology* 1986; **6**: 482.
23 Cimmuno CV. Cholesterolosis. *Radiology* 1960; **74**: 432.
24 Cobden I, Lendrum R, Venables CLO *et al.* Gallstones presenting as mental and physical debility in the elderly. *Lancet* 1984; **i**: 1062.
25 Cotton PB. The problem of pain after cholecystectomy in *Imaging in Hepatobiliary Disease* eds. JS Dooley, R Dick, M Viamonte Jr, S Sherlock. 1987; Blackwell Scientific Publications, Oxford, p. 126.
26 Craig O. Hepato-colic fistula. *Br. J. Radiol.* 1965; **38**: 801.
27 Crumplin MKH, Jenkinson LR, Kassab JY *et al.* Management of gallstones in a district general hospital. *Br. J. Surg.* 1985; **72**: 428.
28 De Lacey G, Gajjar B, Twomey B *et al.* Should

cholecystography or ultrasound be the primary investigation for gallbladder disease? *Lancet* 1984; **i**: 205.

29 Devine RM, Farnell MB, Mucha P Jr. Acute cholecystitis as a complication in surgical patients. *Arch. Surg.* 1984; **119**: 1389.

30 Diehl AK, Beral V. Cholecystectomy and changing mortality from gallbladder cancer. *Lancet* 1981; **i**: 187.

31 Di Padova C, Di Padova F, Montorsi W *et al.* Methyl tert-butyl ether fails to dissolve retained radiolucent common bile duct stones. *Gastroenterology* 1986; **91**: 1296.

32 Dooley JS, Hamilton-Miller JMT, Brumfitt W *et al.* Antibiotics in the treatment of biliary infection. *Gut* 1984; **25**: 988.

33 Dowling RH. The enterohepatic circulation. *Gastroenterology* 1972; **62**: 122.

34 Eggermont AM, Laméris JS, Jeekel J. Ultrasound-guided percutaneous transhepatic cholecystostomy for acute acalculous cholecystitis. *Arch. Surg.* 1985; **120**: 1354.

35 Erlinger S, Go AL, Husson J-M *et al.* Franco-Belgian Cooperative Study of ursodeoxycholic acid in the medical dissolution of gallstones: a double-blind, randomized, dose-response study, and comparison with chenodeoxycholic acid. *Hepatology* 1984; **4**: 308.

36 Flanchbaum L, Majerus TC, Cox EF. Acute post-traumatic acalculous cholecystitis. *Am. J. Surg.* 1985; **150**: 252.

37 Fox MS, Wilk PJ, Weissmann HS *et al.* Acute acalculous cholecystitis. *Surg. Gynecol. Obstet.* 1984; **159**: 13.

38 French EB, Robb WAT. Biliary and renal colic. *Br. med. J.* 1963; **ii**: 135.

39 Friedman GD, Kannel WB, Dawber TR. The epidemiology of gallbladder disease: observations in the Framingham study. *J. chron. Dis.* 1966; **19**: 273.

40 Friedman GD, Goldhaber MK, Queensbury CP Jr. Cholecystectomy and large bowel cancer. *Lancet* 1987; **1**: 906.

41 Fromm H. Gallstone dissolution therapy. Current status and future prospects. *Gastroenterology* 1986; **91**: 1560.

42 Gallinger S, Taylor RD, Harvey PRC *et al.* Effect of mucous glycoprotein on nucleation time of human bile. *Gastroenterology* 1985; **89**: 648.

43 Gallinger S, Harvey RG, Petrunka CN *et al.* Biliary proteins and the nucleation defect in cholesterol cholelithiasis. *Gastroenterology* 1987; **92**: 867.

44 Gilat T, Feldman C, Halpern Z *et al.* An increased familial frequency of gallstones. *Gastroenterology* 1983; **84**: 242.

45 Gitelson S, Schwartz A, Fraenkel M *et al.* Gallbladder dysfunction in diabetes mellitus. The diabetic neurogenic gallbladder. *Diabetes* 1963; **12**: 308.

46 Glenn F. Retained calculi within the biliary duct system. *Ann. Surg.* 1974; **179**: 528.

47 Glenn F, Becker CG. Acute acalculous cholecystitis. *Ann. Surg.* 1982; **195**: 131.

48 Goldstein F, Thornton JJ, Szydlowski T. Biliary tract dysfunction in giardiasis. *Am. J. dig. Dis.* 1978; **23**: 559.

49 Goodman ZD, Ishak KG. Xanthogranulomatous cholecystitis. *Am. J. surg. Path.* 1981; **5**: 653.

50 Griffen WO Jr, Bivins BA, Rogers EL *et al.* Cholecystokinin cholecystography in the diagnosis of gall bladder disease. *Ann. Surg.* 1980; **191**: 636.

51 Gunn AA, Foubister G. Biliary surgery: a five year follow-up. *Ann. R. Coll. Surg.* 1978; **23**: 292.

52 Halpern Z, Dudley MA, Kibe A *et al.* Rapid vesicle formation and aggregation in abnormal human biles. A time-lapse video-enhanced contrast microscopy study. *Gastroenterology* 1986; **90**: 875.

53 Hauer-Jensen M, Karesen R, Nygaard K *et al.* Predictive ability of choledocholithiasis indicators. A prospective evaluation. *Ann. Surg.* 1985; **202**: 64.

54 Herlin P, Ericsson M, Holmin T *et al.* Acute acalculous cholecystitis following trauma. *Br. J. Surg.* 1982; **69**: 475.

55 Holan KR, Holzbach RT, Hermann RE *et al.* Nucleation time: a key factor in the pathogenesis of cholesterol gallstone disease. *Gastroenterology* 1979; **77**: 611.

56 Holzbach RT, Marsh M, Olszewski M *et al.* Cholesterol solubility in bile: evidence that supersaturated bile is frequent in healthy man. *J. clin. Invest.* 1973; **52**: 1467.

57 Holzbach RT. Recent progress in understanding cholesterol crystal nucleation as a precursor to human gallstone formation. *Hepatology* 1986; **6**: 1403.

58 Hopkins SF, Bivins BA, Griffen WO Jr. The problem of the cystic duct remnant. *Surg. Gynecol. Obstet.* 1979; **148**: 531.

59 Hunt DR, Blumgart LH. Iatrogenic choledochoduodenal fistula: an unsuspected cause of postcholecystectomy symptoms. *Br. J. Surg.* 1980; **67**: 10.

60 Jacyna MR, Bouchier IAD. Cholesterolosis: a physical cause of 'functional' disorder. *Br. Med. J.* 1987; **295**: 619.

61 Kerstein MD, McSwain NE. Spontaneous rupture of the common bile duct. *Am. J. Gastroenterol.* 1985; **80**: 469.

62 Kibe A, Holzbach RT, LaRusso NF *et al.* Inhibition of cholesterol crystal formation by apolipoproteins in supersaturated model bile. *Science* 1984; **225**: 514.

63 Keshavarzian A, Dunne M, Iber FL. Gallbladder volume and emptying in insulin requiring male diabetics. *Dig. Dis. Sci.* 1987; **32**: 824.

64 Kirtley JA Jr, Holcomb GW Jr. Surgical management of diseases of the gallbladder and common bile duct in children and adolescents. *Am. J. Surg.* 1966; **111**: 39.

65 Klimberg S, Hawkins I, Vogel SB. Percutaneous cholecystostomy for acute cholecystitis in high-risk patients. *Am. J. Surg.* 1987; **153**: 125.

66 Kurtz RJ, Heimann TM, Kurtz AB. Gallstone ileus: a diagnostic problem. *Am. J. Surg.* 1983; **146**: 314.

67 Lee SS, Wasiljew BK, Lee M-J. Gallstones in women younger than thirty. *J. clin. Gastroenterol.* 1987; **9**: 65.

68 Lee SP, Nicholls JF. Nature and composition of biliary sludge. *Gastroenterology* 1986; **90**: 677.

69 Lees W, Mitchell JE. Bile peritonitis in infancy. *Arch. Dis. Child.* 1966; **41**: 188.

70 Lennard TWJ, Farndon JR, Taylor RMR. Acalculous biliary pain: diagnosis and selection for cholecystectomy using the cholecystokinin test for pain reproduction. *Br. J. Surg.* 1984; **71**: 868.

71 Lindberg EF, Grinnan GLB, Smith L. Acalculous cholecystitis in Viet Nam casualties. *Ann. Surg.* 1970; **171**: 152.

72 Li Volsi VA, Perzin KH, Porter M. Polyarteritis nodosa of the gall bladder presenting as acute cholecystitis. *Gastroenterology* 1973; **65**: 115.

73 Loria P, Carulli N, Medici G *et al.* Effect of ursocholic acid on bile lipid secretion and composition. *Gastroenterology* 1986; **90**: 865.

74 Malet PF, Takabayashi A, Trotman BW *et al.* Black and brown pigment gallstones differ in microstructure and microcomposition. *Hepatology* 1984; **4**: 227.

75 Malet PF, Williamson CE, Trotman BW *et al.* Composition of pigmented centers of cholesterol gallstones. *Hepatology* 1986; **6**: 477.

76 Maringhini A, Moreau J, Melton J III *et al.* Gallstones, gallbladder cancer, and other gastrointestinal malignancies. An epidemiologic study in Rochester, Minnesota. *Ann. intern. Med.* 1987; **107**: 30.

77 May RE, Strong R. Acute emphysematous cholecystitis. *Br. J. Surg.* 1971; **58**: 453.

78 McClure J, Banerjee SS, Schofield PS. Crohn's disease of the gall bladder. *J. clin. Pathol.* 1984; **37**: 516.

79 McGahan JP, Walter JP. Diagnostic percutaneous aspiration of the gallbladder. *Radiology* 1985; **155**: 619.

80 McSherry CK, Ferstenberg H, Calhoun WF *et al.* The natural history of diagnosed gallstone disease in symptomatic and asymptomatic patients. *Ann. Surg.* 1985; **202**: 59.

81 Meredith TJ, Williams GV, Maton PN *et al.* Retrospective comparison of 'cheno' and 'urso' in the medical treatment of gallstones. *Gut* 1982; **23**: 382.

82 Mirizzi PL. Sindrome del conducto hepatico. I. *Int. Chir.* 1948; **8**: 731.

83 Mok HYI, Druffel ERM, Rampone WH. Chronology of cholelithiasis. Dating gallstones from atmospheric radiocarbon produced by nuclear bomb explosions. *N. Engl. J. Med.* 1986; **314**: 1075.

84 Nagase M, Hikasa Y, Soloway RD *et al.* Gallstones in western Japan: factors affecting the prevalence of intrahepatic gallstones. *Gastroenterology* 1980; **78**: 684.

85 Nakayama F. Quantitative microanalysis of gallstones. *J. Lab. clin. Med.* 1968; **72**: 602.

86 Nelson PE, Moyer TP, Thistle JL. Dissolution of calcium bilirubinate (CaB) and calcium carbonate ($CaCO_3$) debris remaining after methyl tert-butyl ether (MTBE) dissolution of cholesterol gallstones (CGS). *Gastroenterology* 1986; **90**: 1751.

87 Neoptolemos JP, Hofmann AF, Moossa AR. Chemical treatment of stones in the biliary tree. *Br. J. Surg.* 1986; **73**: 515.

88 Nicholas P, Rinaudo PA, Conn HO. Increased incidence of cholelithiasis in Laennec's cirrhosis. A postmortem evaluation of pathogenesis. *Gastroenterology* 1972; **63**: 112.

89 Nobusawa S, Adachi T, Miyazaki A *et al.* A case report of biliary peritonitis—spontaneous perforation of an intrahepatic duct. *Am. J. Gastroenterol.* 1986; **81**: 568.

90 Orlando R, Gleason E, Drezner AD. Acute acalculous cholecystitis in the critically ill patient. *Am. J. Surg.* 1983; **145**: 472.

91 Palmer KR, Hofmann AF. Intraductal mono-octanoin for the direct dissolution of bile duct stones: experience in 343 patients. *Gut* 1986; **27**: 196.

92 Park Y-H, Igimi H, Carey MC. Dissolution of human cholesterol gallstones in simulated cheno-deoxycholate-rich and ursodeoxycholate-rich biles. *Gastroenterology* 1984; **87**: 150.

93 Pattinson NR, Chapman BA. Distribution of biliary cholesterol between mixed micelles and non-micelles in relation to fasting and feeding in humans. *Gastroenterology* 1986; **91**: 697.

94 Pellegrini CA. Asymptomatic gallstones. Does diabetes mellitus make a difference? *Gastroenterology* 1986; **91**: 245.

95 Persemlidis D, Panveliwalla D, Kimball A. Effects of clofibrate and of oral contraceptives on biliary lipid composition and bile acid kinetics in man. *Gastroenterology* 1973; **64**: 782.

96 Pessa ME, Hawkins IF, Vogel SB. The treatment of acute cholangitis. Percutaneous transhepatic biliary drainage before definitive therapy. *Ann.*

Surg. 1987; **205**: 389.

97 Pixley F, Wilson D, McPherson K *et al.* Effect of vegetarianism on development of gallstones in women. *Br. Med. J.* 1985; **291**: 11.

98 Ransohoff DF, Gracie WA, Wolfenson LB *et al.* Prophylactic cholecystectomy or expectant management for silent gallstones. *Ann. intern. Med.* 1983; **99**: 199.

99 Ravo B, Epstein H, La Mendola S *et al.* The Mirizzi syndrome: pre-operative diagnosis by sonography and transhepatic cholangiography. *Am. J. Gastroenterol.* 1986; **81**: 688.

100 Reuben A, Maton PN, Murphy GM *et al.* Bile lipid secretion in obese and non-obese individuals with and without gallstones. *Clin. Sci.* 1985; **69**: 71.

101 Riemann JF, Seuberth K, Demling L. Mechanical lithotripsy of common bile duct stones. *Gastrointest. Endoscopy* 1985; **31**: 207.

102 Roberts KM, Parsons MA. Xanthogranulomatous cholecystitis: clinico-pathological study of 13 cases. *J. clin. Pathol.* 1987; **40**: 412.

103 Roslyn JJ, Pitt HA, Mann LL *et al.* Gall bladder disease in patients on long-term parenteral nutrition. *Gastroenterology* 1983; **84**: 148.

104 Roslyn JJ, Thompson JE, Darvin H *et al.* Risk factors for gallbladder perforation. *Am. J. Gastroenterol.* 1987; **82**: 636.

105 Ross PE, Kouroumalis E, Clarke A *et al.* Cholesteryl esters in human gall bladder bile and mucosa. *Clin. Chim. Acta* 1984; **144**: 145.

106 Sackmann M, Delius M, Sauerbruch T *et al.* Extracorporeal shock-wave lithotripsy of gall bladder calculi. *J. Hepatol.* 1987; **5**: S58.

107 Safaie-Shirazi S, Zike WL, Printen KJ. Spontaneous enterobiliary fistulas. *Surg. Gynecol. Obstet.* 1973; **137**: 769.

108 Sauerbruch T, Delius M, Paumgartner G *et al.* Fragmentation of gallstones by extracorporeal shock-waves. *N. Engl. J. Med.* 1986; **314**: 818.

109 Schmidt FR, McCarthy JD. Variations in total serum bilirubin and alkaline phosphatase in the normal post-operative cholecystectomy course. *Am. J. Surg.* 1972; **124**: 794.

110 Schneiderman DJ, Cello JP, Laing FC. Papillary stenosis and sclerosing cholangitis in the acquired immunodeficiency syndrome. *Ann. intern. Med.* 1987; **106**: 546.

111 Schoenfield LJ, Grundy SM, Hofmann AF *et al.* The National Cooperative Gallstone Study viewed by its investigators. *Gastroenterology* 1983; **84**: 644.

112 Schottenfeld D, Winiwar SJ. Cholecystectomy and colorectal cancer. *Gastroenterology* 1983; **85**: 966.

113 Schwesinger WH, Kurtin WE, Levine BA *et al.* Cirrhosis and alcoholism as pathogenetic factors

114 Scragg RKR, McMichael AJ, Baghurst PA. Diet, alcohol and relative weight in gallstone disease: a case-control study. *Br. med. J.* 1984; **288**: 1113.

115 Shaffer E, Small DM. Biliary lipid secretion in cholesterol gallstone disease. *J. clin. Invest.* 1977; **59**: 828.

116 Shea WJ, Demas BE, Goldberg HI *et al.* Sclerosing cholangitis associated with hepatic arterial FUDR chemotherapy: radiographic-histologic correlation. *Am. J. Roentgenol.* 1986; **146**: 717.

117 Siegel JH, Tone P, Menikeim D. Gallstone pancreatitis: pathogenesis and clinical forms—the emerging role of endoscopic management. *Am. J. Gastroenterol.* 1986; **81**: 774.

118 Silverman MA, Greenberg RE, Bank S. Cholescystokinin receptor antagonists: a review. *Am. J. Gastroenterol.* 1987; **82**: 703.

119 Simi M, Loriga P, Basoli A *et al.* Intrahepatic lithiasis. Study of thirty-six cases and review of the literature. *Am. J. Surg.* 1979; **137**: 317.

120 Smith BF, LaMont JT. The central issue of cholesterol gallstones. *Hepatology* 1986; **6**: 529.

121 Smith AC, Schapiro RH, Kelsey PB *et al.* Successful treatment of non-healing biliary cutaneous fistulas with biliary stents. *Gastroenterology* 1986; **90**: 764.

122 Somjen GJ, Gilat T. Contribution of vesicular and micellar carriers to cholesterol transport in human bile. *J. Lipid Res.* 1985; **26**: 699.

123 Staritz M, Floth A, Rambow A *et al.* Shock-wave lithotripsy of gallstones with second-generation device without conventional water bath. *Lancet* 1987; **ii**: 155 (letter).

124 Staritz M, Rambow A, Floth A *et al.* Fragmentation of giant common bile duct stones by extracorporeal shock-wave lithotripsy (device of the second generation). *J. Hepatol.* 1987; **5**: S63.

125 Sutor DJ, Wooley SE. A statistical survey of the composition of gallstones in eight countries. *Gut* 1971; **12**: 55.

126 Suzuki Y, Kobayashi A, Ohto M *et al.* Bacteriological study of transhepatically aspirated bile. *Dig. Dis. Sci.* 1984; **29**: 109.

127 Tanaka M, Ikeda S, Matsumoto S *et al.* Manometric diagnosis of sphincter of Oddi spasm as a cause of postcholecystectomy pain and treatment by endoscopic sphincterotomy. *Ann. Surg.* 1985; **202**: 712.

128 Tanaka K, Shimada M, Hattori M *et al.* Sjorgen's syndrome with abnormal manifestations of the gall bladder and central nervous system. *J. pediatr. Gastroenterol. Nutr.* 1985; **4**: 148.

129 Taylor TV, Armstrong CP. Migration of gallstones. *Br. Med. J.* 1987; **294**: 1320.

130 Thatcher BS, Sivak MV Jr, Tedesco FJ *et al.* Endos-

copic sphincterotomy for suspected dysfunction of the sphincter of Oddi. *Gastrointest. Endosc.* 1987; **33**: 91.

131 Thistle JL, Cleary PA, Lachin JM *et al.* The natural history of untreated cholelithiasis during the National Cooperative Gallstone Study (NCGS). *Gastroenterology* 1982; **82**: 1197.

132 Thomas WEG, Thornton JR, Thompson MH. Staphylococcal acalculous cholecystitis. *Br. J. Surg.* 1981; **68**: 136.

133 Thornton J, Symes C. Heaton K. Moderate alcohol reduces bile cholesterol saturation and raises HDL cholesterol. *Lancet* 1983; **ii**: 819.

134 Tint GS, Salen G, Shefer S. Effect of ursodeoxycholic acid and chenodeoxycholic acid on cholesterol and bile acid metabolism. *Gastroenterology* 1986; **91**: 1007.

135 Tokyo Cooperative Gallstone Study Group. Efficacy and indications of ursodeoxycholic acid treatment for dissolving gallstones: a multicenter double-blind trial. *Gastroenterology* 1980; **78**: 542.

136 Toouli J, Roberts-Thomson IC, Dent J *et al.* Manometric disorders in patients with suspected sphincter of Oddi dysfunction. *Gastroenterology* 1985; **88**: 1243.

137 Trotman BW, Soloway RD. Pigment gallstone disease: summary of the National Institutes of Health International Workshop. *Hepatology* 1982; **2**: 879.

138 Ulloa N, Garrido J, Nervi F. Ultracentrifugal isolation of vesicular carriers of biliary cholesterol in native human and rat bile. *Hepatology* 1987; **7**: 235.

139 Upp JR Jr, Nealon WH, Singh P *et al.* Correlation of cholecystokinin receptors with gallbladder contractility in patients with gallstones. *Ann. Surg.* 1987; **205**: 641.

140 Van Hillo M, van der Vliet JA, Wiggers T *et al.* Gallstone obstruction of the intestine: an analysis of ten patients and a review of the literature. *Surgery* 1987; **101**: 273.

141 Vlahcevic ZR, Bell CC Jr, Buhac I *et al.* Diminished bile acid pool size in patients with gallstones. *Gastroenterology* 1970; **59**: 165.

142 Vlahcevic ZR, Bell CC Jr, Gregory DH *et al.* Relationship of bile acid pool size to the formation of lithogenic bile in female Indians of the southwest. *Gastroenterology* 1972; **62**: 73.

143 Way LW. The National Cooperative Gallstone Study and chenodiol. *Gastroenterology* 1983; **84**: 648.

144 Yoshida J, Donahue PE, Nyhus LM. Hemobilia: review of recent experience with a worldwide problem. *Am. J. Gastroenterol.* 1987; **82**: 448.

145 Zakko SF, Hofmann AF, Schteingart C *et al.* Percutaneous gall bladder stone dissolution using a microprocessor assisted solvent transfer (MAST) system. *Gastroenterology* 1987; **92**: 1794.

32 · Benign Stricture of the Bile Ducts

Benign strictures of the common bile duct in 97% of cases follow biliary tract surgery, usually cholecystectomy. Various factors contribute. Oedema or haemorrhage surrounding the inflamed gallbladder, especially if contracted, makes the bile ducts difficult to distinguish from adjacent structures, and this may be heightened by aberrant anatomical relations. The bile ducts may thus be ligated, sectioned or perforated by suture material. Prolonged T-tube drainage of the common bile duct, cholecystotomy, rough probing of the bile duct for calculi and attempts at operative cholangiography, especially with a normal sized duct, have resulted in stricture formation. A calculus in the common bile duct is an insufficient cause. Bile leakage after biliary operations may form peri-ductal abscesses with constriction of the adjoining duct.

The bile duct depends for its blood supply on the peri-biliary plexus coming from the hepatic artery [12]. Interference with this, especially in the lower and supraduodenal portion, can be followed by stricture formation. This can follow hepatic transplantation or resection of the pancreatic head. Where necessary, the bile duct should be divided proximally as near the ampulla as possible where the blood supply is better.

Excision of a choledochus cyst or a benign tumour of the bile ducts can be so difficult that stricture formation is inevitable.

A benign stricture can follow trauma, a perforated or penetrating duodenal ulcer, chronic sclerosing or relapsing pancreatitis [6], benign bile duct tumours and primary sclerosing cholangitis (Chapter 15).

Anomalies of the right hepatic duct or cystic duct increase the risk of major bile duct injury.

Benign strictures are also being recognized with no obvious cause.

PATHOLOGICAL CHANGES

The duct is usually partially injured, the occlusion develops slowly and a chronic obliterative cholangitis leads to a stricture about 2 cm long. The stricture is usually found in the common hepatic duct or right hepatic duct where the cystic duct has been adherent at the union of the cystic and common hepatic ducts (fig. 32.1) or less frequently in the supraduodenal portion of the duct.

The bile duct above the stricture is grossly dilated and thickened, and below, the duct is represented by a fibrous cord difficult to identify at operation. The bile duct dilatation extends into the liver and depends on the completeness of the obstruction.

The contained bile is viscid and usually infected, resembling biliary mud. Small calculi sometimes extend even into the intra-hepatic branches of the bile ducts.

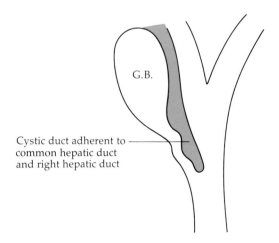

G.B.

Cystic duct adherent to common hepatic duct and right hepatic duct

Fig. 32.1. Biliary stricture may be produced by dissection of adherent cystic duct from the common hepatic and right hepatic ducts.

The liver shows cholestasis. Biliary cirrhosis develops with time. The spleen enlarges and shows chronic infection and portal hypertension.

CLINICAL FEATURES

The condition is more common in females, because they have more biliary surgery. Seventy per cent are less than 50 years old.

If the main bile ducts have been completely divided, jaundice of cholestatic type appears 3–7 days post-operatively. Alternatively, an external biliary fistula develops. Such a fistula, for even a few days, suggests that biliary stricture will follow. The fistula may drain intermittently, with episodes of jaundice when it is closed and subsidence of jaundice when it is draining. When the fistula finally closes, jaundice is continuous.

Post-operative biliary peritonitis with pain and fever is another early method of presentation.

More often the bile duct injury is partial. Insidious jaundice develops early after operation but it may be 3–4 months before jaundice of variable intensity is apparent. This is the period of slow, constrictive cholangitis with stones forming above the stricture (fig. 32.3).

Intermittent attacks of cholangitis with or without jaundice accompany all grades of biliary stricture. The cholangitis is marked by pyrexia, sometimes very high, with a rigor, sweating and epigastric pain followed by pruritus, darkening of the urine, and pallor of the faeces (*Charcot's intermittent biliary fever*). Milder episodes are also seen which can be anicteric.

Sub-hepatic abscess after biliary surgery is another indication of developing stricture formation.

Persistent dull pain may be experienced in the epigastrium.

With time, the patient becomes pigmented (fig. 32.2), with clubbing of the fingers. Skin xanthomas are a rare late development. The liver is firm, extending almost to the umbilicus.

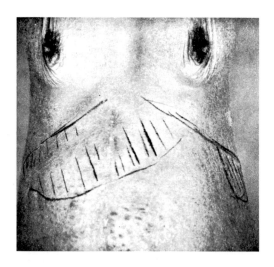

Fig. 32.2. Traumatic stricture of bile duct. Pigmented abdomen with scars of many surgical explorations. Hepatosplenomegaly.

The old gallbladder incision is tender. The spleen becomes palpable.

Liver failure is late and terminal. Gastro-intestinal bleeding due to portal hypertension is late. Peptic ulcers may bleed.

The patients become increasingly introspective as the months pass. They keep the most detailed notes of their symptoms and, perhaps understandably, become querulous and suspicious of their medical advisers.

Secondary sclerosing cholangitis follows contact of the bile duct mucosa with infected duodenal contents (*sump syndrome*) even if the obstruction has been relieved by a biliary-enteric anastomosis.

INVESTIGATIONS

Serum biochemistry is that of intermittent, chronic cholestasis. The serum bilirubin level is moderately increased. The alkaline phosphatase (γ-glutamyl transpeptidase) and bile acid levels may be raised even if the serum bilirubin value is normal.

Radiology. A plain film may show air in the biliary tree (fig. 29.6) and sometimes the actual site of stricture. ERCP is very useful in diagnosis but may fail if there has been a previous

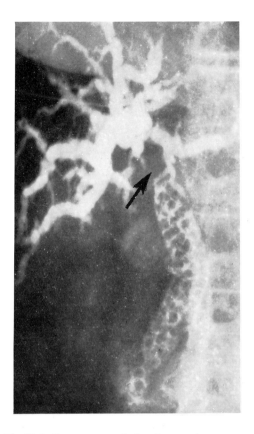

Fig. 32.3. Percutaneous cholangiogram shows dilated common bile duct, full of radio-translucent gallstones. The stricture in the common hepatic duct is marked by an arrow. The intra-hepatic bile ducts are dilated and irregular.

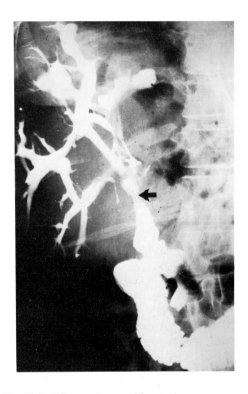

Fig. 32.4. Biliary stricture with patent choledochojejunostomy (arrow). Repeated attacks of cholangitis have led to secondary sclerosing cholangitis shown by irregular stenosis and dilatation of the intra-hepatic bile ducts.

attempt at repair by a choledochojejunostomy. Percutaneous cholangiography (fig. 32.3) may fail if the obstruction is partial and the intra-hepatic ducts are sclerotic or contain stones. Such patients are usually anicteric between the attacks of cholangitis. Secondary sclerosing cholangitis is shown in long-standing cases (fig. 32.4).

Cholangiographic demonstration of the anatomy of the biliary system is of inestimable value to the surgeon. If possible, barium meals should be avoided as the contrast material may regurgitate into the biliary tree and severe cholangitis can result.

Duodenal intubation reveals a heavy growth of *E. coli* and other enteric organisms. Similar organisms may be recovered from the blood and urine during a bout of cholangitis.

The heavy growth of organisms in the upper small intestine may lead to a 'blind loop' syndrome [11].

Haematological findings include a mild, normochromic, normocytic anaemia. A moderate leucocytosis accompanies the febrile episodes.

DIAGNOSIS

The distinction from residual or new bile duct calculi may be impossible; indeed, stricture, biliary sludge and stones may co-exist (fig. 32.3) Stones, usually brown pigment, related to cholangitis form in the duct above the stricture.

Distinction must be made from post-cholecystectomy functional symptoms. An elevated serum alkaline phosphatase level is a good index of continuing biliary obstruction.

Liver biopsy takes second place to visualizing the biliary tract radiologically. Histological changes range from mild cholangitis to a fully developed biliary cirrhosis.

PROGNOSIS

This has been revolutionized by the advent of invasive radiology with balloon dilatation of strictures and the introduction of percutaneously and endoscopically placed stents.

Chances of a successful surgical repair depend on the length of bile duct available for an anastomosis, the time since the injury and the skill and experience of the surgeon. Secondary sclerosing cholangitis is usually irreversible but secondary biliary cirrhosis should not be a contraindication to further reconstructive procedures.

Surgeons who are especially experienced and skilled in the operation will achieve the best results. Operative and post-operative mortality is 13%, usually due to liver failure or haemorrhage [14]. The transected or ischaemic duct wall readily forms scar tissue and results in failure to achieve satisfactory operative results [5]. Re-stenosis is therefore frequent. About 25% will need a second operation. Of those recurring, two-thirds do so within two years and 90% by five years [9]. If the patient remains symptom-free for four years post-operatively, there is a 90% chance of complete cure. This happy result lessens with the number of operations, but *can* follow many attempts at repair.

Since hepato-cellular failure is late, liver function will improve and the portal venous pressure will fall if biliary obstruction can be relieved. If the patient is continuously jaundiced or suffering repeated attacks of cholangitis, cirrhosis is inevitable and death in liver failure follows in 5—12 years [13].

However many previous attempts at relieving the biliary obstruction have been made, a further effort should always be made, if not surgically by an expert, then by dilatation or trans-hepatic or endoscopic stent placement.

TREATMENT (fig. 32.5)

Prevention

The majority of strictures would be prevented if cholecystectomy were less popular, performed only by experienced surgeons, and if the ducts were not dissected in the presence of acute cholecystitis. No structure must be clamped or divided until the anatomy has been defined. If any doubt exists, a cholecystotomy, whether percutaneous, trans-hepatic or surgical, and biliary drainage are indicated. Important technical points include good exposure, adequate relaxation and a dry operative field. The cystic artery must be ligated *before* the cystic duct is tied. Traction on the gallbladder should be avoided. If diagnosed at the time of surgery the duct should be repaired by end-to-end anastomosis [2]. If the length of duct is insufficient, a Roux-en-Y choledochojejunostomy may be performed [1].

The lateral aspect of the common or right hepatic duct is usually injured where the cystic duct has been dissected from it (fig. 32.1).

Medical

Antibiotics will largely be ineffective if there is cholangitis and biliary obstruction, and, with their continued usage, the causative organisms become resistant. They should, therefore, be reserved for the acute attack of cholangitis or pre-operatively. Supplementary vitamins should include vitamins A, D, E and K, if necessary, intramuscularly and ascorbic acid orally. Anaemia should be corrected. If the patient has a biliary fistula, particular attention must be paid to the electrolyte balance.

Balloon dilatation of biliary strictures

The balloon may be introduced percutaneously (trans-hepatically) or via the endoscope.

The *trans-hepatic* approach uses a 22-gauge

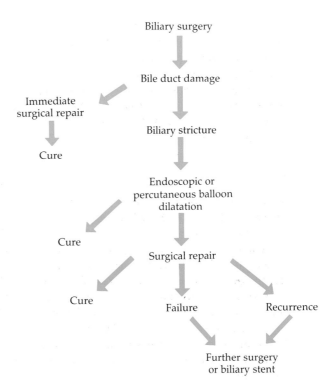

Fig. 32.5. The management of benign biliary stricture.

needle with guide and catheter. Contrast in the balloon or radioopaque bands incorporated in the catheter ensure correct placement. The 6- or 8-mm balloon is inflated for approximately 1½ to 2 minutes and the procedure may be repeated two to four times with 30-second pauses between inflations (fig. 32.7). Following the dilatation, a percutaneous catheter with numerous holes is placed through the stricture for combined internal and external drainage. It is removed as soon as possible. Dilatation may be repeated. It can be a preliminary to surgery or to stenting. Over successive weeks, progressively larger stents are inserted until a 16 to 20 French diameter stent is in position [4].

Endoscopic balloon dilatation usually requires a preliminary papillotomy and a side-viewing endoscope is used. Complications include bile duct perforation (fig. 32.7) [3].

Indications include post-operative biliary stricture, bilio-enteric anastomotic strictures, ampullary stenosis, sclerosing cholangitis, chronic pancreatisis and rarely, neoplasms of

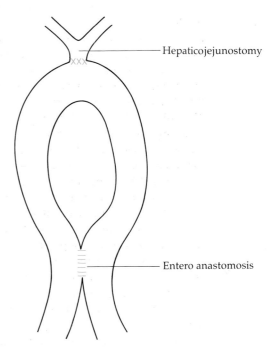

Fig. 32.6. Repair of high biliary stricture by hepaticojejunostomy and entero-anastomosis.

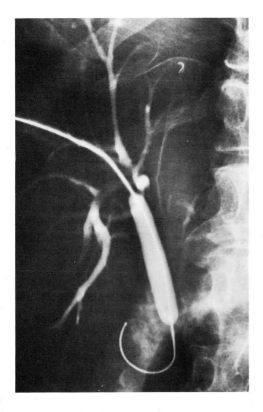

Fig. 32.7. A balloon, introduced trans-hepatically, has been inflated to dilate a benign biliary stricture.

the ampulla. Long dense fibrous strictures may not dilate or may re-stenose within a matter of days.

Biliary dilatation may be used to dilate high strictures before the insertion of a stent.

Operative

Operations should be undertaken under antibiotic cover as soon as possible after the original bile duct injury, before obliterative cholangitis, adhesion formation and secondary changes in the liver have added to the risk and technical difficulties [8]. The surgeon attempting the first repair carries a great responsibility because failure reduces the chance of subsequent cure. The best surgeon should therefore be the first to operate rather than each intervention being undertaken by one of greater skill and reputation than his predecessor.

The operation chosen will depend mainly on two factors—the site and length of the stricture and the amount of duct available for repair. Any operation must provide excision of the stricture with mucosal apposition between the duct lining and the intestinal mucosa. The anastomosis must be as large as possible and not under tension. An entero-anastomosis must be done if there is any risk of ascending infection from the bowel.

Even if sufficient duct is available proximally, excision of the stricture and end-to-end anastomosis of the duct is rarely performed. Differences between the calibre of the duct above and below the stricture are too great for a satisfactory anastomosis.

The usual operation is anastomosing the proximal bile duct to the intestine. An entero-anastomosis is added to minimize reflux from the intestines which would lead to cholangitis. The usual operation is therefore between proximal duct into a Roux-en-Y segment of jejunum, (*choledochojejunostomy*). In the case of high stricture, the hepatic duct is used (*hepatico-jejunostomy*) (fig. 32.6). The duration of splinting the anastomosis is controversial; some recommend at least six months and preferably twelve [10, 14]. Others put a limit of six weeks to three months. In the case of high strictures, changeable trans-hepatic silastic stents may be used and changed as required [10].

Silastic stents can be introduced through a stricture by open operation, through the liver or via the endoscope from below (see Chapter 29). These stents tend to occlude from biliary sediment and stones. It is possible to change the stent without further surgery, either trans-hepatically or via the endoscope.

Long-term access to the stricture may be gained by the subcutaneous fixation of the afferent loop of the Roux-en-Y loop used for biliary-enteric anastomosis. Percutaneous puncture allows simple cholangiography and if necessary, further stricture dilatation [7].

Portal hypertension may be controlled by repairing the stricture, otherwise a porta–caval shunt must be performed later. This may be exceedingly difficult due to the adhesions from previous repairs and a spleno-renal or mesenterico-caval anastomosis may be the only one possible.

The outcome following surgical correction of bile duct stricture depends on the degree of cholangitis, pericholedochitis and scarring and the quality of the duct to be anastomosed. It also depends on the number of previous corrective procedures and the time interval between the injury and the surgical repair. The higher the anatomic location of the stricture the less the chance of a successful result. The presence of hepato-cellular failure is ominous. Finally, the outcome depends on the experience and judgement of the surgeon, endoscopist and radiologist in selecting and performing the most suitable corrective procedure.

References

1 Besson A. The Roux-Y loop in modern digestive tract surgery. *Am. J. Surg.* 1985; **149:** 656.
2 Browder IW, Dowling JB, Koontz KK *et al.* Early management of operative injuries of the extra hepatic biliary tract. *Ann. Surg.* 1987; **205:** 649.
3 Foutch PG, Sivak MV Jr. Therapeutic endoscopic balloon dilatation of the extrahepatic biliary ducts. *Am. J. Gastroenterol.* 1985; **80:** 575.
4 Gallacher DJ, Kadir S, Kaufman SL *et al.* Non-operative management of benign postoperative biliary strictures. *Radiology* 1985; **156:** 625.
5 Glenn F. Iatrogenic injuries to the biliary system. *Surg. Gynecol. Obstet.* 1978; **146:** 430.
6 Lygidakis NJ. Biliary stricture as a complication of chronic relapsing pancreatitis. *Am. J. Surg.* 1983; **145:** 804.
7 Hutson DG, Russell E, Schiff E *et al.* Balloon dilatation of biliary strictures through a choledochojejuno-cutaneous fistula. *Ann. Surg.* 1984; **199:** 637.
8 Mathison O, Bergan A, Flatmark A. Iatrogenic bile duct injuries. *World J. Surg.* 1987; **11:** 392.
9 Pellegrini CA, Thomas MJ, Way LW. Recurrent biliary stricture. Patterns of recurrence and outcome of surgical therapy. *Am. J. Surg.* 1984; **147:** 175.
10 Pitt HA, Miyamoto T, Parapatis SK *et al.* Factors influencing outcome in patients with postoperative biliary strictures. *Am. J. Surg.* 1982; **144:** 14.
11 Scott AJ, Khan GA. Origin of bacteria in bileduct bile. *Lancet* 1967; **ii:** 790.
12 Terblanche J, Allison HF, Northover JMA. An ischemic basis for biliary strictures. *Surgery* 1983; **94:** 52.
13 Turner MD, Sherlock S. The prognosis of biliary stricture. *Gut* 1962; **3:** 94.
14 Warren KW, Jefferson MF. Prevention and repair of strictures of the extra-hepatic bile ducts. *Surg. Clin. N. Am.* 1973; **53:** 1169.

33 · Diseases of the Ampulla of Vater and Pancreas

Carcinoma in the region of the ampulla of Vater

The region of the head of the pancreas is a common site for carcinoma. The tumour may arise in the head of the pancreas (acinar), the ampullary region (papillary, originating in the lower end of bile duct or main hepatic bile duct) or rarely from the duodenum. Tumours arising from any of these sites have the same overall effect (fig. 33.1), and will be considered as a group. They are often termed 'cancer of the head of the pancreas'. However, the prognosis is very different. 87% of patients with carcinoma of the ampulla and 47% of those with malignancy of the duodenum have a potentially operable tumour compared with only 22% of those arising in the head of the pancreas [17].

Aetiological factors include cigarette smoking and previous partial gastrectomy [14]. There is no consistent relationship to coffee drinking or alcohol intake.

PATHOLOGY

The tumour rarely exceeds 3.5 cm in diameter. It may be difficult to recognize macroscopically. The site of origin is often obscure. Tumours arising from the ampulla tend to be polypoid and soft, whereas the acinar tumours are infiltrative, large and firm.

Histologically, the tumour is an adenocarcinoma, whether arising from pancreatic duct, acini or bile duct. The ampullary tumours have a papillary arrangement and are often of low-grade malignancy; fibrosis is prominent.

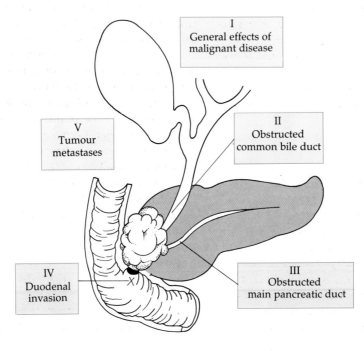

Fig. 33.1. The effects of carcinoma in the ampullary region. **I** General effects of malignant disease—weakness and weight loss. **II** Obstructed common bile duct. Dilated gallbladder and bile ducts—jaundice, hepatomegaly, pruritus. **III** Obstructed main pancreatic duct—fibrous atrophy of pancreas, steatorrhoea and occasional glycosuria. **IV** Duodenal invasion. Barium meal changes—occasional duodenal obstruction, positive stool occult blood, occasional melaena. **V** Tumour metastases. Nerves—back and epigastric pain; regional glands, liver, lungs, peritoneum.

The cell of origin is probably ductal [6].

Obstruction of common bile duct

This results from direct invasion causing a scirrhous reaction, from annular stenosis, and from tumour tissue filling the lumen. The duct may also be compressed by the tumour mass.

Functional obstruction due to involvement of nerves in the wall of the bile duct [9] may explain the occasional spontaneous relief of the jaundice. Sloughing of the surface of the tumour allows bile to reach the duodenum.

The bile ducts dilate and the gallbladder enlarges. An ascending cholangitis in the obstructed ducts is rare. The liver and other tissues show the changes of cholestasis.

Pancreatic changes

The main pancreatic duct may be obstructed as it enters the ampulla. The ducts and acini distal to the obstruction dilate and later rupture, causing focal areas of pancreatitis and fat necrosis. Later all the acinar tissue is replaced by fibrous tissue. Occasionally, particularly in the acinar type, fat necrosis and suppuration may occur in and around the pancreas.

Widespread venous thromboses (thrombophlebitis migrans) are reported in 27.6% of tumours of the head of the pancreas and 50% of the body and tail.

Glycosuria is related to interference with release of insulin from the pancreas. Diabetes mellitus is found in 40%.

Spread of the tumour

Direct extension in the wall of the bile duct and infiltration through the head of the pancreas is common with the acinar although not with the ampullary type. The second part of the duodenum may be invaded, with ulceration of the mucosa and secondary haemorrhage. The splenic and portal veins may be invaded and may thrombose with resultant splenomegaly. Peritoneal involvement is uncommon.

Involvement of regional nodes is found in approximately a third of operated cases. Perineural lymphatic spread is found in 84% of 83 cases of cancer of the pancreas [9]. Bloodborne metastases, with secondaries in liver and lungs, follow invasion of the splenic or portal veins.

CLINICAL FEATURES [12]

Both sexes are affected, but males more frequently than females in a ratio of 2:1. The sufferer is usually between 50 and 69 years old.

The clinical picture is a composite one of cholestasis, pancreatic and biliary insufficiency, and the general and local effects of a malignant tumour (fig. 33.1).

Jaundice is of gradual onset and progressively deepening but ampullary neoplasms can cause mild and intermittent jaundice. Cholangitis is unusual although occasionally fever does follow cholangitis above the obstruction.

Cancer of the head of the pancreas is not painless. Pain is experienced in the back, the epigastrium and right upper quadrant, usually as a continuous distress worse at night and sometimes ameliorated by crouching. It may be aggravated by eating.

Weakness and weight loss are progressive and have usually continued for at least three months before jaundice develops.

Although frank steatorrhoea is rare, the patient often complains of a change in the bowel habit, usually diarrhoea.

Vomiting and intestinal obstruction may follow invasion of the second part of the duodenum. More often ulceration of the duodenum can erode a vessel with haematemesis or, more commonly, occult bleeding. Ampullary lesions tend to present with jaundice, often intermittent. Tumours outside the ampullary area present early with vomiting of pyloric type but without jaundice.

Difficulty in making a diagnosis may make the patient depressed. It then becomes easy to believe, mistakenly, that the patient is psychoneurotic.

Examination. The patient is jaundiced and shows evidence of recent weight loss. Theoreti-

695

cally, the gallbladder should be enlarged and palpable (*Courvoisier's law*). In practice, the gallbladder is only felt in about half the patients, although at subsequent laparotomy a dilated gallbladder is found in three-quarters. The liver is enlarged with a sharp, smooth, firm edge. Hepatic metastases are rarely detected. The pancreatic tumour is impalpable.

The spleen is palpable if involvement of the splenic vein has caused thrombosis. Peritoneal invasion is followed by ascites.

General lymphatic metastases are more usual with cancer of the body rather than head of the pancreas. Occasionally, however, axillary, cervical and inguinal glands may be enlarged and Virchow's gland in the left supra-clavicular fossa may be palpable.

Occasionally, widespread venous thromboses simulate thrombophlebitis migrans.

Very rarely, small tender nodules of fat necrosis occur in the subcutaneous tissues, especially in the back of the neck. Release of pancreatic enzymes into the joints may simulate rheumatoid arthritis.

INVESTIGATIONS

Glycosuria occurs in 15–20% and with it there is an impaired oral glucose tolerance test.

Blood biochemistry. The serum alkaline phosphatase level is greatly raised. The serum amylase and lipase concentrations are sometimes persistently elevated in carcinoma of the ampullary region. Hypoproteinaemia with, later, peripheral oedema may be found.

There are no reliable serum tumour markers.

Radiology

A barium meal may show alterations in duodenal motility with deep indentations. The duodenal mucosa may show constant irregularity due to infiltration by growth (fig. 33.2). A dilated common bile duct may produce a duodenal impression in the immediate post-bulbar region or in the bulb itself.

Stenosis of the duodenum may be total or partial and the proximal loop may be dilated (fig. 33.2).

The medial aspect of the second part of the duodenum may be deformed so that it looks like a reversed number three.

Enlargement and widening of the duodenal loop suggests a large tumour which is more commonly acinar than ampullary. With large tumours, the stomach is displaced forwards and to the left, and the transverse colon downwards.

Ultrasound and CT scanning. May be used to demonstrate a mass in the head of the pancreas. CT may be preferable as ultrasound may be ruined by intestinal gases, the image, particularly of the pancreas, is better and it is more easily interpreted by clinicians (Chapter 29).

Percutaneous guided fine *needle aspiration* of the pancreas is safe and has a sensitivity of about 75%. There is a risk of track dissemination [18].

ERCP is helpful in demonstrating the pancreatic and bile ducts and allowing biopsy of any ampullary lesion [10]. ERCP is also useful in determining the anatomical origin of the tumour [17]. *Vascular radiology* is essential to establish patency of splenic, portal and superior mesenteric veins [2]. Splenic vein encasement is a contraindication to extensive pancreatic surgery.

Duodenoscopy may be used to visualize the growth and allow a biopsy.

A chest radiograph may reveal metastases.

Haematology. Anaemia is mild or absent. The leucocyte count may be normal or raised, with a relative increase in polymorphonuclear leucocytes. The erythrocyte sedimentation rate is usually raised.

DIFFERENTIAL DIAGNOSIS

The diagnosis must be considered in any patient over 40 years with progressive or even intermittent cholestasis. The suspicion would be strengthened by persistent or unexplained abdominal pain, weakness and weight loss, diarrhoea, glycosuria, positive faecal occult

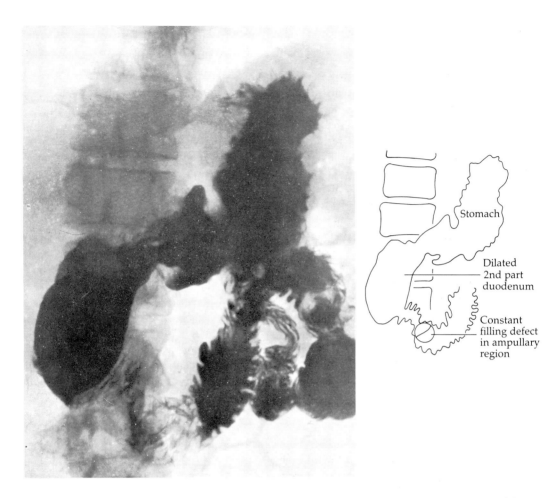

Fig. 33.2. Barium meal shows dilated duodenum and constant mucosal irregularity in the second part of the duodenum.

blood, hepatomegaly, a palpable spleen or thrombophlebitis migrans.

The distinction from jaundice due to other causes is presented in table 12.2.

PROGNOSIS

The prognosis of ampullary carcinoma is grave. The acinar type carries a worse prognosis than the ductal type, for the tumour is less operable and regional lymph glands are involved earlier. The ampullary type is smaller, it obstructs the common bile duct sooner and diagnosis is earlier. Carcinoma of the duodenum has the best prognosis.

Staging of ampullary carcinomas shows 85% five-year survival if the tumour has not spread beyond the muscle of the sphincter of Oddi and only 11−25% if extension is greater [29].

If the early post-operative deaths are excluded, results of palliative or radical surgery show an average life expectancy for carcinoma of the head of the pancreas of 6.2 months, for carcinoma of the ampulla of Vater of 18.5 months, for carcinoma of the common bile duct of 12.7 months and for carcinoma of the duodenum of 35 months. The mean survival for resectable pancreatic ductule adeno-carcinoma is 20.4 months, and for those un-resectable, 6.7 months [27]. Earlier diagnosis is imperative.

Duration of symptoms unfortunately gives little indication of the extent of disease.

Peri-operative mortality and major post-operative complications are falling [11]. Nevertheless, the outlook is grim. Only 23 of 912 patients survived three years and only two of these could be considered cures [7].

Total pancreatectomy does not lead to longer survival than for the more limited Whipple procedure [8].

TREATMENT

The treatment of tumours of the ampullary region is usually surgical: either an attempted removal or palliative anastomosis between the gallbladder and gastrointestinal tract. Difficulties in removal arise because of the inaccessibility of the pancreas on the posterior wall of the abdomen in the vicinity of vital structures. The operability rate is therefore very low.

The usual procedure is *pancreatico-duodenectomy* (Whipple's operation) which is performed in one stage with removal of related regional lymph nodes, the entire duodenum and the distal third of stomach [28]. The continuity of the biliary passages is restored by anastomosis of the common bile duct with the jejunum. The continuity of the intestinal tract is restored by gastrojejunostomy [12].

Frozen section examination of the resection margins is mandatory. The survival is 20.3 months if all the tumour is removed [27], 12.9 months where resection margin shows tumour, and 6.2 months for a palliative bypass. A palliative operation if the tumour is left behind is no better than a bypass.

The mortality of pancreatico-duodenectomy for ampullary carcinoma is 3.4−10% [27]. Removal is most likely to be possible if the tumour is a small, papillary one situated at the ampulla.

Palliative procedures

Choledochojejunostomy plus gastroenterostomy offer the best palliation of jaundice and vomiting.

Trans-hepatic or endoscopic insertion of a stent through the tumour (fig. 33.3) into the duodenum avoids operation [21] and is particularly applicable to old, poor-risk patients, especially when a large, clearly inoperable pancreatic mass has been imaged (Chapter 29) or where extensive metastatic disease is present [13]. 70% of patients with carcinoma of the head of the pancreas are unfit for bypass surgery. Endoscopic placement is preferable because of the complications (liver puncture, haemorrhage, bile leaks) accompaning the percutaneous technique [22] . If an endoscopic insertion fails, a guide wire can be introduced percutaneously and be manipulated through the growth and retrieved with the endoscope [19]. The stent is then fed through the endoscope over the guide wire and across the biliary stricture. Unfortunately stents may block due to the development of adherent bacterial bio-film with deposition of crystals [22]. They can be replaced. As a last resort, external biliary drainage should be performed. No patient with carcinoma of the pancreas should die jaundiced and with intolerable itching. None of these palliative procedures prolongs life.

The complications and 30-day mortality are similar for permanent biliary endoprosthesis or bypass surgery [4]. Survival time for the prosthesis is 19 weeks and for a surgical bypass 15 weeks.

Pruritus is relieved with cholestynamine or, if biliary obstruction is complete, by stanozolol (see Chapter 13).

Benign villous adenoma of the ampulla of Vater [24]

This leads to biliary colic and obstructive jaundice. It is usually confused with ampullary carcinoma and is diagnosed by frozen sections at surgery. It is treated by submucosal excision.

Chronic pancreatitis

Pancreatitis, usually of alcoholic aetiology, can cause narrowing of the intra-pancreatic portion of the common bile duct [3, 20]. The resultant

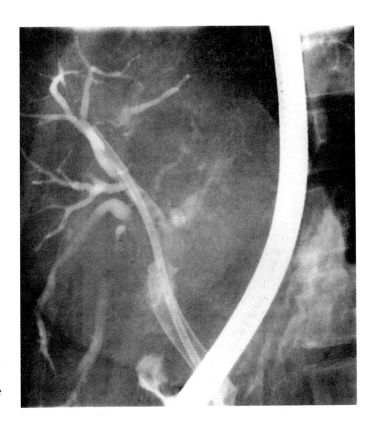

Fig. 33.3. Endoscopic steel stent insertion through a malignant bile duct carcinoma.

cholestasis may be transient during exacerbations of acute pancreatitis. It is presumably related to oedema and swelling of the pancreas. More persistent cholestasis follows encasement of the intra-and peri-pancreatic bile ducts in a progressively fibrotic pancreatitis. Cysts of the head of the pancreas and abscesses can also cause biliary obstruction and persistent cholestasis.

Bile duct stenosis affects about 8% of patients with chronic alcoholic pancreatitis and this figure would be higher if more cholangiograms were done. It should be suspected if the serum alkaline phosphatase is more than twice elevated for longer than one month. ERCP shows a smooth narrowing of the lower end of the common bile duct, sometimes adopting a 'bent knee' configuration (fig. 33.4). The main pancreatic duct may be tortuous, irregular and dilated. Calcification may be present in the pancreas.

Liver biopsy shows portal fibrosis [15], features of biliary obstruction, and sometimes biliary cirrhosis. The features of alcoholic liver disease are unusual.

Splenic vein thrombosis is a complication of chronic pancreatitis [16].

MANAGEMENT

Early diagnosis is essential as biliary cirrhosis and acute cholangitis can develop in the absence of clinical jaundice [25].

The patient must abstain completely from alcohol.

The place of surgery is controversial. In general, patients do well without biliary drainage if a simple stricture is shown [25]. Acute cholangitis, biliary cirrhosis and protracted jaundice are absolute indications for surgery [26]. Choledochoenterostomy is the usual procedure [5, 25].

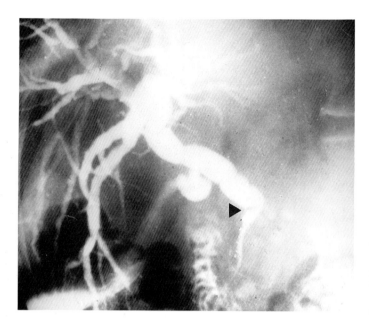

Fig. 33.4. Endoscopic retrograde pancreato-cholangiography in a patient with calcific alcoholic chronic pancreatitis. Note the 'bent knee' narrowing of the distal common bile duct (arrow).

OBSTRUCTION OF THE COMMON BILE DUCT BY ENLARGED LYMPH GLANDS IN THE PORTAL FISSURE

The association is extremely rare, the enlarged glands are nearly always metastatic, frequently from a primary in the alimentary tract, lung or breast, or from a hepato-cellular carcinoma. Where malignant glands in the porta hepatis are associated with deep jaundice the main bile ducts are usually being invaded rather than compressed. Alternatively the secondary deposits in the hepatic parenchyma may invade the bile ducts, causing obstruction.

Portal fissure glands may be enlarged in non-malignant conditions, but the bile ducts usually escape compression. Jaundice in infections such as tuberculosis, sarcoidosis or infectious mononucleosis is not obstructive but due to direct hepatic involvement and to haemolysis.

Glandular enlargement in the reticuloses does, very rarely, cause obstruction to the common bile duct, but jaundice complicating these diseases is more often due to hepatic parenchymal involvement, to increased haemolysis or is of obscure cholestatic type.

OTHER CAUSES OF EXTRINSIC PRESSURE ON THE COMMON BILE DUCT

Duodenal peptic ulceration

This is an extremely rare cause of obstructive jaundice. Perforation, so that the ulcer impinges against the bile duct or causes adhesive peritonitis, may rarely cause biliary obstruction and this can also follow interstitial contraction as the ulcer heals.

Duodenal diverticulum

Diverticula of the duodenum are often found near the ampulla of Vater, but rarely cause obstruction to the bile ducts. When they do so, obstruction is partial and jaundice intermittent.

References

1 Afroudakis A, Kaplowitz N. Liver histopathology in chronic common bile duct stenosis due to chronic alcoholic pancreatitis. *Hepatology* 1981; **1**: 65.

2 Allison DJ. State of the art: assessment of the

operability of malignant lesions of the biliary tree. In *Imaging in Hepatobiliary Disease* Eds J.S. Dooley, R. Dick, M. Viamonte Jr & S. Sherlock. Blackwell Scientific Publications, Oxford, 1987; p. 15.

3 Aranha GV, Prinz RA, Freeark RJ *et al.* The spectrum of biliary tract obstruction from chronic pancreatitis. *Arch. Surg.* 1984; **119**: 595.

4 Bornman PC, Harries-Jones EP, Tobias R *et al.* Prospective controlled trial of transhepatic biliary endoprosthesis versus bypass surgery for incurable carcinoma of head of pancreas. *Lancet* 1986; **i**: 61.

5 Carter DC. Pancreatitis and the biliary tree: the continuing problem. *Am. J. Surg.* 1988; **155**: 10.

6 Chen J, Baithun SI, Ramsay MA. Histogenesis of pancreatic carcinomas: a study based on 248 cases. *J. Pathol.* 1985; **146**: 65.

7 Connolly MM, Dawson PJ, Michelassi F *et al.* Survival in 1001 patients with carcinoma of the pancreas. *Ann. Surg.* 1987; **206**: 366.

8 Coutsoftides T, Macdonald J, Shibata HR. Carcinoma of the pancreas and periampullary region: a 41 year experience. *Ann. Surg.* 1977; **186**: 730.

9 Drapiewski JF. Carcinoma of the pancreas: a study of neoplastic invasion of nerves and its possible clinical significance. *Am. J. clin. Pathol.* 1944; **14**: 549.

10 Freeny PC, Marks WM, Ball TJ. Impact of high-resolution computed tomography of the pancreas on utilization of endoscopic retrograde cholangiopancreatography and angiography. *Radiology* 1982; **142**: 35.

11 Grace PA, Pitt HA, Tompkins RK *et al.* Decreased morbidity and mortality after pancreatoduodenectomy. *Am. J. Surg.* 1986; **151**: 141.

12 Hermann RE, Cooperman AM. Current concepts in cancer. Carcinoma of the pancreas. *N. Engl. J. Med.* 1979; **301**: 482.

13 Huibregtse K, Katon RM, Coene PP *et al.* Endoscopic palliative treatment in pancreatic cancer. *Gastrointest. Endosc.* 1986; **32**: 334.

14 Mack TM, Yu MC, Hanisch R *et al.* Pancreas cancer and smoking, beverage consumption, and past medical history. *J. Nat. Cancer Inst.* 1986; **76**: 49.

15 Morgan MY, Sherlock S, Scheuer PJ. Portal fibrosis in the livers of alcoholic patients. *Gut* 1978; **19**: 1015.

16 Nishiyama T, Iwao N, Myose H *et al.* Splenic vein thrombosis as a consequence of chronic pancreatitis: a study of three cases. *Am. J. Gastroenterol.* 1986; **81**: 1193.

17 Nix GAJJ, Van Overbeeke IC, Wilson JHP *et al.* ERCP diagnosis of tumors in the region of the head of the pancreas. Analysis of criteria and computer-aided diagnosis. *Dig. Dis. Sci.* 1988; **33**: 577.

18 Rashleigh-Belcher HJC, Russell RCG, Lees WR. Cutaneous seeding of pancreatic carcinoma by fine-needle aspiration biopsy. *Br. J. Radiol.* 1986; **59**: 182.

19 Robertson DAF, Ayres R, Hacking CN *et al.* Experience with a combined percutaneous and endoscopic approach to stent insertion in malignant obstructive jaundice. *Lancet* 1987; **ii**: 1449.

20 Scott J, Summerfield JA, Elias E *et al.* Chronic pancreatitis: a cause of cholestasis. *Gut* 1977; **18**: 196.

21 Siegel JH, Snady H. The significance of endoscopically placed prostheses in the management of biliary obstruction due to carcinoma of the pancreas: results of nonoperative decompression in 277 patients. *Am. J. Gastroenterol.* 1986; **81**: 634.

22 Speer AG, Cotton PB, Rode J *et al.* Biliary stent blockage with bacterial biofilm. A light and electron microscopy study. *Ann. intern. Med.* 1988; **108**: 546.

23 Speer AG, Cotton PB, Russell RCG *et al.* Randomized trial of endoscopic versus percutaneous stent insertion in malignant obstructive jaundice. *Lancet* 1987; **ii**: 57.

24 Sobol S, Cooperman AM. Villous adenoma of the ampulla of Vater; an unusual case of biliary colic and obstructive jaundice. *Gastroenterology* 1978; **75**: 107.

25 Stabile BE, Calabria R, Wilson SE *et al.* Stricture of the common bile duct from chronic pancreatitis. *Surg. Gynec. Obstet.* 1987; **165**: 121.

26 Stahl TJ, Allen MO'C, Ansel HJ *et al.* Partial biliary obstruction caused by chronic pancreatitis: an appraisal of indications for surgical biliary drainage. *Ann. Surg.* 1988; **207**: 26.

27 Warren KW, Christophi C, Armendariz R *et al.* Current trends in the diagnosis and treatment of carcinoma of the pancreas. *Am. J. Surg.* 1983; **145**: 813.

28 Whipple AO. Present-day surgery of the pancreas (Biglow Lecture). *N. Engl. J. Med.* 1942; **226**: 515.

29 Yamaguchi K, Enjoji M. Carcinoma of the ampulla of Vater. A clinico-pathologic study and pathologic staging of 109 cases of carcinoma and 5 cases of adenoma. *Cancer* 1987; **59**: 506.

34 · Tumours of the Gallbladder and Bile Ducts

Benign tumours of the gallbladder

PAPILLOMA

Multiple, small, papillomatous tumours, consisting of hypertrophied villi laden with cholesterol esters, may be found in as many as 80% of surgically removed gallbladders. They are often associated with cholesterosis.

Papillomas are seen in about 0.3% of cholecystograms. In a functioning gallbladder they appear as concave filling defects, pointing towards the centre on the lateral wall. They are about 5–10 mm in diameter and may be multiple. They are differentiated from gallstones by their fixed position.

ADENOMA

These very rare, small, single tumours are usually fundal, where they form a semi-solid or cystic papillary mass. Adenoma is usually a symptom free, incidental finding.

Detached tumour particles may cause biliary colic [21].

In cholecystograms, an adenoma is usually seen at the fundus as a small circular or semi-circular translucent filling defect, the gallbladder being well filled.

Carcinoma of the gallbladder

This is an uncommon neoplasm. Gallstones co-exist in about 75% and chronic cholecystitis is a frequent association. There is no definite evidence of a causal relationship. Whatever causes gallstones predisposes to cancer.

The calcified (porcelain) gallbladder is particularly likely to become cancerous [23]. The common gallbladder papillomas are not pre-cancerous. It may complicate ulcerative colitis. An anomalous pancreatico-biliary ductal union, greater than 15 mm from the papilla of Vater, is associated with congenital cystic dilatation of the common bile ducts and with gallbladder carcinoma [14]. Regurgitation of pancreatic juice may be tumorigenic.

Papillary adenocarcinoma commences as a wart-like excrescence [4]. It grows slowly into, rather than through, the wall until a fungating mass fills the gallbladder. Mucoid change is associated with more rapid growth, early metastasis and gelatinous peritoneal carcinomatosis. *Squamous cell carcinoma and scirrhous* forms are recognized. *The anaplastic type* is particularly malignant. The most common tumour is a differentiated adenocarcinoma which may be papillary [12]. Composite tumours (adeno-carcinoma, carcinoid [28], and globlet cell) are described [18].

The tumour usually arises in the fundus or neck, but rapid spread may make the original site difficult to locate. The rich lymphatic and venous drainage of the gallbladder allows rapid spread to related lymph nodes, causing cholestatic jaundice and widespread dissemination. The liver bed is invaded and there is local spread to the duodenum, stomach and colon resulting in fistulae or external compression.

Clinical. The patient is usually an elderly, white female [4], complaining of pain in the right upper quadrant, nausea, vomiting, weight loss and jaundice [12].

Examination reveals a hard and sometimes tender mass in the gallbladder area. Intrahepatic metastases are not usually palpable. The abdomen is distended and gelatinous peritoneal carcinomatosis may prevent individual organs being defined.

Serum, urine and *faeces* show the changes of cholestatic jaundice.

Liver biopsy shows the histological picture of biliary obstruction but does not indicate the cause, because intra-hepatic mestastases are uncommon. *ERCP* may be helpful, but may fail to show the tumour. *CT scanning and ultrasound* may be useful in defining the right upper quadrant mass and any metastases. *Angiography* shows displacement of hepatic and portal blood vessels.

PROGNOSIS

This is hopeless because the majority are inoperable at the time of diagnosis [6]. The only long-term survivors are those in whom the tumour was found incidentally at the time of cholecystectomy for gallstones (carcinoma *in situ*). Mean survival from diagnosis is 4.5 months [12]. The papillary type has the best prognosis, as the growth is inwards rather than through the gallbladder wall and spread is later.

TREATMENT

Cholecystectomy has been recommended for all patients with gallstones in an effort to prevent the development of carcinoma in the gallbladder. This seems drastic for a common condition, and would lead to a large number of unnecessary cholecystectomies. The preoperative diagnosis of carcinoma of the gallbladder should not preclude laparotomy although the results of surgical treatment are disappointing.

Endoscopically or percutaneously placed biliary prostheses may be of palliative value.

Partial hepatectomy has been attempted but with unsatisfactory results.

Leiomyosarcoma is exceedingly rare. Scanning shows a dilated gallbladder with an irregularly thickened wall and polypoid intrusion into the lumen [20].

Carcinoid tumours can very rarely involve the gallbladder and extra-hepatic bile ducts [13]. The argentaffin reaction is positive in tumour cells.

Benign tumours of the extra-hepatic bile ducts

These extremely rare tumours usually remain undetected until there is evidence of biliary obstruction and cholangitis. They are rarely diagnosed pre-operatively.

Recognition is important as resection is curative.

Papilloma is a polypoid tumour which projects into the lumen of the common bile duct. It is a small, soft, vascular tumour, which may be sessile or pedunculated. The tumours may be single or multiple; they may be cystic. Occasionally they undergo malignant change [19]. Cholangiography may show a smooth mass projecting into the bile ducts.

Mucus secretion from the tumour can cause obstructive cholangitis [26].

Adenomyoma can be found anywhere in the biliary tract. It is firm and well circumscribed and varies in size up to 15 cm in diameter. It is cured by resection [7].

Cystadenoma may present as a large pedunculated mass extending into the common bile duct [29]. Resection is usually possible.

Fibroma is small and firm and causes early bile duct obstruction.

Granular cell tumour is of mesenchymal origin. It affects young women, usually black, causing cholestasis [5]. It must be distinguished from cholangiocarcinoma or localised sclerosing cholangitis. Tumours are uniformly resectable and curable.

Carcinoma of the bile ducts (cholangiocarcinoma)

Carcinoma of the bile ducts seems to be increasing. This must in part reflect wider application of newer diagnostic imaging and cholangiographic techniques. Diagnosis of site of origin and spread are more exact. Surgery has made few advances largely because of the inaccessibility of the tumour but the enthusiastic invasive radiologist and endoscopist make sure that no patient dies with jaundice and/or pruritus.

Carcinoma may arise at any point in the biliary tree from small intra-hepatic bile ducts to the common bile duct. The histology of the tumour is the same whatever the site of origin. The clinical picture and treatment differ according to the site. It is often difficult at surgery or autopsy to be sure of the exact origin.

ASSOCIATIONS

Bile duct cancers are associated with ulcerative colitis with or without sclerosing cholangitis involving extra-hepatic bile ducts (Chapter 15).

All members of the congenital fibropolycystic family may be complicated by adenocarcinoma (Chapter 30). These include congenital hepatic fibrosis, cystic dilatation (Caroli's syndrome), choledochal cysts, polycystic liver and von Meyenburg complexes. Cholangiocarcinoma may be associated with biliary cirrhosis due to biliary atresia.

The liver fluke infestations of the orient may be complicated by cholangiocarcinoma. In the Far East (China, Hong Kong, Korea, Japan), where *Clonorchis sinensis* is prevalent, cholangiocarcinoma accounts for 20% of primary liver tumours. These arise in the heavily parasitized bile ducts near the hilum.

Opisthorchis viverrini infestation is important in Thailand, Laos, and Western Malaysia [16].

In New York an association has been shown between hepato-biliary cancer and the typhoid carrier state [31].

The role of gallstones is uncertain.

Bile duct cancers are not closely associated with cirrhosis unless it is of the biliary type [22].

PATHOLOGY

The confluence of cystic duct with main hepatic duct or the right and left main hepatic ducts at the porta hepatis are common sites of origin and the tumour extends into the liver. It causes complete obstruction of the extra-hepatic bile ducts with intra-hepatic biliary dilatation and enlargement of the liver. The gallbladder is collapsed and flaccid. If the tumour is restricted to one hepatic duct, biliary obstruction is incomplete and jaundice absent. The lobe of the liver drained by this duct atrophies and the other hypertrophies.

In the common bile duct the tumour presents as a firm nodule or plaque which causes an annular stricture which may ulcerate. It spreads along the bile duct and through its wall.

Local and distant metastases, even at autopsy, are found in only about half of the patients. They involve peritoneum, abdominal lymph nodes, diaphragm, liver or gallbladder [32]. Blood vessel invasion is rare and extra-abdominal spread is unusual.

Compression of the portal vein can lead to lobar atrophy [27].

Histologically the tumour is usually a mucus-secreting adenocarcinoma with cuboidal or columnar epithelium and abundant fibrous stroma (fig. 34.1). Spread along neural sheaths may be noted.

CLINICAL FEATURES [32]

This tumour tends to occur in the older age group, patients being about 60 years old (fig. 34.2). Slightly more males than females are affected.

Jaundice is the usual presenting feature, to be followed by pruritus—a point of distinction from primary biliary cirrhosis. Jaundice may be delayed if only one main duct is involved. The trend of the serum bilirubin level is always upward, but periods of clearing of jaundice are found in up to 50% (fig. 34.3) [15].

Pain, usually epigastric and mild, is present in about one-half of patients. Diarrhoea may be related to steatorrhoea. Weakness and weight loss, usually 14–28 pounds, are marked.

The condition may be associated with chronic ulcerative colitis, often following long-standing cholestasis due to sclerosing cholangitis.

Examination. Jaundice is deep. The patient is usually afebrile until terminally. Cholangitis is unusual unless the bile ducts have been interfered with surgically [32].

The liver is very large and smooth, extending

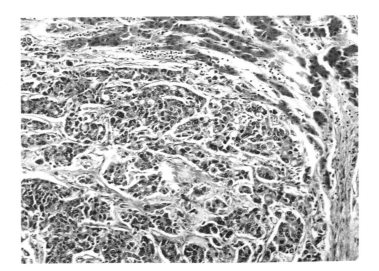

Fig. 34.1. Bile duct carcinoma: a papillary fibrous stroma in seen. (Stained H & E, ×40.)

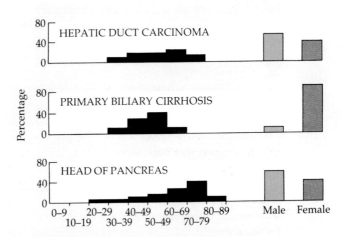

Fig. 34.2. Age distribution of hepatic duct carcinoma compared with primary biliary cirrhosis and carcinoma of the head of the pancreas (Whelton *et al.* 1969).

5–12 cm below the costal margin. The spleen is not felt. Ascites is unusual.

INVESTIGATIONS

Serum biochemical findings are those of cholestatic jaundice. The serum bilirubin level is very high and fluctuations may reflect incomplete obstruction and primary involvement of one hepatic duct.

The serum mitochondrial antibody test is negative and α-fetoprotein is not increased.

The *faeces* are pale and fatty and occult blood is often present. *Glycosuria* is absent.

Anaemia may be greater than that seen with ampullary carcinoma; the explanation is unknown—it is not due to blood loss. The leucocyte count is high–normal with increased polymorphs.

Hepatic biopsy shows the features of large bile duct obstruction. Tumour tissue is not obtained. It is extremely difficult to get histological proof of malignancy. Attempts may be made at obtaining material for cytology at the

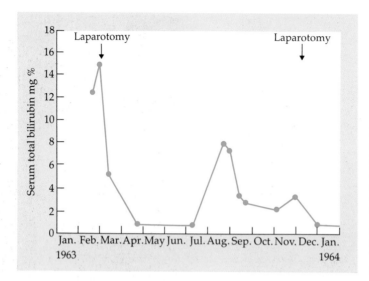

Fig. 34.3. This shows fluctuations in serum bilirubin following laparotomy in a patient with carcinoma of the junction of the hepatic duct. At the initial laparotomy, the tumour was not detected and no procedure other than liver biopsy was performed. The serum bilirubin fell to normal and remained there for some months. At the second operation a bile duct carcinoma was found (Whelton *et al.* 1969).

time of percutaneous or endoscopic cholangiography, but they often fail.

SCANNING

Isotope scans show a defect at the hilum of the liver. This is mainly due to dilated intra-hepatic bile ducts, and rarely to the tumour itself.

Ultrasound is particularly helpful and shows dilated intra-hepatic bile ducts. It can sometimes identify the tumour mass.

CT scans show intra-hepatic biliary dilatation; the tumour is difficult to demonstrate as it is isodense with the rest of the liver. Biliary ductal spread of the sclerosing cholangioma-carcinoma is impossible to determine by CT. *MR imaging* may be more useful [10].

CHOLANGIOGRAPHY

Endoscopic or percutaneous cholangiography, or both, is essential, and should be performed in all patients with the picture of cholestasis and dilated intra-hepatic ducts shown by ultrasound or CT.

Transpapillary forceps biopsy at the time of ERCP may reveal tumour. Endoscopic ultrasound is useful in assessing the extent of the tumour [8].

Endoscopic retrograde. The normal common

bile duct and gallbladder are visualized and the obstruction at the hilum identified (fig. 34.4).

Percutaneous. This is usually successful. The obstruction is shown as a blunt or nipple-like termination (fig. 34.5). Intra-hepatic bile ducts are always dilated. In some instances, intubation of both right and left duct systems may be necessary to outline the obstruction accurately.

DIAGNOSIS (table 34.1)

The clinical diagnosis is likely to be carcinoma of the ampullary region, which is the more common condition. Even at operation after palpation of the hilum and after operative cholangiography through the common bile duct or gallbladder the diagnosis may still be in doubt. The significance of a large, green liver with a collapsed gallbladder may not be realized.

Intra-hepatic cholangiocarcinoma is more difficult to diagnose. CT shows a single homogeneous, low attenuation mass [24]. Multiple lesions and calcification may be seen. Distinction from hepato-cellular carcinoma may be difficult. Hepatic venous and portal venous involvement are rare.

Primary biliary cirrhosis must be excluded (table 34.1). This is usually easy if cholangiography has been done. Careful interpretation

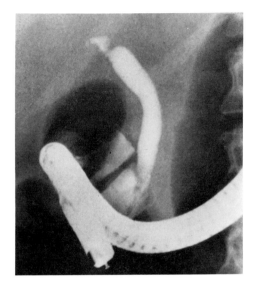

Fig. 34.4. Carcinoma of bile ducts at the hilum of the liver. ERCP shows a common bile duct of normal calibre terminating in an irregular obstruction.

of hepatic biopsies together with a negative mitochondrial antibody make the distinction certain.

Differentiation from chronic cholestatic drug jaundice depends on the history, the mode of onset, and hepatic histology.

Differentiation from primary sclerosing cholangitis can be extremely difficult, particularly as the two conditions may co-exist (Chapter 17). Endoscopic or percutaneous cholangiography is essential.

Hepato-cellular disease may be mimicked by the fluctuating jaundice.

PROGNOSIS

This is ultimately fatal but the tumour is slow growing and metastasizes late so that survival is surprisingly long, particularly if the jaundice can be relieved. Mean survival in one series of 23 patients was 14.4 months [30]. It can be as long as five-and-a-half years. The tumour kills by its site, making it inoperable, rather than by its malignancy. Death is due to hepato-cellular failure and infection, usually suppurative cholangitis and septicaemia. Massive invasion of

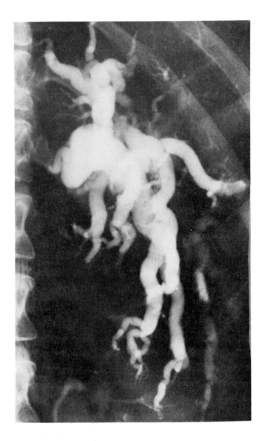

Fig. 34.5. Same patient as in fig. 34.4—a percutaneous trans-hepatic cholangiography shows gross dilatation of intra-hepatic bile ducts and no contrast material enters the common bile duct.

Table 34.1. Chronic cholestais

Type	Diagnostic points	M test
Primary biliary	Females Hepatic histology	+
Chronic chlorpromazine	Acute onset Drug ingestion Hepatic histology	±
Sclerosing cholangitis	Long-standing colitis ERCP	–
Carcinoma hepatic ducts	Deep jaundice Hepatic histology Cholangiography	–

the liver by tumour or extra-hepatic metastases [15] rarely causes death. The prognosis is relatively good so that hepatic transplantation is rarely indicated.

Prognosis depends on the site of the tumour. Those distally placed are more likely to be resectable than those at the hilum. The histologically differentiated do better than the undifferentiated. Polypoid cancers have the best prognosis.

TREATMENT

Surgery

All patients should be operated on if the general condition permits. The resectability rate is only 20%.

Imaging is aimed at establishing whether, after surgical removal, a viable unit of liver remains [2, 30]. This must contain a biliary radicle large enough to anastomose to bowel, a normal portal vein and hepatic arterial branch. Digital vascular imaging CT and endoscopic and percutaneous cholangiography are essential pre-operative procedures.

Tumours of the lower bile duct may be resected with a one-year survival of about 60%. More distal tumours may be resected by local or major liver surgery including excision of the whole bifurcation of the common hepatic duct, lobectomy if necessary and bilateral hepaticojejunostomy. The liver may need to be split back to the vena cava. In one large series, 18 of 94 cholangiocarcinomas at the confluence of hepatic ducts were resected with a hospital mortality of 11%, and mean duration of survival of 17 months [3]. The remaining 72 patients were unresectable and treated by palliation with a hospital mortality of 33% and a mean survival of 8.5 months. The poorer prognosis could be related to the tumour being more advanced so making resection impossible.

Palliation

A stent is introduced through the tumour so allowing biliary drainage into the duodenum.

The stent, made of percuflex and polyurethane or steel, is introduced by a trans-hepatic technique into the bile ducts over a guide wire (Chapters 29, 33). Complications include cholangitis, obstruction and dislocation of the tube [17]. Mean survival is 20 weeks. Endoscopic insertion of the stent is equally satisfactory (25).

Such palliative procedures can restore the patient to a good state of health for a long time.

Internal radiotherapy, using ^{192}iridium wire or radium needles may be combined with biliary drainage [11]. It is probably of little value.

External radiotherapy, and cytotoxic drugs are ineffective.

Symptomatic treatment is that of chronic cholestasis (Chapter 14).

Hepatic transplantation gives poor results, recurrence of the tumour is usual (see Chapter 35).

References

1 Alexander F, Rossi RL, O'Bryan M *et al.* Biliary carcinoma: a review of 109 cases. *Am. J. Surg.* 1984; **147**: 503.
2 Allison DJ. State of the art: assessment of the operability of malignant lesions of the biliary tree. In *Imaging in Hepatobiliary Disease*. eds J.S. Dooley, R. Dick, M Viamonte Jr & S. Sherlock. Blackwell Scientific Publications, Oxford, 1987; p. 15.
3 Blumgart LH, Hadjis NS, Benjamin IS *et al.* Surgical approaches to cholangiocarcinoma at confluence of hepatic ducts. *Lancet* 1984; **i**: 66.
4 Brandt-Rauf PW, Pincus M, Adelson S. Cancer of the gallbladder: a review of 43 cases. *Hum. Pathol.* 1982; **13**: 48.
5 Butterly LF, Schapiro RH, LaMuraglia GM *et al.* Biliary granular cell tumor: a little-known curable bile duct neoplasm of young people. *Surgery* 1988; **103**: 328.
6 Collier NA, Carr D, Hemingway A *et al.* Preoperative diagnosis and its effect on the treatment of carcinoma of the gallbladder. *Surg. Gynecol. Obstet.* 1984; **159**: 465.
7 Cook DJ, Salena BJ, Vincic LM. Adenomyoma of the common bile duct. *Am. J. Gastroenterol.* 1988; **83**: 432.
8 Dancygier H, Rösch T, Lorenz R *et al.* Preoperative staging of a distal common bile duct tumour by endoscopic ultrasound. *Gastroenterology* 1988; **95**: 219.

9 Dooley JS, Dick R, George P *et al.* Percutaneous transhepatic endoprosthesis for bile duct obstruction: complications and results. *Gastroenterology* 1984; **86**: 905.

10 Dooms GC, Kerlan RK, Hricak H *et al.* Cholangiocarcinoma: imaging by MR. *Radiology* 1986; **159**: 89.

11 Fletcher MS, Brinkley D, Dawson JL *et al.* Treatment of hilar carcinoma by bile drainage combined with internal radiotherapy using 192-iridium wire. *Br. J. Surg.* 1983; **70**: 733.

12 Hamrick RE Jr, Liner FJ, Hastings PR *et al.* Primary carcinoma of the gallbladder. *Ann. Surg.* 1982; **195**: 270.

13 Jutte DL, Bell RH Jr, Penn I *et al.* Carcinoid tumor of the biliary system. Case report and literature review. *Dig. Dis. Sci.* 1987; **32**: 763.

14 Kimura K, Ohto M, Saisho H *et al.* Association of gallbladder carcinoma and anomalous pancreaticobiliary ductal union. *Gastroenterology* 1985; **89**: 1258.

15 Klatskin G. Adenocarcinoma of the hepatic duct at its bifurcation within the porta hepatis. An unusual tumour with distinctive clinical and pathological features. *Am. J. Med.* 1965; **38**: 24.

16 Kurathong S, Lerdverasirikul P, Wongpaitoon V *et al.* Opisthorchis Viverrini infection and cholangiocarcinoma. A prospective, case-controlled study. *Gastroenterology* 1985; **89**: 151.

17 Lammer J, Neumayer K. Biliary drainage endoprostheses: experience with 201 placements. *Radiology* 1986; **159**: 625.

18 Muto Y, Okamoto K, Uchimura M. Composite tumor (ordinary adenocarcinoma, typical carcinoid, and goblet cell adenocarcinoid) of the gallbladder: a variety of composite tumor. *Am. J. Gastroenterol.* 1984; **79**: 645.

19 Neumann RD, Livolsi VA, Rosenthal NS *et al.* Adenocarcinoma in biliary papillomatosis. *Gastroenterology* 1976; **70**: 779.

20 Newmark H III, Kliewer K, Curtis A *et al.* Primary leiomyosarcoma of gallbladder seen on computed tomography and ultrasound. *Am. J. Gastroenterol.* 1986; **81**: 202.

21 Niv Y, Kosakov K, Shcolnik B. Fragile papilloma (papillary adenoma) of the gallbladder. A cause of recurrent biliary colic. *Gastroenterology* 1986; **91**: 999.

22 Okuda K. Kubo Y, Okazaki N *et al.* Clinical aspects of intrahepatic bile duct carcinoma including hilar carcinoma: a study of 57 autopsy-proven cases. *Cancer* 1977; **39**: 232.

23 Polk HC. Carcinoma and calcified gallbladder. *Gastroenterology* 1966; **50**: 582.

24 Ros PR, Buck JL, Goodman ZD *et al.* Intrahepatic cholangiocarcinoma: radiologic—pathologic correlation. *Radiology* 1988; **167**: 689.

25 Siegel JH, Daniel SJ. Endoscopic and fluoroscopic transpapillary placement of a large caliber biliary endoprosthesis. *Am. J. Gastroenterol.* 1984; **79**: 461.

26 Styne P, Warren GH, Kumpe DA *et al.* Obstructive cholangitis secondary to mucus secreted by a solitary papillary bile duct tumor. *Gastroenterology* 1986; **90**: 748.

27 Takayasu K, Muramatsu Y, Shima Y *et al.* Hepatic lobar atrophy following obstruction of the ipsilateral portal vein from hilar cholangiocarcinoma. *Radiology* 1986; **160**: 389.

28 Van Steenbergen W, Fevery J, Vanstapel MJ *et al.* Case report: fourteen-year follow-up of an apudoma of the bile ducts at the hilum of the liver. *Gastroenterology* 1983; **84**: 1585.

29 Van Steenbergen W, Ponette E, Marchal G *et al.* Cystadenoma of the common bile duct demonstrated by endoscopic retrograde cholangiography: an uncommon cause of extrahepatic obstruction. *Am. J. Gastroenterol.* 1984; **79**: 466.

30 Voyles CR, Bowley NJ, Allison DJ *et al.* Carcinoma of the proximal extrahepatic biliary tree: radiologic assessment and therapeutic alternatives. *Ann. Surg.* 1983; **197**: 188.

31 Welton JC, Marr JS, Friedman SM. Association between hepatobiliary cancer and typhoid carrier state. *Lancet* 1979; **i**: 791.

32 Whelton MJ, Petrelli M, George P *et al.* Carcinoma at the junction of the main hepatic ducts. *Q. J. Med.* 1969; **28**: 211.

35 · Hepatic Transplantation

In 1955, Welch performed the first transplantation of the liver in dogs [61]. In 1963, Starzl and his group carried out the first successful hepatic transplant in man [49]. Since then, a total of some 4000 transplants have been performed, about 3000 in the United States and 1000 elsewhere [3, 4, 7, 8, 28, 29]. The number is escalating because the one-year survival has improved from 32% in 1979 to 80% in 1988, with a five-year survival of 60 to 70% [36]. These improved results can be related to more careful patient selection with greater emphasis on nutritional status [23], to better surgical techniques and post-operative care, and to greater willingness to re-transplant after rejection (table 35.1). Better immunosuppression, particularly with cyclosporin, has contributed.

Selection of patients (table 35.2)

The patient should suffer from irreversible, progressive liver disease for which there is no acceptable alternative therapy. The patient and his family must understand the magnitude of the undertaking and be prepared to face the difficult early post-operative period and life-long immuno-suppression. The choice of the time for transplant is one of the most difficult decisions for a hepatologist and for the patient and his family. It should be a team one.

Table 35.1. Factors improving survival in liver transplantation

Better patient selection
Improved donor-organ harvesting
Veno−venous bypass during surgery
Improved immunosuppression
Re-transplantation easier

The patient must not be moribund. The best candidate is one that is stable at home; the worst is in intensive care.

Candidates (table 35.2)

In Europe, the pattern of primary indications for liver transplantation is changing (fig. 35.1) [4]. The main indication is cirrhosis, including primary biliary cirrhosis. More patients with acute and subacute hepatic failure and with biliary atresia are being included and fewer with cancer.

NON-ALCOHOLIC CIRRHOSIS

It is particularly difficult to select the right time

Table 35.2. Candidates for hepatic transplantation

Cirrhosis
  'Cryptogenic'
  Primary biliary
Extra-hepatic biliary atresia
Primary sclerosing cholangitis
Subacute hepatic necrosis
Chronic portal−systemic encephalopathy
Budd−Chiari syndrome

Inherited metabolic diseases
α_1-antitrypsin deficiency
Wilson's disease
Homozygous hypercholesterolaemia
Haemophilia (with complicating cirrhosis)
Glycogenosis I and IV
Tyrosinaemia
Crigler−Najjar hyperbilirubinaemia type 1
Protoporphyria

Relative contraindications
Advanced alcoholic liver disease
HBsAg (HBeAg) positive
Hepatic tumours

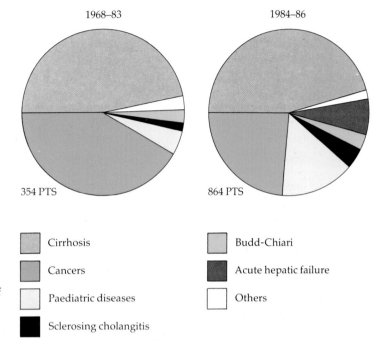

1968–83

1984–86

354 PTS

864 PTS

Fig. 35.1. Changing patterns of primary indications for liver transplantation (Bismuth *et al.* 1987).

Cirrhosis

Cancers

Paediatric diseases

Sclerosing cholangitis

Budd-Chiari

Acute hepatic failure

Others

for the operation. The patient must not be moribund so that the transplant will fail, or capable of leading a relatively normal life for a long period so that the transplant is unnecessary. Indications include a prothrombin time more than 5 seconds prolonged, serum albumin concentration less than 30 g/l, intractable ascites, encephalopathy and bleeding varices.

In general, the patients are poor operative risks because of impaired blood coagulation and portal hypertension, so that blood loss is great. The technical difficulties are, in general, greater when cirrhosis is present, particularly when the liver is small and difficult to remove. Nevertheless, results are improving, the one-year survival increasing from 31% in 1980, to 65% in 1984. Survival is much the same for all forms of cirrhosis.

Transplantation is being performed for end-stage *autoimmune chronic active hepatitis* with cirrhosis, and also for the major side effects of corticosteroid therapy such as bone thinning and recurrent infections. There is only one report of a possible recurrence of the liver disease post-transplant [40].

Non-A, non-B virus-related cirrhosis cannot be diagnosed at present, and the outlook after hepatic transplantation is uncertain.

It seems probable than many instances of post-transplant hepatitis are due to non-A, non-B hepatitis, either occurring in the new liver or transmitted by a blood transfusion.

Aplastic anaemia can complicate liver transplantation for acute non-A, non-B hepatitis [53]. This may be due to the successful transplant permitting a more frequent expression of aplastic anaemia, a known complication of acute non-A, non-B hepatitis.

PRIMARY BILIARY CIRRHOSIS
(see Chapter 14)

This is a prime indication as the end-stage can be predicted with reasonable certainty and hepato-cellular function tends to be maintained. One-year survival after transplantation is now 75% [15]. A patient with primary biliary cirrhosis and primary pulmonary hypertension had a triple-transplant of liver, lung and heart and was well one year later [58].

PRIMARY SCLEROSING CHOLANGITIS

Sepsis and previous biliary surgery provide technical problems. Nevertheless, the results of transplantation are good, one-year survival being 70% and five-year, 57% (see Chapter 15) [31]. Cholangiocarcinoma is a complication which greatly reduces long-term survival.

EXTRA-HEPATIC BILIARY ATRESIA

Children with this condition do particularly well after transplant, and the quality of life is excellent (Chapter 24). Survival at one year is over 80%, and at five years more than 75% [38].

The Kasai procedure may be regarded as a method to 'buy time' until the baby is large enough to tolerate transplantation. It does however, expose the patient to cholangitis and to greater technical difficulties in the operation.

Viral and bacterial immunization is particularly important before children have a transplant.

ACUTE AND SUBACUTE HEPATIC FAILURE

Transplantation is more often indicated in the subacute (onset after 15−90 days) than in the fulminant (onset less than 2 weeks) as the latter carries a better prognosis.

The best indications for transplantation include a serum factor V level less than 20%, a serum creatinine greater than 100 mg, grade IV coma and a young age. Problems in finding a suitable donor at the right time means the liver used tends to be of poor quality, too large, and not of compatible blood group. Nevertheless, 65 hepatic transplants have been performed in four centres on patients with fulminant hepatic failure including acute A, B, non-A, non-B, and drug-related disease (Chapter 8). The overall survival was 46%. Transplantation is rarely necessary in acetaminophen (paracetamol) overdose or isoniazid hepatitis.

Chronic hepatitis B and Delta virus infection

Results of hepatic transplantation are poor, es-pecially if the patient is hepatitis BV DNA positive (Chapter 17). If the patient is HBV-DNA negative, the new liver may not become reinfected.

The use of antiviral therapy and large doses of immunoglobulin pre- and post-transplant is controversial and the value is not established.

Poor results are perhaps due to extra-hepatic replication of virus and to reactivation of hepatitis B infection related to immunosuppressive therapy. Hepatitis B infection of the graft developed in all eight patients with chronic hepatitis B surviving two months following transplant [12].

Hepatic transplantation has been disappointing in delta infected patients with recurrence of the disease usual (see Chapter 17).

Alcoholic liver disease

There is little enthusiasm for giving a new liver to the patient with advanced alcoholic cirrhosis, particularly if another alcohol-related disease, such as cerebral cortical atrophy or pancreatitis, might be present. However, if the candidate has been abstinent for at least six months, the case must be considered on merit [51]. In the West, these patients are likely to provide the largest number of candidates for transplant.

HEPATIC MALIGNANT DISEASE

Perhaps the greatest disappointment of hepatic transplantation has been the results in patients with liver tumours despite all preoperative attempts at identifying extra-hepatic spread [22]. Patients with cancer have the lowest operative mortality, but the worst long-term survival. Carcinomatosis is the usual cause of death. Tumour recurs in 60%, perhaps because of the immunosuppressants necessary to prevent rejection. The peri-operative survival is 76%, but the one-year survival only 50% and two-year survival 31% [4]. There is an occasional dramatic success when a small hepato-cellular carcinoma is discovered by imaging and increased alpha-fetoprotein values [36]. Transplantation for hepato-cellular carcinoma should only be considered for small (4—5 cm) tumours without multilobular growth. One-year survival is 50%, and two-year, 25%.

The best candidates may be those with fibro-lamellar carcinoma in whom the tumour is localized to the liver and cirrhosis is absent. Epithelioid haemangio-endothelioma presents as multiple focal lesions in both lobes of an otherwise normal liver. It can be successfully treated by liver transplantation [42].

Cholangiocarcinoma has proved an unsatifactory indication as tumour recurrence is seen in 75% and death occurs within twelve months [22].

BUDD–CHIARI SYNDROME

Although liver transplants have been performed apparently with success, recurrence of thrombosis is likely especially if, as is usually the case, there is underlying myloproliferative disease. Difficulties will be encountered if previous shunt surgery has been performed necessitating portal vein grafting.

INHERITED METABOLIC DISEASES

Liver homografts retain their original metabolic specificity. Consequently, liver transplantation is used for patients with inborn errors of metabolism which result from defects in hepatic function. Patients suffering from these conditions are good candidates. They are young and cirrhosis, with its accompanying portal hypertension, may be absent, facilitating the technical side of the operation. Selection depends on the prognosis and the likelihood of the later complication of primary liver tumours.

α_1-Antitrypsin deficiency

This may present as cholestasis in the neonate to be followed in early childhood by a relentlessly progressive cirrhosis [21]. The one-year survival after transplant is now approximately 68%. The α_1-antitrypsin serum phenotype remains that of the (normal) donor. The lung disease stabilizes after the transplant. Advanced

pulmonary disease is a contraindication unless both lungs and liver are transplanted. The risk of hepato-cellular cancer has gone following transplant.

Wilson's disease

Liver transplants have to be considered in patients presenting with the clinical picture of fulminant hepatitis; in young cirrhotic patients with severe hepatic decompensation who have failed to improve after three months' adequate D-penicillamine treatment; and in effectively treated patients who have developed severe hepatic decompensation following discontinuance of penicillamine [52]. The one-year survival after transplant is about 68%. Copper metabolism returns to normal.

Neurological manifestations reverse at varying rates [39].

Homozygous type IIA familial hypercholesterolaemia

This is treated by heart—liver transplant. The operation can be done in two stages (using different donors), the cardiac operation first and then the liver [32]. Serum cholesterol values fall markedly [2], and the metabolic defect is cured [54].

Haemophilia A

The hepatic transplant is performed for the end-stage non-A, non-B cirrhosis [5, 17]. Production of Factor VIII is maintained post-transplant. This procedure is not recommended as a cure for haemophilia, but only for any associated end-stage liver disease. AIDS infection would be a contraindication to transplant.

Primary Hyperoxaluria type I

A combined kidney—liver transplant is used [59].

Crigler—Najjar type I

Hepatic transplantation is performed when the serum bilirubin level is very high and cannot be controlled by phototherapy [25].

Hereditary tyrosinaemia

Hepatic transplantation renders the patient free of the metabolic defect and of any complicating hepato-cellular carcinoma [55].

Protoporphyria

Transplantation is done at the stage of jaundice and cirrhosis. The procedure is not curative and the porphyrins accumulate slowly in the transplanted liver [16].

Hepatic transplantation has been successfully performed for *glycogen storage disease types I and IV* [30].

Byler's disease is an indication for transplant.

Absolute and relative contraindications (table 35.3)

Absolute

Active sepsis outside the hepato-biliary tree contraindicates the operation as the one-year survival falls to about 40%. Metastatic malignancy is a clear contraindication. Advanced cardiopulmonary disease contraindicates the operation, particularly with advanced hypoxaemia such as a pulmonary arterio—venous shunt. This renders the operation and post-operative care almost impossible.

Transplant should not be done if the patient cannot comprehend the magnitude of the undertaking and the exceptional physical and psychological commitment required [28, 29].

Active alcoholism contraindicates transplant.

AIDS infection is an absolute contra-indication.

Relative

Many of the features formerly regarded as ab-

Table 35.3. Absolute and relative contraindications to liver transplantation

Absolute
  Psycho-physical-social inability to tolerate the procedure
  Active sepsis
  Metastatic malignancy
  Cholangiocarcinoma
  Active alcoholism
  AIDS
  Diffuse portal vein thrombosis
  Advanced cardio-pulmonary disease
Relative
  Advanced age
  Prior porta—caval shunt
  Portal vein thrombosis (localized)
  Prior complex hepato-biliary surgery
  HBV-DNA positive
  Renal impairment

solute contraindications are becoming relative as techniques and the selection of patients improve.

Age. Children do particularly well but a donor liver is difficult to obtain. There is no absolute contraindication on account of advanced age and transplants have been performed up to age 77 [51]. However, with rare exceptions, age should not exceed 60. The cardiac status of the older patient must be assessed pre-transplant and also their nutritional condition considered.

Anatomical considerations. Previous porta—caval shunts may make the operation impossible, a selective spleno—renal shunt may be feasible, if absolutely necessary, before a transplant.

In general, portal vein thrombosis contraindicates the operation.

Previous complex surgery in the upper abdomen may make the transplant technically impossible.

General preparation of the patient

A standard protocol must be filled in. The procedure is discussed fully with patients and relatives and consent given.

The usual clinical, biochemical and serological investigation of any patient with liver disease is detailed and, in particular, such information as previous haemorrhages, pre-coma and ascites. The synthetic functions of the liver, such as serum albumin and prothrombin are helpful prognostically.

Blood group, HLA and DR antigens are recorded.

In patients with malignant disease, metastases must be sought by all possible techniques.

The hepatic arterial tree must be visualized and any anatomical abnormality, including an aberrant origin of the hepatic artery and a pre-duodenal portal vein, must be noted. The portal vein and the inferior vena cava must be seen, since obstruction to either is usually a contra-indication to transplantation. A selective right renal arteriogram is also performed as failure to recognize a high right kidney may result in unavoidable right nephrectomy. Demonstration of the bile ducts pre-operatively is performed by cholangiography, usually endoscopic but percutaneous when endoscopic fails. Ultrasound and CT scanning are routine.

The pre-transplant medical 'work-up' takes about ten days. It includes psychiatric counselling and confirmation of the diagnosis. The patient may wait up to three months for a suitable donor liver and, during this period, intensive psycho-social support is necessary. Patients, particularly children, often die while waiting for a suitable liver. For every three paediatric patients transplanted, one dies waiting, and for every five adults, one succumbs before the liver arrives [8].

THE DONOR

Informed consent in writing has to be given by the relatives. The donor is characteristically between 2 months and 45 years of age, a victim of brain injury which has resulted in brain death. Cardiovascular and respiratory functions are sustained artificially by mechanical ventilation. The recovery of livers, and other vital organs, from heart-beating cadavers minimizes the ischaemia which occurs at normal body temperatures and is a major contribution to graft success. The donor should suffer from no other disease. Routine biochemical tests of liver function should be normal at the time of donation. The donor should not have had periods of prolonged hypotension or anoxia.

There is a significant advantage for ABO donor—recipient identity [19]. Although ABO blood group-incompatible grafts have functioned for years this practice should be limited to emergency situations or transplants in small children where the supply of donors is severely limited. Vanishing bileducts in the chronic rejection reaction may be related to HLA-DR mismatch, and if possible this should be avoided [13].

The operative details of the donor and recipient operation are discussed elsewhere [8, 46, 47, 50]. The hepatic structures are dissected and the liver is pre-cooled through the splenic vein with Ringer's lactate and 1000 ml of the University of Wisconsin (UW) solution perfused through the aorta and portal vein [24]. A cannula in the distal inferior vena cava provides a vent for venous outflow. After removal, the cold liver is further flushed with an additional 1000 ml UW solution through the hepatic artery and portal vein and stored in this solution in a plastic bag on ice in a portable cooler. This routine has extended the preservation time to 11—20 hours so that the recipient operation may be semi-elective and not performed at unsocial hours. The same surgeon can perform both donor and recipient procedures.

If possible, and particularly for elective procedures, the size and shape of the donor liver should be matched to that of the recipient. It must certainly not be larger, and if possible should be smaller. Occasionally a small-sized liver is transplanted into a larger patient. This is remedied by the recipient liver increasing in size at the rate of about 70 ml per day until it achieves the volume consistent with that expected for the recipient's size, age and sex [57].

The recipient operation (fig 35.2)

The average operative time is 7.6 (4−15) hours. An average of 17 (2−220) packed cells are transfused [7, 8]. A cell-saver is useful, saving approximately a third of the blood lost into the abdominal cavity which is aspirated, repeatedly washed and the red cells resuspended and infused.

The hilar structures and the vena cava above and below the liver are dissected, cross-clamping and dividing the various vessels just as the liver is removed.

During the implantation of the new liver, it is necessary to occlude the splenic and vena caval circulations. During this anhepatic phase, the use of a pump-driven veno−venous bypass prevents pooling in the lower part of the body and so splanchnic congestion. The cannulas are placed in the inferior vena cava (via the femoral vein) and in the portal vein running to the subclavian vein [45].

The veno−venous bypass allows increased operative time, less bleeding, and an easier technique.

All vascular anastomoses are completed before opening the blood supply to the liver. Portal vein thrombosis must be excluded. Hepatic arterial anomalies are frequent, and vessel grafts from the donor should be available for arterial reconstructions as necessary [44].

The usual order of anastomoses is (1) supra-hepatic vena cava, (2) intra-hepatic vena cava, (3) portal vein, (4) hepatic artery and (5) biliary system. The bile duct is usually reconstructed by choledochocholedochostomy with a T-tube stent. If the recipient bile duct is diseased or absent, end-to-side choledochojejunostomy in Roux-en-Y fashion is chosen. Before closing the abdomen, the surgeon usually waits a period of about one hour so that any remaining bleeding points may be identified and closed. The patient should be kept in the operating room until prothrombin time and partial thromboplastin time are almost normal.

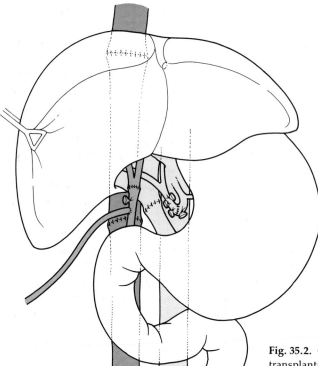

Fig. 35.2. Completed orthotopic liver transplantation. Biliary tract reconstruction is by choledochojejunostomy (Starzl *et al.* 1982).

AUXILIARY HETEROTROPIC AND SEGMENTAL LIVER TRANSPLANTATION

The left lobe of the donor liver is excised and the right lobe anastomosed to the portal vein and aorta of the recipient. The technique has the advantage of less extensive surgery and less blood loss. The donor liver hypertrophies perhaps due to release of growth factors following hepatectomy and the recipient's own liver atrophies [63].

Segmental, (reduced size), adult livers have been used for children because of the difficulties in obtaining a suitable child-sized graft [3].

Immunosuppression

Multiple therapy is usually given which varies from centre to centre.

Cyclosporine is usually included. Improved results for renal and hepatic transplantation have been attributed to its use, although this has not been proved. Side-effects include renal and hepatic dysfunction, hypertension, hirsuties, tremor, gingival hypertrophy and lymphoma. It is costly, has a narrow therapeutic index and its use has to be monitored carefully. Trough blood levels have to be taken, initially frequently and then at regular intervals. The aim is 200−300 ng-ml. The dose is based on the nephrotoxicity of the drug.

Cyclosporine may be given pre-transplant in a dose of 17.5 mg/kg by mouth, or 5 mg/kg intravenously if oral intake is not possible. It is combined with methylprednisolone 20 mg/kg intravenously. After transplant, the patients receive cyclosporine, 5 mg/kg per day intravenously in divided doses, until oral intake is adequate when 17 mg/kg per day orally is continued in divided doses, together with intravenous methyl-prednisolone 10 mg/kg per day initially, tapering to 0.3 mg/kg per day by the end of the first week. When oral intake is possible, it is continued by mouth [7, 8]. Other centres do not used cyclosporine pre-transplant, but prescribe 1.5 mg/kg azathioprine together with 1 mg/kg methyl prednisolone, starting cyclosporine only when renal function is adequate [64]. Long-term maintenance is usually with 5−10 mg cyclosporine mg/kg/day. However, serious side-effects, particularly renal impairment and/or hypertension may necessitate reducing the dose and indeed, replacing cyclosporine with azathioprine [37].

POST-OPERATIVE COURSE

This is not easy, particularly in the adult. The patient is in hospital about 60 days, 15 or so of them in intensive care. Further surgery such as draining abscesses, biliary reconstruction or control of bleeding may be necessary.

Aggressive re-transplantation may reduce the early mortality. This is required in 20−25% of patients [46]. The main indications are primary graft failure, hepatic arterial thrombosis and chronic rejection, often with CMV infection. Renal dialysis may be required.

Factors determining an adverse result include poor pre-transplant nutrition, a raised serum creatinine level and severe coagulation abnormalities. Poor results are related also to the amount of blood products required during surgery, the need for renal dialysis post-transplant and severe rejection. The operation is easier in those without cirrhosis and portal hypertension, where the peri-operative mortality is less.

The causes of death are surgical—technical complications, either immediate or late, biliary leaks, and hepatic rejection, with or without infections often related to the large doses of immunosuppressants necessary to prevent rejection.

The quality of life in adult survivors is usually good: 85% return to their previous occupation, and two women have had subsequent normal pregnancies. A Royal Free male patient with primary biliary cirrhosis has recently completed 90 lengths of a sponsored charity swim 18 months after hepatic transplantation. More than 87% of paediatric survivors are fully rehabilitated and free of medical problems except those associated with follow-up care and recognition and control of rejection. Normal growth, both physical and psychosocial, is usual.

Post-transplantation complications
(table 35.4)

The three major problems are:
1 early technical failures (days 1 to 5);
2 infections (days 3 to 14 and on); and
3 rejection (from 5 to 10 days).

The presenting features of all three are very similar, namely large, firm, tender liver, increasing jaundice and fever and leucocytosis. Specialist investigations must be available to make the correct diagnosis. These include CT and US imaging [27], HIDA scanning, angiography [68], percutaneous and endoscopic cholangiography [67] and liver biopsy [48]. Specialist infectious disease assistance is necessary.

Primary graft failure. The transplantation of a 'bad' liver, usually due to inadequate preservation, is marked by continued serum transaminase elevations, deepening jaundice, scanty bile output, hyperkalaemia and hypoglycaemia. Re-transplantation is the only treatment and should not be delayed in the hope that things will improve.

Technical complications. These are most frequent in children with small vessels and bile ducts. Ultrasound and CT are particularly useful in demonstrating abscesses and infarcts, biliary dilatation, thrombosed portal vein or inferior vena cava and fluid collections of blood, bile or pus. Guided biopsy allows aspiration of fluid collections.

Bleeding: this is suspected by abdominal swelling, blood from abdominal drains, increasing pulse rate, decreasing blood pressure and falling haemoglobin levels. It is more likely if removal of a diseased liver has left a raw area on the diaphragm or if there have been adhesions from previous surgery or infection. Treatment is usually by transfusion and re-operation if necessary.

Hepatic artery thrombosis. This is marked by clinical deterioration, fever, and bacteriaemia. Occasionally, large hepatic infarcts are found which become infected. Loss of the hepatic artery supply may result in necrosis of the complete donor bile duct. Diagnosis is made

Table 35.4. Complications of liver transplantation

Time post-transplant	Complication
First 5 days	Graft failure
	Technical
	Bleeding
	Hepatic artery thrombosis
	Bile leaks
	Portal vein thrombosis
	Renal failure
	Pulmonary
From 3 days	Infections
	Abscess (cholestasis)
	CNS toxicity
From 5 days	Acute graft rejection
From 6 weeks	Chronic graft rejection
	Vanishing bile ducts
	Hepatic vasculitis
From 4 weeks	Chronic opportunist infections
	Biliary strictures
Months	Bone disease
	Ectopic calcification
	Hypertension in children

by angiography, including Doppler real-time ultrasonography. Re-transplantation is the only treatment.

Other biliary tract complications. These include bile leaks, malposition of T-tubes and bile duct obstruction, usually due to stricture. Placement of the biliary anastomosis too distally may be responsible by interfering with the blood supply to the bile duct. HIDA scans are useful in detecting bile leaks. Some strictures respond to trans-hepatic or endoscopic stenting, dilatation or biliary drainage. Others require re-operation. Accumulations of bile may be drained percutaneously, under scanning guidance.

Sludging in the bile ducts is prevented by careful flushing of the biliary tree during the harvesting of the liver.

Portal vein thrombosis. This results from a technical error in the anastomosis. It is recognized by real-time ultrasound or angiography. Doppler ultrasound may show luminal irregularities in the portal vein.

Renal failure. Oliguria is virtually constant post-transplant, but in some patients renal failure is more serious. The causes are many, and include pre-existing kidney disease, hypotension and shock, sepsis, nephrotoxic antibiotics and cyclosporine. Dialysis may be necessary. If renal failure is associated with severe graft rejection or overwhelming infection, dialysis does not improve survival.

Pulmonary complications. Mechanical factors contribute to pulmonary complications. Air passing through an abnormal pulmonary vasculature can cause cerebral air emboli. The right diaphragm is paralysed and right lower lobe atelectasis is common. This is treated by physiotherapy, and, if necessary, therapeutic bronchoscopy. In one series, 20% of patients underwent bronchoscopy and this was repeated until complete resolution of the atelectasis [26]. Pleural effusion is virtually constant and in about 18% aspiration is necessary [66]. About 18.7% have pulmonary infections, including pneumonia, empyaema, and lung abscesses. The causes are frequently opportunist.

During and after the operation, circulatory overload may lead to pulmonary oedema.

Intra—pulmonary shunting and a reduced ventilation—perfusion ratio, together with an increased cardiac output are found in cirrhosis (Chapter 6). These are normalized post-transplant, suggesting their functional nature ('*hepato-pulmonary syndrome*') [14].

INFECTIONS

Each patient has, on average, 2.5 infections episodes. These may be primary, reactivation, or related to opportunistic organisms; they may be fatal [10, 18]. The infections are largely related to immunosuppression not so much with corticosteroids, but with azathioprine and cyclosporine, and particularly anti-lymphocyte serum, monoclonal OKT3 and anti-thymocyte globulin.

Cytomegalovirus (CMV). This infection is a virtually constant complication of liver transplantation but may not always be clinically evident. It may be primary, infection coming from transfused blood or the donor liver, or may be a secondary reactivation. It is usually benign, but 20% are symptomatic.

The infection presents one to four months post-transplant, and continues for months or even years in those with poor graft function who require heavy immunosuppression. The picture is of a mononucleosis-like syndrome with fever and increased transaminases. The lungs are particularly involved in the severely affected. The infection depresses host defences. Chronic infection is associated with the vanishing bile duct syndrome.

Liver biopsy shows typical intranuclear inclusions. Bile duct atypia and mild endothelialitis are absent. The liver biopsy may be cultured, but the results take three weeks. Earlier diagnosis may be made by monoclonal antibodies or by detection of early antigen fluorescent foci in cell culture (DEAFF).

Rapid diagnosis of the primary, but not the secondary CMV infection, can be made by *in situ* hybridization for CMV-DNA in liver biopsy specimens [34, 35].

Ideally, CMV infection could be prevented by using seronegative blood for transfusion and seronegative organ donors. Anti-CMV immune globulin is also being used.

The treatment of the severe infection is by gancyclovir. Chronic CMV infection may be an indication for re-transplant.

Herpes simplex virus: this infection is common and usually related to immunosuppression-induced reactivation. It may be asymptomatic or present as herpes labialis, tracheobronchitis and bronchopneumonia. It responds to intravenous acyclovir.

Similarly, *Epstein—Barr virus infection* may reactivate and the affects are similar to those of CMV.

Fungal, or *nocardial infections* are opportunistic. They cause a respiratory illness with disseminated candidiasis, aspergillosis and cryptococcosis. Systemic antiviral therapy is required. The effects of this on the liver are difficult to distinguish from those of the fungus.

REJECTION

Immunologically, the liver is a privileged organ with regard to transplantation, having a higher resistance to immunological attack than other organs. The liver cell probably carries fewer surface antigens. Nevertheless, episodes of acute rejection of varying severity are virtually constant.

Acute rejection is seen 5–10 days after transplant. The patient feels ill, there is a mild pyrexia and tachycardia. The liver is enlarged and tender. Serum bilirubin, transaminase and prothrombin time increase. The diagnosis is confirmed by liver biopsy. This should be compared with the appearances of the donor liver biopsied at the time of transplantation. Rejection is shown by the classical triad of portal inflammation, bile duct damage and endothelialitis (fig. 35.3) [48]. These three features, but not the individual ones, are specific and mimicked only by graft-versus-host disease. Arteritis and hepato-cellular necrosis may also be seen. Follow-up biopsies may show eosinophilis, resembling a drug reaction and infarct-like areas of necrosis, perhaps secondary to portal venous obstruction by lymphocytes.

CT shows a low attenuation region around peripheral portal tracts (peri-portal collar). This corresponds to lymphocytic infiltration [60].

Very rarely, the acute rejection reaction may continue as full graft-versus-host disease [6].

Rejection is treated by three bolus injections of methyl prednisolone 1 g each intravenously, followed, if necessary, by monoclonal OKT3 [9]. If the patient responds to this treatment, azathioprine 1–2 mg/kg per day is added. Retransplant is the only treatment for continued rejection. The patient rarely dies of acute rejection, but the increased immunosuppression opens the door to multiple infections.

Chronic rejection. The onset is from six weeks to nine months post-transplant but usually within the first three months. It is marked by progressive cholestasis.

Bile ducts are progressively damaged and ultimately disappear. The mechanism seems to be immunological (fig. 35.4). There is aberrant expression of HLA Class 11 antigens on bile ducts. Donor–recipient HLA Class 1 mismatch with class 1 antigen expression on bile ducts is contributory [13].

Histologically, a progressive, non-suppurative cholangitis culminates in disappearance of interlobular bile ducts; the bile duct epithelium is penetrated by mononuclear cells, resulting in focal necrosis and rupture of the epithelium. Larger arteries (not seen in a needle biopsy) show subintimal foam cells, intimal sclerosis and intimal hyperplasia [12]. These arterial lesions must contribute to the bile duct damage.

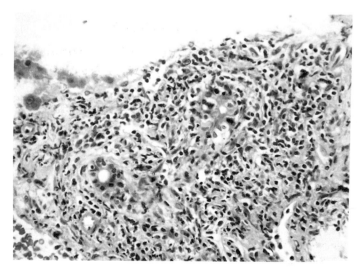

Fig. 35.3. Acute rejection: a damaged bile duct infiltrated with lymphocytes is seen in a densely infiltrated portal tract. (Stained H & E, ×100.)

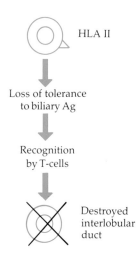

HLA II

Loss of tolerance
to biliary Ag

Recognition
by T-cells

Destroyed
interlobular
duct

Fig. 35.4. Possible mechanism of bile duct damage in hepatic rejection (graft-versus-host disease).

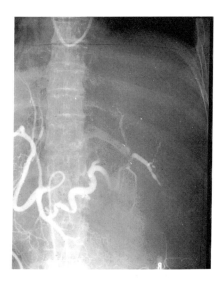

Fig. 35.5. Chronic rejection: coeliac angiogram shows possible pruning of intrahepatic arterial tree. Filling did not improve later in the series (Sherlock & Dick, 1986).

Hepatic angiography shows markedly narrowed hepatic arteries with no peripheral filling and often with branch vessel occlusions (fig. 35.5) [62]. Major hepatic arterial occlusions lead to biliary duct stricturing shown by cholangiography. Cytomegalovious cholangitis can also lead to the sclerosing cholangitis picture. Major biliary stricturing can be treated by endoscopic or trans-hepatic balloon dilatation.

Chronic rejection is not reversed by increasing the immunosuppression. Re-transplant is the only effective treatment.

CENTRAL NERVOUS SYSTEM TOXICITY

Severe central nervous changes can follow liver transplantation [1, 11]. Half the patients show fits, children being more susceptible than adults [1]. Cyclosporine-associated fits are well documented. Phenytoin controls them, but this induces (accelerates) cyclosporine metabolism.

Central pontine myelinosis is related to sudden alterations in serum electrolytes, perhaps in combination with cyclosporine. The CT scan shows white matter lucencies.

Cyclosporine is a highly lipophilic drug which is bound to lipoprotein fractions in the blood. Patients with low serum cholesterol values are at particular risk of central nervous system toxicity after the transplant [1].

Cerebral infarction is related to perioperative hypotension, or air/microthrombus embolism.

Psychosis may complicate high dose steroid treatment for rejection. Cerebral abscess is part of the general infection.

BONE DISEASE

Patients having liver transplants usually have some previous degree of hepatic osteodystrophy. The bones deteriorate post-transplant with vertebral collapse in 38% during the second three months [20]. The cause is multifactorial and includes cholestasis, corticosteroid therapy and bed rest.

ECTOPIC SOFT TISSUE CALCIFICATION [33]

This can develop diffusely and is associated with respiratory insufficiency and bone fractures. It is secondary to hypocalcaemia due to citrate infused in fresh frozen plasma, and in addition renal failure and secondary hyper-parathyroidism. Tissue injury and administration of exogenous calcium lead to the soft-tissue calcium deposition.

DRUG-RELATED HEPATIC COMPLICATIONS

Cyclosporine and azathioprine can be cholestatic. This is dose-dependent and careful monitoring of blood levels is important.

The future

Hepatic transplantation is a tremendous undertaking that does not begin or end with the surgery. It can only be performed in special centres, prepared and able to provide facilities. These include not only skilled surgeons and operating theatre staff, but also hepatologists, intensive care facilities and, among others, well staffed departments of nephrology, infectious disease and immunology. Blood bank demands are considerable. The patient and his family need psychiatric and social support. There must be a back-up programme to procure organs. The work load is considerable. The survivor requires life-long medical and surgical supervision, together with costly drugs, both immunosuppressive and antibiotic.

It is not surprising, therefore, that the cost of hepatic transplantation is high—varying from centre to centre—but about $50 000–100 000 for the preoperative work up, the operation and the immediate post-operative care. This sum must be weighed against the not inconsiderable outlay on a patient with end-stage liver disease being treated by conventional methods.

Technical advances, the training of more transplant teams and less costly immunosuppression will lower the cost.

In one centre, the mean cost was $92 866 for the first year after transplant, and most patients were fully rehabilitated. This compares with $45 643 for the hospital costs of the last year of life of patients with liver disease who would have been candidates for transplantation had circumstances permitted [65].

References

1 Adams DH, Ponsford S, Gunson B et al. Neurological complications following liver transplantation. Lancet 1987; i: 949.
2 Bilheimer DW, Goldstein JL, Grundy SM et al. Liver transplantation to provide low-density-lipoprotein receptors and lower plasma cholesterol in a child with homozygous familial hypocholesterolema. N. Engl. J. Med. 1984; 311: 1638.
3 Bismuth H, Houssin D. Reduced sized orthotopic liver graft in hepatic transplantation in children. Surgery 1984; 95: 367.
4 Bismuth H, Castaing D, Ericzon BG et al. Hepatic transplantation in Europe. First report of the European liver transplant registry. Lancet 1987; ii: 674.
5 Bontempo FA, Lewis JH, Gorenc TJ et al. Liver transplantation in hemophilia. Blood 1987; 69: 1721.
6 Burdick JF, Vogelsang GB, Smith WJ et al. Severe graft-versus-host disease in a liver-transplant recipient. N. Engl. J. Med. 1988; 318: 689.
7 Busittil RW. Liver transplantation today. Ann. intern. Med. 1986; 104: 377.
8 Busittil RW, Colonna JO II, Hiatt JR et al. The first 100 liver transplants at UCLA. Ann. Surg. 1987; 206: 387.
9 Colonna JO II, Goldstein LI, Brems JJ et al. A prospective study on the use of monoclonal anti-T3-cell antibody (OTK3) to treat steroid-resistant liver transplant rejection. Arch. Surg. 1987; 122: 1120.
10 Colonna JO II, Winston DJ, Brill JE et al. Infectious complications in liver transplantation. Arch. Surg. 1988; 123: 360.
11 De Groen PC, Aksamit MD, Rahela J et al. Central nervous system toxicity after liver transplantation. N. Engl. J. Med. 1987; 317: 861.
12 Demetris AJ, Lasky S, Van Thiel DH et al. Pathology of hepatic transplantation: a review of 62 adult allograft recipients immunosuppressed with a cyclosporine/steroid regimen. Am. J. Pathol. 1985; 118: 151.
13 Donaldson PT, Alexander GJM, O'Grady J et al. Evidence for an immune response to HLA class 1 antigens in the vanishing bile duct syndrome after liver transplantation. Lancet 1987; i: 945.
14 Eriksson LS, Soderman C, Wahren J et al. Is hypoxemia in cirrhotic patients due to a functional 'hepato-pulmonary syndrome'? J. Hepatol. 1988; 7 suppl 1: S29.
15 Esquivel CO, Van Thiel DH, Demetris AJ et al. Transplantation for primary biliary cirrhosis. Gastroenterology 1988; 94: 1207.
16 Flye MW, Jendrisak MD. Liver transplantation in the child. World J. Surg. 1986; 10: 432.

17 Gibas A, Dienstag JL, Schafer AI *et al.* Cure of hemophilia A by orthotopic liver transplantation. *Gastroenterology* 1988; **95**: 192.

18 Goldstein LI. Postoperative problems. *Ann. intern. Med.* 1986; **104**: 377.

19 Gordon RD, Iwatsuki S, Esquivel CO *et al.* Liver transplantation across ABO blood groups. *Surgery* 1986; **100**: 342.

20 Haagsma EB, Thijn CJP, Post JG *et al.* Bone disease after orthotopic liver transplantation. *J. Hepatol.* 1988; **6**: 94.

21 Hood JM, Koep LJ, Peters RL *et al.* Liver transplantation for advanced liver disease with alpha-1-antitrypsin deficiency. *N. Engl. J. Med.* 1980; **302**: 272.

22 Iwatsuki S, Gordon RD, Shaw BW *et al.* Role of liver transplantation in cancer therapy. *Ann. Surg.* 1985; **202**: 401.

23 Jenkins RL, Bosari S, Khettry U *et al.* Survival from hepatic transplantation. Relationship of protein synthesis to histological abnormalities in patient selection and postoperative management. *Ann. Surg.* 1986; **204**: 364.

24 Kalayoglu M, Sollinger HW, Stratta RJ, *et al.* Extended preservation of the liver for clinical transplantation. *Lancet* 1988; **i**: 617.

25 Kaufman SS, Wood RP, Shaw BW Jr, *et al.* Orthotopic liver transplantation for type 1 Crigler–Najjar syndrome. *Hepatology* 1986; **6**: 1259.

26 Krowka MF, Cortese DA. Pulmonary aspects of chronic liver disease and liver transplantation. *Mayo Clin. Proc.* 1985; **60**: 407.

27 Letourneau JG, Day DL, Ascher NL *et al.* Abdominal sonography after hepatic transplantation: results in 36 patients. *Am. J. Roentgenol.* 1987; **149**: 299.

28 Letourneau JG, Day DL, Maile CW. Liver allograft transplantation: postoperative CT findings. *Am. J. Roentgenol.* 1987; **148**: 1099.

29 Maddrey WC, Van Thiel DH. Liver transplantation: an overview. *Hepatology* 1988; **8**: 948.

30 Maddrey WC (ed). *Transplantation of the liver.* Elsevier, New York, 1988.

31 Malatack JJ, Finegold DN, Iwatsuki S *et al.* Liver transplantation for type 1 glycogen storage disease. *Lancet* 1983; **i**: 1073.

32 Marsh JW, Iwatsuki S, Makowka L *et al.* Orthotopic liver transplantation for primary sclerosing cholangitis. *Ann. Surg.* 1988; **207**: 21.

33 Mora NP, Cienfuegos JA, Ardaiz J *et al.* Special operative events in the first case of liver grafting after heart transplantation. *Surgery* 1988; **103**: 264.

34 Munoz SJ, Nagelberg SB, Green PJ. *et al.* Ectopic soft tissue calcium deposition following liver transplantation. *Hepatology* 1988; **8**: 476.

35 Naoumov NV, Alexander GJM, O'Grady JG *et al.* Rapid diagnosis of cytomegalovirus infection by in-situ hybridisation in liver grafts. *Lancet* 1988; **i**: 1361.

36 O'Grady JG, Polson RT, Rolles K *et al.* Liver transplantation for malignant disease: results in 93 consecutive patients. *Ann. Surg.* 1988 (in press).

37 Perkins JD, Sterioff S, Wiesner RH *et al.* Conversion from standard cyclosporine to low dose cyclosporine and azathioprine therapy as treatment for cyclosporine-related complications in liver transplant patients. *Transplant Proc.* 1987; **19**: 2434.

38 Pettit BJ, Zitelli BJ, Rowe MI. Analysis of patients with biliary atresia coming to liver transplantation. *J. Pediatr. Surg.* 1984; **19**: 779.

39 Polson RJ, Rolles K, Calne RY *et al.* Reversal of severe neurological manifestations of Wilson's disease following orthotopic liver transplantation. *Q. J. Med.* 1987; **64**: 685.

40 Rolles K, Williams R, Neuberger J *et al.* The Cambridge and King's College Hospital experience of liver transplantation (1968–1983). *Hepatology* 1984; **4**: 50S.

41 Scharschmidt BF. Human liver transplantation: an analysis of 819 patients from eight centres. In *Recent Advances in Hepatology*, 2nd edn, eds. HC Thomas & EA Jones. Churchill-Livingstone, Edinburgh, 1986.

42 Scoazec J-V, Lamy P, Degott C *et al.* Epithelioid hemangioendothelioma of the liver. *Gastroenterology* 1988; **94**: 1447.

43 Seltman HJ, Dekker A, Van Thiel DH *et al.* Budd–Chiari syndrome recurring in a transplanted liver. *Gastroenterology* 1983; **84**: 640.

44 Shaw BW Jr, Iwatsuki S, Starzl TE. Alternative methods of arterialization of the hepatic graft. *Surg. Gynecol. Obstet.* 1984; **159**: 490.

45 Shaw BW Jr, Martin DJ, Marquez JM *et al.* Venous bypass in clinical liver transplantation. *Ann. Surg.* 1984; **200**: 524.

46 Shaw BW, Gordon RD, Iwatsuki S. Retransplantation of the liver. *Semin. Liver Dis.* 1985; **5**: 394.

47 Shaw BW Jr, Wood RP. The operative procedures. In *Transplantation of the Liver*, Ed. W.C. Maddrey, Elsevier, New York, 1988; p. 87.

48 Snover DC, Sibley RK, Freese DK *et al.* Orthotopic liver transplantation: a pathological study of 63 serial liver biopsies from 17 patients with special reference to the diagnostic features and natural history of rejection. *Hepatology* 1984; **4**: 1212.

49 Starzl TE, Marchioro TL, von Kaulla KN *et al.* Homotransplantation of the liver in humans. *Surg. Gynecol. Obstet.* 1963; **117**: 659.

50 Starzl TE, Iwatsuki S, Esquivel CO *et al.* Refinements in the surgical technique of liver transplantation. *Semin. Liv. Dis.* 1985; **5**: 349.

51 Starzl TE, van Thiel D, Tzakis AG. Orthotopic liver transplantation for alcoholic cirrhosis. *J. Am.*

Med. Assoc. 1988; **260**: 2542.

52 Sternlieb I. Wilson's disease: indications for liver transplants. *Hepatology* 1984; **4**: 15S.

53 Tzakis AG, Arditi M, Whitington PF *et al.* Aplastic anemia complicating orthotopic liver transplantation for non-A, non-B hepatitis. *N. Engl. J. Med.* 1988; **319**: 393.

54 Valdivielso P, Escolar JL, Cuervas-Mons V *et al.* Heart and liver transplantation in a patient with familial hypercholesterolemia. *Ann. intern. Med.* 1988; **108**: 204.

55 Van Thiel DH, Tarter R, Gavaler JS *et al.* Liver transplantation in adults: an analysis of costs and benefits at the University of Pittsburgh. *Gastroenterology* 1986; **90**: 211.

56 Van Thiel DH, Gartner LM, Thorp FK *et al.* Resolution of the clinical features of tyrosinemia following orthotopic liver transplantation for hepatoma. *J. Hepatol.* 1986; **3**: 42.

57 Van Thiel DH, Gavaler JS, Kam I *et al.* Rapid growth of an intact human liver transplanted into a recipient larger than the donor. *Gastroenterology* 1987; **93**: 1414.

58 Wallwork J, Williams R, Calne RY. Transplantation of liver heart and lungs for primary biliary cirrhosis and primary pulmonary hypertension. *Lancet* 1987; **ii**: 182.

59 Watts RWE, Calne RY, Rolles K *et al.* Successful treatment of primary biliary hyperoxaluria type 1 by combined hepatic and renal transplantation.

Lancet 1987; **ii**: 474.

60 Wechsler RJ, Munoz SJ, Needleman L *et al.* The periportal collar: a CT sign of liver transplant rejection. *Radiology* 1987; **165**: 57.

61 Welch CS. A note on transplantation of the whole liver in dogs. *Transplant. Bull.* 1955; **2**: 54.

62 White RM, Zajko AB, Demetris AJ *et al.* Liver transplant rejection. Angiographic findings in 35 patients. *Am. J. Roentgenol.* 1987; **148**: 1095.

63 Willemse PJA, Ausema L, van Peski J *et al.* Liver hypertrophy and atrophy after auxiliary partial liver transplantation for chronic end-stage liver disease. *J. Hepatol.* 1988; **7** suppl 1: S 85.

64 Williams R, Calne RY, Rolles K *et al.* Current results with orthotopic liver grafting in Cambridge/King's College Hospital series. *Br. med. J.* 1985; **290**: 49.

65 Williams JW, Vera S, Evans LS. Socioeconomic aspects of hepatic transplantation. *Am. J. Gastroenterol.* 1987; **82**: 1115.

66 Wood RP, Shaw BW Jr, Starzl TE. Extrahepatic complications of liver transplantation. *Semin. Liver Dis.* 1985; **5**: 377.

67 Zajko AB, Campbell WI, Bron KM *et al.* Cholangiography and interventional biliary radiology in adult liver transplantation. *Am. J. Roentgenol.* 1985; **144**: 127.

68 Zajko AB, Bron KM, Starzl TE *et al.* Angiography of liver transplantation patients. *Radiology* 1985; **157**: 305.

Index

continued on 596

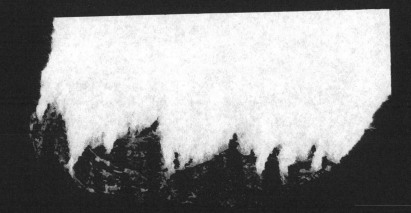

LEEDS BECKETT UNIVERSITY
LIBRARY
DISCARDED

70 0060087 7